PREFIXES AND SUFFIXES

laryng, laryngo-. The larynx
latero-. Side
lepto-. Small; soft
leuko-. White
-lite, -lith. A stone; a calculus
lith-. A stone
-logia, -logy. Science of; study of
-lysis. Setting free; disintegration
macro-. Large; long; big
mal-. Bad; poor; evil
med-, medi-. Middle
mega, megal-. Large; great
-megalia, megaly. Large; great; extreme
melan-, melano-. Black
mes-, meso-. Middle
meta-. Beyond; over; between; change, or transposition
-meter. Measure
metra, metro-. The uterus
micro-. Small
mio-. Less; smaller
mono-. Single
multi-. Many
my, myo-. Muscle
myel, myelo-. Marrow
myxa, myxo-. Mucus
neo-. New
nephr, nephra, nephro-. Kidney
neu, neuro-. Nerve
niter, nitro-. Nitrogen
non-, not-. No
nucleo-. Nucleus
ob-. Against
oculo-. The eye
-ode, oil. Form; shape; resemblance
odont-. A tooth
-oid. Form; shape; resemblance
oligo-. Few
-oma. A tumor
omo-. Shoulder
o-. An egg; ovum
oophoron-. Ovary
opisth-. Backward
orchid-. Testicle
ortho-. Straight; normal
os-. A mouth; a bone
-osis. Condition; disease; intensive
oste, osteo-. A bone
-ostomosis, ostomy. To furnish with a mouth or an outlet
-otomy. Cutting
oxy-. Sharp; acid
pachy-. Thick
pan-. All; entire
para-. Alongside of

path-, -path, -pathy. Disease; suffering
-penia. Lack
per-. Excessive; through
peri-. Around
-phobia. Fear
-phylaxis. Protection
-plasm. To mold
-plastic. Molded; indicates restoration of lost or badly formed features
-plegia. A stroke
plur-. More
pneu-. Relating to the air or lungs
poly-. Much; many
post-. After
pre-. Before
pro-. Before; in behalf of
proto-. First
pseud-, pseudo-. False
psych-. The soul; the mind
py-, pyo-. Pus
re-. Back; again
retro-. Backward
-rhage, -rhagia. Hemorrhage; flow
-rhaphy. A suturing or stitching
-rhea. To flow; indicates discharge
sacchar-. Sugar
sacro-. Sacrum
salping, salpingo-. A tube; relating to a fallopian tube
sarco-. Flesh
sclero-. Hard; relating to the sclera
-sclerosis. Dryness; hardness
-scopy. To see
semi-. Half
-stomosis, -stomy. To furnish with a mouth or outlet
sub-. Under
super, supra-. Above
syn-. With; together
tele-. Distant; far
tetra-. Four
thio-. Sulfur
thyro-. Thyroid gland
-tomy. Cutting
trans-. Across
tri-. Three
-trophic. Relating to nourishment
tropho-. Relating to nutrition
uni-. One
-uria. Relating to the urine
urino, uro-. Relating to the urine or urinary organs
vaso-. A vessel
venter, ventro-. The abdomen
xanth-. Yellow

P9-DDR-827

BOOKS OF RELATED INTEREST

The Radiology Wordbook
Theresa Indovina, CMA, RMA
Wilburta Q. Lindh, CMA
About 500 pp, April 1990

Taber's Cyclopedic Medical Dictionary 16th Edition
Edited by Clayton L. Thomas, M.D, MPH
2,401 pp, 1989

Computer Applications for the Medical Office:
MedicalCare® Basic Management System
Barbara A. Gylys, BS, MEd, CMA-A
About 400 pp, June 1990

Medical Terminology: A Systems Approach 2nd Edition
Barbara A. Gylys, BS, MEd, CMA-A
Mary Ellen Wedding, MEd, CMA, MT(ASCP)
470 pp, 1988

Book of Abbreviations
Sara Lu Mitchell, CMT
About 500 pp, Fall 1990

Medical Terminology: Exercises in Etymology 2nd Edition
Charles W. Dunmore, PhD
Rita M. Fleischer, PhD
305 pp, 1985

Diseases of the Human Body
Carol D. Warden-Tampara, PhD, CMA-A
Marcia A. Lewis, RN, MA, EdD, CMA-AC
391 pp, 1989

AIDS and the Allied Health Professions
Joyce W. Hopp, PhD, MPH
Elizabeth Rogers, EdD, PT
311 pp, 1989

Taber's®

MEDICAL WORD BOOK

WITH PRONUNCIATIONS

based on Taber's Cyclopedic Medical Dictionary, 16th Edition
as edited by Clayton L. Thomas, M.D., M.P.H.

compiled and edited by
M. Katherine Rice, Managing Editor, Dictionary
Dena R. Vardara, Assistant Dictionary Editor
F. A. Davis Company

F. A. DAVIS COMPANY 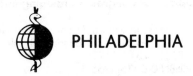 PHILADELPHIA

Copyright © 1990 by F. A. Davis Company

All rights reserved. This book is protected by copyright. No part of it may be repro-
duced, stored in a retrieval system, or transmitted in any form or by any means, electronic, mechanical, photocopying, recording, or otherwise, without written permission
from the publisher.

PRINTED IN THE UNITED STATES OF AMERICA

Last digit indicates print number   10   9   8   7   6   5   4   3   2   1

Library of Congress Cataloging-in-Publication Data

Taber's medical word book with pronunciations.
  1. Medicine—Dictionaries. I. Title. [DNLM: 1. Nomenclature. W 15 T113]
R121.T1813 1990   610'.3   90-2948
ISBN 0-8036-8265-4

INTRODUCTION

For fifty years, *Taber's Cyclopedic Medical Dictionary* has served the health care community more prolifically and usefully than any single title in print. The omnipresence of this wealth of information has become synonymous with the relentless pursuit of better health.

And now, with the advent of database publishing, *Taber's* has spawned the *Taber's Medical Word Book with Pronunciations*. Even at fifty, parenthood suits *Taber's* well. This is the first medical word book to offer pronunciations, and the first medical word book to offer etymologies, and the 55,000 entries and subentries have been organized conveniently in alphabetical as opposed to subject order.

Taber's Medical Word Book has exactly the same entries found in *Taber's* recently published 16th edition, which boasts the widest variety of medical terms found in any one source. Sixteen nursing and allied health specialists were consulted to cover such areas as Radiology, Physical Therapy, Occupational Therapy, Medical Technology, Critical Care, Psychiatry, Community Health, and Dental Technology. Because *Taber's* is depended upon in every corner of the health care system, *Taber's* editors must be cognizant of all the specialized vocabularies.

Taber's Medical Word Book is especially meant to serve the medical transcriptionists, whose role has become even more significant as the need to document more thoroughly and accurately has grown. (n.b. The Managing Editor, of the dictionary/word book, Ms. M. Katherine Rice, was formerly a medical transcriptionist and Assistant to the Executive Director of the American Association for Medical Transcription.) Medical office support personnel should benefit greatly from the unique presentation of this word book. Medically oriented courses offered by classics departments should appreciate the inclusion of etymologies.

Many thanks go to Ms. M. Katherine Rice and Ms. Dena Vardara for bringing this dream to life. Not only did they extract information from the *Taber's* database in an efficiently expeditious manner, but their backgrounds helped give us the confidence to choose this special format. This project, of course, would not be possible without the *Taber's* dictionary and its editor, Clayton L. Thomas, M.D., M.P.H., who has been instrumental in keeping *Taber's* the preeminent medical reference in the world today.

Robert H. Craven, Jr.
President

FEATURES AND THEIR USE

Taber's Medical Word Book with Pronunciations is more than just a word book of medical terms. In addition to listing medical words, it lists conceptual terms vital to the practitioner and student of Nursing and Allied Health. All who work in fields related to health care will find *Taber's Medical Word Book with Pronunciations* a comprehensive resource tool.

Vocabulary: The vocabulary is taken from *Taber's Cyclopedic Medical Dictionary*, 16th edition, recently updated to meet the ongoing needs of those in the Nursing and Allied Health professions. New entries reflect the many changes in the health care professions, approaches to patient care, and aspects of law and ethics.

Pronunciation: More than 95 percent of the main entries are spelled phonetically. Pronunciations are given as simply as possible with most long and short vowels marked diacritically and secondary accents indicated. *Diacritics* are marks over or under vowels. Only two diacritics are used in *Taber's Medical Word Book*: the macron ˉ showing the long sound of vowels, as the a in rāte, e in rēbirth, i in īsle, o in ōver, and u in ūnite; and the breve ˘ showing the short sound of vowels, as the a in ăpple, e in ĕver, i in ĭt, o in nŏt, and u in cŭt. *Accents* are marks used to indicate stress upon certain syllables. A single accent ′ is called a primary accent. A double accent ″ is called a secondary accent; it indicates less stress upon a syllable than that given by a primary accent. This difference in stress can be seen in the word an″es-the′si-a.

Spelling: Many words formerly hyphenated are now listed as one word (corticosteroid, gastrointestinal); diphthongs are eliminated where possible; and American rather than British forms are used.

Biographies: For eponymic terms a brief biography is included in brackets immediately following the pronunciation.

Etymology: The etymology for 90 percent of the main entries is presented in brackets following the entry. The major sources of medical terminology are Latin and Greek. Abbreviations: Amerind, American Indian; AS, Anglo Saxon; Fr., French; Ger., German; Gr., Greek; L., Latin; LL., Late Latin; MD., Middle Dutch; ME., Middle English; NL, New Latin; O.Fr., Old French; and Sp., Spanish.

Alphabetical order: Main entries are alphabetized letter by letter, regardless of spaces that may occur between the words. A comma marks the end of an entry for alphabetical purposes; e.g., **ear, external** precedes **earache** as well as **ear dust**. For alphabetical purposes in eponymic terms, the **'s** is ignored, e.g., **Albini's nodules** precedes **albinism**.

Subentries: Subentries are listed under the noun they modify (such as *labor, premature* or *technician, emergency medical*), indented from the main entry.

Abbreviations: Standard abbreviations are included and are listed alphabetically throughout the text. Additional abbreviations used for charting and prescription writing are listed in the Appendix.

Adapted from Thomas, C. L. (ed.): *Taber's Cyclopedic Medical Dictionary*, ed. 16, F. A. Davis, Philadelphia, 1989, p. xi.

A

α Alpha

Å angstrom unit

A₂ aortic second sound

a accommodation; ampere; anode; anterior; aqua; area; artery

ā ante [L., before]

a-, an- [Gr., not]

A.A., a.a. achievement age; Alcoholics Anonymous; amino acid; arteriae

a̅a̅ [Gr. ana, of each]

A.A.A. American Academy of Allergists; American Association of Anatomists

A.A.A.S. American Association for the Advancement of Science

A.A.C.N. American Association of Critical-Care Nurses; American Association of Colleges of Nursing

A.A.F.P. American Academy of Family Practice

A.A.G.P. American Academy of General Practice

AAL anterior axillary line

A.A.M.A. American Association of Medical Assistants

A.A.M.D. American Association on Mental Deficiency

A.A.M.I. Association for the Advancement of Medical Instrumentation

AAMT American Association for Medical Transcription

A.A.N. American Academy of Nursing

A.A.N.A. American Association of Nurse Anesthetists

A.A.N.N. American Association of Neurological Nurses

A.A.O.H.N. American Association of Occupational Health Nurses

A.A.P. American Academy of Pediatrics; American Association of Pathologists

A.A.P.A. American Academy of Physician Assistants

Aaron's sign (ăr'ŏns) [Charles D. Aaron, U.S. physician, 1866–1951]

A.A.R.T. American Association for Respiratory Therapy

AAS atomic absorption spectroscopy

AASECT American Association of Sex Educators, Counselors, and Therapists

ab antibody

ab- [L. ab, from]

Abadie's sign (ă-bă-dēz') [Charles A. Abadie, Fr. ophthalmologist, 1842–1932; Jean Abadie, Fr. neurologist, 1873–1946]

abaissement (ă-bās' mŏn) [Fr., a lowering]

abalienation (ăb-āl"yĕn-ā' shŭn) [L. abalienare, to separate from]

A band

abandonment

abaptiston (ă"băp-tĭs'tŏn) [Gr. abaptistos, not dipped]

abarognosis (ăb"ăr-ŏg-nō'sĭs) [Gr. a-, not, + baros, weight, + gnosis, knowledge]

abarthrosis (ăb-ăr-thrō'sĭs) [L. ab, from, + Gr. arthron, joint, + osis, condition]

abarticular [" + articulus, joint]

abarticulation

abasia (ă-bā'zē-ă) [Gr. a-, not, + basis, step]

　　a.-astasia

　　a. atactica

　　a., choreic

　　a., paralytic

　　a., paroxysmal trepidant

　　a., spastic

　　a., trembling; a. trepidans

abasic (ă-bā'sĭk)

abate (ă-bāt') [L. ab, from, + battere, to beat]

abatement (ă-bāt'mĕnt)
abatic (ă-băt'ĭk)
abaxial, abaxile (ăb-ăk'sē-al, -sĭl) [L.
ab, from, + axis, axis]
**Abbé-Zeiss apparatus, counting
cell hemocytometer** [Ernest Abbé,
Ger. physicist, 1840–1905; Carl
Zeiss, Ger. optician, 1816–1888]
Abbott's method [Edville G. Abbott,
U.S. orthopedic surgeon, 1870–
1938]
Abbott-Miller tube [W. Osler Abbott,
U.S. physician, 1902–1943; T. Grier
Miller, U.S. physician, b. 1886]
ABC antigen-binding capacity
abdomen (ăb-dō'mĕn, ăb'dō-mĕn) [L.,
belly]
  a., acute
  a., boat-shaped
  a., carinate
  a., navicular
  a. obstipum
  a., pendulous
  a., scaphoid
  a., surgical
abdominal (ăb-dŏm'ĭ-năl)
abdominal cavity
abdominal crisis
abdominal decompression
abdominal examination
abdominal gestation
abdominalgia (ăb-dŏm-ĭn-ăl'jē-ă) [L.
abdomen, belly, + Gr. algos,
pain]
abdominal inguinal ring
abdominal quadrants
abdominal reflexes
abdominal regions
abdominal rings
abdominal section
abdomino- (ăb-dŏm'ĭ-nō)
abdominocardiac reflex (ăb-dŏm"ĭ-
nō-kăr'dĕ-ăk)
abdominocentesis (ăb-dŏm"ĭ-nō-
sĕn-tē'sĭs) [L. abdomen, belly, +
Gr. kentesis, puncture]
abdominocystic [" + Gr. kystis,
bladder]

abdominogenital (ăb-dŏm"ĭ-nō-jĕn'ĭ-
tăl)
abdominohysterectomy [" +
Gr. hystera, womb, + ektome, ex-
cision]
abdominohysterotomy (ăb-dŏm"ĭ-
nō-hĭs-tĕr-ŏt'ō-mē) [" + " +
tome, a cutting, slice]
abdominoperineal
abdominoplasty
abdominoscopy (ăb-dŏm"ĭ-nŏs'kō-
pē) [" + Gr. skopein, to examine]
abdominoscrotal [" + scrotum,
bag]
abdominoscrotal muscle
abdominothoracic (ăb-dŏm"ĭ-nō-thō-
ră'sĭk) [" + Gr. thorax, chest]
abdominothoracic arch
abdominouterotomy (ăb-dŏm"ĭ-nō-
ū-tĕr-ŏt'ō-mē) [" + uterus, womb,
+ Gr. tome, a cutting, slice]
abdominovaginal (ăb-dŏm"ĭ-nō-văj'ĭ-
năl) [" + vagina, sheath]
abdominovesical (ăb-dŏm"ĭ-nō-vĕs'ĭ-
kăl) [" + vesica, bladder]
abdominovesical pouch
abducens (ăb-dū'sĕnz) [L., drawing
away]
  a. labiorum
  a. oculi
abducens muscle
abducens nerve
abducent (ăb-dū'sĕnt) [L. abducens,
drawing away]
abducent nerve
abduct (ăb-dŭkt') [L. abductus, led
away]
abduction (ăb-dŭk'shŭn)
abductor (ăb-dŭk'tor)
abenteric (ăb-ĕn-tĕr'ĭk) [L. ab, from,
+ Gr. enteron, intestine]
Abernethy, John (ăb'ĕr-nē"thē) [Brit.
surgeon, 1764–1831]
  A.'s fascia
  A.'s sarcoma
aberrant (ăb-ĕr'ănt) [L. ab, from, +
errare, to wander]
aberrant conduction

aberrant pyramidal tract
aberratio (ăb-ĕr-ā'shē-ō) [L.]
  a. lactis
  a. testis
aberration (ăb-ĕr-ā'shŭn) [L. ab, from, + errare, to wander]
  a., chromatic
  a., chromosomal
  a., diopteric
  a., distantial
  a., lateral
  a., longitudinal
  a., mental
  a., spherical
aberrometer (ăb"ĕr-ŏm'ĕ-tĕr) [L. ab, from, + errare, to wander, + Gr. metron, measure]
abetalipoproteinemia (ā-bā"tă-lĭp"ō-prō" tēn-ē'mē-ă) [Gr. a-, not, + β + lipos, fat, + protos, first, + haima, blood]
abevacuation (ăb-ē-văk"ū-ā'shŭn) [L. ab, from, + evacuare, to empty]
abeyance (ă-bā'ăns) [O. Fr.]
ABGs arterial blood gases
abient (ăb'ē-ĕnt)
ability
  a., verbal
abiogenesis (ăb-ē-ō-jĕn'ĕ-sĭs) [Gr. a-, not, + bios, life, + genesis, generation, birth]
abiogenetic, abiogenous (ăb-ē-ō-jĕ-nĕt'ĭk, ăb-ē-ŏj'ĭ-nŭs)
abiologic, abiological (ā-bī-ō-lŏj'ĭk, -ăl)
abiosis (ăb-ē-ō'sĭs) [Gr. a-, not, + bios, life, + osis, condition]
abiotic (ăb-ē-ŏt'ĭk)
abiotrophy (ăb-ē-ŏt'rō-fē) [" + " + trophe, nourishment]
abirritant (ăb-ĭr'ĭ-tănt) [L. ab, from, + irritare, to irritate]
abirritation (ăb"ĭr-rĭ-tā'shŭn)
ablactation (ăb-lăk-tā'shŭn) [L. ab, from, + lactatio, suckling]
ablate (ăb-lāt') [L. ablatus, taken away]
ablatio (ăb-lā'shē-ō) [L., carrying away]
  a. placentae
  a. retinae
ablation (ăb-lā'shŭn) [L. ab, from, + latus, carried]
-able
ablepharia (ăb-lĕ-fā'rē-ă) [Gr. a-, not, + blepharon, eyelid]
ablepharon (ă-blĕf'ă-rŏn)
ablepharous (ă-blĕf'ă-rŭs)
ablephary (ă-blĕf'ă-rē)
ablepsia (ă-blĕp'sē-ă) [Gr. a-, not, + blepein, to see]
abluent (ăb'lū-ĕnt) [L. ab, from, + luens, washing]
ablution (ăb-lū'shŭn)
ablutomania (ă-blū"tō-mā'nē-ă) [L. ablutio, a washing, + Gr. mania, frenzy]
abnerval [L. ab, from, + nervus, nerve]
abnormal (ăb-nor'măl) [" + norma, rule]
abnormality (ăb"nor-măl'ĭ-tē)
abnormity (ăb-nor'mĭ-tē)
abocclusion (ăb"ŏ-kloo'zhŭn)
aborad (ăb-ō'răd) [" + oris, mouth]
aboral (ăb-ō'răl)
abort (ă-bort') [L. abortare, to miscarry]
abortient (ă-bor'shĕnt) [L. abortio, abortion]
abortifacient (ă-bor-tĭ-fā'shĕnt) [" + facere, to make]
abortion (ă-bor'shŭn) [L. abortio]
  a., accidental
  a., ampullar
  a., artificial
  a., cervical
  a., complete
  a., criminal
  a., elective
  a., habitual
  a., imminent
  a., incomplete
  a., induced
  a., inevitable
  a., infected
  a., missed

a., nontherapeutic
a., septic
a., spontaneous
a., therapeutic
a., threatened
a., tubal
abortionist (ă-bor′shŭn-ĭst)
abortive (ă-bor′tĭv) [L. *abortivus*]
abortus (ă-bor′tŭs) [L.]
aboulia (ă-boo′lē-ă) [Gr. *a-*, not, + *boule*, will]
ABP arterial blood pressure
abrachia (ă-brā′kē-ă) [″ + *brachion*, arm]
abrachiocephalia (ă-brā″kē-ō-sĕ-fā′lē-ă) [″ + ″ + *kephale*, head]
abradant (ă-brād′ĕnt)
abrade (ă-brād′) [L. *ab*, from, + *radere*, to scrape]
abrasion (ă-brā′zhŭn) [″ + *radere*, to scrape]
abrasive
abreaction (ăb″rē-ăk′shŭn) [″ + *re*, again, + *actus*, acting]
abruptio (ă-brŭp′shē-ō) [L. *abruptus*]
  a. placentae
ABS absolute
abscess (ăb′sĕs) [L. *abscessus*, a going away]
  a., acute
  a., alveolar
  a., amebic
  a., anorectal
  a., apical
  a., appendiceal, appendicular
  a., arthrifluent
  a., atheromatous
  a., axillary
  a., Bartholin
  a., bicameral
  a., bile duct
  a., bilharziasis
  a., biliary
  a., blind
  a., bone
  a., brain
  a., breast

a., Brodie's
a., bursal
a., canalicular
a., caseous
a., cerebral
a., cheesy
a., cholangitic
a., chronic
a., circumscribed
a., circumtonsillar
a., cold
a., collar-button
a., deep
a., dental
a., dentoalveolar
a., diffuse
a., dry
a., embolic
a., emphysematous
a., endamebic; a.,entamebic
a., epidural
a., epiploic
a., extradural
a., fecal
a., filarial
a., follicular
a., frontal
a., fungal
a., gangrenous
a., gas
a., gingival
a., glandular
a., gravitation
a., helminthic
a., hematic
a., hemorrhagic
a., hepatic
a., hot
a., hypostatic
a., idiopathic
a., iliac
a., intracranial
a., intradural
a., intramammary
a., intramastoid
a., ischiorectal
a., kidney
a., lacrimal

a., lacunar
a., lateral; a., lateral alveolar
a., liver
a., lumbar
a., lung
a., lymphatic
a., mammary
a., marginal
a., mastoid
a., mediastinal
a., metastatic
a., migrating
a.'s, miliary
a., milk
a., mother
a., multiple
a., nocardial
a., orbital
a., ossifluent
a., otic cerebral
a., palatal
a., palmar
a., pancreatic
a., parafrenal
a., parametric; a., parametritic
a., paranephric; a., paranephritic
a., parapancreatic
a., parapharyngeal
a., parietal
a., parotid
a., pelvic
a., pelvirectal
a., perianal
a., periapical
a., pericemental
a., pericoronal
a., peridental
a., perinephric
a., periodontal
a., peripleuritic
a., periproctic
a., perirectal
a., perirenal
a., peritoneal
a., peritonsillar
a., periureteral
a., periurethral
a., perivesical

a., phlegmonous
a., pneumococcic
a., postcecal
a., postmammary
a., prelacrimal
a., premammary
a., primary
a., prostatic
a., protozoal
a., psoas
a., pulmonary
a., pulp
a., pyemic
a., rectal
a., renal
a., residual
a., retrocecal
a., retromammary
a., retroperitoneal
a., retropharyngeal
a., retrovesical
a., root
a., sacrococcygeal
a., satellite
a., scrofulous
a., secondary
a., septicemic
a.'s, shirt-stud
a., spermatic
a., spinal
a., splenic
a., stercoral; a.,stercoraceous
a., sterile
a., stitch
a., streptococcal
a., subaponeurotic
a., subarachnoid
a., subareolar
a., subdiaphragmatic
a., subdural
a., subepidermal
a., subfascial
a., subgaleal
a., submammary
a., subpectoral
a., subperiosteal
a., subperitoneal
a., subphrenic

a., subscapular
a., subungual
a., sudoriparous
a., superficial
a., suprahepatic
a., sympathetic
a., syphilitic
a., thecal
a., thymus
a., tonsillar
a., tooth
a., traumatic
a., tropical
a., tuberculous
a., tubo-ovarian
a., tympanitic
a., tympanocervical
a., tympanomastoid
a., urethral
a., urinary
a., urinous
a., verminous
a., wandering
a., warm
a., worm
abscissa (ăb-sĭs'ă) [L. *abscindere*, to cut off]
abscission (ăb-sĭ'zhŭn) [L. *abscindere*, to cut off]
absconsio (ăb-skŏn'sē-ō) [L.]
abscopal (ăb-skŏ'păl)
absence (ăb'sĕnz)
absence seizure
absentia epileptica (ăb-sĕn'shē-ă) [L., absence]
abs. feb. [L.] *absente febre*, in the absence of fever
Absidia (ăb-sĭd'ē-ă)
absinthe, absinth (ăb'sĭnth) [L. *absinthium*, wormwood]
absinthism (ăb'sĭn-thĭzm)
absolute
absolute alcohol
absolute scale
absolute temperature
absolute zero
absorb (ăb-sorb') [L. *absorbere*, to suck in]

absorbance (ăb-sor'băns)
absorbefacient (ăb-sor"bĕ-fā'shĕnt) [" + *facere*, to make]
absorbent (ăb-sor'bĕnt)
absorptiometer (ăb-sorp"shē-ŏm'ĕ-tĕr) [L. *absorptio*, absorption, + Gr. *metron*, measure]
absorption (ăb-sorp'shŭn) [L. *absorptio*]
    a., colon
    a., cutaneous
    a., disjunctive
    a., external
    a., mouth
    a., parenteral
    a., pathologic
    a., percutaneous
    a., protein
    a., small intestine
    a., stomach
absorption lines
absorption spectrum
absorptive (ăb-sorp'tĭv)
abstinence (ăb'stĭ-nĕns) [L. *abstinere*, to abstain]
abstinence syndrome
abstract (ăb'străkt, ăb-străkt') [L. *abstrahere*, to draw away]
abstraction (ăb-străk'shŭn)
abterminal (ăb-tĕr'mĭ-năl) [L. *ab*, from, + *terminus*, end]
abulia (ă-bū'lē-ă) [Gr. *a-*, not, + *boule*, will]
abuse (ă-būs') [L. *abusus*, using up]
    a., aged
    a., child
    a., drug
    a., spouse
abutment (ă-bŭt'mĕnt) [Fr. *abouter*, to place end to end]
A.C. acromioclavicular; adrenal cortex; air conduction; alternating current; anodal closure; atriocarotid; auriculocarotid; axiocervical
Ac actinium
a.c. [L.] *ante cibum*, before meals
acacia (ă-kā'shē-ă)
acalculia (ă-kăl-kū'lē-ă) [Gr. *a-*, not,

+ L. *calculare*, to reckon]
acampsia (ă-kămp′sē-ă) [″ + *kamptein*, to bend]
acantha [Gr. *akantha*, thorn]
acanthamebiasis (ă-kăn″thă-mē-bī′ă-sĭs)
acanthesthesia (ă-kăn″thĕs-thē′zē-ă) [″ + *aisthesis*, feeling, perception]
Acanthia lectularia (ă-kăn′thē-ă lĕk-tū-lā′rē-ă)
acanthiomeatal line
acanthion [Gr. *akanthion*, little thorn]
acantho- [Gr. *akantha*, thorn]
Acanthocephala (ă-kăn″thō-sĕf′ă-lă) [″ + *kephale*, head]
acanthocephaliasis (ă-kăn″thō-sĕf-ă-lī′ă-sĭs)
Acanthocheilonema perstans (ă-kăn″thō-kī″lō-nē′mă pĕr′stăns)
acanthocyte (ă-kăn′thō-sīt″) [Gr. *akantha*, thorn, + *kytos*, cell]
acanthocytosis (ă-kăn″thō-sī-tō′sĭs) [″ + ″ + *osis*, condition]
acanthoid (ă-kăn′thoyd) [″ + *eidos*, form, shape]
acanthokeratodermia (ă-kăn″thō-kĕr″ă-tō-dĕr′mē-ă) [″ + *keras*, horn, + *derma*, skin]
acantholysis (ă-kăn-thŏl′ĭ-sĭs) [″ + *lysis*, dissolution]
  a. bullosa
acanthoma (ăk″ăn-thō′mă) [″ + *oma*, tumor]
  a. adenoides cysticum
acanthopelvis, acanthopelyx (ă-kăn″thō-pĕl′vĭs, -pĕl′ĭks) [″ + *pelyx*, pelvis]
acanthosis (ăk″ăn-thō′sĭs) [″ + *osis*, condition]
  a. nigricans
acanthotic (ăk″ăn-thŏt′ĭk)
acapnia (ă-kăp′nē-ă) [Gr. *akapnos*, smokeless]
acapnial (ă-căp′nē-ăl)
acarbia (ă-kăr′bē-ă)
acardia (ă-kăr′dē-ă) [Gr. *a-*, not, + *kardia*, heart]
acardiac (ă-kăr′dē-ăk)

acardiacus (ă-kăr-dī′ă-kŭs)
acardiotrophia (ă-kăr″dē-ō-trō′fē-a) [″ + ″ + *trophe*, nutrition]
acardius
acariasis (ăk″ă-rī′ă-sĭs) [L. *acarus*, mite, + Gr. *-iasis*, state or condition of]
  a., demodectic
  a., psoroptic
  a., sarcoptic
acaricide (ă-kăr′ĭ-sīd) [″ + *caedere*, to kill]
acarid, acaridan (ăk′ă-rĭd, ă-kăr′ĭ-dăn) [L. *acarus*, mite]
acaridiasis (ă-kăr″ĭ-dī′ă-sĭs) [″ + Gr. *-iasis*, state or condition of]
Acarina (ăk″ă-rī′nă)
acarinosis (ă-kăr″ĭ-nō′sĭs) [L. *acarus*, mite, + Gr. *osis*, condition]
acarodermatitis (ăk″ă-rō-dĕr″mă-tī′tĭs) [″ + Gr. *derma*, skin, + *itis*, inflammation]
acaroid (ăk′ă-royd) [″ + Gr. *eidos*, form, shape]
acarology (ăk″ă-rŏl′ō-jē) [″ + Gr. *logos*, word, reason]
acarophobia (ăk″ăr-ō-fō′bē-ă) [″ + Gr. *phobos*, fear]
Acarus (ăk′ăr-ŭs) [L., mite]
  A. folliculorum
  A. scabiei
acarus [L.]
acaryote (ă-kăr′ē-ōt) [Gr. *a-*, not, + *karyon*, nucleus]
acatalasia (ă″kăt-ă-lā′zē-ă)
acataleptic (ă-kăt″ă-lĕp′tĭk)
acatamathesia (ă-kăt″ă-mă-thē′zē-ă) [Gr. *a-*, not, + *katamathesis*, understanding]
acataphasia (ă-kăt″ă-fā′zē-ă) [″ + *kataphasis*, affirmation]
acatastasia (ă-kăt-ăs-tā′zē-ă) [Gr. *akatastasis*, disorder]
acathexis (ă″kă-thĕks′ĭs) [Gr. *a-*, not, + *kathexis*, retention]
acathisia (ă″kă-thĭz′ē-ă) [″ + *kathisis*, sitting]
acaudal, acaudate (ă-kaw′dăl, -dāt) [″ + L. *cauda*, tail]

ACC *anodal closure contraction*
acc. *accommodation*
accelerated idioventricular rhythm
acceleration (ăk-sĕl″ĕr-ā′shŭn) [L. *accelerans*, hastening]
  a., angular
  a., central
  a., centripetal
  a., linear
  a., negative
  a., positive
  a., standard, of free fall
accelerator (ăk-sĕl′ĕr-ā″tor)
accelerator nerves
accelerator reflexes
accentuation (ăk-sĕn″chū-ā′shŭn) [L. *accentus*, accent]
acceptance
acceptor (ăk-sĕp′tor) [L. *accipere*, to accept]
  a., hydrogen
  a., oxygen
accessorius (ăk″sĕs-ō′rē-ŭs) [L., supplementary]
accessory (ăk-sĕs′ō-rē)
accessory muscles of respiration
accessory nerve
accessory sign
accident (ăk′sĭ-dĕnt) [L. *accidens*, happening]
  a., cerebrovascular
  a., radiation
  a., serum
accidental (ăk″sĭ-dĕn′tăl)
accident-prone
accipiter (ăk-sīp′ĭ-tĕr) [L., a hawk]
ACCI *anodal closure clonus*
acclimation, acclimatization (ăk-lĭ-mā′shŭn, ă-klī″mă-tĭ-zā′shŭn) [Fr. *acclimater*, acclimate]
acclimatize (ăk-klī′mă-tīz)
accommodation (ă-kŏm″ō-dā′shŭn) [L. *accommodare*, to suit]
  a., absolute
  a., amplitude of
  a., binocular
  a., excessive
  a., histologic

  a., mechanism
  a., negative
  a., positive
  a., range of
  a., relative
  a., spasm of
  a., subnormal
  a., synaptic
accommodation reflex
accommodative iridoplegia (ă-kŏm′ō-dā″tĭv ĭr″ĭ-dō-plē′jē-ă)
accouchement (ă-koosh-mŏn′) [Fr.]
  a. forcé
accoucheur, accoucheuse (ă-kooshŭr′, ă-koo-shĕz′) [Fr.]
accountability
accreditation
accrementition (ăk″rĕ-mĕn-tĭsh′ŭn) [L. *accrescere*, to increase]
accretio (ă-krē′shē-ō) [L.]
  a. cordis
accretion (ă-krē′shŭn) [L. *accrescere*, accrue]
acculturation
accuracy
ACD *absolute cardiac dullness*
AC/DC
ACD sol. *citric acid, trisodium citrate, dextrose solution*
ACE *adrenal cortical extract*
Ace bandage
acedia (ă-sē′dē-ă) [Gr. *a-*, not, + *kedos*, care]
acenesthesia (ă-sĕn″ĕs-thē′zē-ă) [″ + *koinos*, common, + *aisthesis*, feeling, perception]
acentric (ă-sĕn′trĭk) [″ + L. *centrum*, center]
A.C.E.P. *American College of Emergency Physicians*
acephalia, acephalism (ă-sĕ-fā′lē-ă, ă-sĕf′ă-lĭzm) [″ + *kephale*, head]
acephalo- (ă-sĕf′ă-lō-) [Gr. *a-*, not, + *kephale*, head]
acephalobrachia (ă-sĕf″ă-lō-brā′kē-ă) [″ + ″ + *brachion*, arm]
acephalocardia (ă-sĕf″ă-lō-kăr′dē-ă) [″ + ″ + *kardia*, heart]

acephalochiria (ă-sĕf"ă-lō-kī'rē-ă) [" + " + cheir, hand]

acephalocyst (ă-sĕf'ă-lō-sĭst) [" + " + kystis, bag]

acephalogastria (ă-sĕf"ă-lō-găs'trē-ă) [" + " + gaster, stomach]

acephalopodia (ă-sĕf"ă-lō-pō'dē-ă) [" + " + pous, foot]

acephalorhachia (ă-sĕf"ă-lō-rā'kē-ă) [" + " + rhachis, spine]

acephalostomia (ă-sĕf"ă-lō-stō'mē-ă) [" + " + stoma, mouth, opening]

acephalothoracia (ă-sĕf"ă-lō-thō-rā'sē-ă) [" + " + thorax, chest]

acephalus (ă-sĕf'ă-lŭs)

acerate (ăs'ĕr-āt) [L. acer]

acerbity (ă-sĕrb'ĭ-tē) [L. acerbus, sharp]

acervuline (ă-sĕr'vū-lĭn) [L. acervulus, a little heap]

acervuloma (ă-sĕr"vū-lō'mă) [" + oma, tumor]

acervulus (ă-sĕr'vū-lŭs) [L.]
a. cerebri

acestoma (ă-sĕs-tō'mă) [" + oma, tumor]

acetabular (ăs"ĕ-tăb'ū-lăr)

acetabulectomy (ăs"ĕ-tăb"ū-lĕk'tō-mē) [L. acetabulum, a little saucer for vinegar, + Gr. ektome, excision]

acetabuloplasty (ăs"ĕ-tăb'ū-lō-plăs"tē) [" + Gr. plassein, to form]

acetabulum (ăs"ĕ-tăb'ū-lŭm) [L., a little saucer for vinegar]

acetal (ăs'ĕ-tăl)

acetaldehyde (ăs"ĕt-ăl'dē-hīd")

acetamide (ăs"ĕt-ăm'īd)

acetaminophen (ă-sĕt"ă-mĭn'ō-fĕn)

acetaminophen poisoning

acetanilid (ăs"ĕ-tăn'ĭ-lĭd)

acetanilid poisoning

acetarsol, acetarsone (ăs"ĕ-tăr'sŏl, -sōn)

acetate (ăs'ĕ-tāt)

acetazolamide (ăs"ĕt-ă-zōl'ă-mīd)

acetic (ă-sē'tĭk) [L. acetum, vinegar]

acetic acid

a.a., glacial

acetic aldehyde

acetify (ă-sĕt'ĭ-fī) [" + fieri, to become]

acetimeter (ă-sē-tĭm'ĕ-tĕr) [" + Gr. metron, measure]

acetoacetic acid (ăs"ē-tō-ă-sē'tĭk)

Acetobacter (ă-sē"tō-băk'tĕr) [L. acetum, vinegar, + Gr. bakterion, little rod]
A. aceti

acetolase (ă-sĕt'ō-lās)

acetohexamide (ăs"ē-tō-hĕks'ă-mīd)

acetoin (ă-sĕt'ō-ĭn)

acetone (ăs'ĕ-tōn)
a. in urine, test for

acetone bodies

acetonemia (ăs"ē-tō-nē'mē-ă) [acetone + Gr. haima, blood]

acetonitrile (ăs"ē-tō-nī'trĭl)

acetonuria (ăs"ē-tō-nū'rē-ă) [acetone + Gr. ouron, urine]

acetophenazine maleate (ăs"ē-tō-fĕn'ă-zēn măl'ē-āt)

acetophenetidin (ăs"ē-tō-fĕ-nĕt'ĭ-dĭn)

acetosoluble (ăs"ē-tō-sŏl'ū-bl)

acetous (ăs'ĕ-tŭs) [L. acetum, vinegar]

acetum (ă-sē'tŭm) [L.]

acetyl (ăs'ĕ-tĭl, ă-sĕt'ĭl) [" + Gr. hyle, matter]
a. CoA

acetylation (ă-sĕt"ĭ-lā'shŭn)

acetylcholine (ăs"ĕ-tĭl-kō'lēn)
a. chloride

acetylcholinesterase (ăs"ĕ-tĭl-kō"lĭn-ĕs'tĕr-ās)

acetylcoenzyme A

acetylcysteine (ăs"ĕ-tĭl-sĭs'tē-ĭn)

acetyldigitoxin (ăs"ĕ-tĭl-dĭj"ĭ-tŏk'sĭn)

acetylene (ă-sĕt'ĭ-lēn)

acetylsalicylic acid (ă-sē"tĭl-săl"ĭ-sĭl'ĭk)

acetylsalicylic acid poisoning

acetyltransferase (ăs"ĕ-tĭl-trăns'fĕr-ās)

ACH adrenocortical hormone

ACh acetylcholine

achalasia (ăk"ă-lā'zē-ă) [Gr. a-, not, + chalasis, relaxation]

a. of the cardia
a., pelvirectal
a., sphincteral
AChE acetylcholinesterase
ache (āk) [AS. acan]
acheilia (ă-kī'lē-ă) [Gr. a-, not, + cheilos, lip]
acheiria (ă-kī'rē-ă) [" + cheir, hand]
acheiropodia (ă-kī"rō-pō'dē-ă) [" + " + pous, foot]
achievement age
Achilles jerk (ă-kĭl'ēz)
Achilles tendon
Achilles tendon reflex
achillobursitis (ă-kĭl"ō-bŭr-sī'tĭs) [Achilles + L. bursa, a pouch, + Gr. itis, inflammation]
achillodynia (ă-kĭl"ō-dĭn'ē-ă) [" + Gr. odyne, pain]
achillorrhaphy (ă-kĭl-or'ă-fē) [" + Gr. rhaphe, seam]
achillotenotomy (ă-kĭl"ō-těn-ŏt'ō-mē) [" + Gr. tenon, tendon, + tome, a cutting, slice]
achillotomy (ă-kĭl-ŏt'ō-mē) [" + tome, a cutting, slice]
achiria (ă-kī'rē-ă) [Gr. a-, not, + cheir, hand]
achlorhydria (ă"klor-hī'drē-ă) [" + chloros, green, + hydor, water]
a., histamine-proved
achloride (ă-klō'rīd)
achloropsia (ă-klō-rŏp'sē-ă) [" + chloros, green, + opsis, sight, appearance, vision]
acholia (ă-kō'lē-ă) [" + chole, bile]
a., pigmentary
acholic (ă-kō'lĭk)
acholuria (ă-kō-lū'rē-ă) [" + chole, bile, + ouron, urine]
achondrogenesis (ă-kŏn"drō-jěn'ē-sĭs) [Gr. a-, not, + chondros, cartilage, + genesis, generation, birth]
achondroplasia (ă-kŏn"drō-plă'sē-ă) [" + " + plasis, a molding]
achroma (ă-krō'mă) [" + chroma, color]

achromasia (ăk"rō-mă'zē-ă) [Gr. achromatos, without color]
achromate (ă-krō'māt) [Gr. a-, not, + chroma, color]
achromatic (ăk"rō-măt'ĭk) [Gr. achromatos, without color]
achromatic lens
achromatin (ă-krō'mă-tĭn)
achromatism (ă-krō'mă-tĭzm") [Gr. a-, not, + chroma, color, + -ismos, condition]
achromatocyte (ăk"rō-măt'ō-sīt) [Gr. achromatos, without color, + kytos, cell]
achromatolysis (ă-krō"mă-tŏl'ĭ-sĭs) [" + lysis, dissolution]
achromatophil (ă"krō-măt'ō-fĭl) [" + philos, love]
achromatopsia (ă-krō"mă-tŏp'sē-ă) [" + opsis, sight, appearance, vision]
achromatosis (ă-krō"mă-tō'sĭs) [" + osis, condition]
achromatous (ă-krō'mă-tŭs)
achromaturia (ă-krō"mă-tū'rē-ă) [" + ouron, urine]
achromia (ă-krō'mē-ă) [Gr. a-, not, + chroma, color]
a., congenital
achromic (ă-krō'mĭk)
achromocyte (ă-krō'mō-sīt) [" + " + kytos, cell]
achromophil (ă-krō'mō-fĭl) [" + " + philos, love]
achromotrichia (ă-krō"mō-trĭk'ē-ă) [" + " + trichia, condition of the hair]
a., nutritional
Achromycin (ăk"rō-mī'sĭn)
achroodextrin (ăk"rō-ō-děks'trĭn) [Gr. achroos, colorless, + dextrin]
achylia (ă-kī'lē-ă) [Gr. a-, not, + chylos, juice]
a. gastrica
a. pancreatica
achylosis (ă"kī-lō'sĭs)
achylous (ă-kī'lŭs) [Gr. achylos, without chyle]

achymia, achymosis (ă-kī'mē-ă, ăk-ĭ-mō'sĭs) [Gr. a-, not, + chymos, juice]

acicular (ă-sĭk'ū-lăr) [L. aciculus, little needle]

acid [L. acidum, acid]
a., acetic
a., acetic, dilute
a., acetic, glacial
a., acetoacetic
a., acetylacetic
a., acetylsalicylic
a., adenylic
a., alginic
a., amino
a., aminoacetic
a., aminobenzoic
a., aminocaproic
a., aminoglutaric
a., aminosalicylic
a., aminosuccinic
a., arachidonic
a., arsonic
a., arylarsonic
a., ascorbic
a., aspartic
a., barbituric
a., benzoic
a., bile
a., boric
a., butyric
a., carbolic
a., carbonic
a., carboxylic
a., chaulmoogric
a., cholic
a., chromic
a., citric
a., deoxyribonucleic
a., desoxyribonucleic
a., diacetic
a., 2-3-dihydroxypropanoic
a., ethanedioic
a., ethanoic
a., ethylenediaminetetraacetic
a., fatty
a., folic
a., formic

a., formiminoglutamic
a., gallic
a., glucuronic
a., glutamic
a., glyceric
a., glycocholic
a., glycuronic
a., hexadecanoic
a., homogentisic
a., hydriodic
a., hydrochloric
a., hydrocyanic
a., hydrosuccinic
a., hydroxy
a., hydroxytoluic
a., imino
a., inorganic
a., lactic
a., linoleic
a., linolenic
a., linolic
a., lysergic
a., malic
a., malonic
a., mandelic
a., methanoic
a., mineral
a., muriatic
a., nicotinic
a., nitric
a., nucleic
a., 9-octadecenoic
a., oleic
a., organic
a., oxalic
a., palmitic
a., pantothenic
a., para-aminobenzoic
a., para-aminosalicylic
a., pectic
a., pentanoic
a., perchloric
a., phenic
a., phenylglycolic
a., phosphoric
a., phosphorous
a., phosphotungstic
a., picric

a., prussic
a., pteroylglutamic
a., pyruvic
a., ribonucleic
a., salicylic
a., saturated fatty
a., silicic
a., stearic
a., succinic
a., sulfonic
a., sulfosalicylic
a., sulfuric
a., sulfurous
a., tannic
a., tartaric
a., taurocholic
a., trichloroacetic
a., 3,4,5-trihydroxybenzoic
a., unsaturated fatty
a., uric
a., valeric
acidaminuria (ăs″ĭd-ăm″ĭ-nū′rē-ă) [L. *acidum*, acid, + *amine* + Gr. *ouron*, urine]
acid-base balance
acidemia (ăs-ĭ-dē′mē-ă) [″ + Gr. *haima*, blood]
acid fallout
acid-fast
acidifiable (ă-sĭd′ĭ-fī″ă-bl) [″ + *fieri*, to be made, + *habilis*, able]
acidification (ă-sĭd″ĭ-fĭ-kā′shŭn) [″ + *factus*, made]
acidifier (ă-sĭd′ĭ-fī″ĕr) [″ + *fieri*, to be made]
acidimeter (ăs″ĭ-dĭm′ĕ-tĕr) [″ + Gr. *metron*, measure]
acidimetry (ăs″ĭ-dĭm′ĕ-trē)
acidism, acidismus (ăs′ĭ-dĭzm, ăs″ĭ-dĭz′mŭs) [L. *acidum*, acid, + Gr. *-ismos*, condition]
acidity (ă-sĭd′ĭ-tē)
    a. of stomach
acidocyte (ăs′ĭ-dō-sīt″) [″ + Gr. *kytos*, cell]
acidocytopenia (ăs″ĭ-dō-sī″tō-pē′nē-ă) [″ + ″ + *penia*, lack]
acidocytosis (ăs″ĭ-dō-sī-tō′sĭs) [″ +

″ + *osis*, condition]
acidophil(e) (ă-sĭd′ō-fĭl, -fīl) [″ + Gr. *philos*, love]
acidophilic (ă-sĭd″ō-fĭl′ĭk)
acidophilus milk (ăs″ĭ-dŏf′ĭ-lŭs)
acidoresistant (ăs″ĭ-dō-rĕ-zĭs′tănt)
acidosic (ăs″ĭ-dō′sĭk)
acidosis (ăs″ĭ-dō′sĭs) [L. *acidum*, acid, + Gr. *osis*, condition]
    a., carbon dioxide
    a., compensated
    a., diabetic
    a., hypercapnic
    a., hyperchloremic
    a., lactic
    a., metabolic
    a., renal
    a., respiratory
acidotic (ăs″ĭ-dŏt′ĭk)
acid poisoning
acid-proof
acid rain
acid salt
acidulate [L. *acidulus*, slightly acid]
acidulous (ă-sĭd′ū-lŭs)
acidum (ăs′ĭ-dŭm) [L.]
aciduria (ăs-ĭd-ū′rē-ă) [L. *acidum*, acid, + Gr. *ouron*, urine]
aciduric (ăs″ĭ-dū′rĭk) [″ + *durare*, to endure]
acies (ā′sē-ēz) [L., edge]
acinar (ăs′ĭ-năr) [L. *acinus*, grape]
acinesia (ăs″ĭ-nē′sē-ă) [Gr. *a-*, not, + *kinesis*, motion]
acinesic, acinetic (ăs-ĭ-nē′sĭk, -nĕt′ĭk)
Acinetobacter (ăs″ĭ-nĕt″ō-băk′tĕr) [Gr. *akinetos*, immovable, + *bakterion*, rod]
acini (ăs′ĭ-nī)
aciniform (ă-sĭn′ĭ-form) [L. *acinus*, grape, + *forma*, shape]
acinitis (ăs″ĭ-nī′tĭs) [″ + Gr. *itis*, inflammation]
acinose (ăs′ĭ-nōs) [L. *acinosus*, grapelike]
acinous (ăs′ĭ-nŭs)
acinus (ăs′ĭ-nŭs) [L., grape]
A.C. joint acromioclavicular joint

ackee (ă'kē)
acladiosis (ăk-lăd"ē-ō'sĭs)
aclasis, aclasia (ăk'lă-sĭs, ă-klā'zē-ă)
[Gr. a-, not, + klasis, a breaking away]
 a., diaphyseal
acleistocardia (ă-klĭs"tō-kăr'dē-ă) [Gr. akleistos, not closed, + kardia, heart]
ACLS Advanced Cardiac Life Support
acme (ăk'mē) [Gr. akme, point]
acne (ăk'nē) [Gr. akme, point]
 a. artificialis
 a. atrophica
 a., bromide
 a. cachecticorum
 a. ciliaris
 a. conglobata
 a., cystic
 a. decalvans
 a. frontalis
 a. fulminans
 a., halogen
 a. indurata
 a., keloid
 a. keratosa
 a. neonatorum
 a. papulosa
 a., petroleum
 a. pustulosa
 a. rosacea
 a., steroid
 a., summer
 a., tropical
 a. urticaria
 a. varioliformis
 a. vulgaris
acnegenic (ăk"nē-jĕn'ĭk) [Gr. akme, point, + gennan, to produce]
acneiform (ăk-nē'ĭ-form) [" + L. forma, shape]
acnemia (ăk-nē'mē-ă) [Gr. a-, not, + kneme, lower leg]
A.C.N.M. American College of Nurse Midwives
A.C.O.G. American College of Obstetricians and Gynecologists
acomia (ă-kō'mē-ă) [Gr. a-, not, + kome, hair]
aconite (ăk'ō-nīt) [Gr. akoniton]
aconitine (ă-kŏn'ĭ-tĭn)
acorea (ă-kō-rē'ă) [Gr. a-, not, + kore, pupil]
acoria (ă-kō'rē-ă) [" + koros, satiety]
acormus (ă-kor'mŭs) [" + kormos, trunk]
acousia (ă-koo'zē-ă) [Gr. akousis, hearing]
acousma (ă-kooz'mă) [Gr. akousma, a thing heard]
acoustic (ă-koos'tĭk) [Gr. akoustikos]
acoustic center
acoustic meatus
acoustic nerve
acousticophobia (ă-koos"tĭ-kō-fō'bē-ă) [Gr. akoustos, heard, + phobos, fear]
acoustics (ă-koos'tĭks)
A.C.P. American College of Physicians; American College of Pathologists
acquired (ă-kwīrd') [L. acquirere, to get]
acquired immune deficiency syndrome
acquisitus (ă-kwĭs'ĭ-tŭs) [L.]
acral (ăk'răl) [Gr. akron, extremity]
acrania (ă-krā'nē-ă) [Gr. a-, not, + kranion, skull]
Acremonium (ăk"rē-mō'nē-ŭm)
acrid (ăk'rĭd) [L. acer, sharp]
acridine (ăk'rĭ-dĭn)
acrimony (ăk'rĭ-mō"nē) [L. acrimonia, pungency]
acrisorcin (ăk-rĭ-sor'sĭn)
acritical (ă-krĭt'ĭ-kăl) [" + kritikos, critical]
acro- (ăk'rō) [Gr. akron, extremity]
acroagnosis (ăk"rō-ăg-nō'sĭs) [" + gnosis, knowledge]
acroanesthesia (ăk"rō-ăn-ĕs-thē'zē-ă) [" + an-, not, + aisthesis, feeling, perception]
acroarthritis (ăk-rō-ăr-thrī'tĭs) [" + arthron, joint, + itis, inflammation]
acroasphyxia (ăk"rō-ăs-fĭk'sē-ă) [" + asphyxia, pulse stoppage]

acroataxia (ăk″rō-ă-tăk′sē-ă) [Gr. *akron*, extremity, + *ataxia*, lack of order]

acroblast (ăk′rō-blăst) [″ + *blastos*, germ]

acrobrachycephaly (ăk″rō-brăk″ĭ-sĕf′ă-lē) [″ + *brachys*, short, + *kephale*, head]

acrobystitis (ăk″rō-bĭs-tī′tĭs) [Gr. *akrobystia*, prepuce, + *itis*, inflammation]

acrocentric (ăk″rō-sĕn′trĭk) [Gr. *akron*, extremity + L. *centrum*, center]

acrocephalia (ăk″rō-sĕf-ă′lē-ă) [″ + *kephale*, head]

acrocephalic (ăk″rō-sĕ-făl′ĭk)

acrocephalosyndactylia, acrocephalosyndactyly (ăk″rō-sĕf″ă-lō-sĭn-dăk-tĭl′ē-ă, -sĭn-dăk′tĭl-ē) [″ + ″ + *syn*, together, + *daktylos*, finger]

acrocephaly (ăk″rō-sĕf′ă-lē) [Gr. *akron*, extremity, + *kephale*, head]

acrochordon (ăk″rō-kor′dŏn) [″ + *chorde*, cord]

acrocinesia, acrocinesis (ăk″rō-sĭn-ē′sē-ă, -sĭs) [″ + *kinesis*, motion]

acrocinetic (ăk″rō-sĭn-ĕt′ĭk)

acrocontracture (ăk″rō-kŏn-trăkt′ūr) [″ + L. *contrahere*, to draw together]

acrocyanosis (ăk″rō-sī-ă-nō′sĭs) [″ + *kyanosis*, dark-blue color]

acrodermatitis (ăk″rō-dĕr-mă-tī′tĭs) [″ + *derma*, skin, + *itis*, inflammation]
   a. chronica atrophicans
   a. continua
   a. enteropathica
   a. hiemalis
   a. perstans

acrodermatosis (ăk″rō-dĕr″mă-tō′sĭs) [Gr. *akron*, extremity, + *derma*, skin, + *osis*, condition]

acrodolichomelia (ăk″rō-dŏl″ĭ-kō-mē′lē-ă) [″ + *dolichos*, long, + *melos*, limb]

acrodynia (ăk″rō-dĭn′ē-ă) [″ + *odyne*, pain]

acrodysesthesia (ăk″rō-dĭs″ĕs-thē′zē-ă) [″ + *dys*, bad, difficult, painful, disordered + *aisthesis*, feeling, perception]

acroesthesia (ăk″rō-ĕs-thē′zē-ă) [″ + *aisthesis*, feeling, perception]

acrogeria (ăk″rō-jĕr′ē-ă) [″ + *geron*, old man]

acrognosis (ăk″rŏg-nō′sĭs) [″ + *gnosis*, knowledge]

acrohyperhidrosis (ăk″rō-hī″pĕr-hī-drō′sĭs) [″ + *hyper*, over, above, excessive, + *hidrosis*, sweating]

acrohypothermy (ăk″rō-hī″pō-thĕr′mē) [″ + *hypo*, under, beneath, below, + *therme*, heat]

acrokeratosis verruciformis (ăk″rō-kĕr″ă-tō′sĭs vĕ-roo′sĭ-for″-mĭs) [″ + *keras*, horn, + *osis*, condition; L. *verruca*, wart, + *forma*, form]

acrokinesia (ăk″rō-kĭn-ē′sē-ă) [″ + *kinesis*, motion]

acrolein (ăk-rō′lē-ĭn) [L. *acer*, acrid, + *oleum*, oil]

acromacria (ăk″rō-măk′rē-ă) [Gr. *akron*, extremity, + *makros*, long]

acromastitis (ăk″rō-măs-tī′tĭs) [″ + *mastos*, breast, + *itis*, inflammation]

acromegaly (ăk″rō-mĕg′ă-lē) [″ + *megas*, big]

acromelalgia (ăk″rō-mĕl-ăl′jē-ă) [Gr. *akron*, extremity, + *melos*, limb, + *algos*, pain]

acromelic (ăk″rō-mĕl′ĭk) [″ + *melos*, limb]

acrometagenesis (ăk″rō-mĕt″ă-jĕn′ē-sĭs) [″ + *meta*, beyond, + *genesis*, generation, birth]

acromial (ăk-rō′mē-ăl) [″ + *omos*, shoulder]

acromial angle

acromial process

acromial reflex

acromicria (ăk″rō-mĭk′rē-ă) [″ + *mikros*, small]

acromioclavicular joint (ă-krō"mē-ŏ-klă-vĭk'ū-lăr) [" + *omos*, shoulder, + L. *clavicula*, small key]

acromiocoracoid (ă-krō"mē-ŏ-kor'ă-koyd) [" + " + *korax*, crow, + *eidos*, form, shape]

acromiohumeral (ăk-rō"mē-ŏ-hū'měr-ăl) [" + " + L. *humerus*, shoulder]

acromion (ă-krō'mē-ŏn) [Gr. *akron*, extremity, + *omos*, shoulder]

acromioscapular (ă-krō"mē-ŏ-skăp'ū-lăr) [" + " + L. *scapula*, shoulder blade]

acromiothoracic (ă-krō"mē-ŏ-thō-răs'ĭk) [" + " + *thorax*, chest]

acromphalus (ăk-rŏm'făl-ŭs) [" + *omphalos*, umbilicus]

acromyotonia, acromyotonus (ăk"rō-mī-ŏ-tō'nē-ă, -ŏt'ō-nŭs) [" + *mys*, muscle, + *tonos*, act of stretching, tension, tone]

acronarcotic (ăk"rō-năr-kŏt'ĭk) [L. *acer*, sharp, + Gr. *narkotikos*, benumbing]

acroneurosis (ăk"rō-nū-rō'sĭs) [Gr. *akron*, extremity, + *neuron*, nerve, + *osis*, condition]

acronym (ăk'rō-nĭm) [" + *onym*, name]

acronyx (ăk'rō-nĭks") [L. *acer*, sharp, + Gr. *onyx*, claw]

acro-osteolysis (ăk"rō-ŏs"tē-ŏl'ĭ-sĭs) [Gr. *akron*, extremity, + *osteon*, bone, + *lysis*, dissolution]

acropachy (ăk'rō-păk"ē) [" + *pachys*, thick]

acropachyderma (ăk"rō-păk"ē-děr'mă) [" + " + *derma*, skin]

acroparalysis (ăk"rō-pă-răl'ĭ-sĭs) [" + *paralyein*, to loosen, disable]

acroparesthesia (ăk"rō-păr-ĕs-thē'zē-ă) [" + *para*, alongside, past, beyond, + *aisthesis*, feeling, perception

acropathology (ăk"rō-pă-thŏl'ō-jē) [" + *pathos*, disease, suffering, + *logos*, word, reason]

acropathy (ă-krŏp'ă-thē) [" + *pathos*, disease, suffering]

acrophobia (ăk-rō-fō'bē-ă) [" + *phobos*, fear]

acroposthitis (ăk"rō-pŏs-thī'tĭs) [Gr. *akroposthis*, prepuce, + *itis*, inflammation]

acroscleroderma (ăk"rō-sklěr-ŏ-děr'mă) [Gr. *akron*, extremity, + *scleros*, hard, + *derma*, skin]

acrosclerosis (ăk"rō-sklěr-ŏ'sĭs) [" + " + *osis*, condition]

acrosome (ăk'rō-sōm) [" + *soma*, body]

acrosphacelus (ăk"rō-sfăs'ĕ-lŭs) [" + *sphakelos*, gangrene]

acroteric (ăk"rō-těr'ĭk) [Gr. *akroterion*, summit]

acrotism (ăk'rō-tĭzm) [Gr. *a-*, not, + *krotos*, striking, + *-ismos*, condition]

acrotrophoneurosis (ăk"rō-trŏf"ō-nū-rō'sĭs) [Gr. *akron*, extremity, + *trophe*, nourishment, + *neuron*, nerve, + *osis*, condition]

acryl(o)-

acrylaldehyde (ăk"rĭl-ăl'dĕ-hīd)

acrylamide (ă-krĭl'ă-mīd)

acrylate (ăk'rĭ-lāt)

acrylic acid (ă-krĭl'ĭk)

acrylic resin

acrylonitrile (ăk"rĭ-lō-nī'trĭl)

A.C.S., ACS American Cancer Society; American Chemical Society; American College of Surgeons; anodal closing sound

A.C.S.M. American College of Sports Medicine

act (ăkt)
   a., compulsive
   a., impulsive

ACTH adrenocorticotropic hormone

actin (ăk'tĭn)

acting out
   a.o., neurotic

actinic (ăk-tĭn'ĭk) [Gr. *aktis*, ray]

actinic burns

actinic dermatitis

actinism (ăk′tĭn-ĭzm)
actinium (ăk-tĭn′ē-ŭm) [Gr. *aktis*, ray]
actino- (ăk′tĭ-nō) [Gr. *aktis*, ray]
Actinobacillus (ăk″tĭ-nō-bă-sĭl′ŭs)
actinochemistry (ăk″tĭ-nō-kĕm′ĭs-trē)
[" + *chemeia*, chemistry]
actinodermatitis (ăk″tĭn-ō-dĕr-mă-
tĭ′tĭs) [" + *derma*, skin, + *itis*,
inflammation]
Actinomyces (ăk″tĭn-ō-mī′sēz) [" +
mykes, fungus]
  A. antibioticus
  A. bovis
  A. israelii
Actinomycetales (ăk″tĭ-nō-mī″sĕ-
tā′lēz)
actinomycete (ăk″tĭ-nō-mī′sēt)
actinomycetic (ăk″tĭ-nō-mī-sēt′ĭk)
actinomycetin (ăk″tĭn-ō-mī-sēt′ĭn)
actinomycin A (ăk″tĭn-ō-mī′sĭn)
actinomycin B
Actinomycin D
actinomycoma (ăk″tĭ-nō-mī-kō′ma)
[Gr. *aktis*, ray, + *mykes*, fungus,
+ *oma*, tumor]
actinomycosis (ăk″tĭn-ō-mī-kō′sĭs)
[" + " + *osis*, condition]
actinomycotic (ăk″tĭn-ō-mī-kŏt′ĭk)
actinon (ăk′tĭn-ŏn) [Gr. *aktis*, ray]
actinoneuritis (ăk″tĭn-ō-nū-rī′tĭs) [" +
neuron, nerve, + *itis*, inflammation]
actinophytosis (ăk″tĭ-nō-fī-tō′sĭs)
[" + *phyton*, plant, + *osis*,
condition]
actinotherapy (ăk″tĭn-ō-thĕr′ă-pē)
[" + *therapeia*, treatment]
action (ăk′shŭn) [L. *actio*]
  a., antagonistic
  a., astringent
  a., bacteriocidal
  a., bacteriostatic
  a., ball-valve
  a., calorigenic
  a., capillary
  a., cumulative
  a., drug
  a., reflex
  a., sparing

  a., specific
  a., specific dynamic
  a., synergistic
  a., thermogenic
  a., trigger
action of arrest
action potential
activate (ăk′tĭ-vāt)
**activated partial thromboplastin
time**
activator (ăk′tĭ-vā″tor)
active motion
active plate activator
active principle
active range of motion
active transport
activities of daily living
activity (ăk-tĭv′ĭ-tē)
  a., optical
activity analysis
actomyosin (ăk″tō-mī′ō-sĭn)
actual (ăk′chū-ăl) [L. *actus*, doing]
actual cautery
acufilopressure (ăk″ū-fĭ′lō-prĕsh″ŭr)
[L. *acus*, needle, + *filum*, thread,
+ *pressura*, pressure]
acuity (ă-kū′ĭ-tē) [L. *acuere*, to sharpen]
  a., visual
acuminate (ă-kū′mĭn-āt) [L. *acuminatus*,
sharpened]
acupressure (ăk′ū-prĕsh″ŭr) [L. *acus*,
needle, + *pressura*, pressure]
acupressure forceps
acupressure needles
acupuncture (ăk″ū-pŭngk′chūr) [" +
punctura, prick]
acus (ā′kŭs) [L., needle]
acusection (ăk″ū-sĕk′shŭn) [" +
secare, to cut]
acusticus (ă-kū′stĭ-kŭs) [Gr. *akoustikos*,
hearing]
acute (ă-kūt′) [L. *acutus*, sharp]
acute care
acutenaculum (ăk″ū-tĕn-ăk′ū-lŭm) [L.
acus, needle, + *tenaculum*,
holder]
**acute necrotizing ulcerative gingi-
vitis**

acute tubular necrosis

acute urethral syndrome

acutorsion (ăk″ū-tor′shŭn) [″ + torsio, twisting]

acyanoblepsia (ă-sī″ă-nō-blĕp′sē-ă) [Gr. a-, not, + kyanos, blue, + blepsis, vision]

acyanopsia (ă-sī″ă-nŏp′sē-ă)

acyanotic (ă-sī″ă-nŏt′ĭk) [″ + kyanos, blue]

acyclic (ă-sī′klĭk)

acyclovir (ă-sī′klō-vĭr)

acyesis (ă″sī-ē′sĭs) [″ + kyesis, pregnancy]

acyl (ăs′ĭl)

acylation (ăs″ĭ-lā′shŭn)

acystia (ă-sĭs′tē-ă) [″ + kystis, bladder]

acystinervia, acystineuria (ă-sĭs″tĭ-nĕr′vē-ă, -nū′rē-ă) [″ + ″ + neuron, nerve]

AD anodal duration; average deviation

ad, ad-, -ad [L., to]

a.d. [L.] auris dextra, right ear

A.D.A. American Dental Association; American Diabetes Association; American Dietetic Association

A.D.A.A. American Dental Assistants Association

adactylia, adactylism, adactyly (ă″dăk-tĭl′ē-ă, ā-dăk′tĭ-lĭzm, -lē) [Gr. a-, not, + daktylos, finger]

adamantine (ăd″ă-măn′tĭn) [Gr. adamantinos]

adamantinoma (ăd″ă-măn″tĭ-nō′mă) [″ + oma, tumor]

adamantoblast (ăd″ă-măn′tō-blăst) [Gr. adamas, hard surface, + blastos, germ]

adamantoblastoma (ăd″ă-măn″tō-blăs-tō′mă) [″ + ″ + oma, tumor]

adamantoma (ăd″ă-măn-tō′mă) [Gr. adamas, hard surface, + oma, tumor]

Adam's apple

Adams-Stokes syndrome [Robert Adams, Irish physician, 1791–1875; William Stokes, Irish physician, 1804–1878]

adaptation (ăd″ăp-tā′shŭn) [L. adaptare, to adjust]

  a., chromatic

  a., dark

  a., light

adapted clothing

adapter (ă-dăp′tĕr)

adaptive device

adaxial (ăd-ăk′sē-ăl) [L. ad, toward, + axis, axis]

ADC anodal duration contraction; axiodistocervical

add. [L.] adde, let there be added

adde (ăd′ē) [L.]

addict (ăd′ĭkt) [L. addictus, given over]

addiction (ă-dĭk′shŭn)

Addis count method (ăd′ĭs) [Thomas Addis, U.S. physician, 1881–1949]

Addison's disease [Thomas Addison, Brit. physician, 1793–1860]

addisonism (ăd′ĭ-sŭn-ĭzm″)

Addison's planes

addition (ă-dĭ′shŭn)

additive (ăd′ĭ-tĭv)

  a., food

adducent (ă-dū′sĕnt) [L. adducere, to bring toward]

adduct (ă-dŭkt′) [L. adductus, brought toward]

adduction (ă-dŭk′shŭn)

  a., convergent-stimulus

adductor (ă-dŭk′tor) [L., a bringer toward]

adductor reflex

adelomorphous (ă-dĕl″ō-mor′fŭs) [Gr. adelos, not seen, + morphe, shape]

adelphotaxis, adelphotaxy (ă-dĕl′fō-tăk″sĭs, -sē) [Gr. adelphos, brother, + taxis, arrangement]

adenalgia (ăd″ĕn-ăl′jē-ă) [Gr. aden, gland, + algos, pain]

adenase (ăd′ĕ-nāz) [″ + -ase, enzyme]

adendric, adendritic (ă-dĕn′drĭk, ă″dĕn-drĭt′ĭk) [Gr. a-, not, + den-

drites, rel. to a tree]

adenectomy (ăd″ĕn-ĕk′tō-mē) [Gr. *aden,* gland, + *ektome,* excision]

adenectopia (ăd″ĕ-nĕk-tō′pē-ă) [″ + ″ + *topos,* place]

adenemphraxis (ăd″ĕ-nĕm-frăk′sĭs) [″ + *emphraxis,* stoppage]

adenia (ă-dē′nē-ă)

adeniform (ă-dĕn′ĭ-form) [″ + L. *forma,* shape]

adenine (ăd′ĕ-nīn)

adenitis (ăd″ĕ-nī′tĭs) [″ + *itis,* inflammation]

adenization (ăd″ĕ-nĭ-zā′shŭn)

adeno- [Gr. *aden,* gland]

adenoacanthoma (ăd″ĕ-nō-ăk″ăn-thō′mă) [″ + *akantha,* thorn, + *oma,* tumor]

adenoameloblastoma (ăd″ĕ-nō-ă-mĕl″ō-blăs-tō′mă) [″ + O. Fr. *amel,* enamel, + Gr. *blastos,* germ, + *oma,* tumor]

adenoblast (ăd′ĕ-nō-blăst) [″ + *blastos,* germ]

adenocarcinoma (ăd″ĕ-nō-kăr″sĭn-ō′mă) [″ + *karkinos,* crab, + *oma,* tumor]
　　a., acinar
　　a., alveolar

adenocele (ăd′ĕ-nō-sēl″) [″ + *kele,* tumor, swelling]

adenocellulitis (ăd″ĕ-nō-sĕl″ū-lī′tĭs) [″ + L. *cella,* small chamber, + Gr. *itis,* inflammation]

adenochondroma (ăd″ĕ-nō-kŏn-drō′mă) [″ + *chondros,* cartilage, + *oma,* tumor]

adenocyst (ăd′ĕ-nō-sĭst″) [″ + *kystis,* sac]

adenocystoma (ăd″ĕ-nō-sĭs-tō′mă) [″ + *kystis,* sac, + *oma,* tumor]

adenodynia (ăd″ĕ-nō-dĭn′ē-ă) [″ + *odyne,* pain]

adenoepithelioma (ăd″ĕ-nō-ĕp″ĭ-thĕl-ē-ō′mă) [″ + *epi,* on, + *thele,* nipple, + *oma,* tumor]

adenofibroma (ăd″ĕ-nō-fĭ-brō′mă) [″ + L. *fibra,* fiber, + Gr. *oma,* tumor]

adenofibrosis (ăd″ĕ-nō-fĭ-brō′sĭs) [″ + ″ + Gr. *osis,* condition]

adenogenous (ăd″ĕ-nŏj′ĕ-nŭs) [″ + *gennan,* to produce]

adenohypophysis (ăd″ĕ-nō-hī-pŏf′ĭ-sĭs) [″ + *hypo,* under, beneath, below, + *phyein,* to grow]

adenoid (ăd′ĕ-noyd) [″ + Gr. *eidos,* form, shape]

adenoidectomy (ăd″ĕ-noyd-ĕk′tō-mē) [″ + ″ + *ektome,* excision]

adenoid hypertrophy

adenoiditis (ăd″ĕ-noyd-ī′tĭs) [″ + ″ + *itis,* inflammation]

adenoids (ăd′ĕ-noyds)

adenoid tissue

adenolipoma (ăd″ĕ-nō-lĭp-ō′mă) [″ + *lipos,* fat, + *oma,* tumor]

adenolymphitis (ăd″ĕ-nō-lĭm-fī′tĭs) [Gr. *aden,* gland, + L. *lympha,* lymph, + Gr. *itis,* inflammation]

adenolymphocele (ăd″ĕ-nō-lĭm′fō-sēl) [″ + ″ + Gr. *kele,* tumor, swelling]

adenolymphoma (ăd″ĕ-nō-lĭm-fō′mă) [″ + ″ + Gr. *oma,* tumor]

adenoma (ăd″ĕ-nō′mă) [″ + *oma,* tumor]
　　a., acidophil(ic)
　　a., basophil(ic)
　　a., chromophobe
　　a., eosinophil(ic)
　　a., fibroid
　　a., follicular
　　a., Hürthle cell
　　a., islet
　　a., langerhansian
　　a., malignant
　　a., papillary
　　a., pituitary
　　a., sebaceous
　　a. sebaceum
　　a., tubular
　　a., villous

adenomalacia (ăd″ĕ-nō-mă-lā′shē-ă) [Gr. *aden,* gland, + *malakia,* softening]

adenomatome (ăd″ĕ-nō′mă-tōm) [″ + oma, tumor, + tome, a cutting, slice]

adenomatosis (ăd″ĕ-nō-mă-tō′sĭs) [″ + oma, tumor, + osis, condition]

adenomatous (ăd″ĕ-nō′mă-tŭs)

adenomere (ăd′ĕ-nō-mēr″) [″ + meros, part]

adenomyoma (ăd″ĕ-nō-mī-ō′mă) [″ + mys, muscle, + oma, tumor]

adenomyometritis (ăd″ĕ-nō-mī″ō-mĕ-trī′tĭs) [″ + ″ + metra, womb, + itis, inflammation]

adenomyosarcoma (ăd″ĕ-nō-mī″ō-săr-kō′mă) [″ + ″ + sarx, flesh, + oma, tumor]

adenomyosis (ăd″ĕ-nō-mī-ō′sĭs) [″ + mys, muscle, + osis, condition]

adenopathy (ăd-ĕ-nŏp′ă-thē) [″ + pathos, disease, suffering]

adenopharyngitis (ăd″ĕ-nō-făr″ĭn-jī′tĭs) [″ + pharynx, throat, + itis, inflammation]

adenophthalmia (ăd″ĕ-nŏf-thăl′mē-ă) [″ + ophthalmos, eye]

adenosarcoma (ăd″ĕ-nō-săr-kō′mă) [″ + sarx, flesh, + oma, tumor]

adenosclerosis (ăd″ĕ-nō-sklĕ-rō′sĭs) [″ + sklerosis, a hardening]

adenose (ăd′ĕ-nōs)

adenosine (ă-dĕn′ō-sēn)
   a. 3′,5′-cyclic monophosphate
   a. diphosphate, a. 5′-diphosphate
   a. monophosphate, a. 5′-mono-phosphate
   a. triphosphate

adenosine triphosphatase (ă-dĕn″ō-sĭn trī-fŏs′fă-tās)

adenosis (ăd″ĕ-nō′sĭs) [Gr. aden, gland, + osis, condition]

adenotome (ăd′ĕ-nō-tōm) [″ + tome, a cutting, slice]

adenotonsillectomy (ăd″ĕ-nō-tŏn″sĭl-lĕk′tō-mē) [″ + L. tonsilla,

almond, + Gr. ektome, excision]

adenous (ăd′ĕ-nŭs)

adenovirus (ăd′ĕ-nō-vī′rŭs)

adenyl (ăd′ĕ-nĭl)
   a. cyclase

adenylate cyclase (ă-dĕn′ĭ-lāt sī′klās)

adenylic acid

adeps (ăd′ĕps) [L.]
   a. benzoinatus
   a. lanae
   a. lanae hydrosus

adermia (ă-dĕr′mē-ă) [Gr. a-, not, + derma, skin]

adermogenesis (ă-dĕr″mō-jĕn′ĕ-sĭs) [″ + ″ + genesis, generation, birth]

ADH antidiuretic hormone

A.D.H.A. American Dental Hygienists' Association

adherence, bacterial (ăd-hēr′ĕns)

adherent (ăd-hē′rĕnt) [L. adhaerere, to stick to]

adhesio (ăd-hē′zē-ō) [L. adhaesio, stuck to]

adhesion (ăd-hē′zhŭn) [L. adhaesio, stuck to]
   a., abdominal
   a., pericardial

adhesiotomy (ăd-hē″zē-ŏt′ō-mē) [L. adhaesio, stuck to, + Gr. tome, a cutting, slice]

adhesive (ăd-hē′sĭv) [L. adhaesio, stuck to]

adhesive inflammation

adhesive tape

adiadochokinesia, adiadochokinesis (ă-dī″ă-dō″kō-kĭ-nē′sē-ă, -nē′sĭs) [Gr. a-, not, + diadochas, successive, + kinesis, motion]

adiaphoresis (ă-dī″ă-fō-rē′sĭs) [″ + diaphorein, to perspire]

adiapneustia (ă″dī-ăp-nū′stē-ă) [″ + diapnein, to breathe through]

adiastole (ă″dī-ăs′tō-lē) [″ + diastole, dilatation]

adiathermancy (ă-dī″ă-thĕr′măn-sē) [″ + dia, through, + therme, heat]

Adie's syndrome (ā'dēz) [W. J. Adie, Brit. neurologist, 1886–1935]
adipectomy (ăd″ĭ-pĕk'tō-mē) [L. *adeps,* fat, + Gr. *ektome,* excision]
adipic (ă-dĭp'ĭk)
adipo-, adip- [L. *adeps,* fat]
adipocele (ăd'ĭ-pō-sēl″) [L. *adeps,* fat, + Gr. *kele,* tumor, swelling]
adipocellular (ăd″ĭ-pō-sĕl'ū-lăr)
adipocere (ăd'ĭ-pō-sēr″) [″ + *cera,* wax]
adipocyte (ăd'ĭ-pō-sīt) [″ + Gr. *kytos,* cell]
adipofibroma [″ + *fibra,* fiber, + Gr. *oma,* tumor]
adipogenous, adipogenic (ăd″ĭ-pŏj'ĕn-ŭs, -pō-jĕn'ĭk) [″ + Gr. *gennan,* to produce]
adipoid (ăd'ĭ-poyd) [L. *adeps,* fat, + Gr. *eidos,* form, shape]
adipokinesis (ăd″ĭ-pō-kī-nē'sīs) [″ + Gr. *kinesis,* motion]
adipokinetic action
adipolysis (ăd″ĭ-pŏl'ĭ-sīs) [″ + Gr. *lysis,* dissolution]
adiponecrosis (ăd″ĭ-pō-nĕ-krō'sīs) [″ + Gr. *nekrosis,* state of death]
adipose [L. *adiposus,* fatty]
adipose capsule
adipose tissue
adiposis (ăd″ĭ-pō'sīs) [″ + Gr. *osis,* condition]
　　a. cerebralis
　　a. dolorosa
　　a. hepatica
adipositis (ăd″ĭ-pō-sī'tīs) [L. *adiposus,* fatty, + Gr. *itis,* inflammation]
adiposity (ăd″ĭ-pŏs'ĭ-tē)
adiposogenital dystrophy (ăd″ĭ-pō″sō-jĕn'ĭ-tăl dĭs'trō-fē) [″ + *genitalis,* to beget, + Gr. *dys,* bad, difficult, painful, disordered, + *trophe,* nourishment]
adiposuria (ăd″ĭ-pō-sū'rē-ă) [″ + Gr. *ouron,* urine]
adipsia, adipsy (ă-dĭp'sē-ă, -sē) [Gr. *a-,* not, + *dipsa,* thirst]

aditus (ăd'ĭ-tŭs) [L.]
　　a. ad antrum
　　a. ad aquaeductum cerebri
　　a. ad infundibulum
　　a. glottidis inferior
　　a. glottidis superior
　　a. laryngis
adjunct (ăd'jŭnkt)
adjuster
adjustment [L. *adjuxtare,* to bring together]
adjustment disorder
adjuvant (ăd'jū-vănt) [L. *adjuvans,* aiding]
　　a., Freund's complete [Jules T. Freund, Hungarian-born U.S. bacteriologist, 1890–1961]
　　a., Freund's incomplete
adjuvant therapy
ADL activities of daily living,
Adler, Alfred [Austrian psychiatrist, 1870–1937]
ad lib. [L.] *ad libitum,* at pleasure; as much as is wanted
A.D.N. Associate Degree in Nursing
ad nauseam (ăd naw'sē-ăm) [L.]
adnerval (ăd-nĕr'văl) [L. *ad.* to, + *nervus,* nerve]
adneural (ăd-nū'răl) [″ + Gr. *neuron,* nerve]
adnexa (ăd-nĕk'să) [L.]
　　a., dental
　　a. oculi
　　a. uteri
adnexal (ăd-nĕk'săl)
adnexitis (ăd″nĕk-sī'tīs) [L. *adnexa,* appendages, + Gr. *itis,* inflammation]
adnexopexy (ăd-nĕks'ō-pĕk″sē) [″ + Gr. *pexis,* fixation]
Ad-OAP Adriamycin (doxorubicin), Oncovin (vincristine), Ara-C (cytarabine), prednisone
adolescence (ăd″ō-lĕs'ĕns) [L. *adolescens*]
adolescent (ăd″ō-lĕs'ĕnt)
adoption (ă-dŏp'shŭn) [L. *ad,* to, + *optare,* to choose]

adoral (ăd-ō'răl) [" + os, mouth]
ADP adenosine diphosphate
adrenal (ăd-rē'năl) [L. ad, to, + ren, kidney]
adrenal crisis
adrenalectomy (ăd-rē"năl-ĕk'tō-mē) [L. ad, to, + ren, kidney, + Gr. ektome, excision]
adrenal gland
Adrenalin (ă-drĕn'ă-lĭn)
adrenaline (ă-drĕn'ă-lēn)
adrenalinemia (ă-drĕn"ă-lĭn-ē'mē-ă) [L. ad, to, + ren, kidney, + Gr. haima, blood]
adrenalinuria (ă-drĕn"ă-lĭn-ū'rē-ă) [" + " + Gr. ouron, urine]
adrenarche (ăd"rĕn-ăr'kē) [" + " + Gr. arche, beginning]
adrenergic (ăd-rĕn-ĕr'jĭk) [" + " + Gr. ergon, work]
adrenergic neuron-blocking agents
adrenitis (ăd"rē-nī'tĭs) [" + " + Gr. itis, inflammation]
adrenoceptive (ă-drē"nō-sĕp'tĭv) [" + " + recipere, to receive]
adrenochrome (ăd"rē'nō-krōm) [" + " + Gr. chroma, color]
adrenocortical (ăd-rē"nō-kor'tĭ-kăl)
adrenocortical hormones
adrenocorticotropic (ăd-rē"nō-kor"tĭ-kō-trōp'ĭk) [" + " + cortex, bark + Gr. tropikos, turning]
adrenocorticotropic hormone
adrenocorticotropin (ăd-rē"nō-kor"tĭ-kō-trōp'ĭn)
adrenogenital (ăd-rē-nō-jĕn'ĭ-tăl) [" + " + genitalis, to beget]
adrenogenital syndrome
adrenogenous (ăd"rĕn-ŏj'ĕ-nŭs) [" + " + Gr. gennan, to produce]
adrenoleukodystrophy (ă-drē"nō-loo"kō-dĭs'trō-fē) [" + " + Gr. leukos, white + dys, bad, difficult, painful, disordered, + trephein, to nourish]
adrenolytic (ăd"rĕn-ō-lĭt'ĭk) [L. ad, to, + ren, kidney, + Gr. lysis, dissolution]
adrenomegaly (ăd-rĕn"ō-mĕg'ă-lē) [" + " + Gr. megas, large]
adrenomimetic (ă-drē"nō-mĭ-mĕt'ĭk) [" + " + Gr. mimetikos, imitating]
adrenopathy (ăd"rĕn-ŏp'ă-thē) [" + " + Gr. pathos, disease, suffering]
adrenopause (ăd-rĕn'ō-pawz) [" + " + Gr. pausis, cessation]
adrenosterone (ăd"rĕ-nŏs'tĕ-rōn)
adrenotoxin (ăd-rē"nō-tŏk'sĭn) [" + " + Gr. toxikon, poison]
adrenotropic (ăd-rē"nō-trŏp'ĭk) [" + " + Gr. tropikos, turning]
Adriamycin
ADS antidiuretic substance
adsorbate (ăd-sor'bāt)
adsorbent (ăd-sor'bĕnt)
adsorption (ăd-sorp'shŭn) [L. ad, to, + sorbere, to suck in]
adsternal (ăd-stĕr'năl) [" + Gr. sternon, chest]
adterminal (ăd-tĕr'mĭ-năl) [" + terminus, boundary]
adtorsion (ăd-tor'shŭn) [" + torsio, twisted]
adult (ă-dŭlt') [L. adultus, grown up]
adulteration (ă-dŭl"tĕr-ă'shŭn) [L. adulterare, to pollute]
adult respiratory distress syndrome (ARDS)
advance (ăd-văns') [Fr. avancer, to set forth]
advanced cardiac life support
advancement (ăd-văns'mĕnt) [Fr. avancer, to set forth]
 a., capsular
adventitia (ăd"vĕn-tĭsh'ē-ă) [L. adventicius, coming from abroad]
adventitious (ăd"vĕn-tĭsh'ŭs)
adverse effects
adverse reactions
adynamia (ăd"ĭ-nā'mē-ă) [Gr. a-, not, + dynamis, strength]
adynamic (ăd"ĭ-năm'ĭk, ă-dī-năm'ĭk)
adynamic ileus

A.E. *above elbow*
Aedes (ă-ē′dēs) [Gr. *aedes*, unpleasant]
   A. aegypti
aeluropsis (ē″lū-rŏp′sĭs) [Gr. *ailouros*, cat, + *opsis*, sight, appearance, vision]
aer- (ĕr) [Gr. *aer*, air]
aerated (ĕr′ā″tĕd)
aeration (ĕr″ā′shŭn)
aeriform (ĕr′ĭ-form) [″ + L. *forma*, shape]
aero- (ĕr′ō)
Aerobacter (ĕr″ō-băk′tĕr) [″ + *bakterion*, little rod]
   A. aerogenes
aerobe (ĕr′ōb) [″ + *bios*, life]
   a., facultative
   a., obligate
aerobic (ĕr-ō′bĭk)
aerobic exercise
aerobic training
aerobion (ĕr″ō′bē-ŏn)
aerobiosis (ĕr″ō-bī-ō′sĭs) [″ + *biosis*, mode of living]
aerocele (ĕr′ō-sēl) [″ + *kele*, tumor, swelling]
aerocolpos (ĕr″ō-kŏl′pŏs) [″ + *kolpos*, vagina]
aerocoly (ĕr″ŏk′ō-lē) [″ + *kolon*, colon]
aerocystoscopy (ĕr″ō-sĭs-tŏs′kō-pē) [″ + *kystis*, bladder, + *skopein*, to examine]
aerodermectasia (ĕr″ō-der″mĕk-tā′zē-ă) [Gr. *aer*, air, + *derma*, skin, + *ektasis*, stretching out]
aerodontalgia (ĕr″ō-dŏnt-ăl′jē-ă) [″ + *odous*, tooth, + *algos*, pain]
aerodontia (ĕr″ō-dŏn′shē-ă)
aerodynamics (ĕr″ō-dĭ-năm′ĭks) [″ + *dynamis*, force]
aeroembolism (ĕr″ō-ĕm′bō-lĭzm) [″ + NL. *embolismus*, intercalary, + *-ismos*, condition]
aeroemphysema (ĕr″ō-ĕm-fĭ-zē′ma) [″ + *emphysema*, an inflation]

aerogen (ĕr′ō-jĕn″) [″ + *gennan*, to produce]
aerogenesis (ĕr″ō-jĕn′ĕ-sĭs) [″ + *genesis*, generation, birth]
aerogenic, aerogenous (ĕr″ō-jĕn′ĭk, -ŏj′ĕn-ŭs)
aerogram (ĕr′ō-grăm″) [″ + *gramma*, letter, piece of writing]
aerohydrotherapy [″ + *hydor*, water, + *therapeia*, treatment]
aeromedical transportation
aerometer (ĕr-ŏm′ĕ-tĕr) [″ + *metron*, measure]
Aeromonas (ĕr″ō-mō′năs)
   A. hydrophilia
aeroneurosis (ĕr″ō-nū-rō′sis) [Gr. *aer*, air, + *neuron*, nerve, + *osis*, condition]
aeropathy (ĕr-ŏp′ă-thē) [″ + *pathos*, disease, suffering]
aeroperitoneum, aeroperitonia (ĕr″ō-pĕr″ĭ-tō-nē′ŭm, -tō′nē-ă) [″ + *peritonaion*, stretched around or over]
aerophagia, aerophagy (ĕr″ō-fā′jē-ă, ĕr″ŏf′ă-jē) [″ + *phagein*, to eat]
aerophilic, aerophilous (ĕr″ō-fĭl′ĭk, -ŏf′ĭ-lŭs) [″ + *philein*, to love]
aerophobia (ĕr-ō-fō′bē-ă) [″ + *phobos*, fear]
aerophore (ĕr′ō-for) [″ + *phoros*, bearing]
aerophyte (ĕr′-ō-fīt) [″ + *phyton*, plant]
aeroplethysmograph (ĕr″ō-plĕ-thĭz′mō-grăf) [″ + *plethysmos*, enlargement, + *graphein*, to write]
aeroscope (ĕr′ō-skōp) [″ + *skopein*, to examine]
aerosinusitis (ĕr″ō-sī″nŭs-ī′tĭs) [″ + L. *sinus*, a hollow, + Gr. *itis*, inflammation]
aerosis (ĕr-ō′sĭs) [″ + *osis*, condition]
aerosol (ĕr′ō-sŏl) [″ + L. *solutio*, solution]
aerosolization (ĕr″ō-sŏl″ĭ-zā′shŭn)
aerosol therapy
aerospace medicine

Aerosporin (ĕr″ō-spō′rĭn)
aerotaxis (ĕr″ō-tăk′sĭs) [Gr. *aer*, air, + *taxis*, arrangement]
aerotherapy (ĕr″ō-thĕr′ă-pē) [″ + *therapeia*, treatment]
aerothermotherapy (ĕr″ō-thĕr″mō-thĕr′ă-pē) [″ + *thermos*, heat, + *therapeia*, treatment]
aerothorax (ĕr″ō-thō′răks) [″ + *thorax*, chest]
aerotitis (ĕr-ō-tī′tĭs) [″ + *ot-*, ear, + *itis*, inflammation]
aerotropism (ĕr-ŏt′rō-pĭzm) [″ + *trope*, a turn, + *-ismos*, condition]
aerourethroscope (ĕr-ō-ū″rē′thrō-skōp″) [″ + *ourethra*, urethra, + *skopein*, to examine]
aerourethroscopy (ĕr″ō-ū″rē-thrŏs′kō-pē)
Aesculapius (ĕs″kū-lā′pē-ŭs)
   A., staff of
aesthetics (ĕs-thĕt′ĭks) [Gr. *aisthesis*, feeling, perception]
afebrile (ă-fĕb′rĭl) [Gr. *a-*, not, + L. *febris*, fever]
affect (ăf′fĕkt) [L. *affectus*, exerting influence on]
affection (ă-fĕk′shŭn)
affective (ă-fĕk′tĭv)
affective disorders
afferent (ăf′ĕr-ĕnt) [L. *ad*, to, + *ferre*, to bear]
afferent nerves
affiliation (ă-fĭl-ē-ā′shŭn) [L. *affiliare*, to take to onself as a son]
affinity (ă-fĭn′ĭ-tē) [L. *affinis*, neighboring]
   a., chemical
   a., elective
   a., selective
afflux (ăf′lŭks) [L. *ad*, to, + *fluere*, to flow]
A fiber
afibrinogenemia (ă-fī″brĭn-ō-jĕ-nē′mē-ă) [Gr. *a-*, not, + L. *fibra*, fiber, + Gr. *gennan*, to produce, + *haima*, blood]
aflatoxicosis (ăf′lă-tŏk″sĭ-kō′sĭs)

aflatoxin (ăf′lă-tŏk′sĭn)
AFP *alpha-fetoprotein*
afteraction
afterbirth
aftercare
aftercataract
aftercurrent
afterdischarge
aftereffect
afterhearing
afterimage
afterimpression
afterload
aftermovement
afterpains
afterperception
afterpotential wave
aftersensation
aftertaste
aftertreatment
aftervision
Ag [L.] *argentum*, silver
against medical advice
agalactia (ăg″ă-lăk′shē-ă) [Gr. *a-*, not, + *gala*, milk]
agalorrhea (ă-găl″ō-rē′ă) [″ + ″ + *rhein*, to flow]
agamic (ă-găm′ĭk) [″ + *gamos*, marriage]
agammaglobulinemia (ă-găm″ă-glŏb″ū-lĭn-ē′mē-ă) [″ + *gamma globulin* + Gr. *haima*, blood]
agamogenesis (ăg″ă-mō-jĕn′ĕ-sĭs) [″ + *gamos*, marriage, + *genesis*, generation, birth]
agar (ā′găr, ăg′ăr) [Malay, gelatin]
agar-agar
agaric (ă-găr′ĭk) [Gr. *agarikon*, a sort of fungus]
agastria (ă-găs′trē-ă) [Gr. *a-*, not, + *gaster*, stomach]
agastric (ă-găst′rĭk)
agathanasia (ăg″ă-thă-nā′zē-ă) [Gr. *aganthos*, good, + *thanatus*, death]
AgCl
age [Fr. *age*, L. *aetas*]
   a., achievement

a., anatomical
a., bone
a., chronological
a., developmental
a., emotional
a., gestational
a., menarcheal
a., mental
a., physiological
aged (ājd', ā'jĕd)
ageism (āj'ĭzm)
agenesia, agenesis (ă"jĕn-ē'sē-ă, ă-jĕn'ĕ-sis) [Gr. a-, not, + genesis, generation, birth]
agenitalism (ă-jĕn'ĭ-tăl-ĭzm) [" + L. genitalis, to beget, + Gr. -ismos, condition]
agent (ā'jĕnt) [L. agere, to do]
Agent Orange
age of consent
agerasia (ā-jĕr-ā'sē-ă) [Gr. a-, not, + geras, old age]
ageusia, ageustia (ă-gū'sē-ă, ă-goos'tē-ă) [" + geusis, taste]
a., central
a., conduction
a., peripheral
agger (ăj'ĕr) [L.]
a. nasi
agglomerate (ă-glŏm'ĕ-rāt) [L. ad, to, + glomerare, to wind into a ball]
agglutinable (ă-gloo'tĭ-nă-bl) [L. agglutinans, gluing]
agglutinant (ă-gloo'tĭ-nănt)
agglutination (ă-gloo"tĭ-nā'shŭn)
agglutinative (ă-gloo'tĭ-nā"tĭv)
agglutinin (ă-gloo'tĭ-nĭn) [L. agglutinans, gluing]
a., anti-Rh
a., cold
a., flagellar
a., group
a., H
a., immune
a., nonspecific
a., O
a., somatic
agglutinogen (ă-gloo-tĭn'ō-jĕn) [L.

agglutinans, gluing, + Gr. gennan, to produce]
a.'s, A and B
a.'s, M and N
a., Rh
agglutinogenic, agglutogenic (ă-gloo"tĭ-nō-jen'ĭk, ă-gloo"tō-jĕn'ĭk)
agglutinoid (ă-gloo'tĭn-oyd) [L. agglutinans, gluing, + Gr. eidos, form, shape]
agglutinophilic (ă-gloo"tĭn-ō-fĭl'ĭk) [" + Gr. philos, love]
agglutinophore (ă-gloo'tĭn-ō-for) [" + Gr. pherein, to bear]
agglutometer (ăg"loo-tŏm'ĕ-tĕr) [" + Gr. metron, measure]
aggregate (ăg'rĕ-gāt) [L. aggregatus, collect]
aggregation (ăg"rĕ-gā'shŭn)
a., cell
a., familial
aggression (ă-grĕsh'ŭn) [L. aggredi, to approach with hostility]
aging (āj'ĭng)
agitated depression
agitation (ăj"ĭ-tā'shŭn) [L. agitare, to drive]
agitographia (ăj"ĭ-tō-grăf'ē-ă) [" + Gr. graphein, to write]
agitophasia (ăj"ĭ-tō-fā'zē-ă) [" + Gr. phasis, utterance]
aglaucopsia, aglaukopsia (ă"glaw-kŏp'sē-ă) [Gr. a-, + glaukos, gleaming, gray, + opsis, sight, appearance, vision]
aglossia (ă-glŏs'ē-ă) [" + glossa, tongue]
aglossostomia (ă"glŏs-ō-stō'mē-ă) [" + " + stoma, mouth, opening]
aglutition (ă-gloo-tĭsh'ŭn) [" + L. glutire, to swallow]
aglycemia (ă"glī-sē'mē-ă) [" + glykys, sweet, + haima, blood]
aglycosuric (ă-glī"kō-sū'rĭk) [" + " + ouron, urine]
agminate(d) (ăg'mĭ-nāt) [L. agmen, a crowd]

agminated follicles
agnathia (ăg-nā′thē-ă) [Gr. a-, not, + gnathos, jaw]
agnea (ăg′nē-ă) [″ + gnosis, knowledge]
AgNO₃
agnogenic (ăg-nō-jĕn′ĭk) [″ + gnosis, knowledge, + gennan, to produce]
agnosia (ăg-nō′zē-ă) [″ + gnosis, knowledge]
   a., auditory
   a., finger
   a., optic
   a., tactile
-agogue (ă-gŏg) [Gr. agogos, leading, inducing]
agonad, agonadal (ă-gō′năd, ă-gŏn′ă-dăl) [Gr. a-, not, + gone, seed]
agonal (ăg′ō-năl) [Gr. agon, a contest]
agonist (ăg′ŏn-ĭst)
agony (ăg′ō-nē)
agoraphobia (ăg″ō-ră-fō′bē-ă) [Gr. agora, marketplace, + phobos, fear]
-agra [Gr. agra, a seizure]
agranulocyte (ă-grăn′ū-lō-sīt) [Gr. a-, not, + L. granulum, granule, + Gr. kytos, cell]
agranulocytic (ă-grăn-ū-lō-sĭt′ĭk)
agranulocytosis (ă-grăn″ū-lō-sī-tō′sĭs) [″ + ″ + ″ + osis, condition]
agranuloplastic (ă-grăn″ū-lō-plăs′tĭk) [″ + L. granulum, granule, + Gr. plastikos, formative]
agranulosis (ă-grăn″ū-lō′sĭs)
agraphia (ă-grăf′ē-ă) [″ + graphein, to write]
   a., absolute
   a., acoustic
   a., amnemonic
   a., atactic
   a., cerebral
   a., mental
   a., motor
   a., optic

   a., verbal
agromania (ăg″rō-mā′nē-ă) [Gr. agros, field, + mania, frenzy]
agrypnia (ă-grĭp′nē-ă) [Gr. agrypnos, sleepless]
agrypnocoma (ă-grĭp″nō-kō′mă) [″ + koma, deep sleep]
agrypnotic (ă″grĭp-nŏt′ĭk)
ague (ā′gū) [Fr. aigu, sharp, acute]
agyria (ă-jī′rē-ă) [Gr. a-, not, + gyros, circle]
ah hypermetropic astigmatism
A.H.A. American Heart Association; American Hospital Association
AHF antihemophilic factor
AHG antihemophilic globulin
Ahlfeld's sign (ăl′fĕlts) [Friedrich Ahlfeld, Ger. obstetrician, 1843–1929]
ahypnia (ă-hĭp′nē-ă) [Gr. a-, not, + hypnos, sleep]
A.I. aortic insufficiency; artificial insemination; axioincisal
aichmophobia (ăk″mō-fō′bē-ă) [Gr. aichme, point, + phobos, fear]
A.I.D. Agency for International Development; artificial insemination by donor
aid (ād)
   a., hearing
AIDS acquired immune deficiency syndrome
AIDS-related complex
A.I.H. artificial insemination by husband
ailment
ailurophobia (ă-lū″rō-fō′bē-ă) [Gr. ailouros, cat, + phobos, fear]
ainhum (ān′hŭm) [African]
air (ār) [Gr. aer, air]
   a., alveolar
   a., complemental
   a., dead space
   a., dead space, mechanical
   a., functional residual
   a., liquid
   a., minimal
   a., reserve
   a., residual
   a., supplemental
   a., tidal

air bed
air bronchogram sign
air cell
air conditioning
air conduction
air curtain
air cushion
air embolism [L. *embolismus*]
air flow, laminar
air-fluidized bed
air gap principle
air hunger
airplane splint
air pollution
air sac
airsickness
air splint
air swallowing
air vesicle
airway
A.K. *above knee*
akaryocyte (ă-kăr′ē-ō-sīt″) [Gr. a-, not, + *karyon*, nucleus, + *kytos*, cell]
akaryote (ă-kăr′ē-ōt) [″ + *karyon*, nucleus]
akatamathesia (ă-kăt″ă-mă-thē′zē-ă) [″ + *katamathesis*, understanding]
akathisia (ăk″ă-thĭ′zē-ă) [″ + *kathisis*, sitting]
akee (ăk′ē, ă-kē′) [Liberian]
akembe (ă-kěm′bē) [African]
akinesia (ă″kĭ-nē′zē-ă) [Gr. a-, not, + *kinesis*, motion]
  a. algera
  a. amnestica
akinetic (ă″kĭ-nět′ĭk)
Al *aluminum*
-al [L.]
ala (ā′lă) [L., wing]
  a. auris
  a. cerebelli
  a. cinerea
  a. cristae galli
  a. lobuli centralis
  a. major ossis sphenoidalis
  a. minor ossis sphenoidalis
  a. nasi

  a. of ethmoid
  a. of ilium
  a. of sacrum
  a. vomeris
alacrima (ā-lăk′rĭ-mă) [Gr. a-, not, + L. *lacrima*, tear]
alalia (ă-lā′lē-ă) [″ + *lalia*, chatter, prattle]
alanine (ăl′ă-nēn)
  a. aminotransferase
alar (ā′lăr) [L. *ala*, wing]
alar artery
alar cartilage
alastrim (ă-lăs′trĭm) [Portuguese *alastrar*, to spread]
alate (ā′lāt) [L. *ala*, wing]
alba [L. *albus*, white]
albedo (ăl-bē′dō) [L.]
  a. retinae
  a. unguium
Albers-Schönberg disease (ăl-bărs-shěrn′bărg) [Heinrich Ernst Albers-Schönberg, Ger. roentgenologist, 1865–1921]
Albert's disease [Eduard Albert, Austrian surgeon, 1841–1900]
albicans [L.]
  a., corpus
albidum (ăl′bĭ-dŭm) [L.]
albiduria [L. *albidus*, white, + Gr. *ouron*, urine]
albidus (ăl′bĭ-dŭs) [L.]
Albini's nodules (ăl-bē′nēz) [Giuseppe Albini, It. physiologist, 1830–1911]
albinism (ăl′bĭn-ĭzm) [L. *albus*, white, + Gr. *-ismos*, condition]
albino (ăl-bī′nō)
albinuria (ăl″bĭ-nū′rē-ă) [″ + Gr. *ouron*, urine]
albocinereous (ăl″bō-sĭn-ē′rē-ŭs) [″ + *cinereus*, gray]
Albright's disease [Fuller Albright, U.S. physician, 1900–1969]
albuginea (ăl-bū-jĭn′ē-ă) [L. from *albus*, white]
  a. corporum cavernosorum
  a. oculi

a. ovarii

a. testis

albugineotomy (ăl″bū-jĭn″ē-ŏt′ō-mē) [*albuginea* + Gr. *tome*, a cutting, slice]

albugineous (ăl″bū-jĭn′ē-ŭs)

albuginitis (ăl″bū-jĭn-ī′tĭs) [″ + Gr. *itis*, inflammation]

albugo (ăl-bū′gō) [L.]

albumen (ăl-bū′měn) [L.]

albumin (ăl-bū′mĭn) [L. *albumen*, white of egg]

a., acid

a., alkali

a., blood

a., circulating

a., derived

a., egg

a., human

a., muscle

a., native

a., serum

a., urinary

a., vegetable

albuminate (ăl-bū′mĭ-nāt)

albuminaturia (ăl-bū″mĭ-nă-tū′rē-ă) [L. *albumen*, white of egg, + Gr. *ouron*, urine]

albuminiferous (ăl-bū″mĭn-ĭf′ĕ-rŭs) [″ + *ferre*, to bear]

albuminimeter (ăl-bū″mĭn-ĭm′ĕ-tĕr) [″ + Gr. *metron*, measure]

albuminiparous (ăl-bū″mĭn-ĭp′ă-rŭs) [″ + *parere*, to beget, produce]

albuminocholia (ăl-bū″mĭ-nō-kō′lē-ă) [″ + Gr. *chole*, bile]

albuminogenous (ăl-bū″mĭn-ŏj′ĕ-nŭs) [″ + Gr. *gennan*, to produce]

albuminoid (ăl-bū′mĭ-noyd″) [″ + Gr. *eidos*, form, shape]

albuminolysis (ăl-bū″mĭn-ŏl′ĭ-sĭs) [″ + Gr. *lysis*, dissolution]

albuminoptysis (ăl-bū-mĭn-ŏp′tĭ-sĭs) [″ + Gr. *ptyein*, to spit]

albuminoreaction (ăl-bū″mĭ-nō-rē-ăk′shŭn) [″ + *re*, again, + *agere*, to act]

albuminorrhea (ăl-bū″mĭ-nō-rē′ă)

[″ + Gr. *rhein*, to flow]

albuminose (ăl-bū′mĭn-ōs)

albuminosis (ăl-bū″mĭ-nō′sĭs) [″ + Gr. *osis*, condition]

albuminous (ăl-bū′mĭ-nŭs)

albumin test

albuminuretic [L. *albumen*, white of egg, + Gr. *ouretikos*, causing urine to flow]

albuminuria (ăl-bū-mĭ-nū′rē-ă) [″ + Gr. *ouron*, urine]

a., cyclic

a., digestive

a., extrarenal or accidental

a., functional

a., intrinsic

a., orthostatic

a., pathological

a., physiological

a., postural

a., renal

a., toxic

a., transient

a., true

albuminuric retinitis (ăl″bū-mĭ-nū′rĭk rĕt″ĭ-nī′tĭs)

albumoscope (ăl-bū′mō-skōp) [″ + Gr. *skopein*, to examine]

albumose (ăl′bū-mōs)

albumosemia (ăl″bū-mō-sē′mē-ă) [″ + Gr. *haima*, blood]

albumosuria (ăl″bū-mō-sū′rē-ă) [″ + Gr. *ouron*, urine]

albus [L.]

Alcaligenes (ăl″kă-lĭj′ĭ-nēz)

A. faecalis

Alcock's canal [Thomas Alcock, London surgeon, 1784–1833]

alcohol (ăl′kō-hŏl) [Arabic *al-koh'l*, something subtle]

a., absolute

a., dehydrated

a., denatured

a., diluted

a., ethyl

a., grain

a., methyl

a., wood

Alcohol, Drug Abuse, and Mental Health Administration
alcoholic (ăl-kō-hŏl′ĭk) [L. *alcoholicus*]
alcoholic fermentation
alcoholic psychosis
Alcoholics Anonymous
alcoholism (ăl′kō-hŏl-ĭzm) [Arabic *al-koh'l*, something subtle, + Gr. *-ismos*, condition]
  a., acute
  a., chronic
alcoholomania (ăl″kō-hŏl″ō-mā′nē-ă) [Arabic *al-koh'l*, something subtle, + Gr. *mania*, frenzy]
alcoholometer (ăl″kō-hŏl-ŏm′ĕ-tĕr) [″ + Gr. *metron*, measure]
alcoholophilia (ăl″kō-hŏl-ō-fĭl′ē-ă) [″ + Gr. *philein*, to love]
alcohol syndrome, fetal
alcoholuria (ăl″kō-hŏl-ū′rē-ă) [″ + Gr. *ouron*, urine]
aldehyde (ăl′dĕ-hīd) [*alcohol dehydrogenatum*]
aldolase (ăl′dō-lās)
aldopentose (ăl″dō-pĕn′tōs)
aldose
aldosterone (ăl-dŏs′tĕr-ōn, ăl″dō-stĕr′ōn)
aldosteronism (ăl″dō-stĕr′ōn-ĭzm″)
  a., primary
  a., secondary
aldrin (ăl′drĭn)
alemmal (ă-lĕm′ăl) [Gr. *a-*, not, + *lemma*, husk]
Aleppo boil
alertness
alethia (ă-lē′thē-ă) [″ + *lethe*, forgetfulness]
aleukemia (ă-loo-kē′mē-ă) [″ + *leukos*, white, + *haima*, blood]
aleukemic (ă″loo-kē′mĭk)
aleukocytosis (ă-loo″kō-sī-tō′sĭs) [″ + *leukos*, white, + *kytos*, cell, + *osis*, condition]
aleuron, aleurone (ăl-oo′rŏn, -rōn) [Gr. *aleuron*, flour]
Alexander-Adams operation [William Alexander, Brit. surgeon, 1844–1919; James A. Adams, Scottish gynecologist, 1857–1930]
alexeteric (ă-lĕk″sĕ-tĕr′ĭk) [Gr. *alexeterios*, able to ward off]
alexia [Gr. *a-*, not, + *lexis*, word]
  a., motor
  a., musical
  a., optic or visual
alexic (ă-lĕks′ĭk)
aleydigism (ă-lī′dĭg-ĭzm)
ALG *antilymphocyte globulin*
algae (ăl′jē) [L. *alga*, seaweed]
algesia (ăl-jē′zē-ă) [Gr. *algesis*, sense of pain]
algesic (ăl-jē′sĭk)
algesichronometer (ăl-jē″zē-krō-nŏm′ĕ-tĕr) [″ + *chronos*, time + *metron*, measure]
algesimeter (ăl″jē-sĭm′ĕ-tĕr) [″ + *metron*, measure]
algesthesia (ăl″jĕs-thē′zē-ă) [Gr. *algos*, pain, + *aisthesis*, feeling, perception]
algetic (ăl-jĕt′ĭk)
-algia (ăl′jē-ă) [Gr.]
algicide (ăl′jĭ-sīd) [L. *alga*, seaweed, + *caedere*, to kill]
algid (ăl′jĭd) [L. *algidus*, cold]
algid stage
alginate (ăl′jĭ-nāt)
alginic acid
algiomotor (ăl″jē-ō-mō′tor) [Gr. *algos*, pain, + L. *motor*, a mover]
algiomuscular (ăl″jē-ō-mŭs′kū-lăr) [″ + L. *musculus*, muscle]
algogenic (ăl-gō-jĕn′ĭk) [″ + *gennan*, to produce; L. *algor*, cold, + Gr. *gennan*, to produce]
algolagnia (ăl″gō-lăg′nē-ă) [Gr. *algos*, pain, + *lagneia*, lust]
  a., active
  a., passive
algolagnist (ăl-gō-lăg′nĭst)
algometer [″ + *metron*, measure]
algophobia (ăl″gō-fō′bē-ă) [″ + *phobos*, fear]
algor (ăl′gor) [L., cold]
  a. mortis

algorithm (ăl'gŏ-rĭthm)
algos (ăl'gōs) [Gr.]
alible (ăl'ĭ-bl) [L. *alibilis*, nutritive]
alicyclic (ăl-ĭ-sī'klĭk)
alien (āl'yĕn)
alienate (āl'yĕn-āt)
alienation (āl″yĕn-ā'shŭn) [L. *alienare*, to make strange]
alienia (ā″lĭ-ē'nē-ă) [Gr. *a-*, not, + L. *lien*, spleen]
aliform (ăl'ĭ-form) [L. *ala*, wing, + *forma*, shape]
aliform process
alignment (ă-līn'mĕnt) [Fr. *aligner*, to put in a straight line]
aliment (ăl'ĭ-mĕnt) [L. *alimentum*, nourishment]
alimentary (ăl″ĭ-mĕn'tăr-ē) [L. *alimentum*, nourishment]
alimentary canal or tract
alimentary duct
alimentation (ăl″ĭ-mĕn-tā'shŭn)
   a., artificial
   a., forced
   a., rectal
alimentotherapy (ăl″ĭ-mĕn″tō-thĕr'ă-pē) [L. *alimentum*, nourishment, + Gr. *therapeia*, treatment]
alinasal [L. *ala*, wing, + *nasus*, nose]
alinement (ă-līn'mĕnt) [Fr. *aligner*, to put in a straight line]
aliphatic (ăl″ĭ-făt'ĭk) [Gr. *aleiphar*, *aleiphatos*, fat, oil]
aliquot (ăl'ĭ-kwŏt) [L. *alius*, other, + *quot*, how many]
alisphenoid (ăl-ĭ-sfē'noyd) [L. *ala*, wing, + Gr. *sphen*, wedge, + *eidos*, form, shape]
alizarin (ă-lĭz'ă-rĭn) [Arabic *ala sara*, extract]
alkalemia (ăl″kă-lē'mē-ă) [Arabic *al-qaliy*, ashes of salt wort, + Gr. *haima*, blood]
alkalescence (ăl″kă-lĕs'ens)
alkalescent (ăl″kă-lĕs'ent)
alkali (ăl'kă-lĭ) [Arabic *al-qaliy*, ashes of salt wort]

   a., corrosive
alkalimeter (ăl″kă-lĭm'ĕ-tĕr) [″ + Gr. *metron*, measure]
alkalimetry (ăl″kă-lĭm'ĕ-trē)
alkaline (ăl'kă-lĭn)
alkaline phosphatase
alkaline reserve
alkaline salts
alkaline tide
alkalinity (ăl″kă-lĭn'ĭ-tē)
alkalinize (ăl'kă-lĭn-īz″)
alkalinuria (ăl″kă-lĭn-ū'rē-ă) [*alkali* + Gr. *ouron*, urine]
alkalipenia (ăl″kă-lĭ-pē'nē-ă) [″ + Gr. *penia*, lack]
alkali poisoning
alkali reserve
alkalitherapy (ăl″kă-lĭ-thĕr'ă-pē) [″ + Gr. *therapeia*, treatment]
alkalization (ă″kă-lĭ-zā'shŭn)
alkalize (ăl'kă-līz)
alkaloid (ăl'kă-loyd) [*alkali* + Gr. *eidos*, form, shape]
   a., synthetic
alkalometry (ăl″kă-lŏm'ĕ-trē) [″ + Gr. *metron*, measure]
alkalosis (ăl″kă-lō'sĭs) [″ + Gr. *osis*, condition]
   a., altitude
   a., compensated
   a., hypochloremic
   a., hypokalemic
   a., metabolic
   a., respiratory
alkalotherapy (ăl″kă-lō-thĕr'ă-pē) [*alkali* + Gr. *therapeia*, treatment]
alkalotic (ăl″kă-lŏt'ĭk)
alkaluria (ăl″kă-lū'rē-ă) [*alkali* + Gr. *ouron*, urine]
alkapton(e) (ăl-kăp'tōn) [″ + Gr. *hapto*, to bind to]
alkaptonuria (ăl″kăp-tō-nū'rē-ă) [*alkapton* + Gr. *ouron*, urine]
alkene (ăl'kēn)
Alkeran
alkyl (ăl'kĭl)
alkylate (ăl'kĭ-lāt)
alkylating agent

alkylation (ăl″kĭ-lā′shŭn)
ALL *acute lymphocytic leukemia*
all- [Gr. *allos*, other]
allachesthesia (ăl″ă-kĕs-thē′zē-ă) [Gr. *allache*, elsewhere, + *aisthesis*, feeling, perception]
allantochorion (ă-lăn″tō-kō′rē-ŏn)
allantoic (ăl″ăn-tō′ĭk)
allantoid [Gr. *allantos*, sausage, + *eidos*, form, shape]
allantoin (ă-lăn′tō-ĭn)
allantoinuria (ă-lăn″tō-ĭn-ū′rē-ă) [*allantoin* + Gr. *ouron*, urine]
allantois (ă-lăn′tō-ĭs) [Gr. *allantos*, sausage, + *eidos*, form, shape]
allayed (ă-lād′)
allele (ă-lēl′, ă-lĕl′) [Gr. *allelon*, of one another]
allelic (ă-lĕl′ĭk)
allelic gene
allelomorph (ă-lē″lō-morf, ă-lĕl′ō-morf) [″ + *morphe*, form]
allelotaxis (ă-lē″lō-tăk′sĭs) [″ + *taxis*, order]
Allen-Doisy test (ăl′ĕn-doy′sē) [Edgar V. Allen, U.S. anatomist, 1892–1943; Edward A. Doisy, U.S. biochemist and physiologist, b. 1893]
Allen-Doisy unit
allenthesis (ă-lĕn′thĕ-sĭs) [Gr. *allos*, other, + *en*, in, + *thesis*, a placing]
allergen (ăl′ĕr-jĕn) [Gr. *allos*, other, + *ergon*, work, + *gennan*, to produce]
allergenic (ăl″ĕr-jĕn′ĭk)
allergic (ă-lĕr′jĭk)
allergization (ăl″ĕr-jĭ-zā′shŭn)
allergy (ăl′ĕr-jē) [Gr. *allos*, other, + *ergon*, work]
a., food
allesthesia (ăl″ĕs-thē′sē-ă) [″ + *aisthesis*, feeling, perception]
alliaceous (ăl″ē-ā′shŭs) [L. *allium*, garlic, + *-aceus*, of a specific kind]
allied health professional
alliesthesia (ăl″ē-ĕs-thē′sē-ă) [Gr. *allios*, changed, + *aisthesis*, feeling, perception]
alliteration (ă-lĭt″ĕr-ā′shŭn) [L. *ad*, to, + *litera* letter]
allo- [Gr. *allos*, other]
alloantigen (ăl″lō-ăn′tĭ-jĕn) [″ + *anti*, against, + *gennan*, to produce]
allobiosis (ăl″ō-bī-ō′sĭs) [″ + *bios*, life]
allochesthesia (ăl″ō-kĕs-thē′zē-ă) [Gr. *allache*, elsewhere, + *aisthesis*, feeling, perception]
allochezia, allochetia (ăl″ō-kē′zē-ă, ăl″ō-kē′shē-ă) [Gr. *allos*, other, + *chezein*, to defecate]
allochiria, allocheiria (ăl″ō-kī′rē-ă) [″ + *cheir*, hand]
allochroism (ăl-ōk′rō-ĭzm, ăl″ō-krō′ĭzm) [″ + *chroa*, color + *-ismos*, condition]
allochromasia (al″ō-krō-mā′sē-ă)
allocinesia (ăl″ō-sĭn-ē′sē-ă) [Gr. *allos*, other, + *kinesis*, motion]
allodiploidy (ăl″ō-dĭp′loy-dē) [″ + *diploe*, fold, + *eidos*, form, shape]
allodynia (ăl″ō-dĭn′ē-ă)
alloeroticism (ăl″ō-ē-rŏt′ĭ-sĭzm)
alloerotism (ăl″ō-ĕr′ō-tĭzm) [″ + *Eros*, god of love]
allogeneic, allogenic (ăl″ō-jĕ-nē′ĭk, ăl″ō-jĕn′ĭk)
allograft (ăl″ō-grăft) [″ + L. *graphium*, stylus]
alloimmune (ăl″ō-ĭm-ūn′) [″ + L. *immunis*, safe]
allokinesis (ăl″ō-kĭ-nē′sĭs) [″ + *kinesis*, motion]
allokinetic (ăl″ō-kĭ-nĕt′ĭk)
allolalia (ăl″ō-lā′lē-ă) [″ + *lalia*, chatter, prattle]
allomerism (ă-lŏm′ĕr-ĭzm) [″ + *meros*, part, + *-ismos*, condition]
allomorphism (ăl″ō-mor′fĭzm) [″ + *morphe*, form, + *-ismos*, condition]
allongement (ăl-ŏnzh-mŏn′) [Fr., elongation]
allopath (ăl′ō-păth)
allopathy (ăl′ŏp′ă-thē) [″ +

pathos, disease, suffering]
allophasis (ăl-ŏf'ă-sĭs) [Gr. allos, other,
+ phasis, utterance]
alloplasia (ăl"ō-plā'zē-ă) [" +
plasis, a molding]
alloplasty (ăl'ō-plăs-tē) [" +
plasis, a molding]
alloploidy (ăl"ō-ploy'dē) [" +
ploos, fold, + eidos, form, shape]
allopolyploidy (ăl"ō-pŏl'ē-ploy-dē)
[" + polys, many, + ploos,
fold, + eidos, form, shape]
allopsychic (ăl-ō-sī'kĭk) [" +
psyche, mind]
allopsychosis [" + " + osis,
condition]
allopurinol (ăl"ō-pū'rĭn-ŏl)
all-or-none law
allotherm (ăl'ō-thĕrm) [" +
therme, heat]
allotoxin (ăl"ō-tŏk'sĭn) [" + toxikon, poison]
allotransplantation (ăl"ō-trăns"plăn-
tā'shŭn) [" + L. trans, through, +
plantare, to plant]
allotriogeustia (ă-lŏt"rē-ō-jūst'ē-ă,
-gū'stē-a) [Gr. allotrios, strange, +
geusis, taste]
allotriophagy (ă-lŏt"rē-ŏf'ă-jē) [" +
phagein, to eat]
allotropic (ăl"ō-trŏp'ĭk) [Gr. allos,
other, + tropos, direction]
allotropism, allotropy (ă-lŏt'rō-
pĭzm, -pē) [" + trope, a turn, +
-ismos, condition]
alloxan (ăl-ŏk'săn) [allantoin +
oxalic]
alloy (ăl'oy, ă-loy') [Fr. aloyer, to com-
bine]
allyl (ăl'ĭl) [L. allium, garlic, + Gr.
hyle, matter]
Alma-Ata Declaration
alochia (ă-lō'kē-ă) [Gr. a-, not, +
lokhos, pert. to childbirth]
aloe (ăl'ō)
aloin (ăl'ō-ĭn)
alopecia (al"ō-pē'shē-ă) [Gr. alopekia,
fox mange]

a. adnata
a. areata
a. capitis totalis
a., cicatricial
a. congenitalis
a. follicularis
a. furfuracea
a. liminaris
a. liminaris frontalis
a., male pattern
a. medicamentosa
a. neurotica
a. pityroides
a. prematura
a. senilis
a. symptomatica
a. totalis
a. toxica
a. universalis
alpha (ăl'fă)
alpha-adrenergic blocking agent
alpha-adrenergic receptor
alpha-1 antitrypsin
alpha-fetoprotein
alpha-globulins
alpha particles, rays
alpha-rhythm
alpha-tocopherol
alpha-wave
Alport's syndrome [Arthur Cecil Alport, S. African physician, 1880–
1959]
ALS amyotrophic lateral sclerosis; antilymphocytic serum
alternans (awl-tĕr'nănz) [L. alternare,
to alternate]
a., pulsus
Alternaria (awl"tĕr-nā'rē-ă)
alternating current
alternative medicine
alternator
alt. hor. [L.] alternis horis, every other
hour
altitude sickness
altricious (ăl-trĭsh'ŭs) [L. altrix, nour-
isher]
alum (ăl'ŭm) [L. alumen]
a., ammonia

a., potassium
aluminosis (ă-loo"mĭn-ō'sĭs) ["   +
Gr. osis, condition]
aluminum
a. acetate
a. ammonia sulfate
a. hydroxide gel
a. potassium sulfate
**alveobronchiolitis, alveobron-
chitis** (ăl"vē-ō-brŏng"kē-ō-lĭ'tĭs,
-brŏng-kī'tĭs) [L. alveolus, small hollow or
cavity,   +   Gr. bronchos, windpipe,
+   itis, inflammation]
alveolalgia (ăl"vē-ō-lăl'jē-ă) ["   +
Gr. algos, pain]
alveolar (ăl-vē'ō-lăr)
alveolar air
alveolar bone
alveolar-capillary block
alveolar duct
alveolar periosteum
alveolar process
alveolar proteinosis
alveolate (ăl-vē'ō-lāt)
alveolectomy (ăl"vē-ō-lĕk'tō-mē) [L.
alveolus, small hollow or cavity,   +
Gr. ektome, excision]
alveoli (ăl-vē'ō-lī) [L.]
a. dentales
a. pulmonis
alveolitis (ăl"vē-ō-lī'tĭs) ["   +   Gr.
itis, inflammation]
a., allergic
alveoloclasia (ăl-vē"ō-lō-klā'sē-ă)
["   +   Gr. klasis, fracture]
alveolodental (ăl-vē"ō-lō-dĕn'tăl)
["   +   dens, tooth]
alveololingual (ăl-vē"ō-lō-lĭng'gwăl)
["   +   lingua, tongue]
alveoloplasty (ăl-vē"ō-lō-plăs'tē)
["   +   Gr. plassein, to form]
alveolotomy (ăl"vē-ō-lŏt'ō-mē) ["   +
Gr. tome, a cutting, slice]
alveolus (ăl-vē'ō-lŭs) [L., small hollow or
cavity]
a. dentalis
a., pulmonary
alveus (ăl'vē-ŭs) [L.]

a. hippocampi
alymphia (ă-lĭm'fē-ă) [Gr. a-, not,   +
L. lympha, lymph]
alymphocytosis (ă-lĭm"fō-sī-tō'sĭs)
["   +   "   +   Gr. kytos, cell,   +
osis, condition]
alymphoplasia (ă"lĭm-fō-plā'zē-ă)
["   +   "   +   Gr. plasis, a devel-
oping]
a., thymic
Alzheimer's disease (ălts'hī-mĕrz)
[Alois Alzheimer, Ger. neurologist,
1864–1915]
Am mixed astigmatism; ametropia
A.M.A. American Medical Association
AMA against medical advice
amaas (ă'măs)
amacrine (ăm'ă-krĭn) [Gr. a-, not,   +
makros, long,   +   is, inos, fiber]
amacrine cell
amalgam (ă-măl'găm) [Gr. malagma,
soft mass]
a., dental
amalgamate (ă-măl'gă-māt")
amalgamation (ă-măl"gă-mā'shŭn)
amalgamator (ă-măl'gă-mā"tor)
amanita (ăm"ă-nī'tă, -nē'tă) [Gr.
amanitai, mushrooms]
amantadine   hydrochloride
(ă-măn'tă-dēn hī"drō-klor'ĭd)
amarthritis (ăm"ăr-thrī'tĭs) [Gr. hama,
at same time,   +   arthron, joint,   +
itis, inflammation]
amastia (ă-măs'tē-ă) ["   +   mastos,
breast]
amaurosis (ăm"aw-rō'sĭs) [Gr., dark-
ening]
a., albuminuric
a., congenital
a., diabetic
a., epileptoid
a. fugax
a., lead
a. partialis fugax
a., reflex
a., saburral
a., toxic
a., uremic

amaurotic (ăm-aw-rŏt′ĭk)

amazia (ă-mā′zē-ă) [Gr. a-, not, + mazos, breast]

ambi- [L. ambi-, on both sides]

ambidextrous (ăm″bĭ-dĕk′strŭs) [″ + dexter, right]

ambient (ăm′bē-ĕnt) [L. ambiens, going around]

ambient noise

ambilateral (ăm″bĭ-lăt′ĕr-ăl) [L. ambi-, on both sides, + latus, side]

ambilevous (ăm-bĭ-lē′vŭs) [″ + laevus, lefthanded]

ambiopia (ăm″bē-ō′pē-ă) [″ + Gr. ops, eye]

ambisexual (ăm″bĭ-sĕks′ū-ăl) [″ + sexus, sex]

ambisinister (ăm″bĭ-sĭn′ĭs-tĕr) [″ + sinister, left]

ambitendency (ăm″bĭ-tĕn′dĕn-sē) [″ + tendere, to stretch]

ambivalence (ăm-bĭv′ă-lĕns) [″ + valentia, strength]

ambivalent (ăm-bĭv′ă-lĕnt)

ambivert (ăm′bĭ-vĕrt) [″ + vertere, to turn]

amblyacousia (ăm″blē-ă-koo′sē-ă) [Gr. amblys, dull, + akousis, hearing]

amblychromasia (ăm″blē-krō-mā′sē-ă) [″ + chroma, color]

amblychromatic (ăm″blē-krō-măt′ĭk)

amblyopia (ăm″blē-ō′pē-ă) [″ + ops, eye]

  a., crossed

  a. ex anopsia

  a., reflex

  a., toxic

  a., uremic

amblyoscope (ăm′blē-ŏ-skōp″) [″ + ″ + skopein, to examine]

ambon (ăm′bŏn) [Gr., edge of a dish]

ambos (ăm′bōs) [Ger.]

Ambu bag (ăm′bū)

ambulance [L. ambulare, to move about]

ambulant, ambulatory (ăm′bū-lănt, -lă-tō″rē)

Ambu simulator

Amcill

Ameba, Amoeba (ă-mē′bă)

ameba, amoeba [Gr. amoibe, change]

amebiasis (ăm″ĕ-bī′ă-sĭs) [″ + -iasis, state or condition of]

  a., hepatic

amebic (ă-mē′bĭk)

amebic carrier state

amebic dysentery

amebic hepatitis

amebicide, amebacide (ă-mē′bĭ-sīd) [Gr. amoibe, change, + L. caedere, to kill]

amebiform (ă-mē′bĭ-form) [″ + L. forma, shape]

amebocyte (ă-mē′bō-sīt″) [″ + kytos, cell]

ameboid (ă-mē′boyd) [″ + eidos, form, shape]

ameboidism (ă-mē′boyd-ĭzm)

ameboid movement

ameboma (ăm″ē-bō′mă) [″ + oma, tumor]

ameburia (ăm″ĕ-bū′rē-ă) [Gr. amoibe, change, + ouron, urine]

amelanotic (ă″mĕl-ă-nŏt′ĭk)

amelia (ă-mē′lē-ă) [Gr. a-, not, + melos, limb]

amelification (ă-mĕl″ĭ-fĭ-kā′shŭn) [O. Fr. amel, enamel, + L. facere, to make]

amelioration (ă-mēl″yō-rā′shŭn) [L. ad, to, + melior, better]

ameloblast (ă-mĕl′ō-blăst) [O. Fr. amel, enamel, + Gr. blastos, germ]

ameloblastoma (ă-mĕl″ō-blăs-tō′mă) [″ + ″ + oma, tumor]

amelodentinal [O. Fr. amel, enamel, + L. dens, dent-, tooth]

amelogenesis (ăm″e-lō-jĕn′ĕ-sĭs) [″ + Gr. genesis, generation, birth]

amelus (ăm′ĕ-lŭs) [Gr. a-, not, + melos, limb]

amenia (ă-mē′nē-ă) [Gr. a-, not, + men, month]

amenorrhea (ă-měn″ō-rē′ă) [″ + ″ + *rhein*, to flow]
   a., dietary
   a., emotional
   a., nutritional
   a., pathologic
   a., physiologic
   a., primary
   a., secondary
   a., stress
amenorrheic (ă-měn″ō-rē′ĭk)
amentia (ă-měn′shē-ă) [L. *ab*, from, + *mens*, mind]
   a. agitata
   a. attonita
   a., nevoid
   a., phenylpyruvic
Americaine
American Sign Language
americium (ăm-ĕr-ĭsh′ē-ŭm)
ametria (ă-mē′trē-ă) [″ + *metra*, uterus]
ametrometer (ăm″ĕ-trŏm′ĕ-tĕr) [*ametropia* + Gr. *metron*, measure]
ametropia (ă″mĕ-trō′pē-ă) [Gr. *ametros*, disproportionate, + *ops*, eye]
AMI *acute myocardial infarction*
amicrobic (ă″mĭ-krō′bĭk) [Gr. *a-*, not, + *mikros*, small, + *bios*, life]
amicroscopic (ă-mī″krō-skŏp′ĭk) [″ + ″ + *skopein*, to examine]
amidase (ăm′ĭ-dās)
amide (ăm′ĭd)
amido-
amidulin (ă-mĭd′ū-lĭn) [Fr. *amidon*, starch]
amikacin sulfate
amimia (ă-mĭm′ē-ă) [Gr. *a-*, not, + *mimos*, mimic]
   a., amnesic
   a., ataxic
amine (ă-mēn′, ăm′ĭn)
amino- (ă-mē′nō, ăm′ĭ-nō)
aminoacetic acid (ăm″ĭn-ō-ă-ā-sē′tĭk)
amino acid
   a.a., essential
   a.a., nonessential
aminoacidemia (ă-mē″nō-, ăm″ĭ-nō-ăs″ĭ-dē′mē-ă) [*amino acid* + Gr. *haima*, blood]
amino acid group
aminoacidopathies (ăm″ĭ-nō-ăs″ĭ-dŏp′ă-thēz) [″ + Gr. *pathos*, disease, suffering]
aminoaciduria (ă-mē″nō-, ăm″ĭ-nō-ăs″ĭ-dū′rē-ă) [″ + Gr. *ouron*, urine]
aminobenzene (ă-mē″nō-, ăm″ĭ-nō-běn′zēn)
aminobenzoic acid
aminocaproic acid
aminoglutethimide (ăm″ĭ-nō-glootěth′ĭ-mīd)
aminohippuric acid, sodium
aminolysis (ăm″ĭ-nŏl′ĭ-sĭs) [*amine* + Gr. *lysis*, dissolution]
aminometradine (ăm″ĭ-nō-mět′rădēn)
aminophylline (ăm-ĭ-nŏf′ĭ-lĭn, ăm″ĭ-nō-fĭl′ĭn)
aminophylline poisoning
aminopterin (ăm-ĭ-nŏp′tĕr-ĭn)
aminopurine (ăm″ĭ-nō-pū′rĭn)
aminopyrine (ăm″ĭn-ō-pī′rĭn)
aminosalicylic acid
aminuria (ăm-ĭ-nū′rē-ă) [*amine* + Gr. *ouron*, urine]
Amitid
amitosis (ăm″ĭ-tō′sĭs) [Gr. *a-*, not, + *mitos*, a thread, + *osis*, condition]
amitotic (ăm″ĭ-tŏt′ĭk)
amitryptyline hydrochloride (ăm″ĭ-trĭp′tĭ-lēn)
AML *acanthiomeatal line; acute myelocytic leukemia*
ammeter (ăm′mĕ-tĕr) [*ampere* + Gr. *metron*, measure]
ammoaciduria (ăm″ō-ăs″ĭ-dū′rē-ă) [*ammonia* + *amino acid* + Gr. *ouron*, urine]
ammonemia (ă-mō-nē′mē-ă) [*ammonia* + Gr. *haima*, blood]
ammonia (ă-mō′nē-ă) [*Ammo*, Egyptian deity near whose temple it was originally obtained]
   a., aromatic spirit of
   a., blood

ammoniacal (ăm″ō-nī′ă-kăl)
ammonia intoxication
ammonia solution, diluted
ammonia solution, strong
ammoniated (ă-mō′nē-āt′d)
ammonia toxicity
ammonia water
ammoniemia (a-mō″nĭ-ē′mē-ă) [*ammonia* + Gr. *haima*, blood]
ammonium (ă-mō′nē-ŭm)
   a. alum
   a. carbonate
   a. chloride
   a. hydroxide
   a., thiosulfate
ammoniuria (ă-mō″nē-ū′rē-ă) [″ + Gr. *ouron*, urine]
ammonotelic (ă-mō″nō-tĕl′ĭk)
amnesia (ăm-nē′zē-ă) [Gr.]
   a., anterograde
   a., auditory
   a., lacunar
   a., retroanterograde
   a., retrograde
   a., tactile
   a., transient global
   a., traumatic
   a., visual
amnesic (ăm-nē′sĭk)
amnesic aphasia
amnestic (ăm-nĕs′tĭk)
amniocentesis (ăm″nē-ō-sĕn-tē′sĭs) [Gr. *amnion*, lamb, + *kentesis*, puncture]
amniochorial, amniochorionic (ăm″nē-ō-kō′rē-ăl, -kō-rē-ŏn′ĭk)
amnioclepsis (ăm″nē-ō-klĕp′sĭs) [″ + *kleptein*, to steal]
amniogenesis (ăm″nē-ō-jĕn′ĕ-sĭs) [″ + *genesis*, generation, birth]
amniography [″ + *graphein*, to write]
amnioinfusion (ăm″nē-ō-ĭn-fū′zhŭn)
amnion (ăm′nē-ŏn) [Gr. *amnion*, lamb]
   a. nodosum
amnionitis (ăm″nē-ō-nī′tĭs) [″ + *itis*, inflammation]
amniorrhea (ăm″nē-or-rē′ă) [″ +

rhein, to flow]
amnioscope (ăm′nē-ō-skōp) [Gr. *amnion*, lamb, + *skopein*, to examine]
   a., suction
amnioscopy
amniote (ăm′nē-ōt)
amniotic (ăm-nē-ŏt′ĭk)
amniotic band syndrome
amniotic cavity
amniotic fluid
amniotic sac
amniotitis (ăm-nē-ō-tī′tĭs) [Gr. *amnion*, lamb, + *itis*, inflammation]
amniotome (ăm′nē-ō-tōm) [″ + Gr. *tome*, a cutting, slice]
amniotomy (ăm″nē-ŏt′ō-mē)
amnitis (ăm-nī′tĭs)
amobarbital (ăm″ō-bar′bĭ-tăl)
   a. sodium
A-mode (amplitude modulation) display
amodiaquine hydrochloride (ăm″ō-dī′ă-kwĭn)
amoeba (ă-mē′ba) [Gr. *amoibe*, change]
amok, amuck (ă-mŏk′, ă-mŭk′) [Malay, to engage furiously in battle]
amor (ā′mor) [L.]
amorphia, amorphism (ă-mor′fē-ă, ă-mor′fĭzm) [Gr. *a-*, not + *morphe*, form]
amorphous (ă-mor′fŭs)
amotio (ă-mō′shē-ō) [L. *amovere*, to move from]
   a. retinae
amoxicillin (ă-mŏks″ĭ-sĭl′ĭn)
Amoxil
AMP *adenosine monophosphate*
amperage (ăm-pēr′ĭj)
ampere (ăm′pēr)
ampere meter
amphetamine (ăm-fĕt′ă-mēn, -mĭn)
   a. sulfate
amphetamine poisoning
amphi- [Gr. *amphi*, on both sides]
amphiarthrosis (ăm″fē-ăr-thrō′sĭs) [″ + Gr. *arthrosis*, joint]
amphiaster (ăm″fē-ăs′tĕr) [″ +

aster, star]
Amphibia (ăm-fĭb′ē-ă) [Gr. *amphibios,* double life]
amphibious (ăm-fĭb′ē-ŭs)
amphiblastula (ăm‴fē-blăs′tū-lă) [Gr. *amphi,* on both sides, + *blastula,* little sprout]
amphibolic (ăm‴fĭ-bŏl′ĭk) [Gr. *amphibolia,* uncertainty]
amphicelous (ăm‴fĭ-sē′lŭs) [Gr. *amphi,* on both sides + *koilos,* hollow]
amphicentric (ăm‴fĭ-sĕn′trĭk) [″ + *kentron,* center]
amphichroic, **amphichromatic** (ăm‴fē-krō′ĭk, -krō-măt′ĭk) [″ + *chroma,* color]
amphicrania (ăm‴fē-krā′nē-ă) [″ + *kranion,* skull]
amphicyte (ăm′fē-sīt) [″ + *kytos,* cell]
amphidiarthrosis (ăm‴fē-dĭ-ăr-thrō′sĭs) [″ + *diarthrosis,* articulation]
amphigony (ăm-fĭg′ō-nē) [″ + *gonos,* offspring, procreation]
amphimixis (ăm‴fē-mĭks′ĭs) [″ + *mixis,* mingling]
amphitheater (ăm‴fĭ-thē′ă-tĕr) [″ + *theatron,* theater]
amphitrichate, **amphitrichous** (ăm-fĭt′rĭ-kāt, -kŭs) [″ + *thrichos,* hair]
ampho- [Gr. *ampho,* both]
amphocyte (ăm′fō-sīt) [″ + *kytos,* cell]
amphodiplopia (ăm-fō-dĭ-plō′pē-ă) [″ + *diploos,* double, + *ops,* vision]
Amphojel (ăm′fō-jĕl)
ampholyte (ăm′fō-līt) [″ + *electrolyte*]
amphopeptone (ăm‴fō-pĕp′tōn)
amphophil, amphophilous (ăm′fō-fĭl, ăm-fŏf′ĭ-lŭs) [″ + *philos,* love]
amphoric (ăm-for′ĭk) [L. *amphoricus*]
amphoricity (ăm‴for-ĭs′ĭ-tē)
amphoriloquy (ăm‴for-ĭl′ō-kwē) [L. *amphora,* jar, + *loqui,* to speak]

amphorophony (ăm‴for-ŏf′ō-nē) [Gr. *amphoreus,* jar, + *phone,* voice]
amphoteric, amphoterous (ăm-fō-tĕr′ĭk, ăm-fŏt′ĕr-ŭs) [Gr. *amphoteros,* both]
amphoteric compound
amphotericin B (ăm‴fō-tĕr′ĭ-sĭn)
amphoteric reaction
amphoterism (ăm-fō′tĕr-ĭzm)
amphoterodiplopia (ăm-fŏt‴ĕr-ō-dĭ-plō′pē-ă) [″ + *diploos,* double, + *ops,* vision]
amphotonic [″ + *tonos,* act of stretching, tension, tone]
amphotony (ăm-fŏt′ō-nē)
ampicillin (ămp‴ĭ-sĭl′ĭn)
    a. sodium
amplification (ăm‴plĭ-fĭ-kā′shŭn) [L. *amplificatio,* making larger]
amplifier (ăm′plĭ-fī′ĕr)
amplitude (ăm′plĭ-tūd) [L. *amplitudo*]
amplitude modulation
ampule (ăm′pūl) [Fr. *ampoule*]
ampulla (ăm-pŭl′lă) [L., little jar]
    a. ductus deferentis
    a. of lacrimal duct
    a. of rectum
    a. of semicircular canal
    a. of semicircular ducts
    a. of uterine tube
    a. of vas deferens
    a. of Vater
ampullitis (ăm‴pŭl-lī′tĭs) [″ + Gr. *itis,* inflammation]
ampullula (ăm-pŭl′ū-lă) [dim. of L. *ampulla*]
amputation (ăm‴pū-tā′shŭn) [L. *amputare,* to cut around]
    a., congenital
    a., double-flap
    a. in contiguity
    a. in continuity
    a., primary
    a., secondary
    a., spontaneous
    a., tertiary
amputee (ăm‴pū-tē′)
A.M.R.A. *American Medical Record As-*

sociation

A.M.T. *American Medical Technologists*

amuck, amok (ă-mŭk′) [Malay *amok*, furious attack]

amusia (ă-mū′sē-ă) [Gr. *amousos*, unmusical]

    a., motor

    a., sensory

Amussat's operation (ăm′ū-săz) [Jean Z. Amussat, Fr. surgeon, 1796–1856]

amychophobia (ă-mī″kŏ-fō′bē-ă) [Gr. *amyche*, scratch, + *phobos*, fear]

amyelencephaly (ă-mī″ĕl-ĕn-sĕf-ă′lē) [Gr. *a-*, not, + *myelos*, marrow, + *enkephalos*, brain]

amyelia (ă-mī-ē′lē-ă) [″ + *myelos*, marrow]

amyelinic (ă-mī″ĕ-lĭn′ĭk)

amyeloneuria (ă-mī″ĕl-ō-nū′rē-ă) [″ + *myelos*, marrow, + *neuron*, nerve]

amyelotrophy (ă-mī″ĕl-ŏt′rō-fē) [″ + ″ + *atrophia*, atrophy]

amyelus (ă-mī′ĕ-lŭs)

amygdala (ă-mĭg′dă-lă) [L., almond]

amygdalin (ă-mĭg′dă-lĭn)

amygdaline (ă-mĭg′dă-lĭn, -lĭn) [L. *amygdalinus*]

amygdaloid (ă-mĭg′dă-loyd) [Gr. *amygdale*, almond, + *eidos*, form, shape]

amygdaloid fossa

amygdaloid tubercle

amygdalolith (ă-mĭg′dă-lō-lĭth″) [″ + *lithos*, stone]

amygdalopathy (ă-mĭg″dă-lŏp′ă-thē) [″ + *pathos*, disease, suffering]

amygdalotome (ă-mĭg′dă-lō-tōm″) [″ + *tome*, a cutting, slice]

amyl (ăm′ĭl) [Gr. *amylon*, starch]

    a. nitrite

amylaceous (ăm″ĭ-lā′shē-ŭs)

amylase (ăm′ĭ-lās) [″ + *-asis*, colloid enzyme]

    a., pancreatic

    a., salivary

    a., vegetable

amylasuria (ăm″ĭ-lās-ū′rē-ă) [″ + *ouron*, urine]

amylemia (ăm″ĭ-lē′mē-ă) [″ + *haima*, blood]

amylodextrin [″ + *dexter*, right]

amylodyspepsia (ăm″ĭ-lō-dĭs-pĕp′sē-ă) [″ + *dys*, bad, difficult, painful, disordered, + *pepsis*, digestion]

amylogenesis (ăm″ĭ-lō-jĕn′ĕ-sĭs) [″ + *genesis*, generation, birth]

amylogenic (ăm″ĭ-lō-jĕn′ĭk) [″ + *gennan*, to produce]

amyloid (ăm′ĭ-loyd) [Gr. *amylon*, starch, + *eidos*, form, shape]

amyloid degeneration

amyloid disease

amyloid kidney

amyloid nephrosis

amyloidosis (ăm″ĭ-loy-dō′sĭs) [Gr. *amylon*, starch, + *eidos*, form, shape, + *osis*, condition]

    a., lichen

    a., localized

    a., primary

    a., secondary

amylolysis (ăm″ĭl-ŏl′ĭ-sĭs) [″ + *lysis*, dissolution]

amylolytic (ăm″ĭl-ō-lĭt′ĭk)

amylolytic enzyme

amylopectin (ăm″ĭl-ō-pĕk′tĭn)

amylophagia (ăm″ĭ-lō-fā′jē-ă) [″ + *phagein*, to eat]

amylopsin (ăm″ĭ-lŏp′sĭn) [″ + *opsis*, sight, appearance, vision]

amylose (ăm′ĭ-lōs) [Gr. *amylon*, starch]

amylosis (ăm″ĭ-lō′sĭs) [″ + *osis*, condition]

amylosuria (ăm″ĭ-lō-sū′rē-ă) [″ + *ouron*, urine]

amylum (ăm′ĭ-lŭm) [Gr. *amylon*, starch]

amyluria [″ + Gr. *ouron*, urine]

amyocardia (ă-mī″ō-kăr′dē-ă) [Gr. *a-*, not, + *mys*, muscle, + *kardia*, heart]

amyoplasia (ă-mī″ō-plā′zē-ă) [″ + ″ + *plassein*, to form]

    a. congenita

amyostasia (ă-mī″ō-stă′sē-ă) [″ +

" + *stasis,* standing still]

amyosthenia (ă-mī″ŏs-thē′nē-ă) [" + " + *sthenos,* strength]

amyosthenic (ă-mī″ŏs-thĕn′ĭk)

amyotaxy (ă-mī″ō-tăks′ē) [" + " + *taxis,* order]

amyotonia (ă-mī″ō-tō′nē-ă) [" + " + *tonos,* act of stretching, tension, tone]

a. congenita

amyotrophia, amyotrophy (ă-mī″ō-trō′fē-ă, ă-mī-ŏt′rō-fē) [" + " + *trophe,* nourishment]

a., progressive spinal

amyotrophic (ă-mī″ō-trŏf′ĭk)

amyotrophic lateral sclerosis

amyous (ăm′ē-ŭs) [" + *mys,* muscle]

Amytal

Amytal Sodium

amyxia (ă-mĭks′ē-ă) [" + *myxa,* mucus]

amyxorrhea (ă-mĭks-ō-rē′ă) [" + " + *rhein,* to flow]

An *actinon; anisometropia; anode; antigen*

an- [Gr.]

A.N.A. *American Nurses' Association*

ana (ăn′ă) [Gr.] *so much of each; antinuclear antibody*

anabasis (ă-năb′ă-sĭs) [Gr., ascent]

anabatic (ăn″ă-băt′ĭk)

anabiosis (ăn″ă-bī-ō′sĭs) [Gr. *anabiosis,* revive]

anabiotic (ăn-ă-bī-ŏt′ĭk)

anabolic (ăn″ă-bŏl′ĭk) [Gr. *anabolikos*]

anabolic agents

anabolin (ă-năb′ō-lĭn)

anabolism (ă-năb′ō-lĭzm) [Gr. *anabole,* a building up, + *-ismos,* condition]

anabolite (ă-năb′ō-līt″)

anabrosis (ăn″ă-brō′sĭs) [Gr.]

anabrotic (ăn″ă-brŏt′ĭk)

anacamptics (ăn″ă-kămp′tĭks) [Gr. *anakamptein,* to bend back]

anacamptometer (ăn″ă-kămp-tŏm′ĕ-tĕr) [Gr. *ana,* up, + *kamptos,* flexi-ble, + *metron,* to measure]

anacatesthesia (ăn″ă-kăt″ĕs-thē′zē-ă) [" + " + *aisthesis,* feeling, perception]

anacatharsis (ăn″ă-kă-thăr′sĭs) [Gr. *anakatharsis,* upward cleansing]

anacathartic (ăn″ă-kă-thăr′tĭk)

anacidity (ăn″ă-sĭd′ĭ-tē) [Gr. *an-,* not, + L. *acidum,* acid]

anaclasis (ă-năk′lă-sĭs) [Gr. *anaklasis,* reflection]

anaclitic (ăn″ă-klĭt′ĭk)

anacrotic (ăn″ă-krŏt′ĭk) [Gr. *ana,* up, + *krotos,* stroke]

anacrotic pulse

anacrotism (ă-năk′rō-tĭzm)

anacusia, anacusis, anakusis (ăn-ă-kū′sē-ă, -sĭs) [Gr. *an-,* not, + *akouein,* to hear]

anadenia (ăn-ă-dē′nē-ă) [" + *aden,* gland]

anadicrotic (ăn″ă-dī-krŏt′ĭk) [Gr. *ana,* up, + *dikrotos,* double beating]

anadicrotism (ăn-ă-dĭk′rō-tĭzm)

anadidymus (ăn″ă-dĭd′ĭ-mŭs) [" + *didymus,* twin]

anadipsia (ăn″ă-dĭp′sē-ă) [Gr. *ana,* intensive, + *dipsa,* thirst]

anadrenalism (ăn″ă-drē′năl-ĭzm) [Gr. *an-,* not, + *adrenal* + Gr. *-ismos,* condition]

anaerobe (ăn′ĕr-ōb) [" + *aer,* air, + *bios,* life]

a., facultative

a., obligatory

anaerobic (ăn″ĕr-ō′bĭk)

anaerobic exercise

anaerobiosis (ăn″ĕr-ō-bī-ō′sĭs) [" + *aer,* air, + *bios,* life, + *osis,* condition]

anagen (ăn′ă-jĕn) [Gr. *ana,* up, + *genesis,* generation, birth]

anakatadidymus (ăn″ă-kăt″ă-dĭd′ĭ-mŭs) [Gr. *ana,* up, + *kala,* down, + *didymos,* twin]

anakusis (ăn″ă-kū′sĭs) [Gr. *an-,* not, + *akouein,* to hear]

anal (ā′năl) [L. *analis*]

anal canal

analepsis (ăn″ă-lĕp′sĭs) [Gr. *analepsis,* a taking up]

analeptic (ăn″ă-lĕp′tĭk) [Gr. *analeptikos,* restorative]

anal erotism

analgesia (ăn-ăl-jē′zē-ă) [Gr. *an-,* not, + *algos,* pain]
 a. algera, a. dolorosa
 a., paretic
 a., patient-controlled

analgesic (ăn″ăl-jē′sĭk)

analgesic nephropathy

analgetic (ăn″ăl-jĕt′ĭk)

analgia (ăn-ăl′jē-ă) [″ + *algos,* pain]

analgic (ăn-ăl′jĭk)

anal incontinence

analog, analogue (ăn′ă-lŏg) [Gr. *analogos,* proportionate]

analogous (ă-năl′ō-gŭs)

analogy (ă-năl′ō-jē) [Gr. *analogos,* proportionate]

anal personality

anal reflex

anal stage

analysand (ăn-ăl′ĭ-zănd)

analysis (ă-năl′ĭ-sĭs) [LL. *ana,* up, back, + Gr. *lysis,* dissolution]
 a., centrifugal
 a., chromatographic
 a., cohort
 a., colorimetric
 a., continuous-flow
 a., densimetric
 a., gastric
 a., qualitative
 a., quantitative
 a., spectrophotometric
 a., volumetric

analysis of variance

analyst (ăn′ă-lĭst) [Gr. *analyein,* to dissolve]

analytic (ăn-ă-lĭt′ĭk) [Gr. *analytikos*]

analytical balance

analyze (ăn′ă-līz) [Gr. *analyein,* to dissolve]

analyzer (ăn′ă-lī″zĕr)

anamnesis (ăn″ăm-nē′sĭs) [Gr. *anamnesis,* recalling]

anamnestic (ăn″ăm-nĕs′tĭk)

anamniotic [Gr. *an-,* not, + *amnion,* amnion]

anancastic (ăn″ăn-kăs′tĭk) [Gr. *anankastos,* compelled]

anangioplasia (ăn-ăn″jē-ō-plā′sē-ă) [Gr. *an-,* not, + *angeion,* vessel, + *plassein,* to form]

anangioplastic (ăn-ăn″jē-ō-plăs′tĭk)

anaphase (ăn′ă-fāz) [″ + *phainein,* to appear]

anaphoresis (ăn″ă-fō-rē′sĭs) [″ + *phoresis,* bearing]

anaphoria (ăn″ă-for′ē-ă) [Gr. *ana,* up, + *phorein,* to carry]

anaphrodisia (ăn-ăf″rō-dĭz′ē-ă) [Gr. *an-,* not, + *aphrodisia,* sexual desire]

anaphrodisiac (ăn″ăf-rō-dĭz′ē-ăk)

anaphrodite (ăn-ăf′rō-dīt)

anaphylactia (ăn″ă-fĭ-lăk′shē-ă) [Gr. *ana,* up, + *phylaxis,* guard]

anaphylactic (ăn″ă-fĭ-lăk′tĭk)

anaphylactic shock

anaphylactogenesis (ăn″ă-fĭ-lăk″tō-jĕn′ĕ-sĭs)

anaphylactogenic (ăn″ă-fĭ-lăk″tō-jĕn′ĭk)

anaphylatoxin (ăn″ă-fĭ-lă-tŏk′sĭn)

anaphylaxis (ăn″ă-fĭ-lăk′sĭs) [″ + *phylaxis,* guard]
 a., active
 a., heterologous
 a., homologous
 a., local
 a., passive

anaplasia (ăn″ă-plā′zē-ă) [″ + *plassein,* to form]

anaplastic (ăn″ă-plăs′tĭk) [″ + *plassein,* to form]

anapnea (ăn″ăp-nē′ă) [Gr. *anapnein,* to breathe again]

anapneic (ăn″ăp-nē′ĭk)

anapophysis (ăn″ă-pŏf′ĭ-sĭs) [Gr. *ana,* back, + *apophysis,* offshoot]

anaptic (ăn-ăp′tĭk) [Gr. *an-,* not, +

aptein, to touch]
anarthria (ăn-ăr'thrē-ă) [" +
arthron, joint]
  a. centralis
  a. literalis
anasarca (ăn"ă-săr'kă) [Gr. *ana,*
through, + *sarkos,* flesh]
anasarcous (ăn"ă-săr'kŭs)
anaspadias (ăn"ă-spă'dē-ăs) [" +
spadon, a rent]
anastole (ăn-ăs'tō-lē) [Gr.]
anastomose (ă-năs'tō-mōs) [Gr. *anas-tomosis,* opening]
anastomosis (ă-năs"tō-mō'sĭs) [Gr.,
opening]
  a., antiperistaltic
  a., arteriovenous
  a., crucial
  a., end-to-end
  a., Galen's
  a., heterocladic
  a., homocladic
  a., Hyrtl's
  a., intestinal
  a., isoperistaltic
  a., Jacobson's
  a., precapillary
  a., Schmidel's
  a., side-to-side
  a., terminoterminal
  a., ureterotubal
  a., ureteroureteral
anastomotic (ă-năs"tō-mŏt'ĭk)
anatomic (ăn"ă-tŏm'ĭk) [Gr. *anatome,*
dissection]
anatomical snuffbox
anatomist (ă-năt'ō-mĭst)
anatomy (ă-năt'ō-mē) [Gr. *anatome,*
dissection]
  a., applied
  a., comparative
  a., descriptive
  a., developmental
  a., gross
  a., macroscopic
  a., microscopic
  a., morbid
  a., pathological

  a., radiological
  a., surface
  a., systematic
  a., topographic
  a., x-ray
anatoxic (ăn"ă-tŏks'ĭk) [Gr. *ana,* back-ward, + *toxikon,* poison]
anatoxin (ăn"ă-tŏks'ĭn)
anatricrotic (ăn"ă-trī-krŏt'ĭk) [Gr. *ana,*
up, + *tresis,* three, + *krotos,*
stroke]
anatricrotism (ăn"ă-trĭk'rō-tĭzm)
anatripsis (ăn"ă-trĭp'sĭs) [" +
tripsis, a rubbing, friction]
anatriptic (ăn"ă-trĭp'tĭk) [" +
tripsis, a rubbing, friction]
anatropia (ăn"ă-trō'pē-ă) [" +
trope, a turning]
Anavar
anaxon(e) (ăn-ăk'sŏn) [Gr. *an-,* not,
+ *axon,* axis]
A.N.C. *Army Nurse Corps*
AnCC *anodal closure contraction*
anchor (ăng'ker) [Gr. *ankyra,* anchor]
anchorage (ăng'kĕr-ĭj)
anchors
ancillary (ăn'sĭl-lār"ē) [L. *ancillaris,*
handmaid]
Ancobon
anconad (ăn'kō-năd) [Gr. *ankon,*
elbow, + L. *ad,* to]
anconagra (ăn"kŏn-ăg'ră) [" +
agra, a seizure]
anconal, anconeal (ăn'kō-năl,
ăn-kō'nē-ăl)
anconal fossa, anconeal fossa
anconeus (ăn-kō'nē-ŭs) [Gr. *ankon,*
elbow]
anconitis (ăn"kō-nī'tĭs) [" + *itis,* in-flammation]
Ancylostoma (ăn"sĭl-ŏs'tō-mă) [Gr.
ankylos, crooked, + *stoma,* mouth,
opening]
  A. braziliense
  A. caninum
  A. duodenale
Ancylostomatidae (ăn"sĭ-lŏs"tō-
măt'ĭ-dē)

ancylostomiasis (ăn"sĭ-lŏs-tō-mī'ă-sĭs) [Gr. *ankylos*, crooked, + *stoma*, mouth, opening, + *-iasis*, state or condition of]

ancyroid (ăn'sĭ-royd) [Gr. *ankyra*, anchor, + *eidos*, form, shape]

Andernach's ossicles (ŏn'dĕr-nŏks) [Johann Winther von Andernach, Ger. physician, 1487 – 1574]

Andersen's disease [Dorothy H. Andersen, U.S. pediatrician, 1901 – 1963]

Andral's decubitus (ăn'drăls) [Gabriel Andral, Fr. physician, 1797 – 1876]

andriatrics (ăn"drē-ăt'rĭks) [Gr. *andros*, man, + *iatreia*, medical treatment]

andro- [Gr. *andros*, man]

androgalactozemia (ăn"drō-găl-ăk"tō-zē'mē-ă) [" + *gala*, milk, + *zemia*, loss]

androgen (ăn'drō-jĕn) [Gr. *andros*, man, + *gennan*, to produce]

androgenic (ăn"drō-jĕn'ĭk)

androgyne (ăn'drō-jīn) [" + *gyne*, woman]

androgynoid (ăn-drŏj'ĭ-noyd) [" + " + *eidos*, form, shape]

androgynous (ăn-drŏj'ĭ-nŭs) [" + *gyne*, woman]

androgynus (ăn-drŏj'ĭ-nŭs)

android (ăn'droyd) [" + *eidos*, form, shape]

andrology (ăn-drŏl'ō-jē) [" + *logos*, word, reason]

andromimetic (ăn"drō-mĭ-mĕt'ĭk) [" + *mimetikos*, imitative]

andromorphous (ăn"drō-mor'fŭs) [" + *morphe*, form]

andropathy (ăn-drŏp'ă-thē) [" + *pathos*, disease, suffering]

androphilic (ăn'drō-fĭl-ĭk) [" + *philos*, love]

androphobia (ăn"drō-fō'bē-ă) [" + *phobos*, fear]

androstane (ăn'drō-stān)

androsterone (ăn"drō-stēr'ōn, ăn-drŏs'tĕr-ōn)

-ane

anecdotal evidence (ăn"ĭk-dōt'l) [Gr. *an*, not + *ekdotos*, given out]

anecdotal records

anechoic room

Anectine

anelectrotonus (ăn"ĕl-ĕk-trŏt'ō-nŭs) [Gr. *ana*, up, + *elektron*, amber, + *tonos*, act of stretching, tension, tone]

Anel's operation (ă-nĕlz') [Dominique Anel, Fr. surgeon, 1679 – 1725]

Anel's probe

anemia (ă-nē'mē-ă) [Gr. *an-*, not, + *haima*, blood]
    a., achlorhydric
    a., addisonian
    a., aplastic
    a., blind loop
    a., chlorotic
    a., congenital hemolytic
    a., Cooley's
    a., crescent cell
    a., deficiency
    a., drepanocytic
    a., erythroblastic
    a., hemolytic
    a., hyperchromic
    a., hypersplenic
    a., hypochromic
    a., hypoplastic
    a., iron-deficiency
    a., Jaksch's
    a., macrocytic
    a., Mediterranean
    a., megaloblastic
    a., microcytic
    a., myelopathic
    a., normochromic
    a., normocytic
    a., nutritional
    a. of chronic disease
    a., pernicious
    a., pure red cell aplasia
    a., septic
    a., sickle cell
    a., splenic
    a., traumatic cardiac hemolytic

anemic (ă-nē'mĭk)
anemic hypoxia
anemophobia (ăn"ĕ-mō-fō'bē-ă) [Gr.
anemos, wind,   +   phobos, fear]
anencephalus (ăn"ĕn-sĕf'ă-lŭs) [Gr.
an-, not,   +   enkephalos, the brain]
anephrogenesis (ă-nĕf"rō-jĕn'ĕ-sĭs)
[Gr. a-, not,   +   nephros, kidney,
  +   genesis, generation, birth]
anergasia (ăn"ĕr-gā'sē-ă) [Gr. an-,
not   +   ergon, work]
anergastic reaction (ăn"ĕr-găs'tĭk)
anergia (ăn-ĕr'jē-ă) ["   +   ergon,
work]
anergic (ăn-ĕr'jĭk)
anergic stupor
anergy (ăn'ĕr-jē)
aneroid (ăn'ĕr-ŏyd) [Gr. a-, not,   +
neron, water,   +   eidos, form,
shape]
anerythroplasia (ăn"ĕ-rĭth"rō-plā'zē-
ă) [Gr. an-, not,   +   erythros, red,
  +   plasis, a molding]
anerythroplastic (ăn"ĕ-rĭth"rō-
plăs'tĭk)
anerythropsia (ăn"ĕ-rī-thrŏp'sē-ă)
["   +   "   +   opsis, sight, appearance, vision]
anesthecinesia,   anesthekinesia
(ăn-ĕs-thē"sĭn-ē'zē-ă,   -kĭ-nē'zē-ă)
["   +   aisthesis, feeling, perception,
  +   kinesis, motion]
anesthesia (ăn"ĕs-thē'zē-ă) ["   +
aisthesis, feeling, perception]
  a., audio
  a., basal
  a., block
  a., bulbar
  a., caudal
  a., central
  a., closed
  a., conduction
  a., crossed
  a., dissociative
  a. dolorosa
  a., electric
  a., endotracheal
  a., frost

  a., general
  a., Gwathmey's
  a., hysterical
  a., ice
  a., infiltration
  a., inhalation
  a., insufflation
  a., local
  a., mixed
  a., neural
  a., neuroleptic
  a., open
  a., peripheral
  a., primary
  a., pudendal
  a., rectal
  a., refrigeration
  a., regional
  a., segmental
  a., sexual
  a., spinal
  a., splanchnic
  a., surgical
  a., tactile
  a., topical
  a., traumatic
  a., twilight
anesthesimeter (ăn-ĕs"thĕ-sĭm'ĕ-tĕr)
[Gr. an-, not,   +   aisthesis, feeling,
perception,   +   metron, measure]
anesthesiologist (ăn"ĕs-thē"zē-ŏl'ō-
jĭst)
anesthesiology (ăn"ĕs-thē"zē-ŏl'ō-jē)
["   +   "   +   logos, word, reason]
anesthetic (ăn"ĕs-thĕt'ĭk)
anesthetist (ă-nĕs'thĕ-tĭst)
anesthetization (ă-nĕs"thĕ-tĭ-zā'shŭn)
anesthetize (ă-nĕs'thĕ-tīz)
anethole (ăn'ĕ-thōl)
anetoderma (ăn"ĕt-ō-dĕr'mă) [Gr.
anetos, relaxed,   +   derma, skin]
aneuploidy (ăn"ū-ploy'dē) [Gr. an-,
not,   +   eu, well,   +   ploos, fold,
  +   eidos, form, shape]
aneurine hydrochloride (ă-nū'rĭn)
aneurysm (ăn'ū-rĭzm) [Gr. aneurysma,
a widening]
  a., aortic

a., arteriovenous
a., atherosclerotic
a., berry
a., cirsoid
a., compound
a., dissecting
a., fusiform
a., mycotic
a., racemose
a., sacculated
a., varicose
a., venous

aneurysmal (ăn"ū-rĭz'măl) [Gr. aneurysma, a widening]
aneurysmectomy (ăn"ū-rĭz-mĕk'tō-mē) [" + ektome, excision]
aneurysmoplasty (ăn"ū-rĭz'mō-plăs"tē) [" + plassein, to form]
aneurysmorrhaphy (ăn"ū-rĭz-mor'ă-fē) [" + rhaphe, seam]
aneurysmotomy (ăn"ū-rĭz-mŏt'ō-mē) [" + tome, a cutting, slice]
A.N.F. American Nurses' Foundation
anfractuosity (ăn-frăk"tū-ŏs'ĭ-tē) [L. anfractus, a winding]
angel dust (PCP)
angel's trumpet [Datura ruaveolens]
angel's wing
Angelucci's syndrome (ăn"jĕ-loo'chēz) [Arnaldo Angelucci, It. ophthalmologist, 1854–1934]
anger (ăng'er) [L. angere, anguish]
angi- (ăn'jē) [Gr. angeion, vessel]
angiasthenia (ăn"jē-ăs-thē'nē-ă) [" + a-, not, + sthenos, strength]
angiectasia, angiectasis (ăn"jē-ĕk-tā'zē-ă, -ĕk'tă-sĭs) [" + ektasis, stretching]
angiectomy (ăn"jē-ĕk'tō-mē) [" + ektome, excision]
angiectopia (ăn"jē-ĕk'tō'pē-ă) [" + ektopos, out of place]
angiemphraxis (ăn"jē-ĕm-frăk'sĭs) [" + emphraxis, stoppage]
angiitis (ăn"jē-ī'tĭs) [" + itis, inflammation]
angina (ăn-jī'nă, ăn'jĭ-nă) [L. angina,

quinsy, from angere, to choke]
a. abdominis
a. acuta
a., agranulocytic
a. cruris
a. decubitus
a. epiglottidea
a. follicularis
a., intestinal
a. laryngea
a. ludovici, a. ludwigii
a., Ludwig's
a. maligna
a., necrotic
a. parotidea
a. pectoris
a., phlegmonous
a., Prinzmetal's
a. simplex
a. streptococcus
a. tonsillaris
a. trachealis
a., unstable
a., variant
a., Vincent's
anginal (ăn'jĭ-nal)
anginiform (ăn-jĭn'ĭ-form) [L. angina, quinsy, + forma, having the form of]
anginoid (ăn'jĭ-noyd) [" + Gr. eidos, form, shape]
anginophobia (ăn"jĭ-nō-fō'bē-ă) [" + Gr. phobos, fear]
anginose (ăn'jĭ-nōs) [L. angina, quinsy]
anginous (ăn'jĭ-nŭs)
angio- (ăn'jē-ō) [Gr. angeion, vessel]
angioataxia (ăn"jē-ō-ă-tăk'sē-ă) [" + ataxia, lack of order]
angioblast (ăn'jē-ō-blăst) [" + blastos, germ]
angioblastoma (ăn"jē-ō-blăs-tō'mă) [" + " + oma, tumor]
angiocardiogram (ăn"jē-ō-kăr'dē-ō-grăm) [" + kardia, heart, + gramma, letter, piece of writing]
angiocardiography (ăn"jē-ō-kăr"dē-ŏg'ră-fē) [" + " + graphein, to write]

angiocardiokinetic (ăn″jē-ō-kăr″dē-ō-kĭ-nĕt′ĭk) [″ + ″ + kinesis, motion]

angiocardiopathy (ăn″jē-ō-kăr″dē-ŏp′ă-thē) [″ + ″ + pathos, disease, suffering]

angiocarditis (ăn″jē-ō-kăr-dī′tĭs) [″ + ″ + itis, inflammation]

angiocavernous (ăn″jē-ō-kăv′ĕr-nŭs) [″ + L. caverna, cavern]

angiocholecystitis (ăn″jē-ō-kō″lē-sĭs-tī′tĭs) [″ + chole, bile, + kystis, bladder, + itis, inflammation]

angiocholitis (ăn″jē-ō-kō-lī′tĭs) [″ + ″ + itis, inflammation]

angiodystrophia (ăn″jē-ō-dĭs-trō′fē-ă) [″ + dys, bad, difficult, painful, disordered, + trophe, nourishment]

angioedema (ăn″jē-ō-ĕ-dē′mă) [″ + oidema, swelling]

angioendothelioma (ăn″jē-ō-ĕn″dō-thē″lē-ō′mă) [″ + endon, within, + thele, nipple, + oma, tumor]

angiofibroma (ăn″jē-ō-fĭ-brō′mă) [″ + L. fibra, fiber, + Gr. oma, tumor]

angiogenesis (ăn″jē-ō-jĕn′ĕ-sĭs) [″ + genesis, generation, birth]

angiogenic (ăn″jē-ō-jĕn′ĭk)

angiogenic factors

angioglioma (ăn″jē-ō-glī-ō′mă) [Gr. angeion, vessel, + glia, glue, + oma, tumor]

angiogram (ăn′jē-ō-grăm) [″ + gramma, letter, piece of writing]
   a., aortic
   a., cardiac
   a., cerebral

angiograph (ăn′jē-ō-grăf″) [″ + graphein, to write]

angiography (ăn″jē-ŏg′ră-fē)
   a., aortic
   a., cardiac
   a., cerebral
   a., coronary
   a., digital subtraction
   a., peripheral
   a., pulmonary
   a., selective
   a., vertebral

angiohyalinosis (ăn″jē-ō-hī″ă-lĭn-ō′sĭs) [Gr. angeion, vessel, + hyalos, glass, + osis, condition]

angiohypertonia (ăn″jē-ō-hī″pĕr-tō′nē-ă) [″ + hyper, over, above, excessive, + tonos, act of stretching, tension, tone]

angiohypotonia (ăn″jē-ō-hī″pō-tō′nē-ă) [″ + hypo, under, beneath, below, + tonos, act of stretching, tension, tone]

angioid (ăn′jē-oyd) [″ + eidos, form, shape]

angioid streaks

angiokeratoma (ăn″jē-ō-kĕr″ă-tō′mă) [″ + keras, horn, + oma, tumor]

angiokinetic (ăn″jē-ō-kĭ-nĕt′ĭk) [″ + kinesis, motion]

angioleukitis (ăn″jē-ō-loo-kī′tĭs) [″ + leukos, white, + itis, inflammation]

angiolipoma (ăn′jē-ō-lĭp-ō′mă) [″ + lipos, fat, + oma, tumor]

angiolith (ăn′jē-ō-lĭth) [″ + lithos, stone]

angiology (ăn″jē-ŏl′ō-jē) [″ + logos, word, reason]

angiolymphitis (ăn″jē-ō-lĭm-fī′tĭs) [″ + L. lympha, lymph, + itis, inflammation]

angiolysis (ăn″jē-ŏl′ĭ-sĭs) [″ + lysis, dissolution]

angioma (ăn″jē-ō′mă) [″ + oma, tumor]
   a., capillary
   a. cavernosum
   a., senile
   a., serpiginous
   a. simplex
   a., stellate
   a., telangiectatic
   a. venosum racemosum

angiomalacia (ăn″jē-ō-mă-lā′sē-ă) [Gr. angeion, vessel, + malakia, softness]

angiomatosis (ăn"jē-ō-mă-tō'sĭs) ["
+ oma, tumor, + osis, condition]
angiomatous (ăn"jē-ō'mă-tŭs)
angiomegaly (ăn"jē-ō-mĕg'ă-lē)
[" + megas, large]
angiometer (ăn"jē-ŏm'ĕ-tĕr) [" +
metron, measure]
angiomyocardiac (ăn"jē-ō-mī"ō-
kăr'dē-ăk) [" + mys, muscle, +
kardia, heart]
angiomyolipoma (ăn"jē-ō-mī"ō-lĭ-
pō'mă) [" + " + lipos, fat,
+ oma, tumor]
angiomyoma (ăn"jē-ō-mī-ō'mă)
[" + " + oma, tumor]
angiomyoneuroma (ăn"jē-ō-mī"ō-
nū-rō'mă) [" + " + neuron,
nerve, + oma, tumor]
angiomyosarcoma (ăn"jē-ō-mī"ō-
săr-kō'mă) [" + " + sarx,
flesh, + oma, tumor]
angioneurectomy (ăn"jē-ō-nū-rĕk'tō-
mē) [" + neuron, nerve, + ektome, excision]
angioneuromyoma (ăn"jē-ō-nū"rō-
mī-ō'mă) [" + " + mys, muscle, + oma, tumor]
angioneurosis (ăn"jē-ō-nū-rō'sĭs)
[" + " + osis, condition]
angioneurotic (ăn"jē-ō-nū-rŏt'ĭk)
angioneurotic edema
angioneurotomy (ăn"jē-ō-nū-rŏt'ō-
mē) [" + " + tome, a cutting,
slice]
angionoma (ăn"jē-ō-nō'mă) [Gr. angeion, vessel, + nome, ulcer]
angioparalysis (ăn"jē-ō-pă-răl'ĭ-sĭs) ["
+ paralyein, to loosen, disable]
angiopathology (ăn"jē-ō-pă-thŏl'ō-
jē) [" + pathos, disease, suffering,
+ logos, word, reason]
angiopathy (ăn-jē-ŏp'ă-thē)
**angiophacomatosis, angiophako-
matosis** (ăn"jē-ō-făk"ō-mă-tō'sis) ["
+ phakos, lens, + oma, tumor,
+ osis, condition]
angioplasty (ăn'jē-ō-plăs"tē) [" +
plassein, to form]

angiopoiesis (ăn"jē-ō-poy-ē'sĭs)
[" + poiein, to make]
angiopoietic (ăn"jē-ō-poy-ĕt'ĭk)
angiopressure (ăn'jē-ō-prĕsh"ŭr)
angiorrhaphy (ăn"jē-or'ă-fē) [" +
rhaphe, seam]
angiorrhexis (ăn"jē-or-ĕk'sĭs) [" +
rhexis, rupture]
angiosarcoma (ăn"jē-ō-săr-kō'mă) ["
+ sarx, flesh, + oma, tumor]
angiosclerosis (ăn"jē-ō-sklĕ-rō'sĭs)
[" + sklerosis, a hardening]
angioscope (ăn'jē-ō-skōp) [" +
skopein, to examine]
angioscotoma (ăn"jē-ō-skō-tō'mă)
[" + skotoma, darkness]
angiosis (ăn"jē-ō'sĭs) [Gr. angeion, vessel, + osis, condition]
angiospasm (ăn'jē-ō-spăzm) [" +
spasmos, a convulsion]
angiospastic (ăn'jē-ō-spăs'tĭk)
angiostaxis (ăn"jē-ō-stăk'sĭs) [" +
staxis, trickling]
angiostenosis (ăn"jē-ō-stĕ-nō'sĭs)
[" + stenoein, to make narrow,
+ osis, condition]
angiosteosis (ăn"jē-ŏs"tē-ō'sĭs) [" +
osteon, bone, + osis, condition]
angiostomy (ăn"jē-ŏs'tō-mē) [" +
stoma, mouth, opening]
angiostrophy (ăn"jē-ŏs'trō-fē) [" +
strophe, twist]
angiosynizesis (ăn"jē-ō-sīn"ĭ-zē'sĭs)
[" + synizesis, contraction]
angiotelectasis (ăn"jē-ō-tĕl-ĕk'tă-sĭs)
[" + telos, end, + ektasis,
stretching out]
angiotenic (ăn"jē-ō-tĕn'ĭk) [" +
teinen, to stretch]
angiotensin (ăn"jē-ō-tĕn'sĭn)
a. I
a. II
a. amide
angiotensinogen (ăn"jē-ō-tĕn-sĭn'ō-
jĕn)
angiotitis (ăn"jē-ō-tī'tĭs) [" + otos,
ear, + itis, inflammation]
angiotome (ăn'jē-ō-tōm") [Gr. an-

geion, vessel, + *tome*, a cutting, slice]
angiotomy (ăn″jē-ŏt″ŏ-mē)
angiotonic (ăn″jē-ō-tŏn′ĭk) [″ + *tonos*, act of stretching, tension, tone]
angiotonin (ăn″jē-ō-tŏn′ĭn)
angiotrophic (ăn″jē-ō-trŏf′ĭk) [″ + *trophe*, nourishment]
angitis (ăn-jī′tĭs) [″ + *itis*, inflammation]
angle (ăng′gl) [L. *angulus*]
  a., acromial
  a., acute
  a., alpha
  a., alveolar
  a., biorbital
  a., cardiophrenic
  a., carrying
  a., cavity
  a., cephalometric
  a., cerebellopontine
  a., costal
  a., costophrenic
  a., craniofacial
  a., facial
  a., flat
  a., gamma
  a., gonial
  a., metafacial
  a., obtuse
  a., occipital
  a. of convergence
  a. of incidence
  a. of iris
  a. of jaw
  a. of Louis
  a. of mandible
  a. of Treitz
  a., ophryospinal
  a., optic
  a., parietal
  a., pontine
  a., pubic
  a., right
  a., sphenoid
  a., sternal
  a., venous
  a., visual

angophrasia (ăn″gō-frā′zē-ă) [Gr. *anchein*, to choke, + *phrasis*, diction]
angor (ăng′gor) [L., strangling]
angor animi (ăng′gor ăn′ĭ-mē) [″ + L. *animus*, soul]
angstrom unit (ŏng′strŭm) [Anders J. Ångström, Swedish physicist, 1814–1874]
angular (ăng′gū-lăr) [L.]
angular artery
angulation (ăng″ū-lā′shŭn)
angulus [L.]
anhaphia (ăn-hă′fē-ă) [Gr. *an-*, not, + *haphe*, touch]
anhedonia (ăn″hē-dō′nē-ă) [″ + *hedone*, pleasure]
anhedonic (ăn″hē-dŏn′ĭk)
anhepatia (ăn-hĕ-pā′shē-ă) [″ + *hepar*, liver]
anhepatic (ăn-hĕ-păt′ĭk)
anhepatogenic (ăn-hĕp″ă-tō-jĕn′ĭk) [″ + *hepar*, liver, + *gennan*, to produce]
anhidrosis (ăn″hī-drō′sĭs) [″ + *hidros*, sweat]
anhidrotic (ăn″hī-drŏt′ĭk)
anhistic, anhistous (ăn-hĭs′tĭk, -hĭs′tŭs) [″ + *histos*, tissue]
anhydrase (ăn″hī′drās) [″ + *hydor*, water, + *-ase*, enzyme]
anhydration (ăn-hī′drā′shŭn) [″ + *hydor*, water]
anhydride (ăn-hī′drīd) [Gr. *an-*, not, + *hydor*, water]
anhydrochloric (ăn-hī-drō-klō′rĭk) [″ + ″ + *chloros*, green]
Anhydron
anhydrous (ăn-hī′drŭs) [″ + *hydor*, water]
anianthinopsy (ăn-ē-ăn′thĭn-ŏp″sē) [″ + *ianthinos*, violet, + *opsis*, sight, appearance, vision]
anicteric (ăn″ĭk-tĕr′ĭk) [″ + *ikteros*, jaundice]
anidrosis (ăn-ī-drō′sĭs) [″ + *hidros*, sweat]
anidrotic (ăn-ī-drŏt′ĭk)
anile (ăn′il, ā′nīl) [L. *anilis*, from *anus*, an

old woman]
anileridine (ăn″ĭ-lĕr′ĭ-dēn)
aniline (ăn′ĭ-lĭn) [Arabic *an-nil*, the indigo plant]
aniline poisoning
anilism (ăn′ĭl-ĭzm) [″ + -*ismos*, condition]
anility (ă-nĭl′ĭ-tē) [L. *anilitas*, from *anus*, an old woman]
anima (ăn′ĭ-mă) [L., soul]
animal (ăn′ĭ-măl) [L. *animalis*, living]
  a., cold-blooded
  a., warm-blooded
animalcule (ăn″ĭ-măl′kūl) [L. *animalculum*, little animal]
animation (ăn-ĭ-mā′shŭn) [L. *animus*, soul]
  a., suspended
animatism (ăn′ĭ-mă-tĭzm)
animi agitatio (ăn′ĭ-mē ă-jĭ-tā′shē-ō) [″ + *agitare*, to turn over]
animism (ăn′ĭ-mĭzm)
animus [L., breath, mind, soul]
anion (ăn′ĭ-ŏn) [Gr. *ana*, up, + *ion*, going]
anion gap
anionic (ăn″ĭ-ŏn′ĭk)
anionic detergent
aniridia (ăn″ĭ-rĭd′ē-ă) [Gr. *an-*, not, + *iris*, bend, turn]
anisakiasis (ăn″ĭs-să-kī′ă-sĭs)
aniseikonia (ăn-īs-ĭ-kō′nē-ă) [Gr. *anisos*, unequal, + *eikon*, image]
anise oil
aniso- (ăn-ī′sō) [Gr. *anisos*, unequal]
anisoaccommodation (ăn-ī″sō-ă-kŏm″mŏ-dā′shŭn) [″ + L. *accommodare*, to suit]
anisochromatic (ăn-ī″sō-krō-măt′ĭk) [″ + *chroma*, color]
anisocoria (ăn-ī″sō-kō′rē-ă) [″ + *kore*, pupil]
anisocytosis (ăn-ī″sō-sī-tō′sĭs) [″ + *kytos*, cell, + *osis*, condition]
anisogamy (ăn″ī-sŏg′ă-mē) [″ + *gamos*, marriage]
anisognathous (ăn″ī-sŏg′nă-thŭs) [″ + *gnathos*, jaw]

anisohypercytosis (ăn-ī″sō-hī″pĕr-sī-tō′sĭs) [″ + *hyper*, over, above, excessive, + *kytos*, cell, + *osis*, condition]
anisohypocytosis (ăn-ī″sō-hī″pō-sī-tō′sĭs) [″ + *hypo*, under, beneath, below, + *kytos*, cell, + *osis*, condition]
anisoiconia (ăn-ī″sō-ĭ-kō′nē-ă) [″ + *eikon*, image]
anisokaryosis (ăn-ī″sō-kăr″ē-ŏ′sĭs) [″ + *karyon*, nucleus, + *osis*, condition]
anisomastia (ăn-ī-sō-măs′tē-ă) [″ + *mastos*, breast]
anisomelia (ăn-ī″sō-mē′lē-ă) [″ + *melos*, limb]
anisometrope (ăn-ī″sō-mĕt′rōp) [Gr. *anisos*, unequal, + *metron*, measure, + *ops*, vision]
anisometropia (ăn-ī″sō-mĕ-trō′pē-ă)
anisometropic (ăn-ī″sō-mĕ-trŏp′ĭk)
anisonormocytosis (ăn-ī″sō-nor″mō-sī-tō′sĭs) [″ + L. *norma*, rule, + Gr. *kytos*, cell, + *osis*, condition]
anisophoria (ăn″ī-sō-fō′rē-ă) [″ + *phoros*, bearing]
anisopia (ăn″ī-sō′pē-ă) [″ + *ops*, vision]
anisopiesis (ăn-ī″sō-pī-ē′sĭs) [″ + *piezein*, to squeeze]
anisosthenic (ăn-ī″sŏs-thĕn′ĭk) [″ + *sthenos*, strength]
anisotonic (ăn-ī″sō-tŏn′ĭk) [″ + *tonos*, act of stretching, tension, tone]
anisotropal (ăn″ī-sŏt′rō-păl) [″ + *tropos*, a turning]
anisotropic (ăn-ī″sō-trŏp′ĭk)
anisotropous (ăn-ī-sŏt′rō-pŭs)
ankh (ăngk) [Egyptian, *life*]
ankle (ăng′kl) [AS. *ancleow*]
ankle bone
ankle clonus
  a.c. reflex
ankle jerk
ankle joint
ankylo- (ăng′kĭ-lō) [Gr. *ankylos*, crooked]

ankyloblepharon (ăng″kĭ-lō-blĕf′ăr-ŏn) [″ + blepharon, eyelid]

ankylochilia (ăng″kĭ-lō-kĭ′lē-a) [″ + cheilos, lip]

ankylocolpos (ăng-kĭ-lō-kŏl′pŏs) [″ + kolpos, vagina]

ankylodactylia (ăng-kĭ-lō-dăk-tĭl′ē-a) [″ + daktylos, finger]

ankyloglossia (ăng″kĭ-lō-glŏs′sē-ă) [″ + glossa, tongue]

ankylopoietic (ăng″kĭ-lō-poy-ĕt′ĭk) [Gr. ankyle, stiff joint, + poiein, to form]

ankyloproctia (ăng″kĭ-lō-prŏk′shē-ă) [Gr. ankylos, crooked, + proktos, anus]

ankylosed

ankylosis (ăng″kĭ-lō′sĭs) [Gr. ankyle, stiff joint, + osis, condition]
  a., artificial
  a., bony
  a., dental
  a., extracapsular
  a., false
  a., fibrous
  a., intracapsular
  a., ligamentous
  a., true

Ankylostoma (ăng″kĭ-lŏs′tō-mă)

ankylostoma (ăng″kĭ-lŏs′tō-mă)

ankylostomiasis (ăng″kĭ-lō-stō-mī′ă-sĭs)

ankylotia (ăng″kĭ-lō′shē-ă) [Gr. ankylos, crooked, + ot-, ear]

ankylotome (ăng′kĭl-ō-tōm, ăng-kĭl′ō-tōm) [″ + tome, a cutting, slice]

ankylurethria (ăng″kĭl-ū-rē′thrē-ă) [″ + ourethra, urethra]

anlage (ŏn′lŏ-jhă) [Ger., a laying on]

annatto (ă-nŏ′tō) [Cariban]

annealing (an-nēl′ĭng) [AS. anaelan, to burn]

annectent (ă-nĕk′tĕnt) [L. annectens, tying or binding to]

Annelida (ă-nĕl′ĭ-dă)

annexa (ă-nĕks′ă) [L. annectere, to tie or bind to]

annexitis (ă-nĕks-ī′tĭs) [″ + Gr. itis, inflammation]

annexopexy (ă-nĕk′sō-pĕk-sē) [″ + Gr. pexis, fixation]

annular (ăn′ū-lăr) [L. annulus, ring]

annulorrhaphy (an″ū-lor′ă-fē) [″ + Gr. rhaphe, seam]

annulus (ăn′ū-lŭs) [L.]

anococcygeal (ă″nō-kŏk-sĭ′jē-al) [L. anus, anus, + Gr. kokkyx, coccyx]

anococcygeal body

anococcygeal ligament

anodal (ăn-ō′dăl) [Gr. ana, up, + hodos, way]

anodal closure contraction

anode (ăn′ōd) [Gr. ana, up, + hodos, way]

anodmia (ăn-ŏd′mē-ă) [Gr. an-, not, + odme, stench]

anodontia (ăn″ō-dŏn′shē-ă) [″ + odous, tooth]

anodyne (ăn′ō-dīn) [″ + odyne, pain]

anodynia (ăn″ō-dĭn′ē-ă)

anoesia (ăn″ō-ē′zē-ă) [Gr. anoesia, want of understanding]

anoetic (ăn″ō-ĕt′ĭk)

anomaloscope (ă-nŏm′ă-lō-skōp″) [Gr. anomalos, irregular, + skopein, to examine]

anomalous (ă-nŏm′ă-lŭs) [Gr. anomalos, uneven]

anomaly (ă-nŏm′ă-lē) [Gr. anomalia, irregularity]
  a., congenital

anomia (a-nō′mē-ă) [Gr. a-, not, + onoma, name]

anomie (ăn′ō-mē)

anonychia (ăn-ō-nĭk′ē-ă) [Gr. an-, not, + onyx, nail]

anoopsia (ăn″ō-ŏp′sē-ă) [Gr. ano, upward, + opsis, sight, appearance, vision]

anoperineal (ā″nō-pĕr-ĭ-nē′ăl)

Anopheles (ă-nŏf′ĕ-lēz) [Gr. anopheles, harmful, useless]

anophoria (ăn-ō-fō′rē-ă) [Gr. ano, upward, + pherein, to bear]

anophthalmia (ăn-ŏf-thăl′mē-ă) [Gr.

an-, not, + *ophthalmos*, eye]
anopia (ăn-ō'pē-ă) [" + *ops*, eye]
anoplasty (ā'nō-plăs"tē) [L. *anus*, anus, + Gr. *plassein*, to form]
Anoplura (an-ō-ploo'ră) [Gr. *anoplos*, unarmed, + *oura*, tail]
anopsia (ăn-ŏp'sē-ă) [" + *opsis*, sight, appearance, vision]
anorchidism (ăn-or'kĭ-dĭzm")
anorchism (ăn-or'kĭzm) [" + *orchis*, testicle, + *-ismos*, condition]
anorectal (ā-nō-rĕk'tăl)
anorectic, anorectous (ăn-ō-rĕk'tĭc, -tŭs) [Gr. *anorektos*, without appetite for]
anorexia (ăn-ō-rĕk'sē-ă) [Gr. *an-*, not, + *orexis*, appetite]
   a. nervosa
anorexigenic (ăn"ō-rĕk"sĭ-jĕn'ĭk) [" + " + *gennan*, to produce]
anorgasmy (ăn-or-găz'mē) [" + *orgasmos*, swelling]
anorthography (ăn"or-thŏg'ră-fē) [" + *orthos*, straight, + *graphein*, to write]
anorthopia (ăn"or-thō'pē-ă) [" + " + *ops*, eye]
anoscope (ā'nō-skōp) [L. *anus*, anus, + Gr. *skopein*, to examine]
anosigmoidoscopy (ā"nō-sĭg"moy-dŏs'kō-pē) [" + Gr. *sigmoeides*, shaped like Greek S, + *skopein*, to examine]
anosmatic (ăn-ŏz-măt'ĭk) [Gr. *an-*, not, + *osme*, smell]
anosmia (ăn-ŏz'mē-ă)
anosmic, anosmous (ăn-ŏz'mĭk, -mŭs)
anosognosia (ăn-ō-sŏg-nō'zē-ă) [" + " + *gnosis*, knowledge]
anosphrasia (ăn-ŏs-frā'zē-ă) [Gr. *an-*, not, + *osphresis*, smell]
anospinal (ā"nō-spī'năl) [L. *anus* + *spina*, thorn]
anostosis (ăn-ŏs-tō'sĭs) [Gr. *an-*, not, + *osteon*, bone, + *osis*, condition]
anotia (ăn-ō'shē-ă) [" + *ours*, ear]
anotropia (ăn"ō-trō'pē-ă) [Gr. *ana*,

up, + *trope*, a turning]
ANOVA *analysis of variance*
anovaginal (ā"nō-văj'ĭ-năl)
anovarism (ăn-ō'văr-ĭzm) [Gr. *an-*, not, + NL. *ovarium*, ovary, + Gr. *-ismos*, condition]
anovesical (ā"nō-vĕs'ĭ-kl) [L. *anus*, anus, + *vesica*, bladder]
anovular, anovulatory (ăn-ŏv'ū-lar, ăn-ŏv'ū-lă-tō"rē) [Gr. *an-*, not, + NL. *ovarium*, ovary]
anovular cycle
anoxemia (ăn-ŏk-sē'mē-ă) [" + *oxygen* + Gr. *haima*, blood]
anoxia (ăn-ŏk'sē-ă) [" + *oxygen*]
   a., altitude
   a., anemic
   a., anoxic
   a., hypokinetic
   a., stagnant
anoxic (ăn-ŏks'ĭk)
ansa (ăn'să) [L., a handle]
   a. cervicalis
   a. hypoglossi
   a. lenticularis
   a. nervorum spinalium
   a. peduncularis
   a. sacralis
   a. subclavia
A.N.S.I. *American National Standards Institute*
ansiform (ăn'sī-form) [L. *ansa*, a handle, + *forma*, shape]
ant- [Gr.]
Antabuse (ăn'tă-būs")
antacid (ănt-ăs'ĭd) [Gr. *anti*, against, + L. *acidum*, acid]
antagonism (ăn-tăg'ō-nĭzm") [Gr. *antagonizesthai*, to struggle against]
   a., bacterial
antagonist (ăn-tăg'ō-nĭst)
   a., dental
   a., muscular
   a., narcotic
antalgesic (ănt-ăl-jē'sĭk) [Gr. *anti*, against, + *algos*, pain]
antalgic (ănt-ăl'jĭk)
antalkaline (ănt-ăl'kă-lĭn, -lĭn) [" +

alkaline]

antaphrodisiac (ănt″ăf-rō-dĭz′ē-ăk) [″ + *aphrodisiakos*, sexual]

antarthritic (ănt″ăr-thrĭt′ĭk) [″ + *arthritikos*, gouty]

antasthenic (ănt″ăs-thĕn′ĭk) [″ + *astheneia*, weakness]

antasthmatic (ănt″ăz-măt′ĭk) [″ + Gr. *asthma*, panting]

antatrophic (ănt″ă-trō′fĭk) [″ + *atrophia*, atrophy]

antazoline phosphate (ăn-tăz′ō-lēn)

ante- [L.]

antebrachium (ăn″tē-brā′kē-ŭm) [L. *ante*, before, + *brachium*, arm]

antecardium (ăn″tē-kăr′dē-ŭm) [″ + Gr. *kardia*, heart]

antecedent (ăn″tē-sē′dĕnt) [L. *antecedere*, to precede]
a., plasma thromboplastin

ante cibum (ăn′tē sē′bŭm) [L.]

antecubital (ăn″tē-kū′bĭ-tăl) [″ + *cubitum*, elbow]

antecubital fossa

antecurvature (ăn″tē-kŭr′vă-tŭr″) [″ + *curvatura*, bend]

antefebrile (an″tē-fē′brĭl, -fē′brĭl, -fĕb′rĭl) [L. *ante*, before, + *febris*, fever]

anteflect (ăn″tē-flĕkt) [″ + *flectere*, to bend]

anteflexion (ăn″tē-flĕk′shŭn)

antegrade (ăn′tē-grād)

antelocation (ăn″tē-lō-kă′shŭn) [″ + *locare*, to place]

antemetic (ănt″ĕ-mĕt′ĭk) [Gr. *anti*, against, + *emetikos*, emetic]

ante mortem (ăn′tē mor′tĕm) [L.]

ante mortem statement

antenatal (ăn″tē-nā′tăl) [″ + *natus*, born]

antenatal diagnosis

antenatal surgery

Antepar

antepartal; ante partum (ăn″tē-păr′tăl, -tŭm) [L.]

antepyretic (ăn″tē-pī-rĕt′ĭk) [L. *ante*, before, + Gr. *pyretos*, fever]

anterior [L.]

anterior chamber

anterior drawer sign

anterior horn cell

antero- [L.]

anteroexternal (ăn″tĕr-ō-ĕks-tĕr′năl) [L. *antero*, anterior, + *externus*, outside]

anterograde [″ + *gradior*, to step]

anteroinferior [″ + *inferior*, below]

anterointernal (ăn″tĕr-ō-ĭn-tĕr′năl) [″ + *internus*, within]

anterolateral [″ + *latus*, side]

anteromedian [″ + *medius*, middle]

anteroposterior [″ + *posterior*, rear]

anterosuperior [″ + *superior*, above]

anteversion (ăn″tē-vĕr′zhŭn) [″ + *vertere*, to turn]

anteverted (an″tē-vĕrt′ĕd)

anthelix (ănt′hē-lĭks, ăn′thē-lĭks) [Gr. *anti*, against, + *helix*, coil]

anthelmintic, anthelminthic, antihelmintic (ănt″hĕl-mĭn′tĭk, -thĭk, ăn″tĭ-hĕl-mĭn′tĭk) [″ + *helmins*, worm]

Anthemis (ăn′thĕm-ĭs)

anthemorrhagic (ănt″hĕm-ō-răj′ĭk) [″ + *haima*, blood, + *rhegnynai*, to burst forth]

anthocyanin (ăn″thō-sī′ă-nĭn) [Gr. *anthos*, flower, + *kyanos*, a blue substance]

Anthomyia (ăn″thō-mī′yă) [″ + *myia*, fly]
A. canicularis

anthophobia (ăn″thō-fō′bē-ă) [″ + *phobos*, fear]

anthracemia (ăn″thră-sē′mē-ă) [Gr. *anthrax*, coal, + *haima*, blood]

anthracene (ăn′thră-sēn)

anthracia (an-thră′sē-ă) [Gr. *anthrax*, coal, carbuncle]

anthracoid (an′thră-koyd) [″ + *eidos*, form, shape]

anthracometer (ăn″thră-kŏm′ĕ-ter)
[″ + metron, measure]
anthraconecrosis (ăn″thră-kō-nĕ-
krŏ′sĭs) [″ + nekrosis, state of
death]
anthracosilicosis (ăn″thră-kō-sĭl″ĭ-
kō′sĭs) [″ + L. silex, flint, + Gr.
osis, condition]
anthracosis (ăn-thră-kō′sĭs) [″ +
osis, condition]
Anthra-Derm
anthralin (ăn′thră-lĭn)
anthrax (ăn′thrăks) [Gr., coal, carbun-
cle]
anthropo- [Gr. anthropos, man]
anthropobiology (ăn″thrō-pō-bī-ŏl′ō-
jē) [″ + bios, life, + logos,
word, reason]
anthropogeny (ăn″thrō-pŏj′ĕ-nē)
[″ + gennan, to produce]
anthropoid (ăn′thrō-poyd) [″ +
eidos, form, shape]
anthropological baseline
anthropology (ăn″thrō-pŏl′ō-jē)
[″ + logos, word, reason]
anthropometer (ăn″thrō-pŏm′ĕ-tĕr)
[″ + metron, measure]
anthropometry (ăn-thrō-pŏm′ĕt-rē)
anthropomorphism (ăn″thrō-pō-
mor′fĭzm) [″ + morphe, form, +
-ismos, condition]
anthropophilic (ăn″thrō-pō-fĭl′ĭk)
[″ + philein, to love]
anthropozoonoses (ăn″thrō-pō-
zō″ō-nō′sĕs) [″ + zoon, animal,
+ nosis, disease]
anti- [Gr.]
antiadrenergic (ăn″tē-ă-drĕn-ĕr′jĭk)
[Gr. anti, against, + L. ad, to, +
ren, kidney, + Gr. ergon, work]
antiagglutinin (ăn″tē-ă-gloo′tĭ-nĭn)
antiamebic (ăn″tē-ă-mē′bĭk) [″ +
amoibe, change]
antianaphylaxis (ăn″tē-ăn-ă-fĭ-
lăks′ĭs) [″ + ana, away from, +
phylaxis, guard]
antiandrogen (ăn″tē-ăn′drō-jĕn)
[″ + androgen]

antianemic (ăn″tē-ă-nē′mĭk)
antiantibody (ăn″tē-ăn′tĭ-bŏd-ē)
[″ + antibody]
antiantitoxin (ăn″tē-ăn″tĭ-tŏk′sin)
[″ + antitoxin]
antiapoplectic (ăn″tē-ăp″ō-plĕk′tĭk)
antiarrhythmic (ăn″tē-ă-rĭth′mĭk) [″
+ a-, not, + rhythmos, rhythm]
antiarthritic (ăn″tē-ăr-thrĭt′ĭk) [″ +
arthritikos, gouty]
antibacterial (ăn″tĭ-băk-tē′rē-ăl)
antibiosis (an″tĭ-bī-ō′sĭs) [″ + bios,
life]
antibiotic (ăn″tĭ-bī-ŏt′ĭk)
    a., bacteriocidal or bactericidal
    a., bacteriostatic
    a., broad-spectrum
antibody (ăn′tĭ-bŏd″ē)
    a., blocking
    a., cross-reacting
    a., fluorescent
    a., maternal
    a., monoclonal
    a., natural
antibody-coated bacteria
antibrachium (ăn″tĭ-brā′kē-ŭm)
antibromic (ăn″tĭ-brō′mĭk) [Gr. anti,
against, + bromos, smell]
antiburnscar garment
anticarcinogenic
anticardium (ăn″tĭ-kăr′dē-ŭm)
anticariogenic
anticarious (ăn″tĭ-kā′rē-ŭs) [″ +
caries, decay]
anticatarrhal (ăn″tĭ-kă-tăr′ăl) [″ +
L. catarrhus, catarrhal]
anticholagogue (ăn″tĭ-kŏl′ă-gŏg) [Gr.
anti, against, + chole, bile, +
agein, to lead forth]
anticholinergic (ăn″tĭ-kō″lĭn-ĕr′jĭk)
anticholinesterase (ăn″tĭ-kō-lĭn-
ĕs′tĕr-ās)
anticipate (ăn-tĭs′ĭ-pāt) [L. ante, before,
+ capere, to take]
anticipatory guidance
anticlinal (ăn″tĭ-klī′năl) [Gr. anti,
against, + klinein, to incline]
anticoagulant (ăn″tĭ-kō-ăg′ū-lănt)

[" + L. *coagulans*, forming clots]
   a. citrate dextrose solution
   a. citrate phosphate dextrose solution
   a. heparin solution
   a. sodium citrate solution

anticodon (ăn″tĭ-kō′dŏn)
anticomplement (ăn″tĭ-kŏm′plĕ-mĕnt)
anticonvulsant (ăn″tĭ-kŏn-vŭl′sănt) [" + L. *convulsio*, pulling together]
antidepressant (ăn″tĭ-dē-prĕs′sănt)
antidiabetic (ăn″tĭ-dī″ă-bĕt′ĭk)
antidiarrheal (ăn″tĭ-dī-ă-rē′ăl)
antidiuretic (ăn″tĭ-dī-ū-rĕt′ĭk) [" + *dia*, intensive, + *ouresis*, urination]
antidiuretic hormone
antidotal (ăn″tĭ-dō′tăl)
antidote (ăn′tĭ-dōt) [Gr. *antidoton*, given against]
   a., chemical
   a., mechanical
   a., physiologic
   a., universal
antidromic (ăn″tĭ-drŏm′ĭk) [Gr. *anti*, against, + *dromos*, running]
antidysenteric (ăn″tĭ-dĭs″ĕn-tĕr′ĭk)
antiemetic (ăn″tĭ-ē-mĕt′ĭk) [" + *emetikos*, inclined to vomit]
antienzyme (ăn″tĭ-ĕn′zīm)
antiepileptic (ăn″tĭ-ĕp″ĭ-lĕp′tĭk)
antiestrogen (ăn″tĭ-ĕs′trō-jĕn)
antifebrile (ăn″tĭ-fē′brĭl, -fē′brĭl, -fĕb′rĭl) [" + L. *febris*, fever]
antifibrinolysin (ăn″tĭ-fī″brĭ-nŏl′ĭ-sĭn) [" + L. *fibra*, fiber, + Gr. *lysis*, dissolution]
antifungal (ăn″tĭ-fŭng′găl)
antigalactic (ăn″tĭ-gă-lăk′tĭk)
antigen (ăn′tĭ-jĕn) [Gr. *anti*, against, + *gennan*, to produce]
   a.'s, histocompatibility
   a., H-Y
antigen-antibody reaction
antigenic (ăn-tĭ-jĕn′ĭk)
antigenic drift
antigenotherapy (ăn″tĭ-jĕn″ō-thĕr′ă-pē)
antiglobulin (ăn″tĭ-glŏb′ū-lĭn)

antigoitrogenic (ăn″tĭ-goy″trō-jĕn′ĭk) [" + L. *guttur*, throat, + Gr. *gennan*, to produce]
antigonorrheic (ăn″tĭ-gŏn″ō-rē′ĭk)
anti-G suit [" + G, gravity]
antihelix (ăn″tĭ-hē′lĭks) [" + Gr. *helix*, coil]
antihemolysin (ăn″tĭ-hē-mŏl′ĭ-sĭn)
antihemophilic factor
Antihemophilic Globulin (AHG)
antihemorrhagic (ăn″tĭ-hĕm-ō-răj′ĭk)
antihidrotic (ăn″tĭ-hī-drŏt′ĭk) [" + *hidrotikos*, sweating]
antihistamine (ăn″tĭ-hĭs′tă-mēn, -mĭn)
antihistamine poisoning
antihistaminic (ăn″tĭ-hĭs″tă-mĭn′ĭk)
antihydropic (ăn″tĭ-hī-drŏp′ĭk) [Gr. *anti*, against, + *hydropikos*, dropsical]
antihypercholesterolemic (ăn″tĭ-hī″pĕr-kō-lĕs″tĕr-ŏl-ē′mĭk) [" + *hyper*, over, above, excessive, + *chole*, bile, + *stereos*, solid, + *haima*, blood]
antihypertensive (ăn″tĭ-hī″pĕr-tĕn′sĭv) [" + " + L. *tensio*, tension]
antihypnotic (ăn″tĭ-hĭp-nŏt′ĭk)
anti-icteric (ăn″tĭ-ĭk-tĕr′ĭk) [" + *ikteros*, jaundice]
anti-immune (ăn″tĭ-ĭ-mūn′)
anti-infectious (ăn″tĭ-ĭn-fĕk′shŭs)
anti-inflammatory (ăn″tĭ-ĭn-flăm′ă-tō-rē)
antiketogenesis (ăn″tĭ-kē-tō-jĕn′ĕ-sĭs) [" + *ketone* + Gr. *genesis*, generation, birth]
antiketogenetic, antiketogenic (ăn″tĭ-kē″tō-jĕ-nĕt′ĭk, -jĕn′ĭk)
antilactase (ăn″tĭ-lăk′tās) [" + *lac*, milk, + *-ase*, enzyme]
antilipemic (ăn″tĭ-lĭ-pē′mĭk)
Antilirium
antilithic (ăn″tĭ-lĭth′ĭk) [" + *lithos*, stone]
antiluetic (ăn″tĭ-loo-ĕt′ĭk) [Gr. *anti*, against, + L. *lues*, pestilence]
antilymphocytic serum (ăn″tĭ-lĭm″fō-sĭt′ĭk)

antilysin (ăn-tĭ-lī′sĭn)

antilysis (ăn-tĭ-lī′sĭs) [″ + *lysis,* dissolution]

antilyssic (ăn-tĭ-lĭs′ĭk) [″ + *lyssa,* frenzy]

antilytic (ăn-tĭ-lĭt′ĭk)

antimalarial (ăn″tĭ-mă-lā′rē-ăl)

antimere (ăn′tĭ-mēr) [″ + *meros,* a part]

antimetabolite (ăn″tĭ-mě-tăb′ō-līt)

antimetropia (ăn″tĭ-mě-trō′pē-ă) [″ + *metron,* measure, + *ops,* eye]

antimicrobial (ăn″tĭ-mī-krō′bē-ăl)

antimicrobial drugs

antimicrobic (ăn″tĭ-mī-krō′bĭk) [″ + *mikros,* small, + *bios,* life]

Antiminth

antimitotic (ăn″tĭ-mī-tŏt′ĭk)

antimonial (ăn″tĭ-mō′nē-ăl)

antimony (ăn′tĭ-mō″nē)

antimony poisoning

antimycotic (ăn″tĭ-mī-kŏt′ĭk) [Gr. *anti,* against, + *mykes,* fungus]

antinarcotic (ăn″tĭ-năr-kŏt′ĭk) [″ + *narkotikos,* benumbing]

antinatriuresis (ăn″tĭ-nā″trĭ-ū-rē′sĭs) [″ + L. *natrium,* sodium, + Gr. *ouresis,* making water]

antinauseant (ăn″tĭ-naw′sē-ănt)

antineoplastic (ăn″tĭ-nē″ō-plăs′tĭk)

antinephritic (ăn″tĭ-ně-frĭt′ĭk)

antineuralgic (ăn″tĭ-nū-răl′jĭk) [″ + *neuron,* nerve, + *algos,* pain]

antineuritic (ăn″tĭ-nū-rĭt′ĭk)

antinuclear (ăn″tĭ-nū′klē-ăr)

antinuclear antibodies

antiodontalgic (ăn″tē-ō″dŏn-tăl′jĭk) [″ + *odous,* tooth, + *algos,* pain]

antiovulatory (ăn″tē-ŏv′ū-lă-tō″rē)

antioxidant (ăn″tē-ŏk′sĭ-dănt)

antioxidation (ăn″tē-ŏk″sĭ-dā′shŭn)

antipaludian (ăn″tĭ-pă-loo′dē-ăn)

antiparalytic (ăn″tĭ-păr-ă-lĭt′ĭk)

antiparasitic (ăn″tĭ-păr-ă-sĭt′ĭk)

antipathic (ăn″tĭ-păth′ĭk) [Gr. *anti,* against, + *pathein,* to feel]

antipathy (ăn-tĭp′ă-thē)

antipedicular (ăn″tĭ-pě-dĭk′ū-lăr)

antiperiodic (ăn″tĭ-pē-rē-ŏd′ĭk) [″ + *periodos,* a circle]

antiperistalsis (ăn″tĭ-pěr″ĭ-stăl′sĭs) [″ + *peri,* around, + *stalsis,* constriction]

antiperistaltic (ăn″tĭ-pěr″ĭ-stăl′tĭk)

antiperspirant (ăn″tĭ-pěr′spī-rănt)

antiphagocytic (ăn″tĭ-făg-ō-sīt′ĭk)

antiphlogistic (ăn″tĭ-flō-jĭs′tĭk) [″ + *phlogistos,* on fire]

antiplasmin (ăn″tĭ-plăz′mĭn)

antiplastic (ăn″tĭ-plăs′tĭk) [″ + *plassein,* to form]

antiplatelet (ăn″tĭ-plāt′lĕt)

antipodal (ăn-tĭp′ō-dăl) [Gr. *antipous,* with feet opposite]

antipraxia (ăn″tĭ-prăk′sē-ă)

antiprostaglandin (ăn″tĭ-prŏs″tă-glăn′dĭn)

antiprostate (ăn″tĭ-prŏs′tāt)

antiprostatitis (ăn″tĭ-prŏs″tă-tī′tĭs)

antiprotease (ăn″tĭ-prō′tē-ās)

antiprotozoal (ăn″tĭ-prō″tō-zō′ăl)

antipruritic (ăn″tĭ-proo-rīt′ĭk)

antipsoriatic (ăn″tĭ-sō″rē-ăt′ĭk) [″ + *psora,* itch]

antiputrefactive (ăn″tĭ-pū″trě-făk′tĭv)

antipyogenic (ăn″tĭ-pī-ō-jěn′ĭk) [″ + ″ + *gennan,* to produce]

antipyresis (ăn″tĭ-pī-rē′sĭs) [″ + *pyretos,* fever]

antipyretic (ăn-tĭ-pī-rĕt′ĭk)

antipyrotic (ăn″tĭ-pī-rŏt′ĭk) [″ + *pyrotikos,* burning]

antirabic (ăn″tĭ-rā′bĭk)

antirachitic (ăn″tĭ-ră-kĭt′ĭk) [″ + *rachitis,* rickets]

antirheumatic (ăn″tĭ-roo-măt′ĭk)

antiricin (ăn″tĭ-rī′sĭn)

antiscabietic (ăn″tĭ-skă″bē-ĕt′ĭk) [Gr. *anti,* against, + L. *scabies,* itch]

antiscorbutic (ăn″tĭ-skor-bū′tĭk) [″ + L. *scorbutus,* scurvy]

antiseborrheic (ăn″tĭ-sĕb″ō-rē′ĭk)

antisecretory (ăn″tĭ-sē-krē′tō-rē)

antiself

antisepsis (ăn″tĭ-sĕp′sĭs) [″ + *sepsis,* decay]

antiseptic (ăn″tĭ-sĕp′tĭk)
antiserum (ăn″tĭ-sē′rŭm)
   a., monovalent
   a., polyvalent
antishock garment
antisialagogue (ăn″tĭ-sī-ăl′ă-gŏg) [Gr. *anti*, against, + *sialon*, saliva, + *agogos*, drawing forth]
antisialic (ăn″tĭ-sī-ăl′ĭk)
antisocial (ăn″tĭ-sō′shăl)
antisocial personality disorder
antispasmodic [″ + *spasmos*, a convulsion]
anti-stain formulary
antistaphylococcic (ăn″tĭ-stăf″ĭ-lō-kŏk′sĭk) [Gr. *anti*, against, + *staphyle*, bunch of grapes, + *cocci*, bacteria]
antistreptococcic (ăn″tĭ-strĕp″tō-kŏk′sĭk)
antistreptolysin (ăn″tĭ-strĕp-tŏl′ĭ-sĭn)
antisudoral (ăn″tĭ-soo′dor-ăl) [″ + L. *sudor*, sweat]
antisudorific (ăn″tĭ-soo″dor-ĭf′ĭk)
antisyphilitic (ăn″tĭ-sĭf″ĭ-lĭt′ĭk) [″ + L. *syphiliticus*, pert. to syphilis]
antitabetic (ăn″tĭ-tă-bĕt′ĭk) [″ + L. *tabes*, wasting disease]
antithenar (ăn-tĭth′ĕn-ăr) [″ + *thenar*, palm]
antithrombotic (ăn″tĭ-thrŏm-bŏt′ĭk)
antithyroid (ăn″tĭ-thī′royd) [″ + *thyreoeides*, thyroid]
antitonic (ăn″tĭ-tŏn′ĭk) [″ + *tonos*, act of stretching, tension, tone]
antitoxic (ăn″tĭ-tŏk′sĭk) [″ + *toxikon*, poison]
antitoxic serum
antitoxigen (ăn″tĭ-tŏk′sĭ-gĕn) [″ + ″ + *gennan*, to produce]
antitoxin (ăn″tĭ-tŏk′sĭn)
antitoxinogen (ăn″tĭ-tŏk-sĭn′ō-jĕn) [Gr. *anti*, against, + *toxikon*, poison, + *gennan*, to produce]
antitragicus (ăn″tĭ-trăj′ĭ-kŭs)
antitragus (ăn″tĭ-trā′gŭs) [″ + L. *tragus*, goat]
antitrichomonal
antitrismus (ăn″tĭ-trĭs′mŭs) [″ +

trismos, grinding]
antitrypsin (ăn″tĭ-trĭp′sĭn)
   a., alpha 1-
antitrypsin deficiency
antitryptic (ăn″tĭ-trĭp′tĭk)
antituberculotic (ăn″tĭ-too-bĕr′kū-lŏt″ĭk)
antitussive (ăn″tĭ-tŭs′ĭv) [Gr. *anti*, against, + L. *tussis*, cough]
   a., centrally acting
antiuratic (ăn″tĭ-ū-răt′ĭk) [″ + L. *uras*, urate]
antivaccinationist (ăn″tĭ-văk″sĭ-nā′shŭn-ĭst)
antivenene (ăn″tĭ-vĕn′ēn)
antivenereal (ăn″tĭ-vĕ-nē′rē-ăl)
antivenin (ăn″tĭ-vĕn′ĭn)
   a., black widow spider
   a., (crotalidae) polyvalent
antivenom (ăn″tĭ-vĕn′ŏm)
antivenomous (ăn″tĭ-vĕn′ō-mŭs)
Antivert
antiviral (ăn″tĭ-vī′răl)
antivitamin
antivivisection (ăn″tĭ-vĭv″ĭ-sĕk′shŭn)
antixenic (ăn″tĭ-zē′nĭk) [Gr. *anti*, against, + *xenos*, strange]
antixerotic (ăn″tĭ-zē-rŏt′ĭk) [″ + *xerosis*, dryness]
antizymotic (ăn″tĭ-zī-mŏt′ĭk) [″ + *zymosis*, fermentation]
antra (ăn′tră) [L.]
antral (ăn′trăl)
antrectomy (ăn-trĕk′tō-mē) [L. *antrum*, cavity, + Gr. *ektome*, excision]
antritis (ăn″trī′tĭs) [″ + Gr. *itis*, inflammation]
antro- [L. *antrum*, cavity]
antroatticotomy (ăn″trō-ăt″ĭ-kŏt′ō-mē) [″ + *atticus*, attic, + Gr. *tome*, a cutting, slice]
antrobuccal (ăn″trō-bŭk′ăl) [″ + *bucca*, cheek]
antrocele (ăn′trō-sēl) [″ + Gr. *kele*, tumor, swelling]
antroduodenectomy (ăn″trō-dū″ō-dē-nĕk′tō-mē) [″ + *duodeni*, twelve, + Gr. *ektome*, excision.]
antronasal (ăn″trō-nā′zăl) [″ +

nasalis, nasal]

antrophore (ăn'trō-for) [″ + Gr. *phorein*, to carry]

antroscope (ăn'trō-skōp) [″ + Gr. *skopein*, to examine]

antroscopy (ăn-trŏs'kō-pē)

antrostomy (ăn-trŏs'tō-mē) [″ + Gr. *stoma*, mouth, opening]

antrotome (ăn'trō-tōm) [″ + Gr. *tome*, a cutting, slice]

antrotomy (ăn″trŏt'ō-mē)

antrotympanic (ăn″trō-tĭm-păn'ĭk) [L. *antrum*, cavity, + Gr. *tympanon*, drum]

antrotympanitis (ăn″trō-tĭm″păn-ī'tĭs) [″ + ″ + *itis*, inflammation]

antrum (ăn'trŭm) [L., cavity]
    a. auris
    a. cardiacum
    a., duodenal
    a., mastoid; a. mastoideum
    a., maxillary
    a. of Highmore
    a., puncture of
    a., pyloric; a. pyloricum
    a., tympanic; a.tympanicum

ANTU

Antuitrin S

Anturane

anuclear (ă-nū'klē-ăr)

ANUG *acute necrotizing ulcerative gingivitis*

anulus (ăn'ū-lŭs) [L.]
    a. abdominalis
    a. femoralis
    a. fibrosus
    a. inguinalis profundus
    a. inguinalis superficialis
    a. tympanicus
    a. umbilicalis
    a. urethralis

anuresis (ăn-ū-rē'sĭs) [Gr. *an-*, not, + *ouresis*, urination]

anuretic (ăn-ū-rĕt'ĭk)

anuria (ăn-ū'rē-ă) [″ + *ouron*, urine]

anus (ā'nŭs) [L.]
    a., artificial
    a., imperforate
    a., vulvovaginal

anvil (ăn'vĭl) [AS. *anfilt*]

anxiety (ăng-zī'ĕ-tē)

anxiety disorders

anxiety neurosis

anxiolytic (ăng″zī-ō-lĭt'ĭk) [L. *anxietas*, anxiety, + Gr. *lysis*, dissolution]

A.O.A. *Alpha Omega Alpha, American Osteopathic Association*

A.O.C. *anodal opening contraction*

AOD *adult-onset diabetes mellitus*

A.O.R.N. *Association of Operating Room Nurses*

aorta (ā-or'tă) [L. from Gr. *aorte*]

aortal (ā-or'tăl)

aortalgia (ā″or-tăl'jē-ă) [L. from Gr. *aorte*, aorta, + *algos*, pain]

aortarctia (ā″or-tărk'shē-ă) [″ + L. *arctare*, to narrow]

aortectasia (ā″or-tĕk-tā'zē-ă) [″ + *ek*, out, + *tasis*, a stretching]

aortectomy (ā″or-tĕk'tō-mē) [″ + *ektome*, excision]

aortic (ā-or'tĭk)

aortic balloon pump

aortic murmur

aortic opening

aortic regurgitation

aortic stenosis

aortic valve

aortitis (ā-or-tī'tĭs) [L. from Gr. *aorte*, aorta, + *itis*, inflammation]

aortoclasia (ā″or-tō-klā'zē-ă) [″ + *klasis*, a breaking]

aortocoronary (ā-or″tō-kor'ō-nă-rē)

aortocoronary bypass

aortogram (ā-or'tō-grăm″) [″ + *gramma*, letter, piece of writing]

aortography (ā″or-tog'ră-fē) [L. from Gr. *aorte*, aorta, + *graphein*, to write]
    a., retrograde
    a., translumbar

aortoiliac (ā-or″tō-ĭl'ē-ăk)

aortolith (ā-or'tō-lĭth) [″ + *lithos*, stone]

aortomalacia (ā-or″tō-mă-lā'shē-ă) [″ + *malakia*, softness]

aortopathy (ā″or-tŏp'a-thē) [″ +

pathos, disease, suffering]

aortoptosia, aortoptosis (ā″or-tŏp-tō′zē-ă, -sĭs) [″ + *ptosis*, fall, falling]

aortorrhaphy (ā″or-tor′ă-fē) [″ + *rhaphe*, seam]

aortosclerosis (ā-or″tō-sklĕr-ō-sĭs) [″ + *skleros*, hard]

aortostenosis (ā-or″tō-stĕn-ō′sĭs) [″ + *stenosis*, act of narrowing]

aortotomy (ā″or-tŏt′ō-mē) [″ + *tome*, a cutting, slice]

AOS anodal opening sound

aosmic (ā-ŏz′mĭk) [Gr. *a-*, not, + *osme*, smell]

A.O.T.A. American Occupational Therapy Association

A.O.T.F. American Occupational Therapy Foundation

A.P. anteroposterior

A.P.A. American Pharmaceutical Association; American Physiotherapy Association; American Psychiatric Association

APACHE acute physiology and chronic health evaluation

apallesthesia (ā-păl″ĕs-thē′zē-ă) [″ + *pallein*, to tremble, + *aisthesis*, feeling, perception]

apancreatic (ā-păn″krē-ăt′ĭk)

aparalytic (ā-păr″ă-lĭt′ĭk) [Gr. *a-*, not, + *paralytikos*]

aparathyrosis (ā-păr″ă-thī-rō′sĭs) [″ + *para*, alongside, past, beyond, + *thyreos*, an oblong shield, + *osis*, condition]

apareunia (ā″păr-ū′nē-ă) [″ + *pareunos*, lying with]

aparthrosis (ăp″ăr-thrō′sĭs) [Gr. *apo*, from, + *arthron*, joint, + *osis*, condition]

apastia (ā-păs′tē-ă) [Gr., fasting]

apathetic (ăp″ă-thĕt′ĭk) [″ + *pathos*, disease, suffering]

apathic (ā-păth′ĭk)

apathism (ăp′ă-thĭzm) [″ + *pathos*, disease, suffering, + *-ismos*, condition]

apathy (ăp′ă-thē) [Gr. *apatheia*]

apatite (ăp′ă-tīt″) [Ger. *Apatit*, "the deceptive stone"]

A.P.C. aspirin, phenacetin, and caffeine

APE anterior pituitary extract

ape

apeidosis (ăp″ī-dō′sĭs) [Gr. *apo*, away, + *eidos*, form, shape]

apellous (ă-pĕl′ŭs) [Gr. *a-*, not, + L. *pellis*, skin]

apenteric (ăp″ĕn-tĕr′ĭk) [Gr. *apo*, from, + *enteron*, intestine]

apepsia (ă-pĕp′sē-ă) [Gr. *a-*, not, + *pepsis*, digesting]

apepsinia (ā″pĕp-sĭn′ē-ă)

aperient (ă-pĕr′ē-ĕnt) [L. *aperiens*, opening]

aperistalsis (ā″pĕr-ĭ-stăl′sĭs) [Gr. *a-*, not, + *peri*, around, + *stalsis*, constriction]

apéritif (ă-pĕr″ĭ-tēf′) [L. *aperire*, to open]

aperitive (ă-pĕr′ĭ-tĭv)

Apert's syndrome (ă-pārz′) [Eugene Apert, Fr. pediatrician, 1868–1940]

apertura (ăp″ĕr-tū′ră) [L.]

aperture (ăp′ĕr-chūr″)

apex (ā′pĕks) [L., tip]
    a. of the lung
    a., root

apex beat

apexcardiogram

apexigraph, apexograph (ā-pĕks′ī-grăf, -ō-graf) [L. *apex*, tip, + Gr. *graphein*, to write]

apex murmur

Apgar score [Virginia Apgar, U.S. anesthesiologist, 1909–1974]

A.P.H.A. American Public Health Association

aphacia (ă-fā′sē-ă)

aphacic (ă-fā′sĭk)

aphagia (ă-fā′jē-ă) [Gr. *a-*, not, + *phagein*, to eat]

aphakia (ă-fā′kē-ă) [″ + *phakos*, lentil]

aphakic (ă-fā′kĭk)

aphalangia (ā″fă-lăn′jē-ă) [″ + *phalanx*, line of battle]

aphanisis (ă-făn'ĭ-sĭs) [Gr. *aphaneia*, disappearance]

aphasia (ă-fā'zē-ă) [Gr. *a-*, not, + *phasis*, utterance]
- a., amnesic
- a., anomic
- a., ataxic
- a., auditory
- a., Broca's
- a., conduction
- a., expressive
- a., fluent
- a., gibberish
- a., global
- a., jargon
- a., mixed
- a., motor
- a., nominal
- a., optic
- a., receptive
- a., semantic
- a., sensory
- a., syntactic
- a., traumatic
- a., visual
- a., Wernicke's

aphasic, aphasiac (ă-fā"zĭk, ă-fā'zē-ăk)

aphasiologist (ă-fā"zē-ŏl'ō-jĭst) [Gr. *a-*, not, + *phasis*, utterance, + *logos*, word, reason]

aphemesthesia (ă-fĕm"ĕs-thē'zē-ă) [" + *pheme*, speech, + *aisthesis*, feeling, perception]

aphemia (ă-fē'mē-ă) [" + *pheme*, speech]

aphephobia (af"ĕ-fō'bē-ă) [Gr. *haphe*, touch, + *phobos*, fear]

apheresis (ă-fĕr'ē-sĭs) [Gr. *aphairesis*, separation]

aphonia (ă-fō'nē-ă) [" + *phone*, voice]
- a., hysterical
- a. paralytica
- a. paranoica
- a., spastic

aphonogelia (ă-fō"nō-jē'lē-ă) [" + *phone*, voice, + *gelos*, laughter]

aphose (ăf'ōz) [" + *phos*, light]

aphrasia (ă-frā'zē-ă) [" + *phrasis*, diction]

aphrodisiac (ăf"rō-dĭz'ē-ăk)

aphthae (ăf'thē) [Gr. *aphtha*, small ulcer]
- a., Bednar's
- a., cachectic

aphthoid (ăf'thoyd)

aphthongia (ăf-thŏn'jē-ă) [Gr. *a-*, not, + *phthongos*, voice]

aphthosis (ăf-thō'sĭs) [Gr. *aphtha*, small ulcer, + *osis*, condition]

aphthous (ăf'thŭs) [Gr. *aphtha*, small ulcer]

aphylactic (ă"fĭ-lăk'tĭk) [Gr. *a-*, not, + *phylaxis*, guard]

aphylaxis (ă-fĭ-lăk'sĭs)

apical (ăp'ĭ-kal, ā'pĭ-kal) [L. *apex*, tip]

apicectomy (ăp"ĭ-sĕk'tō-mē) [L. *apex*, tip, + Gr. *ektome*, excision]

apices (ā'pĭ-sēz, ăp'ĭ-sēz) [L.]

apicitis (ăp-ĭ-sī'tĭs) [L. *apices*, tips, + Gr. *itis*, inflammation]

apicoectomy (ăp-ĭ-kō-ĕk'tō-mē) [L. *apex*, tip, + Gr. *ektome*, excision]

apicolocator (ă"pĭ-kō-lō'kă-tor) [" + *locare*, to place]

apicolysis (ăp"ĭ-kŏl'ĭ-sĭs) [" + Gr. *lysis*, dissolution]

apicostomy (ăp"ĭ-kŏs'tō-mē) [L. *apex*, tip, + Gr. *stoma*, mouth, opening]

apicotomy (ăp"ĭ-kŏt'ō-mē) [L. *apex*, tip, + Gr. *tome*, a cutting, slice]

apinealism (ă-pĭn'ē-ăl-ĭzm) [Gr. *a-*, not, + L. *pinea*, pine cone, + Gr. *-ismos*, condition]

apituitarism (ă"pĭ-tū'ĭ-tăr-ĭzm) [" + L. *pituita*, phlegm, + *-ismos*, condition]

A.P.L.

aplanatic lens (ă"plă-năt'ĭk lĕnz) [" + *planetos*, wandering]

aplasia (ă-plă'zē-ă) [" + *plasis*, a developing]
- a. axialis extracorticalis congenita
- a. cutis congenita
- a., gonadal

aplastic (ă-plăs'tĭk) [" + *plastikos*, shaped]

aplastic anemia

A.P.M.A. American Podiatric Medical Association

apnea (ăp-nē'ă) [" + *pnoe*, breathing]
    a., sleep

apnea alarm mattress

apneic oxygenation

apneumatic (ăp"nū-măt'ĭk) [Gr. *a-*, not, + *pneuma*, air]

apneumatosis (ăp"nū-mă-tō'sĭs) [" + " + *osis*, condition]

apneumia (ăp-nū'mē-ă) [" + *pneumon*, lung]

apneusis (ăp-nū'sĭs)

apo- (ăp'ō) [Gr. *apo*, from]

apocamnosis (ăp"ō-kăm-nō'sĭs) [Gr. *apokamnein*, to grow weary]

apochromatic lens (ăp"ō-krō-măt'ĭk)

apocoptic (ăp-ō-kŏp'tĭk)

apocrine (ăp'ō-krēn, -krĭn, -krĭn) [Gr. *apo*, from, + *krinein*, to separate]

apocrine sweat glands

apocrustic (ăp"ō-krŭs'tĭk) [Gr. *apokroustikos*, able to ward off]

apodal (ă-pō'dăl) [Gr. *a-*, not, + *pous*, foot]

apodemialgia (ăp"ō-dē"mē-ăl'jē-ă) [Gr. *apodemia*, away from home, + *algos*, pain]

apodia (ă-pō'dē-ă) [Gr. *a-*, not, + *pous*, foot]

apoenzyme (ăp-ō-ĕn'zīm)

apoferritin (ăp"ō-fĕr'ĭ-tĭn)

apogee (ăp'ō-jē) [Gr. *apo*, from, + *gaia*, earth]

apokamnosis (ăp"ō-kăm-nō'sĭs)

apolar (ă-pō'lăr) [Gr. *a-*, not, + *polos*, pole]

apolepsis (ăp"ō-lĕp'sĭs) [Gr. *apolepsis*, a leaving off]

apolipoprotein

apomorphine (ăp"ō-mor'fēn) [Gr. *apo*, from, + *morphine*]
    a. hydrochloride

aponeurology (ăp"ō-nū-rŏl'ō-jē)

[" + *neuron*, nerve, tendon, + *logos*, word, reason]

aponeurorrhaphy (ăp"ō-nū-ror'ă-fē) [" + " + *rhaphe*, seam]

aponeurosis (ăp"ō-nū-rō'sĭs) [" + *neuron*, nerve, tendon]
    a., epicranial
    a., lingual
    a., palatine
    a., pharyngeal
    a., plantar

aponeurositis (ăp"ō-nū-rō-sī'tĭs) [" + " + *itis*, inflammation]

aponeurotic (ăp"ō-nū-rŏt'ĭk) [" + *neuron*, nerve, tendon]

aponeurotome (ăp"ō-nū'rō-tōm) [" + " + *tome*, a cutting, slice]

aponeurotomy (ăp"ō-nū-rŏt'ō-mē)

aponia (ă-pōn'ē-ă) [Gr. *a-*, not, + *ponos*, toil, pain]

aponic (ă-pŏn'ĭk)

apophyseal, apophysial (ăp"ō-fĭz'ē-ăl) [" + *physis*, growth]

apophysis (ă-pŏf'ĭ-sĭs) [Gr. *apophysis*, off-shoot]
    a., basilar
    a., lenticular
    a. of Ingrassia
    a. of Rau, a. raviana
    a., temporal

apophysitis (ă-pŏf"ĭ-sī'tĭs) [" + *physis*, growth, + *itis*, inflammation]

apoplectic (ăp"ō-plĕk'tĭk) [Gr. *apoplektikos*, crippled by stroke]

apoplectiform (ăp"ō-plĕk'tĭ-form) [Gr. *apoplexia*, to cripple by a stroke, + L. *forma*, form]

apoplectoid (ăp"ō-plĕk'toyd) [" + *eidos*, form, shape]

apoplexia (ăp"ō-plĕk'sē-ă) [Gr. *apoplessein*, to cripple by a stroke]
    a. uteri

apoplexy (ăp'ō-plĕk"sē) [Gr. *apoplessein*, to cripple by a stroke]

apoptosis (ă-pŏp-tō'sĭs, ă-pō-tō'sĭs) [Gr. *apo*, from, + *ptosis*, fall, falling]

aporepressor (ăp"ō-rē-prĕs'or)
aposia (ă-pō'zē-ă) [Gr. a-, not, +
posis, drink]
aposthia (ă-pŏs'thē-ă) [Gr. a-, not,
+ posthe, foreskin]
apotemnophilia (ăp"ō-tĕm"nō-fĕl'ē-
ă) [Gr. apo, away, + temnein, to
cut, + philein, to love]
apothanasia (ăp"ō-thă-nā'zē-ă) [Gr.
apo, away, + thanatos, death]
**apothecaries' weights and mea-
sures**
apothecary (ă-pŏth'ĕ-kā-rē) [Gr.
apotheke, storing place]
apothem, apotheme (ăp'ō-thĕm,
-thĕm) [Gr. apo, from, + thema,
deposit]
apotripsis (ăp"ō-trĭp'sĭs) [Gr. apotri-
bein, to abrade]
apparatus (ăp"ă-rā'tŭs, -răt'ŭs) [L. ap-
parare, to prepare]
  a., acoustic
  a., biliary
  a., Clover's
  a., Fell-O'Dwyer's
  a., Golgi
  a., juxtaglomerular
  a., lacrimal
  a., respiratory
  a., sound-conducting
  a., sound-perceiving
  a., urogenital
  a., vocal
appendage (ă-pĕn'dĭj)
  a., atrial
  a., auricular
  a.'s of the eye
  a.'s of the fetus
  a.'s of the skin
  a., uterine
appendalgia (ăp"ĕn-dăl'jē-ă) [L. appendere, hang to, + Gr. algos,
pain]
appendectomy (ăp"ĕn-dĕk'tō-mē)
[" + Gr. ektome, excision]
  a., incidental
appendical, appendiceal (ă-pĕn'dĭ-
kăl, ăp-ĕn-dĭs'ē-ăl)

appendical reflex
appendicectasis (ă-pĕn"dĭ-sĕk'tă-sĭs)
[L. appendere, hang to, + Gr. ektasis, a stretching]
appendicectomy (ă-pĕn"dĭ-sĕk'tō-
mē) [" + Gr. ektome, excision]
appendices (ă-pĕn'dĭ-sēz)
appendicitis (ă-pĕn"dĭ-sī'tĭs) [L. appendere, hang to, + Gr. itis, inflamma-
tion]
  a., acute
  a., chronic
  a., gangrenous
appendicoenterostomy (ă-pĕn"dĭk-
ō-ĕn"tĕr-ŏs'tō-mē) [L. appendere, hang
to, + Gr. enteron, intestine, +
stoma, mouth, opening]
appendicolithiasis (ă-pĕn"dĭ-kō"lĭ-
thī'ă-sĭs) [" + Gr. lithos, stone, +
-iasis, state or condition of]
appendicolysis (ă-pĕn"dĭ-kŏl'ĭ-sĭs)
[" + Gr. lysis, dissolution]
appendicopathy (ă-pĕn"dĭ-kŏp'ă-
thē) [" + Gr. pathos, disease, suf-
fering]
  a. oxyurica
appendicostomy (ă-pĕn"dĭ-kŏs'tō-
mē) [" + Gr. stoma, mouth, open-
ing]
appendicular (ăp"ĕn-dĭk'ū-lăr) [L. appendere, to hang to]
appendicular skeleton
appendix (ă-pĕn'dĭks) [L.]
  a., atrial
  a., auricular
  a., ensiform
  a. epididymidis
  a. epiploica
  a. testis
  a., ventricular
  a. vermiformis
  a., vesicular
  a., xiphoid
apperception (ăp"ĕr-sĕp'shŭn) [L. ad,
to, + percipere, to perceive]
apperceptive (ăp"ĕr-sĕp'tĭv)
appestat (ăp'ĕ-stăt) [L. appetitus, longing for, + Gr. states, stand]

appetence, appetency (ăp'ĕ-tĕns, -tĕn-sē) [L. appetere, to strive for]
appetite (ăp'ĕ-tīt) [L. appetitus, longing for]
  a., perverted
appetizer (ăp'ĕ-tī"zĕr)
applanation (ăp"lă-nā'shŭn) [L. ad, toward, + planare, to flatten]
applanometer (ăp"lă-nŏm'ĕ-tĕr) [" + planum, plane, + Gr. metron, measure]
apple, Adam's
apple packer's epistaxis
apple picker's disease
apple sorter's disease
appliance (ă-plī'ăns)
applicator (ăp'lĭ-kā"tor) [L. applicare, to attach]
apposition (ăp"ō-zĭ'shŭn) [L. ad, toward, + ponere, to place]
approach (ă-prōch')
approximal (ă-prŏk'sĭ-măl) [" + proximus, nearest]
approximate (ă-prŏk'sĭ-māt) [" + proximare, to come near]
apraxia (ă-prăk'sē-ă) [Gr. a-, not, + praxis, action]
  a., akinetic
  a., amnesic
  a., constructional
  a., developmental
  a., dressing
  a., ideational
  a., motor
  a., sensory
apraxic
Apresoline Hydrochloride
aproctia (ă-prŏk'shē-ă) [Gr. a-, not, + proktos, anus]
apron (ā'prŏn) [O. Fr. naperon, cloth]
  a., Hottentot
  a., lead
aprosody (ă-prŏs'ō-dē) [Gr. a- not, + prosodia, voice modulation]
aprosopia (ăp"rō-sō'pē-ă) [" + prosopon, face]
apselaphesia (ăp"sĕl-ă-fē'zē-ă) [" + pselaphesis, feeling]

APT alum-precipitated toxoid
A.P.T.A. American Physical Therapy Association
aptitude (ăp'tĭ-tūd)
aptitude test
aptyalia, aptyalism (ăp"tē-ā'lē-ă, ăp-tē'ă-lĭzm, ă-tī'ă-lĭzm) [" + ptyalon, saliva]
APUD cells amine precursor uptake and decarboxylation
apulmonism (ă-pool'mŏn-ĭzm) [Gr. a-, not, + L. pulmo, lung, + Gr. -ismos, condition]
apus (ā'pŭs) [" + pous, foot]
apyetous (ă-pī-'ĕ-tŭs) [" + pyesis, suppuration]
apyknomorphous (ă-pĭk"nō-mor'fŭs) [" + pyknos, thick, + morphe, form]
apyogenous (ā-pī-ŏj'ĕn-ŭs) [" + pyon, pus, + genos, origin]
apyous (ă-pī'ŭs)
apyretic (ā-pī-rĕt'ĭk) [" + pyretos, fever]
apyrexia (ā-pī-rĕks'ē-ă) [" + pyrexis, feverishness]
apyrogenetic, apyrogenic (ā"pī-rō-jĕ-nĕt'ĭk, -jĕn'ĭk) [" + " + genos, origin]
AQ achievement quotient
aq. [L.] aqua, water
aqua (awk'wă) [L.]
  a. aerata
  a. ammonia
  a. calcariae
  a. camphorae
  a. destillata
  a. fervens
  a. fontana
  a. fortis
  a. labyrinthi
  a., medicated
  a. oculi
  a. pura
  a. purificata
  a. regia
  a. rosea
  a. sterilisata

a. tepida
Aquamephyton
aquanaut (ă'kwă-nawt)
aquaphobia (ăk"wă-fō'bē-ă) [" + Gr. *phobos,* fear]
Aquaplast
aquapuncture (ăk"wă-pŭngk'chŭr) [" + *punctura,* prick]
Aquatensen
aquatic
aqueduct (ăk'wĕ-dŭkt") [" + *ductus,* duct]
a., cerebral
a., vestibular
aqueductus (ăk"wĕ-dŭk'tŭs)
a. cerebri
a. cochleae
a. Fallopii
a. Sylvii
a. vestibuli
aqueous (ā'kwē-ŭs) [L. *aqua,* water]
aqueous chambers
aqueous humor
aquiparous (ăk-wĭp'ă-rŭs) [" + L. *parere,* to beget, produce]
AR *achievement ratio; alarm reaction*
Ar *argon*
ara-A
arabinose (ă-răb'ĭ-nōs)
arabinosuria (ă-răb"ĭ-nō-sū'rē-ă) [*arabinose* + Gr. *ouron,* urine]
Ara-C
arachidonic acid (ă-răk"ĭ-dŏn'ĭk)
arachnid (ă-răk'nĭd)
Arachnida (ă-răk'nĭ-dă) [Gr. *arachne,* spider]
arachnidism (ă-răk'nĭd-ĭzm) [" + *eidos,* form, shape, + *-ismos,* condition]
arachnitis (ă"răk-nī'tĭs) [" + *itis,* inflammation]
arachnodactyly (ă-răk"nō-dăk'tĭl-ē) [" + *dactylos,* finger]
arachnoid (ă-răk'noyd) [" + *eidos,* form, shape]
a., cranial
a., spinal
arachnoidea (ă-răk-noyd'ē-ă)

a. encephali
a. spinalis
arachnoidism (ă-răk'noyd-ĭzm) [Gr. *arachne,* spider, + *eidos,* form, shape, + *-ismos,* condition]
arachnoiditis (ă-răk"noyd-ī'tĭs) [" + *eidos,* form, shape, + *itis,* inflammation]
arachnoid membrane
arachnoid villi
arachnolysin (ă-răk-nŏl'ĭ-sĭn) [" + *lysis,* dissolution]
arachnophobia (ă-răk"nō-fō'bē-ă) [" + *phobos,* fear]
Aralen Hydrochloride
Aralen Phosphate
Aramine
Aran-Duchenne disease (ăr-ŏn'dū-shĕn)
araneous (ă-rā'nē-ŭs) [L. *aranea,* cobweb]
Arantius' body, nodule (ăr-ăn'shē-ŭs) [Julius Caesar Arantius, It. anatomist and physician, 1530 – 1589]
arborescent (ăr"bor-ĕs'ĕnt) [L. *arborescere,* to become a tree]
arborization (ăr"bor-ī-zā'shŭn) [L. *arbor,* tree]
arbor vitae (ăr'bor vī'tē) [L. *arbor,* tree, + *vita,* life]
arboviruses (ăr"bō-vī'rŭs-ĕs) [*arthropod-borne viruses*]
ARC *AIDS-related complex*
arc (ărk) [L. *arcus,* bow]
a., reflex
arcade (ăr-kād)
a., Flint's
arcanum (ăr-kā'nŭm) [L. *arcanum,* a secret]
arcate (ăr'kăt) [L. *arcatus,* bow-shaped]
arc eyes
arch-, arche-, archi- [Gr. *arche,* beginning]
arch [L. *arcus,* a bow]
a., abdominothoracic
a., alveolar
a., aortic; a. of the aorta
a.'s, aortic

a., axillary
a.'s, branchial
a., carotid
a., costal
a., crural
a., deep crural
a., dental
a., femoral
a., glossopalatine
a., hemal
a., hyoid
a., Langer's
a., longitudinal
a., mandibular
a., maxillary
a., nasal
a., neural
a.'s of Corti
a.'s of foot
a., palmar
a.'s, pharyngeal
a., pharyngopalatine
a., plantar
a., pubic
a., pulmonary
a., superciliary
a., supraorbital
a., tarsal
a., thyrohyoid
a., transverse
a., vertebral
a.'s, visceral
a., zygomatic
archenteron (ărk-ĕn'tĕr-ŏn) [Gr. arche, beginning, + enteron, intestine]
archeokinetic (ăr"kē-ŏ-kĭ-nĕt'ĭk) [" + kinetikos, concerning movement]
archetype (ăr'kĕ-tīp) [" + typos, model]
archiblast (ăr'kĭ-blăst) [" + blastos, a germ, bud]
archiblastic (ăr"kĭ-blăs'tĭk)
archiblastoma (ăr"kĭ-blăs-tō'mă) [" + blastos, germ, + oma, tumor]
archigaster (ăr'kĭ-găs"tĕr) [" + gaster, belly]
archinephron (ăr"kĭ-nĕf'rŏn) [" + nephros, kidney]

archineuron (ăr-kĭ-nū'rŏn) [" + neuron, nerve, tendon]
archipallium (ăr"kĭ-păl'ē-ŭm) [" + L. pallium, a cloak]
archiplasm (ăr'kĭ-plăzm) [" + LL. plasma, form, mold]
archistome (ăr'kĭ-stōm) [" + stoma, mouth, opening]
architectural barrier
architis (ăr-kī'tĭs) [Gr. archos, anus, + itis, inflammation]
archo- [Gr. archos, rectum]
arch width
arciform (ăr'sĭ-form) [L. arcus, bow, + forma, shape]
arctation (ărk-tā'shŭn) [L. arctatus, pressing together]
arcuate (ăr'kū-āt) [L. arcuatus, bowed]
arcuation (ăr-kū-ā'shŭn)
arcus (ăr'kŭs) [L. arcus, a bow]
a. alveolaris mandibulae
a. alveolaris maxillae
a. dentalis
a. juvenilis
a. plantaris
a. senilis
ARD acute respiratory disease (or distress
ardanesthesia (ăr"dăn-ĕs-thē'zē-ă) [L. ardor, heat, + Gr. an-, not, + aisthesis, feeling, perception]
ardor (ăr'dor) [L., heat]
a. urinae
a. veneris
ARDS adult respiratory distress syndrome
area (ā'rē-ă) [L. area, an open space]
a., acoustic
a., association
a., auditory
a., body surface
a., Broca's
a.'s, Brodmann's
a. germinativa
a., Kiesselbach's
a., macular
a., mitral
a., occipital
a. pellucida

a., Rolando's
a., silent
a., vestibular
areata,   **areatus**   (ă″rē-ā′tă,
ă″rē-ā′tŭs)
areflexia (ă″rē-flĕk′sē-ă) [Gr. *a-*, not,
+ L. *reflectere*, to bend back]
arenaceous (ăr″ĕ-nā′sē-ŭs) [L. *arena-
ceus,* sandy]
arenation (ă″rĕ-nā′shŭn) [L. *arena,*
sand]
arenaviridae
arenaviruses (ă″rē-nă-vī′rŭs-ĕs)
[" + *virus,* poison]
arenoid (ăr′ĕ-noyd) [" + Gr.
eidos, form, shape]
areola (ă-rē′ō-lă) [L. *areola,* a small
space]
a. mammae
a. papillaris
a., second
a. umbilicalis
areolar (ă-rē′ō-lăr)
areolar glands
areolar tissue
areolitis (ăr″ē-ō-lī′tĭs) [" + Gr. *itis,*
inflammation]
areometer (ă-rē-ŏm′ĕ-tĕr) [Gr. *araios,*
thin, + *metron,* a measure]
arevareva (ăr-ē″vā-rā′vă) [Tahitian,
skin rash]
ARF *acute respiratory failure*
Arfonad
argamblyopia (ăr″găm-blē-ō′pē-ă)
[Gr. *argos,* idle, + *amblus,* dulled,
+ *ops,* eye]
Argasidae (ăr-găs′ĭ-dī) [Gr. *argeeis,*
shining]
argentaffin, argentaffine (ăr-jĕnt′ă-
fĭn) [L. *argentum,* silver, + *affinis,*
associated with]
argentaffinoma (ăr″jĕn-tăf″ĭ-nō′mă)
[" + " + Gr. *oma,* tumor]
argentum (ăr-jĕn′tŭm) [L.]
arginase (ăr′jĭ-nās)
arginine (ăr′jĭ-nēn, -nĭn) [L. *argentum,*
silver]
a. glutamate
a. hydrochloride

a., suberyl
argininosuccinic acid (ăr″jĭ-nī″nō-sŭk-
sĭn′ĭk)
argininosuccinicaciduria (ăr″jĭn-ĭn-ō-
sŭk-sĭn″ĭk-ăs-ĭ-dū′rē-ă)
argon (ăr′gŏn) [Gr. *argos,* inactive]
Argyll Robertson pupil (ăr-gĭl′
rŏb′ĕrt-sŏn) [Douglas Argyll Robertson,
Scottish   ophthalmologist,   1837–
1909]
argyria, argyriasis (ăr-jĭr′ē-ă, ăr″jĭ-
rī′ă-sĭs) [Gr. *argyros,* silver]
argyric (ăr-jĭr′ĭk)
argyrism (ăr′jĭr-ĭzm) [Gr. *argyros,* silver]
Argyrol (ăr′jĭ-rŏl)
argyrophil (ăr-jĭ′rō-fĭl) [" + *philos,*
love]
argyrosis (ăr″jĭ-rō′sĭs) [" + *osis,*
condition]
arhinia
arhythmia
Arias-Stella reaction [Javier Arias-
Stella, Peruvian pathologist, b. 1924]
ariboflavinosis (ă-rī″bō-flā″vĭn-ō′sĭs)
[Gr. *a-*, not, + *riboflavin* +
Gr. *osis,* condition]
Aristocort
Aristocort Acetonide
Aristocort Forte Parenteral
aristogenics (ă-rĭs″tō-jĕn′ĭks) [Gr. *ar-
istos,* best, + *gennan,* to produce]
Aristospan
arithmetic mean
arkyochrome (ăr′kē-ō-krōm) [Gr.
arkys, net, + *chroma,* color]
arkyostichochrome (ar″kē-ō-stĭk′ō-
krōm) [" + *stichos,* row, +
chroma, color]
Arlidin
arm
a., bird
a., brawny
a., Saturday-night
armamentarium (ăr″mă-mĕn-tā′rē-
ŭm) [L. *armamentum,* implement]
armature (ăr′mă-tūr) [L. *armatura,*
equipment]
arm board
armpit

Arneth, Joseph (ăr′nāt)
[Ger. physician, 1873 – 1955]
    A.'s classification of neutrophils
    A.'s formula
Arnold, Friedrich [Ger. anatomist,
    1803 – 1890]
    A.'s canal
    A.'s ganglion
    A.'s nerve
Arnold-Chiari deformity (ăr′nōlt-
    kē′ă-rē) [Julius Arnold, Ger. patholo-
    gist, 1835 – 1915; Hans Chiari, Ger.
    pathologist, 1851 – 1916]
AROM   *active range of motion*
aroma (ă-rō′mă) [Gr. *aroma*, spice]
aromatic (ăr″ō-măt′ĭk)
aromatic ammonia spirit
aromatic compounds
aromatic elixir
arousal
arrachement (ă-răsh-mŏn′) [Fr., ex-
    traction]
array (ă-rā′)
array detector
arrectores pilorum (ă″rĕk-tō′rĕz
    pĭl-ō′rŭm) [L. *arrectores*, raisers, +
    pilus, hair]
arrest (ă-rĕst′)
    a., cardiac
    a., epiphysial
    a., pelvic
    a., respiratory
    a., sinus
arrhenoblastoma (ă-rē″nō-blăs-
    tō′mă) [Gr. *arren*, male, +   *blastos*,
    germ, +   *oma*, tumor]
arrhinia (ă-rĭn′ē-ă) [Gr. *a-*, not, +
    rhis, nose]
arrhythmia (ă-rĭth′mē-ă) [″ +
    rhythmos, rhythm]
    a., cardiac
    a., sinus
arrhythmic (ă-rĭth′mĭk)
A.R.R.T.   *American Registry of Radio-*
    logic Technologists
arseniasis (ăr″sĕ-nī′ă-sĭs) [L. *arsenium*,
    arsenic, +   *-iasis*, state or condition
    of]

arsenic (ăr′sĕ-nĭk) [L. *arsenicum*]
    a. trioxide
    a., white
arsenical (ăr-sĕn′ĭ-kăl)
arsenic-fast
arsenicism (ăr-sĕn′ĭ-sĭzm) [L. *arsenicum*,
    arsenic, +   Gr. *-ismos*, condition]
arsenicophagy (ăr″sĕn-ĭ-kŏf′ă-jē)
    [″ +   *phagein*, to eat]
arsenic poisoning
arsenionization (ăr″sĕn-ī″ŏn-ĭ-
    zā′shŭn)
arsenium (ăr-sē′nē-ŭm) [L.]
arsenoresistant (ăr-sĕn″ō-rē-zĭs′tănt)
    [L. *arsenium*, arsenic, +   *resistare*,
    to withstand]
arsenotherapy (ăr″sĕ-nō-thĕr′ă-pē)
    [″ +   Gr. *therapeia*, treatment]
arsenous (ăr′sĕ-nŭs) [L. *arsenium*, arse-
    nic]
arsenous hydride
arsenous powder
arsine (ăr′sĕn)
arsphenamine (ărs-fĕn′ă-mēn)
Artane
artefact (ăr′tĕ-făkt) [L. *ars*, art, +
    factus, made]
arterectomy (ăr″tĕ-rĕk′tō-mē) [Gr. *ar-*
    teria, artery, +   *ektome*, excision]
arteria (ăr″tē′rē-ă)
arterial (ăr-tē′rē-ăl)
arterial bleeding
arterial blood gases
arterial circulation
arterial line
arterial varix
arteriectasis, arteriectasia (ăr″tĕ-
    rē-ĕk′tă-sĭs, -ĕk-tā′zē-ă) [″ +   *ek-*
    tasis, a stretching out]
arteriectomy (ăr″tĕ-rē-ĕk′tō-mē)
    [″ +   *ektome*, excision]
arterio- [Gr. *arteria*, artery]
arterioatony (ăr-tē″rē-ō-ăt′ō-nē)
    [″ +   *atonia*, languor]
arteriocapillary (ăr-tē″rē-ō-kăp′ĭ-
    lăr″ē) [″ +   L. *capillus*, like hair]
arteriocapillary fibrosis
arteriofibrosis (ăr-tē″rē-ō-fĭ-brō′sĭs)

[" + L. *fibra*, fiber, + Gr. *osis*, condition]

arteriogram (ăr″tē-rē-ō-grăm) [" + *gramma*, letter, piece of writing]

arteriography (ăr″tē-rē-ŏg′ră-fē) [" + *graphein*, to write]

arteriola (ăr-tē″rē-ō′lă) [L.]
- a. macularis inferior
- a. macularis superior
- a. medialis retinae
- a. nasalis retinae inferior
- a. nasalis retinae superior
- a. recta
- a. temporalis retinae inferior
- a. temporalis retinae superior

arteriole (ăr-tē′rē-ōl) [L. *arteriola*]

arteriolith (ăr-tē′rē-ō-lĭth) [" + Gr. *lithos*, stone]

arteriolitis (ăr-tēr″ē-ō-lī′tĭs) [" + Gr. *itis*, inflammation]

arteriology (ăr-tē″rē-ŏl′ō-jē) [" + Gr. *logos*, word, reason]

arteriolonecrosis (ăr-tē″rē-ō″lō-nĕ-krō′sĭs) [" + Gr. *nekrosis*, state of death]

arteriolosclerosis (ăr-tē″rē-ō″lō-sklĕ-rō′sĭs) [L. *arteriola*, small artery, + Gr. *sklerosis*, a hardening]

arteriolosclerotic (ăr-tē″rē-ō″lō-sklĕ-rŏt′ĭk)

arteriomotor (ăr-tē″rē-ō-mō′tor) [Gr. *arteria*, artery, + L. *movere*, to move]

arteriomyomatosis (ăr-tē″rē-ō-mī″ō-mă-tō′sĭs) [" + *mys*, muscle, + *oma*, tumor, + *osis*, condition]

arterionecrosis (ăr-tē″rē-ō-nĕ-krō′sĭs) [" + *nekrosis*, state of death]

arteriopathy (ăr″tē-rē-ŏp′ă-thē) [" + *pathos*, disease, suffering]

arterioplasty (ăr-tē″rē-ō-plăs′tē) [" + *plassein*, to form]

arteriopressor (ăr-tē″rē-ō-prĕs′or) [" + L. *pressura*, force]

arteriorrhaphy (ăr-tē″rē-or′ă-fē) [" + *rhaphe*, seam]

arteriorrhexis (ăr-tē″rē-ō-rĕk′sĭs) [" + *rhexis*, rupture]

arteriosclerosis (ăr-tē″rē-ō-sklĕ-rō′sĭs) [" + *sklerosis*, a hardening]
- a., hypertensive
- a., medial
- a., Mönckeberg's
- a., nodular
- a. obliterans
- a., senile

arteriosclerotic (ăr-tē″rē-ō-sklĕ-rŏt′ĭk)

arteriospasm (ăr-tē′rē-ō-spăzm″) [Gr. *arteria*, artery, + *spasmos*, a convulsion]

arteriostenosis (ăr-tē″rē-ō-stĕ-nō′sĭs) [" + *stenosis*, act of narrowing]

arteriostosis (ăr-tē″rē-ŏs-tō′sĭs) [" + *osteon*, bone, + *osis*, condition]

arteriostrepsis (ăr-tē″rē-ō-strĕp′sĭs) [" + *strepsis*, a twisting]

arteriosympathectomy (ăr-tē″rē-ō-sĭm″pă-thĕk′tō-mē) [" + *sympatheia*, suffer with, + *ektome*, excision]

arteriotomy (ăr″tē-rē-ŏt′ō-mē)

arteriotony (ăr-tē″rē-ŏt′ō-nē) [" + *tonos*, act of stretching, tension, tone]

arteriovenous (ăr-tē″rē-ō-vē′nŭs) [" + L. *vena*, a vein]

arterioversion (ăr-tē″rē-ō-vĕr′shŭn) [" + L. *versio*, a turning]

arteritis (ăr″tē-rī′tĭs) [" + *itis*, inflammation]
- a., cranial
- a., giant cell
- a., granulomatous
- a. nodosa
- a. obliterans
- a., rheumatic
- a., rheumatoid
- a., temporal

artery (ăr′tĕr-ē) [Gr. *arteria*, windpipe]
- a., coiled
- a., elastic
- a., end
- a., muscular
- a., sheathed
- a., spiral
- a., terminal

arthral (ăr′thrăl)

arthralgia (ăr-thrăl′jē-ă) [″   +   *algos*, pain]
a. saturnina
arthrectomy (ăr-thrĕk′tō-mē) [″   +   *ektome*, excision]
arthredema (ăr-thrĕ-dē′mă) [″   +   *oidema*, a swelling]
arthrempyesis (ăr″thrĕm-pī-ē′sĭs) [″   +   *empyesis*, suppuration]
arthresthesia (ăr″thrĕs-thē′zē-ă) [″   +   *aisthesis*, feeling, perception]
arthritic (ăr-thrĭt′ĭk)
arthritide (ăr′thrĭ-tĭd)
arthritides (ăr-thrĭt′ĭ-dēz)
arthritis (ăr-thrī′tĭs) [″   +   *itis*, inflammation]
a., acute secondary
a., acute suppurative
a., allergic
a., atrophic
a. deformans
a., degenerative
a., gonorrheal
a., gouty
a., hypertrophic
a., juvenile rheumatoid
a., neurogenic
a., neurotrophic
a., osteo-
a., palindromic
a., psoriatic
a., rheumatoid
a., suppurative
a., syphilitic
a., tuberculous
arthro- [Gr. *arthron*, joint]
arthrobacterium (ăr″thrō-băk-tē′rē-ŭm) [″   +   *bakterion*, little staff]
arthrocace (ăr-thrŏk′ă-sē) [″   +   *kake*, badness]
arthrocele (ăr′thrō-sēl) [″   +   *kele*, tumor, swelling]
arthrocentesis (ăr″thrō-sĕn-tē′sĭs) [″   +   *kentesis*, a puncture]
arthrochondritis (ăr″thrō-kŏn-drī′tĭs) [″   +   *chondros*, cartilage,   +   *itis*, inflammation]
arthroclasia (ăr″thrō-klă′zē-ă) [″   +   *klasis*, a breaking]
arthrodesis (ăr-thrō-dē′sĭs) [″   +   *desis*, binding]
arthrodia (ăr-thrō′dē-ă) [Gr.]
arthrodynia (ăr″thrō-dĭn′ē-ă) [Gr. *arthron*, joint,   +   *odyne*, pain]
arthrodysplasia (ăr″thrō-dĭs-plă′zē-ă) [″   +   *dys*, bad, difficult, painful, disordered,   +   *plassein*, to form]
arthroempyesis (ăr″thrō-ĕm-pī-ē′sĭs) [″   +   *empyesis*, suppuration]
arthroendoscopy (ăr″thrō-ĕn-dŏs′kō-pē) [″   +   *endon*, within,   +   *skopein*, to examine]
arthrogram (ăr′thrō-grăm) [″   +   *gramma*, letter, piece of writing]
arthrography (ăr-thrŏg′ră-fē) [″   +   *graphein*, to write]
arthrogryposis (ăr″thrō-grī-pō′sĭs) [″   +   *grypos*, curved,   +   *osis*, condition]
a. multiplex congenita
arthrokleisis (ăr″thrō-klī′sĭs) [″   +   *kleisis*, a closure]
arthrolith (ăr′thrō-lĭth) [″   +   *lithos*, stone]
arthrology (ăr-thrŏl′ō-jē) [Gr. *arthron*, joint,   +   *logos*, word, reason]
arthrolysis (ăr-thrŏl′ĭ-sĭs) [″   +   *lysis*, dissolution]
arthromeningitis (ăr″thrō-mĕn″ĭn-jī′tĭs) [″   +   *meninx*, membrane,   +   *itis*, inflammation]
arthrometer (ăr-thrŏm′ĕ-ter) [″   +   *metron*, measure]
arthroneuralgia (ăr″thrō-nū-răl′jē-ă) [″   +   *neuron*, nerve,   +   *algos*, pain]
arthropathology (ăr″thrō-pă-thol′ō-jē) [″   +   *pathos*, disease, suffering,   +   *logos*, word, reason]
arthropathy (ăr-thrŏp′ă-thē) [″   +   *pathos*, disease, suffering]
a., Charcot's
a., inflammatory
a., Jaccoud
arthrophyte (ăr′thrō-fīt) [Gr. *arthron*, joint,   +   *phyton*, growth]

arthroplasty (ăr′thrō-plăs″tē) [″ + *plassein*, to form]

arthropneumoroentgenography (ăr″thrō-nū″mō-rĕnt-gĕn-ŏg′ră-fē) [″ + *pneuma*, air, + *roentgen*, + *graphein*, to write]

arthropod (ăr″thrō-pŏd)

Arthropoda (ăr-thrŏp′ō-dă) [″ + *pous*, foot]

arthropyosis (ăr″thrō-pī-ō′sĭs) [″ + *pyosis*, suppuration]

arthrorheumatism (ăr″thrō-roo′mă-tĭzm) [″ + *rheumatismos*, flux]

arthrorrhagia (ăr″thrō-rā′jē-ă) [″ + *rhegnynai*, to burst forth]

arthrosclerosis [Gr. *arthron*, joint, + *sklerosis*, a hardening]

arthroscope (ăr′thrō-skōp) [″ + *skopein*, to examine]

arthroscopy (ăr-thrŏs′kō-pē)

arthrosis (ăr-thrō′sĭs) [″ + *osis*, condition]

arthrospore (ăr′thrō-spor) [″ + *sporos*, seed]

arthrosteitis (ăr″thrōs-tē-ī′tĭs) [″ + *osteon*, bone, + *itis*, inflammation]

arthrostenosis (ăr″-thrō-stĕ-nō′sĭs) [″ + *stenosis*, act of narrowing]

arthrostomy (ăr-thrŏs′tō-mē) [″ + *stoma*, mouth, opening]

arthrosynovitis (ăr″thrō-sĭn″ō-vī′tĭs) [″ + L. *synovia*, joint fluid, + Gr. *itis*, inflammation]

arthrotome (ăr′thrō-tōm) [″ + *tome*, a cutting, slice]

arthrotomy (ăr-thrŏt′ō-mē)

arthrous (ăr′thrŭs) [Gr. *arthron*, joint]

arthroxesis (ăr-thrŏk′sĭ-sĭs) [″ + *xexis*, scraping]

Arthus reaction or phenomenon (ăr-toos′) [Maurice Arthus, Fr. physiologist, 1862–1945]

artichoke factor

articular (ăr-tĭk′ū-lăr) [L. *articularis*]

articulate (ăr-tĭk′ū-lāt, -lăt) [L. *articulatus*, jointed]

articulated (ăr-tĭk′ū-lāt-ĕd)

articulatio (ăr-tĭk″ū-lā′shē-ō) [L.]

articulation
a., apophyseal
a., articulator
a., confluent
a., dental

articulator (ăr-tĭk′ū-lā″tor)

articulo mortis (ăr-tĭk′ū-lō″ mor′tĭs) [L.]

articulus (ăr-tĭk′ū-lŭs) [L.]

artifact, artefact (ăr′tĭ-făkt, ăr′tĕ-făkt) [L. *ars*, art, + *facere*, to make]

artificial (ăr″tĭ-fĭsh′ăl)

artificial assists

artificial hyperemia

artificial impregnation

artificial insemination
a.i., donor
a.i., husband

artificial intelligence

artificial pneumothorax

artificial respiration

artisan's cramp

aryepiglottic (ăr″ē-ĕp″ĭ-glŏt′ĭk) [Gr. *arytaina*, ladle, + *epi*, upon, + *glottis*, tongue]

aryl-
a. group

arytenoid (ăr″ĭ-tĕ′noyd) [Gr. *arytaina*, ladle, + *eidos*, form, shape]

arytenoidectomy (ăr″ĭ-tĕ″noyd-ĕk′tō-mē) [″ + ″ + *ektome*, excision]

arytenoiditis (ăr-ĭt″ē-noy-dī′tĭs) [″ + *itis*, inflammation]

arytenoidopexy (ăr″ĭ-tĕ-noy′dō-pĕk″sē) [″ + ″ + *pexis*, fixation]

Arzberger's pear (ărz′bĕr-gĕrz) [Friedrich Arzberger, Austrian physicist, 1833–1905]

AS [L.] *auris sinistra*, left ear; *aortic stenosis*

As *arsenic*; *astigmatic*; *astigmatism*

ASA *acetylsalicylic acid*

asafetida, asafoetida (ăs-ă-fĕt′ĭd-ă) [L. *asa*, gum, + *foetida*, smelly]

ASAHP *American Society of Allied Health Professions*

ASAP *as soon as possible*

asaphia (ă-săf'ē-ă, ă-sā'fē-ă) [Gr. asapheia, obscurity]
asbestiform (ăs-bĕs'tĭ-form) [Gr. asbestos, unquenchable, + L. forma, appearance]
asbestos (ăs-bĕs'tōs) [Gr. asbestos, unquenchable]
asbestosis (ăs"bĕ-stō'sĭs) [" + osis, condition]
ascariasis (ăs"kă-rī'ă-sĭs) [Gr. askaris, pinworm, + -iasis, state or condition of]
ascaricide (ăs-kăr'ĭ-sīd) [" + L. caedere, to kill]
ascarides (ăs-kăr'ĭ-dēz)
Ascaris (ăs'kă-rĭs)
   A. lumbricoides
ascaris
Aschheim-Zondek test (ăsh'hīm-tsŏn'dĕk) [Selmar Aschheim, Ger. gynecologist, 1878–1965; Bernhardt Zondeck, Ger. gynecologist, 1891–1966]
Aschner's phenomenon, reflex, sign (ăsh'nĕrz) [Bernhard Aschner, Austrian gynecologist, 1883–1960]
Aschoff, Ludwig (ăsh'ŏf) [Ger. pathologist, 1866–1942]
   A.'s bodies
   A.'s cells
   A.'s nodules
asci (ăs'ī)
ascia (ăs'ē-ă, ăs'kē-ă) [L. ascia, ax]
ascites (ă-sī'tēz) [Gr. askitēs from askos, wineskin, bladder, belly]
   a. chylosus
ascitic (ă-sĭt'ĭk)
ascitic fluid
Ascoli's reaction, test (ăs-kō'lēz) [Alberto Ascoli, It. serologist, 1877–1957]
Ascomycetes (ăs"kō-mī-sē'tēz) [Gr. askos, leather bag, + mykes, fungus]
ascorbic acid (ăs-kor'bĭk) [Gr. a-, not, + L. scorbutus, scurvy]
ascospore (ăs'kō-spor) [Gr. askos, leather bag, + sporos, seed]

ascus (ăs'kŭs) [Gr. askos, leather bag]
-ase
asemia, asemasia (ă-sē'mē-ă, ăs"ī-mā'zē-ă) [Gr. a-, not, + semasia, the giving of a sign]
asepsis (ā-sĕp'sĭs) [" + sepesthai, to decay]
aseptic (ă-sĕp'tĭk)
aseptic-antiseptic [Gr. a-, not, + sepsis, decay, + anti, against, + sepsis, decay]
aseptic technique
Asepto syringe
asexual (ā-sĕk'shū-ăl) [" + L. sexualis, having sex]
asexualization (ā-sĕk"shū-ăl-ĭ-zā'shŭn)
ash (ăsh) [AS. aesc, ash]
ASHD arteriosclerotic heart disease
asialia (ă"sī-ā'lē-ă, ă"sē-ā'lē-a) [" + sialon, spittle]
Asiatic cholera
asiderosis (ă"sĭd-ĕ-rō'sĭs) [" + sideros, iron, + osis, condition]
ASIS anterior superior iliac spine
asitia (ă-sĭsh'ē-ă) [" + sitos, food]
ASLO antistreptolysin-O
A.S.M.T. American Society for Medical Technology
asocial (ā-sō'shĭl)
asoma (ā-sō'mă) [Gr. a-, not, + soma, body]
asonia (ă-sō'nē-ă) [" + L. sonus, sound]
asparaginase (ăs-păr'ă-jĭn-āz)
asparagine (ăs-păr'ă-jĭn)
Asparagus (ă-spăr'ă-gŭs) [Gr. asparagos]
aspartame (ă-spăr'tām)
aspartate aminotransferase (ă-spăr'tāt)
aspartic acid
aspastic (ă-spăs'tĭk) [Gr. a-, not, + spastikos, drawing]
aspecific (ă-spē-sĭf'ĭk)
aspect (ăs'pĕkt) [L. aspectus, a view]
aspergillin (ăs"pĕr-jĭl'ĭn)
aspergillosis (ăs"pĕr-jĭl-ō'sĭs) [asper-

gillus + Gr. *osis*, condition]
   a., aural
   a., pulmonary
Aspergillus (ăs″pĕr-jĭl′ŭs) [L. *aspergere*, to sprinkle]
   A. auricularis
   A. barbae
   A. bouffardi
   A. bronchialis
   A. clavatus
   A. concentricus
   A. flavus
   A. fumigatus
   A. glaucus
   A. mucoroides
   A. nidulans
   A. niger
   A. ochraceus
   A. pictor
   A. repens
aspermatic (ă-spĕr-măt′ĭk) [Gr. *a-*, not, + *sperma*, seed]
aspermatism (ă-spĕr′mă-tĭzm) [″ + ″ + *-ismos*, condition]
aspermatogenesis (ă-spĕr″mă-tō-jĕn′ĕ-sĭs) [″ + ″ + *genesis*, generation, birth]
aspermia (ă-spĕr′mē-ă) [″ + *sperma*, seed]
aspermous (ă-spĕr′mŭs)
asperous (ăs′pĕr-us) [L. *asper*, rough]
aspersion (ăs-pĕr′zhŭn) [L. *aspersio*, sprinkling]
asphalgesia (ăs″făl-jē′zē-ă) [Gr. *asphe-*, self, + *algos*, pain]
asphyctic, asphyctous (ăs-fĭk′tĭk, -tŭs) [Gr. *a-*, not, + *sphyxis*, pulse]
asphyxia (ăs-fĭk′sē-ă) [″ + *sphyxis*, pulse]
   a. carbonica
   a., fetal
   a. livida
   a., local
   a. neonatorum
   a. pallida
asphyxial (ăs-fĭk′sē-ăl)
asphyxiant (ăs-fĭk′sē-ănt)
asphyxiate (ăs-fĭk′sē-āt)

asphyxiation (ăs-fĭk″sē-ā′shŭn)
aspidium (ăs-pĭd′ē-ŭm) [Gr. *aspidion*, little shield]
   a. oleoresin
aspirate (ăs′pĭ-rāt) [L. *ad*, to, + *spirare*, to breathe]
aspiration (ăs-pĭ-rā′shŭn)
aspirator (ăs′pĭ-rā-tor)
aspirin (ăs′pĕr-ĭn)
aspirin poisoning
asplenia (ă-splē′nē-ă) [Gr. *a-*, not, + L. *splen*, spleen]
asporogenic (ăs″pō-rō-jĕn′ĭk) [″ + *sporos*, seed, + *gennan*, to produce]
asporous (ă-spō′rŭs)
A.S.R.T. American Society of Radiologic Technologists
assault (ă-sawlt′) [L. *assultus*, having assailed]
   a., sexual
assay (ă-sā′, ăs′ā) [O. Fr. *assai*, trial]
   a., biological
assessment, nursing
assident (ăs′ĭ-dĕnt) [L. *assidere*, to sit by]
assimilable (ă-sĭm′ĭ-lă-bl) [L. *ad*, to + *similare*, to make like]
assimilate (ă-sĭm′ĭ-lāt)
assimilation (ă-sĭm″ĭ-lā′shŭn)
assistant
   a., dental
assisted circulation
associated movements
association [L. *ad*, to + *socius*, companion]
   a., controlled
   a., free
   a., induced
association areas
association center
association neuron
association of ideas
association test
association time
assonance (ăs′ō-năns) [L. *assonans*, answering with some sound]
Ast. *astigmatism*

astasia (ă-stā′zē-ă) [Gr. a-, not, +
stasis, standing still]
  a. -abasia
astatine (ăs′tă-tēn, -tĭn) [Gr. astatos,
unstable]
asteatosis (ăs″tē-ă-tō′sĭs) [Gr. a-, not,
+ stear, tallow, + osis, condi-
tion]
  a. cutis
aster (ăs′tĕr) [Gr., star]
astereognosis (ă-stĕr″ē-ŏg-nō′sĭs)
[Gr. a-, not, + stereos, solid, +
gnosis, knowledge]
asterion (ăs-tē′rē-ŏn) [Gr., starlike]
asterixis (ăs″tĕr-ĭk′sĭs) [Gr. a-, not, +
sterixis, fixed position]
asternal (ā-stĕr′năl) [″ + sternon,
chest]
asternia (ă-stĕr′nē-ă)
asteroid (ăs′tĕr-oyd) [Gr. aster, star,
+ eidos, form, shape]
asthenia (ăs-thē′nē-ă) [Gr. asthenes,
without strength]
  a., neurocirculatory
asthenic (ăs-thĕn′ĭk)
asthenobiosis (ăs-thĕ″nō-bī-ō′sĭs) [Gr.
asthenes, without strength, + bios,
life, + osis, condition]
asthenocoria (ăs-thē″nō-kō′rē-ă)
[″ + kore, pupil]
asthenometer (ăs″thĕ-nŏm′ĕ-ter)
[″ + metron, measure]
asthenope (ăs′thĕ-nōp) [″ +
opsis, sight, appearance, vision]
asthenopia (ăs″thĕ-nō′pē-ă)
  a., accommodative
  a., muscular
  a., nervous
  a., photogenous
asthenopic (ăs″thĕ-nŏp′ĭk)
asthenospermia (ăs″thĕ-nō-spĕr′mē-
ă) [″ + sperma, seed]
asthenoxia [″ + oxygen]
asthma (ăz′mă) [Gr., panting]
  a., bronchial
  a., cardiac
  a., exercise-induced
  a., extrinsic
  a., intrinsic

  a., nonatopic
  a., thymic
asthmatic (ăz-măt′ĭk) [L. asthmaticus]
astigmatic (ăs″tĭg-măt′ĭk)
astigmatism (ă-stĭg′mă-tĭzm) [Gr. a-,
not, + stigma, point, +
-ismos, condition]
  a., compound
  a., index
  a., mixed
  a., simple
astigmatometer (ăs″tĭg-mă-tŏm′ĕ-tĕr)
[″ + stigma, point, + metron,
measure]
astigmatoscope (ăs″tĭg-măt′ō-skōp)[″
+ ″ + skopein, to examine]
astigmatoscopy (ă-stĭg″mă-tŏs′kō-
pē)
astigmia (ă-stĭg′mē-ă)
astigmometer (ăs″tĭg-mŏm′ĕ-tĕr)
astigmoscope (ăs-tĭg′mō-skōp)
astomatous, astomous (ăs-tōm′ă-
tŭs, ăs′tō-mŭs) [Gr. a-, not, +
stoma, mouth, opening]
astomia (ă-stō′mē-ă)
astragalectomy (ăs″trăg-ă-lĕk′tō-mē)
[astragalus + Gr. ektome, exci-
sion]
astragalus (ă-străg′ă-lŭs) [Gr. astragalos, ball of the ankle joint]
astraphobia (ăs-tră-fō′bē-ă) [Gr. as-
trape, lightning, + phobos, fear]
astrict (ă-strĭkt′) [L. astringere, to bind
fast]
astriction (ă-strĭk′shŭn)
astringent (ă-strĭn′jĕnt) [L. astringere, to
bind fast]
astro- [Gr. astron, star]
astrobiology
astroblast (ăs′trō-blăst) [″ + Gr.
blastos, germ]
astroblastoma (ăs″trō-blăs-tō′mă)
[″ + ″ + oma, tumor]
astrocyte (ăs′trō-sīt) [″ + kytos,
cell]
astrocytoma (ăs″trō-sī-tō′mă) [″ +
″ + oma, tumor]
astroglia (ăs-trŏg′lē-ă) [″ + glia,
glue]

astrokinetic motions (ăs"trō-kǐ-nĕt'ǐk) [" + *kinesis,* motion]

astrophobia (ăs"trō-fō'bē-ă) [" + *phobos,* fear]

astrosphere (ăs'trō-sfēr) [" + *sphaira,* sphere]

astrostatic (ăs"trō-stăt'ǐk) [" + *statikos,* standing]

asyllabia (ă"sǐl-ā'bē-ă) [Gr. *a-,* not, + *syllabe,* syllable]

asylum (ă-sī'lŭm) [Gr. *asylon,* sanctuary]

asymbolia (ă-, ă-sǐm-bō'lē-ă) [Gr. *a-,* not, + *symbolon,* a sign]

asymmetry (ă-sǐm'ĕ-trē) [" + *symmetria,* symmetry]

asymphytous (ă-sǐm'fǐ-tŭs) [" + *symphysis,* a growing together]

asymptomatic (ā"sǐmp-tō-măt'ǐk) [" + *symptoma,* occurrence]

asynchronism (ă-sǐn'krō-nǐzm) [" + *syn,* together, + *chronos,* time, + *-ismos,* condition]

asynclitism (ă-sǐn'klǐ-tǐzm) [" + *synklinein,* to lean together, + *-ismos,* condition]
　a., anterior
　a., posterior

asyndesis (ă-sǐn'dē-sǐs) [Gr. *a-,* not, + *syn,* together, + *desis,* binding]

asynechia (ă"sǐ-nēk'ē-ă) [" + *synecheia,* continuity]

asynergia, asynergy (ă-sǐn-ĕr'jē-ă, ă-sǐn'ĕr-jē) [" + Gr. *synergia,* cooperation]

asynovia (ă-sǐn-ō'vē-ă) [" + *syn,* with, + *oon,* egg]

asyntaxia (ă"sǐn-tăk'sē-ă) [" + *syntaxis,* orderly arrangement]

asystematic (ă-sǐs"tĕ-măt'ǐk) [" + LL. *systema,* arrangement]

asystole, asystolia (ă-sǐs'tō-lē, ă"sǐs-tō'lē-ă) [" + *systole,* contraction]

At *astatine*

Atabrine Hydrochloride (ăt'ă-brǐn)

atactic (ă-tăk'tǐk) [Gr. *ataktos,* disorderly]

atactiform (ă-tăk'tǐ-form) [" + L. *forma,* form]

ataractic (ăt"ă-răk'tǐk) [Gr. *ataraktos,* quiet]

Atarax

ataraxia, ataraxy (ăt"ă-răk'sē-ă, -sē) [Gr. *ataraktos,* quiet]

atavism (ăt'ă-vǐzm) [L. *atavus,* ancestor, + Gr. *-ismos,* condition]

atavistic (ăt-ă-vǐs'tǐk)

ataxaphasia (ă-tăk"să-fā'zē-ă) [Gr. *ataxia,* lack of order, + *phasis,* utterance]

ataxia (ă-tăk'sē-ă) [Gr., lack of order fr. *ataktos,* disorderly]
　a., alcoholic
　a., autonomic
　a., Briquet's
　a., Bruns'
　a., bulbar
　a., cerebellar
　a., choreic
　a., Friedreich's
　a., hereditary cerebellar
　a., hereditary spinal
　a., hysterical
　a., locomotor
　a., Marie's
　a., motor
　a., sensory
　a., spinal
　a., static
　a. -telangiectasia

ataxiagram (ă-tăk'sē-ă-grăm) [Gr. *ataxia,* lack of order, + *gramma,* letter, piece of writing]

ataxiagraph (ă-tăk'sē-ă-grăf) [" + *graphein,* to write]

ataxiameter (ă-tăk"sē-ăm'ĕ-tĕr) [" + *metron,* measure]

ataxiamnesia (ă-tăk"sē-ăm-nē'zē-ă) [" + *amnesia,* forgetfulness]

ataxiaphasia (ă-tăk"sē-ă-fā'zē-ă) [" + *phasis,* utterance]

ataxic, ataxial (ă-tăk'sǐk, ă-tăk'sē-ăl)

ataxophemia (ă-tăk"sō-fē'mē-ă) [" + *pheme,* speech]

ataxophobia (ă-tăk"sō-fō'bē-ă) [" + *phobos,* fear]

A.T.B.C.B. *Architectural and Transportation Barriers Compliance Board*

atelectasis (ăt″ĕ-lĕk′tă-sĭs) [Gr. *ateles*, imperfect, + *ektasis*, expansion]

atelencephalia (ăt-ĕl″ĕn-sĕ-fā′lē-ă) [Gr. *ateleia*, incompleteness, + *enkephalos*, brain]

atelia (ă-tē′lē-ă) [Gr. *ateleia*, incompleteness]

ateliosis (ă-tē″lē-ō′sĭs) [Gr. *a-*, not, + *teleios*, complete, + *osis*, condition]

ateliotic (ă-tē″lē-ŏt′ĭk)

atelo- (ăt′ĕ-lō) [Gr. *ateles*, imperfect]

atelocardia (ăt″ĕ-lō-kăr′dē-ă) [″ + *kardia*, heart]

atelocephaly (ăt″ĕ-lō-sĕf′ă-lē) [″ + *kephale*, head]

atelocheilia (ăt″ĕ-lō-kī′lē-ă) [″ + *cheilos*, lip]

atelocheiria (ăt″ĕ-lō-kī′rē-ă) [″ + *cheir*, hand]

ateloencephalia (ăt″ĕ-lō-ĕn″sĕ-fā′lē-ă)

ateloglossia (ăt″ĕ-lō-glŏs′ē-ă) [″ + *glossa*, tongue]

atelognathia (ăt″ĕ-lŏg-nā′thē-ă) [″ + *gnathos*, jaw]

atelomyelia (ăt″ĕ-lō-mī-ē′lē-ă) [″ + *myelos*, marrow]

atelopodia (ăt″ĕ-lō-pō′dē-ă) [″ + *pous*, foot]

ateloprosopia (ăt″ĕ-lō-prō-sō′pē-ă) [″ + *prosopon*, face]

atelorhachidia (ăt″ĕ-lō-ră-kĭd′ē-ă) [″ + *rhachis*, spine]

atelostomia (ăt″ĕ-lō-stō′mē-ă) [″ + *stoma*, mouth, opening]

athelia (ă-thē′lē-ă) [Gr. *a-*, not, + *thele*, nipple]

athermic, athermous (ă-thĕr′mĭk, -mŭs) [″ + *therme*, heat]

athermosystaltic (ă-thĕr″mō-sĭs-tăl′tĭk) [″ + ″ + *systaltikos*, drawing together]

atherogenesis (ăth″ĕr-ō-jĕn′ĕ-sĭs) [Gr. *athere*, porridge, + *genesis*, generation, birth]

atheroma (ăth″ĕr-ō′mă) [″ + *oma*, tumor]

atheromatosis (ăth″ĕr-ō″mă-tō′sĭs)

atheromatous (ăth″ĕr-ō′mă-tŭs)

atheronecrosis (ăth″ĕr-ō″nĕ-krō′sĭs) [″ + *nekrosis*, state of death]

atherosclerosis (ăth″ĕr-ō″sklĕ-rō′sĭs) [″ + Gr. *sklerosis*, a hardening]

athetoid (ăth′ĕ-toyd) [Gr. *athetos*, not fixed, + *eidos*, form, shape]

athetosis (ăth-ĕ-tō′sĭs) [″ + *osis*, condition]

athlete's foot

athrepsia, athrepsy (ă-thrĕp′sē-ă, -sē) [Gr. *a-*, not, + *threpsis*, nourishment]

athreptic (ă-thrĕp′tĭk)

athrombia (ă-thrŏm′bē-ă) [″ + *thrombos*, a clot]

Athrombin-K

athymia (ă-thī′mē-ă) [″ + *thymos*, mind, spirit]

athymic (ă-thī′mĭk)

athymism (ă-thī′mĭzm) [″ + ″ + *-ismos*, condition]

athyrea (ă-thī′rē-ă)

athyreosis (ă-thī″rē-ō′sĭs) [″ + *thyreos*, shield, + *eidos*, form, shape, + *osis*, condition]

athyria (ă-thī′rē-ă)

athyroidemia (ăth″ĭ-roy-, ă-thī″roy-dē′mē-ă) [″ + ″ + ″ + *haima*, blood]

athyroidism (ă-thī′roy-dĭzm) [″ + ″ + ″ + *-ismos*, condition]

athyrosis (ă-thī-rō′sĭs)

atlantad (ăt-lăn′tăd)

atlantal (ăt-lăn′tăl)

atlantoaxial (ăt-lăn″tō-ăk′sē-ăl) [Gr. *atlas*, a support, + L. *axis*, a pivot]

atlantodidymus (ăt-lăn″tō-dĭd′ĭ-mŭs) [″ + *didymus*, twin]

atlanto-occipital (ăt-lăn″tō-ŏk-sĭp′ĭ-tăl) [″ + L. *occipitalis*, occipital]

atlas (ăt′lăs) [Gr.]

atloaxoid (ăt″lō-ăk′soyd) [″ + L. *axis*, a pivot, + Gr. *eidos*, form, shape]

atlodidymus (ăt-lō-dĭd′ĭ-mŭs) [″ + Gr. *didymos*, twin]

atm. *atmosphere; atmospheric*
atmo- [Gr. *atmos*, vapor or steam]
atmosphere (ăt′mŏs-fēr) [″ +
sphaira, sphere]
atmospheric (ăt″mŏs-fēr′ĭk)
ATN *acute tubular necrosis*
at. no. *atomic number*
ATNR *asymmetrical tonic neck reflex*
atocia (ăt-ō′sē-ă) [Gr. *a-*, not, +
tokos, birth]
atom (ăt′ŏm) [Gr. *atomos*, indivisible]
  a., tagged
atomic (ă-tŏm′ĭk)
atomic number
atomic theory
atomic weight
atomization (ăt″ŏm-ĭ-zā′shŭn)
atomize (ăt′ŏm-īz)
atomizer (ăt′ŏm-ī-zĕr)
atonic (ă-tŏn′ĭk) [″ + *tonos*, act of
stretching, tension, tone]
atonicity (ăt-ō-nĭs′ĭ-tē)
atony (ăt′ō-nē) [″ + *tonos*, act of
stretching, tension, tone]
  a., gastric
atopen (ăt′ō-pĕn) [″ + *topos*,
place]
atopic (ă-tŏp′ĭk)
atopognosis (ă-tŏp″ŏg-nō′sĭs) [″ +
topos, place, + *gnosis*, knowl-
edge]
atopy (ăt′ō-pē) [Gr. *atopia*, strange-
ness]
atoxic [Gr. *a-*, not, + *toxikon*, poi-
son]
ATP *adenosine triphosphate*
ATPase *adenosine triphosphatase*
atraumatic (ā″traw-măt′ĭk) [Gr. *a-*, not,
+ *traumatikos*, relating to injury]
atremia (ă-trē′mē-ă) [″ + *tremein*,
to tremble]
atresia (ă-trē′zē-ă) [″ + *tresis*, a
perforation]
  a., anal; a., ani
  a., aortic
  a., biliary
  a., duodenal
  a., esophageal

  a., follicular
  a., intestinal
  a., mitral
  a., prepyloric
  a., pulmonary
  a., tricuspid
  a., urethral
  a., vaginal
atresic (ă-trē′zĭk)
atreto- (ă-trē′tō) [Gr. *atretos*, imperfor-
ate]
atria (ā′trē-ă)
atrial (ā′trē-ăl)
atrial fibrillation
atrial flutter
atrial natriuretic factor
atrichia (ă-trĭk′ē-ă) [Gr. *a-*, not, +
thrix, hair]
atrichosis (ă-trĭ-kō′sĭs) [″ + ″ +
osis, condition]
atrichous (ă-trĭk′ŭs)
atrionector (ăt″rē-ō-nĕk′tor) [L. *atrium*,
corridor, + *nector*, connector]
atrioseptopexy (ā″trē-ō-sĕp′tō-
pĕk″sē) [″ + *saeptum*, a partition,
+ Gr. *pexis*, fixation]
atriotome (ā′trē-ō-tōm) [″ + Gr.
tome, a cutting, slice]
atrioventricular (ā″trē-ō-vĕn-trĭk′ū-
lăr) [″ + *ventriculus*, ventricle]
atrioventricular bundle
atrioventricularis communis
(ā″trē-ō-vĕn-trĭk″ū-lā′rĭs kŏ-mū′nĭs)
atriplicism (ă-trĭp′lĭ-sĭzm)
atrium (ā′trē-ŭm) [L., corridor]
  a. of ear
  a. of heart
  a. of lungs
Atromid-S
atrophia (ă-trō′fē-ă) [Gr.]
atrophic (ă-trō′fĭk)
atrophied (ăt′rō-fēd)
atrophoderma (ăt″rō-fō-dĕr′mă) [Gr.
a-, not + *trophe*, nourishment,
+ *derma*, skin]
atrophodermatosis (ăt-rō″fō-dĕr-
mă-tō′sĭs) [″ + ″ + ″ +
osis, condition]

atrophy (ăt'rō-fē) [Gr. *atrophia*]
 a., acute yellow
 a., compression
 a., correlated
 a., Cruveilhier's
 a., healed yellow
 a., Hoffmann's
 a., Landouzy-Déjérine
 a., muscular
 a., myelopathic
 a., myotonic
 a. of disuse
 a., optic
 a., pathologic
 a., peroneal muscular
 a., physiologic
 a., progressive muscular
 a., Sudeck's [P.H.M. Sudeck, Ger.
   surgeon, 1866–1938]
 a., trophoneurotic
 a., unilateral facial
 a., white
atropine sulfate (ăt'rō-pēn sŭl'fāt)
atropine sulfate poisoning
atropinism, atropism (ăt'rō-pĭn-ĭzm,
  -pĭzm)
atropinization (ăt-rō"pĭn-ĭ-zā'shŭn)
Atropisol
attachment (ă-tăch'mĕnt)
 a., epithelial
attack (ă-tăk') [Fr. *attaquer*, join]
attendant
attention [L. *attendere*, to wait upon]
attention deficit disorder
attention reflex
attenuant (ă-tĕn'ū-ănt) [L. *attenuare*, to
  thin]
attenuate (ă-tĕn'ū-āt)
attenuated (ă-tĕn'ū-āt'd)
attenuation (ă-tĕn"ū-ā'shŭn)
Attenuvax
attic (ăt'ĭk) [L. *atticus*]
attic disease
atticitis (ăt"ĭ-sī'tĭs) [L. *atticus*, attic, +
  Gr. *itis*, inflammation]
atticoantrotomy (ăt"ĭ-kō-ăn-trŏt'ō-
  mē) [" + Gr. *antron*, cave, +
  tome, a cutting, slice]

atticotomy (ăt"ĭ-kŏt'ō-mē) [" +
  Gr. *tome*, a cutting, slice]
attitude [LL. *aptitudo*, fitness]
 a., crucifixion
 a., defense
 a., fetal
 a., forced
 a., frozen
 a., illogical
 a., passional
 a., stereotyped
atto [Danish, *atten*, eighteen]
attolens (ă-tōl'ĕnz) [L.]
attraction (ă-trăk'shŭn) [L. *attrahere*, to
  draw toward]
 a., capillary
 a., chemical
 a., molecular
attrition (ă-trĭsh'ŭn) [L. *attritio*, a rubbing
  against]
at. wt. *atomic weight*
atypia (ă-tĭp'ē-ă) [Gr. *a-*, not, +
  typos, type]
atypical (ă-tĭp'ĭ-kăl) [" + *typikos*,
  pert. to type]
A.U. *ångström unit*
Au [L.] *aurum*, gold
Aub-Dubois table (awb-dū-boy') [Jo-
  seph C. Aub, U.S. physician, 1890–
  1973; Eugene F. Dubois, U.S. physician, 1882–1959]
audible
audible sound
audile (aw'dĭl)
audioanesthesia (aw"dē-ō-ăn"ĕs-
  thē'zē-ă) [L. *audire*, to hear, + Gr.
  an-, not, + *aisthesis*, feeling, per-
  ception]
audiogenic (aw-dē-ō-jĕn'ĭk) [" +
  Gr. *genesis*, generation, birth]
audiogram (aw'dē-ō-grăm") [" +
  Gr. *gramma*, letter, piece of writing]
audiologist
audiology (aw"dē-ŏl'ō-jē) [" +
  Gr. *logos*, word, reason]
audiometer (aw"dē-ŏm'ĕ-tĕr) [" +
  Gr. *metron*, measure]
audiometry (aw"dē-ŏm'ĕ-trē)

a., averaged electroencephalic

audiphone (aw′dĭ-fōn) [L. *audire*, to hear, + Gr. *phone*, voice]

audition (aw-dĭ′shŭn) [L. *auditio*, hearing]

    a., chromatic
    a., colored
    a., gustatory
    a., mental

auditive (aw′dĭ-tĭv)

audito-oculogyric reflex (aw″dĭt-ō-ŏk″ū-lō-jī′rĭk)

auditory (aw′dĭ-tō″rē) [L. *auditorius*]

auditory bulb

auditory canal

auditory evoked response

auditory muscles

auditory nerve

auditory ossicles

auditory placode

auditory reflex

auditory teeth

auditory tube

Auenbrugger's sign (ow-ĕn-broog′ĕrz) [Leopold Joseph Auenbrugger, Austrian physician, 1722–1809]

Auerbach's plexus (ow′ĕr-bǎks) [Leopold Auerbach, Ger. anatomist, 1828–1897]

Auer's bodies (ow′ĕrz) [John Auer, U.S. physician, 1875–1948]

Aufrecht's sign (owf′rĕkhts) [Emanuel Aufrecht, Ger. physician, 1844–1933]

augment (awg-mĕnt′) [L. *augmentum*, increase]

augmentation (awg″mĕn-tā′shŭn)

augnathus (awg-nā′thŭs) [Gr. *au*, again, + *gnathos*, jaw]

aula (aw′lǎ) [Gr. *aule*, hall]

aura (aw′rǎ) [L., breeze]

aural (aw′rǎl) [L. *auris*, the ear]

aurantiasis cutis (aw″rǎn-tī′ǎ-sīs kū′tĭs) [L. *aurantium*, orange, + Gr. *-iasis*, state or condition of; L. *cutis*, skin]

Aureomycin (aw″rē-ō-mī′sĭn)

auriasis (aw-rī′ǎ-sīs) [L. *aurum*, gold, + Gr. *-iasis*, state or condition of]

auric (aw′rĭk) [L. *aurum*, gold]

auricle (aw′rĭ-kl)

auricula (aw-rĭk′ū-lǎ) [L., little ear]

auricular (aw-rĭk′ū-lǎr)

auriculare (aw-rĭk″ū-lā′rē)

auriculocervical nerve reflex (aw-rĭk″ū-lō-sĕr′vĭk′l) [L. *auricula*, little ear, + *cervicalis*, pert. to the neck]

auriculocranial (aw-rĭk″ū-lō-krā′nē-ǎl) [″ + *cranialis*, pert. to the skull]

auriculopalpebral reflex (aw-rĭk″ū-lō-pǎl′pĕb-rǎl) [″ + *palpebra*, eyelid]

auriculotemporal (aw-rĭk″ū-lō-tĕm′pŏ-rǎl) [″ + *temporalis*, pert. to the temples]

auriform (aw′rĭ-form) [L. *auris*, ear, + *forma*, shape]

auris (aw′rĭs) [L.]

    a. dextra
    a. externa
    a. interna
    a. media
    a. sinistra

auriscalp, auriscalpium (aw′rĭ-skǎlp, aw″rĭ-skǎl′pē-ŭm) [″ + *scalpere*, to scrape]

auriscope (aw′rĭ-skōp) [″ + Gr. *skopein*, to examine]

aurotherapy (aw″rō-thĕr′ǎ-pē) [L. *aurum*, gold, + Gr. *therapeia*, treatment]

aurum (aw′rŭm) [L.]

auscult (aws-kŭlt′)

auscultate (aws′kŭl-tāt) [L. *auscultare*, listen to]

auscultation (aws″kŭl-tā′shŭn)

    a., immediate
    a., mediate

auscultatory (aws-kŭl′tǎ-tō″rē)

auscultatory percussion

auscultoplectrum (aws-kŭl″tō-plĕk′trŭm) [L. *auscultare*, listen to, + Gr. *plektron*, hammer]

Austin Flint murmur [Austin Flint, U.S. physician, 1812–1886]

Australia antigen

autacoid (aw′tǎ-koyd) [Gr. *autos*, self,

+ *akos*, remedy, + *eidos*, form, shape]

autarcesis (aw-tăr'sĭ-sĭs, aw"tăr-sē'sĭs) [" + *arkein*, to ward off]

autarcetic (awt"ăr-sĕt'ĭk)

autechoscope (aw-tĕk'ō-skōp) [" + *echos*, sound, + *skopein*, to examine]

autism (aw'tĭzm) [Gr. *autos*, self, + *-ismos*, condition]
a., infantile

auto- [Gr. *autos*, self]

autoactivation (aw"tō-ăk"tĭ-vā'shŭn) [" + L. *agere*, to act]

autoagglutination (aw"tō-ă-gloo"tĭ-nā'shŭn) [" + L. *agglutinare*, adhere to]

autoagglutinin (aw"tō-ă-glū'tĭ-nĭn)

autoallergy (aw"tō-ăl'ĕr-jē)

autoamputation (aw"tō-ăm"pū-tā'shŭn)

autoanalysis (aw"tō-ă-năl'ĭ-sĭs) [" + *analyein*, to dissolve]

Autoanalyzer (aw"tō-ăn'ă-līz"ĕr)

autoantibody (aw"tō-ăn'tĭ-bŏd"ē) [" + *anti*, against, + AS, *bodig*, body]

autoantigen (aw"tō-ăn'tĭ-jĕn) [" + " + *gennan*, to produce]

autoantitoxin (aw"tō-ăn"tĭ-tŏk'sĭn) [" + " + *toxikon*, poison]

autoblast (aw'tō-blăst) [" + *blastos*, germ]

autocatalysis (aw"tō-kă-tăl'ĭ-sĭs) [" + *katalyein*, to dissolve]

autocatharsis (aw-tō-kă-thăr'sĭs) [" + *katharsis*, to cleanse, purify]

autochthonous (aw-tŏk'thō-nŭs) [Gr. *autos*, self, + *chthon*, earth]

autocinesia, autocinesis (aw"tō-sĭ-nē'sē-ă, -nē'sĭs) [" + *kinesis*, motion]

autoclasis (aw"tŏk'lă-sĭs) [" + *klasis*, a breaking]

autoclave (aw'tō-klāv) [" + L. *clavis*, key]

autocrine factor

autocystoplasty (aw"tō-sĭs'tō-plăs"tē) [" + *kystis*, bladder, + *plassein*, to mold]

autocytolysin (aw"tō-sī-tŏl'ĭ-sĭn) [" + *kytos*, cell, + *lysis*, dissolution]

autocytolysis (aw"tō-sī-tŏl'ĭ-sĭs)

autodermic (aw"tō-dĕr'mĭk) [" + *derma*, skin]

autodigestion (aw"tō-dī-jĕs'chŭn) [" + L. *digestio*, a taking apart]

autodiploid (aw"tō-dĭp'loyd) [" + *diploe*, fold, + *eidos*, form, shape]

autodrainage (aw"tō-drān'ĭj) [" + AS. *dreahnian*, drain]

autoecholalia (aw"tō-ĕk-ō-lā'lē-ă) [" + *echo*, echo, + *lalia*, chatter, prattle]

autoecic (aw-tē'sĭk) [" + *oikos*, house]

autoerotism (aw"tō-ē-rŏt'ĭsm) [Gr. *autos*, self, + *erotikos*, rel. to love]

autoexamination (aw"tō-ĕg-zăm"ĭ-nā'shŭn) [" + L. *examinare*, to examine]

autofundoscope (aw"tō-fŭn'dō-skōp) [" + L. *fundus*, bottom, + Gr. *skopein*, to examine]

autogenesis (aw-tō-jĕn'ĕ-sĭs) [" + *genesis*, generation, birth]

autogenetic, autogenic (aw-tō-jĕ-nĕt'ĭk, aw-tō-jĕn'ĭk)

autogenous (aw-tŏj'ĕ-nŭs)

autograft (aw'tō-grăft) [" + L. *graphium*, stylus]

autohemagglutination (aw"tō-hĕm"ă-glū"tĭ-nā'shŭn)

autohemic (aw"tō-hē'mĭk) [" + *haima*, blood]

autohemolysin (aw"tō-hē-mŏl'ĭ-sĭn) [" + " + *lysis*, dissolution]

autohemolysis (aw"tō-hē-mŏl'ĭ-sĭs)

autohemotherapy (aw"tō-hē"mō-thĕr'ă-pē) [" + *haima*, blood, + *therapeia*, treatment]

autohypnosis (aw"tō-hĭp-nō'sĭs)

autoimmune disease (aw"tō-ĭm-mūn') [" + L. *immunis*, safe]

autoimmunity (aw"tō-ĭm-mū'nĭ-tē)

autoimmunization (aw"tō-ĭm"ū-nĭ-zā'

shŭn)

autoinfection (aw″tō-ĭn-fĕk′shŭn) [Gr. *autos*, self, + L. *inficere*, to taint]

autoinfusion (aw″tō-ĭn-fū′zhŭn) [″ + L. *in*, into, + *fundere*, to pour]

autoinoculation (aw″tō-ĭn-ŏk″ū-lā′shŭn) [″ + L. *inoculare*, to ingraft]

autointoxication (aw″tō-ĭn-tŏk″sĭ-kā′shŭn) [″ + L. *in*, into, + Gr. *toxikon*, poison]

autoisolysin (aw″tō-ī-sŏl′ĭ-sĭn) [″ + *isos*, equal, + *lysis*, dissolution]

autokeratoplasty (aw″tō-kĕr′ă-tō-plăs″tē) [″ + *keras*, harm, + *plassein*, to form]

autokinesis (aw″tō-kī-nē′sĭs) [″ + *kinesis*, motion]

autokinetic (aw″tō-kī-nĕt′ĭk)

autolesion (aw′tō-lē″zhŭn) [″ + L. *laedere*, to wound]

autologous (aw-tŏl′ō-gŭs) [″ + *logos*, word, reason]

autologous blood transfusion

autolysate (aw-tŏl′ĭ-sāt) [″ + *lysis*, dissolution]

autolysin (aw-tŏl′ĭ-sĭn)

autolysis (aw-tŏl′ĭ-sĭs)

autolytic (aw″tō-lĭt′ĭk)

automatic [Gr. *automatos*, self-acting]

automatism (aw-tŏm′ă-tĭzm) [″ + *-ismos*, condition]

autonomic (aw-tō-nŏm′ĭk) [″ + *nomos*, law]

autonomic hyperreflexia

autonomic nervous system

autonomous (aw-tŏn′ō-mŭs)

autonomy (aw-tŏn′ō-mē) [Gr. *autos*, self, + *nomos*, law]

autophagia, autophagy (aw″tō-fā′jē-ă, aw-tŏf′ă-jē) [″ + *phagein*, to eat]

autophil (aw′tō-fĭl) [″ + *philein*, to love]

autophilia (aw-tō-fĭl′ē-ă)

autophobia (aw″tō-fō′bē-ă) [″ + *phobos*, fear]

autophony (aw-tŏf′ō-nē) [″ + *phone*, voice]

autoplasmotherapy (aw″tō-plăs″mō-thĕr′ă-pē) [″ + LL. *plasma*, form, mold, + *therapeia*, treatment]

autoplastic (aw″tō-plăs′tĭk) [″ + *plassein*, to form]

autoplasty (aw′tō-plăs″tē)

autoploidy (aw″tō-ploy′dē)

autopolyploidy (aw″tō-pŏl′ē-ploy″dē) [″ + *polys*, many, + *ploos*, fold, + *eidos*, form, shape]

autoprecipitin (aw″tō-prē-sĭp′ĭ-tĭn) [Gr. *autos*, self, + L. *praecipitare*, to cast down]

autopsy (aw′tŏp-sē)
  a., psychological

autopsychic (aw″tō-sī′kĭk) [″ + *psyche*, soul]

autopsychosis (aw″tō-sī-kō′sĭs) [″ + *psyche*, soul]

autopyotherapy (aw″tō-pī″ō-thĕr′ă-pē) [″ + *pyon*, pus, + *therapeia*, treatment]

autoradiogram

autoradiograph (aw″tō-rā′dē-ō-grăf)

autoradiography

autoregulation (aw″tō-rĕg″ū-lā′shŭn)

autoreinfusion (aw″tō-rē″ĭn-fū′zhŭn) [″ + L. *re*, back, + *in*, into, + *fundere*, to pour]

autosensitization (aw″tō-sĕn″sĭ-tĭ-zā′shŭn)

autosepticemia (aw″tō-sĕp″tĭ-sē′mē-ă) [″ + *septos*, rotten, + *haima*, blood]

autoserodiagnosis (aw″tō-sē″rō-dī-ăg-nō′sĭs) [″ + L. *serum*, whey, + Gr. *dia*, through, + *gnosis*, knowledge]

autoserotherapy (aw″tō-sē″rō-thĕr′ă-pē) [″ + ″ + Gr. *therapeia*, treatment]

autoserous (aw″tō-sē′rŭs)

autoserum (aw″tō-sē′rŭm)

autosite (aw′tō-sīt) [Gr. *autos*, self, + *sitos*, food]

autosmia (aw-tŏz′mē-ă) [″ + *osme*, smell]

autosomatognosis (aw"tō-sō"mă-tŏg-nō'sĭs) [" + soma, body, + gnosis, knowledge]

autosome (aw'tō-sōm) [" + soma, body]

autosplenectomy (aw"tō-splĕn-ĕk'tō-mē) [" + splen, spleen, + ektome, excision]

autostimulation (aw"tō-stĭm"ū-lā'shŭn)

autosuggestibility (aw"tō-sŭg-jĕs"tĭ-bĭl'ĭ-tē) [" + L. suggerere, to suggest]

autosuggestion (aw"tō-sŭg-jĕs'chŭn)

autotemnous (aw"tō-tĕm'nŭs) [" + temnein, to divide]

autotherapy (aw"tō-thĕr'ă-pē) [" + therapeia, treatment]

autotomography (aw"tō-tō-mŏg'ră-fē) [" + Gr. tomos, slice, section, + graphein, to write]

autotopagnosia (aw"tō-tŏp-ăg-nō'zē-ă) [" + topos, place, + a-, not, + gnosis, knowledge]

autotoxemia, autotoxicosis (aw"tō-tŏk-sē'mē-ă, aw"tō-tŏk"sĭ-kō'sĭs) [" + toxikon, poison, + haima, blood; " + toxikon, poison, + osis, condition]

autotoxin (aw"tō-tŏk'sĭn)

autotransfusion (aw"tō-trăns-fū'zhŭn) [" + L. trans, across, + fundere, pour]

autotransplantation (aw"tō-trăns"plăn-tā'shŭn) [" + " + plantare, to plant]

autotrophic (aw"tō-trō'fĭk) [" + trophe, nourishment]

autotuberculin (aw"tō-tū-bĕr'kū-lĭn) [" + L. tuberculum, a small swelling]

autovaccination (aw"tō-văk"sĭ-nā'shŭn) [" + vacca, cow]

autovaccine (aw"tō-văk'sēn)

autoxidation (aw"tŏk-sĭ-dā'shŭn) [" + oxys, sharp, + gennan, to produce]

auxetic (awk-sĕt'ĭk) [Gr. auxe, increase]

auxiliary (ăwg-zĭl'ē-air-ē) [L. auxiliarius, help]
a., dental

auxin [Gr. auxe, increase]

auxocyte (awk'sō-sīt) [Gr. auxanu, to increase, + kytos, cell]

auxotroph (awk'sō-trōf) [" + trophe, nutrition]

A-V atrioventricular

availability

avalanche theory [Fr. avaler, to descend]

avalvular (ă-văl'vū-lăr)

avascular (ă-văs'kū-lăr) [Gr. a-, not, + L. vasculum, little vessel]

avascularization (ă-văs"kū-lăr-ĭ-zā'shŭn)

Avazyme

A-V block

A-V bundle

Avellis' paralysis syndrome [George Avellis, Ger. laryngologist, 1864–1916]

Aventyl Hydrochloride

average

aversion therapy

aviation medicine

aviation physiology

avidin (ăv'ĭ-dĭn) [L. avidus, greedy]

avidity

avirulent (ă-vĭr'ū-lĕnt) [Gr. a-, not, + L. virus, poison]

avitaminosis (ā-vī"tă-mĭ-nō'sĭs) [" + vitamin + osis, condition]

avitaminotic (ā-vī-tăm-ĭn-ŏt'ĭk)

avivement (ă-vēv-mŏn') [Fr.]

Avlosulfon

Avogadro's law (ŏv-ō-gŏd'rōs) [Amadeo Avogadro, It. physicist, 1776–1856]

Avogadro's number

avoidance (ă-voyd'ăns)

avoirdupois measure (ăv"ĕr-dĕ-poyz') [Fr., to have weight]

avulsion (ă-vŭl'shŭn) [Gr. a-, not, + L. vellere, to pull]

axanthopsia (ăk"săn-thŏp'sē-ă) [" + xanthos, yellow, + opsis, sight, appearance, vision]

axenic (ă-zĕn′ĭk) [″ + *xenos*, stranger]

axial (ăk′sē-ăl) [L. *axis*, axle]

axial line

axial skeleton

axifugal (ăks-ĭf′ū-găl) [″ + *fugere*, to flee]

axilemma (ăk″sĭ-lĕm′ă) [″ + Gr. *lemma*, husk]

axilla (ăk-sĭl′ă) [L. *axilla*]

axilla conformer

axillary (ăk′sĭ-lār-ē)

axillofemoral bypass graft (ăk″sĭl-ō-fĕm′or-ăl)

axio- (ăk′sē-ō) [L. *axis*, axle]

axiobuccal (ăk″sē-ō-bŭk′kăl) [L. *axis*, axle, + *bucca*, cheek]

axioincisal (ăk″sē-ō-ĭn-sī′zăl) [″ + *incisor*, a cutter]

axiolabial (ăk″sē-ō-lā′bē-ăl) [″ + *labialis*, pert. to the lips]

axiolingual (ăk″sē-ō-lĭng′gwăl) [″ + *lingua*, tongue]

axiomesial (ăk″sē-ō-mē′zē-ăl) [″ + Gr. *mesos*, middle]

axio-occlusal (ăk″sē-ō-ō-klū′zăl) [″ + *occlusio*, closure]

axioplasm (ăk′sē-ō-plăzm) [″ + LL. *plasma*, form, mold]

axiopulpal (ăk″sē-ō-pŭl′păl) [″ + *pulpa*, pulp]

axipetal (ăk-sĭp′ĕt-ăl) [L. *axis*, axle, + *petere*, to seek]

axis [L.]

    a., basicranial

    a., basifacial

    a., binauricular

    a., cardiac

    a., celiac

    a., cerebrospinal

    a., condylar

    a., frontal

    a., hinge

    a., neural

    a., optic

    a., principal

    a., sagittal

    a., visual

axis cylinder

axis deviation

axis traction

axo- [Gr. *axon*, axis]

axodendrite (ăk″sō-dĕn′drīt) [″ + *dendron*, tree]

axofugal (ăk-sŏf′ū-găl) [″ + L. *fugere*, to flee]

axolemma (ăk″sō-lĕm′ă) [″ + *lemma*, husk]

axolysis (ăk-sŏl′ĭ-sĭs) [″ + *lysis*, dissolution]

axometer (ăk-sŏm′ĕ-tĕr) [″ + *metron*, measure]

axon, axone (ăk′sŏn, -sōn) [Gr. *axon*, axis]

axoneme (ăk′sō-nēm) [″ + *nema*, a thread]

axoneuron (ăk-sō-nū′rŏn) [″ + *neuron*, nerve]

axonometer (ăk-sō-nŏm′ĕ-tĕr) [″ + *metron*, measure]

axonotmesis (ăk″sŏn-ŏt-mē′sĭs) [″ + *tmesis*, incision]

axon reflex

axopetal (ăk-sŏp′ĕ-tăl) [″ + L. *petere*, to seek]

axoplasm (ăk′sō-plăzm) [″ + LL. *plasma*, form, mold]

axospongium (ăk-sō-spŏn′jē-ŭm) [″ + *spongos*, sponge]

Ayerza's syndrome (ō-yĕr′thŏz) [Abel Ayerza, Brazilian physician, 1861–1918]

Az *azote*

azalein (ă-zā′lē-ĭn) [L. *azalea*, azalea)

Azapen

azathioprine (ā″ză-thī′ō-prēn)

Azima battery [Fern J. Cramer-Azima, contemporary Canadian psychologist]

azo-

azo compounds

azoic (ă-zō′ĭk) [Gr. *a-*, not, + *zoe*, life]

Azolid

azoospermia (ă-zō-ō-spĕr′mē-ă) [″ + *zoon*, animal, + *sperma*, seed]

Azorean disease (ā-zor′ē-ăn)
azotation (ăz″ō-tā′shŭn)
azote (ăz′ōt) [″ + zoe, life]
azotemia (ăz″ō-tē′mē-ă) [″ + ″ + haima, blood]
azotenesis (ăz-ō-tĕ-nē′sĭs)
azotification (ăz-ō″tĭ-fĭ-kā′shŭn)
azotized (ăz′ō-tīzd)
Azotobacter (ā-zō″tō-băk′tĕr)
azoturia (ăz″ō-tū′rē-ă) [″ + ″ + ouron, urine]
Azulfidine
azure lunulae (ăz′ŭr loo′nū-lē) [O. Fr. azur, blue, + L. lunula, little moon]

azurophil(e) (ăz-ū′rō-fĭl) [″ + Gr. philein, to love]
azurophilia (ăz″ū-rō-fĭl′ē-ă)
azygography (ăz″ĭ-gŏg′ră-fē) [Gr. a-, not, + zygon, yoke, + graphein, to write]
azygos (ăz′ĭ-gŏs) [″ + zygon, yoke]
azygos vein
azygous (ăz′ĭ-gŭs)
azymia (ă-zī′mē-ă) [″ + zyme, ferment]
azymic, azymous (ā-zī′mĭk, -mŭs, ăz′ĭ-mŭs)

B

β Beta

B *Bacillus; Balantidium; barometric; base; bath; behavior; boron; buccal*

B.A. *Bachelor of Arts*

Ba *barium*

Babbitt metal (băb′ĭt) [Isaac Babbitt, U.S. inventor, 1799–1862]

Babcock's operation (băb′kŏks) [William Wayne Babcock, U.S. surgeon, 1872–1963]

Babcock's test [Stephen Moulton Babcock, U.S. chemist, 1843–1931]

Babès-Ernst granules (bä′băz-ĕrnst) [Victor Babès, Rumanian bacteriologist, 1854–1926; Paul Ernst, Ger. pathologist, 1859–1937]

Babesia (bă-bē′zē-ă) [Victor Babès]
  B. bigemina
  B. bovis

babesiosis (bă-bē-zē-ō′sĭs)

Babinski's reflex (bă-bĭn′skēz) [Joseph Babinski, Fr. neurologist, 1857–1932]

Babinski's sign

baby [ME. *babie*]
  b., battered
  b., blue
  b., collodion

bacampicillin hydrochloride

bacca (băk′ă) [L.]

bacciform (băk′sĭ-form) [″ + *forma,* form]

Bacid

Bacillaceae (băs-ĭ-lā′sē-ē)

bacillar, bacillary (băs′ĭl-ăr, băs′ĭl-ăr-ē)

bacille Calmette-Guérin (bă-sēl′)

bacillemia (băs-ĭ-lē′mē-ă) [L. *bacillus,* rod, + Gr. *haima,* blood]

bacilli (bă-sĭl′ī)

bacilliform (bă-sĭl′ĭ-form) [″ + *forma,* form]

bacillophobia (băs″ĭ-lō-fō′bē-ă) [″ + Gr. *phobos,* fear]

bacillosis (băs″ĭ-lō′sĭs) [″ + Gr. *osis,* condition]

bacilluria (băs″ĭ-lū′rē-ă) [″ + Gr. *ouron,* urine]

Bacillus (bă-sĭl′ŭs) [L.]
  B. anthracis
  B. subtilis

bacillus
  b., abortus
  b., acid-fast
  b., Bang's
  b. cereus
  b., cholerae
  b., comma
  b., diphtheria
  b., Döderlein's
  b., Ducrey's
  b., Flexner's
  b., Friedländer's
  b., gas
  b., Hansen's
  b., Klebs-Loeffler
  b., Koch-Weeks
  b. licheniformis
  b. melaninogenicus
  b., Morax-Axenfeld
  b., Pfeiffer's
  b., Shiga
  b., Sonne
  b., tubercle
  b., typhoid

bacitracin (băs-ĭ-trā′sĭn)
  b., zinc

back

backache

backbone

backcross

backflow

background radiation
backrest
backup
bacteremia (băk-tĕr-ē′mē-ă) [Gr. *bak-terion*, rod, + *haima*, blood]
bacteria (băk-tē′rē-ă) [Gr. *bakterion*, rod]
 b., antibody-coated
bacterial antagonism
bacterial resistance
bactericidal (băk″tĕr-ĭ-sī′dăl)
bactericide (băk-tĕr′ĭ-sīd) [Gr. *bacterion*, rod, + L. *cida* fr. *caedere*, to kill]
bactericidin
bacterid (băk′tĕr-ĭd)
bacteriemia (băk-tĕr-ē-ē′mē-ă) [″ + *haima*, blood]
bacterio- (băk-tē′rē-ō)
bacterioagglutinin (băk-tē″rē-ō-ă-gloo′tĭ-nĭn) [″ + L. *agglutinans*, gluing]
bacteriocidal (băk″tĕr-ē-ō-sī′dăl)
bacteriocin (băk-tē′rē-ō-sĭn)
bacteriocinogen (băk-tē″rē-ō-sĭn′ō-gĕn)
bacterioclasis (băk-tē″rē-ōk′lă-sĭs) [″ + *klasis*, breaking]
bacteriogenic (băk-tē″rē-ō-jĕn′ĭk) [″ + *gennan*, to produce]
bacteriohemagglutinin (băk-tē″rē-ō-hĕm″ă-gloo′tĭ-nĭn) [″ + *haima*, blood, + L. *agglutinans*, gluing]
bacteriohemolysin (băk-tē″rē-ō-hē-mŏl′ĭ-sĭn) [″ + ″ + *lysis*, dissolution]
bacterioid (băk-tĕr′ē-oyd) [″ + *eidos*, form, shape]
bacteriologic, **bacteriological** [″ + *logos*, word, reason]
bacteriologist
bacteriology
bacteriolysin (băk-tē″rē-ŏl′ĭ-sĭn) [″ + *lysis*, dissolution]
bacteriolysis (băk-tē″rē-ŏl′ĭ-sĭs)
bacteriolytic (băk-tē″rē-ō-lĭt′ĭk)
bacteriophage (băk-tē′rē-ō-fāj″) [Gr. *bakterion*, rod, + *phagein*, to eat]

bacteriophagia (băk-tē″rē-ō-fā′jē-ă)
bacteriophytoma (băk-tē″rē-ō-fĭ-tō′mă) [″ + *phyton*, plant, + *oma*, tumor]
bacterioprecipitin (băk-tē″rē-ō-prē-sĭp′ĭ-tĭn)
bacterioprotein (băk-tē″rē-ō-prō′tē-ĭn)
bacteriopsonin (băk-tē″rē-ŏp′sō-nĭn)
bacteriosis (băk-tē″rē-ō′sĭs) [″ + *osis*, condition]
bacteriostasis (băk-tē″rē-ŏs′tă-sĭs) [″ + *stasis*, standing still]
bacteriostatic (băk-tē-rē-ō-stăt′ĭk)
bacteriotoxic (băk-tē″rē-ō-tŏk′sĭk)
bacteriotoxin (băk-tē″rē-ō-tŏk′sĭn) [″ + *toxikon*, poison]
bacteriotropin (băk-tē″rē-ŏt′rō-pĭn) [″ + *tropos*, a turn]
bacteristatic
Bacterium (băk-tē′rē-ŭm)
 B. aerogenes
 B. aertrycke
 B. ambiguus
 B. cholerae suis
 B. coli
 B. paratyphi (Type A)
 B. paratyphi (Type B)
 B. tularense
 B. (Eberthella) typhi
 B. typhosum
bacterium
bacteriuria (băk-tē″rē-ū′rē-ă) [Gr. *bakterion*, rod, + *ouron*, urine]
 b., significant
bacteroid (băk′tĕr-oyd) [″ + *eidos*, form, shape]
Bacteroides (băk-tĕr-oyd′ēz)
Bactocill
baculiform (băk-ū′lĭ-form) [L. *baculum*, rod, + *forma*, shape]
bad breath
bag [ME. *bagge*]
 b. of waters
 b., Politzer's
bagassosis (băg-ă-sō′sĭs) [Sp. *bagazo*, husks, + Gr. *osis*, condition]
baker [AS. *bacan*, cook by dry heat]

Baker's cyst [William M. Baker, Brit. surgeon, 1839 – 1896]

baker leg

BAL British anti-lewisite

balance (băl'ăns) [L. bilanx]
   b., acid-base
   b., analytical
   b., electrolyte
   b., fluid
   b., nitrogen

balance beam

balance board

balanic (bă-lăn'ĭk) [Gr. balanos, glans]

balanitis (băl-ă-nī'tĭs) [" + itis, inflammation]

balano- (băl'ă-nō) [Gr. balanos, glans]

balanoblennorrhea (băl"ă-nō-blĕn"ō-rē'ă) [" + blennos, mucus, + rhein, to flow]

balanocele (băl'ă-nō-sēl") [" + kele, tumor, swelling]

balanoplasty (băl'ă-nō-plăs"tē) [" + plassein, to form]

balanoposthitis (băl"ă-nō-pŏs-thī'tĭs) [" + posthe, prepuce, + itis, inflammation]

balanopreputial (băl"ă-nō-prē-pū'shē-ăl)

balanorrhagia (băl"ă-nō-rā'jē-ă) [" + rhegnynai, burst forth]

balanorrhea (băl-ăn-ō-rē'ă) [" + rhein, to flow]

balantidial (băl-ăn-tĭd'ē-ăl)

balantidiasis (băl"ăn-tĭ-dī'ă-sĭs)

Balantidium (băl-ăn-tĭd'ē-ŭm) [Gr. balantidion, a bag]
   B. coli

balanus (băl'ă-nŭs) [Gr. balanos, glans]

baldness [ME. ballede, without hair]
   b., male pattern

Balkan frame

Balke test [Bruno Balke, contemporary Ger.-born U.S. physician]

ball
   b., hair
   b. of foot
   b. of thumb
   b. thrombus

ball-and-socket joint

ball bearing feeder

ballism, ballismus (băl'ĭzm, bă-lĭz'mŭs) [Gr. ballismos, jumping about]

ballistics (bă-lĭs'tĭks) [Gr. ballein, to throw]

ballistocardiograph (bă-lĭs"tō-kăr'dē-ō-grăf) [" + kardia, heart, + graphein, to write]

balloon [It. ballone, great ball]

balloon bezoar

ballooning
   b., intragastric

ballottable (bă-lŏt'ă-bl)

ballottement (băl-ŏt-mŏn') [Fr. balloter, to toss about]

ball-valve action

balm [Gr. balsamon, balsam]
   b. of Gilead

balneology (băl-nē-ŏl'ō-jē) [L. balneum, bath, + Gr. logos, word, reason]

balneotherapy, balneotherapeutics (băl"nē-ō-thĕr'ă-pē, -thĕr"ă-pū'tĭks) [" + Gr. therapeia, treatment]

balsam (bawl'săm) [Gr. balsamon, balsam]
   b. of Peru

Balser's fatty necrosis (băl'zĕrs) [W. Balser, 19th-century Ger. physician]

bamboo spine

Bancroft's filariasis [Joseph Bancroft, Brit. physician, 1836 – 1894]

band

bandage [ME. bande, a band]
   b., abdomen
   b., Ace
   b., amputation-stump
   b., ankle
   b., axilla
   b., back
   b., Barton
   b., breast
   b., butterfly
   b., buttocks
   b., capeline

b., chest
b., circular
b., cohesive
b., cravat
b., cravat elbow
b., cravat, for clenched fist
b., cravat, for fracture of clavicle
b., cravat, sling
b., crucial
b., demigauntlet
b., ear
b.'s, elastic
b., Esmarch
b., eye
b., figure-of-eight
b., finger
b., foot
b., forearm
b., four-tailed
b., Fricke's
b., groin
b., hand
b., head
b., heel
b., hip
b., immovable
b., impregnated
b., knee
b., knotted
b., leg
b., Maissonneuve's
b., many-tailed
b., Martin's
b., neck
b., oblique
b., plaster
b., postoperative
b., pressure
b., protective
b., quadrangular
b., recurrent
b., reversed
b., roller
b., rubber
b., Scultetus
b., shoulder
b., spica
b., spiral reverse

b., suspensory
b., T
b., tailed
b., toe
b., triangular
b., Velpeau
bandage roller
Bandl's ring (băn'd'ls) [Ludwig Bandl, Ger. obstetrician, 1842 – 1892]
bandwidth
bandy leg
bank
   b., sperm
Banthine
Banting, Sir Frederick Grant [Canadian scientist, 1891 – 1941]
Banti's syndrome (băn'tēz) [Guido Banti, It. physician, 1852 – 1925]
bar
bar, median
baragnosis (băr-ăg-nō'sĭs) [Gr. *baros*, weight, + *a-*, not, + *gnosis*, knowledge]
barber's itch
barbital (băr'bĭ-tăl)
   b., sodium
barbital poisoning
barbiturates (băr-bĭt'ū-rāts, băr-bĭ-tū'rāts)
barbotage (băr-bō-tŏzh') [Fr. *barboter*, to dabble]
barbula hirci (băr'bū-lă hĭr'sĭ) [L. *barbula*, little beard, + *hircus*, goat]
baresthesia (băr-ĕs-thē'zē-ă) [Gr. *baros*, weight, + *aisthesis*, feeling, perception]
baresthesiometer (băr"ĕs-thē"zē-ŏm'ĕ-tĕr) [" + " + *metron*, measure]
bariatrics (băr"ē-ă'trĭks) [" + *iatrike*, medical treatment]
barium (bă'rē-ŭm)
   b. sulfate
barium compounds
barium enema
   b.e., double contrast
barium meal
barium swallow

barium test
bark [Old Norse *börkr*]
Barlow's disease [Sir Thomas Barlow, Brit. physician, 1845–1945]
baro- [Gr. *baros*, weight]
barognosis (băr-ŏg-nō'sĭs) [" + *gnosis*, knowledge]
baroreceptor (băr″ō-rē-sĕp'tor)
baroreflexes (băr″ō-rē'flĕk-sĕs) [" + L. *reflexus*, to bend, turn]
baroscope (băr'ō-skōp) [" + *skopein*, to examine]
barosinusitis (băr″ō-sī″nū-sī'tĭs) [Gr. *baros*, weight, + L. *sinus*, curve, + Gr. *itis*, inflammation]
barospirator (băr″ō-spī'rā-tor) [" + L. *spirare*, to breathe]
barostat
barotaxis (băr″ō-tăk'sĭs) [" + *taxis*, turning]
barotitis (băr″ō-tī'tĭs) [" + *otos*, ear, + *itis*, inflammation]
barotrauma (băr″ō-traw'mă) [" + *trauma*, wound]
barotropism (băr-ŏt'rō-pĭzm) [" + *trope*, turning]
Barr body [Murray L. Barr, Canadian anatomist, b. 1908]
barrel chest
barren [O. Fr. *barhaine*, unproductive]
barrier [O. Fr. *barriere*]
   b., blood-brain
   b., placental
   b., primary radiation
   b., secondary radiation
barrier-free design
barrier layer cell
Bartholin's abscess (băr'tō-lĭnz) [Casper Bartholin, Dan. anatomist, 1655–1738]
Bartholin's cyst
Bartholin's ducts
Bartholin's gland
bartholinitis (băr″tō-lĭn-ī'tĭs) [Bartholin + Gr. *itis*, inflammation]
Barton, Clara [U.S. nurse, 1821–1912]
Bartonella (băr″tō-nĕl'ă) [A. L. Barton,

S. Amer. physician, 1871–1950]
   B. bacilliformis
bartonellosis (băr″tō-nĕl-ō'sĭs) [*Bartonella* + Gr. *osis*, condition]
Bartter's syndrome [F.C. Bartter, U.S. physician, b. 1914]
Baruch's law (băr'ooks) [Simon Baruch, U.S. physician, 1840–1921]
bary- [Gr. *barys*, heavy]
baryglossia (băr-ĭ-glŏs'ē-ă) [Gr. *barys*, heavy, + *glossa*, tongue]
barylalia (băr-ĭ-lā'lē-ă) [" + *lalia*, chatter, prattle]
baryphonia (băr″ĭ-fō'nē-ă) [" + *phone*, voice]
basad (bā'săd) [Gr. *basis*, base, + L. *ad*, toward]
basal (bā'săl)
basal ganglia
basal lamina
basal metabolic rate
basal metabolism
basal ridge
basal temperature chart
base [Gr. *basis*, base]
   b., cavity or b., cement
   b., denture
   b. of radiographic film
baseball finger
Basedow's disease (băz'ē-dōz) [Karl A. von Basedow, Ger. physician, 1799–1854]
baseline (bās'lĭn)
basement lamina [Gr. *basis*, base, + L. *lamina*, thin plate]
basement membrane
base pair
baseplate (bās'plāt)
basi-, basio- [Gr. *basis*, base]
basial (bās'sē-ăl) [L. *basialis*]
basiarachnoiditis (bā″sē-ă-răk″noy-dī'tĭs) [Gr. *basis*, base, + *arachne*, spider, + *eidos*, form, shape, + *itis*, inflammation]
BASIC *Beginner's All-Purpose Symbolic Instruction Code*
basic
basic life support

basicranial axis (bā"sē-krā'nē-ăl) ["
+ *kranion*, skull, + *axis*, pivot]
basic salt
Basidiomycetes (bă-sĭd"ē-ō-mī-
sē'tēz)
basifacial axis (bā-sē-fā'shăl) ["   +
L. *facies*, face, + Gr. *axis*, pivot]
basihyal (bā"sē-hī'ăl) ["   + *oeides*,
hyoid]
basilar (băs'ĭ-lăr) [L. *basilaris*]
basilateral (bā"sē-lăt'ĕr-ăl) ["   +
L. *lateralis*, pert. to the side]
basilemma (bā"sē-lĕm'ă) [Gr. *basis*,
base, + *lemma*, husk]
basilic (bă-sĭl'ĭk) [L. *basilicus*]
basilic vein
basiloma (băs-ĭ-lō'mă) [Gr. *basis*,
base, + *oma*, tumor]
basin
    b., emesis
basio- [Gr. *basis*, base]
basioccipital bone (bā"sē-ŏk-sĭp'ĭ-tăl)
["   + L. *occiput*, head]
basion (bā'sē-ŏn)
basiphobia (bā"sē-fō'bē-ă) [Gr. *basis*,
a stepping, + *phobos*, fear]
basirhinal (bā-sē-rī'năl) [Gr. *basis*,
base, + *rhis*, nose]
basis (bā'sĭs) [L., Gr.]
basisphenoid (bā-sē-sfē'noyd) ["   +
sphen, wedge, + *eidos*, form,
shape]
basket [ME.]
basket cells
basophil(e) (bā'sō-fĭl, -fīl) ["   + *philein*, to love]
basophilia (bā-sō-fĭl'ē-ă)
basophilic (bā-sō-fĭl'ĭk)
basophilism (bā-sŏf'ĭ-lĭzm)
    b., pituitary
basophobia (băs-ō-fō'bē-ă) [Gr.
basis, a stepping, + *phobos*, fear]
bass deafness
Bassini's operation (bă-sē'nēz)
[Edoardo Bassini, It. surgeon, 1844–
1924]
bastard [O. Fr. *batard*]
bath [AS. *baeth*]

b., acid
b., air
b., alcohol
b., alkaline
b., alum
b., antipyretic
b., aromatic
b., astringent
b., bed
b., bland
b., blanket
b., box
b., bran
b., brine
b., bubble
b., carbon dioxide
b., cold
b., colloid
b., continuous
b., contrast
b., earth
b., emollient
b., foam
b., foot
b., full
b., glycerin
b., herb
b., hip
b., hot
b., hot air
b., hyperthermal
b., kinetotherapeutic
b., lukewarm
b., medicated
b., milk
b., mud
b., mustard
b., Nauheim
b., needle
b., neutral
b., neutral sitz
b., oatmeal
b., oxygen
b., paraffin
b., powdered borax
b., saline
b., sauna
b., seawater

b., sedative
b., sheet
b., shower
b., sitz
b., sponge
b., starch
b., steam
b., stimulating
b., sulfur
b., sun
b., sweat
b., towel
b., vapor
b., whirlpool
bathophobia (băth″ō-fō′bē-ă) [Gr. *bathos*, deep, + *phobos*, fear]
bathyanesthesia (băth-ē-ăn″ĕs-thē′zē-ă) [″ + *an-*, not, + *aisthesis*, feeling, perception]
bathycardia (băth″ē-kăr′dē-ă) [″ + *kardia*, heart]
bathyesthesia (băth″ē-ĕs-thē′zē-ă) [″ + *aisthesis*, feeling, perception]
bathyhyperesthesia (băth-ē-hī″pĕr-ĕs-thē′zē-ă) [″ + *hyper*, over, above, excessive, + *aisthesis*, feeling, perception]
bathyhypesthesia (băth″ē-hīp″ĕs-thē′zē-ă) [″ + *hypo*, under, beneath, below, + *aisthesis*, feeling, perception]
battered child syndrome
battered woman syndrome
battery [Fr. *battre*, to beat]
Baudelocque's diameter (bōd-lŏks′) [Jean Louis Baudelocque, Sr., Fr. obstetrician, 1746–1810]
Baudelocque's method
baud rate (bawd) [named for Jean M. Émile Baudot, Fr. engineer, 1845–1903]
Baumé scales (bō-mā′) [Antoine Baumé, Fr. chemist, 1728–1805]
bay (bā)
Bayes' theorem [Thomas Bayes, Brit. mathematician, 1702–1761]
bayonet leg
Bazin's disease (bă-zăz′) [Antoine P.

E. Bazin, Fr. dermatologist, 1807–1878]
B cells
BCG *bacille Calmette-Guérin*
BCG vaccine
b.d. [L.] *bis die*, twice a day
bdellometer (dĕl-ŏm′ĕ-tĕr) [Gr. *bdella*, leech, + *metron*, measure]
B.E. barium enema; below elbow
Be beryllium
beaded (bēd′ĕd)
beads, rachitic
beaker (bē′kĕr)
beam
beard
bearing down
beat [AS. *beatan*, to strike]
b., apex
b., capture
b., ectopic
b., escape
b., forced
b., premature
Beau's lines (bōz) [J. H. S. Beau, Fr. physician, 1806–1865]
Bechterew's (also Bekhterev's) reflex (bĕk′tĕr-ĕvs) [Vladimir Mikhailovich von Bechterew, Russ. neurologist, 1857–1927]
beclomethasone dipropionate
becquerel (bĕk′rĕl) [Antoine Henri Becquerel, Fr. physicist, 1852–1908]
bed [AS. *bedd*]
b., air
b., air-fluidized
b., capillary
b., circular
b., float
b., flotation
b., fracture
b., Gatch
b., hydrostatic
b., kinetic
b., metabolic
b., nail
b., open
b., recovery
b., surgical

b., tilt
b., water
bed blocking
bed blocks
bedbug
bedfast
bedlam [From Hospital of St. Mary of Bethlehem, pronounced Bedlem in ME.]
Bednar's aphthae [Alois Bednar, physician in Vienna, 1816–1888]
bedpan [AS. *bedd*, bed, + *panna*, flat vessel]
bedrest
bedridden
bedsore [AS. *bedd*, bed, + *sare*, open wound]
bedwetting
Beer's operation [Georg Joseph Beer, Ger. ophthalmologist, 1763–1821]
bee sting [AS. *beo*, bee, + *stingan*, to pierce]
beeswax (bēz'wăks)
beeturia (bēt-ū'rē-ă)
behavior [ME. *behaven*, to hold oneself in a certain way]
behavioral science
behaviorism
behavior modification
Behçet's syndrome (bā'sĕts) [Hulusi Behçet, Turkish dermatologist, 1889–1948]
bejel (bĕj'ĕl)
bel (bĕl)
belch [AS. *baelcan*, to eructate]
belching
belemnoid (bē-lĕm'noyd) [Gr. *belemnon*, dart, + *eidos*, form, shape]
Bell, Sir Charles [Scottish physiologist and surgeon, 1774–1842]
B.'s law
B.- Magendie's law
B.'s nerve
B.'s palsy
belladonna (bĕl"ă-dòn'ă) [It., beautiful lady]
b. leaf
belladonna and atropine poisons

Bellini's tubule (bĕ-lē'nēz) [Lorenzo Bellini, It. anatomist, 1643–1704]
bell-metal resonance
Bellocq's cannula (bĕl-ŏks') [Jean J. Bellocq, Fr. surgeon, 1732–1807]
belly [AS. *baelg*, bag]
bellyache
belly button
belonephobia (bĕl"ō-nĕ-fō'bē-ă) [Gr. *belone*, needle, + *phobos*, fear]
belonoid (bĕl'ō-noyd) [" + *eidos*, form, shape]
belonoskiascopy (bĕl"ō-nō-skī-ăs'kō-pē) [" + *skia*, shadow, + *skopein*, to examine]
Benadryl (bĕn'ă-drĭl)
Bence Jones protein [Henry Bence Jones, Brit. physician, 1813–1873]
Bender's Visual Motor Gestalt test [Lauretta Bender, N.Y. psychiatrist, b. 1897]
Bendopa
bendroflumethiazide (bĕn"drō-floo"mĕ-thī'ă-zīd)
bends
Benedict's solution (bĕn'ĕ-dĭkts) [Stanley R. Benedict, U.S. chemist, 1844–1936]
Benedict's test
Benedikt's syndrome [Moritz Benedikt, Austrian physician, 1835–1920]
benefit
Benemid
benign (bē-nīn') [L. *benignus*, mild]
benign prostatic hypertrophy
Bennett double-ring splint
bentonite (bĕn'tòn-īt) [Fort Benton, U.S.]
Bentyl
benzaldehyde (bĕn-zăl'dĕ-hīd)
benzalkonium chloride (bĕnz"ăl-kō'nē-ŭm klō'rĭd)
Benzedrine (bĕn'zĕ-drēn)
benzene, benzin, benzine (bĕn'zēn, bĕn-zēn', bĕn'zĭn) [*benz*(oin) + Gr. *ene*, suffix used in chemistry to denote unsaturated compound]
benzestrol (bĕn-zĕs'trŏl)

benzethonium chloride (bĕn″zĕ-thō′nē-ŭm)

benzidine (bĕn′zĭ-dĭn)

benzoate (bĕn′zō-āt)

benzocaine (bĕn′zō-kān)

benzodiazepine (bĕn″zō-dī-ăz′ĕ-pēn)

benzoic acid

benzoin (bĕn′zoyn, -zō-ĭn) [Fr. benjoin]

benzol

benzonatate (bĕn-zō′nă-tāt)

benzoylpas calcium

benzoyl peroxide

benzthiazide (bĕnz-thī′ă-zīd)

benztropine mesylate (bĕnz′trō-pēn)

benzyl

b. benzoate

benzylpenicillin procaine (bĕn″zĭl-pĕn-ĭ-sĭl′ĭn)

Bérard's aneurysm (bā-rărz′) [Auguste Bérard, Fr. surgeon, 1802–1846]

Béraud's valve (bā-rōz′) [Bruno J.J. Béraud, Fr. surgeon, 1823–1865]

berdache (bĕr-dăsh′) [Fr.]

bereavement

beriberi (bĕr′ē-bĕr′ē) [Singhalese beri, weakness]

Berkefeld filter (bĕr′kĕ-fĕld) [Wilhelm Berkefeld, Ger. manufacturer, 1836–1897]

berkelium (bĕrk′lē-ŭm) [U. of California at Berkeley, where first produced]

berloque dermatitis (bĕr′lŏck) [Fr., charm for a watch or bracelet]

Bernard's duct (bĕr-nărz′) [Claude Bernard, Fr. physiologist, 1813–1878]

Bernard's glandular layer

Bertin, columns of (bĕr′tăn) [Exupère Joseph Bertin, Fr. anatomist, 1712–1781]

Bertin's ligament

berylliosis (bĕr″ĭl-lē-ō′sĭs) [beryllium + Gr. osis, condition]

beryllium (bĕ-rĭl′ē-ŭm) [Gr. beryllos, beryl]

bestiality (bĕs-tē-ăl′ĭ-tē) [L. bestia, beast]

beta (bā′tă)

beta-adrenergic blocking agent

beta-adrenergic receptor

beta cells

betacism (bā′tă-sĭzm) [Gr. beta, the letter b, + -ismos, condition]

Betadine

betaine hydrochloride (bē′tă-ĭn) [L. beta, beet]

beta-lactamase resistance

Betalin S

betamethasone (bā″tă-mĕth′ă-sōn)

Betapar

beta particles, rays

beta subunit

betatron (bā′tă-trŏn)

betazole hydrochloride (bā′tă-zōl)

bethanechol chloride (bĕ-thā′nĕ-kŏl)

Betz cells [Vladimir A. Betz, Russ. anatomist, 1834–1894]

bevel (bĕv′ĕl)

bezoar (bē′zor) [Arabic bazahr, protecting against poison]

b., balloon

BFP biologically false positive

Bi bismuth

bi- (bī) [L. bis, twice]

biarticular (bī″ăr-tĭk′ū-lăr) [″ + articulus, joint]

bias (bī′ŭs)

bibasic (bī-bā′sĭk) [″ + Gr. basis, foundation]

bibliomania (bĭb″lē-ō-mā′nē-ă) [Gr. biblion, book, + mania, madness]

bibliotherapy (bĭb″lē-ō-thĕr′ă-pē) [″ + therapeia, treatment]

bibulous (bĭb′ū-lŭs) [L. bibulus, from bibere, to drink]

bicameral (bī-kăm′ĕr-ăl) [L. bis, twice, + Gr. kamara, vault]

bicapsular (bī-kăp′sū-lăr) [″ + capsula, container]

bicarbonate (bī-kăr′bō-nāt)

b., blood

bicellular (bī-sĕl′ū-lăr) [″ + cellularis, little cell]

biceps (bī'sĕps) [" + *caput*, head]
  b. brachii
  b. femoris
biceps reflex
Bichat, Marie François X. (bē-shä')
[Fr. physiologist and anatomist, 1771 –
1802]
  B.'s canal
  B.'s fat ball
  B.'s fissure
  B.'s ligament
  B.'s tunic
bichloride of mercury (bī-klō'rīd)
bicipital (bī-sīp'ī-tăl) [L. *biceps*, two
heads]
BiCNU
biconcave (bī-kŏn'kāv) [L. *bis*, twice,
+ *concavus*, concave]
biconvex (bī-kŏn'vĕks) [" + *con-vexus*, rounded raised surface]
bicornate, bicornis (bī-kor'nāt, -nĭs)
[" + *cornutus*, horned]
bicornis uterus
bicoronal (bī"kō-rō'năl) [" + Gr.
korone, crown]
bicorporate (bī-kor'ŏ-rāt) [" +
corpus, body]
bicuspid (bī-kŭs'pĭd) [" + *cuspis*,
point]
bicuspid tooth
bicuspid valve
bicycle ergometer
b.i.d. [L.] *bis in die*, twice daily
bidet (bē-dā') [Fr., a small horse]
biduous (bĭd'ū-ŭs) [L. *bis*, twice, +
dies, a day]
Bielschowsky disease (bē"ĕl-shō'skē) [Max Bielschowsky, Ger. neur-opathologist, 1869 – 1940]
bifacial (bī-fā'shē-ăl) [" + *facies*,
face]
bifid (bī'fĭd) [" + *findere*, to cleave]
bifid spine
bifid tongue
bifocal (bī-fō'kăl) [" + *focus*,
hearth]
bifocal glasses
bifurcate, bifurcated (bī'fŭr-kāt['d],

bī-fŭr'kāt['d]) [" + *furca*, fork]
bifurcation (bī-fŭr-kā'shŭn)
bigemina (bī-jĕm'ī-nă) [L.]
bigeminal (bī-jĕm'ī-năl) [L. *bigeminum*,
twin]
bigeminal pulse
bigeminum (bī-jĕm'ī-nŭm) [L.]
bigeminy (bī-jĕm'ī-nē)
  b., junctional
  b., nodal
  b., ventricular
bi-ischial
bilabe (bī'lāb) [L. *bis*, twice, + *la-bium*, lip]
bilateral (bī-lăt'ĕr-ăl) [" + *latus*,
side]
bilateral carotid body resection
bilateralism (bī-lăt'ĕr-ăl-ĭzm) ["
+ " + Gr. *-ismos*, condition]
bilateral symmetry
bilayer
  b., lipid
bile (bīl) [L. *bilis*, bile]
  b., cystic
  b., hepatic
bile acids
bile ducts
bile pigments
bile salts
Bilharzia (bĭl-hăr'zē-ă) [Theodor M. Bil-harz, Ger. helminthologist, 1825 –
1862]
bilharzial, bilharzic (bĭl-hăr'zē-ăl,
-zĭk)
bilharziasis (bĭl"hăr-zī'ă-sĭs)
bili- [L. *bilis*]
biliary (bĭl'ē-ār-ē)
biliary calculus
biliary colic
biliary tract
bilicyanin (bĭl"ī-sī'ă-nĭn) [L. *bilis*, bile,
+ *cyaneus*, blue]
biliflavin (bĭl"ī-flā'vĭn) [" + *flavus*,
yellow]
bilifulvin (bĭl"ī-fŭl'vĭn) [" + *fulvus*,
tawny]
bilifuscin (bĭl"ī-fŭs'ĭn) [" + *fuscus*,
brown]

biligenesis (bĭl″ĭ-jĕn′ĕ-sĭs) [″ + Gr. *genesis*, generation, birth]

biligenetic, biligenic (bĭl″ĭ-jĕn-ĕt′ĭk, -jĕn′ĭk) [″ + Gr. *gennan*, to produce]

bilihumin (bĭl″ĭ-hū′mĭn) [″ + *humus*, earth]

bilineurine (bĭl″ĭ-nū′rĭn) [″ + Gr. *neuron*, nerve]

bilious (bĭl′yŭs) [L. *bilosus*]

bilious fever

biliousness (bĭl′yŭs-nĕs)

biliprasin (bĭl″ĭ-prā′sĭn) [″ + Gr. *prason*, green]

bilirachia (bĭl-ĭ-rā′kē-ă) [″ + Gr. *rhachis*, spine]

bilirubin (bĭl-ĭ-roo′bĭn) [″ + *ruber*, red]
   b., direct
   b., indirect

bilirubinate (bĭl-ĭ-roo′bĭn-āt)

bilirubinemia (bĭl″ĭ-roo-bĭn-ē′mē-ă) [″ + *ruber*, red, + Gr. *haima*, blood]

bilirubinuria (bĭl″ĭ-roo-bĭn-ū′rē-ă) [″ + ″ + Gr. *ouron*, urine]

biliuria (bĭl-ĭ-ū′rē-ă)

biliverdin (bĭl-ĭ-vĕr′dĭn) [″ + L. *viridis*, green]

billion [Fr. *bi*, two, + *million*, million]

Billroth's operation(s) [C. A. Theodore Billroth, Austrian surgeon, 1829–1894]

bilobate (bī-lō′bāt) [L. *bis*, twice, + *lobus*, lobe]

bilobular (bī-lŏb′ū-lăr)

bilocular (bī-lŏk′ū-lăr) [″ + *loculus*, cell]

bimanual (bī-măn′ū-ăl) [″ + *manus*, hand]

bimaxillary (bī-măk′sĭ-lĕr″ē) [″ + *maxilla*, jawbone]

bimodal (bī-mō′dăl) [″ + *modus*, mode]

binary (bī′năr-ē) [L. *binarius*, of two]

binary acid

binary code

binary digit

binary gas

binary system

binaural (bĭn-aw′răl) [L. *bis*, twice, + *auris*, ear]

binauricular (bĭn″aw-rĭk′ū-lăr) [″ + *auricula*, little ear]

binder (bīnd′ĕr) [AS. *bindan*, to tie up]
   b., abdominal
   b., chest
   b., double-T
   b., obstetrical
   b., Scultetus [Johann Schultes (Scultetus), Ger. surgeon, 1595–1645]
   b., T
   b., towel

binocular (bĭn-ŏk′ū-lăr) [L. *bis*, twice, + *oculus*, eye]

binocular vision

binomial (bī-nō′mē-ăl) [″ + *nomen*, name]

binotic (bĭn-ŏt′ĭk) [″ + Gr. *ous*, ear]

binovular (bĭn-ŏv′ū-lăr) [″ + *ovum*, egg]

binuclear, binucleate (bī-nū′klē-ăr, -āt) [″ + *nucleus*, kernel]

bio- [Gr. *bios*, life]

bioactive

bioassay (bī″ō-ăs′ā) [″ + O. Fr. *asaier*, to try]

bioastronautics (bī″ō-ăs″trō-naw′tĭks)

bioavailability (bī″ō-ă-văl″ă-bĭl′ĭ-tē)

biocatalyst (bī-ō-kăt′ă-lĭst) [″ + *katalyein*, to dissolve]

biocenosis (bī″ō-sĕn-ō′sĭs) [″ + *koinos*, shared in common, + *osis*, condition]

biochemical marker

biochemistry [″ + *chemeia*, chemistry]

biochemorphology (bī″ō-kĕ-mor-fŏl′ō-jē) [″ + ″ + *morphe*, shape, + *logos*, word, reason]

biocide (bī′ō-sīd) [″ + L. *caedere*, to kill]

bioclimatology (bī″ō-klī-mă-tŏl′ō-jē) [″ + *klima*, climate, + *logos*,

word, reason]
biocolloid (bī"ō-kŏl'oyd) [" + *kollodes*, glutinous]
biodegradable
biodegradation (bī"ō-dĕg"rĕ-dā'shŭn)
biodynamics (bī"ō-dī-năm'ĭks) [Gr. *bios*, life, + *dynamis*, force]
bioelectronics (bī"ō-ē"lĕk-trŏn'ĭks)
bioenergetics (bī"ō-ĕn"ĕr-jĕt'ĭks)
biofeedback
biogenesis (bī"ō-jĕn'ĕ-sĭs) [" + *genesis*, generation, birth]
biogenetic
biogenic amines
biohazard
biokinetics (bī"ō-kĭ-nĕt'ĭks) [" + *kinetikos*, moving]
biologic, biological [" + *logos*, word, reason]
biological degradation
biological rhythms
biologicals
biological warfare
biologic half-life
biologist
biology (bī-ŏl'ō-jē) [Gr. *bios*, life, + *logos*, word, reason]
bioluminescence (bī"ō-loo"mĭ-nĕs'ĕns) [" + L. *lumen*, light]
biolysis (bī-ŏl'ĭ-sĭs) [" + *lysis*, dissolution]
biolytic (bī-ō-lĭt'ĭk)
biomass (bī'ō-măs) [" + L. *massa*, mass]
biome (bī'ōm) [" + *oma*, tumor]
biomechanics (bī"ō-mĕ-kăn'ĭks)
biomedical
biomedical engineering
biometeorology (bī"ō-mē"tē-or-ŏl'ō-jē) [" + *meteoros*, raised from off the ground, + *logos*, word, reason]
biometrics (bī"ō-mĕt'rĭks)
biometry (bī-ŏm'ĕ-trē) [" + *metron*, measure]
biomicroscope (bī"ō-mī'krō-skōp)
bion (bī'ŏn) [Gr. *bios*, life]

bionergy (bī-ŏn'ĕr-jē) [" + *ergon*, work]
bionics (bī-ŏn'ĭks)
bionomics (bī"ō-nŏm'ĭks) [" + *nomos*, law]
bionomy (bī-ŏn'ō-mē)
bionosis (bī-ō-nō'sĭs) [" + *nosos*, disease]
biophagism, biophagy (bī-ŏf'ă-jĭzm, -ă-jē) [" + *phagein*, to eat]
biophotometer (bī"ō-fō-tŏm'ĕ-tĕr) [" + *photos*, light, + *metron*, measure]
biophysics (bī"ō-fĭz'ĭks) [" + *physikos*, natural]
bioplasm (bī'ō-plăzm) [" + LL. *plasma*, form, mold]
biopsy (bī'ŏp-sē) [" + *opsis*, sight, appearance, vision]
  b., aspiration
  b., liver
  b., muscle
  b., needle
  b., punch
biopterin (bī-ŏp'tĕr-ĭn)
biorhythms (bī"ō-rĭth'ŭms) [" + *rhythmos*, rhythm]
bios (bī'ŏs) [Gr., life]
bioscience (bī"ō-sī'ĕns) [" + L. *scientia*, knowledge]
-biosis (bī'ōs-ĭs)
biospectrometry (bī"ō-spĕk-trŏm'ĕ-trē) [" + L. *spectrum*, image, + Gr. *metron*, measure]
biospectroscopy (bī"ō-spĕk-trŏs'kō-pē) [" + " + Gr. *skopein*, to examine]
biosphere (bī'ō-sfēr") [" + *sphaira*, ball]
biostatics (bī'ō-stăt'ĭks) [" + *statikos*, standing]
biostatistics
biosynthesis (bī"ō-sĭn'thĕ-sĭs) [" + *synthesis*, a putting together]
biota (bī-ō'tă) [Gr. *bios*, life]
biotaxis, biotaxy (bī"ō-tăk'sĭs, -sē) [" + *taxis*, arrangement]
Biot's breathing (bē-ōz') [Camille

Biot, Fr. physician, b. 1878]
biotechnology
biotelemetry (bī"ō-těl-ěm'ě-trē) [Gr. *bios*, life, + *tele*, distant, + *metron*, measure]
biotics (bī-ŏt'ĭks) [Gr. *biotikos*, living]
biotin (bī'ō-tĭn)
biotomy (bī-ŏt'ō-mē) [Gr. *bios*, life, + *tome*, a cutting, slice]
biotoxin (bī-ō-tŏk'sĭn) [" + *toxikon*, poison]
biotransformation
biotype (bī'ō-tīp) [" + *typos*, mark]
biovular twins [L. *bis*, twice, + *ovum*, egg]
bipara (bĭp'ă-ră) [" + *parere*, to beget, produce]
biparasitic (bī"păr-ă-sĭt'ĭk) [" + Gr. *para*, alongside, past, beyond, + *sitos*, food]
biparental (bī"pă-rĕn'tăl) [" + *parere*, to beget, produce]
biparietal (bī"pă-rī'ĕ-tăl)
biparous (bĭp'ă-rŭs)
bipartite patella
biped (bī'pĕd) [" + *pes*, foot]
bipenniform (bī-pĕn'ĭ-form) [" + *penna*, feather, + *forma*, shape]
biperforate (bī-pĕr'fō-rāt) [" + *perforatus*, pierced with holes]
biperiden (bī-pĕr'ĭ-dĕn)
biplane
bipolar (bī-pōl'ăr) [" + *polus*, a pole]
bipolar affective disorder
biramous (bī-rā'mŭs) [" + *ramus*, a branch]
bird-breeder's lung
birefractive, birefringent (bī"rē-frăk'tĭv, -frĭn'jĕnt) [" + *refrangere*, to break up]
birth [Old Norse *burdhr*]
    b., complete
    b., cross
    b., dry
    b., live
    b., multiple
    b., premature

birth canal
birth certificate
birth control
birth control pill
birth defect
birthing chair
birth injury
birthmark
birth palsy
birth rate
birth trauma
birth weight
bisacodyl (bĭs-ăk'ō-dĭl; bĭs"ă-kō'dĭl)
bisacromial (bĭs"ă-krō'mē-ăl) [L. *bis*, twice, + Gr. *akron*, point, + *omos*, shoulder]
bisection (bī-sĕk'shŭn) [" + *sectio*, a cutting]
bisexual (bī-sĕks'ū-ăl) [" + *sexus*, sex]
bisferious (bĭs-fĕr'ē-ŭs) [" + *ferire*, to beat]
bishydroxycoumarin (bĭs"hī-drŏk"sē-koo'mă-rĭn)
bisiliac (bĭs-ĭl'ē-ăk) [" + *ilium*, ilium]
bis in die [L.] Twice in a day
bismuth (bĭz'mŭth) [Ger. *Wismuth*, white mass]
    b. subcarbonate
    b. subgallate
    b. subnitrate
bismuth poisoning
bisulfate (bī-sŭl'fāt)
bit
bite (bīt) [AS. *bitan*, to bite]
    b., balanced
    b., close, closed
    b., end-to-end
    b., open
    b., over
    b., under
bitelock
bitemporal (bī-tĕm'pō-răl) [L. *bis*, twice, + *temporalis*, pert. to a temple]
biteplate (bīt'plāt)
bites or stings
bitewing radiograph

Bitot's spots (bē'tōz) [Pierre A. Bitot, Fr. physician, 1822–1888]
bitrochanteric (bī"trō-kăn-tĕr'ĭk)
bitter (bĭt'ĕr) [AS. *biter,* strong]
bituminosis (bĭ-tū"mĭ-nō'sĭs)
biuret (bī'ū-rĕt) [L. *bis,* twice, + *urea*]
biuret test
bivalent (bī-vā'lĕnt) [" + *valens,* powerful]
biventer (bī-vĕn'tĕr) [" + *venter,* belly]
biventral (bī-vĕn'trăl)
bizygomatic (bī"zī-gō-măt'ĭk)
Bjerrum's screen (byĕr'oomz) [Jamik Bjerrum, Dan. ophthalmologist, 1827–1892]
Bjerrum's sign
B.K. *below knee*
Bk *berkelium*
black (blăk) [AS. *blaec*]
black death
black eye
blackhead
black lung
black measles
blackout
black vomit
blackwater fever
black widow
bladder (blăd'dĕr) [AS. *blaedre*]
   b., atony of
   b., autonomous
   b., exstrophy of
   b., hypertonic
   b., irritable
   b., nervous
   b., neurogenic
   b., spastic
   b., urinary
bladder drill
bladder training
bladder worm
blanch (blănch)
blanch test, blanching t.
bland [L. *blandus*]
bland diet
Blandin's glands (blŏn-dănz') [Phi-

lippe F. Blandin, Fr. surgeon, 1798–1849]
blanket, hypothermia
blast [AS. *bloest,* a puff of wind]
-blast [Gr. *blastos,* germ]
blastema (blăs-tē'mă) [Gr. *blastema,* sprout]
blastid (blăs'tĭd) [Gr. *blastos,* germ]
blasto- [Gr. *blastos,* germ]
blastocele, blastocoele (blăs'tō-sēl) [" + *koilos,* hollow]
blastochyle (blăs'tō-kĭl) [" + *chylos,* juice]
blastocyst (blăs'tō-sĭst) [" + *kystis,* bag]
blastocyte (blăs'tō-sīt) [" + *kytos,* cell]
blastocytoma (blăs-tō-sī-tō'mă) [" + " + *oma,* tumor]
blastoderm (blăs'tō-dĕrm) [" + *derma,* skin]
blastodermic vesicle
blastodisk (blăs'tō-dĭsk) [" + *diskos,* disk]
blastogenesis (blăs"tō-jĕn'ĕ-sĭs) [" + *genesis,* generation, birth]
blastokinin (blăs"tō-kĭ'nĭn)
blastolysis (blăs-tŏl'ĭ-sĭs) [" + *lysis,* dissolution]
blastoma (blăs-tō'mă) [" + *oma,* tumor]
blastomere (blăs'tō-mēr) [" + *meros,* a part]
blastomerotomy (blăs"tō-mēr-ŏt'ō-mē) [" + " + *tome,* a cutting, slice]
Blastomyces (blăst-ō-mī'sēz) [Gr. *blastos,* germ, + *mykes,* fungus]
   B. brasiliensis
   B. dermatitidis
blastomycete (blăs"tō-mī'sēt)
blastomycosis (blăs"tō-mī-kō'sĭs) [" + *mykes,* fungus, + *osis,* condition]
   b., keloidal
   b., North American
   b., South American
blastopore (blăs'tō-por) [" +

poros, passage]
blastospore (blăs'tō-spor) [" + *sporos,* seed]
blastula (blăs'tū-lă) [L.]
Blatta (blăt'ă) [L.]
  B. germanica
  B. orientalis
bleaching
bleaching powder
bleb (blĕb)
bleeder [AS. *bledan,* to bleed]
bleeder's disease
bleeding [AS. *bledan,* to bleed]
  b., arterial
  b., breakthrough
  b., occult
  b., venous
bleeding time
blenn-, blenno- [Gr. *blennos,* mucus]
blennadenitis (blĕn"ăd-ĕ-nī'tĭs) [" + *aden,* gland, + *itis,* inflammation]
blennemesis (blĕn-ĕm'ĕ-sĭs) [" + *emesis,* vomiting]
blennogenic, **blennogenous** (blĕn"ō-jĕn'ĭk, blĕn-ŏj'ĕ-nŭs) [" + *gennan,* to produce]
blennoid (blĕn'oyd) [" + *eidos,* form, shape]
blennometritis (blĕn"ō-mĕ-trī'tĭs) [" + *metra,* womb, + *itis,* inflammation]
blennophthalmia (blĕn"ŏf-thăl'mē-ă) [" + *ophthalmos,* eye]
blennorrhagia (blĕn"ō-rā'jē-ă) [" + *rhegnynai,* to break forth]
blennorrhea (blĕn"ō-rē'ă) [Gr. *blennos,* mucus, + *rhein,* to flow]
  b., inclusion
  b. neonatorum
blennostasis (blĕn-ŏs'tă-sĭs) [" + *stasis,* standing still]
blennostatic
blennothorax (blĕn"ō-thō'răks) [" + *thorax,* chest]
blennuria (blĕn-ū'rē-ă) [" + *ouron,* urine]
Blenoxane
bleomycin (blē-ō-mī'sĭn)

  b., sulfate, sterile
blepharadenitis (blĕf"ăr-ăd-ĕ-nī'tĭs) [Gr. *blepharon,* eyelid, + *aden,* gland, + *itis,* inflammation]
blepharal (blĕf'ăr-ăl)
blepharectomy (blĕf"ă-rĕk'tō-mē) [" + *ektome,* excision]
blepharedema (blĕf"ăr-ĕ-dē'mă) [" + *oidema,* swelling]
blepharism [" + *-ismos,* condition]
blepharitis (blĕf"ăr-ī'tĭs) [" + *itis,* inflammation]
  b. angularis
  b. ciliaris
  b. marginalis
  b. parasitica
  b. squamosa
  b. ulcerosa
blepharo- [Gr. *blepharon,* eyelid]
blepharoadenitis (blĕf"ăr-ō-ăd"ĕ-nī'tĭs) [" + *aden,* gland, + *itis,* inflammation]
blepharoadenoma (blĕf"ăr-ō-ăd-ĕ-nō'mă) [" + " + *oma,* tumor]
blepharoatheroma (blĕf"ăr-ō-ăth"ĕ-rō'mă) [" + *athere,* thick fluid, + *oma,* tumor]
blepharochalasis (blĕf"ăr-ō-kăl'ă-sĭs) [" + *chalasis,* relaxation]
blepharochromhidrosis (blĕf"ă-rō-krŏm-hī-drō'sĭs) [" + *chroma,* color, + *hidros,* sweat, + *osis,* condition]
blepharoclonus (blĕf"ă-rŏk'lō-nŭs) [" + *klonos,* tumult]
blepharoconjunctivitis (blĕf"ă-rō-kŏn-jŭnk"tĭ-vī'tĭs) [" + L. *conjungere,* to join together, + Gr. *itis,* inflammation]
blepharodiastasis (blĕf-ă-rō-dī-ăs'tă-sĭs) [" + *diastasis,* separation]
blepharoncus (blĕf"ă-rŏn'kŭs) [" + *onkos,* bulk, mass]
blepharopachynsis (blĕf"ă-rō-pă-kĭn'sĭs) [" + *pachynsis,* thickening]
blepharophimosis (blĕf"ă-rō-fĭ-mō'sĭs) [" + *phimosis,* narrowing]

blepharoplast (blĕf'ă-rō-plăst)
blepharoplasty (blĕf'ă-rō-plăs"tē)
blepharoplegia (blĕf"ă-rō-plē'jē-ă)
[Gr. *blepharon,* eyelid, + *plege,* a
stroke]
blepharoptosis (blĕf"ă-rō-tō'sĭs)
[" + *ptosis,* fall, falling]
blepharopyorrhea (blĕf"ă-rō-pī-ō-
rē'ă) [" + *pyon,* pus, + *rhein,*
to flow]
blepharorrhaphy (blĕf"ă-ror'ă-fē)
[" + *rhaphe,* seam]
blepharorrhea (blĕf"ă-rō-rē'ă) [" +
rhein, to flow]
blepharospasm (blĕf'ă-rō-spăsm)
[" + *spasmos,* a convulsion]
  b., essential
blepharosphincterectomy
(blĕf"ă-rō-sfĭnk"tĕr-ĕk'tō-mē) [" +
sphinkter, band, + *ektome,* exci-
sion]
blepharostat (blĕf'ă-rō-stăt) [" +
histanai, cause to stand]
blepharostenosis (blĕf"ă-rō-stĕn-
ō'sĭs) [" + *stenosis,* act of narrow-
ing]
blepharosynechia (blĕf"ă-rō-sĭ-
nē'kē-ă) [" + *synecheia,* a holding
together]
blepharotomy (blĕf-ă-rŏt'ō-mē)
[" + *tome,* a cutting, slice]
blepsopathia (blĕp"sō-păth'ē-ă) [Gr.
blepsis, sight, + *pathos,* disease,
suffering]
Bleuler, Eugen [Swiss psychiatrist,
1857–1939]
blind [AS.]
blindness
  b., amnesic color
  b., color
  b., cortical
  b., day
  b., eclipse
  b., hysterical
  b., legal
  b., letter
  b., night
  b., psychic

  b., snow
  b., transient
  b., word
blind sight
blind spot
blink
blink reflex
blister [MD. *bluyster,* a swelling]
  b., blood
  b., fever
  b., fly
bloated (blōt'ĕd) [AS. *blout*]
block [MD. *blok,* trunk of a tree]
  b., air
  b., atrioventricular
  b., bite
  b., ear
  b., field
  b., heart
  b., mandibular
  b., neuromuscular
  b., paravertebral
  b., second division
  b., sinoatrial
  b., spinal
  b., ventricular
blockade (blŏk-ād')
blocker
blocking
blocking factors
blood [AS. *blod*]
  b., clotting of
  b., cord
  b., defibrinated
  b., occult
  b., sludged
  b., transfusion of a single unit
  b., unit of
  b., vessels
blood bank
blood-brain barrier
blood cell
blood cell casts
blood clot
blood component therapy
blood corpuscles
blood count
  b.c., differential

blood crossmatching
blood donor
blood dust
blood gas analysis
blood gases
blood groups
bloodless
bloodletting
blood levels
blood platelets
blood poisoning
blood pressure
   b.p., central
   b.p., diastolic
   b.p., direct measurement of
   b.p., indirect measurement of
   b.p., mean
   b.p., negative
   b.p., normal
   b.p., systolic
blood pressure monitor
bloodshot
blood shunting
blood smear
bloodstream
blood sugar
blood test
blood transfusion
   b.t., autologous
blood typing
blood urea nitrogen
blood vessels
blood warmer
bloody sweat
bloody weeping
blotch
blowfly
blowpipe
BLS basic life support
blue [O. Fr. bleu]
blue baby
bluebottle flies
Blue Cross
Blue Shield
Blumberg's sign (blŭm'bĕrgs) [Jacob Moritz Blumberg, Ger. surgeon and gynecologist, 1873–1955]
Blumenbach's clivus (bloo'mĕn-

bawks) [Johann F. Blumenbach, Ger. physiologist and anthropologist, 1752–1840]
blush [AS. blyscan, to be red]
B-lymphocytes
B.M.A. British Medical Association
B-mode (brightness mode) display
B.M.R. basal metabolic rate
B.M.S. Bachelor of Medical Science
BNA Basle Nomina Anatomica
board
   b., back
board certification
board certified
board eligible
Boas' point (bō'ăz) [Ismar I. Boas, Ger. physician, 1858–1938]
Bochdalek's ganglion (bŏk'dăl-ĕks) [Victor Bochdalek, Czech. anatomist, 1801–1883]
bode plot (bōd)
Bodo (bō'dō)
body [AS. bodig]
   b., acetone
   b., amygdaloid
   b., aortic
   b., asbestosis
   b.'s, Aschoff
   b., Barr
   b., basal
   b., carotid
   b., chromaffin
   b.'s, chromophilous
   b., ciliary
   b., coccygeal
   b.'s, Donovan
   b., foreign
   b., geniculate, lateral
   b., geniculate, medial
   b., Heinz
   b., Hensen's
   b., inclusion
   b., ketone
   b.'s, Leishman-Donovan
   b., malpighian
   b., mammillary
   b., medullary
   b.'s, Negri

b.'s, Nissl
b., olivary
b., pacchionian
b., perineal
b., pineal
b., pituitary
b., polar
b., postbranchial
b., psammoma
b.'s, quadrigeminal
b., restiform
b., striate
b., trachoma
b., vertebral
b., vitreous
b., wolffian
body cavities
body composition
body fluids
body image
body language
body mass index
body mechanics
"body packer" syndrome
body rocking
body section radiography
body snatching
body surface area
body type
Boeck's sarcoid (běks) [Caesar P. M. Boeck, Norwegian physician, 1845–1917]
Boerhaave syndrome (boor'hă-vě) [H. Boerhaave, Dutch physician, 1668–1738]
boil [AS. *byl*, a swelling]
boiling
boiling point
bolometer (bō-lŏm'ě-těr) [Gr. *bole*, a ray, + *metron*, measure]
bolus (bō'lŭs) [L., from Gr. *bolos*, a lump]
b., alimentary
bombesin (bŏm'bě-sĭn)
bond
bonding, male-male or female-female
bonding, mother-infant
bone [AS. *ban*, bone]

b., alveolar
b., ankle
b., breast
b., brittle
b., cancellous
b., cartilage
b., cavalry
b., collar
b., compact
b., cotyloid
b., cranial
b., dermal
b., endochondral
b., incarial
b., incisive
b., innominate
b., intracartilaginous
b., ivory
b., marble
b., membrane
b., perichondral or -chondrial
b., periosteal
b., ping pong
b., replacement
b., sesamoid
b., spongy
b., sutural
b., thigh
b., wormian
b., woven
bone age
bone cell
bone cyst
bone graft
bonelet
bone marrow
bone marrow transplant
Bonine (bō'nēn)
bony
booster (boo'stěr)
boot
borate (bō'rāt)
borated
borax (bor'ăks) [L., from Arabic, from Persian *burah*]
borborygmus (bor"bō-rĭg'mŭs) [Gr. *borborygmos*, rumbling in the bowels]
border (bor'děr)

b., brush
b., striated
borderline
Bordetella (bor"dĕ-tĕl'lă) [Jules Bordet, Belg. physician, bacteriologist, and physiologist, 1870 – 1961]
B. pertussis
boredom
boric acid
boric acid poisoning
borism
Bornholm disease (born'hōm) [named for the Danish island Bornholm]
boroglycerin (bor"ō-glĭs'ĕr-ĭn)
boroglycerol (bor"ō-glĭs'ĕr-ŏl)
boron [borax + carbon]
Borrelia (bor-rē'lē-ă)
B. duttonii
B. recurrentis
boss [O. Fr. boce, a swelling]
bosselated (bŏs'ĕ-lāt-ĕd)
Boston arm
Botallo's duct (bō-tăl'ōz) [Leonardo Botallo, It. anatomist, 1530 – 1600]
botany (bŏt'n-ē) [Gr. botanikos, pertaining to plants]
botfly (bŏt'flĭ)
botryoid (bŏt'rē-oyd) [Gr. botrys, bunch of grapes, + eidos, form, shape]
botuliform (bŏt-ū'lĭ-form) [L. botulus, sausage, + forma, shape]
botulin (bŏt'chū-lĭn)
botulinic acid
botulism (bŏt'ū-lĭzm) [" + Gr. -ismos, condition]
b., infant
bouba (boo'bă)
Bouchut's respiration (boo-shooz') [Jean A. E. Bouchut, Fr. physician, 1818 – 1891]
Bouchut's tubes
bougie (boo'zhē) [Fr. bougie, candle]
bouillon (boo-, bool-yŏn') [Fr.]
bouquet (boo-kā') [Fr., nosegay]
bourdonnement (boor-dŏn-mŏn') [Fr.]
boutonnière (boo-tŏn-yār') [Fr., buttonhole]

boutonnière deformity
boutons terminaux (boo-tŏn' tĕr-mĭnō') [Fr., terminal buttons]
bovine (bō'vīn) [L. bovinus]
bowel [O. Fr. boel, intestine]
bowel movement
bowleg (bō'lĕg)
Bowman's capsule (bō'măns) [Sir William Bowman, Brit. physician, 1816 – 1892]
Bowman's glands
Bowman's membrane
boxing
box-note
box splint
Boyer's bursa (bwă-yāz') [Baron Alexis de Boyer, Fr. surgeon, 1757 – 1833]
Boyer's cyst
Boyle's law [Robert Boyle, Brit. physicist, 1627 – 1691]
Bozeman-Fritsch **catheter** (bōz'măn-frĭtch) [Nathan Bozeman, U.S. surgeon, 1825 – 1905; Heinrich Fritsch, Ger. gynecologist, 1844 – 1915]
B.P. blood pressure; British Pharmacopoeia
b.p. boiling point
BPD biparietal diameter
BPH benign prostatic hypertrophy
Bq becquerel
Br bromine; Brucella
brace (brās)
brachia (brā'kē-ă)
brachial (brā'kē-ăl) [L. brachiolis]
brachial artery
brachialgia (brā"kē-ăl'jē-ă) [" + Gr. algos, pain]
brachialis (brā"kē-ăl'ĭs) [L. brachialis, brachial]
brachial plexus
brachial veins
brachiocephalic (brā"kē-ō-sĕ-făl'ĭk) [L. brachium, arm, + Gr. kephale, head]
brachiocrural (brā"kē-ō-kroo'răl) [" + L. cruralis, pert. to the leg]

brachiocubital (brā″kē-ō-kū′bĭ-tăl) [″ + L. cubitus, forearm]

brachiocyllosis (brā″kē-ō-sĭl-ō′sĭs) [″ + kyllosis, a crooking]

brachioradialis (brā″kē-ō-rā″dē-ă′lĭs) [″ + radialis, radius]

brachium (brā′kē-ŭm) [L., arm, from Gr. brakhion, shorter, hence "upper arm" as opposed to longer forearm]
   b. conjunctivum
   b. pontis

brachy- [Gr. brachys, short]

brachybasia (brăk-ē-bā′sē-ă) [″ + basis, walking]

brachycardia (brăk-ē-kăr′dē-ă) [″ + kardia, heart]

brachycephalic, brachycephalous (brăk″ē-sĕ-făl′ĭk, -sef′ă-lŭs) [″ + kephale, head]

brachycheilia (brăk″ē-kī′lē-ă) [″ + cheilos, lip]

brachydactylia (brăk″ē-dăk-tĭl′ē-ă) [″ + daktylos, finger]

brachygnathia (brăk-ĭg-nā′thē-ă) [″ + gnathos, jaw]

brachymetropia (brăk″ē-mĕ-trō′pē-ă) [″ + metron, measure, + opsis, sight, appearance, vision]

brachymorphic (brăk″ē-mor′fĭk) [″ + morphe, form]

brachyphalangia (brăk″ē-fă-lăn′jē-ă) [″ + phalanx, line of battle]

brachystasis (bră-kĭs′tă-sĭs) [″ + stasis, standing still]

brachytherapy (brăk″ē-thĕr′ă-pē) [″ + therapeia, treatment]

bracket

Bradford frame [Edward H. Bradford, U.S. orthopedic surgeon, 1848–1926]

brady- [Gr. bradys, slow]

bradyacusia (brăd″ē-ă-koo′sē-ă) [″ + akouein, to hear]

bradyarrhythmia (brăd″ē-ă-rĭth′mē-ă) [″ + a-, not, + rhythmos, rhythm]

bradycardia (brăd″ē-kăr′dē-ă) [″ + kardia, heart]
   b., sinus

bradycrotic (brăd″ē-krŏt′ĭk) [″ + krotos, pulsation]

bradydiastole (brăd″ē-dĭ-ăs′tō-lē) [″ + diastole, dilatation]

bradyecoia (brăd″ē-ē-koy′ă) [Gr. bradyekoos, slow of hearing]

bradyesthesia (brăd″ē-ĕs-thē′zē-ă) [″ + aisthesis, feeling, perception]

bradyglossia (brăd″ē-glŏs′ē-ă) [″ + glossa, tongue]

bradykinesia (brăd″ē-kĭ-nē′sē-ă) [″ + kinesis, motion]

bradykinin (brăd″ē-kī′nĭn)

bradylalia (brăd″ē-lā′lē-ă) [″ + lalia, chatter, prattle]

bradylexia (brăd″ē-lĕks′ē-ă) [Gr. bradys, slow, + lexis, word]

bradylogia (brăd″ē-lō′jē-ă) [″ + logos, word, reason]

bradyphagia (brăd″ē-fā′jē-ă) [″ + phagein, to eat]

bradyphrasia (brăd″ē-frā′zē-ă) [″ + phrasis, diction]

bradypnea (brăd″ĭp-nē′ă, brăd″ĭ-nē′ă) [″ + pnoe, breathing]

bradyrhythmia (brăd″ē-rĭth′mē-ă) [″ + rhythmos, rhythm]

bradyspermatism (brăd-ē-spĕr′mă-tĭzm) [″ + sperma, semen + -ismos, condition]

bradysphygmia (brăd″ē-sfĭg′mē-ă) [″ + sphygmos, pulse]

bradystalsis (brăd″ē-stăl′sĭs) [″ + stalsis, constriction]

bradytachycardia (brăd″ē-tăk″ē-kăr′dē-ă) [″ + tachys, swift, + kardia, heart]

bradytocia (brăd″ē-tō′sē-ă) [″ + tokos, childbirth]

bradyuria (brăd″ē-ū′rē-ă) [″ + ouron, urine]

braille (brāl) [Louis Braille, blind Fr. educator, 1809–1852]

brain (brān) [AS. braegen]

brain death

brain edema

brain fever

brain implant
Brain's reflex [W. Russell Brain, Brit. physician, 1895–1966]
brain sand
brain scan
brain stem
brainstorm
brain swelling
brain tumor
brainwashing
bran
branch
branchial (brăng'kē-ăl) [L. *branchia*, gills]
branchial arches
branchial clefts
branchial grooves
branchial muscles
branchiogenic,   branchiogenous (brăng"kē-ō-jĕn'ĭk, brăng"kē-ŏj'ĕ-nŭs) [L. *branchia*, gills, + Gr. *gennan*, to produce]
branchioma (brăng"kē-ō'mă) [" + Gr. *oma*, tumor]
branchiomeric (brăng"kē-ō-mĕr'ĭk) [" + Gr. *meros*, part]
Brandt-Andrews maneuver
brandy
Branhamella (Neisseria) catarrhalis (brăn"hă-mĕl'ă)
brash
   b., water
brass poisoning
brawny induration
Braxton Hicks sign [John Braxton Hicks, Brit. gynecologist, 1823–1897]
Brazelton Neonatal Assessment Scale [T. Berry Brazelton, American pediatrician, b. 1918]
break
breakbone fever
breakdown, nervous
breast [AS. *breost*]
   b., chicken
   b., self-examination of
breast cancer
breast pump
breath (brĕth) [AS. *braeth*, odor]

Breathalyzer (brĕth'ă-lĭ-zĕr)
breathing
   b., asthmatic
   b., bronchial
   b., Cheyne-Stokes
   b., cog-wheel
   b., continuous positive-pressure
   b., intermittent positive-pressure
   b., Kussmaul
   b., shallow
breech [AS. *brec*, buttocks]
breech presentation
breeze
bregma (brĕg'mă) [Gr., front of head]
bregmatic
bregmocardiac reflex (brĕg"mō-kăr'dē-ăk) [Gr. *bregma*, front of head, + *kardia*, heart]
brei (brī) [Gr., pulp]
Breisky's disease (brī'skēz) [August Breisky, Ger. gynecologist, 1832–1889]
Brenner's tumor [Fritz Brenner, Ger. pathologist, 1877–1969]
Breokinase
Brethine
brevicollis (brĕv"ĭ-kŏl'ĭs) [L. *brevis*, short, + *collum*, neck]
brevilineal (brĕv-ĭ-lĭn'ē-ăl) [L. *brevis*, short, + *linea*, line]
Brevital Sodium
Bricanyl
bridge (brĭj) [AS. *brycg*]
   b. of nose
bridgework (brĭj'work)
   b., fixed
   b., removable
bridle (brī'dl)
Bright's disease [Richard Bright, Brit. physician, 1789–1858]
brightness gain
brim
Briquet's syndrome [Paul Briquet, Fr. physician, 1796–1881]
brisement (brēz-mŏn') [Fr., crushing]
Brissaud's reflex (brĭs-sōz') [Edouard Brissaud, Fr. physician, 1852–1909]
Bristamycin

British antilewisite
British Pharmacopoeia
British thermal unit
brittle diabetes
broach (brōch) [ME. *broche,* pointed rod]
Broadbent's sign [Sir William Henry Broadbent, Brit. physician, 1835–1907]
Broca's area (brō'kăs) [Pierre Paul Broca, Fr. surgeon, 1824–1880]
Brodie's abscess [Sir Benjamin Collins Brodie, Brit. surgeon, 1783–1862]
brom-, bromo- [Gr. *bromos,* stench]
bromelain (brō'mĕ-lān)
bromide (brō'mīd) [Gr. *bromos,* stench]
bromide poisoning
bromidrosiphobia (brō"mĭd-rō-sī-fō'bē-ă) [" + *hidros,* sweat, + *phobos,* fear]
bromidrosis, bromhidrosis (brō"mĭ-drō'sĭs)
bromine (brō'mēn, -mĭn) [Gr. *bromos,* stench]
bromism, brominism (brō'mĭzm, brō'mĭn-ĭzm) [" + *-ismos,* condition]
bromocriptine mesylate (brō"mō-krĭp'tēn)
bromoderma (brō"mō-dĕr'mă) [" + *derma,* skin]
bromodiphenhydramine hydrochloride (brō"mō-dī"fĕn-hī'dră-mēn)
bromoiodism (brō"mō-ī'ŏ-dĭzm) [" + *ioeides,* violet colored, + *-ismos,* condition]
bromomania (brō"mō-mā'nē-ă) [" + *mania,* insanity]
bromomenorrhea (brō"mō-mĕn-ō-rē'ă) [" + *men,* month, + *rhein,* to flow]
bromopnea (brōm"ŏp-nē'ă) [" + *pnoe,* breath]
brompheniramine maleate (brōm"fĕn-ĭr'ă-mēn)
Brompton's cocktail [Brompton Chest Hospital, England]
bronchadenitis (brŏng"kăd-ē-nī'tĭs) [Gr. *bronchos,* windpipe, + *aden,*

gland, + *itis,* inflammation]
bronchi (brŏng'kī) [L.]
  b., foreign bodies in
bronchial (brŏng'kē-ăl)
bronchial crises
bronchial glands
bronchial tree
bronchial tubes
bronchial washing
bronchiarctia (brŏng"kē-ărk'shē-ă) [Gr. *bronchos,* windpipe + L. *arctare,* to compress]
bronchiectasis (brŏng"kē-ĕk'tă-sĭs) [" + *ektasis,* dilatation]
bronchiloquy (brŏng-kĭl'ō-kwē) [" + L. *loqui,* to speak]
bronchiocele (brŏng'kē-ō-sēl) [" + *kele,* tumor, swelling]
bronchiogenic (brŏng"kē-ō-jĕn'ĭk) [" + *gennan,* to produce]
bronchiole (brŏng'kē-ōl) [L. *bronchiolus,* air passage]
  b., respiratory
  b., terminal
bronchiolectasis (brŏng"kē-ō-lĕk'tă-sĭs) [" + Gr. *ektasis,* dilatation]
bronchiolitis (brŏng"kē-ō-lī'tĭs) [" + Gr. *itis,* inflammation]
  b. exudativa
  b., vesicular
bronchiolus (brŏng-kē-ō-lŭs) [L.]
bronchiospasm (brŏng'kē-ō-spăzm) [Gr. *bronchos,* windpipe, + *spasmos,* a convulsion]
bronchiostenosis (brŏng"kē-ō-stĕn-ō'sĭs) [" + *stenosis,* act of narrowing]
bronchitis (brŏng-kī'tĭs) [" + *itis,* inflammation]
  b., acute
  b., chronic
  b., plastic
  b., putrid
  b., vegetal
bronchium (brŏng'kē-ŭm) [Gr. *bronchos,* windpipe]
broncho-, bronch- [Gr. *bronchos,* windpipe]

bronchoadenitis (brŏng"kō-ăd"ē-nī'tĭs) [" + aden, gland, + itis, inflammation]

bronchoalveolar (brŏn"kō-ăl-vē'ō-lăr) [" + alveolus, small hollow]

bronchoblennorrhea (brŏng"kō-blĕn"ō-rē'ă) [" + blennos, mucus, + rhein, to flow]

bronchocele (brŏng'kō-sēl) [" + kele, tumor, swelling]

bronchoconstriction (brŏng"kō-kŏn-strĭk'shŭn) [" + L. constringere, to draw together]

bronchodilatation (brŏng"kō-dĭl-ă-tā'shŭn) [" + L. dilatare, to open]

bronchoedema (brŏng"kō-ĕ-dē'mă) [" + oidema, swelling]

bronchoesophageal (brŏng"kō-ĕ-sŏf"ă-jē'ăl) [" + oisophagos, gullet]

bronchofiberscope (brŏng"kō-fī'bĕr-skōp) [" + L. fibra, fiber, + Gr. skopein, to examine]

bronchogenic (brŏng-kō-jĕn'ĭk) [" + gennan, to produce]

bronchogram (brŏng'kō-grăm) [" + gramma, letter, piece of writing]

bronchography (brŏng-kŏg'ră-fē) [" + graphein, to write]

broncholith (brŏng'kō-lĭth) [" + lithos, stone]

broncholithiasis (brŏng"kō-lĭth-ī'ă-sĭs) [" + lithos, stone, + -iasis, state or condition of]

bronchomotor (brŏng"kō-mō'tor) [" + L. motus, moving]

bronchomycosis (brŏng"kō-mī-kō'sĭs) [" + mykes, fungus, + osis, condition]

bronchopathy (brŏng-kŏp'ă-thē) [" + pathos, disease, suffering]

bronchophony (brŏng-kŏf'ō-nē) [" + phone, voice]

bronchoplasty (brŏng'kō-plăs"tē) [" + plassein, to form]

bronchoplegia (brŏng"kō-plē'jē-ă) [" + plege, stroke]

bronchopleural (brŏng"kō-ploor'ăl) [" + pleura, side, rib]

bronchopneumonia (brŏng"kō-nū-mō'nē-ă) [" + pneumonia, lung inflammation]

bronchopulmonary (brŏng"kō-pŭl'mō-nă-rē) [Gr. bronchos, windpipe, + L. pulmonarius, pert. to lung]

bronchopulmonary lavage

bronchorrhagia (brŏng"kor-ā'jē-ă) [" + rhegnynai, to break forth]

bronchorrhaphy (brŏng-kor'ă-fē) [" + rhaphe, seam]

bronchorrhea (brŏng-kō-rē'ă) [" + rhein, to flow]

bronchorrhoncus (brŏng"kor-ŏn'kŭs) [" + rhonchos, snore]

bronchoscope (brŏng'kō-skōp) [" + skopein, to examine]

bronchoscopy (brŏng-kŏs'kō-pē)

bronchosinusitis (brŏng"kō-sī"nŭs-ī'tĭs) [" + L. sinus, a hollow, + Gr. itis, inflammation]

bronchospasm (brŏng'kō-spăzm) [" + spasmos, a convulsion]

bronchospirochetosis (brŏng"kō-spī"rō-kē-tō'sĭs) [" + speira, coil, + chaite, wavy hair, + osis, condition]

bronchospirometer (brŏng"kō-spī-rŏm'ě-tĕr) [" + L. spirare, to breathe, + Gr. metron, measure]

bronchostaxis (brŏng"kō-stăk'sĭs) [" + staxis, dripping]

bronchostenosis (brŏng"kō-stĕn-ō'sĭs) [" + stenosis, act of narrowing]

bronchostomy (brŏng-kŏs'tō-mē) [" + stoma, mouth, opening]

bronchotomy (brŏng-kŏt'ō-mē) [" + tome, a cutting, slice]

bronchotracheal (brŏng"kō-trā'kē-ăl) [" + trachea, rough]

bronchovesicular (brŏng"kō-vě-sĭk'ū-lăr) [" + L. vesicula, a tiny bladder]

bronchus (brŏng'kŭs) [Gr. bronchos, windpipe]

Bronkaid Mist

Bronkephrine

Bronkosol
brontophobia (brŏn"tō-fō'bē-ă) [Gr. *bronte*, thunder, + *phobos*, fear]
bronzed skin
brood capsule
brooding
broth [ME.]
brow
brownian movement (brow'nē-ăn) [Robert Brown, Brit. botanist, 1773–1858]
Brown-Séquard's   **syndrome** (brown'sā-kărz') [Charles E. Brown-Séquard, Fr. physician, 1818–1894]
brow presentation
Brucella (broo-sĕl'ă) [Sir David Bruce, Brit. bacteriologist, 1855–1931]
brucellar
brucellin (broo-sĕl'ĭn)
brucellosis (broo"sĕl-ō'sĭs) [*Brucella* + Gr. *osis*, condition]
Bruch's membrane (brooks) [Karl W. L. Bruch, Ger. anatomist, 1819–1884]
brucine (broo'sēn, broo'sĭn) [J. Bruce, African traveler, 1730–1794]
Bruck's disease (brooks) [Alfred Bruck, Ger. physician, b. 1865]
bruise (brooz) [O. Fr. *bruiser*, to break]
   b. of head, chest, and abdomen
   b., stone
bruissement (broo-ēs-mŏn') [Fr., droning noise]
bruit (brwē, broot') [Fr., noise]
   b., placental
Brunner's glands (brŭn'ĕrz) [Johann C. Brunner, Swiss anatomist, 1653–1727]
brush
   b., tooth-
brush border
Brushfield spots [T. Brushfield, Brit. physician, 1858–1937]
brushing
bruxism (brŭk'sĭzm) [Gr. *brychein*, to grind the teeth, + *-ismos*, condition]
Bryant's traction [Sir Thomas Bryant, Brit. surgeon, 1828–1914]

Bryrel
B.S. *Bachelor of Science; Bachelor of Surgery*
BSE *breast self-examination*
B.S.N. *Bachelor of Science in Nursing*
BTU *British thermal unit*
bubo (boo'bō) [Gr. *boubon*, groin, swollen gland]
   b., axillary
   b., indolent
   b., inguinal
   b., pestilential
   b., venereal
bubonadenitis (boo-bŏn-ăd-ĕ-nī'tĭs) [" + *aden*, gland, + *itis*, inflammation]
bubonic plague [" + L. *plaga*, stroke, wound]
bucardia (bū-kăr'dē-ă) [Gr. *bous*, ox, + *kardia*, heart]
bucca (bŭk'ă) [L., cheek]
buccal (bŭk'ăl)
buccal cavity
buccal fat pad
buccal glands
buccinatolabialis (bŭk"sĭn-ă-tō-lā"bē-ă'lĭs) [L. *buccinator*, trumpeter, + *labialis*, pert. to the lips]
buccinator (bŭk'sĭn-ā-tor)
buccoaxiocervical (bŭk"kō-ăk"sē-ō-sĕr'vĭ-kăl)
buccocervical (bŭk"kō-sĕr'vĭ-kăl)
buccodistal (bŭk"kō-dĭs'tăl)
buccogingival (bŭk"kō-jĭn'jĭ-văl)
buccolabial (bŭk"kō-lā'bē-ăl)
buccolingual (bŭk"kō-lĭng'gwăl)
buccomesial (bŭk"kō-mē'zē-ăl)
bucco-occlusal (bŭk"kō-ō-kloo'săl)
buccopharyngeal (bŭk"kō-fă-rĭn'jē-ăl)
buccopulpal (bŭk"kō-pŭl'păl)
buccoversion (bŭk"kō-vĕr'zhŭn) [L. *bucca*, cheek, + *versio*, turning]
buccula (bŭk'ū-lă) [L., a little cheek]
Buck's extension [Gurdon Buck, U.S. surgeon, 1807–1877]
Buck's traction
Bucky diaphragm [Gustav P. Bucky,

Ger.-born U.S. roentgenologist, 1880–1963]
buclizine hydrochloride (bū'klĭ-zēn)
bucnemia (bŭk-nē'mē-ă) [Gr. *bous*, ox, + *kneme*, leg]
bud [ME. *budde*, to swell]
  b., taste
  b., tooth
budding
Buerger's disease (bŭr'gĕrz) [Leo Buerger, U.S. physician, 1879–1943]
bufa-, bufo- (bū'fă, bū'fō) [L. *bufo*, toad]
buffalo hump
buffer (bŭf'ĕr) [ME. *buffe*, to deaden shock of]
  b., blood
buffy coat
bufotoxin [L. *bufo*, toad, + Gr. *toxikon*, poison]
bug
  b., assassin
  b., bed
  b., kissing
  b., red
bulb [L. *bulbus*, bulbous root; Gr. *bolbos*]
  b., aortic
  b., duodenal
  b., hair
  b. of the eye
  b. of the urethra
  b. of the vestibule
  b., olfactory
  b., terminal, of Krause
bulbar
bulbar paralysis
bulbiform (bŭl'bĭ-form) [" + *forma*, shape]
bulbitis (bŭl-bī'tĭs) [" + Gr. *itis*, inflammation]
bulbocavernosus (bŭl"bō-kăv"ĕr-nō'sŭs) [" + *cavernosus*, hollow]
bulbocavernosus reflex
bulboid (bŭl'boyd) [" + Gr. *eidos*, form, shape]
bulbomimic reflex (bŭl"bō-mĭm'ĭk) [" + Gr. *mimikos*, imitator]

bulbonuclear (bŭl"bō-nū'klē-ăr) [" + *nucleus*, kernel]
bulbospongiosus (bŭl"bō-spŏn"jē-ō'sŭs)
bulbospongiosus reflex
bulbourethral glands (bŭl"bō-ū-rē'thrăl) [" + Gr. *ourethra*, urethra]
bulbous (bŭl'bŭs) [L. *bulbus*]
bulbus [L.; Gr. *bolbos*]
  b. corpus spongiosum
  b. vestibuli
bulesis (bŭ-lē'sĭs) [Gr. *boulesis*, a willing]
bulimia (bū-lĭm'ē-ă) [L.]
bulimic
bulk
bulla (bŭl'lă) [L., a bubble]
  b. ethmoidalis
  b. ossea
bullet wound
bullous (bŭl'ŭs) [L. *bulla*, bubble]
BUN blood urea nitrogen
bundle
  b., Arnold's
  b., atrioventricular
  b. of His
  b. of Türck
  b., Schultze's
bundle branch block
  b.b.b., left
  b.b.b., right
bunion (bŭn'yŭn)
Bunnell block
Bunsen burner (bŭn'sĕn) [Robert W. E. von Bunsen, Ger. chemist, 1811–1899]
Bunyaviridae (bŭn"yă-vĭr'ĭ-dē)
buphthalmia, buphthalmos (bŭf-thăl'mē-ă, -mōs) [Gr. *bous*, ox, + *ophthalmos*, eye]
bur, burr (bŭr)
Burdach's tract (boor'dăks) [Karl F. Burdach, Ger. physiologist, 1776–1847]
buret, burette (bū-rĕt') [Fr.]
Burkitt's lymphoma [D. P. Burkitt, Ugandan physician, b. 1911]
burn [AS. *baernan*, to burn]
  b., acid

b., alkali
b., brush
b., chemical
b., electric
b., fireworks
b., flash
b., gunpowder
b., inhalation
b. of eye
b., radiation
b., respiratory
b., thermal
b., x-ray
Burnett's syndrome [Charles Burnett, U.S. physician, 1913–1967]
burning foot syndrome
burnish (bĕr′nĭsh)
burnisher (bĕr′nĭsh-ĕr)
burnout
   b., radiographic
   b., wax
Buro-sol Concentrate
Burow's solution [Karl A. Burow, Ger. surgeon, 1809–1874]
burr
burrow (bŭr′rō)
burrowing
bursa (bŭr′să) [Gr., a leather sack]
   b., Achilles
   b., adventitious
   b., olecranon
   b., omental
   b., patellar
   b., pharyngeal
   b., subacromial
bursae (bŭr′sē)
bursal (bŭr′săl)
bursalis (bŭr-săl′ĭs) [L., pert. to a bursa]
bursectomy (bŭr-sĕk′tō-mē) [″ + ektome, excision]
bursitis (bŭr-sī′tĭs) [″ + itis, inflammation]
bursolith (bŭr′sō-lĭth) [″ + lithos, stone]
bursopathy (bŭr-sŏp′ă-thē) [″ + pathos, disease, suffering]

bursotomy (bŭr-sŏt′ō-mē) [″ + tome, a cutting, slice]
bursula (bŭr′sū-lă) [L., little sack]
   b. testium
Burton's line (bŭr′tŏns) [Henry Burton, Brit. physician, 1799–1849]
bus (bŭs)
busulfan (bū-sŭl′făn)
butacaine sulfate (bū′tă-kān)
butamben (bū-tăm′bĕn)
butane (bū′tān)
Butazolidin (bū″tă-zŏl′ĭ-dĭn)
Butisol Sodium (bū′tĭ-sŏl sō′dē-ŭm)
butt [ME. butte, end]
butterfly
butterfly rash
buttocks (bŭt′ŭks) [AS. buttuc, end]
button (bŭt′n)
button aid
buttonhole
button suture
butyl aminobenzoate (bū′tĭl ăm″ĭ-nō-bĕn′zō-āt)
butylene (bū′tĭ-lēn)
butyraceous (bū″tĭ-rā′shŭs) [L. butyrum, butter]
butyrate (bū″tĭ-rāt)
butyric acid (bū-tĭr′ĭk) [L. butyrum, butter]
butyrin (bū′tĭr-ĭn)
butyroid (bū′tĭ-royd) [″ + eidos, form, shape]
butyrometer (bū″tĭ-rŏm′ĕ-tĕr) [″ + metron, measure]
butyrophenone (bū″tĭ-rō-fē′nōn)
butyrous (bū′tĭ-rŭs)
bypass
bysma (bĭs′mă) [Gr., plug]
byssinosis (bĭs″ĭ-nō′sĭs) [Gr. byssos, cotton, + osis, condition]
byssocausis (bĭs″ō-kaw′sĭs) [″ + kausis, burning]
byssoid (bĭs′oyd) [″ + eidos, form, shape]
byte (bīt)

C

C *carbon; calorie* (if not capitalized); *Celsius; centigrade;* [L.] *centum,* one hundred; *circa,* about; *clonus; closure; compound; congius* (gallon); [L.] *cum,* with; *kilocalorie* (when capitalized)

¹⁴C *radioactive carbon*

Ca *calcium;cathode*

CABG *coronary artery bypass graft*

Cabot's ring bodies (kăb'ŏts) [Richard C. Cabot, U.S. physician, 1868–1939]

cac-, caci-, caco- [Gr. *kakos,* bad]

CaC₂ *calcium carbide*

cacanthrax (kăk-ăn'thrăks) [" + *anthrax,* carbuncle]

cacao (kă-kā'ō, kă-kaw'ō) [Mex.-Sp. from Nahuatl *cacahuatl,* cacao beans]

cachectic (kă-kĕk'tĭk) [Gr. *kakos,* bad, + *hexis,* condition]

cachectins

cachet (kă-shā') [Fr., a seal]

cachexia (kă-kĕks'ē-ă) [Gr. *kakos,* bad, + *hexis,* condition]

    c., cancerous

    c. hypophysiopriva

    c., lymphatic

    c., malarial

    c., pituitary

    c., strumipriva

cachinnation (kăk-ĭ-nā'shŭn) [L. *cachinnare,* to laugh aloud]

CaCl₂ *calcium chloride*

caco-, cac-, caci- [Gr. *kakos,* bad]

CaCO₃ *calcium carbonate*

CaC₂O₄ *calcium oxalate*

cacodylate (kăk'ō-dĭl-āt)

cacogenesis (kăk"ō-jĕn'ĕ-sĭs) [" + *genesis,* generation, birth]

cacogenic (kăk"ō-jĕn'ĭk)

cacogeusia (kăk"ō-gū'sē-ă) [" + *geusis,* taste]

cacoplastic (kăk"ō-plăs'tĭk) [" + *plastikos,* formed]

cacorhythmic (kăk"ō-rĭth'mĭk) [" + *rhythmos,* rhythm]

cacosmia (kă-kŏz'mē-ă) [" + *osme,* smell]

cacotrophy (kăk-ŏt'rō-fē) [" + *trophe,* nourishment]

cacumen (kăk-ū'mĕn) [L. *cacumen,* summit]

CAD *computer-assisted design; coronary artery disease*

cadaver (kă-dăv'ĕr) [L. *cadere,* to fall, die]

cadaveric (kă-dăv'ĕr-ĭk)

cadaverine (kă-dăv'ĕr-ĭn)

cadaverous (kă-dăv'ĕr-ŭs)

cadence (kā'dĕns)

cadmiosis (kăd-mē-ō'sĭs)

cadmium (kăd'mē-ŭm) [L. *cadmia,* calamine]

caduca (kă-dū'kă) [L. *caducus,* falling]

caduceus (kă-dū'sē-ŭs) [L., a herald's wand]

caelotherapy (sē"lō-thĕr'ă-pē) [L. *caelum,* heaven, + Gr. *therapeia,* treatment]

café au lait spot

Cafergot

caffeine (kăf'ēn, kă-fēn')

    c. and sodium benzoate

    c. and sodium salicylate

    c., citrate

caffeine poisoning

caffeinism (kăf'ēn-ĭzm)

Caffey, John (kăf'fē) [U.S. pediatrician, 1895–1966]

    C.'s disease

cage, Faraday

cage, thoracic

C.A.H.E.A. *Committee on Allied Health*

Education and Accreditation

cainotophobia (kī-nō″tō-fō′bē-ă) [Gr. *kainotes*, novelty, + *phobos*, fear]

caisson disease (kā′sŏn) [Fr. *caisse*, a box]

caked breast

Cal *large Calorie*

cal *small calorie*

calamine (kăl′ă-mīn)

calamus scriptorius [L.]

calcaneal, calcanean (kăl-kā′nē-ăl, -ăn) [L. *calcaneus*, heel]

calcaneoapophysitis (kăl-kā″nē-ō-ă-pŏf″ĕ-zī′tĭs) [″ + Gr. *apophysis*, offshoot, + *itis*, inflammation]

calcaneocuboid (kăl-kā″nē-ō-kū′boyd) [″ + Gr. *kubos*, cube, + *eidos*, form, shape]

calcaneodynia (kăl-kā″nē-ō-dĭn′ē-ă) [″ + Gr. *odyne*, pain]

calcaneofibular (kăl-kā″nē-ō-fĭb′ū-lăr) [″ + *fibula*, pin]

calcaneonavicular (kăl-kā″nē-ō-nă-vĭk′ū-lăr) [″ + *navicula*, boat]

calcaneoscaphoid (kăl-kā″nē-ō-skā′foyd) [″ + Gr. *skaphe*, skiff, + *eidos*, form, shape]

calcaneotibial (kăl-kā″nē-ō-tĭb′ē-ăl) [″ + *tibia*, shinbone]

calcaneum (kăl-kā′nē-ŭm) [L. *calcaneus*, heel]

calcaneus (kăl-kā′nē-ŭs) [L.]

calcanodynia (kăl″kăn-ō-dĭn′ē-ă) [″ + Gr. *odyne*, pain]

calcar (kăl′kăr) [L., a spur]

c. avis

c. femorale

c. pedis

calcareous (kăl-kā′rē-ŭs) [L. *calcarius*, of lime]

calcarine (kăl′kăr-īn) [L. *calcar*, spur]

calcariuria (kăl-kăr″ē-ū′rē-ă) [L. *calcarius*, of lime, + Gr. *ouron*, urine]

calcaroid (kăl′kăr-oyd) [L. *calcar*, spur, + Gr. *eidos*, form, shape]

calcemia (kăl-sē′mē-ă) [L. *calx*, lime, + Gr. *haima*, blood]

calcic (kăl′sĭk) [L. *calcarius*]

calcicosis (kăl″sĭ-kō′sĭs) [L. *calx*, lime,

+ Gr. *osis*, condition]

calciferol (kăl-sĭf′ĕr-ŏl)

calciferous (kăl-sĭf′ĕr-ŭs) [″ + *ferre*, to carry]

calcific (kăl-sĭf′ĭk) [″ + *facere*, to make]

calcification (kăl″sĭ-fĭ-kā′shŭn)

c., arterial

c., metastatic

c., Mönckeberg's

calcific tendinitis

calcigerous (kăl-sĭj′ĕr-ŭs) [″ + *gerere*, to bear]

Calcimar

calcination (kăl″sĭ-nā′shŭn) [L. *calcinare*, to char]

calcine (kăl′sīn)

calcinosis (kăl″sĭ-nō′sĭs) [L. *calx*, lime, + Gr. *osis*, condition]

c. circumscripta

calcipectic (kăl″sĭ-pĕk′tĭk) [″ + Gr. *pexis*, fixation]

calcipenia (kăl″sĭ-pē′nē-ă) [″ + Gr. *penia*, lack]

calcipexis, calcipexy (kăl″sĭ-pĕk′sĭs, -pĕk′sē) [″ + Gr. *pexis*, fixation]

calciphylaxis (kăl″sĭ-fĭ-lăk′sĭs) [″ + Gr. *phylaxis*, guard]

calciprivia (kăl″sĭ-prĭv′ē-ă) [″ + *privus*, without]

calcitonin (kăl″sĭ-tō′nĭn)

calcium (kăl′sē-ŭm) [L. *calx*, lime]

c. carbonate, precipitated

c. chloride

c. cyclamate

c. disodium edetate

c. gluconate

c. glycerophosphate

c. hydroxide

c. lactate

c. levulinate

c. mandelate

c. oxalate

c. oxide

c. pantothenate

c. phosphate, precipitated

c. saccharin

c. sulfate

c., total serum

c. tungstate
calcium antagonists
calcium channel blockers
Calcium Disodium Versenate
calciuria (kăl″sē-ū′rē-ă) [″ + Gr. *ouron*, urine]
calcophorous (kăl-kŏf′or-ŭs) [″ + Gr. *phoros*, bearing]
calcospherite (kăl″kŏ-sfē′rīt) [″ + Gr. *sphaira*, sphere]
calculary (kăl′kū-lā-rē) [L. *calculus*, pebble]
calculi (kăl′kū-lī)
calculifragous (kăl″kū-lĭf′ră-gŭs) [″ + *frangere*, to break]
calculogenesis (kăl″kū-lō-jĕn′ĕ-sĭs) [″ + Gr. *genesis*, generation, birth]
calculosis (kăl″kū-lō′sĭs) [″ + *osis*, condition]
calculous (kăl′kū-lŭs)
calculus (kăl′kū-lŭs) [L., pebble]
   c., biliary
   c., dental
   c., hemic
   c., pancreatic
   c., renal
   c., salivary
   c., urinary
   c., vesical
calefacient (kăl″ĕ-fā′shĕnt) [L. *calere*, to be warm, + *facere*, to make]
calf (kăf) [AS. *cealf*]
caliber (kăl′ĭ-bĕr) [Fr. *calibre*, diameter of bore of gun]
calibration (kăl-ĭ-brā′shŭn)
calibrator (kăl′ĭ-brā-tor)
caliceal (kăl″ĭ-sē′ăl) [Gr. *kalyx*, cup of a flower]
calicectasis (kăl″ĭ-sĕk′tă-sĭs) [″ + *ektasis*, dilatation]
calices
caliculus (kă-lĭk′ū-lŭs) [L., small cup]
   c. gustatorius
   c. ophthalmicus
caliectasis (kăl″ē-ĕk′tă-sĭs) [Gr. *kalyx*, cup of a flower, + *ektasis*, dilatation]
californium (kăl″ĭ-for′nē-ŭm) [Named for California, the state and university

where it was first discovered in 1950]
caligo (kă-lī′gō) [L., darkness]
caliper(s) (kăl′ĭ-pĕr) [Fr. *calibre*, diameter of bore of gun]
calisthenics (kăl″ĭs-thĕn′ĭks) [Gr. *kalos*, beautiful, + *sthenos*, strength]
calix (kā′lĭks) [Gr. *kalyx*, cup of a flower]
Calliphora vomitoria (kă-lĭf′ĕr-ă)
callisection [L. *callus*, hardened skin, + *sectio*, a cutting]
callomania (kăl″ō-mā′nē-ă) [Gr. *kalos*, beautiful, + *mania*, madness]
callosal (kă-lō′săl) [L. *callus*, hardened skin]
callosity, callositas (kă-lŏs′ĭ-tē, -ĭ-tăs) [L. *callosus*, hard]
callosomarginal (kă-lō″sō-măr′jĭ-năl) [L. *callus*, hardened skin, + *margo*, margin]
callosum (kă-lō′sŭm) [L. *callosus*, hard]
callous (kăl′ŭs)
callus (kăl′ŭs) [L., hardened skin]
   c., definitive
   c., provisional
calmative (kă′-, kăl′mă-tĭv)
Calmette's reaction (kăl-mĕtz′) [Albert Leon Charles Calmette, Fr. bacteriologist, 1863–1933]
calmodulins
calomel (kăl′ō-mĕl) [Gr. *kalos*, beautiful, + *melas*, black]
calor (kā′lor) [L., heat]
calorescence (kăl″or-ĕs′ĕns)
Calori's bursa (kăl-ō′rēz) [Luigi Calori, It. anatomist, 1807–1896]
caloric (kă-lor′ĭk) [L. *calor*, heat]
caloricity (kăl″or-ĭs′ĭ-tē)
calorie (kăl′ō-rē) [L. *calor*, heat]
   c., gram
   c., kilogram
   c., large
   c., small
calorifacient (kă-lor″ĭ-fā′shĕnt) [L. *calor*, heat, + *faciens*, making]
calorific (kăl″ō-rĭf′ĭk)
calorigenic (kă-lor″ĭ-jĕn′ĭk) [″ + Gr. *gennan*, to produce]
calorimeter (kăl″ō-rĭm′ĕ-tĕr) [″ + Gr. *metron*, measure]

c., bomb
c., respiration
calorimetry (kăl″ō-rĭm′ĕ-trē)
caloripuncture (kăl″ō-rĭ-pŭnk′chūr)
calory
calvaria (kăl-vā′rē-ă) [L., skull]
Calvé-Perthes disease (kăl-vā′pĕr′tās) [Jacques Calvé, Fr. orthopedist, 1875–1954; Georg C. Perthes, Ger. surgeon, 1869–1927]
calvities (kăl-vĭsh′ē-ēz) [L. *calvus,* bald]
calx (kălks) [L.]
c. chlorinata
c. sulfurata
calyces
calyciform (kă-lĭs′ĭ-form) [Gr. *kalyx,* cup of a flower, + L. *forma,* shape]
Calymmatobacterium granulomatis (kă-lĭm″mă-tō-băk-tē′rē-ŭm)
calyx (kā′lĭx) [Gr. *kalyx,* cup of a flower]
camera (kăm′ĕr-ă) [Gr. *kamara,* vault]
c. anterior bulbi
c. posterior bulbi
camisole (kăm′ĭ-sōl) [Fr., little shirt]
camomile
Camoquin Hydrochloride
CAMP *cyclic adenosine monophosphate*
camphor (kăm′for) [Malay, *kapur,* chalk]
camphorated
camphorated oil
camphoromania (kăm-for-ō-mā′nē-ă) [″ + Gr. *mania,* madness]
camphor poisoning
campimeter (kămp-ĭm′ĕ-tĕr) [L. *campus,* field, + Gr. *metron,* measure]
campimetry (kămp-ĭm′ĕ-trē)
campospasm (kăm′pō-spăzm)
camptocormia (kămp″tō-kor′mē-ă) [Gr. *kamptos,* flexible, + *kormos,* trunk]
camptodactylia (kămp″tō-dăk-tĭl′ē-ă) [″ + *dactylos,* finger]
camptomelic dwarfism
camptospasm (kămp′tō-spăzm) [″ + *spasmos,* a convulsion]

Campylobacter (kăm′pĭ-lō-băk′tĕr) [Gr. *kampylos,* curved, + *bakterion,* little rod]
C. fetus
C. jejuni
Canadian Nurses' Association
Canadian Nurses' Association Testing Service
canal (kă-năl′) [L. *canalis,* channel]
c., adductor
c., Alcock's
c., alimentary
c.'s, alveolar
c., alveolar, inferior
c., anal
c., auditory, external
c., auditory, internal
c., birth
c., carotid
c., central
c., cervical
c., cochlear, spiral
c., condylar
c., craniopharyngeal
c.'s dental
c.'s, ethmoidal
c., facial
c., femoral
c., gastric
c.'s, haversian
c., hyaloid
c., hypoglossal
c., incisive
c., infraorbital
c., inguinal
c., intestinal
c., lacrimal
c., mandibular
c., maxillary
c., medullary
c., nasolacrimal
c., Nuck's
c., nutrient
c., obturator
c., optic
c., pharyngeal
c., portal
c., pterygoid

c., pterygopalatine
c., pudendal
c., pulp
c., root
c., sacral
c., Schlemm's
c.'s, semicircular, bony
c.'s, semicircular, membranous
c., spinal
c., spiral, cochlear
c., spiral, of the modiolus
c., uterine
c., uterocervical
c., uterovaginal
c., vaginal
c., vertebral
c.'s, Volkmann's
canalicular (kăn″ă-lĭk′ū-lăr) [L. canali-cularis]
canaliculus (kăn″ă-lĭk′ū-lŭs) [L.]
canalis (kă-nā′lĭs) [L., channel]
canalization (kăn″ăl-ī-zā′shŭn)
canavanine (kă-năv′ă-nīn)
cancellated (kăn′sĕ-lāt″ĕd) [L. can-cellus, lattice]
cancelli (kăn-sĕl′ī)
cancellous (kăn′sĕl-ŭs)
cancellus (kăn-sĕl′ŭs) [L.]
cancer (kăn′sĕr) [L., crab, creeping ulcer]
c., bone
c., hard
c., lip
c., scirrhous
cancer cell
cancer clusters
cancer grading and staging
cancericidal (kăn″sĕr-ĭ-sī′dăl) [L. cancer, crab, + cida fr. caedere, to kill]
cancerigenic (kăn″sĕr-ĭ-jĕn′ĭk) [″ + Gr. gennan, to produce]
cancerogenic (kăn″sĕr-ō-jĕn′ĭk) [″ + Gr. gennan, to produce]
cancerophobia [″ + Gr. phobos, fear]
cancerous
cancra (kăng′kră)

cancriform (kăng′krĭ-form) [″ + forma, appearance]
cancroid (kăng′kroyd) [″ + Gr. eidos, form, shape]
cancrum (kăng′krŭm) [L. cancer, crab, creeping ulcer]
c. nasi
c. oris
c. pudendi
candela (kăn-dĕl′ă) [L. candela, candle]
candicidin (kăn″dĭ-sī′dĭn)
Candida (kăn′dĭ-dă) [L. candidus, glowing white]
C. albicans
candidiasis (kăn″dĭ-dī′ă-sīs)
candle [L. candela]
cane
canescent (kă-nĕs′ĕnt) [L. canus, gray]
cane sugar
canine (kā′nīn) [L. caninus, dog]
canities (kăn-ĭsh′ē-ēz) [L., gray hair]
c. unguium
canker (kăng′kĕr) [L. cancer, crab, creeping ulcer]
cannabis (kăn′ă-bĭs) [Gr. kannabis, hemp]
cannibalism
cannula (kăn′ū-lă) [L., a small reed]
c., nasal
cannulate (kăn′ū-lāt)
canthal (kăn′thăl) [Gr. kanthos, corner of the eye]
cantharidal (kăn-thăr′ĭ-dăl) [Gr. kanth-aris, beetle, + eidos, form, shape]
cantharides (kăn-thăr′ĭ-dēz)
Cantharis (kăn′thă-rĭs)
canthectomy (kăn-thĕk′tō-mē) [Gr. kanthos, corner of the eye, + ek-tome, excision]
canthi (kăn′thī)
canthitis (kăn-thī′tĭs) [″ + itis, in-flammation]
cantholysis (kăn-thŏl′ĭ-sĭs) [″ + lysis, dissolution]
canthoplasty (kăn′thō-plăs″tē) [″ + plassein, to form]
canthorrhaphy (kăn-thor′ă-fē) [″ + rhaphe, seam]

canthotomy (kăn-thŏt′ō-mē) [″ + tome, a cutting, slice]
canthus (kăn′thŭs) [Gr. kanthos, corner of the eye]
Cantil
CaO calcium oxide
Ca(OH)₂ calcium hydroxide
cap (kăp) [LL. cappa, hood]
   c., cradle
   c., knee
capacitance (kă-păs′ĭ-tăns) [L. capacitas, holding]
capacitation (kă-păs″ĭ-tā′shŭn)
capacitor (kă-păs′ĭ-tor)
capacity
CAPD continuous ambulatory peritoneal dialysis
capeline (kăp′ĕ-lĭn) [Fr., a hat]
Capgras' syndrome [Jean Marie Joseph Capgras, Fr. psychiatrist, 1873–1950]
capillarectasia (kăp″ĭ-lăr″ĕk-tā′sē-ă) [L. capillaris, hairlike, + Gr. ektasis, dilatation]
Capillaria (căp″ĭ-lăr′ē-ă)
   C. philippinensis
capillariasis (kăp″ĭ-lă-rī′ă-sĭs) [Capillaria + Gr. -iasis, state or condition of]
capillaries (kăp′ĭ-lā″rēz)
capillariography (kăp″ĭ-lăr″ē-ŏg′ră-fē) [L. cappillaris, hairlike, + Gr. graphein, to write]
capillaritis (kăp″ĭ-lăr-ī′tĭs) [″ + Gr. itis, inflammation]
capillarity (kăp″ĭ-lăr′ĭ-tē)
capillaropathy (kăp″ĭ-lăr-ŏp′ă-thē) [″ + Gr. pathos, disease, suffering]
capillaroscopy (kăp″ĭ-lăr-ŏs′kō-pē) [″ + Gr. skopein, to examine]
capillary (kăp′ĭ-lăr″ē) [L. capillaris, hairlike]
   c.'s, arterial
   c.'s, bile
   c.'s, blood
   c.'s, lymphatic
   c.'s venous
capillary attraction

capillary permeability
capillus (kă-pĭl′ŭs) [L., a hair]
capital [L. capitalis]
capitate (kăp′ĭ-tāt) [L. caput, head]
capitation fee (kăp″ĭ-tā′shŭn)
capitatum (kăp″ĭ-tā′tŭm)
capitellum (kăp″ĭ-tĕl′ŭm) [L., small head]
capitula [L.]
capitular (kă-pĭt′ū-lăr)
capitulum (kă-pĭt′ū-lŭm, kă-pĭch′ū-lŭm) [L., small head]
   c. fibulae
   c. humeri
   c. mallei
   c. stapedis
Caplan's syndrome [Anthony Caplan, Brit. physician, 1907–1976]
capnophilic (kăp-nō-fĭl′ĭk) [Gr. kapnos, smoke, + philein, to love]
capotement (kă-pōt-mŏn′) [Fr.]
Capoten
capping (kăp′ĭng)
capreomycin sulfate
capsicum (kăp′sĭ-kŭm)
capsid (kăp′sĭd)
capsitis (kăp-sī′tĭs) [L. capsa, box, + Gr. itis, inflammation]
capsomer (kăp′sō-mĕr) [″ + Gr. meros, part]
capsula [L., little box]
   c. articularis
   c. bulbi
   c. fibrosa perivascularis
   c. glomeruli
   c. lentis
capsulae (căp′sū-lē) [L.]
capsular
capsulation
capsule [L. capsula, little box]
   c., articular
   c., auditory
   c., bacterial
   c., Bowman's
   c., cartilage
   c., Glisson's
   c., glomerular
   c., joint

c., lens
c., nasal; c., optic; c., otic
c. of kidney
c. of Tenon
c., renal
c., suprarenal
c., temporomandibular joint
capsulectomy (kăp″sū-lĕk′tō-mē) [L. *capsula*, little box, + Gr. *ektome*, excision]
capsulitis (kăp″sū-lī′tĭs) [″ + Gr. *itis*, inflammation]
capsulociliary (kăp″sū-lō-sĭl′ē-ĕr-ē) [″ + *ciliaris*, pert. to the eyelashes]
capsulolenticular (kăp″sū-lō-lĕn-tĭk′ū-lăr) [″ + *lenticularis*, pert. to a lens]
capsuloplasty (kăp′sū-lō-plăs″tē) [″ + Gr. *plassein*, to mold]
capsulorrhaphy (kăp″sū-lor′ă-fē) [″ + Gr. *rhaphe*, seam]
capsulotome (kăp′sū-lō-tōm″) [″ + Gr. *tome*, a cutting, slice]
capsulotomy (kăp″sū-lŏt′ō-mē)
captopril
capture
c., ventricular
caput (kā′pŭt, kăp′ŭt) [L.]
c. gallinaginis
c. medusae
c. succedaneum
caramel (kăr′ă-mĕl, kăr′mĕl)
carbachol (kăr′bă-kōl)
carbamazepine (kăr-bă-măz′ĕ-pēn)
carbamide (kăr′bă-mīd, kăr-băm′ĭd)
carbaminohemoglobin (kăr-băm″ĭ-nō-hē″mō-glō′bĭn)
carbarsone (kăr′băr-sōn)
carbenicillin indanyl sodium (kăr″bĕn-ĭ-sĭl′ĭn)
carbidopa (kăr″bĭ-dō′pă)
carbinoxamine maleate (kăr″bĭn-ŏk′să-mēn)
Carbocaine
carbohydrase (kăr″bō-hī′drās)
carbohydrate (kăr″bō-hī′drāt) [L. *carbo*, carbon, + Gr. *hydor*, water]
carbohydrate loading

carbolic acid [L. *carbo*, carbon, + *oleum*, oil]
carbolism (kăr′bŏl-ĭzm)
carbolize (kăr′bŏl-īz)
carboluria (kăr″bō-lū′rē-ă) [″ + *oleum*, oil, + Gr. *ouron*, urine]
carbon [L. *carbo*, carbon]
carbon-14
carbonate (kăr′bŏn-āt) [L. *carbo*, carbon]
c. of soda
carbon dioxide
carbon dioxide combining power
carbon dioxide inhalation
carbon dioxide poisoning
carbon dioxide solid therapy
carbon dioxide test
carbonemia (kăr″bō-nē′mē-ă) [L. *carbo*, carbon, + Gr. *haima*, blood]
carbonic
c. acid
c. anhydrase
carbonize (kăr′bŏn-īz)
carbon monoxide
carbon monoxide poisoning
carbon tetrachloride (tĕt″ră-klō′rīd)
carbon tetrachloride poisoning
carbonuria (kăr″bō-nū′rē-ă) [L. *carbo*, carbon, + Gr. *ouron*, urine]
carbonyl (kăr′bŏn-ĭl) [″ + Gr. *hyle*, matter]
Carbowax
carboxyhemoglobin (kăr-bŏk″sē-hē″mō-glō′bĭn) [″ + Gr. *oxys*, acid, + *haima*, blood, + L. *globus*, sphere]
carboxyl (kăr-bŏk′sĭl)
carboxylase (kăr-bŏk′sī-lās)
carboxylation
carboxylic acids
carboxylmethylcellulose sodium
carbuncle, carbunculus (kăr′bŭng″k′l, kărbŭng′kū-lŭs) [L. *carbunculus*, small glowing ember]
carbuncular
carbunculosis (kăr-bŭng″kū-lō′sĭs) [″ + Gr. *osis*, condition]

carbutamide (kăr-bū'tă-mīd)
carcass (kăr'kăs)
carcinelcosis (kăr"sĭ-něl-kō'sĭs) [Gr.
karkinos, crab, + helkosis, ulceration]
carcinoembryonic **antigens**
(kăr"sĭn-ō-ĕm"brē-ŏn'ĭk)
carcinogen (kăr'sĭn-, kăr-sĭn'ō-jĕn)
c., chemical
carcinogenesis (kăr"sĭ-nō-jĕn'ĕ-sĭs)
[" + genesis, generation, birth]
carcinogenic (kăr"sĭ-nō-jĕn'ĭk)
carcinoid (kăr'sĭ-noid) [" + eidos,
form, shape]
carcinoid syndrome
carcinolysis (kăr"sĭ-nŏl'ĭ-sĭs) [Gr. karkinos, crab, + lysis, dissolution]
carcinolytic (kăr"sĭ-nō-lĭt'ĭk)
carcinoma (kăr"sĭ-nō'mă) [" +
oma, tumor]
c., alveolar cell
c., basal cell
c., bronchogenic
c., chorionic
c., cylindrical
c., embryonal
c., epidermoid
c., giant cell
c., glandular
c. in situ
c., lipomatous
c., medullary
c., melanotic
c., mucinous
c., oat cell
c., scirrhous
c., squamous-cell
carcinomatophobia (kăr"sĭ-nō"mă-
tō-fō'bē-ă) [Gr. karkinos, crab, +
oma, tumor, + phobos, fear]
carcinomatosis (kăr"sĭ-nō"mă-tō'sĭs)
[" + " + osis, condition]
carcinophilia (kăr"sĭ-nō-fĭl'ē-ă) [" +
philos, love]
carcinosarcoma (kăr"sĭ-nō-săr-kō'mă)
[" + sarx, flesh, + oma,
tumor]
c., embryonal

carcinosis (kăr"sĭ-nō'sĭs) [" + osis,
condition]
cardamom, cardamon [Gr. karda-
momon]
Cardarelli's sign (kăr"dă-rĕl'lēz) [An-
tonio Cardarelli, It. physician, 1831 –
1926]
cardia (kăr'dē-ă) [Gr. kardia, heart]
cardiac (kăr'dē-ăk) [L. cardiacus]
cardiac arrest
cardiac arrhythmia
cardiac atrophy
cardiac catheterization
cardiac compensation
cardiac cycle
cardiac failure
cardiac hypertrophy
cardiac insufficiency
cardiac massage
cardiac monitor
cardiac output
cardiac plexus
cardiac reflex
cardiac reserve
cardialgia (kăr"dē-ăl'jē-ă) [Gr. kardia,
heart, + algos, pain]
cardiaortic (kăr"dē-ā-or'tĭk) [" +
aorte, aorta]
cardiasthenia (kăr"dē-ăs-thē'nē-ă)
[" + astheneia, weakness]
cardiasthma (kăr"dē-ăz'mă) [" +
asthma, panting]
cardiectasia, cardiectasis (kăr"dē-
ĕk-tā'sē-ă, -ĕk'tă-sĭs) [" + ektasis,
dilatation]
cardiectomy (kăr"dē-ĕk'tō-mē) [" +
ektome, excision]
Cardilate
cardinal [LL. cardinalis, important]
cardio- [Gr. kardia, heart]
cardioaccelerator (kăr"dē-ō-ăk-
sĕl'ĕr-ă-tor) [" + L. accelerare, to
hasten]
cardioactive (kăr"dē-ō-ăk'tĭv) [" +
L. activus, acting]
cardioangiography (kăr"dē-ō-ăn"jē-
ŏg'ră-fē) [" + angeion, vessel,
+ graphein, to write]

cardioangiology (kăr″dē-ō-ăn″jē-ŏl′ō-jē) [″ + ″ + logos, word, reason]

cardioaortic (kăr″dē-ō-ā-or′tĭk) [″ + aorte, aorta]

cardiocatheterization (kăr″dē-ō-kăth″ĕ-tĕr-ĭ-zā′shŭn)

cardiocele (kăr′dē-ō-sēl) [″ + kele, tumor, swelling]

cardiocentesis (kăr″dē-ō-sĕn-tē′sĭs) [″ + kentesis, puncture]

cardiochalasia (kăr″dē-ō-kă-lā′zē-ă) [″ + chalasis, relaxation]

cardiocirrhosis (kăr″dē-ō-sĭr-rō′sĭs) [″ + kirrhos, orange-yellow, + osis, condition]

cardiodiaphragmatic (kăr″dē-ō-dī″ă-frăg-măt′ĭk)

cardiodilator (kăr″dē-ō-dī′lă-tor) [″ + L. dilatare, to enlarge]

cardiodynamics (kăr″dē-ō-dī-năm′ĭks)

cardiodynia kăr″dē-ō-dĭn′ē-ă) [Gr. kardia, heart, + odyne, pain]

cardioesophageal

cardioesophageal reflux

cardiogenesis (kăr″dē-ō-jĕn′ĕ-sĭs) [″ + genesis, generation, birth]

cardiogenic (kăr″dē-ō-jĕn′ĭk) [″ + gennan, to produce]

cardiogenic shock

cardiogram (kăr′dē-ō-grăm″) [″ + gramma, letter, piece of writing]

cardiograph (kăr′dē-ō-grăf″) [″ + graphein, to write]

cardiographic (kăr″dē-ō-grăf′ĭk)

cardiography (kăr″dē-ŏg′ră-fē)

cardiohepatic (kăr″dē-ō-hĕ-păt′ĭk) [″ + hepatos, liver]

cardiohepatomegaly (kăr″dē-ō-hĕp″ă-tō-mĕg′ă-lē) [″ + ″ + megas, large]

cardioinhibitory (kăr″dē-ō-ĭn-hĭb′ĭ-tō-rē) [″ + L. inhibere, to check]

cardiokinetic (kăr″dē-ō-kī-nĕt′ĭk) [″ + kinesis, motion]

cardiokymography

cardiolipin (kăr″dē-ō-lĭp′ĭn) [″ + lipos, fat]

cardiolith (kăr′dē-ō-lĭth″) [″ + lithos, stone]

cardiologist (kăr-dē-ŏl′ō-jĭst) [″ + logos, word, reason]

cardiology (kăr-dē-ŏl′ō-jē)

cardiolysin (kăr″dē-ŏl′ĭ-sĭn) [″ + lysis, dissolution]

cardiolysis (kăr-dē-ŏl′ĭ-sĭs)

cardiomalacia (kăr″dē-ō-mă-lā′shē-ă) [Gr. kardia, heart, + malakia, softening]

cardiomegaly (kăr″dē-ō-mĕg′ă-lē) [″ + megas, large]

cardiomotility (kăr″dē-ō-mō-tĭl′ĭ-tē) [″ + L. motilis, moving]

cardiomyoliposis (kăr″dē-ō-mī″ō-lĭp-ō′sĭs) [″ + mys, muscle, + lipos, fat, + osis, condition]

cardiomyopathy (kăr″dē-ō-mī-ŏp′ă-thē) [″ + ″ + pathos, disease, suffering]

   c., alcoholic

   c., congestive

   c., constrictive

   c., parasitic

   c., restrictive

cardiomyopexy (kăr″dē-ō-mī′ō-pĕk″sē) [″ + ″ + pexis, fixation]

cardiomyotomy

cardionecrosis (kăr″dē-ō-nĕ-krō′sĭs) [″ + nekrosis, state of death]

cardionecteur, cardionector (kăr″dē-ō-nĕk′tĕr) [″ + L. nektor, joiner]

cardionephric (kăr″dē-ō-nĕf′rĭk) [″ + nephros, kidney]

cardioneural (kăr″dē-ō-nū′răl) [″ + neuron, nerve]

cardioneurosis (kăr″dē-ō-nū-rō′sĭs) [″ + ″ + osis, condition]

cardiopathy (kăr″dē-ŏp′ă-thē) [″ + pathos, disease, suffering]

cardiopericarditis (kăr″dē-ō-pĕr″ĭ-kăr-dī′tĭs) [″ + peri, around, + kardia, heart, + itis, inflammation]

cardiophobia (kăr″dē-ō-fō′bē-ă) [″ + phobos, fear]

cardiophone (kăr′dē-ō-fōn) [″ + *phone,* voice]

cardioplasty (kăr″dē-ō-plăs′tē) [″ + *plassein,* to form]

cardioplegia (kăr″dē-ō-plē′jē-ă) [″ + *plege,* stroke]

cardiopneumatic (kăr″dē-ō-nū-măt′ĭk) [″ + *pneuma,* air]

cardiopneumograph (kăr″dē-ō-nū′mō-grăf) [″ + ″ + *graphein,* to write]

cardioptosis (kăr″dē-ŏp-tō′sĭs) [″ + *ptosis,* fall, falling]

cardiopulmonary (kăr″dē-ō-pŭl′mō-nĕr-ē) [″ + L. *pulmo,* lung]

cardiopulmonary arrest

cardiopulmonary resuscitation

cardiopuncture [″ + L. *punctura,* prick]

cardiopyloric (kăr″dē-ō-pī-lor′ĭk) [″ + *pyloros,* gatekeeper]

cardiorenal (kăr″dē-ō-rē′năl) [Gr. *kardia,* heart, + L. *renalis,* pert. to kidney]

cardiorrhaphy (kăr″dē-or′ă-fē) [″ + *rhaphe,* seam]

cardiorrhexis (kăr″dē-ō-rĕk′sĭs) [″ + *rhexis,* rupture]

cardiosclerosis (kăr″dē-ō-sklĕ-rō′sĭs) [″ + *sklerosis,* a hardening]

cardioscope (kăr′dē-ō-skōp) [″ + *skopein,* to examine]

cardioscopy (kăr″dē-ŏs′kō-pē)

cardiospasm (kăr′dē-ō-spăzm) [″ + *spasmos,* a convulsion]

cardiosphygmograph (kăr″dē-ō-sfĭg′mō-grăf) [″ + *sphygmos,* throb, + *graphein,* to write]

cardiosymphysis (kăr″dē-ō-sĭm′fĭ-sĭs) [″ + *symphysis,* growing together]

cardiotachometer (kăr″dē-ō-tăk-ŏm′ĕ-tĕr) [Gr. *kardia,* heart, + *tachos,* speed, + *metron,* measure]

cardiotherapy (kăr″dē-ō-thĕr′ă-pē) [″ + *therapeia,* treatment]

cardiothyrotoxicosis (kăr″dē-ō-thī″rō-tŏk″sĭ-kō′sĭs) [″ + *thyreos,* shield, + *toxikon,* poison, + *osis,* condition]

cardiotomy (kăr″dē-ŏt′ō-mē) [″ + *tome,* a cutting, slice]

cardiotonic (kăr″dē-ō-tŏn′ĭk) [″ + *tonos,* act of stretching, tension, tone]

cardiotoxic (kăr″dē-ō-tŏk′sĭk) [″ + *toxikon,* poison]

cardiovalvulitis (kăr″dē-ō-văl″vū-lī′tĭs) [″ + L. *valvula,* valve, + Gr. *itis,* inflammation]

cardiovalvulotome (kăr″dē-ō-văl′vū-lō-tōm″) [″ + ″ + Gr. *tome,* a cutting, slice]

cardiovascular (kăr″dē-ō-văs′kū-lăr) [″ + L. *vasculum,* small vessel]

cardiovascular reflex

cardiovasology (kăr″dē-ō-văs-ŏl′ō-jē) [″ + L. *vas,* vessel, + Gr. *logos,* word, reason]

cardioversion (kăr′dē-ō-vĕr″zhŭn) [″ + L. *versio,* a turning]

cardioverter (kăr′dē-ō-vĕr″tĕr)

carditis (kăr-dī′tĭs) [″ + *itis,* inflammation]
  c., Coxsackie
  c., rheumatic

Cardrase

C.A.R.F. *Commission on Accreditation of Rehabilitation Facilities*

caries (kăr′ēz, kăr′ĭ-ēz) [L., rottenness]
  c., arrested
  c., bottle mouth
  c., classification of
  c., dental
  c., necrotic
  c., radiation
  c., rampant
  c. sicca
  c., spinal

carina (kă-rī′nă) [L., keel of a boat]
  c. nasi
  c. tracheae
  c. urethralis

carinae (kă-rī′nē) [L.]

carinate (kăr′ĭ-nāt) [L. *carina,* keel of a boat]

cariogenesis (kăr″ē-ō-jĕn′ĕ-sĭs) [L.

caries, rottenness, + Gr. *genesis*, generation, birth]

cariogenic (kǎ″rē-ō-jĕn′ĭk) [″ + Gr. *gennan*, to produce]

carious (kǎ′rē-ŭs)

carisoprodol (kǎr″ĭ-sō-prō′dŏl)

carminative (kǎr-mĭn′ǎ-tĭv) [L. *carminativus*, cleanse]

carmustine

carnal (kǎr′nǎl) [L. *carnalis*, flesh]

carnal knowledge

carneous (kǎr′nē-ŭs) [L. *carneus*, fleshy]

carnitine (kǎr′nĭ-tĭn)

carnivore (kǎr′nĭ-vor)

carnivorous (kǎr-nĭv′ō-rŭs) [L. *carnivorus*]

carnophobia (kǎr″nō-fō′bē-ǎ) [″ + Gr. *phobos*, fear]

carnose (kǎr′nōs)

carnosine (kǎr′nō-sĭn)

carnosity (kǎr-nŏs′ĭ-tē) [L. *carnositas*, fleshiness]

carotenase (kǎr-ŏt′ĕ-nās) [Gr. *karoton*, carrot]

carotene (kǎr′ō-tēn) [Gr. *karoton*]

carotenemia (kǎr″ō-tĕ-nē′mē-ǎ) [″ + *haima*, blood]

carotenoid (kǎ-rŏt′ĕ-noyd) [″ + *eidos*, form, shape]

carotenosis [″ + *osis*, condition]

carotic (kǎ-rŏt′ĭk) [Gr. *karos*, deep sleep]

caroticotympanic (kǎ-rŏt″ĭ-kō-tĭm-pǎn′ĭk)

carotid (kǎ-rŏt′ĭd) [Gr. *karos*, deep sleep]

carotid body

carotid sinus

carotid siphon

carotidynia (kǎr-ŏt″ĭ-dĭn′ē-ǎ) [″ + *odyne*, pain]

carotin [Gr. *karoton*, carrot]

carotinase

carotinemia

carpal [Gr. *karpalis*]

carpale (kǎr-pǎ′lē) [Gr. *karpos*]

carpal tunnel

carpal tunnel syndrome

carpectomy (kǎr-pĕk′tō-mē) [″ + *ektome*, excision]

carphenazine maleate (kǎr-fĕn′ǎ-zēn)

carphologia, carphology (kǎr-fō-lō′jē-ǎ, -fŏl′ō-jē) [Gr. *karphos*, dry twig, + *legein*, to pluck]

carpo- [Gr. *karpos*]

carpometacarpal [″ + *meta*, beyond, + *karpos*, wrist]

carpopedal (kǎr″pō-pēd′ǎl) [″ + L. *ped*, foot]

carpopedal spasm

carpoptosis (kǎr″pŏp-tō′sĭs) [″ + *ptosis*, fall, falling]

carpus (kǎr′pŭs) [L.]

carrageen, carragheen (kǎr′ǎ-gēn)

Carrel-Dakin treatment (kǎr-ĕl′dǎ′kĭn) [Alexis Carrel, Fr.-U.S. surgeon, 1873–1944; Henry D. Dakin, U.S. chemist, 1880–1952]

carrier [O. Fr. *carier*, to bear]
   c., active
   c., convalescent
   c., genetic
   c., healthy
   c., incubatory
   c., intermittent
   c., passive

carrier-free (kǎr′ē-ĕr-frē)

Carrion's disease (kǎr-ē-ōnz′) [Daniel A. Carrion, a Peruvian student who lost his life after voluntarily taking an injection, 1850–1885]

car sickness

cartilage (kǎr′tĭ-lĭj) [L. *cartilago*, wickerwork]
   c., articular
   c., costal
   c., fibrous
   c., hyaline
   c., semilunar
   c., thyroid
   c., yellow

cartilaginification (kǎr″tĭ-lǎ-jĭn″ĭ-fĭ-kǎ′shŭn) [″ + *facere*, to make]

cartilaginoid (kǎr″tĭ-lǎj′ĭ-noyd) [″ + Gr. *eidos*, form, shape]

cartilaginous (kăr"tĭ-lăj'ĭ-nŭs)
cartilago (kăr"tĭ-lă'gō) [L.]
caruncle (kăr'ŭng-kl) [L. *caruncula*, small flesh]
   c., lacrimal
   c., sublingual
   c., urethral
caruncula (kăr-ŭng'kū-lă) [L.]
   c. hymenales
carver
   c., amalgam
   c., wax
cary-, caryo- [Gr. *karyon*, nucleus]
cascade (kăs-kād')
cascara sagrada (kăs-kăr'ă să-gră'dă)
case [L. *casus*, happening]
caseate (kā'sē-āt) [L. *caseus*, cheese]
caseation (kā"sē-ā'shŭn)
case control
case-control study
casefinding
case history
casein (kā'sē-ĭn) [L. *caseus*, cheese]
caseinogen (kā-sē-ĭn'ō-jĕn) [" + Gr. *gennan*, to produce]
caseous (kā'sē-ŭs)
CaSO₄ *calcium sulfate*
Casoni's reaction (kă-sō'nēz) [Tomaso Casoni, It. physician, 1880 – 1933]
cassette (kă-sĕt') [Fr., little box]
cast [ME. *casten*, to carry]
   c., blood
   c., body
   c., bronchial
   c., epithelial
   c., fatty
   c., fibrinous
   c., granular
   c., hyaline
   c., pseudo-
   c., pus
   c., urinary
   c., uterine
   c., waxy
Castellani's paint (kăs-tĕl-ăn'ēz) [Aldo Castellani, It. physician, 1878 – 1971]

Castle's intrinsic factor [William Bosworth Castle, U.S. physician and educator, b. 1897]
castor oil
castrate (kăs'trāt) [L. *castrare*, to prune]
castrated
castration (kăs-trā'shŭn)
   c., female
   c., male
   c., parasitic
castration anxiety or complex
casualty (kăz'ū-ăl-tē) [L. *casualis*, accidental]
casuistics (kăz-ū-ĭs'tĭks) [L. *casus*, chance]
cat
cata- [Gr. *kata*, down]
catabasis (kă-tăb'ă-sĭs) [Gr. *kata*, down, + *basis*, going]
catabatic (kăt-ă-băt'ĭk)
catabolic (kăt"ă-bŏl'ĭk)
catabolin (kă-tăb'ō-lĭn)
catabolism (kă-tăb'ō-lĭzm) [Gr. *katabole*, a casting down, + *-ismos*, condition]
catabolite (kă-tăb'ō-līt)
catacrotic (kăt"ă-krŏt'ĭk) [" + *krotos*, beat]
catacrotism (kă-tăk'rō-tĭzm) [" + " + *-ismos*, condition]
catadicrotic (kăt"ă-dĭ-krŏt'ĭk) [" + *dis*, twice, + *krotos*, beat]
catadicrotism (kăt"ă-dĭ'krō-tĭzm) [" + " + " + *-ismos*, condition]
catadioptric (kăt"ă-dĭ-ŏp'trĭk) [" + *diopsesthai*, to see through]
catagen (kăt'ă-jĕn) [" + *gennan*, to produce]
catagenesis (kăt"ă-jĕn'ĕ-sĭs) [" + *genesis*, generation, birth]
catalase (kăt'ă-lās)
catalepsy (kăt'ă-lĕp"sē) [Gr. *kata*, down, + *lepsis*, seizure]
cataleptic
cataleptiform (kăt-ă-lĕp'tĭ-form) [" + *lepsis*, seizure, + L. *forma*, shape]
cataleptoid (kăt"ă-lĕp'toyd) [" + " + *eidos*, form, shape]

catalysis (kă-tăl′ĭ-sĭs) [Gr. *katalyein*, to dissolve]

catalyst (kăt′ă-lĭst)

catalytic (kăt-ă-lĭt′ĭk) [Gr. *katalytikos*]

catalyze (kăt′ă-līz) [Gr. *katalyein*, to dissolve]

catalyzer (kăt′ă-lī-zĕr)

catamenia (kăt-ă-mē′nē-ă) [Gr. *kata*, according to, + *men*, month]

catamenial (kăt′′ă-mēn′ē-ăl)

catamnesis (kăt-ăm-nē′sĭs) [Gr. *kata*, down, + *mneme*, memory]

cataphasia (kăt-ă-fā′zē-ă) [″ + *phasis*, utterance]

cataphora (kă-tăf′ō-ră) [Gr. *kataphora*]

cataphoresis (kăt′′ă-fō-rē′sĭs) [Gr. *kata*, down, + *phoresis*, being carried]

cataphoria (kăt′′ă-fō′rē-ă) [″ + *pherein*, to bear]

cataphoric

cataphrenia (kăt′′ă-frē′nē-ă) [″ + *phrein*, mind]

cataphylaxis (kăt′′ă-fĭ-lăk′sĭs) [″ + *phylaxis*, guard]

cataplasia, cataplasis (kăt′′ă-plā′zē-ă, kă-tăp′lă-sĭs) [″ + *plassein*, to form]

cataplasm (kăt′ă-plăzm) [L. *cataplasma*]

cataplectic (kăt-ă-plĕk′tĭk) [″ + *plexis*, stroke]

cataplexy, cataplexia (kăt′ă-plĕks-ē, kăt-ă-plĕk′sē-ă)

Catapres

cataract (kăt′ă-răkt) [L. *cataracta*, waterfall]
  c., capsular
  c., hypermature
  c., immature
  c., lenticular
  c., morgagnian
  c., overripe
  c., radiation
  c., ripe
  c., senile

cataractogenic (kăt′′ă-răk′′tō-jĕn′ĭk) [L. *cataracta*, waterfall, + Gr. *gen-*

nan, to produce]

catarrh (kă-tăr′) [Gr. *katarrhein*, to flow down]
  c., dry

catarrhal (kă-tăr′ăl)

catatonia (kăt-ă-tō′nē-ă) [″ + *tonos*, act of stretching, tension, tone]
  c., Stauder's

catatonic

catatricrotic (kăt′′ă-trī-krŏt′ĭk) [″ + *treis*, three, + *krotos*, beat]

catatricrotism (kăt′′ă-trī′krō-tĭzm)

catatropia (kăt′′ă-trō′pē-ă) [″ + *tropos*, turning]

catchment area

cat-cry syndrome

catecholamines (kăt′′ē-kōl′ă-mēns)

catelectrotonus (kăt′′ē-lĕk-trŏt′ō-nŭs) [″ + *elektron*, amber, + *tonos*, act of stretching, tension, tone]

catenating (kăt′ĕn-āt′′ĭng) [L. *catena*, chain]

catenoid (kăt′ĕ-noyd) [″ + Gr. *eidos*, form, shape]

caterpillar sting

catfish sting

catgut
  c., chromic

catharsis (kă-thăr′sĭs) [Gr. *katharsis*, to cleanse, purify]

cathartic (kă-thăr′tĭk) [Gr. *kathartikos*, purging]

cathepsins (kă-thĕp′sĭns)

cathepsis (kă-thĕp′sĭs) [Gr. *kathepsis*, boiling down]

catheresis (kăth-ĕ-rē′sĭs) [Gr. *kathairesis*, destruction]

catheter (kăth′ĕ-tĕr) [Gr. *katheter*, something inserted]
  c., arterial
  c., cardiac
  c., central
  c., central venous
  c., condom
  c., double-channel
  c., elbowed
  c., eustachian
  c., female
  c., Foley

c., indwelling
c., intra-aortic
c., intravenous
c., Karman
c., male
c., pacing
c., prostatic
c., pulmonary artery
c., self-retaining
c., suprapubic
c., Swan-Ganz
c., Tenckhoff peritoneal
c., triple-lumen
c., vertebrated
c., winged

catheter fever
catheterization (kăth"ē-těr-ĭ-zā'shŭn) [Gr. katheterismos]
c., cardiac
c., urinary bladder
catheterize (kăth'ē-těr-īz)
cathexis (kă-thěk'sĭs) [Gr. kathexis, retention]
cathodal (kăth'ō-dăl) [Gr. kathodos, downward path]
cathode (kăth'ōd)
cathode stream
cathodic (kă-thŏd'ĭk)
cation (kăt'ĭ-ŏn) [Gr. kation, descending]
catlin (kăt'lĭn)
catoptric (kă-tŏp'trĭk) [Gr. katoptrikos, reflecting]
catoptrophobia (kăt"ŏp-trō-fō'bē-ă) [Gr. katoptron, mirror, + phobos, fear]
CAT scan
cat scratch disease
cat scratch fever
cat's eye pupil
cat's eye reflex
Caucasian
caucasoid
cauda (kaw'dă) [L.]
c. epididymidis
c. equina
c. helicis
c. pancreatis

c. striati
caudad (kaw'dăd) [L. cauda, tail, + ad, toward]
caudal (kawd'ăl) [L. caudalis]
caudate (kaw'dăt) [L. caudatus]
caudation (kaw-dā'shŭn) [L. cauda, tail]
caudocephalad (kaw-dō-sěf'ă-lăd) [" + Gr. kephale, head, + L. ad, toward]
caul (kawl) [O. Fr. cale, a small cap]
cauliflower ear
causalgia (kaw-săl'jē-ă) [" + algos, pain]
cause [L. causa]
c., antecedent
c., determining
c., predisposing
c., proximate
c., remote
c., ultimate
caustic (kaw'stĭk) [Gr. kaustikos, capable of burning]
cauterant (kaw'těr-ănt) [Gr. kauter, a burner]
cauterization (kaw"těr-ĭ-zā'shŭn) [Gr. kauteriazein, to burn]
c., chemical
c., electrical
cauterize (kaw'těr-īz)
cautery (kaw'těr-ē) [Gr. kauter, a burner]
cava (kā'vă)
caval (kā'văl)
cavalry bone
cavern (kăv'ěrn)
cavernitis (kăv"ěr-nī'tĭs) [L. caverna, hollow, + Gr. itis, inflammation]
cavernoma (kăv"ěr-nō'mă) [" + Gr. oma, tumor]
cavernositis (kăv"ěr-nō-sī'tĭs) [" + Gr. itis, inflammation]
cavernous (kăv'ěr-nŭs) [L. caverna, a hollow]
cavitary (kăv'ĭ-tā"rē)
cavitation [L. cavitas, hollow]
cavitis (kă-vī'tĭs) [" + Gr. itis, inflammation]
cavity (kăv'ĭ-tē) [L. cavitas, hollow]

c., abdominal
c., alveolar
c., amniotic
c., articular
c., body
c., buccal
c., cotyloid
c., cranial
c., dental
c., glenoid
c., oral
c., pelvic
c., pericardial
c., peritoneal
c., peritoneal, lesser
c., pleural
c., pulp
c., Rosenmüller's
c., serous
c., splanchnic
c., tympanic
c., uterine
cavity classification
cavity preparation
cavum (kā'vŭm) [L. *cavus*, a hollow]
c. abdominis
c. conchae
c. mediastinale
c. medullare
c. oris
c. pelvis
c. septi pellucidi
c. trigeminale
c. tympani
c. uteri
cavus (kā'vŭs) [L., hollow]
cayenne pepper (kī-ĕn', kā-ĕn')
C bar
CBC *complete blood count*
C.C. *chief complaint; Commission Certified*
cc *cubic centimeter*
CCl₃·CHO $CCl_3 \cdot CHO$ *chloral*
CCl₄ CCl_4 *carbon tetrachloride*
CCNU
CCRN
C.C.U. *coronary care unit*
Cd *cadmium*

CDC *Centers for Disease Control*
Ce *cerium*
cebocephalus (sē"bō-sĕf'ǎ-lŭs) [Gr. *kebos*, monkey, + *kephale*, head]
cecal (sē'kǎl) [L. *caecalis*, pert. to blindness]
cecectomy (sē-sĕk'tō-mē) [L. *caecum*, blindness, + Gr. *ektome*, excision]
cecitis (sē-sī'tĭs) [" + Gr. *itis*, inflammation]
cecocolopexy (sē"kō-kō'lō-pĕk"sē) [" + Gr. *kolon*, colon, + *pexis*, fixation]
cecocolostomy (sē"kō-kō-lŏs'tō-mē) [" + " + *stoma*, mouth, opening]
cecoileostomy (sē"kō-ĭl"ē-ŏs'tō-mē) [" + *ileum*, ileum, + Gr. *stoma*, mouth, opening]
Cecon
cecopexy (sē'kō-pĕk"sē) [" + Gr. *pexis*, fixation]
cecoplication (sē"kō-plī-kā'shŭn) [" + *plica*, fold]
cecoptosis (sē"kŏp-tō'sĭs) [" + Gr. *ptosis*, fall, falling]
cecosigmoidostomy (sē"kō-sĭg"moyd-ŏs'tō-mē) [" + Gr. *sigmoeides*, shaped like Gr. letter S, + *stoma*, mouth, opening]
cecostomy (sē-kŏs'tō-mē) [" + Gr. *stoma*, mouth, opening]
cecotomy (sē-kŏt'ō-mē) [" + Gr. *tome*, a cutting, slice]
cecum (sē'kŭm) [L. *caecum*, blindness]
Cedilanid
Cedilanid-D
Cefadyl
cefamandole nafate
cefoxitin sodium
Celbenin
-cele [Gr. *kele*, tumor, swelling; *koilia*, cavity, belly]
Celestone
celiac (sē'lē-ǎk) [Gr. *koilia*, cavity, belly]
celiac artery
celiac disease
celiac plexus

celiectomy (sē″lē-ěk′tō-mē) [″ + *ektome*, excision]

celiocentesis (sē″lē-ō-sěn-tē′sĭs) [″ + *kentesis*, puncture]

celiocolpotomy (sē″lē-ō-kōl-pŏt′ō-mē) [″ + *kolpos*, vagina, + *tome*, a cutting, slice]

celioenterotomy (sē″lē-ō-ěn″těr-ŏt′ō-mē) [″ + *enteron*, intestine, + *tome*, a cutting, slice]

celiogastrostomy (sē″lē-ō-gǎs-trŏs′tō-mē) [″ + *gaster*, stomach, + *stoma*, mouth, opening]

celiogastrotomy (sē″lē-ō-gǎs-trŏt′ō-mē) [Gr. *koilia*, cavity, belly, + *gaster*, stomach, + *tome*, a cutting, slice]

celiohysterectomy (sē″lē-ō-hĭs-těr-ěk′tō-mē) [″ + *hystera*, womb, + *ektome*, excision]

celiohysterotomy (sē″lē-ō-hĭs″těr-ŏt′ō-mē) [″ + ″ + *tome*, a cutting, slice]

celioma (sē-lē-ō′mǎ) [″ + *oma*, tumor]

celiomyalgia (sē″lē-ō-mī-ǎl′gē-ǎ) [″ + *mys*, muscle, + *algos*, pain]

celiomyomectomy (sē″lē-ō-mī″ō-měk′tō-mē) [″ + ″ + *oma*, tumor, + *ektome*, excision]

celiomyomotomy (sē″lē-ō-mī″ō-mŏt′ō-mē) [″ + ″ + ″ + *tome*, a cutting, slice]

celiomyositis (sē″lē-ō-mī″ō-sī′tĭs) [″ + ″ + *itis*, inflammation]

celioparacentesis (sē″lē-ō-pǎr″ǎ-sěn-tē′sĭs) [″ + *para*, alongside, past, beyond, + *kentesis*, puncture]

celiopathy (sē″lē-ŏp′ǎ-thē) [″ + *pathos*, disease, suffering]

celiorrhaphy (sē″lē-or′ǎ-fē) [″ + *rhaphe*, seam]

celiosalpingectomy (sē″lē-ō-sǎl″pĭn-jěk′tō-mē) [″ + *salpinx*, tube, + *ektome*, excision]

celioscope (sē′lē-ō-skōp) [″ + *sko-pein*, to examine]

celioscopy (sē″lē-ŏs′kō-pē)

celiotomy (sē″lē-ŏt′ō-mē) [″ + *tome*, a cutting, slice]
c., vaginal

celitis (sē-lī′tĭs) [″ + *itis*, inflammation]

cell [L. *cella*, a chamber]
c., acidophil
c., acinar
c., adipose
c., adventitial
c.'s, alpha
c.'s, argentaffin
c., band
c., basal
c., basket
c., basophil
c.'s, beta
c.'s, Betz
c., bipolar
c., blast
c., blood
c.'s, capsule
c., castration
c., centroacinar
c.'s, chief
c.'s, chromaffin
c., cleavage
c.'s, clue
c., columnar
c., cone
c., cuboid
c., daughter
c., endothelial
c., epithelial
c., ethmoidal
c., fat
c.'s, foam
c., ganglion
c., giant
c., glia
c., goblet
c., Golgi's
c.'s, granule
c., gustatory
c., HeLa
c., horizontal

c.'s, Hürthle
c., hybridoma
c., interstitial
c.'s, islet
c.'s, juxtaglomerular
c., Kupffer
c., L.E. *(lupus erythematosus)*
c.'s, Leydig's
c., littoral
c., lutein
c., mast
c.'s, mastoid
c.'s, microglia
c., mother
c., mucous
c., myeloma
c.'s, natural killer
c., nerve
c.'s, neuroglia
c., Niemann-Pick
c., olfactory
c., oxyntic
c., parent
c.'s, phalangeal
c., pigment
c.'s, plasma
c., prickle
c.'s, primordial
c., Purkinje's
c., pus
c., pyramidal
c., red
c., reticular
c.'s, reticuloendothelial
c., Rieder
c., rod
c.'s, rosette
c.'s, Rouget
c.'s, satellite
c., segmented
c., sensory
c.'s, septal
c., Sertoli
c., sickle
c., signet-ring
c., somatic
c., spider
c., squamous

c., stellate
c.'s, Sternberg-Reed; c.'s, Reed-Sternberg
c., stipple
c.'s, sympathicotrophic
c.'s, sympathochromaffin
c., target
c., tart
c., taste
c., totipotent
c., Touton giant
c., Türk's irritation
c., Tzanck
c., undifferentiated
c., visual
c., wandering
c., white
c.'s, zymogenic
cell bank
cell culture
cell cycle
cell division
cell-free
cell growth cycle
cell kill
cell kinetics
cell mass
cell membrane
cellobiose (sĕl″ō-bī′ōs)
cellophane (sĕl′ō-fān)
cell organelle
cell receptor
cellucidal (sĕl″ū-sī′dăl) [L. *cella*, a chamber, + *cida* fr. *caedere*, to kill]
cellula (sĕl′ū-lă) [L., little cell]
cellular (sĕl′ū-lăr)
cellular immunity
cellulase (sĕl′ū-lās)
cellulifugal (sĕl″ū-lĭf′ū-găl) [″ + *fugere*, to flee]
cellulipetal (sĕl″ū-lĭp′ĭ-tăl) [″ + *petere*, to seek]
cellulitis (sĕl-ū-lī′tĭs) [″ + Gr. *itis*, inflammation]
c., pelvic
cellulofibrous (sĕl″ū-lō-fī′brŭs) [″ + *fibra*, fiber]

celluloneuritis (sĕl"ū-lō-nū-rī'tĭs) [" + Gr. *neuron*, nerve, + *itis*, inflammation]
   c., acute anterior
cellulose (sĕl'ū-lōs) [L. *cellula*, little cell]
   c., oxidized
   c., sodium, carboxymethyl
cellulotoxic (sĕl"ū-lō-tŏk'sĭk) [" + Gr. *toxikon*, poison]
cell wall
celo- [Gr. *kele*, tumor, swelling; *koilia*, cavity, belly]
celology (sē-lŏl'ō-jē) [Gr. *kele*, tumor, swelling, + *logos*, word, reason]
celom, celoma (sē'lŏm, sē-lō'mă) [Gr. *koiloma*, a hollow]
celoschisis (sē-lŏs'kī-sĭs) [Gr. *koilia*, cavity, belly, + *schisis*, cleavage]
celoscope (sē'lō-skōp) [" + *skopein*, to examine]
celosomia (sē-lō-sō'mē-ă) [" + *soma*, body]
celozoic [" + *zoon*, animal]
Celsius scale (sĕl'sē-ŭs) [Anders Celsius, Swedish astronomer, 1701–1744]
cement (sē-mĕnt')
cementicle (sē-mĕn'tĭ-kl)
cementitis (sē"mĕn-tī'tĭs) [L. *cementum*, cement, + Gr. *itis*, inflammation]
cementoblast (sē-mĕn'tō-blăst) [" + Gr. *blastos*, germ]
cementoclasia (sē-mĕn"tō-klā'sē-ă) [" + Gr. *klasis*, breaking]
cementoclast (sē-mĕn'tō-klăst)
cementogenesis (sē-mĕn"tō-jĕn'ĕ-sĭs) [" + Gr. *genesis*, generation, birth]
cementoid (sē"mĕn'toyd) [" + Gr. *eidos*, form, shape]
cementoma (sē"mĕn-tō'mă) [" + Gr. *oma*, tumor]
cementum (sē-mĕn'tŭm) [L.]
cenesthesia (sē"nĕs-thē'zē-ă) [Gr. *koinos*, common, + *aisthesis*, feeling, perception]
cenesthesic, cenesthetic
cenesthopathia, cenesthopathy (sē-nĕs-, sĕn-ĕs-thō-păth'ē-ă, -thŏp'ă-thē) [" + " + *pathos*, disease, suffering]
Cenolate
cenosis (sĕn-ō', sē-nō'sĭs) [Gr. *kenos*, empty, + *osis*, condition]
cenosite (sĕn'ō-, sē'nō-sīt) [Gr. *koinos*, common, + *sitos*, food]
cenotic (sĕn-ŏt', sē-nŏt'ĭk) [Gr. *kenos*, empty]
cenotophobia (sĕn"ō-, sē"nō-tō-fō'bē-ă) [Gr. *kainotes*, novelty, + *phobos*, fear]
cenotype (sē'nō-, sĕn'ō-tīp) [" + *typos*, a type]
censor (sĕn'sĕr) [L. *censor*, judge]
center (sĕn'tĕr) [L. *centrum*, center]
   c., apneustic
   c., auditory
   c., autonomic
   c., Broca's
   c., burn
   c., cardioaccelerator
   c., cardioinhibitory
   c., chondrification
   c., ciliospinal
   c., community health
   c.'s, defecation
   c., deglutition
   c., epiotic
   c., feeding
   c., germinal
   c., gustatory
   c.'s, heat-regulating
   c., higher
   c., lower
   c., medullary
   c., micturition
   c., motor cortical
   c., neighborhood health
   c., nerve
   c., ossification
   c., pneumotaxic
   c., psychocortical
   c., reflex
   c., respiratory
   c., satiety
   c., speech
   c., suicide prevention

c., taste
c., temperature
c., thermoregulatory
c., trophic
c., vasoconstrictor
c., vasodilator
c., vasomotor
c., visual
c., Wernicke's
c., word

Centers for Disease Control

centesis (sĕn-tē'sĭs) [Gr. *kentesis*, puncture]

centigrade (sĕn'tĭ-grăd) [L. *centum*, a hundred, + *gradus*, a step]

centigram (sĕn'tĭ-grăm) [" + Gr. *gramma*, a small weight]

centiliter (sĕn'tĭ-lē-tĕr) [" + Gr. *litra*, measure of wt.]

centimeter (sĕn'tĭ-mē-tĕr) [" + Gr. *metron*, measure]

centinormal (sĕn'tĭ-nor'măl) [" + *norma*, rule]

centipede (sĕn'tĭ-pēd") [" + *pes*, foot]

centipoise (sĕn'tĭ-poyz)

centrad (sĕn'trăd) [Gr. *kentron*, center, + L. *ad*, toward]

central (sĕn'trăl)

central core disease

central I.V. line

central line

central nervous system

centraphose (sĕn'tră-fōz) [Gr. *kentron*, center, + *a*, not + *phos*, light]

centre

centriciput (sĕn-trĭs'ĭ-pŭt) [" + L. *caput*, head]

centrifugal (sĕn-trĭf'ū-găl) [" + L. *fugere*, to flee]

centrifugal force

centrifuge (sĕn'trĭ-fūj)
c., human

centrilobular (sĕn"trĭ-lŏb'ū-lăr)

centriole (sĕn'trē-ōl)

centripetal (sĕn-trĭp'ĕ-tăl) [" + L. *petere*, to seek]

centrocyte (sĕn'trō-sīt) [" + *kytos*, cell]

centrodesmus (sĕn-trō-dĕz'mŭs) [Gr. *kentron*, center, + *desmos*, a band]

centrolecithal (sĕn"trō-lĕs'ĭ-thăl) [" + *lekithos*, yoke]

centromere (sĕn'trō-mēr) [" + *meros*, part]

centrophose (sĕn'trō-fōz) [" + *phos*, light]

centrosclerosis (sĕn"trō-sklĕ-rō'sĭs) [" + *sklerosis*, a hardening]

centrosome (sĕn'trō-sōm) [" + *soma*, body]

centrosphere (sĕn'trō-sfēr) [" + *sphaira*, sphere]

centrostaltic (sĕn"trō-stăl'tĭk) [" + *stellein*, send forth]

centrum (sĕn'trŭm) [L.]
c. semiovale
c. tendineum

cephalad (sĕf'ă-lăd) [Gr. *kephale*, head, + L. *ad*, toward]

cephalalgia (sĕf-ă-lăl'jē-ă) [" + *algos*, pain]

cephalalgic (sĕf-ăl-ăl'jĭk)

cephalea (sĕf-ă-lē'ă) [Gr. *kephale*, head]

cephaledema (sĕf"ăl-ĕ-dē'mă) [" + *oidema*, swelling]

cephalexin (sĕf"ă-lĕk'sĭn)

cephalhematocele (sĕf"ăl-hē-măt'ō-sēl) [" + *haima*, blood, + *kele*, tumor, swelling]

cephalhematoma (sĕf"ăl-hē"mă-tō'mă) [" + " + *oma*, tumor]

cephalic (sĕ-făl'ĭk) [L. *cephalicus*]

cephalic index

cephalin (sĕf'ă-lĭn) [Gr. *kephale*, head]

cephalitis (sĕf"ăl-ī'tĭs) [" + *itis*, inflammation]

cephalocaudal pattern of development

cephalocele (sĕf'ă-lō-sēl) [" + *kele*, tumor, swelling]

cephalocentesis (sĕf"ă-lō-sĕn-tē'sĭs) [" + *kentesis*, puncture]

cephalodynia (sĕf"ă-lō-dĭn'ē-ă) [" + *odyne*, pain]
cephaloglycin (sĕf"ă-lō-glī'sĭn)
cephalogyric (sĕf"ă-lō-jī'rĭk) [" + *gyros*, a turn]
cephalohemometer (sĕf"ă-lō-hē-mŏm'ĕ-tĕr) [" + *haima*, blood, + *metron*, measure]
cephalomenia (sĕf"ă-lō-mē'nē-ă) [" + *men*, month]
cephalomeningitis (sĕf"ă-lō-mĕn"ĭn-jī'tĭs) [" + *meninx*, membrane, + *itis*, inflammation]
cephalometer (sĕf-ă-lŏm'ĕ-tĕr) [" + *metron*, measure]
cephalometry (sĕf"ă-lŏm'ĕ-trē)
cephalomotor (sĕf"ă-lō-mō'tor) [Gr. *kephale*, head, + L. *motus*, motion]
cephalone (sĕf'ă-lōn) [" + *on*, being]
cephalonia (sĕf"ă-lō'nē-ă)
cephalopathy (sĕf"ă-lŏp'ă-thē) [" + *pathos*, disease, suffering]
cephalopelvic (sĕf"ă-lō-pĕl'vĭk)
cephaloplegia (sĕf"ă-lō-plē'jē-ă) [" + *plege*, stroke]
cephalorhachidian (sĕf"ă-lō-ră-kĭd'ē-ăn) [" + *rhachis*, spine]
cephaloridine (sĕf"ă-lor'ĭ-dēn)
cephaloscope (sĕf'ă-lō-skōp) [" + *skopein*, to examine]
cephalosporin (sĕf"ă-lō-spor'ĭn)
cephalothin sodium (sĕf'ă-lō-thĭn")
cephalothoracic (sĕf"ă-lō-thō-răs'ĭk) [" + *thorakos*, chest]
cephalothoracopagus (sĕf"ă-lō-thō"ră-kŏp'ă-gŭs) [" + " + *pagos*, thing fixed]
cephalotome (sĕf'ă-lō-tōm) [" + *tome*, a cutting, slice]
cephalotomy (sĕf-ă-lŏt'ō-mē)
cephalotrypesis (sĕf"ă-lō-trĭp-ē'sĭs) [" + *trypesis*, a boring]
cephapirin sodium (sĕf-ă-pī'rĭn)
Cephulac
ceptor (sĕp'tor) [L. *receptor*, receiver]
  c., chemical
  c., contact
  c., distance
cera (sē'ră) [L.]
  c. alba
  c. flava
ceramics, dental [Gr. *keramos*, potter's clay]
ceramide (sĕr'ă-mĭd)
  c. oligosaccharides
ceramodontia (sē-răm"ō-dŏn'sheē-ă) [Gr. *keramos*, potter's clay, + *odous*, tooth]
cerate ceratum (sē'rāt) [L. *ceratum*]
ceratocele (sĕr'ă-tō-sēl) [Gr. *keras*, horn, + *kele*, tumor, swelling]
ceratotome (sĕ-răt'ō-tōm) [" + *tome*, a cutting, slice]
cercaria (sĕr-kā'rē-ă) [Gr. *kerkos*, tail]
cercaricide
cerclage (sār-klŏzh') [Fr., hooping]
  c., cervical
Cercomonas (sĕr-kŏm'ō-năs) [Gr. *kerkos*, tail, + *monas*, unit]
cercomoniasis (sĕr"kō-mō-nī'ă-sĭs)
cercus (sĕr'kŭs) [L., tail]
cerea flexibilitas (sē'rē-ă flĕk"sĭ-bĭl'ĭ-tăs) [L. *cera*, wax, + *flexibilitas*, flexibility]
cereals [L. *cerealis*, of grain]
cerebellar (sĕr-ĕ-bĕl'ăr) [L., little brain]
cerebellifugal (sĕr"ĕ-bĕl-ĭ-fū'găl) [" + *fugere*, to flee]
cerebellipetal (sĕr"ĕ-bĕl-lĭp'ĭ-tăl) [" + *petere*, to seek]
cerebellitis (sĕr"ĕ-bĕl-ī'tĭs) [" + Gr. *itis*, inflammation]
cerebellospinal (sĕr"ĕ-bĕl-ō-spī'năl) [" + *spina*, thorn]
cerebellum (sĕr-ĕ-bĕl'ŭm) [L.]
cerebral (sĕr'ĕ-brăl, sĕ-rē'brăl) [L. *cerebrum*, brain]
cerebral anoxia
cerebral hemorrhage
cerebral palsy
cerebral palsy feeder
cerebration (sĕr"ĕ-brā'shŭn) [L. *cerebratio*, brain activity]
cerebrifugal (sĕr"ĕ-brĭf'ū-găl) [L. *cerebrum*, brain, + *fugere*, to flee]

cerebripetal (sĕr″ĕ-brĭp′ĕ-tăl) [″ + petere, to seek]

cerebritis (sĕr″ĕ-brī′tĭs) [″ + Gr. itis, inflammation]

cerebroid (sĕr′ĕ-broyd) [″ + Gr. eidos, form, shape]

cerebromalacia (sĕr″ĕ-brō″mă-lā′shē-ă) [″ + Gr. malakia, softening]

cerebromedullary (sĕr″ĕ-brō-mĕd′ū-lă-rē)

cerebromeningitis (sĕr″ĕ-brō-mĕn″ĭn-jī′tĭs) [″ + Gr. meninx, membrane, + itis, inflammation]

cerebropathy (sĕr-ĕ-brŏp′ă-thē) [″ + pathos, disease, suffering]

cerebrophysiology (sĕr″ĕ-brō-fīz-ĕ-ŏl′ō-jē) [″ + Gr. physis, nature, + logos, word, reason]

cerebropontile (sĕr″ĕ-brō-pŏn′tĭl) [″ + pons, bridge]

cerebropsychosis (sĕr″ĕ-brō″sī-kō′sĭs) [″ + psyche, soul, mind, + osis, condition]

cerebrosclerosis (sĕr″ĕ-brō″sklĕ-rō′sĭs) [″ + Gr. sklerosis, a hardening]

cerebroscope (sĕr-ĕ′brō-skōp) [″ + Gr. skopein, to examine]

cerebroscopic (sĕr-ĕ″brō-skŏp′ĭk)

cerebroscopy (sĕr-ĕ-brŏs′kō-pē) [″ + Gr. skopein, to examine]

cerebrose (sĕr′ĕ-brōs)

cerebroside (sĕr′ĕ-brō-sīd″)

cerebrosidosis (sĕr″ĕ-brō″sī-dō′sĭs)

cerebrosis (sĕr″ĕ-brō′sĭs) [L. cerebrum, brain, + Gr. osis, condition]

cerebrospinal (sĕr″ĕ-brō-spī′năl) [″ + spina, thorn]

cerebrospinal axis

cerebrospinal fever

cerebrospinal fluid

cerebrospinal ganglia

cerebrospinal nerves

cerebrospinal puncture

cerebrosuria (sĕr″ĕ-brō-sū′rē-ă) [L. cerebrum, brain, + Gr. ouron, urine]

cerebrotomy (sĕr″ĕ-brŏt′ō-mē) [″ + Gr. tome, a cutting, slice]

cerebrovascular (sĕr″ĕ-brō-văs′kū-lăr) [″ + vasculum, vessel]

cerebrovascular accident

cerebrum (sĕr′ĕ-brŭm, sĕr-ē′brŭm) [L.]

Cerespan

cerium (sē′rē-ŭm) [L.]

ceroid (sē′royd)

ceroma (sē-rō′mă) [L. cera, wax, + Gr. oma, tumor]

ceroplasty (sē′rō-plăs″tē) [″ + Gr. plassein, to mold]

certifiable (sĕr″tĭ-fī′ă-b'l)

certification (sĕr″tĭ-fĭ-kā′shŭn)

ceruloderma (sĕ-roo″lō-dĕr′mă) [L. caeruleus, dark blue, + Gr. derma, skin]

ceruloplasmin (sĕ-roo″lō-plăz′mĭn)

cerumen (sĕ-roo′mĕn) [L. cera, wax]

ceruminal (sĕ-roo′mĭ-năl)

ceruminolysis (sĕ-roo″mī-nŏl′ĭ-sĭs)

ceruminolytic agent (sĕ-roo″mī-nō-lĭt′ĭk)

ceruminosis (sĕ-roo″mī-nō′sĭs) [″ + Gr. osis, condition]

ceruminous (sĕ-roo′mī-nŭs)

ceruminous glands

ceruse (sē′roos) [L. cerussa]

cervical (sĕr′vĭ-kăl) [L. cervicalis]

cervical cap

cervical nerves

cervical plexus

cervical ribs

cervical spondylosis

cervical vertebrae

cervicectomy (sĕr″vĭ-sĕk′tō-mē) [L. cervix, neck, + Gr. ektome, excision]

cervices

cervicitis (sĕr-vĭ-sī′tĭs) [″ + Gr. itis, inflammation]

cervico- (sĕr′vĭ-kō) [L. cervix]

cervicobrachial (sĕr″vĭ-kō-brā′kē-ăl) [″ + Gr. brachion, arm]

cervicocolpitis (sĕr″vĭ-kō-kŏl-pī′tĭs) [″ + Gr. kolpos, vagina, + itis, inflammation]

cervicodynia (sĕr″vĭ-kō-dĭn′ē-ă [″ +

Gr. *odyne*, pain]
cervicofacial (sĕr″vĭ-kō-fā′shē-ăl)
[″ + *facies*, face]
cervicovaginitis (sĕr″vĭ-kō-văj″ĭ-nī′tĭs)
[″ + *vagina*, sheath, + Gr.
itis, inflammation]
cervicovesical (sĕr″vĭ-kō-vĕs′ĭ-kăl)
[″ + *vesica*, bladder]
cervix (sĕr′vĭks) [L.]
c. uteri
c. vesicae
c.e.s. *central excitatory state*
cesarean hysterectomy (sē-sār′ē-
ăn) [L. *caesarea*, cut]
cesarean section
c.s., cervical
c.s., classic
c.s., extraperitoneal
c.s., low transverse
c.s., postmortem
cesarotomy (sēz″ă-rŏt′ō-mē) [″ +
Gr. *tome*, a cutting, slice]
cesium (sē′zē-ŭm) [L. *caesius*, sky blue]
cesspool
Cestan-Chenais syndrome (sĕs-
tăn′shĕn-ā′) [Raymond Cestan, Fr. neurologist, 1872–1934; Louis J.
Chenais, Fr. physician, 1872–1950]
Cestoda (sĕs-tōd′ă) [Gr. *kestos*, girdle]
cestode (sĕs′tōd) [″ + *eidos*, form,
shape]
cestodiasis (sĕs″tō-dī′ă-sĭs) [″ + ″
+ *-iasis*, state or condition of]
cestoid (sĕs′toyd) [″ + *eidos*, form,
shape]
Cestoidea (sĕs-toy′dē-ă)
Cetacort
Cetamide
Cetane
cetylpyridinium chloride
CF *Christmas factor; citrovorum factor*
Cf *Californium*
C.F.T. *complement fixation test*
C.G.S. *centimeter-gram-second*
CH₄ *methane*
C₂H₂ *acetylene*
C₂H₄ *ethylene*
C₆H₆ *benzene*

Chaddock's reflexes (chăd′ŏks)
[Charles G. Chaddock, U.S. neurologist, 1861–1936]
chafe (chāf) [O. Fr. *chaufer*, to warm]
chafing (chāf′ĭng)
Chagas' disease (chăg′ăs) [Carlos
Chagas, Braz. physician, 1879–
1934]
chain (chān) [O. Fr. *chaine*, chain]
c., food
chaining (chān′ĭng)
chair, birthing
chalasia (kă-lā′zē-ă) [Gr. *chalasis*, re-
laxation]
chalazion (kă-lā′zē-ŏn) [Gr. *khalaza*,
hailstone]
chalcosis (kăl-kō′sĭs) [Gr. *chalkos*, copper, + *osis*, condition]
chalice cell (chăl′ĭs) [Gr. *kalyx*, cup of a
flower]
chalicosis (kăl-ĭ-kō′sĭs) [Gr. *chalix*, lime-
stone, + *osis*, condition]
chalinoplasty (kăl′ĭ-nō-plăs″tē) [Gr.
chalinos, corner of mouth, + *plassein*, to mold]
challenge (chăl′ĕnj)
chalone (kăl′ōn) [Gr. *chalan*, to relax]
chamber (chăm′bĕr) [Gr. *kamara*,
vault]
c., altitude
c., anterior
c., aqueous
c., Boyden
c., hyperbaric
c., low pressure
c., posterior
c., pulp
c., vitreous
chamomile, camomile (kăm′ĕ-mĭl)
[Gr. *khamaemelon*, earth apple]
chancre (shăng′kĕr) [Fr., ulcer]
c., hard
c., simple
c., soft
c., true
chancroid (shăng′kroyd) [″ + Gr.
eidos, form, shape]
chancrous (shăng′krŭs)

change, fatty
change of life
channel
chapped (chăpt) [ME. *chappen*]
character (kăr'ăk-tĕr)
  c., acquired
  c., anal
  c., dominant
  c., primary sex
  c., recessive
  c., secondary sex
  c., sex-conditioned
  c., sex-limited
  c., sex-linked
characteristic (kăr"ăk-tĕr-ĭs'tĭk)
characteristic radiation
charbon (shăr-bŏn') [Fr., coal]
charcoal (chăr'kōl) [ME. *charcole*]
Charcot's joint (shăr-kōz') [Jean M.
  Charcot, Fr. neurologist, 1825–1893]
Charcot-Leyden crystals (shăr-
  kō'lī'dĕn) [Charcot; Ernest V. von Leyden, Ger. physician, 1832–1910]
Charcot-Marie-Tooth disease
  [Charcot; Pierre Marie, Fr. neurologist,
  1853–1940; Howard Tooth, Brit.
  physician, 1856–1926]
Charcot's triad
charge
  c., customary and reasonable
charlatan (shăr'lă-tăn) [It. *ciarlatano*]
charlatanry (shăr'lă-tăn-rē)
Charles' law (shărl) [Jacques A. C.
  Charles, Fr. physicist, 1746–1823]
charleyhorse
chart [L. *charta*, paper]
  c., dental
charta (kăr'tă) [L.]
charting
  c., dental
chartula (kăr'tū-lă) [L., small piece of
  paper]
chasma (kăz'mă) [Gr., a cleft]
chaude-pisse (shōd-pēs') [Fr.]
chauffage (shō-fŏzh') [O. Fr. *chaufer*,
  to heat]
chaulmoogra oil, chaulmugra,
  chaulmaugra (chŏl-moo'grŭ, chŏl-

mŏ'grŭ) [Bengali *caulmugra*]
Chaussier's areola (shō-sē-āz') [Fran-
  çois Chaussier, Fr. physician, 1746–
  1828]
chavicine (chăv'ĭ-sēn)
CHB *complete heart block*
Ch.B. *Bachelor of Surgery*
CHD *coronary heart disease*
check [O. Fr. *eschec*]
check bite
check-up
Chédiak-Higashi syndrome
  (shē'dē-ăk-hē-gă'shē) [A. Chédiak and
  O. Higashi, contemporary Cuban and
  Japanese physicians, respectively]
cheek [AS. *ceace*]
cheekbone
cheek retractor
cheilectomy (kī-lĕk'tō-mē) [Gr. *cheilos*,
  lip, + *ektome*, excision]
cheilectropion (kī"lĕk-trō'pē-ŏn)
  [" + *ektrope*, a turning aside]
cheilitis (kī-lī'tĭs) [" + *itis*, inflamma-
  tion]
  c. actinica
  c. exfoliativa
  c. glandularis
  c. venenata
cheilognathopalatoschisis (kī"lō-
  nā"thō-păl-ă-tŏs'kī-sĭs) [" +
  gnathos, jaw, + L. *palatum*, palate, + Gr. *schisis*, cleavage]
cheilophagia (kī"lō-fā'jē-ă) [" +
  phagein, to eat]
cheiloplasty (kī'lō-plăs"tē) [" +
  plassein, to form]
cheilorrhaphy (kī-lor'ă-fē) [" +
  rhaphe, seam]
cheiloschisis (kī-lŏs'kī-sĭs) [" +
  schisis, cleavage]
cheilosis (kī-lō'sĭs) [" + *osis*, condi-
  tion]
cheilostomatoplasty (kī"lō-stō-
  măt'ō-plăs"tē) [" + *stoma*, mouth,
  opening, + *plassein*, to form]
cheilotomy, chilotomy (kī-lŏt'ō-mē)
  [" + *tome*, a cutting, slice]
cheirognostic (kī"rŏg-nŏs'tĭk) [Gr.

cheir, hand, **+** *gnostikos,* knowing]
cheirology (kī-rŏl'ō-jē) [" **+** *logos,*
word, reason]
cheirospasm (kī'rō-spăsm) [" **+**
Gr. *spasmos,* a convulsion]
chelate (kē'lāt) [Gr. *chele,* claw]
chelating agent
chelation (kē-lā'shŭn) [Gr. *chele,* claw]
cheloid (kē'loyd) [Gr. *kele,* tumor, swelling, **+** *eidos,* form, shape]
chemabrasion (kĕm-ă-brā'shŭn)
chemexfoliation (kĕm'ĕks-fō'lē-
ā"shŭn)
chemical [Gr. *chemeia,* chemistry]
Chemical Abstract Service
chemical bond
chemical change
chemical compound
chemical element
chemical reflex
chemical warfare
chemiluminescence (kĕm"ĭ-loo"mĭ-
nĕs'ĕns)
chemise (shĕ-mēz') [LL. *camisa,* linen
shirt]
chemist (kĕm'ĭst)
chemistry [Gr. *chemeia,* chemistry]
   c., analytical
   c., biological
   c., general
   c., inorganic
   c., nuclear
   c., organic
   c., pathological
   c., pharmaceutical
   c., physical
   c., physiological
chemobiotic (kē"mō-bī-ŏt'ĭk)
chemocautery (kĕm"ō-kaw'tĕr-ē) [Gr.
chemeia, chemistry, **+** *kauterion,*
branding iron]
chemoceptor (kĕm'ō-sĕp-tĕr)
chemocoagulation (kē"mō-kō-ăg"ū-
lā'shŭn) [" **+** L. *coaglutio,* coagula-
tion]
chemodectoma (kē"mō-dĕk-tō'mă)
[" **+** *dektikos,* receptive, **+**
oma, tumor]

chemoluminescence (kē"mō-loo"mĭ-
nĕs'ĕns)
chemolysis (kē-mŏl'ĭ-sĭs) [" **+** *lysis,*
dissolution]
chemonucleolysis (kĕm"ō-nū-klē-ŏl'ĭ-
sĭs)
chemopallidectomy (kē"mō-păl"ĭ-
dĕk'tō-mē) [" **+** L. *pallidum,* globus
pallidus, **+** Gr. *ektome,* excision]
chemoprophylaxis (kē"mō-prō"fĭ-
lăk'sĭs)
chemopsychiatry (kē"mō-sī-kī'ă-trē)
chemoreceptor (kē"mō-rē-sĕp'tor)
[" **+** L. *recipere,* to receive]
chemoreflex (kē"mō-rē'flĕks) [" **+**
L. *reflectere,* to bend back]
chemoresistance (kē"mō-rē-zĭs'tăns)
chemosensitive (kē"mō-sĕn'sĭ-tĭv)
chemosensory (kē"mō-sĕn'sō-rē)
chemoserotherapy (kē"mō-sē"rō-
thĕr'ă-pē)
chemosis (kē-mō'sĭs) [Gr. *cheme,* cock-
leshell, **+** *osis,* condition]
chemosmosis (kē"mŏs-mō'sĭs)
chemosterilant (kē"mō-stĕr'ĭ-lănt)
chemosurgery
chemosynthesis (kē"mō-sĭn'thĕ-sĭs)
chemotactic (kē"mō-tăk'tĭk)
chemotaxis (kē"mō-tăk'sĭs) [Gr. *chemeia,* chemistry, **+** *taxis,* arrange-
ment]
chemothalamectomy (kē"mō-thăl-ă-
mĕk'tō-mē)
chemotherapeutic index
chemotherapy (kē"mō-thĕr'ă-pē)
[" **+** *therapeia,* treatment]
   c., combination
chemotic (kē-mŏt'ĭk)
chemotropism (kē-mŏt'rō-pĭzm)
[" **+** *tropos,* a turning]
chenodeoxycholic acid
chenopodium oil (kĕn-ō-pō'dē-ŭm)
[Gr. *chen,* goose, **+** *pous,* foot]
cherophobia (kē"rō-fō'bē-ă) [Gr.
chairein, to rejoice, **+** *phobos,*
fear]
cherry-red spot
cherubism (chĕr'ū-bĭzm)

chest [AS. *cest,* a box]
   c., emphysematous
   c., flail
   c., flat
   c., pigeon
chestnut, horse
chest prominences and depressions
chest P.T. *chest physical therapy*
chest regions
chest thump
Cheyne-Stokes respiration (chān'stōks') [John Cheyne, Scot. physician, 1777–1836; William Stokes, Irish physician, 1804–1878]
CHF *congestive heart failure*
Chiari's deformity (kē-ǎr'ēz)
Chiari-Frommel syndrome (kē-ǎr'ē-frŏm'měl) [H. Chiari, Austrian pathologist, 1851–1916; R. Frommel, Ger. gynecologist, 1854–1912]
chiasm, chiasma (kī'ǎzm, kī-ǎz'mǎ) [Gr. *khiasma,* cross]
   c., optic
chickenpox
chief complaint(s)
chiggers (chĭg'ěrs)
chigo, chigre (chē'gō, chē'grǎ) [Sp.]
chikungunya virus
chilblain (chĭl'blān) [AS. *cele,* cold, + *blegen,* to puff]
child [AS. *cild,* child]
child abuse
childbed
childbed fever
childbirth
   c., natural
   c., prepared
child neglect
childproof
chilectropion (kī"lěk-trō'pē-ŏn) [Gr. *cheilos,* lip, + *ektrope,* turning out]
chilitis (kī-lī'tĭs) [" + *itis,* inflammation]
chill (chĭl) [AS. *cele,* cold]
   c., nervous
chilo-, cheilo- [Gr. *cheilos,* lip]
chiloangioscopy (kī"lō-ǎn"jē-ŏs'kō-pē) [" + *angeion,* vessel, + *skopein,* to examine]
Chilomastix mesnili (kī"lō-mǎs'tĭks měs-nĭl'ē)
chimera (kī-mē'rǎ)
chimney sweeps' cancer
chimpanzee (chĭm-pǎn'zē)
chin [AS. *cin,* chin]
China clay
Chinese restaurant syndrome
chin jerk
chin reflex
chip
chiragra (kī-rǎg'rǎ) [Gr. *cheir,* hand, + *agra,* seizure]
chiralgia (kī-rǎl'jē-ǎ) [" + *algos,* pain]
   c. paresthetica
chirismus (kī-rĭs'mŭs)
chirognostic (kī"rŏg-nŏs'tĭk) [" + *gnostikos,* knowing]
chirokinesthesia (kī"rō-kĭn"ěs-thē'zē-ǎ) [" + *kinesis,* motion, + *aisthesis,* feeling, perception]
chiromegaly (kī"rō-měg'ǎ-lē) [" + *megas,* large]
chiroplasty (kī'rō-plǎs"tē) [" + *plassein,* to form]
chiropodist (kī-rŏp'ō-dĭst, kī-) [" + *pous,* foot]
chiropody (kī-rŏp'ō-dē)
chiropractic (kī"rō-prǎk'tĭk) [Gr. *cheir,* hand, + *prattein,* to do]
chiropractor
chirospasm (kī'rō-spǎzm) [" + *spasmos,* a convulsion]
chirurgery, chirurgia (kī-rŭr'jěr-ē, kī-rŭr'gē-ǎ)
chisel (chĭs'l)
chi-square (kī-skwār)
chitin (kī'tĭn) [Gr. *chiton,* tunic]
chitinous (kī'tĭ-nŭs)
Chlamydia (klǎ-mĭd'ē-ǎ) [Gr. *chlamys,* cloak]
chloasma (klō-ǎz'mǎ) [Gr. *chloazein,* to be green]
   c., gravidarum
   c., idiopathic

c., symptomatic

c. traumaticum

c. uterinum

chloracne (klor-ăk′nē)

chloral (klō′răl) [Gr. *chloras*, green]

chloral hydrate

chloral hydrate poisoning

chlorambucil (klō-răm′bū-sĭl)

chloramines (klō′ră-mīns)

chloramphenicol (klō″răm-fĕn′ĭ-kŏl)

chlorate (klō′rāt)

chlorbutanol

chlorbutol

chlorcyclizine hydrochloride

chlordane (klor′dăn)

chlordantoin (klor-dăn′tō-ĭn)

chlordiazepoxide hydrochloride (klor″dī-ăz″ĕ-pŏk′sīd)

chloremia (klō-rē′mē-ă) [Gr. *chloros*, green, + *haima*, blood]

chlorhexidene gluconate (klor-hĕk′sĭ-dēn)

chlorhydria (klor-hī′drē-ă) [″ + *hydor*, water]

chloride (klō′rīd) [Gr. *chloros*, green]

chloridemia (klō″rĭ-dē′mē-ă) [″ + *haima*, blood]

chloride poisoning

chloridimeter (klor-ĭ-dim′ĕ-tur)

chloriduria (klō″rĭ-dū′rē-ă) [″ + *ouron*, urine]

chlorinated (klō′rĭn-ā-tĕd)

chlorinated lime

chlorination (klō″rĭ-nā′shŭn)

chlorine (klō′rēn) [Gr. *chloros*, green]

chlorine preparations

chlorite (klō′rīt)

chlormerodrin Hg 197 (klor-mĕr′ō-drĭn)

chlormerodrin Hg 203

chloroazodin (klor-ō-ăz′ō-dĭn)

chlorobutanol (klō-rō-bū′tă-nŏl)

chloroform (klō′rō-form) [Gr. *chloros*, green, + L. *forma*, form]

chloroformism (klō′rō-form″ĭzm)

chloroleukemia (klō″rō-loo-kē′mē-ă) [″ + *leukos*, white, + *haima*, blood]

chloroma (klō-rō′mă) [″ + *oma*, tumor]

Chloromycetin (klō″rō-mī-sē′tĭn)

chloropenia (klō″rō-pē′nē-ă) [″ + *penia*, lack]

chloropenic (klō″rō-pēn′ĭk)

chlorophane (klō′rō-fān) [″ + *phainein*, to show]

chlorophenothane (klō″rō-fĕn′ō-thān)

chlorophyll, chlorophyl (klō′rō-fĭl) [″ + *phyllon*, leaf]

chloropia, chloropsia (klō-rō′pē-ă, klō-rŏp′sē-ă) [″ + *opsis*, sight, appearance, vision]

chloroplast, chloroplastid (klō′rō-plăst, klō″rō-plăs′tĭd) [″ + *plastos*, formed]

chloroprivic (klō″rō-prĭv′ĭk) [″ + L. *privare*, to deprive of]

chloroprocaine hydrochloride (klō″rō-prō′kăn)

chloroquine hydrochloride (klō′rō-kwīn)

chlorosis (klō-rō′sĭs) [″ + *osis*, condition]

chlorothiazide sodium (klō″rō-thī′ă-zīd)

chlorothymol (klō″rō-thī′mōl)

chlorotic (klō-rŏt′ĭk)

chlorotrianisene (klō″rō-trī-ăn′ĭ-sēn)

chlorpheniramine maleate (klor″fĕn-ĭr′ă-mēn)

chlorphenoxamine hydrochloride (klor″fĕn-ŏk′să-mēn)

chlorpromazine (klor-prō′mă-zēn)

chlorpromazine poisoning

chlorpropamide (klor-prō′pă-mīd)

chlorprothixene (klor-prō-thĭks′ēn)

chlorquinaldol (klor-kwĭn′ăl-dŏl)

chlortetracycline hydrochloride (klor″tĕt-ră-sī′klēn)

chlorthalidone (klor-thăl′ĭ-dōn)

Chlor-Trimeton

chlorzoxazone (klor-zŏk′să-zōn)

Ch.M. *chirurgiae magister*, Master of Surgery

choana (kō′ă-nă) [Gr. *choane*, funnel]

choanoid (kō'ăn-oyd) [" + *eidos*, form, shape]

choke [ME. *choken*]

choked disk

chokes

choke-saver

choking [ME. *choken*, to suffocate]

choking on food

cholagogue (kō'lă-gŏg) [Gr. *chole*, bile, + *agein*, to lead forth]

Cholan-DH

cholangiectasis (kō-lăn"jē-ĕk'tă-sĭs) [" + *angeion*, vessel, + *ektasis*, dilatation]

cholangiocarcinoma (kō-lăn"jē-ō-kăr"sĭ-nō'mă) [" + " + *karkinos*, crab, + *oma*, tumor]

cholangioenterostomy (kō-lăn"jē-ō-ĕn"tĕr-ŏs'tō-mē) [" + " + *enteron*, intestine, + *stoma*, mouth, opening]

cholangiogastrostomy (kō-lăn"jē-ō-găs-trŏs'tō-mē) [" + " + *gaster*, stomach, + *stoma*, mouth, opening]

cholangiography (kō-lăn"jē-ŏg'ră-fē) [" + " + *graphein*, to write]

cholangiole (kō-lăn'jē-ōl) [" + " + *ole*, dim. suffix]

cholangiolitis (kō-lăn"jē-ō-lī'tĭs) [" + " + " + Gr. *itis*, inflammation]

cholangioma (kō-lăn-jē-ō'mă) [" + *angeion*, vessel, + *oma*, tumor]

cholangiostomy (kō"lăn-jē-ŏs'tō-mē) [" + " + *stoma*, mouth, opening]

cholangiotomy (kō"lăn-jē-ŏt'ō-mē) [" + " + *tome*, a cutting, slice]

cholangitis (kō"lăn-jī'tĭs) [" + *angeion*, vessel, + *itis*, inflammation]

cholanopoiesis (kō"lă-nō-poy-ē'sĭs) [Gr. *chole*, bile, + *ano*, upward, + *poiesis*, making]

cholate (kō'lāt)

cholecalciferol (ko"lē-kăl-sĭf'ĕr-ŏl)

cholecyst (kō'lē-sĭst) [" + *kystis*, bladder]

cholecystagogue (kō"lē-sĭs'tă-gŏg)

[" + " + *agogos*, leader]

cholecystalgia (kō"lē-sĭs-tăl'jē-ă) [" + " + *algos*, pain]

cholecystangiography (kō"lē-sĭs"tăn-jē-ŏg'ră-fē) [" + " + *angeion*, vessel, + *graphein*, to write]

cholecystectasia (kō"lē-sĭs-tĕk-tā'zē-ă) [" + " + *ektasis*, dilatation]

cholecystectomy (kō"lē-sĭs-tĕk'tō-mē) [" + " + *ektome*, excision]

cholecystenterorrhaphy (kō"lē-sĭs-tĕn"tĕr-or'ă-fē) [" + " + *enteron*, intestine, + *rhaphe*, seam]

cholecystenterostomy (kō"lē-sĭs-tĕn"tĕr-ŏs'tō-mē) [" + " + *enteron*, intestine, + *stoma*, mouth, opening]

cholecystic (kō"lē-sĭs'tĭk)

cholecystitis (kō"lē-sĭs-tī'tĭs) [Gr. *chole*, bile, + *kystis*, bladder, + *itis*, inflammation]

cholecystnephrostomy (kō"lē-sĭst"nē-frŏs'tō-mē) [" + *kystis*, bladder, + *nephros*, kidney, + *stoma*, mouth, opening]

cholecystocolostomy (kō"lē-sĭs"tō-kō-lŏs'tō-mē) [" + " + *kolon*, colon, + *stoma*, mouth, opening]

cholecystocolotomy (kō"lē-sĭs"tō-kō-lŏt'ō-mē) [" + " + " + *tome*, a cutting, slice]

cholecystoduodenostomy (kō"lē-sĭs"tō-dū"ō-dē-nŏs'tō-mē) [" + " + L. *duodeni*, twelve, + Gr. *stoma*, mouth, opening]

cholecystogastrostomy (kō"lē-sĭs"tō-găs-trŏs'tō-mē [" + " + *gaster*, belly, + *stoma*, mouth, opening]

cholecystogram (kō"lē-sĭs'tō-grăm) [" + " + *gramma*, letter, piece of writing]

cholecystography (kō"lē-sĭs-tŏg'ră-fē) [" + " + *graphein*, to write]

cholecystoileostomy (kō"lē-sĭs"tō-ĭl-ē-ŏs'tō-mē) [" + *kystis*, bladder,

+ L. *ileum*, ileum, + Gr. *stoma*, mouth, opening]

cholecystojejunostomy (kō″lē-sĭs″tō-jĕ-jū-nŏs′tō-mē) [″ + ″ + L. *jejunum*, empty, + Gr. *stoma*, mouth, opening]

cholecystokinin (kō″lē-sĭs″tō-kī′nĭn) [″ + ″ + *kinein*, to move]

cholecystolithiasis (kō″lē-sĭs″tō-lĭ-thī′ă-sĭs) [″ + ″ + *lithos*, stone, + *-iasis*, state or condition of]

cholecystolithotripsy (kō″lē-sĭs″tō-lĭth′ō-trĭp″sē) [″ + ″ + ″ + *tripsis*, a rubbing, friction]

cholecystomy (kō″lē-sĭs′tō-mē) [Gr. *chole*, bile, + *kystis*, bladder, + *tome*, a cutting, slice]

cholecystopathy (kō″lē-sĭs-tŏp′ă-thē) [″ + ″ + *pathos*, disease, suffering]

cholecystopexy (kō″lē-sĭs′tō-pĕk″sē) [″ + ″ + *pexis*, fixation]

cholecystoptosis (kō″lē-sĭs-tō-tō′sĭs) [″ + ″ + *ptosis*, fall, falling]

cholecystorrhaphy (kō″lē-sĭs-tor′ă-fē) [″ + *kystis*, bladder, + *rhaphe*, seam]

cholecystostomy (kō″lē-sĭs-tŏs′tō-mē) [″ + ″ + *stoma*, mouth, opening]

cholecystotomy (kō″lē-sĭs-tŏt′ō-mē) [″ + ″ + *tome*, a cutting, slice]

choledochal (kō-lē-dŏk′ăl) [″ + *dochos*, receptacle]

choledochectasia (kō-lĕd″ō-kĕk-tā′zē-ă) [″ + ″ + *ektasis*, distention]

choledochectomy (kō-lĕd″ō-kĕk′tō-mē) [″ + ″ + *ektome*, excision]

choledochitis (kō″lē-dō-kī′tĭs) [″ + ″ + *itis*, inflammation]

choledochoduodenostomy (kō-lĕd″ō-kō-dū-ō-dē-nŏs′tō-mē) [″ + ″ + L. *duodeni*, twelve, + Gr. *stoma*, mouth, opening]

choledochoenterostomy (kō-lĕd″ō-kō-ĕn-tĕr-ŏs′tō-mē) [″ + ″ + *enteron*, intestine, + *stoma*, mouth,

opening]

choledochography (kō-lĕd″ō-kŏg′ră-fē) [″ + *dochos*, receptacle, + *graphein*, to write]

choledochojejunostomy (kō-lĕd″ō-kō-jĕ-jū-nŏs′tō-mē) [″ + ″ + L. *jejunum*, empty, + Gr. *stoma*, mouth, opening]

choledocholith (kō-lĕd′ō-kō-lĭth″) [″ + ″ + *lithos*, stone]

choledocholithiasis (kō-lĕd″ō-kō-lĭ-thī′ă-sĭs) [″ + ″ + *lithos*, stone, + *-iasis*, state or condition of]

choledocholithotomy (kō-lĕd″ō-kō-lĭth-ŏt′ō-mē) [″ + ″ + ″ + *tome*, a cutting, slice]

choledocholithotripsy (kō-lĕd′ō-kō-lĭth″ō-trĭp-sē) [″ + ″ + ″ + *tripsis*, a rubbing, friction]

choledochoplasty (kō-lĕd′ō-kō-plăs″tē) [Gr. *chole*, bile, + *dochos*, receptacle, + *plassein*, to form]

choledochorrhaphy (kō-lĕd″ō-kor′ă-fē) [″ + ″ + *rhaphe*, seam]

choledochostomy (kō-lĕd″ō-kŏs′tō-mē) [″ + ″ + *stoma*, mouth, opening]

choledochotomy (kō″lĕd-ō-kŏt′ō-mē) [″ + ″ + *tome*, a cutting, slice]

choledochus (kō-lĕd′ō-kŭs) [″ + *dochos*, receptacle]

choleic (kō-lē′ĭk)

cholelith (kō′lē-lĭth) [″ + *lithos*, stone]

cholelithiasis (kō″lē-lĭ-thī′ă-sĭs) [″ + *-iasis*, state or condition of]

cholelithic (kō″lē-lĭth′ĭk)

cholelithotomy (kō″lē-lĭ-thŏt′ō-mē) [″ + *lithos*, stone, + *tome*, a cutting, slice]

cholelithotripsy, cholelithotrity (kō″lē-lĭth′ō-trĭp-sē, kō″lē-lĭ-thŏt′rĭ-tē) [″ + ″ + *tripsis*, a rubbing, friction]

cholemesis (kō-lĕm′ĕ-sĭs) [″ + *emein*, to vomit]

cholemia (kō-lē′mē-ă) [″ + *haima*, blood]

cholepathia (kō″lē-păth′ē-ă) [″ +

pathos, disease, suffering]
  c. spastica
choleperitoneum (kō″lē-pĕr″ĭ-tō-
nē′ŭm) [″ + peri, around, +
teinein, to stretch]
cholepoiesis (kō″lē-poy-ē′sĭs) [″ +
poiein, to make]
cholera (kŏl′ĕr-ă) [L. cholera, bilious di-
arrhea]
  c. sicca
choleragen (kŏl′ĕr-ă-gĕn)
cholerase (kŏl′ĕr-ās)
choleresis (kŏl-ĕr-ē′sĭs, kō-lĕr′ĕ-sĭs)
[Gr. chole, bile, + hairesis, re-
moval]
choleretic (kŏl-ĕr-ĕt′ĭk)
choleric (kŏl′ĕr-ĭk)
choleriform (kŏl-ĕr′ĭ-form) [L. cholera,
+ forma, shape]
cholerigenous, cholerigenic (kŏl-ĕr-
ĭj′ĕn-ŭs, kŏl″ĕr-ĭ-jĕn′ĭk) [″ + Gr.
gennan, to produce]
cholerine (kŏl′ĕr-ĭn)
choleroid (kŏl′ĕr-oyd) [″ + Gr.
eidos, form, shape]
choleromania (kŏl″ĕr-ō-mā′nē-ă)
[″ + Gr. mania, madness]
cholerophobia (kŏl″ĕr-ō-fō′bē-ă)
[″ + Gr. phobos, fear]
cholestasia (kō″lē-stā′zē-ă) [Gr. chole,
bile, + stasis, standing still]
cholestatic
cholesteatoma (kō″lē-stē″ă-tō′mă)
[″ + steatos, fat, + oma, tumor]
cholesteremia, cholesterolemia
(kō-lĕs″tĕ-rē′mē-ă, kō-lĕs″tĕr-ŏl-ē′mē-
ă) [″ + stereos, solid, +
haima, blood]
cholesterin (kō-lĕs′tĕr-ĭn)
cholesterinemia (kō-lĕs″tĕr-ĭn-
ē′mē-ă)
cholesterinuria (kō-lĕs″tĕr-ĭn-ū′rē-ă) [″
+ stereos, solid, + ouron, urine]
cholesterohydrothorax (kō-lĕs″tĕr-
ō-hī″drō-thō′răks) [″ + ″ +
hydor, water, + thorax, chest]
cholesterol (kō-lĕs′tĕr-ŏl) [″ +
stereos, solid]

cholesteroluria (kō-lĕs″tĕr-ŏl-ū′rē-ă)
[″ + ″ + ouron, urine]
cholesterosis (kō-lĕs-tĕr-ō′sĭs) [″ +
″ + osis, condition]
cholestyramine resin (kō″lē-stī′ră-
mĭn)
choletelin (kō-lĕt′ĕl-ĭn) [″ + telos,
end]
choletherapy (kō″lē-thĕr′ă-pē) [″ +
therapeia, treatment]
choleuria (kō″lē-ū′rē-ă) [″ +
ouron, urine]
choleverdin (kō″lē-vĕr′dĭn) [″ + L.
viridis, green]
cholic acid (kō′lĭk)
choline (kō′lĭn, -lēn) [Gr. chole, bile]
cholinergic (kō″lĭn-ĕr′jĭk) [″ +
ergon, work]
cholinergic fibers
cholinesterase (kō″lĭn-ĕs′tĕr-ās)
cholinoceptive (kō″lĭn-ō-sĕp′tĭv)
[″ + L. receptor, receiver]
cholinolytic (kō″lĭn-ō-lĭt′ĭk) [″ +
lysis, dissolution]
cholinomimetic (kō″lĭ-nō-mĭ-mĕt′ĭk)
[″ + mimetikos, imitating]
cholochrome (kō′lō-krōm) [″ +
chroma, color]
chologenic (kō″lō-jĕn′ĭk) [″ + gennan, to produce]
cholohemothorax (kō″lō-hĕm″ō-
thō′răks) [″ + haima, blood, +
thorax, chest]
chololith (kŏl′ō-lĭth) [″ + lithos,
stone]
chololithiasis (kŏl″ō-lĭth-ī′ăs-ĭs) [″ +
″ + -iasis, state or condition of]
cholorrhea (kŏl″ō-rē′ă) [″ + rhein,
to flow]
Choloxin
choluria (kō-lū′rē-ă) [″ + ouron,
urine]
chondral (kŏn′drăl) [Gr. chondros, car-
tilage]
chondralgia (kŏn-drăl′jē-ă) [″ +
algos, pain]
chondralloplasia (kŏn″drăl-ō-plā′zē-
ă) [″ + allos, other, + plas-

sein, to form]

chondrectomy (kŏn-drĕk'tō-mē)
[" + *ektome,* excision]

chondric (kŏn'drĭk) [Gr. *chondros,* cartilage]

chondrification (kŏn-drĭ-fĭ-kā'shŭn)
[" + L. *facere,* to make]

chondrigen (kŏn'drĭ-jĕn) [" + *gennan,* to produce]

chondrin (kŏn'drĭn) [Gr. *chondros,* cartilage]

chondritis (kŏn-drī'tĭs) [" + *itis,* inflammation]

chondroadenoma (kŏn"drō-ăd-ē-nō'mă) [" + *aden,* gland, + *oma,* tumor]

chondroangioma (kŏn"drō-ăn-jē-ō'ma) [" + *angeion,* vessel, + *oma,* tumor]

chondroblast (kŏn'drō-blăst) [" + *blastos,* germ]

chondroblastoma (kŏn"drō-blăs-tō'mă) [" + " + *oma,* tumor]

chondrocalcinosis (kŏn"drō-kăl"sĭn-ō'sĭs) [" + L. *calx,* lime, + Gr. *osis,* condition]

chondroclast (kŏn'drō-klăst) [" + *klastos,* broken into bits]

chondrocostal (kŏn"drō-kŏs'tăl) [" + L. *costa,* rib]

chondrocranium (kŏn-drō-krā'nē-ŭm) [" + *kranion,* head]

chondrocyte (kŏn'drō-sīt) [" + *kytos,* cell]

chondrodermatitis nodularis chronica helicis

chondrodynia (kŏn"drō-dĭn'ē-ă) [" + *odyne,* pain]

chondrodysplasia (kŏn"drō-dĭs-plā'zē-ă) [" + Gr. *dys,* bad, difficult, painful, disordered, + *plasis,* a molding]

chondrodystrophy (kŏn"drō-dĭs'trō-fē) [" + " + *trophe,* nourishment]

chondroendothelioma (kŏn"drō-ĕn"dō-thē"lē-ō'mă) [" + *endon,* within, + *thele,* nipple, +

oma, tumor]

chondroepiphysitis (kŏn"drō-ĕp"ĭ-fĭz-ī'tĭs) [" + *epiphysis,* a growing on, + *itis,* inflammation]

chondrofibroma (kŏn"drō-fĭ-brō'mă) [" + L. *fibra,* fiber, + Gr. *oma,* tumor]

chondrogen (kŏn'drō-jĕn) [Gr. *chondros,* cartilage, + *gennan,* to produce]

chondrogenesis (kŏn"drō-jĕn'ĕ-sĭs) [" + *genesis,* generation, birth]

chondrogenic (kŏn"drō-jĕn'ĭk)

chondroid (kŏn'droyd) [" + *eidos,* form, shape]

chondroitin (kŏn-drō'ĭ-tĭn)

chondrolipoma (kŏn-drō-lĭp-ō'mă) [" + *lipos,* fat, + *oma,* tumor]

chondrology (kŏn-drŏl'ō-jē) [" + *logos,* word, reason]

chondrolysis (kŏn-drŏl'ĭ-sĭs) [" + *lysis,* dissolution]

chondroma (kŏn-drō'mă) [" + *oma,* tumor]

chondromalacia (kŏn-drō-măl-ā'shē-ă) [" + *malakia,* softness]

chondromatosis (kŏn"drō-mă-tō'sĭs) [" + *oma,* tumor, + *osis,* condition]

chondromatous (kŏn-drŏm'ă-tŭs) [" + *oma,* tumor]

chondromucin (kŏn"drō-mū'sĭn)

chondromucoid (kŏn"drō-mū'koyd) [" + L. *mucus,* mucus, + Gr. *eidos,* form, shape]

chondromucoprotein (kŏn"drō-mū"kō-prō'tē-ĭn) [" + " + *protos,* first]

chondromyoma (kŏn"drō-mī-ō'mă) [" + *mys,* muscle, + *oma,* tumor]

chondromyxoma (kŏn"drō-mĭks-ō'mă) [" + *myxa,* mucus, + *oma,* tumor]

chondromyxosarcoma (kŏn-drō-mĭk"sō-săr-kō'mă) [" + " + *sarx,* flesh, + *oma,* tumor]

chondro-osseus (kŏn"drō-ŏs'ē-ŭs) [" + L. *osseus,* bony]

chondro-osteodystrophy (kŏn"drō-

ŏs"tē-ō-dĭs'trō-fē) [" + *osteon*,
bone, + *dys*, bad, difficult, painful,
disordered, + *trophe*, nourish-
ment]
chondropathology   (kŏn"drō-pă-
thŏl'ō-jē) [Gr. *chondros*, cartilage, +
pathos, disease, suffering, +
logos, word, reason]
chondropathy (kŏn-drŏp'ă-thē)
chondroplasia   (kŏn"drō-plā'zē-ă)
[" + *plassein*, to mold]
chondroplast (kŏn'drō-plăst)
chondroplasty   (kŏn'drō-plăs"tē)
[" + *plassein*, to mold]
chondroporosis   (kŏn"drō-pō-rō'sĭs)
[" + *poros*, passage]
chondroproteins   (kŏn-drō-prō'tē-ĭns)
[" + *protos*, first]
chondrosarcoma   (kŏn-drō-săr-kō'mă)
[" + *sarx*, flesh, + *oma*,
tumor]
chondrosin (kŏn'drō-sĭn)
chondrosis (kŏn-drō'sĭs) [" + *osis*,
condition]
chondrosternal   (kŏn"drō-stĕr'năl)
[" + *sternon*, chest]
chondrosternoplasty   (kŏn"drō-
stĕr'nō-plăs"tē) [" + " + *plassein*, to mold]
chondrotome (kŏn'drō-tōm) [" +
tome, a cutting, slice]
chondrotomy (kŏn-drŏt'ō-mē)
chondroxiphoid   (kŏn"drō-zī'foyd)
[" + *xiphos*, sword, + *eidos*,
form, shape]
Chondrus [NL. fr. Gr. *chondros*, grain,
cartilage]
Chopart's amputation   (shō-pärz')
[François Chopart, Fr. surgeon, 1743–
1795]
chorda (kor'dă) [Gr. *chorde*, cord]
    c. dorsalis
    c. gubernaculum
    c. obliqua
    c. tympani
    c. umbilicalis
    c. vocalis
    c. willisii

chordae tendineae   (kor'dē tĕn-
dĭn'ē-ē)
chordal (kor'dăl)
Chordata (kor-dā'tă) [LL., notochord]
chordee (kor-dē') [Fr., corded]
chorditis (kor-dī'tĭs) [Gr. *chorde*, cord,
    + *itis*, inflammation]
    c. nodosa
chordoma (kor-dō'mă) [" + *oma*,
tumor] .
chordotomy (kor-dŏt'ō-mē) [" +
tome, a cutting, slice]
chorea (kō-rē'ă) [Gr. *choreia*, dance]
    c., acute
    c., Bergeron's
    c., chronic
    c., electric
    c., epidemic
    c., gravidarum
    c., Henoch's
    c., hereditary
    c., Huntington
    c., hyoscine
    c., mimetic
    c. minor
    c., posthemiplegic
    c., senile
    c., Sydenham's
choreal (kō-rē'al, kō'rē-ăl)
choreic (kō-rē'ĭk)
choreiform (kō-rē'ĭ-form) [Gr. *choreia*,
dance, + L. *forma*, form]
choreoathetoid   (kō"rē-ō-ăth'ĕ-toyd)
[" + *athetos*, not fixed, +
eidos, form, shape]
choreoathetosis   (kō"rē-ō-ăth"ĕ-
tō'sĭs) [" + " + *osis*, condition]
choreomania   (kō"rē-ō-mă'nē-ă)
[" + *mania*, madness]
choreophrasia (kō-rē"ō-frā'zē-ă) ["
    + *a-*, not, + *phrasis*, diction]
chorioadenoma   (kō"rē-ō-ăd"ĕn-
ō'mă) [Gr. *chorion*, outer membrane
enclosing an embryo, + *aden*,
gland, + *oma*, tumor]
    c. destruens
chorioallantois (kō"rē-ō-ă-lăn'tō-ĭs)
chorioamnionitis (kō"rē-ō-ăm"nē-ō-

nī′tĭs) [″ + *amnion*, lamb, + *itis*, inflammation]

chorioangioma (kō″rē-ō-ăn-jē-ō′mă) [″ + *angeion*, vessel, + *oma*, tumor]

choriocapillaris (kō″rē-ō-kăp-ĭl-lā′rĭs) [Gr. *choroeides*, resembling a membrane, + L. *capillaris*, hairlike]

choriocarcinoma (kō″rē-ō-kăr″sĭ-nō′mă) [Gr. *chorion*, chorion, + *karkinoma*, cancer]

choriocele (kō′rē-ō-sēl) [Gr. *choroeides*, resembling a membrane, + *kele*, tumor, swelling]

chorioepithelioma (kō″rē-ō-ĕp″ĭ-thē″lē-ō′mă)

choriogenesis (kō″rē-ō-jĕn′ĕ-sĭs) [Gr. *chorion*, chorion, + *genesis*, generation, birth]

chorioid (kō′rē-oyd)

chorioma (kō″rē-ō′mă) [″ + *oma*, tumor]

choriomeningitis (kō″rē-ō-mĕn″ĭn-jī′tĭs) [″ + *meninx*, membrane, + *itis*, inflammation]
   c., lymphocytic

chorion (kō′rē-ŏn) [Gr.]
   c. frondosum
   c. laeve

chorionepithelioma (kō″rē-ŏn-ĕp″ĭ-thē″lē-ō′mă) [″ + *epi*, on, + *thele*, nipple, + *oma*, tumor]

chorionic (kō-rē-ŏn′ĭk)

chorionic plate

chorionic villi

chorionic villus sampling

chorionitis (kō″rē-ŏn-ī′tĭs) [″ + *itis*, inflammation]

chorioretinal (kō″rē-ō-rĕt′ĭ-năl)

chorioretinitis (kō″rē-ō-rĕt″ĭn-ī′tĭs) [Gr. *chorioeides*, skinlike, + L. *rete*, network, + Gr. *itis*, inflammation]

chorista (kō-rĭs′tă) [Gr. *choristos*, separated]

choristoma (kō-rĭs-tō′mă) [″ + *oma*, tumor]

choroid (kō′royd) [Gr. *chorioeides*, skinlike]

choroideremia (kō-roy-dĕr-ē′mē-ă)

[″ + *eremia*, destitution]

choroiditis (kō″royd-ī′tĭs) [″ + *itis*, inflammation]
   c., anterior
   c., areolar
   c., central
   c., diffuse
   c., exudative
   c. guttata senilis
   c., metastatic
   c., suppurative
   c., Tay's

choroidocyclitis (kō-roy″dō-sĭk-lī′tĭs) [Gr. *chorioeides*, skinlike, + *kyklos*, a circle, + *itis*, inflammation]

choroidoiritis (kō-royd″ō-ī-rī′tĭs) [″ + *iris*, bend, turn, + *itis*, inflammation]

choroidopathy (kō″roy-dŏp′ă-thē) [″ + *pathos*, disease, suffering]

choroidoretinitis (kō-royd″ō-rĕt″ĭn-ī′tĭs) [″ + L. *rete*, network, + Gr. *itis*, inflammation]

choromania (kō″rō-mā′nē-ă) [Gr. *choros*, dance, + *mania*, madness]

Christian Science

Christian-Weber disease [Henry A. Christian, U.S. physician, 1876 – 1951; Frederick P. Weber, Brit. physician, 1863 – 1962]

Christmas disease [*Christmas*, name of the first patient with the disease who was studied]

Christmas factor

chromaffin (krō-măf′ĭn) [Gr. *chroma*, color, + L. *affinis*, having affinity for]

chromaffin cells

chromaffinoma (krō″măf-ĭ-nō′mă) [″ + ″ + Gr. *oma*, tumor]

chromaffinopathy (krō″măf-ĭn-ŏp′ă-thē) [″ + ″ + Gr. *pathos*, disease, suffering]

chromaffin reaction

chromaffin system

chromaphil (krō′mă-fĭl) [″ + *philein*, to love]

chromate (krō′māt) [Gr. *chromatos*, color]

chromatic (krō-măt′ĭk)

chromatid (krō′mă-tĭd)
chromatin (krō′mă-tĭn) [Gr. _chroma,_ color]
   c., sex
chromatin-negative
chromatinolysis (krō″mă-tĭn-ŏl′ĭ-sĭs) [″ + _lysis,_ dissolution]
chromatinorrhexis (krō″mă-tĭn-or-rĕk′sĭs) [″ + _rhexis,_ rupture]
chromatin-positive
chromatism (krō′mă-tĭzm) [″ + _-ismos,_ condition]
chromatogenous (krō″mă-tŏj′ĕn-ŭs) [″ + _gennan,_ to produce]
chromatogram (krō-măt′ō-grăm) [″ + _gramma,_ letter, piece of writing]
chromatography (krō″mă-tŏg′ră-fē) [″ + _graphein,_ to write]
   c., adsorption
   c., column
   c., gas
   c., gas-liquid
   c., high-performance liquid
   c., paper
   c., partition
   c., thin layer
chromatoid (krō′mă-toyd) [Gr. _chroma,_ color, + _eidos,_ form, shape]
chromatokinesis (krō″mă-tō-kĭ-nē′sĭs) [″ + _kinesis,_ motion]
chromatolysis (krō″mă-tŏl′ĭ-sĭs) [″ + _lysis,_ dissolution]
chromatometer (krō-mă-tŏm′ĕt-ĕr) [″ + _metron,_ measure]
chromatophil, **chromatophilic** (krō′mă-tō-fĭl″, krō″mă-tō-fĭl′ĭk) [″ + _philein,_ to love]
chromatophore (krō-măt′ō-for) [″ + _phoros,_ bearing]
chromatopsia (krō″mă-tŏp′sē-ă) [″ + _opsis,_ sight, appearance, vision]
chromatoptometry (krō″măt-ŏp-tŏm′ĕ-trē) [″ + _optos,_ visible, + _metron,_ measure]
chromatosis (krō″mă-tō′sĭs) [″ + _osis,_ condition]
chromaturia (krō-mă-tū′rē-ă) [″ + _ouron,_ urine]

chromesthesia (krō″mĕs-thē′zē-ă) [″ + _aisthesis,_ feeling, perception]
chromicize (krō′mĭ-sīz)
chromidiosis (krō-mĭd-ē-ō′sĭs)
chromidium (krō-mĭd′ē-ŭm) [″ + _-idion,_ a dim. termination]
chromidrosis, **chromhidrosis** (krō″mĭd-rō′sĭs) [″ + _hidros,_ sweat]
chromium (krō′mē-ŭm) [L., color]
chromium poisoning
chromoblast (krō′mō-blăst) [Gr. _chroma,_ color, + _blastos,_ germ]
chromocenter (krō′mō-sĕn″tĕr) [″ + _kentros,_ middle]
chromocrinia (krō″mō-krĭn′ē-ă) [″ + _krinein,_ to separate]
chromocystoscopy (krō″mō-sĭs-tŏs′kō-pē) [″ + _kystis,_ bladder, + _skopein,_ to examine]
chromocyte (krō′mō-sīt) [″ + _kytos,_ cell]
chromocytometer (krō″mō-sī-tŏm′ĕt-ĕr) [″ + ″ + _metron,_ measure]
chromodacryorrhea (krō″mō-dăk″rē-ō-rē′ă) [″ + _dacryon,_ tear, + _rhein,_ to flow]
chromogen (krō′mō-jĕn) [″ + _gennan,_ to produce]
chromogenesis (krō″mō-jĕn′ĕ-sĭs) [″ + _genesis,_ generation, birth]
chromogenic (krō″mō-jĕn′ĭk)
chromolipoid (krō″mō-lĭp′oyd) [″ + _lipos,_ fat, + _eidos,_ form, shape]
chromolysis (krō-mŏl′ĭ-sĭs) [″ + _lysis,_ dissolution]
chromomere (krō′mō-mēr) [Gr. _chroma,_ color, + _meros,_ part]
chromometer (krō-mŏm′ĕ-tĕr) [″ + _metron,_ measure]
chromometry (krō-mŏm′ĕt-rē)
chromomycosis (krō″mō-mī-kō′sĭs) [″ + _myxa,_ mucus, + _osis,_ condition]
chromoparic (krō-mō-păr′ĭk) [″ + L. _parere,_ to beget, produce]
chromopexic, **chromopectic** (krō″mō-pĕk′sĭk, -pĕk′tĭk) [″ + _pexis,_ fixation]
chromophane (krō′mō-fān) [″ +

phainein, to show]

chromophil(e) (krō'mō-fĭl, -fīl) [" + *philein*, to love]

chromophilic,   chromophilous (krō-mō-fĭl'ĭk, krō-mŏf'ĭl-ŭs)

chromophobe (krō'mō-fōb) [" + *phobos*, fear]

chromophobia (krō"mō-fō'bē-ă)

chromophobic (krō-mō-fō'bĭk)

chromophore (krō'mō-for) [" + *pherein*, to bear]

chromophoric (krō"mō-for'ĭk) [" + *pherein*, to bear]

chromophose (krō'mō-fōz) [" + *phos*, light]

chromophytosis (krō"mō-fī-tō'sĭs) [" + *phyton*, plant, + *osis*, condition]

chromoplasm (krō'mō-plăzm) [" + LL. *plasma*, form, mold]

chromoplastid [" + *plastos*, formed]

chromoprotein (krō"mō-prō'tē-ĭn) [" + *protos*, first]

chromopsia [" + *opsis*, sight, appearance, vision]

chromoptometer (krō"mŏp-tŏm'ĕ-tĕr) [" + *opsis*, sight, appearance, vision, + *metron*, measure]

chromoradiometer [" + L. *radius*, ray, + Gr. *metron*, measure]

chromoscope (krō'mō-skōp) [" + *skopein*, to examine]

chromoscopy (krō-mŏs'kō-pē)

chromosome (krō'mō-sōm) [Gr. *chroma*, color, + *soma*, body]
  c., accessory
  c.'s, banded
  c., bivalent
  c.'s, giant
  c., Philadelphia; c., Ph[1]
  c., sex
  c., somatic
  c., X
  c., Y

chromotherapy (krō"mō-thĕr'ă-pē) [Gr. *chroma*, color, + *therapeia*, treatment]

chromotoxic (krō"mō-tŏk'sĭk) [" + *toxikon*, poison]

chromotrichia (krō"mō-trĭk'ē-ă) [" + *thrix*, hair]

chromotropic (krō"mō-trŏp'ĭk) [" + *tropikos*, turning]

chromoureteroscopy (krō"mō-ū-rē"tĕr-ŏs'kō-pē) [" + *oureter*, ureter, + *skopein*, to examine]

chronaxie (krō'năk-sē) [Gr. *chronos*, time, + *axia*, value]

chronaximeter (krō"năk-sĭm'ĕt-ĕr) [" + " + *metron*, measure]

chronic [Gr. *chronos*, time]

chronic bacterial prostatitis

chronic granulomatous disease

chronicity (krŏn-ĭs'ĭt-ē)

chronic obstructive lung disease

chronobiology (krŏn"ō-bī-ŏl'ō-jē) [Gr. *chronos*, time, + *bios*, life, + *logos*, word, reason]

chronognosis (krŏn"ŏg-nō'sĭs) [" + *gnosis*, knowledge]

chronograph (krŏn'ō-grăf) [" + *graphein*, to write]

chronological (krŏn"ō-lŏj'ĭ-kăl) [" + *logos*, word, reason]

chronoscope (krŏn'ō-skōp) [" + *skopein*, to examine]

chronotaraxis (krō-nō-tăr-ăk'sĭs) [" + *taraxis*, without order]

chronotropic (krŏn"ō-trŏp'ĭk) [" + *tropikos*, turning]

chronotropism [" + " + *-ismos*, condition]
  c., negative
  c., positive

chrysarobin (krĭs"ă-rō'bĭn) [Gr. *chrysos*, gold, + Brazilian *araraba*, bark]

chrysiasis (krī-sī'ă-sĭs)

chrysoderma (krĭs"ō-dĕr'mă) [" + *derma*, skin]

chrysotherapy (krĭs"ō-thĕr'ă-pē) [" + *therapeia*, treatment]

Chvostek's sign (vŏs'tĕks) [Franz Chvostek, Austrian surgeon, 1835–1884]

chylangioma (kī"lăn-jē-ō'mă) [Gr.

chylos, juice, + angeion, vessel, + oma, tumor]

chyle (kīl) [Gr. *chylos*, juice]

chylemia (kī-lē′mē-ă) [" + *haima*, blood]

chylifacient (kī″lĭ-fā′shěnt) [" + L. *facere*, to make]

chylifaction, chylification (kī-lĭ-făk′shŭn, kī-lĭ-fĭ-kā′shŭn)

chylifactive (kī-lĭ-făk′tĭv)

chyliferous (kī-lĭf′ěr-ŭs) [" + L. *ferre*, to carry]

chyliform (kī′lĭ-form) [" + L. *forma*, shape]

chylocele (kī′lō-sēl) [" + *kele*, tumor, swelling]

chyloderma (kī″lō-děr′mă) [" + *derma*, skin]

chylology (kī-lŏl′ō-jē) [" + *logos*, word, reason]

chylomediastinum (kī″lō-mē″dē-ăs-tī′nŭm) [" + L. *mediastinum*, median]

chylomicron (kī″lō-mī′krŏn) [" + *mikros*, small]

chylopericardium (kī″lō-pěr″ĭ-kăr′dē-ŭm) [" + L. *peri*, around, + Gr. *kardia*, heart]

chyloperitoneum (kī″lō-pěr″ĭ-tō-nē′ŭm) [" + *peritonaion*, stretched around or over]

chylophoric (kī″lō-for′ĭk) [" + *phoros*, bearing]

chylopneumothorax (kī″lō-nū″mō-thō′răks) [" + *pneumon*, lung, + *thorax*, chest]

chylopoiesis (kī″lō-poy-ē′sĭs) [" + *poiesis*, production]

chylorrhea (kī″lō-rē′ă) [Gr. *chylos*, juice, + *rhein*, to flow]

chylothorax [" + *thorax*, chest]

chylous (kī′lŭs)

chyluria (kī-lū′rē-ă) [" + *ouron*, urine]

chymase (kī′mās)

chyme (kīm) [Gr. *chymos*, juice]

chymopapain (kī-mō-pă′pā-ĭn)

chymosin (kī′mō-sĭn) [Gr. *chymos*, juice]

chymotrypsin (kī″mō-trĭp′sĭn) [" +

tryein, to rub, + *pepsis*, digestion]

C.I. chemotherapeutic index; color index

Ci curie

cib. [L.] *cibus*, food

cibisotome (sĭ-bĭs′ō-tōm) [Gr. *kibisis*, pouch, + *tome*, a cutting, slice]

cibophobia (sī″bō-fō′bē-ă) [L. *cibus*, food, + Gr. *phobos*, fear]

cicatricial (sĭk″ă-trĭsh′ăl) [L. *cicatrix*, scar]

cicatricotomy (sĭk″ă-trĭk-ŏt′ō-mē) [" + Gr. *tome*, a cutting, slice]

cicatrix (sĭk′ă-trĭks, sĭk-ā′trĭks) [L.]

cicatrizant (sĭk-ăt′rĭ-zănt) [L. *cicatrix*, scar]

cicatrization (sĭk″ă-trĭ-zā′shŭn)

cicatrize (sĭk′ă-trīz)

cicutism (sĭk′ū-tĭzm)

cigarette

ciguatera (sē″gwă-tā′ră) [Sp. Amer. from W. Indies *cigua*, sea snail]

ciguatoxin (sē″gwă-tŏk′sĭn)

cilia (sĭl′ē-ă) [L., eyelids]
    c., immotile, syndrome

ciliariscope (sĭl″ē-ă′rĭ-skōp) [L. *ciliaris*, pert. to eyelid, + Gr. *skopein*, to examine]

ciliarotomy (sĭl″ē-ă-rŏt′ō-mē) [" + Gr. *tome*, a cutting, slice]

ciliary (sĭl′ē-ěr″ē) [L. *ciliaris*, pert. to eyelid]

ciliary apparatus

ciliary arteries

ciliary body

ciliary ganglion

ciliary glands

ciliary muscle

ciliary nerves, long

ciliary nerves, short

ciliary processes

ciliary reflex

Ciliata (sĭl″ē-ă′tă)

ciliate (sĭl′ē-āt) [L. *cilia*, eyelids]

ciliated (sĭl′ē-ă-těd)

ciliated epithelium

ciliectomy (sĭl″ē-ěk′tō-mē) [" + Gr. *ektome*, excision]

ciliogenesis (sĭl″ē-ō-jěn′ě-sĭs)

ciliospinal (sĭl″ē-ō-spī′năl) [" +

spinalis, pert. to a spine]
ciliospinal center
ciliospinal reflex
ciliostatic (sĭl"ē-ō-stăt'ĭk) [" + Gr. *statos,* placed]
ciliotomy (sĭl"ē-ŏt'ō-mē) [" + Gr. *tome,* a cutting, slice]
ciliotoxicity
cilium (sĭl'ē-ŭm) [L.]
cillosis (sĭl-ō'sĭs) [L.]
cimbia (sĭm'bē-ă) [L.]
cimetidine
Cimex lectularius (sī'mĕks lĕk-tū-lā'rē-ŭs)
cimicosis (sĭm"ĭ-kō'sĭs)
cinchona (sĭn-kō'nă, -chō'nă) [Sp. *cinchon,* Countess of Cinchon]
cinchonism (sĭn'kŏn-ĭzm) [" + Gr. *-ismos,* condition]
cinchophen (sĭn'kō-fĕn)
cinclisis (sĭn'klĭ-sĭs) [Gr. *kinklisis,* a wagging]
cincture sensation (sĭnk'chūr) [L. *cinctura,* girdle]
cineangiocardiography (sĭn"ē-ăn"jē-ō-kăr"dē-ŏg'ră-fē) [Gr. *kinesis,* motion, + *angeion,* vessel, + *kardia,* heart, + *graphein,* to write]
    c., radionuclide
cinecystourethrogram (sĭn-ē-sĭs"tō-ū-rē'thrō-grăm)
cinefluorography (sĭn"ē-floo"or-ŏg'ră-fē)
cinematics (sĭn"ē-măt'ĭks) [Gr. *kinema,* motion]
cinematoradiography (sĭn"ē-măt-ō-rā"dē-ŏg'ră-fē) [" + L. *radius,* ray, + Gr. *graphein,* to write]
cinemicrography (sĭn"ē-mī-krŏg'ră-fē) [Gr. *kinesis,* motion, + *mikros,* small, + *graphein,* to write]
cineplastics (sĭn"ē-plăs'tĭks) [" + *plassein,* to form]
cineraceous (sĭn-ē-rā'shŭs) [L. *cinis,* ashes]
cineradiography (sĭn"ē-rā"dē-ŏg'ră-fē) [Gr. *kinesis,* motion, + L. *radius,*

ray, + Gr. *graphein,* to write]
cinerea (sĭn-ē'rē-ă) [L. *cinereus,* ashen-hued]
cinereal (sĭn-ē'rē-ăl)
cineritious (sĭn"ĕr-ĭsh'ŭs) [L. *cineritius,* ashen]
cinesi- [Gr. *kinesis,* motion]
cineurography (sĭn"ē-ū-rŏg'ră-fē) [Gr. *kinesis,* motion, + *ouron,* urine, + *graphein,* to write]
cingulotomy (sĭn'gū-lŏt'ō-mē) [L. *cingulum,* girdle, + Gr. *tome,* a cutting, slice]
cingulum (sĭn'gū-lŭm) [L., girdle]
cinnamon
cinoxacin
CinQuin
cion (sī'ŏn) [Gr. *kion,* pillar]
circa (sĭr'kă) [L.]
circadian (sĭr"kă-dē'ăn, sĭr-kā'dē-ăn) [L. *circa,* about, + *dies,* day]
circinate (sĕr'sĭ-nāt) [L. *circinatus,* made round]
circle [L. *circulus,* a little ring]
    c. of diffusion
    c. of Willis
Circ-O-Lectric bed
circuit (sĕr'kĭt) [L. *circuire,* to go around]
circular [L. *circularis*]
circulation [L. *circulatio*]
    c., bile salts
    c., blood
    c., collateral
    c., coronary
    c., extracorporeal
    c., fetal
    c., lymph
    c., portal
    c., pulmonary
    c., systemic
    c., venous
circulation rate
circulation time
circulatory
circulatory collapse
circulatory failure
circulatory overload
circulatory system

circulus (sĕr'kū-lŭs) [L.]
circum- [L.]
circumarticular (sĕr″kŭm-ăr-tĭk'ū-lăr)
[L. *circum*, around, + *articulus*,
small joint]
circumcision (sĕr″kŭm-sĭ'zhŭn) [L. *cir-
cumcisio*, a cutting around]
c., ritual
circumclusion (sĕr″kŭm-klū'zhŭn) [L. *cir-
cumcludere*, to shut in]
circumcorneal (sĕr″kŭm-kor'nē-ăl) [L.
circum, around, + *corneus*, horny]
circumduction (sĕr″kŭm-dŭk'shŭn)
[″ + *ducere*, to lead]
circumference (sĕr-kŭm'fĕr-ĕns)
[″ + *ferre*, to bear]
circumferential (sĕr″kŭm-fĕr-ĕn'shăl)
circumflex (sĕr'kŭm-flĕks) [″ +
flectere, to bend]
circuminsular (sĕr″kŭm-ĭn'sū-lăr) [″ +
insula, island]
circumlental (sĕr″kŭm-lĕn'tăl) [″ +
lens, lens]
circumnuclear (sĕr″kŭm-nū'klē-ăr)
[″ + *nucleus*, kernel]
circumocular (sĕr″kŭm-ŏk'ū-lăr) [″ +
oculus, eye]
circumoral (sĕr″kŭm-ō'răl) [L. *circum*,
around, + *os*, mouth]
circumoral pallor
circumorbital (sĕr″kŭm-or'bĭt-ăl)
[″ + *orbita*, orbit]
circumpolarization (sĕr″kŭm-pō″lăr-ĭ-
zā'shŭn) [″ + *polaris*, polar]
circumrenal (sĕr″kŭm-rē'năl) [″ +
renalis, pert. to kidney]
circumscribed (sĕr'kŭm-skrīb'd) [″ +
scribere, to write]
circumstantiality (sĕr″kŭm-stăn″shē-
ăl'ĭ-tē) [L. *circum*, around, + *stare*,
to stand]
circumvallate (sĕr″kŭm-văl'āt) [″ +
vallare, to wall]
circumvallate papillae
circumvascular (sĕr″kŭm-văs'kū-lăr)
[″ + *vasculum*, vessel]
cirrhosis (sĭ-rō'sĭs) [Gr. *kirrhos*, orange
yellow, + *osis*, condition]

c., alcoholic
c., atrophic
c., biliary
c., cardiac
c., fatty
c., hypertrophic
c., infantile
c., macronodular
c., metabolic
c., micronodular
c., obstructive biliary
c., primary biliary
c., syphilitic
c., toxic
c., zooparasitic
cirrhotic (sĭ-rŏt'ĭk)
cirsectomy (sĕr-sĕk'tō-mē) [Gr. *kirsos*,
varix, + *ektome*, excision]
cirsoid (sĕr'soyd) [″ + *eidos*, form,
shape]
cirsomphalos (sĕr-sŏm'fă-lōs) [″ +
omphalos, navel]
cirsotome (sĕr'sō-tōm) [″ + *tome*,
a cutting, slice]
cirsotomy (sĕr-sŏt'ō-mē)
C.I.S. central inhibitory state
cis (sĭs) [L., on the same side]
cisplatin (sĭs'plă-tĭn)
cissa (sĭs'ă) [Gr. *kissa*]
cistern (sĭs'tĕrn)
cisterna [L.]
c. chyli
c. subarachnoidalis
cisternal (sĭs-tĕr'năl)
cisternal puncture
cisvestitism (sĭs-vĕs'tĭ-tĭzm) [L. *cis*, on
the same side, + *vestitus*, dressed,
+ Gr. *-ismos*, condition]
Citanest
Citelli's syndrome (chē-tĕl'ēz) [Salva-
tore Citelli, It. laryngologist, 1875–
1947]
citrate (sĭt'rāt, sī'trāt)
citrated (sĭt'rāt-ĕd)
citrate solution
citric acid
citric acid cycle
citronella (sĭt″rŏn-ĕl'ă)

citrovorum factor
citrulline (sĭt-rŭl′lĭn)
citrullinemia (sĭt-rŭl″lĭ-nē′mē-ă)
citrullinuria (sĭt-rŭl″lĭ-nū′rē-ă)
Cl *chlorine; chloride; clavicle; Clostridium*
cladosporiosis (klăd″ō-spō-rē-ō′sĭs) [Gr. *klados*, branch, + *sporos*, seed, + *osis*, condition]
Cladosporium
clairvoyance (klăr-voy′ăns) [Fr.]
clamp (klămp) [MD. *klampe*, metal clasp]
    c., rubber-dam
clang [L. *clangere*, to peal]
clap
clapotage, clapotement (klă″pō-täzh′, klă-pŏt-maw′) [Fr.]
clapping (klăp′ĭng)
Clapton's lines
clarificant (klăr-ĭf′ĭk-ănt) [L. *clarus*, clear, + *facere*, to make]
clarification (klăr″ĭ-fĭ-kā′shŭn)
Clark's rule
Clarke, Jacob A. L. [Brit. anatomist, 1817–1880]
    C.'s bodies
    C.'s column
Clarke-Hadfield syndrome [Cecil Clarke; Geoffrey Hadfield, Brit. pathologist, b. 1899]
clasmatocyte (klăz-măt′ō-sīt) [Gr. *klasma*, fragment, + *kytos*, cell]
clasmatodendrosis (klăz-măt″ō-dĕn-drō′sĭs) [″ + *dendron*, tree, + *osis*, condition]
clasmatosis (klăz″mă-tō′sĭs) [″ + *osis*, condition]
clasp (klăsp)
clasp-knife rigidity
class [L. *classis*, division]
classification (klăs″sĭ-fĭ-kā′shŭn)
    c., plant or animal
clastic (klăs′tĭk) [Gr. *klastos*, broken]
clastogenic (klăs′tō-jĕn″ĭc) [″ + *gennan*, to produce]
clastothrix (klăs′tō-thrĭks) [″ + *thrix*, hair]
Claude's syndrome (klawdz) [Henri

Claude, Fr. psychiatrist, 1869–1945]
claudication (klaw-dĭ-kā′shŭn) [L. *claudicare*, to limp]
    c., intermittent
    c., venous
Claudius' cells (klaw′dē-ŭs) [Friedrich Claudius, Austrian anatomist, 1822–1869]
Claudius' fossa
claustrophilia (klaws-trō-fĭl′ē-ă) [L. *claustrum*, a barrier, + Gr. *philein*, to love]
claustrophobia (klaws-trō-fō′bē-ă) [″ + Gr. *phobos*, fear]
claustrum (klŏs′trŭm) [L.]
clausura (klaw-sū′ră) [L.]
clava (klā′vă) [L., club]
clavate (klā′vāt)
clavicle (klăv′ĭ-k′l) [L. *clavicula*, little key]
    c., dislocation of
    c., fracture of
clavicotomy (klăv″ĭ-kŏt′ō-mē) [″ + Gr. *tome*, a cutting, slice]
clavicular (klă-vĭk′ū-lăr)
clavus (klā′vŭs) [L., nail]
clawfoot
clawhand
claw toe
Clayton gas
clean-catch method
cleaning, ultrasonic
clean room
clearance
clearing agent
cleavage (klē′vĕj) [AS. *cleofian*, to cleave]
cleavage cell
cleavage lines
cleft (klĕft) [ME. *clift*, crevice]
    c., alveolar
    c., branchial
    c., facial
cleft cheek
cleft foot
cleft hand
cleft lip
cleft palate
cleft sternum

cleft tongue
cleido- (klī'dō) [L. *clavis*, key]
cleidocostal (klī"dō-kŏs'tăl) [" + *costa*, rib]
cleidorrhexis (klī"dō-rĕk'sĭs) [" + Gr. *rhexis*, rupture]
cleidotomy (klī-dŏt'ō-mē) [" + Gr. *tome*, a cutting, slice]
clemastine fumarate (klĕm'ăs-tēn)
clenching (klĕnch'ĭng)
cleptomania (klĕp"tō-mā'nē-ă)
click (klĭk)
clidinium bromide (klĭ-dĭn'ē-ŭm)
client
climacteric (klĭ-măk'tĕr-ĭk, klĭ-măk-tĕr'ĭk) [Gr. *klimakter*, a rung of a ladder]
climatology, medical [Gr. *klima*, sloping surface of the earth, + *logos*, word, reason]
climatotherapy (klī"măt-ō-thĕr'ăp-ē) [" + *therapeia*, treatment]
climax (klī'măks) [Gr. *klimax*, ladder]
clindamycin hydrochloride (klĭn"dă-mī'sĭn)
clinic (klĭn'ĭk) [Gr. *klinikos*, pert. to a bed]
clinical
clinical analysis
clinical judgment
clinical pathology
clinical thermometer
clinical trial
clinician (klĭn-ĭsh'ăn) [Gr. *klinikos*, pert. to a bed]
  c., nurse
clinicopathologic (klĭn"ĭ-kō-pă"thō-lŏj'ĭk)
clinicopathologic conference
clinocephaly (klī"nō-sĕf'ă-lē) [Gr. *klinein*, to bend, + *kephale*, head]
clinodactyly (klī"nō-dăk'tĭ-lē) [" + *daktylos*, finger]
clinoid (klī'noyd) [Gr. *kline*, bed, + *eidos*, form, shape]
clinoid processes
clinometer (klī-nŏm'ĕ-tĕr) [Gr. *klinein*, to slope, + *metron*, measure]
clinoscope (klī'nō-skōp) [" + *skopein*, to examine]

clinostatism (klī'nō-stăt"ĭzm)
clip
cliseometer (klĭs"ē-ŏm'ĕt-ĕr) [Gr. *klisis*, inclination, + *metron*, measure]
Clistin
clithrophobia (klĭth"rō-fō'bē-ă) [Gr. *kleithria*, keyhole, + *phobos*, fear]
clition (klĭt'ē-ōn) [Gr. *kleitys*, slope]
clitoridectomy (klī"tō-rĭd-ĕk'tō-mē) [Gr. *kleitoris*, clitoris, + *ektome*, excision]
clitoriditis (klī"tō-rĭd-ī'tĭs) [" + *itis*, inflammation]
clitoridotomy (klī"tō-rĭd-ŏt'ō-mē) [" + *tome*, a cutting, slice]
clitoris (klī'tō-rĭs, klĭt'ō-rĭs) [Gr. *kleitoris*]
clitoris crises
clitorism (klī'tō-rĭzm)
clitoritis (klī"tō-rī'tĭs)
clitoromegaly (klī"tō-rō-mĕg'ă-lē) [" + *megas*, large]
clivus (klī'vŭs) [L., a slope]
  c. blumenbachii
clo
cloaca (klō-ā'kă) [L. *cloaca*, a sewer]
clobetasol propionate
clock [LL. *clocca*]
  c., biological
clofazimine (klō-fă'zĭ-mēn)
clofibrate (klō-fī'brāt)
Clomid
clomiphene citrate (klō'mĭ-fēn)
clonal (klōn'ăl)
clonazepam (klō-năz'ĕ-păm)
clone (klōn) [Gr. *klon*, a cutting used for propagation]
clonic (klŏn'ĭk) [Gr. *klonos*, turmoil]
clonicity (klŏn-ĭs'ĭ-tē)
clonicotonic (klŏn"ĭ-kō-tŏn'ĭk) [Gr. *klonos*, turmoil, + *tonikos*, tonic]
clonic spasm
clonidine hydrochloride (klō'nĭ-dēn)
clonism, clonismus (klōn'ĭzm, klō-nĭz'mŭs) [" + *-ismos*, condition]
clonograph (klŏn'ō-grăf)
clonorchiasis (klō"nor-kī'ă-sĭs)
Clonorchis sinensis (klō-nor'kĭs sĭ-nĕn'sĭs)

clonospasm (klŏn'ō-spăzm) [" + spasmos, a convulsion]

clonus (klō'nŭs)

Cloquet's canal (klō-kāz') [Jules Germain Cloquet, Fr. surgeon, 1790–1883]

Clos-O-Mat

Clostridium (klō-strĭd'ē-ŭm) [Gr. kloster, spindle]
  C. botulinum
  C. chauvoei
  C. difficile
  C. histolyticum
  C. novyi
  C. perfringens
  C. septicum
  C. sporogenes
  C. tetani
  C. welchii

closure (klō'shŭr)

clot (klŏt) [AS. clott, lump]
  c., agony
  c., antemortem
  c., blood
  c., chicken fat
  c., currant jelly
  c., distal
  c., external
  c., heart
  c., internal
  c., laminated
  c., muscle
  c., passive
  c., plastic
  c., postmortem
  c., proximal
  c., stratified

clothes louse

clothing [AS. clath, cloth]

clotrimazole (klō-trĭm'ă-zōl)

clotting

clouding of consciousness

cloudy swelling

cloven spine

clove oil [L. clavus, a nail or spike]

clownism (klown'ĭzm)

cloxacillin sodium (klŏks"ă-sĭl'ĭn)

Cloxapen

clubbing (klŭb'ĭng)

clubfoot

clubhand

clue cells

clump (klŭmp) [AS. clympre, a lump]

clumping [AS. clympre, a lump]

clunes (kloo'nēz) [L.]

cluster headache

cluttering (klŭt'ĕr-ĭng)

Clutton's joint [Henry Hugh Clutton, Brit. surgeon, 1850–1909]

clysis (klī'sĭs) [Gr. klyzein, to wash]

clysma (klĭs'mă) [Gr. klysma, a drenching]

clyster (klĭs'tĕr) [Gr. klyster, syringe]

C.M. chirurgiae magister

Cm curium

cm centimeter

c/m counts per minute

cm² square centimeter

cm³ cubic centimeter

C.M.A. Canadian Medical Association

CMI cell-mediated immunity

c/min counts per minute

c.mm cubic millimeter

CMRR common mode rejection ratio

CMT certified medical transcriptionist

CN cyanogen

C.N.A. Canadian Nurses' Association

cnemial (nē'mē-ăl)

cnemis (nē'mĭs) [Gr. knemis, legging]

cnemitis (nē-mī'tĭs) [" + itis, inflammation]

cnemoscoliosis (nē"mō-skō"lē-ō'sĭs) [" + skoliosis, crookedness]

C.N.M. certified nurse-midwife

CNS central nervous system; clinical nurse specialist

CO carbon monoxide; cardiac output

CO₂ carbon dioxide

CO₂ therapy

Co cobalt

CoA coenzyme A

coacervate (kō-ăs'ĕr-vāt) [L. coacervatus, heaped up]

coadaptation (kō"ăd-ăp-tā'shŭn)

coadunation (kō"ăd-ū-nā'shŭn) [L. co-, together, + ad, to, + unus, one]

coagglutination (kō"ă-gloo"tĭn-ā'shŭn) [L. *coagulare*, to curdle]

coagula (kō-ăg'ū-lă) [L.]

coagulability (kō-ăg"ū-lă-bĭl'ĭ-tē)

coagulable (kō-ăg'ū-lă-b'l)

coagulant (kō-ăg'ū-lănt) [L. *coagulans*, congealing]

coagulase (kō-ăg'ū-lāz) [L. *coagulum*, blood clot]

coagulate (kō-ăg'ū-lāt) [L. *coagulare*, to congeal]

coagulated

coagulated proteins

coagulation (kō-ăg"ū-lā'shŭn) [L. *coagulatio*, clotting]

coagulation factors

coagulation time

coagulative (kō-ăg'ū-lā"tĭv)

coagulometer (kō-ăg"ū-lŏm'ĕt-ĕr) [L. *coagulare*, to congeal, + Gr. *metron*, measure]

coagulopathy (kō-ăg"ū-lŏp'ă-thē) [" + Gr. *pathos*, disease, suffering]

　c., consumption

coagulum (kō-ăg'ū-lŭm) [L.]

coalesce (kō-ăl-ĕs') [L. *coalescere*]

coalescence (kō-ă-lĕs'ĕns)

coal tar

coal worker's pneumoconiosis

coapt (kō'ăpt) [L. *coaptare*, to fit together]

coaptation (kō"ăp-tā'shŭn) [L. *coaptare*, to fit together]

coarctate (kō-ărk'tāt) [L. *coarctare*, to tighten]

coarctation (kō"ărk-tā'shŭn)

　c. of aorta

coarctotomy (kō"ărk-tŏt'ō-mē) [" + Gr. *tome*, a cutting, slice]

coat [L. *cotta*, a tunic]

C.O.A.T.S. *Comprehensive Occupational Assessment and Training System*

Coats' disease [George Coats, Brit. ophthalmologist, 1876–1915]

cobalamin (kō-băl'ă-mĭn)

cobalamin concentrate

cobalt (kō'bălt)

cobalt-57

cobalt-60

cobra (kō'bră)

cobra venom solution

COBS *cesarean-obtained barrier-sustained*

coca (kō'kă)

cocaine hydrochloride (kō-kān', kō'kān)

cocaine hydrochloride poisoning

cocainism (kō'kăn-ĭzm)

cocainization (kō"kăn-ĭ-zā'shŭn)

cocainomania (kō"kăn-ō-mā'nē-ă)

cocarboxylase (kō"kăr-bŏk'sĭ-lās)

cocarcinogen (kō-kăr'sĭ-nō-jĕn")

coccal (kŏk'ăl)

cocci (kŏk'sī)

Coccidia (kŏk-sīd'ē-ă) [Gr. *kokkos*, berry]

coccidian (kŏk-sīd'ē-ăn)

Coccidioides

coccidioidin (kŏk"sĭd-ē-oy'dĭn)

coccidioidomycosis (kŏk-sĭd"ĭ-oyd-ō-mī-kō'sĭs) [" + *eidos*, form, shape, + *mykes*, fungus, + *osis*, condition]

coccidiosis (kŏk-sĭd-ē-ō'sĭs) [" + *osis*, condition]

coccobacilli (kŏk"ō-bă-sĭl'ī)

coccobacteria (kŏk"ō-băk-tē'rē-ă)

coccogenous (kŏk-ŏj'ĕn-ŭs) [Gr. *kokkos*, berry, + *gennan*, to produce]

coccoid (kŏk'oyd) [" + *eidos*, form, shape]

coccus (kŏk'ŭs) [Gr. *kokkos*, berry]

coccyalgia, coccydynia (kŏk"sē-ăl'jē-ă, kŏk"sē-dĭn'ē-ă) [Gr. *kokkyx*, coccyx, + *algos*, pain; " + *odyne*, pain]

coccygeal (kŏk-sĭj'ē-ăl)

coccygeal body

coccygeal nerves

coccygectomy (kŏk"sī-jĕk'tō-mē) [" + *ektome*, excision]

coccygeus (kŏk-sĭj'ē-ŭs)

coccygodynia (kŏk-sī-gō-dĭn'ē-ă) [" + *odyne*, pain]

coccyx (kŏk'sĭks) [Gr. *kokkyx*, coccyx]

cochineal (kŏch'ĭn-ēl) [L. *coccinus*, scarlet]

cochlea (kŏk'lē-ă) [Gr. *kokhlos,* land snail]

cochlear (kŏk'lē-ăr)

cochleare (kŏk"lē-ā'rē) [L., spoon]

cochleariform (kŏk"lē-ār'ĭ-form) [" + L. *forma,* shape]

cochlear implant

cochlear nerve

cochleitis (kŏk"lē-ī'tĭs) [Gr. *kokhlos,* land snail, + *itis,* inflammation]

cochleo-orbicular reflex (kŏk"lē-ō-or-bĭk'ū-lăr)

cochleopalpebral reflex (kŏk"lē-ō-păl'pē-brăl)

cochleovestibular (kŏk"lē-ō-vĕs-tĭb'ū-lăr) [" + L. *vestibulum,* vestibule]

cochlitis (kŏk-lī'tĭs) [" + *itis,* inflammation]

cockroach [Sp. *cucaracha*]

cocktail (kŏk'tāl)
   c., lytic

cock-up splint

cock-up toe

cocoa butter

coconsciousness (kō-kŏn'shŭs-nĕs)

cocontraction (kō"kŏn-trăk'shŭn)

coconut "water" [Sp. and Port. *coco,* coconut, + Eng. *nut*]

Coco-Quinine

coctolabile (kŏk"tō-lā'bĭl) [L. *coctus,* cooked, + *labilis,* perishable]

coctoprecipitin (kŏk"tō-prē-sĭp'ĭt-ĭn) [" + *praecipitare,* to cast down]

coctostabile (kŏk"tō-stā'bĭl) [" + *stabilis,* resisting]

code (kōd)
   c., genetic
   c., triplet

Code for Nurses

codeine (kō'dēn) [Gr. *kodeia,* poppy-head]
   c. phosphate
   c. sulfate

codeine poisoning

cod liver oil

codon (kō'dŏn)

Codroxomin

coefficient (kō"ē-fĭsh'ĕnt) [L. *co-,* to-gether, + *efficere,* to produce]
   c., isotonic
   c. of absorption

Coelenterata (sē-lĕn"tĕr-ā'tă) [Gr. *koilos,* hollow, + *enteron,* intestine]

coelom (sē'lŏm) [Gr. *koiloma,* a cavity]
   c., extraembryonic

coenocyte (sē'nō-sīt, sĕn'ō-sīt) [Gr. *koinos,* common, + *kytos,* cell]

coenzyme (kō-ĕn'zīm) [L. *co-,* together, + Gr. *en,* in, + *zyme,* leaven]

coenzyme A

coetaneous (kō"ē-tā'nē-ŭs) [" + *aetas,* age]

coexcitation (kō-ĕk-sī-tā'shŭn) [" + *excitare,* to arouse]

cofactor (kō'făk-tor)

coferment (kō-fĕr'mĕnt) [" + *fermentum,* leaven]

coffee

coffee-ground vomitus

Cogan's syndrome (kō'găns) [David G. Cogan, U.S. ophthalmologist, b. 1908]

Cogentin

cognition (kŏg-nĭsh'ŭn) [L. *cognoscere,* to know]

cogwheeling

cogwheel respiration

coherent (kō-hēr'ĕnt) [L. *cohaerere,* to stick together]

cohesion (kō-hē'zhŭn)

cohesive (kō-hē'sĭv)

Cohnheim's areas (kōn'hīmz) [Julius Friedrich Cohnheim, Ger. pathologist, 1839–1884]

Cohnheim's theory

cohort

cohort study

coil (koyl)

coilonychia (koy"lō-nĭk'ē-ă) [Gr. *koilos,* hollow, + *onyx,* nail]

coin counting

coin test

coital (kō'ĭ-tăl)

coition (kō-ĭsh'ŭn) [L. *coire,* to come together]

coitophobia (kō"ĭ-tō-fō'bē-ă) [" +

Gr. *phobos*, fear]
coitus (kō′ĭ-tŭs)
   c. à la vache
   c. interruptus
   c. reservatus
   c. Saxonius
col (kŏl)
Cola (kō′lă) [W. African *kola*]
Colace
colalgia (kō-lăl′jē-ă) [Gr. *kolon*, colon,
   + *algos*, pain]
colation (kō-lā′shŭn) [L. *colare*, to strain]
colauxe (kŏl-ăwk′sē) [Gr. *kolon*, colon,
   + *auxe*, increase]
colchicine (kŏl′chĭ-sĭn)
COLD *chronic obstructive lung disease*
cold [AS. *ceald*, cold]
   c., chest
   c., common
cold agglutinin
cold agglutinin disease
cold cream
cold pack
cold pressor test
cold sore
coldspray
colectomy (kō-lĕk′tō-mē) [Gr. *kolon*,
   colon, + *ektome*, excision]
coleocystitis (kō″lē-ō-sĭs-tī′tĭs) [Gr.
   koleos, sheath, + *kystis*, bladder,
   + *itis*, inflammation]
coleoptosis (kō″lē-ŏp-tō′sĭs) [″ +
   ptosis, fall, falling]
coleotomy (kō″lē-ŏt′ō-mē) [″ +
   tome, a cutting, slice]
colestipol hydrochloride (kō-lĕs′tĭ-
   pōl)
colibacillemia (kō″lĭ-băs-ĭl-lē′mē-ă)
   [Gr. *kolon*, colon, + L. *bacillus*, little rod, + Gr. *haima*, blood]
colibacillosis (kō″lĭ-băs-ĭ-lō′sĭs) [″ +
   ″ + Gr. *osis*, condition]
colibacilluria (kō-lĭ-băs-ĭl-ū′rē-ă)
   [″ + ″ + Gr. *ouron*, urine]
colibacillus (kō″lĭ-bă-sĭl′ŭs) [″ + L.
   bacillus, little rod]
colic (kŏl′ĭk) [Gr. *kolikos*, pert. to the
   colon]

   c., biliary
   c., infantile
   c., intestinal
   c., lead
   c., menstrual
   c., renal
   c., uterine
colica (kŏl′ĭ-kă) [L.]
colicin (kŏl′ĭ-sĭn)
colicky (kŏl′ĭk-ē)
colicolitis (kō″lĭ-kō-lī′tĭs) [Gr. *kolon*,
   colon, + *kolon*, colon, + *itis*,
   inflammation]
colicoplegia (kō″lĭ-kō-plē′jē-ă) [″ +
   plege, stroke]
colicystitis (kō″lĭ-sĭs-tī′tĭs) [″ +
   kystis, bladder, + *itis*, inflamma-
   tion]
colicystopyelitis (kō-lĭ-sĭs″tō-pī″ĕ-lī′tĭs)
   [″ + ″ + *pyelos*, pelvis, +
   itis, inflammation]
coliform (kō′lĭ-form) [″ + L. *forma*,
   form]
colilysin (kō-lĭl′ĭ-sĭn) [″ + *lysis*, dis-
   solution]
colinephritis (kō″lĭ-nē-frī′tĭs) [″ +
   nephros, kidney, + *itis*, inflamma-
   tion]
colipase
coliplication (kō″lĭ-plĭ-kā′shŭn) [″ +
   L. *plica*, fold]
colipuncture (kō′lĭ-pŭnk″chūr) [″ +
   L. *punctura*, prick]
colipyuria (kō″lĭ-pī-ū′rē-ă) [″ +
   pyon, pus, + *ouron*, urine]
colisepsis [″ + *sepsis*, decay]
colistimethate sodium, sterile
   (kō-lĭs″tĭ-mĕth′āt)
colistin sulfate (kō-lĭs′tĭn)
colitis (kō-lī′tĭs) [″ + *itis*, inflamma-
   tion]
   c., amebic
   c., mucous
   c., pseudomembranous
   c., ulcerative
colitoxemia (kō″lĭ-tŏk-sē′mē-ă) [Gr.
   kolon, colon, + *toxikon*, poison,
   + *haima*, blood]

colitoxicosis (kō″lǐ-tŏk″sǐ-kō′sǐs) [″ + ″ + osis, condition]

colitoxin (kō″lǐ-tŏk′sǐn) [″ + toxikon, poison]

coliuria (kō″lǐ-ū′rē-ȧ) [″ + ouron, urine]

colla (kŏl′lȧ)

collagen (kŏl′ȧ-jěn) [Gr. kolla, glue, + gennan, to produce]

collagenase (kŏl-lăj′ě-nās) [″ + ″ + -ase, enzyme]

collagenation (kŏl-lăj″ě-nā′shŭn)

collagenic (kŏl″ȧ-jěn′ĭk)

collagenoblast (kŏl-lăj′ě-nō-blăst) [″ + ″ + blastos, germ]

collagenolysis (kŏl″ȧ-jěn-ŏl′ĭ-sĭs) [″ + ″ + lysis, dissolution]

collagenosis (kŏl-lăj″ě-nō′sĭs) [″ + ″ + osis, condition]

collagen vascular diseases

collapse [L. collapsus, fallen to pieces]
   c., circulatory
   c. of lung

collapsing

collapsing pulse

collapsotherapy (kŏ-lăp″sō-thěr′ȧ-pē) [L. collapsus, fallen to pieces, + Gr. therapeia, treatment]

collar (kŏl′ȧr) [L. collum, neck]
   c. of Venus

collarbone

collateral (kŏ-lăt′ěr-ȧl) [L. con, together, + lateralis, pert. to a side]

collateral circulation

collateral eminence

collateral fissure

collateral ganglia

collaterals

collateral trigone

collecting tubules

Colles' fascia (kŏl′ēz) [Abraham Colles, Ir. surgeon, 1773–1843]

Colles' fracture

colliculectomy (kŏl-lĭk″ū-lěk′tō-mē) [L. colliculus, mound, + Gr. ektome, excision]

colliculitis (kŏl-lĭk″ū-lī′tĭs) [″ + Gr. itis, inflammation]

colliculus (kŏl-lĭk′ū-lŭs) [L.]
   c. bulbi; c. bulbi intermedius
   c. cervicalis
   c. inferior
   c. seminalis
   c. superior
   c. urethralis

collimation (kŏl″ĭ-mā′shŭn) [L. collineare, to align]

collimator (kŏl′ĭ-mā″tur) [L. collineare, to align, direct, aim]

colliquation (kŏl″ĭ-kwā′shŭn) [L. con, together, + liquare, to melt]

coliquative (kŏ-lĭk′wȧ-tĭv)

collodion (kō-lō′dē-ŏn) [Gr. kollodes, resembling glue]
   c., flexible
   c., salicylic acid

colloid (kŏl′oyd) [Gr. kollodes, glutinous]
   c., thyroid

colloidal (kŏl-loyd′ȧl)

colloidal dispersion

colloid chemistry

colloid cyst

colloid degeneration

colloidin (kŏl-loy′dĭn)

colloidoclasia (kŏl-oyd″ō-klā′sē-ȧ) [″ + klasis, fracture]

colloidopexy (kŏl-oyd′ō-pěk″sē) [″ + pexis, fixation]

colloid suspension

colloma (kŏ-lō′mȧ) [Gr. kolla, glue, + oma, tumor]

collonema (kŏl″ō-nē′mȧ) [″ + nema, yarn]

collopexia (kŏl″ō-pěk′sē-ȧ) [L. collum, neck, + Gr. pexis, fixation]

collum (kŏl′lŭm) [L.]

collyrium (kō-lĭr′ē-ŭm) [Gr. kollyrion, eye salve]

coloboma (kŏl″ō-bō′mȧ) [Gr. koloboma, a mutilation]

colocecostomy (kō″lō-sē-kŏs′tō-mē) [Gr. kolon, colon, + L. caecum, blindness, + Gr. stoma, mouth, opening]

colocentesis (kō″lō-sěn-tē′sĭs) [″ +

kentesis, puncture]

colocholecystostomy (kō″lō-kō″lē-sĭs-tŏs′tō-mē) [″ + *chole,* bile, + *kystis,* bladder, + *stoma,* mouth, opening]

coloclysis, coloclyster (kō-lŏk′lĭ-sĭs, kō″lō-klĭs′tĕr) [″ + *klysis,* a washing]

colocolostomy (kō″lō-kō-lŏs′tō-mē) [″ + *kolon,* colon, + *stoma,* mouth, opening]

colocutaneous (kō″lō-kū-tā′nē-ŭs) [″ + L. *cutis,* skin]

colocynth (kŏl′ō-sĭnth) [Gr. *kolokynthe,* fruit of *Citrullus colocynthis*]

coloenteritis (kŏ″lō-ĕn″tĕr-ī′tĭs) [Gr. *kolon,* colon, + *enteron,* intestine, + *itis,* inflammation]

colofixation (kō″lō-fĭk-sā′shŭn)

Cologel

colon [L.; Gr. *kolon*]
　　c., bacteria of
　　c., irritable
　　c., toxic dilatation of

colonalgia (kō″lŏn-ăl′jē-ă) [Gr. *kolon,* colon, + *algos,* pain]

colonic (kō-lŏn′ĭk)

colonic irrigation

colonitis (kō-lŏn-ī′tĭs) [″ + *itis,* inflammation]

colonization (kŏl″ō-nī-zā′shŭn)

colonometer (kŏl″ŏn-ŏm′ĕ-tĕr) [L. *colonia,* colony, + Gr. *metron,* measure]

colonopathy (kō″lō-nŏp′ă-thē) [Gr. *kolon,* colon, + *pathos,* disease, suffering]

colonopexy (kō-lŏn′ō-pĕk″sē) [″ + *pexis,* fixation]

colonorrhagia (kō″lŏn-ō-rā′jē-ă) [″ + *rhegnynai,* to burst forth]

colonorrhea (kō″lŏn-ō-rē′ă) [″ + *rhein,* to flow]

colonoscope (kō-lŏn′ō-skōp) [″ + *skopein,* to examine]

colonoscopy (kō″lŏn-ŏs′kō-pē)

colony (kŏl′ō-nē) [L. *colonia*]

colony counter

colony-stimulating factor

colopexostomy (kō″lō-pĕks-ŏs′tō-mē) [Gr. *kolon,* colon, + *pexis,* fixation, + *stoma,* mouth, opening]

colopexotomy (kō″lō-pĕks-ŏt′ō-mē) [″ + ″ + *tome,* a cutting, slice]

colopexy, colopexia (kō′lō-pĕk″sē, -pĕks′ē-ă)

coloplication (kō″lō-plĭ-kā′shŭn) [″ + L. *plica,* fold]

coloproctectomy (kō″lō-prŏk-tĕk′tō-mē) [″ + *proktos,* anus, + *ektome,* excision]

coloproctitis [″ + ″ + *itis,* inflammation]

coloproctostomy (kō″lō-prŏk-tŏs′tō-mē) [″ + ″ + *stoma,* mouth, opening]

coloptosia (kō″lŏp-tō′sē-ă) [″ + *ptosis,* fall, falling]

coloptosis (kō-lŏp-tō′sĭs)

colopuncture (kō′lō-pŭnk-chŭr) [″ + L. *punctura,* prick]

color [L.]
　　c.'s, primary

color blindness

color deficient

colorectitis (kō″lō-rĕk-tī′tĭs) [Gr. *kolon,* colon, + L. *rectum,* straight, + Gr. *itis,* inflammation]

colorectostomy (kō″lō-rĕk-tŏs′tō-mē) [″ + ″ + Gr. *stoma,* mouth, opening]

colorectum (kŏl″ō-rĕk′tŭm)

color gustation

color hearing

colorimeter (kŭl″or-ĭm′ĕ-tĕr) [L. *color,* color, + Gr. *metron,* measure]

color index

colorrhaphy (kō-lor′ă-fē) [Gr. *kolon,* colon, + *rhaphe,* seam]

color sense

coloscopy (kō-lŏs′kō-pē)

colosigmoidostomy (kō″lō-sĭg″moy-dŏs′tō-mē) [″ + *sigmoeides,* shaped like Gr. S, + *stoma,* mouth, opening]

colostomy (kō-lŏs′tō-mē) [Gr. *kolon,*

colon, + *stoma*, mouth, opening]
c., double barrel
c., terminal
c., wet
colostrorrhea (kō-lŏs"trō-rē'ă) [L. *colostrum*, colostrum, + Gr. *rhein*, to flow]
colostrum [L.]
colotomy (kō-lŏt'ō-mē) [Gr. *kolon*, colon, + *tome*, a cutting, slice]
colovaginal (kō"lō-văj'ĭ-năl)
colovesical (kō"lō-vĕs'ĭ-kăl)
colpalgia (kŏl-păl'jē-ă) [Gr. *kolpos*, vagina, + *algos*, pain]
colpatresia (kŏl-pă-trē'zē-ă) [" + *a-*, not, + *tresis*, a perforation]
colpectasia (kŏl-pĕk-tā'sē-ă) [" + *ektasis*, distention]
colpectomy (kŏl-pĕk'tō-mē) [" + *ektome*, excision]
colpeurynter (kŏl'pū-rĭn"tĕr) [" + *eurynein*, to dilate]
colpeurysis (kŏl-pū'rĭs-ĭs)
colpitis (kŏl-pī'tĭs) [" + *itis*, inflammation]
colpocele (kŏl'pō-sēl) [" + *kele*, tumor, swelling]
colpoceliotomy (kŏl"pō-sē"lē-ŏt'ō-mē) [" + *koilia*, cavity, belly, + *tome*, a cutting, slice]
colpocleisis (kŏl"pō-klī'sĭs) [" + *kleisis*, a closure]
colpocystitis (kŏl"pō-sĭs-tī'tĭs) [" + *kystis*, bladder, + *itis*, inflammation]
colpocystocele (kŏl"pō-sĭs'tō-sēl) [" + *kystis*, bladder, + *kele*, tumor, swelling]
colpocystoplasty (kŏl"pō-sĭs'tō-plăs"tē) [" + " + *plassein*, to form]
colpocystosyrinx (kŏl"pō-sĭs-tō-sĭr'ĭnks) [" + " + *syrinx*, fistula]
colpocystotomy (kŏl"pō-sĭs-tŏt'ō-mē) [" + " + *tome*, a cutting, slice]
colpocytology (kŏl"pō-sī-tŏl'ō-jē) [" + *kytos*, cell, + *logos*, word, reason]

colpodynia (kŏl"pō-dĭn'ē-ă) [Gr. *kolpos*, vagina, + *odyne*, pain]
colpohyperplasia (kŏl"pō-hī-pĕr-plā'zē-ă) [" + *hyper*, over, above, excessive, + *plasis*, a forming]
c. cystica
colpomicroscope (kŏl"pō-mī'krō-skōp) [" + *mikros*, small, + *skopein*, to view]
colpomyomectomy (kŏl"pō-mī"ō-mĕk'tō-mē) [" + *mys*, muscle, + *oma*, tumor, + *ektome*, excision]
colpomyomotomy (kŏl"pō-mī"ō-mŏt'ō-mē) [" + " + " + *tome*, a cutting, slice]
colpoperineoplasty (kŏl"pō-pĕr"ĭn-ē'ō-plăs"tē) [" + *perinaion*, perineum, + *plassein*, to form]
colpoperineorrhaphy (kŏl"pō-pĕr"ĭn-ē-or'ră-fē) [" + " + *rhaphe*, seam]
colpopexy (kŏl'pō-pĕk"sē) [" + *pexis*, fixation]
colpoplasty (kŏl'pō-plăs"tē) [" + *plassein*, to form]
colpoptosis (kŏl"pŏp-tō'sĭs) [" + *ptosis*, fall, falling]
colporrhagia (kŏl"pō-rā'jē-ă) [" + *rhegnynai*, to burst forth]
colporrhaphy (kŏl-por'ă-fē) [" + *rhaphe*, seam]
colporrhexis (kŏl"pō-rĕk'sĭs) [" + *rhexis*, rupture]
colposcope (kŏl'pō-skōp) [" + *skopein*, to examine]
colposcopy (kŏl-pŏs'kō-pē)
colpospasm, colpospasmus (kŏl"pō-spăzm, kŏl"pō-spăz'mŭs) [Gr. *kolpos*, vagina, + *spasmos*, a convulsion]
colpostat (kŏl'pō-stăt) [" + *statikos*, standing]
colpostenosis (kŏl"pō-stĕn-ō'sĭs) [" + *stenosis*, act of narrowing]
colpostenotomy (kŏl"pō-stĕn-ŏt'ō-mē) [" + " + *tome*, a cutting, slice]
colpotherm (kŏl'pō-thĕrm) [" + *therme*, heat]

colpotomy (kŏl-pŏt'ō-mē) [" + *tome*, a cutting, slice]

colpoureterocystotomy (kŏl"pō-ū-rē"tĕr-ō-sĭs-tŏt'ō-mē) [" + *oureter*, ureter, + *kystis*, bladder, + *tome*, a cutting, slice]

colpoureterotomy (kŏl"pō-ū-rē"tĕr-ŏt'ō-mē) [" + " + *tome*, a cutting, slice]

colpoxerosis (kŏl"pō-zē-rō'sĭs) [" + *xerosis*, dryness]

columbium

columella (kŏl"ū-mĕl'lă) [L., small column]

   c. cochleae

   c. nasi

column (kŏl'ŭm) [L. *columna*, pillar]

   c., anal

   c., anterior

   c., Clarke's

   c., fornix

   c., gray

   c., lateral

   c. of Burdach

   c. of Goll

   c. of Gowers

   c. of Morgagni

   c., posterior

   c., rectal

   c., renal

   c., spinal

   c., vertebral

   c., vesicular

columna (kō-lŭm'na) [L.]

   c. carnea

   c. nasi

   c. rugarum vaginae

   c. vaginalis

columnar layer

columning (kŏl'ŭm-ĭng)

Coly-Mycin M

Coly-Mycin S Oral

coma (kō'mă) [Gr. *koma*, deep sleep]

   c., alcoholic

   c., apoplectic

   c., barbiturate

   c., diabetic

   c., hepatic

   c., hypoglycemic

   c., irreversible

   c., Kussmaul's

   c., uremic

   c., vigil

coma scale

comatose (kō'mă-tōs)

combustion (kŏm-bŭst'yŭn)

comedo (kŏm'ē-dō) [L. *comedere*, to eat up]

comes (kō'mēz) [L., companion]

Comfolax

comma bacillus

comma tract of Schultze

commensal (kō-mĕn'săl) [L. *com-*, together, + *mensa*, table]

commensalism (kō-mĕn'săl-ĭzm")

comminute (kŏm'ĭ-nūt) [L. *com-*, together, + *minuere*, to crumble]

comminuted fracture

comminution (kŏm"ĭ-nū'shŭn) [L. *comminutio*, crumbling]

commissura (kŏm"mĭ-sū'ră) [L.]

commissural (kŏm-mĭs'ū-răl)

commissure (kŏm'ĭ-shūr) [L. *commissura*, a joining together]

   c., anterior cerebral

   c., anterior gray

   c., anterior white

   c., of fornix

   c., posterior, of brain

   c., posterior, of spinal cord

commissurorrhaphy (kŏm"ĭ-shūr-or'ă-fē) [" + Gr. *rhaphe*, seam]

commissurotomy (kŏm"ĭ-shūr-ŏt'ō-mē) [" + Gr. *tome*, a cutting, slice]

commitment (kō-mĭt'mĕnt)

common bile duct

commotio (kō-mō'shē-ō) [L. *commotio*, a disturbance]

   c. retinae

   c. spinalis

commune (kŏm'yoon)

communicable disease

communicans (kō-mū'nĕ-kănz) [L. *communicare*, to connect with]

communication board

communicator

communis (kŏ-mū′nĭs) [L.]
community medicine
Comolli's sign (kō-mōl′lēz) [Antonio Comolli, It. pathologist, b. 1879]
compact [L. *compactus,* joined together]
compact bone
compaction (kŏm-păk′shŭn)
comparative anatomy
compartmental syndrome
compatibility [L. *compati,* to sympathize with]
compatible
Compazine
compensating
compensation [L. *cum,* with, + *pensare,* to weigh]
    c., failure of
competence (kŏm′pĕ-tĕns)
competition (kŏm″pĕ-tĭsh′ŭn)
complaint (kŏm-plānt′)
complement (kŏm′plĕ-mĕnt) [L. *complere,* to complete]
complemental, complementary
    c. air
    c. colors
complementarity
complement fixation
complementophil (kŏm″plĕ-mĕnt′ō-fĭl) [″ + Gr. *philein,* to love]
complex [L. *complexus,* woven together]
    c., castration
    c., Electra
    c., Ghon
    c., Golgi
    c., inferiority
    c., Oedipus
    c., superiority
complexion (kŏm-plĕk′shŭn)
complexus (kŏm-plĕk′sŭs) [L.]
compliance (kŏm-plī′ăns)
    c., pulmonary
complication [L. *cum,* with, + *plicare,* to fold]
component
component blood therapy
compos mentis (kŏm″pŭs mĕn′tĭs) [L.]

compound [L. *componere,* to place together]
    c., dental
    c., inorganic
    c., organic
compound astigmatism
compound fracture
compound microscope
compress (kŏm′prĕs); (kŏm-prĕs′) [L. *compressus,* squeezed together]
    c., chest
    c., cold
    c., forehead
    c., hot
    c., wet
compressed spectral array
compression (kŏm-prĕsh′ŭn) [L. *compressio,* a compression]
    c., cerebral
    c., digital
    c., myelitis
compression gloves
compressor
    c., air
compulsion (kŏm-pŭl′shŭn) [L. *compulsio,* compulsion]
compulsion neurosis
compulsive (kŏm-pŭl′sĭv)
compulsive ideas
compulsory (kŏm-pŭl′sor-ē)
computer
    c., digital
computer-assisted design
computer interface
con- [L.] *together with*
conarium (kō-nā′rē-ŭm) [L.]
conation (kō-nā′shŭn) [L. *conatio,* an attempt]
conative (kŏn′ă-tĭv)
concanavalin A (kŏn″kă-năv′ĭ-lĭn)
concatenation (kŏn-kăt″ĭ-nā′shŭn) [L. *con,* together, + *catena,* chain]
Concato's disease (kŏn-kŏ′tōs) [Luigi M. Concato, It. physician, 1825–1882]
concave (kŏn′kāv, kŏn-kāv′) [″ + *cavus,* hollow]
concavity (kŏn-kăv′ĭ-tē)

concavoconcave (kŏn-kā″vō-kŏn′kāv)
[″ + cavus, hollow, + con,
with, + cavus, hollow]
concavoconvex (kŏn-kā″vō-kŏn′vĕks)
[″ + ″ + convexus, vaulted]
conceive (kŏn-sēv′) [L. concipere, to
take to oneself]
concentration (kŏn-sĕn-trā′shŭn) [L.
con, together with, + centrum,
center]
  c., hydrogen ion
  c., minimum inhibitory
concentric (kŏn-sĕn′trĭk) [″ + centrum, center]
concept (kŏn′sĕpt) [L. conceptum,
something understood]
conception (kŏn-sĕp′shŭn)
conceptus (kŏn-sĕp′tŭs)
concha (kŏng′kă) [Gr. konche, shell]
  c. auriculae
  c. bullosa
  c., nasal
  c. sphenoidalis
conchitis (kŏng-kī′tĭs) [″ + itis, in-
flammation]
conchoidal (kŏng-koy′dăl) [″ +
eidos, form, shape]
conchoscope (kŏng′kō-skōp) [″ +
skopein, to examine]
conchotome (kŏng′kō-tōm) [″ +
tome, a cutting, slice]
conchotomy (kŏng-kŏt′ō-mē)
concoction (kŏn-kŏk′shŭn) [L. con, with,
+ coquere, to cook]
concomitant (kŏn-kŏm′ĭ-tănt) [″ +
comes, companion]
concordance (kŏn-kor′dăns)
concrement (kŏn′krē-mĕnt) [L. concre-
mentum]
concrescence (kŏn-krĕs′ĕns) [L. con,
with, + crescere, to grow]
concrete (kŏn′krēt, kŏn-krēt′) [L. con-
cretus, solid]
concretio cordis (kŏn-krē′shē-ō
kor′dĭs)
concretion (kŏn-krē′shŭn) [″ + crescere, to grow]
concubitus (kŏn-kū′bĭ-tŭs) [L.]

concussion (kŏn-kŭsh′ŭn) [L. concussus,
shaken violently]
  c. of brain
  c. of labyrinth
  c., spinal
condensation (kŏn″dĕn-sā′shŭn)
[″ + densare, to make thick]
condenser (kŏn-dĕn′sĕr)
  c., electrical
  c., substage
condiment (kŏn′dĭ-mĕnt) [L. condire, to
pickle]
condition
conditioned reflex
conditioning (kŏn-dĭsh′ŭn-ĭng)
  c., operant
condom (kŏn′dŭm) [L. condus, a recep-
tacle]
  c., instructions for use
conductance (kŏn-dŭk′tăns) [L. condu-
cere, to lead]
conduction (kŏn-dŭk′shŭn)
  c., bone
conduction system, cardiac
conductivity (kŏn″dŭk-tĭv′ĭ-tē)
conductor (kŏn-dŭk′tor)
conduit (kŏn′doo-ĭt)
  c., ileal
condylar (kŏn′dĭ-lăr) [Gr. kondylos,
knuckle]
condylarthrosis (kŏn″dĭl-ăr-thrō′sĭs)
[″ + arthrosis, a joint]
condyle (kŏn′dĭl) [Gr. kondylos,
knuckle]
condylectomy (kŏn″dĭ-lĕk′tō-mē)
[″ + ektome, excision]
condylion (kŏn-dĭl′ē-ŏn) [Gr. kondy-
lion, knob]
condyloid (kŏn′dĭ-loyd) [Gr. kondylos,
knuckle, + eidos, form, shape]
condyloid process
condyloid tubercle
condyloma (kŏn″dĭ-lō′mă) [Gr. kondy-
loma, wart]
  c. acuminatum
  c. latum
condylomatous (kŏn″dĭ-lō′mă-tŭs)
condylotomy (kŏn″dĭ-lŏt′ō-mē) [Gr.

kondylos, knuckle, + *tome,* a cutting, slice]
condylus (kŏn′dĭ-lŭs)
cone (kōn) [Gr. *konos,* cone]
   c., ocular
   c., retinal
cone of light
conexus (kŏ-nĕk′sŭs) [L.]
confabulation (kŏn-făb″ū-lā′shŭn) [L. *confabulari,* to talk together]
confectio, confection (kŏn-fĕk′shē-ō, -shŭn) [L. *conficere,* to prepare]
confidentiality
configuration (kŏn-fĭg″ū-rā′shŭn)
confinement (kŏn-fīn′mĕnt) [O. Fr. *confiner,* to restrain in a place]
conflict (kŏn′flĭkt) [L. *confligere,* to contend]
confluence of sinuses
confluent (kŏn′floo-ĕnt) [L. *confluere,* to run together]
conformation (kŏn″for-mā′shŭn)
confrontation (kŏn″frŭn-tā′shŭn) [L. *con,* together with, + *frons,* face]
confusion (kŏn-fū′zhŭn)
   c., mental
congelation (kŏn″jĕ-lā′shŭn) [L. *congelare,* to freeze]
congener (kŏn′jĕn-ĕr) [L. *con,* together, + *genus,* race]
congenerous (kŏn-jĕn′ĕr-ŭs)
congenital (kŏn-jĕn′ĭ-tăl) [L. *congenitus,* born together]
congenital anomaly
congested (kŏn-jĕs′tĕd) [L. *congerere,* to heap together]
congestion
   c., active
   c., passive
   c., pulmonary
congestive (kŏn-jĕs′tĭv)
congius (kŏn′jē-ŭs) [L.]
conglobate (kŏn′glō-bāt) [L. *con,* together, + *globare,* to make round]
conglobation (kŏn″glō-bā′shŭn)
conglomerate (kŏn-glŏm′ĕr-āt) [″ + *glomerare,* to heap]
conglutin (kŏn-gloo′tĭn) [L. *conglutin-*

are, to glue together]
conglutinant (kŏn-gloo′tĭ-nănt)
conglutinate (kŏn-gloo′tĭ-nāt)
conglutination (kŏn-gloo″tĭn-ā′shŭn)
coniasis (kō-nī′ă-sĭs) [Gr. *konis,* dust, + *-iasis,* state or condition of]
conidia (kō-nĭd′ē-ă)
conidiophore (kŏn-ĭd′ē-ō-for) [″ + *phoros,* bearing]
coniofibrosis (kō″nē-ō-fī-brō′sĭs) [Gr. *konis,* dust, + L. *fibra,* fiber, + Gr. *osis,* condition]
coniology (kō-nē-ŏl′ō-jē) [″ + *logos,* word, reason]
coniosis (kō″nē-ō′sĭs) [″ + *osis,* condition]
coniosporosis (kō″nē-ō-spō-rō′sĭs) [″ + *sporos,* seed, + *osis,* condition]
coniotomy (kō″nē-ŏt′ō-mē) [Gr. *konos,* cone, + *tome,* a cutting, slice]
conization (kŏn″ĭ-zā′shŭn) [Gr. *konos,* cone]
conjugata (kŏn″jū-gā′tă) [L. *conjugatus,* yoked together]
   c. vera
conjugate (kŏn′jū-gāt)
   c. deviation
   c., diagonal
   c. diameter
   c., external
   c., true
conjugation (kŏn″jū-gā′shŭn)
conjunctiva (kŏn″jŭnk-tī′vă, kŏn-jŭnk′tĭ-vă) [L. *conjungere,* to join together]
conjunctival reflex
conjunctivitis (kŏ-jŭnk″tĭ-vī′tĭs) [″ + Gr. *itis,* inflammation]
   c., actinic
   c., acute contagious
   c., angular, of Morax-Axenfeld
   c., catarrhal
   c., epidemic hemorrhagic
   c., follicular
   c., gonorrheal
   c., granular
   c., inclusion
   c., membranous

c. of newborn
c., phlyctenular
c., purulent
c., vernal
conjunctivoma (kŏn-jŭnk"tĭ-vō'mă) [L. conjungere, to join together, + Gr. oma, tumor]
conjunctivoplasty (kŏn"jŭnk-tĭ'vō-plăs"tē) [" + Gr. plassein, to form]
connective [L. connectere, to bind together]
connective tissue
connective tissue diseases
Conn's syndrome [J. W. Conn, U.S. physician, b. 1907]
conoid (kō'noyd) [Gr. konos, cone, + eidos, form, shape]
conoid ligament
conoid tubercle
consanguinity (kŏn"săn-gwĭn'ĭ-tē) [L. consanguinitas, kinship]
conscience (kon'shŭntz)
conscious (kŏn'shŭs) [L. conscius, aware]
consciousness
c., clouding of
c., cosmic
c., disintegration of
c., levels of
consensual (kŏn-sĕn'shū-ăl) [L. consensus, agreement]
consensual light index
consensual light reflex
consensual reflex
consent
c., implied
c., informed
consenting adult
conservative (kŏn-sĕr'vă-tĭv) [L. conservare, to preserve]
consolidation (kŏn-sŏl-ĭ-dā'shŭn) [L. consolidare, to make firm]
constant (kŏn'stănt) [L. constans, standing together]
constellation (kŏn"stĕl-lā'shŭn) [L. con, together, + stella, star]
constipation (kŏn"stĭ-pā'shŭn) [L. constipare, to press together]

c., atonic
c., obstructive
c., spastic
constitution [L. constituere, to establish]
constitutional
constitutional disease
constriction [L. con, together, + stringere, to draw]
constrictor
constructive metabolism
consultant [L. consultare, to counsel]
consultation
consummation
consumption (kŏn-sŭmp'shŭn) [L. consumere, to waste away]
consumption-coagulopathy
consumptive
contact [L. con, with, + tangere, to touch]
c., complete
c., direct
c., indirect
c., mediate
c., occlusal
c., proximal; c., proximate
contactant (kŏn-tăk'tănt)
contact dermatitis
contact lens
c.l., bifocal
c.l., hard
c.l., soft
contact surface
contagion (kŏn-tā'jŭn) [L. contingere, to touch]
contagious (kŏn-tā'jŭs)
contagious pustular dermatitis
contagium (kŏn-tā'jē-ŭm) [L.]
containers, care and handling of
contaminant (kŏn-tăm'ĭ-nănt)
contaminate (kŏn-tăm'ĭ-nāt) [L. contaminare, to render impure]
contamination
c., radiation
content
contiguity (kŏn"tĭ-gū'ĭ-tē) [L. contiguus, touching]
c., amputation in
c., law of

c., solution of

continence (kŏn′tĭ-nĕns) [L. *continere*, to hold together]

continent (kŏn′tĭ-nĕnt)

continued (kŏn-tĭn′ūd)

continuity (kŏn″tĭ-nū′ĭ-tē) [L. *continuus*, continued]

   c., amputation in

   c., solution of

continuous (kŏn-tĭn′ū-ŭs) [L. *continere*, to hold together]

continuous spectrum

continuous subcutaneous insulin infusion

contortion (kŏn-tor′shŭn) [L. *contorquere*, to twist together]

contour (kŏn′toor) [It. *contornare*, to go around]

   c., gingival

   c., gingival denture

contoured (kŏn′toord)

contra- [L.] *opposite or against*

contra-aperture [L. *contra*, against, + *apertura*, opening]

contraception (kŏn″tră-sĕp′shŭn) [″ + *conceptio*, a conceiving]

contraceptive (kŏn″tră-sĕp′tĭv)

contract (kŏn-trăkt′) [L. *contrahere*, to draw together]

contractile (kŏn-trăk′tĭl)

contractility (kŏn-trăk-tĭl′ĭ-tē)

contraction (kŏn-trăk′shŭn)

   c., Braxton Hicks

   c., carpopedal

   c., Dupuytren's [Baron G. Dupuytren, Fr. surgeon, 1777–1835]

   c., isometric

   c., isotonic

   c., postural

   c., tetanic

   c., tonic

contraction stress test

contracture (kŏn-trăk′chūr) [L. *contractura*]

   c., Dupuytren's

   c., functional

   c., ischemic

   c., physiological

c., Volkmann's

contrafissura (kŏn″tră-fĭ-shū′ră) [L. *contra*, against, + *fissura*, fissure]

contraindication (kŏn″tră-ĭn-dĭ-kā′shŭn) [″ + *indicare*, to point out]

contralateral (kŏn″tră-lăt′ĕr-ăl) [″ + *latus*, side]

contralateral reflexes

contrast (kŏn′trăst)

contrast medium

contrast sprays

contravolitional (kŏn″tră-vō-lĭ′shŭn-ăl) [L. *contra*, against, + *velle*, to wish]

contrecoup (kŏn-tr-koo′) [Fr., counterblow]

contrecoup injury

contrectation (kŏn″trĕk-tā′shŭn) [L. *contrectare*, to handle]

control (kŏn-trōl′) [L. *contra*, against, + *rotulus*, little wheel]

controlled substance act

contrude (kŏn-trood′) [L. *con*, with, + *trudere*, to thrust]

contrusion (kŏn-troo′zhŭn)

contuse (kŏn-tooz′) [L. *contundere*, to bruise]

contusion (kŏn-too′zhŭn)

conus (kō′nŭs) [Gr. *konos*]

   c. arteriosus

   c. medullaris

convalescence (kŏn″văl-ĕs′ĕns) [L. *convalescere*, to become strong]

convalescent

convalescent diet

convection (kŏn-vĕk′shŭn) [L. *convehere*, to convey]

convergence (kŏn-vĕr′jĕns) [L. *con*, with, + *vergere*, to incline]

convergent (kŏn-vĕr′jĕnt)

conversion (kŏn-vĕr′zhŭn) [L. *convertere*, to turn round]

conversion reaction

conversion symptom

convex (kŏn′vĕks, kŏn-vĕks′) [L. *convexus*, vaulted, arched]

convexoconcave (kŏn-vĕk″sō-kŏn′kăv, -kŏn-kăv′) [″ + *concavus*,

vaulted hollow]
convexoconvex [" + *convexus*, arched]
convolute (kŏn'vō-loot) [L. *convolvere*, to roll together]
convoluted
convoluted tubule
convolution (kŏn"vō-loo'shŭn) [L. *convolvere*, to roll together]
  c., angular
  c.'s, annectant
  c., anterior choroid
  c., anterior orbital
  c., Arnold's
  c., ascending frontal
  c., ascending parietal
  c., Broca's
  c., callosal
  c.'s, cerebral
  c., cuneate
  c., dentate
  c.'s, exterior olfactory
  c., hippocampal
  c., inferior frontal
  c., inferior occipital
  c., insular
  c.'s, intestinal
  c., marginal
  c., middle frontal
  c., middle occipital
  c., middle temporosphenoidal
  c.'s, occipitotemporal
  c. of the corpus callosum
  c. of the sylvian fissure
  c., olfactory
  c.'s, orbital
  c.'s, parietal
  c., posterior orbital
  c., second frontal
  c., superior frontal
  c., superior occipital
  c., superior parietal
  c., superior temporosphenoidal
  c., supramarginal
  c., transverse orbital
  c., uncinate
convulsant (kŏn-vŭl'sănt) [L. *convellere*, to pull together]

convulsant poisons
convulsion (kŏn-vŭl'shŭn)
  c., clonic
  c., febrile
  c., hysterical
  c., mimetic
  c., oscillating
  c., puerperal
  c., salaam
  c., tonic
  c., toxic
  c., uremic
convulsive (kŏn-vŭl'sĭv)
convulsive reflex
convulsive tic
cooking [L. *coquere*, to cook]
Cooley's anemia [Thomas Cooley, U.S. pediatrician, 1871–1945]
Coombs' test [R. R. A. Coombs, Brit. immunologist, b. 1921]
coordination (kō-or"dĭn-ā'shŭn) [L. co-, same, + *ordinare*, to arrange]
COPD *chronic obstructive pulmonary disease*
cope (kōp) [ME. *caupen*, to contend with]
coping
copodyskinesia (kō"pō-dĭs"kĭn-ē'sē-ă) [Gr. *kopos*, fatigue, + *dys*, bad, difficult, painful, disordered, + *kinesis*, motion]
copolymer (kō-pŏl'ĭ-mĕr)
copper [L. *cuprum*]
copperas (kŏp'ĕr-ăs)
copperhead
copper sulfate
copper sulfate poisoning
copremesis (kŏp-rĕm'ĕ-sĭs) [Gr. *kopros*, dung, + *emesis*, vomiting]
coproantibody (kŏp"rō-ăn'tĭ-bŏd"ē)
coprolagnia (kŏp"rō-lăg'nē-ă) [" + *lagneia*, lust]
coprolalia (kŏp"rō-lā'lē-ă) [" + *lalia*, chatter, prattle]
coprolith (kŏp'rō-lĭth) [" + *lithos*, stone]
coprology (kŏp-rŏl'ō-jē) [" + *logos*, word, reason]

coproma (kŏp-rō′mă)
coprophagy (kŏp-rŏf′ă-jē) [″ +
phagein, to eat]
coprophilia (kŏp″rō-fil′ē-ă) [″ +
philein, to love]
coprophilic
coprophobia (kŏp″rō-fō′bē-ă) [″ +
phobos, fear]
coproporphyria (kŏp″rō-por-fir′ē-ă)
[″ + porphyra, purple]
coproporphyrin (kŏp″rō-por′fir-ĭn)
coproporphyrinuria (kŏp″rō-por″fir-
ĭn-ū′rē-ă)
coprostanol (kŏp″rō-stā′nŏl)
coprozoa (kŏp″rō-zō′ă) [″ +
zoon, animal]
coprozoic (kŏp″rō-zō′ĭk)
copula (kŏp′ū-lă) [L., link]
copulation (kŏp″ū-lā′shŭn) [L. copula-
tio]
cor (kor) [L.]
   c. pulmonale
coracoacromial (kor″ă-kō-ă-krō′mē-
ăl) [Gr. korax, raven, + akron,
point, + omos, shoulder]
coracoid (kor′ă-koyd) [″ + eidos,
form, shape]
coracoid process
cord [Gr. khorde]
   c., spermatic
   c., spinal
   c., umbilical
   c., vocal
cordal (kor′dăl)
cordate (kor′dāt) [L. cor, heart]
cord bladder
cordectomy (kor-dĕk′tō-mē) [Gr.
khorde, cord, + ektome, excision]
cordiform (kor′dĭ-form) [L. cor, heart,
+ forma, shape]
corditis (kor-dī′tĭs) [Gr. khorde, cord,
+ itis, inflammation]
cordopexy (kor′dō-pĕk″sē) [″ +
pexis, fixation]
cordotomy (kor-dŏt′ō-mē) [″ +
tome, a cutting, slice]
Cordran
core (kor)

coreclisis (kor″ē-klī′sĭs) [Gr. kore, pupil
of the eye, + kleisis, closure]
corectasia, corectasis (kor-ĕk-tā′zē-
ă, -ĕk′tă-sĭs) [″ + ektasis, dilata-
tion]
corectome (kō-rĕk′tōm) [″ + ektome, excision]
corectomy (kō-rĕk′tō-mē)
corectopia (kor-ĕk-tō′pē-ă) [″ +
ek, out of, + topos, place]
coredialysis (kō″rē-dī-ăl′ĭ-sĭs) [″ +
dia, through, + lysis, dissolution]
corediastasis (kor″ē-dī-ăs′tă-sĭs)
[″ + diastasis, a standing apart]
corelysis (kor-ĕl′ĭ-sĭs) [″ + lysis,
dissolution]
coremorphosis (kor″ē-mor-fō′sĭs)
[″ + morphe, form, + osis,
condition]
coreometer (kō″rē-ŏm′ē-tĕr) [″ +
metron, measure]
coreometry (kō″rē-ŏm′ē-trē)
coreoplasty (kō′rē-ō-plăs″tē) [″ +
plassein, to form]
corepressor (kō″rē-prĕs′sor)
corestenoma (kor″ē-stĕn-ō′mă) [″ +
stenoma, contraction]
   c. congenitum
core temperature
coretomedialysis (kor″ĕt-ō-mē-dē-
ăl′ĭ-sĭs) [″ + tome, a cutting, slice,
+ dia, through, + lysis, dissolu-
tion]
coretomy (kō-rĕt′ō-mē) [″ + tome,
a cutting, slice]
Cori cycle (kō′rē) [Carl F. Cori, U.S.
pharmacologist and biochemist,
1896–1984; Gerty T. Cori, U.S. biochemist, 1896–1957]
corium (kō′rē-ŭm) [L., skin]
corm (korm) [Gr. kormos, a trimmed tree
trunk]
corn [L. cornu, horn]
cornea (kor′nē-ă) [L. corneus, horny]
corneal
corneal impression
corneal reflex
corneal transplant

corneitis (kor″nē-ī′tĭs) [L. *corneus*, horny, + Gr. *itis*, inflammation]
Cornell Medical Index
corneoblepharon (kor″nē-ō-blĕf′ă-rŏn) [″ + Gr. *blepharon*, eyelid]
corneoiritis (kor″nē-ō-ī-rī′tĭs) [L. *corneus*, horny, + Gr. *iris*, bend, turn, + *itis*, inflammation]
corneomandibular **reflex** (kor″nē-ō-măn-dĭb′ū-lăr)
corneosclera (kor″nē-ō-sklē′ră) [L. *corneus*, horny, + *skleros*, hard]
corneous (kor′nē-ŭs) [L. *corneus*]
corneous layer
corneum (kor′nē-ŭm) [L., horny]
corniculate (kor-nĭk′ū-lāt)
corniculum (kor-nĭk′ū-lŭm) [L., little horn]
cornification (kor″nĭ-fĭ-kā′shŭn) [″ + *facere*, to make]
cornified (kor′nĭ-fīd)
cornu (kor′nū) [L., horn]
    c. ammonis
    c. anterius
    c. coccygeum
    c. cutaneum
    c. inferius
    c. of the hyoid
    c. of the sacrum
    c. posterius
cornua (kor′nū-ă)
cornual (kor′nū-ăl)
corona (kŏ-rō′nă) [Gr. *korone*, crown]
    c. capitis
    c. ciliaris
    c. dentis
    c. glandis
    c. radiata
    c. veneris
coronal (kō-rō′năl)
coronal plane
coronal suture
coronary (kor′ō-nă-rē) [L. *coronarius*, pert. to a crown or circle]
coronary angiography
coronary arteries
coronary artery disease
coronary artery spasm
coronary blood flow

coronary bypass
coronary care unit
coronary heart disease
coronary occlusion
coronary plexus
coronary sinus
coronary thrombosis
coronaviruses (kor″ō-nă-vī′rŭs-ĕs) [L. *corona*, crown, + *virus*, poison]
coroner (kor′ō-nĕr) [L. *corona*, crown]
coronoid (kor′ō-noyd) [Gr. *korone*, something curved, kind of crown, + *eidos*, form, shape]
coronoidectomy (kor″ō-noy-dĕk′tō-mē) [″ + ″ + *ektome*, excision]
coronoid fossa
coronoid process
coroparelcysis (kor″ō-păr-ĕl′sĭ-sĭs) [Gr. *kore*, pupil, + *parelkein*, to draw aside]
coroscopy (kō-rŏs′kō-pē) [″ + *skopein*, to examine]
corotomy (kō-rŏt′ō-mē) [″ + *tome*, a cutting, slice]
corpora (kor′pō-ră)
    c. arantii
    c. arenacea
    c. olivaria
    c. paraaortica
    c. quadrigemina
corporeal (kor-pō′rē-ăl)
corpse (korps) [L. *corpus*, body]
corpsman (kor′măn)
corpulence (kor′pū-lĕns) [L. *corpulentia*]
corpulent (kor′pū-lĕnt)
cor pulmonale
corpus (kor′pŭs) [L., body]
    c. albicans
    c. amygdaloideum
    c. amylaceum
    c. annulare
    c. callosum
    c. cavernosum
    c. cavernosum penis
    c. cerebellum
    c. ciliare
    c. dentale

c. fimbriatum
c. flavum
c. fornicis
c. geniculatum
c. hemorrhagicum
c. highmorianum
c. interpedunculare
c. luteum
c. Luysii
c. mammillare
c. restiforme
c. rhomboidale
c. spongiosum
c. striatum
c. subthalamicum
c. trapezoideum
c. vitreum
c. wolffianum
corpuscle (kor'pŭs-ĕl) [L. *corpusculum*, little body]
 c., axile; c., axis
 c., blood
 c., bone
 c., cancroid
 c., cartilage
 c., chromophil
 c.'s, chyle
 c., colloid
 c., colostrum
 c.'s, corneal
 c.'s, Drysdale's
 c.'s, genital
 c., ghost
 c.'s, Gierke's
 c.'s, Golgi-Mazzoni
 c.'s, Hassall's
 c.'s, Krause's
 c., lymph
 c., malpighian
 c.'s, Mazzoni's
 c.'s, Meissner's
 c.'s, milk
 c., pacinian
 c., phantom
 c., Purkinje's
 c., red
 c., renal
 c.'s, reticulated

c., splenic
c., tactile
c., terminal
c.'s, thymic
c., white
corpuscular (kor-pŭs'kū-lăr)
corpusculum (kŏr-pŭs'kū-lŭm) [L., little body]
correction
corrective (kŏ-rĕk'tĭv) [L. *corrigere*, to correct]
correlation (kor"ĕ-lā'shŭn) [L. *com-*, together, + *relatio*, relation]
correspondence
 c., retinal
corresponding
corresponding points of retina
Corrigan's pulse (kor'ĭ-găns) [Sir Dominic J. Corrigan, Ir. physician, 1802–1880]
corrosion (kŏ-rō'zhŭn) [L *corrodere*, to corrode]
corrosive (kŏ-rō'sĭv)
corrosive alkalies
corrosive poisoning
corrugator (kor'ū-gā"tor) [L. *con*, together, + *rugare*, to wrinkle]
Cortef
Cortef Acetate
Cortenema
cortex (kor'tĕks) [L., rind]
 c., adrenal
 c., cerebellar
 c., cerebral
 c., interpretive
 c., renal
 c., temporal
Corti, Alfonso (kor'tē) It. anatomist, 1822–1888
 C., canal of
 C.'s membrane
 C., organ of
cortiadrenal (kor"tē-ăd-rē'năl) [L. *cortex*, rind, + *ad*, toward, + *ren*, kidney]
cortical (kor'tĭ-kăl)
corticate (kor'tĭ-kāt)
corticectomy (kor"tĭ-sĕk'tō-mē) ["   +

Gr. *ektome*, excision]
cortices (kor″tĭ-sēz)
corticifugal (kor″tĭ-sĭf′ū-găl) [L. *cortex*, rind, + *fugere*, to flee]
corticipetal (kor″tĭ-sĭp′ĕ-tăl) [″ + *petere*, to seek]
corticoadrenal (kor″tĭ-kō-ăd-rē′năl) [″ + *ad*, toward, + *ren*, kidney]
corticoafferent (kor″tĭ-kō-ăf′fĕr-ĕnt) [″ + *adferre*, to bear to]
corticobulbar (kor″tĭ-kō-bŭl′băr) [″ + *bulbus*, bulb]
corticoefferent (kor″tĭ-kō-ĕf′-ĕr-ĕnt) [″ + *effere*, to bring out of]
corticoid (kor′tĭ-koyd) [″ + Gr. *eidos*, form, shape]
corticopeduncular (kor″tĭ-kō-pĕ-dŭng′kū-lăr) [″ + *pedunculus*, little foot]
corticopleuritis (kor″tĭ-kō-ploo-rī′tĭs) [″ + Gr. *pleura*, rib, + *itis*, inflammation]
corticopontine (kor″tĭ-kō-pŏn′tīn) [″ + *pons*, bridge]
corticospinal (kor″tĭ-kō-spī′năl) [″ + *spina*, thorn]
corticosteroid (kor″tĭ-kō-stĕr′oyd)
corticosterone (kor″tĭ-kŏs′tĕ-rōn)
corticothalamic (kor″tĭ-kō-thă-lăm′ĭk) [″ + Gr. *thalamos*, chamber]
corticotrophic, corticotropic (kor″tĭ-kō-trŏf′ĭk, -trŏp′ĭk) [″ + Gr. *trophe*, nourishment; ″ + Gr. *trope*, a turn]
corticotrophin, corticotropin (kor″tĭ-kō-trō′fĭn, -trō′pĭn)
corticotrophin releasing factor
cortin (kor′tĭn) [L. *cortex*, rind]
cortisol (kor′tĭ-sŏl)
cortisone (kor′tĭ-sōn)
Cortone Acetate
Cortril
Cortril Acetate-AS
Cortrophin
Cortrophin Zinc ACTH
Cortrosyn
coruscation (kō-rŭs-kā′shŭn) [L. *coruscare*, to glitter]

corybantism (kor″ĭ-băn′tĭzm) [Gr. *Korybas*, a priest of Cybele who accompanied the goddess, during her travels, with music and wild dancing, + *-ismos*, condition]
Corynebacterium (kō-rī″nē-băk-tē′rē-ŭm) [Gr. *coryne*, a club, + *bacterion*, a small rod]
　C. diphtheriae
　C. vaginale
coryza (kō-rī′ză) [Gr. *koryza*, catarrh]
cosensitize (kō-sĕn′sī-tīz) [L. *con*, with, + *sensitivus*, sensitive]
Cosmegen
cosmetic (kŏz-mĕt′ĭk)
cosmetic surgery
cosmic (kŏz′mĭk) [Gr. *kosmos*, order, the universe]
costa (kŏs′tă) [L.]
　c. fluctuans
　c. spuria
　c. vera
costal (kŏs′tăl)
costal cartilage
costalgia (kŏs-tăl′jē-ă) [L. *costa*, rib, + Gr. *algos*, pain]
costal pit
costectomy (kŏs-tĕk′tō-mē) [″ + Gr. *ektome*, excision]
Costen's syndrome [James B. Costen, U.S. otolaryngologist, 1895–1961]
costive (kŏs′tĭv) [L. *constipare*, to press together]
costiveness (kŏs′tĭv-nĕs)
costocervical (kŏs″tō-sĕr′vĭ-kăl)
costochondral (kŏs″tō-kŏn′drăl) [L. *costa*, rib, + Gr. *chondros*, cartilage]
costoclavicular (kŏs″tō-klă-vĭk′ū-lăr) [″ + *clavicula*, a little key]
costocoracoid (kŏs″tō-kor′ă-koyd) [″ + Gr. *korax*, crow, + *eidos*, form, shape]
costophrenic [″ + Gr. *phren*, diaphragm]
costopneumopexy (kŏs″tō-nū′mō-pĕk″sē) [″ + Gr. *pneumon*, lung,

+ *pexis*, fixation]

costosternal (kŏs"tō-stĕr'năl) [" + Gr. *sternon*, chest]

costosternoplasty (kŏs"tō-stĕr'nō-plăs"tē) [" + " + *plassein*, to form]

costotome (kŏs'tō-tōm) [" + Gr. *tome*, a cutting, slice]

costotomy (kŏs-tŏt'ō-mē)

costotransverse (kŏs"tō-trăns-vĕrs') [" + *transvertere*, to turn across]

costovertebral (kŏs"tō-vĕr'tĕ-brăl) [" + *vertebra*, joint]

costoxiphoid (kŏs"tō-zī'foyd) [" + Gr. *xiphos*, sword, + *eidos*, form, shape]

cosyntropin (kō-sĭn-trō'pĭn)

C.O.T.A. certified occupational therapy assistant

Cotazym

cotinine

cotton [ME. *cotoun*, from Arabic *qutn*, cotton]

c., purified

c., styptic

cotton-wool spot

co-twin (kō-twĭn)

cotyledon (kŏt"ĭ-lē'dŏn) [Gr. *kotyledon*, hollow of a cup]

cotyloid (kŏt'ĭ-loyd) [Gr. *kotyloeides*, cup-shaped]

cotyloid cavity

couching (kow'chĭng) [Fr. *coucher*, to lay down]

cough (kawf) [ME. *coughen*]

c., aneurysmal

c., asthmatic

c., brassy

c., bronchial

c., diphtherial

c., dry

c., ear

c., effective

c., hacking

c., harsh

c., moist

c., paroxysmal

c., productive

c., pulmonary

c., reflex

c., uterine

c., whooping

coulomb (koo'lŏm, -lōm) [Charles A. de Coulomb, Fr. physicist, 1736–1806]

Coumadin

counseling

count

counter (kown'tĕr)

c., Coulter

c., Geiger

c., scintillation

counteract (kown"tĕr-ăkt')

counteraction (kown"tĕr-ăk'shŭn)

countercurrent exchanger

counterextension (kown"tĕr-ĕks-tĕn'shŭn) [L. *contra*, against, + *extendere*, to extend]

counterimmunoelectrophoresis (kown"tĕr-ĭm"ū-nō-ē-lĕk"trō-fō-rē'sĭs) [" + *immunis*, safe, + Gr. *elektron*, amber, + *phoresis*, bearing]

counterincision (kown"tĕr-ĭn-sĭzh'ŭn) [" + *incisio*, incision]

counterirritant (kown"tĕr-ĭr'ĭ-tănt) [" + *irritare*, to excite]

counterirritation (kown"tĕr-ĭr"ĭ-tā'shŭn)

counteropening (kown"tĕr-ō'pĕn-ĭng) [L. *contra*, against, + AS. *open*, open]

counterpressure instrument

counterpulsation, intra-aortic balloon

counterpuncture [" + *punctura*, prick]

countershock

counterstain (kown'tĕr-stān)

countertraction (kown"tĕr-trăk'shŭn)

countertransference (kown"tĕr-trăns-fĕr'ĕns)

coup de soleil (kū-dă-sŏ-lā') [Fr.]

couple

coupling (kŭp'lĭng)

course, courses (kors, kor'sĕs) [L. *cursus*, a flowing]

Courvoisier's law (koor-vwă'zē-āz) [Ludwig Courvoisier, Fr. surgeon, 1843–1918]

couvade (koo-vǎd')
Couvelaire uterus [Alexandre Couvelaire, Fr. obstetrician, 1873–1948]
covalence, covalent (kō-vǎl'ĕns, -ĕnt)
covariance (kō-vā'rē-ǎns)
covariant (kō-vā'rē-ănt)
cover
cover glass, cover slip
Cowden's disease [Cowden, family name of first patient described]
Cowling's rule
Cowper's glands [William Cowper, Brit. anatomist, 1666–1709]
cowperitis (kow"pĕr-ī'tĭs) [Cowper + Gr. *itis*, inflammation]
cowpox (kow'poks)
coxa (kŏk'sǎ) [L.]
  c. plana
  c. valga
  c. vara
coxalgia (kŏk-sǎl'jē-ǎ) [L. *coxa*, hip, + Gr. *algos*, pain]
coxarthrosis (kŏks"ărth-rō'sĭs) [" + Gr. *arthron*, joint, + *osis*, condition]
Coxiella (kŏk"sē-ĕl'lǎ) [Herald R. Cox, U.S. bacteriologist, b. 1907]
  C. burnetii [Cox; Sir Frank Macfarlane Burnet, Australian Nobel prize winner, b. 1899]
coxitis (kŏk-sī'tĭs) [L. *coxa*, hip, + Gr. *itis*, inflammation]
coxodynia (kŏk"sō-dĭn'ē-ǎ) [" + Gr. *odyne*, pain]
coxofemoral (kŏk"sō-fĕm'ō-rǎl) [" + *femur*, thigh]
coxotuberculosis (kŏk"sō-tū-bĕr"kū-lō'sĭs) [" + *tuberculum*, a little swelling, + *osis*, condition]
coxsackievirus (kŏk-sǎk'ē-vī"rŭs) [Coxsackie, a city in N.Y., + L. *virus*, poison]
cozymase (kō-zī'mās)
C.P. candle power; cerebral palsy; chemically pure
C.P.A. Canadian Physiotherapy Association
CPAP continuous positive air pressure
CPK creatine phosphokinase

c.p.m. counts per minute
CPPV continuous positive pressure ventilation
CPR cardiopulmonary resuscitation
C.P.S. cycles per second
CR conditioned reflex
C.R. crown-rump; central ray
Cr chromium
crab louse
"crack"
cracked pot sound
cradle [AS. *cradel*]
cradle cap
cramp [ME. *crampe*]
cranial (krā'nē-ǎl) [L. *cranialis*]
cranial bones
cranial nerves
craniectomy (krā-nē-ĕk'tō-mē) [Gr. *kranion*, skull, + *ektome*, excision]
cranio- [Gr. *kranion*, L. *cranium*, skull]
cranioacromial (krā"nē-ō-ǎ-krō'mē-ǎl) [Gr. *kranion*, skull, + *akron*, extremity]
craniocaudal (krā"nē-ō-kawd'ǎl) [" + L. *cauda*, tail]
craniocele (krā'nē-ō-sēl) [" + *kele*, tumor, swelling]
craniocerebral (krā"nē-ō-sĕr-ē'brǎl) [" + L. *cerebrum*, brain]
cranioclasis (krā"nē-ŏk'lǎ-sĭs) [" + *klasis*, fracture]
cranioclast (krā'nē-ō-klǎst) [" + *klastos*, broken]
cranioclasty (krā'nē-ō-klǎs"tē)
craniocleidodysostosis (krā"nē-ō-klī"dō-dĭs-ŏs-tō'sĭs) [" + *kleis*, clavicle, + *dys*, bad, difficult, painful, disordered, + *osteon*, bone, + *osis*, condition]
craniodidymus (krā"nē-ō-dĭd'ĭ-mŭs) [" + *didymos*, twin]
craniofacial (krā"nē-ō-fā'shǎl)
craniograph (krā-'nē-ō-grǎf) [" + *graphein*, to write]
craniology (krā"nē-ŏl'ō-jē) [" + *logos*, word, reason]
craniomalacia (krā-nē-ō-mǎ-lā'shē-ǎ) [" + *malakia*, softening]
craniometer (krā-nē-ŏm'ĕ-tĕr) [" +

metron, measure]
craniometric points
craniometry (krā-nē-ŏm'ĕ-trē) [" + *metron*, measure]
craniopagus (krā-nē-ŏp'ă-gŭs) [" + *pagos*, a fixed or solid thing]
craniopharyngeal (krā"nē-ō-făr-ĭn'jē-ăl) [" + *pharynx*, throat]
craniopharyngioma (krā"nē-ō-făr-ĭn-jē-ō'mă) [" + " + *oma*, tumor]
cranioplasty (krā'nē-ō-plăs-tē) [" + *plassein*, to form]
craniopuncture (krā'nē-ō-pŭnk"chŭr) [" + L. *punctura*, prick]
craniorhachischisis (krā"nē-ō-ră-kĭs'kĭ-sĭs) [" + *rhachis*, spine, + *schizein*, to split]
craniosacral (krā"nē-ō-sā'krăl)
cranioschisis (krā"nē-ŏs'kĭ-sĭs) [" + *schizein*, to split]
craniosclerosis (krā"nē-ō-sklĕ-rō'sĭs) [" + *skleros*, hard, + *osis*, condition]
cranioscopy (krā"nē-ŏs'kō-pē) [" + *skopein*, to examine]
craniospinal (krā'nē-ō-spī'năl)
craniostenosis (krā"nē-ō-stē-nō'sĭs) [" + *stenosis*, act of narrowing]
craniostosis (krā-nē-ŏs-tō'sĭs) [" + *osteon*, bone, + *osis*, condition]
craniosynostosis (krā"nē-ō-sĭn"ŏs-tō'sĭs) [" + *syn*, together, + *osteon*, bone, + *osis*, condition]
craniotabes (krā"nē-ō-tā'bēz) [" + L. *tabes*, wasting disease]
craniotome (krā'nē-ō-tōm) [" + *tome*, a cutting, slice]
craniotomy (krā-nē-ŏt'ō-mē)
craniotonoscopy (krā"nē-ō-tō-nŏs'kō-pē) [" + *tonos*, act of stretching, tension, tone, + *skopein*, to examine]
craniotrypesis (krā"nē-ō-trī-pē'sĭs) [" + Gr. *trypesis*, a boring]
craniotympanic (krā"nē-ō-tĭm-păn'ĭk) [" + *tympanon*, kettle-drum]
cranium (krā'nē-ŭm) [L.]
crapulent, crapulous (L. *crapula*, ex-cessive drinking]

crater (krā'tĕr)
crateriform (krā-tĕr'ĭ-form) [Gr. *krater*, bowl, + L. *forma*, shape]
cravat bandage (kră-văt') [Fr. *cravate*, a necktie]
crazing
crazy bone
C-reactive protein
cream of tartar
crease (krēs) [ME. *crest*, crest]
  c., gluteofemoral
creatinase (krē-ăt'ĭn-ās) [Gr. *kreas*, flesh, + *-ase*, enzyme]
creatine (krē'ă-tĭn) [Gr. *kreas*, flesh]
creatine kinase
creatinemia (krē"ă-tĭn-ē'mē-ă) [" + *haima*, blood]
creatinine (krē-ăt'ĭn-ĭn) [Gr. *kreas*, flesh]
creatinine phosphokinase
creatinuria (krē-ă"tĭn-ū'rē-ă) [" + *ouron*, urine]
creatorrhea (krē"ă-tō-rē'ă) [" + *rhein*, to flow]
Credé's method (krā-dāz') [Karl S. F. Credé, Ger. gynecologist, 1819–1892]
cremains [contraction of cremated remains]
cremaster (krē-măs'tĕr) [L., to suspend]
cremasteric (krē-măs'tĕr-ĭk)
cremasteric fascia
cremasteric reflex
cremate (krē'māt) [L. *crematio*, a burning]
crematorium (krē"mă-tō'rē-ŭm) [L.]
crenate (krē'nāt) [L. *crenatus*]
crenation (krē-nā'shŭn)
crenocyte (krē'nō-sīt)
creosote (krē'ō-sōt) [Gr. *kreas*, flesh, + *sozein*, to preserve]
crepitant (krĕp'ĭ-tănt) [L. *crepitare*]
crepitation (krĕp-ĭ-tā'shŭn)
crepitus (krĕp'ĭ-tŭs) [L.]
  c. redux
crepuscular (krē-pŭs'kū-lăr) [L. *crepusculum*, twilight]

crescent (krĕs'ĕnt) [L. *crescens*]
  c., articular
  c., myopic
  c. of Giannuzzi
crescent bodies
crescentic (krĕs-ĕn'tĭk)
Crescormon
cresol (krē'sŏl)
cresomania, croesomania (krē"sō-mā'nē-ă) [Croesus, wealthy king of Lydia, 6th century B.C.]
crest [L. *crista*, crest]
  c., alveolar
CREST syndrome [Calcinosis, Raynaud's (phenomenon), Esophageal (dysfunction), Sclerodactyly, Telangiectasia]
cretin (krē'tĭn) [Fr.]
cretinism (krē'tĭn-ĭzm) [" + Gr. *-ismos*, condition]
cretinoid (krē'tĭ-noyd) [" + Gr. *eidos*, form, shape]
cretinous (krē'tĭ-nŭs)
crevice (krĕv'ĭs) [Fr. *crever*, to break]
  c., gingival
crevicular (krĕv-ĭk'ū-lăr)
CRF *corticotrophin-releasing factor*
crib (krĭb) [AS. *cribbe*, manger]
cribbing (krĭb'ĭng)
crib death
cribrate (krĭb'rāt) [L. *cribratus*]
cribration (krĭb-rā'shŭn)
cribriform (krĭb'rĭ-form) [L. *cribrum*, a sieve, + *forma*, form]
cribriform fascia
cribriform plate
crick
cricoarytenoid (krī"kō-ă-rĭt'ĕn-oyd) [Gr. *krikos*, ring, + *arytaina*, pitcher, + *eidos*, form, shape]
cricoderma (krī-kō-dĕr'mă) [" + *derma*, skin]
cricoid (krī'koyd) [" + *eidos*, form, shape]
cricoid cartilage
cricoidectomy (krī"koyd-ĕk'tō-mē) [" + " + *ektome*, excision]
cricoidynia (krī-koy-dĭn'ē-ă) [" + "

+ *odyne*, pain]
cricopharyngeal (krī"kō-făr-ĭn'jē-ăl) [" + *pharynx*, throat]
cricothyroid (krī-kō-thī'royd) [" + *thyreos*, shield, + *eidos*, form, shape]
cricothyrotomy (krī"kō-thī-rŏt'ō-mē) [" + " + *tome*, a cutting, slice]
cricotomy (krī-kŏt'ō-mē) [" + *tome*, a cutting, slice]
cricotracheotomy (krī"kō-trā"kē-ŏt'ō-mē) [" + *tracheia*, windpipe, + *tome*, a cutting, slice]
cri du chat syndrome (krē-dū-shă)
Crigler-Najjar syndrome (krēg'lĕr-nă'hăr) [John F. Crigler, U.S. physician, b. 1919; Victor A. Najjar, U.S. physician, b. 1914]
criminal [L. *crimen*, crime]
criminology (krĭm"ĭ-nŏl'ō-jē)
crinogenic (krĭn"ō-jĕn'ĭk) [Gr. *krinein*, to secrete, + *gennan*, to produce]
cripple
crisis (krī'sĭs) [Gr. *krisis*, turning point]
  c., abdominal
  c., addisonian
  c., celiac
  c., Dietl's
  c., salt-losing
  c., sickle cell
  c., tabetic
  c., thyroid
  c., true
crisis intervention
crispation (krĭs-pā'shŭn) [L. *crispare*, to curl]
crista (krĭs'tă) [L.]
  c. ampullaris
  c. galli
  c. lacrimalis posterior
  c. spiralis
criterion (krī-tē'rē-ŏn) [Gr. *kriterion*, a means for judging]
critical (krĭt'ĭ-kăl) [Gr. *kritikos*, critical]
critical period
CRNA *certified registered nurse anesthetist*
crocodile tears

Crohn's disease (krōnz) [Burrill B. Crohn, U.S. gastroenterologist, b. 1884]
cromolyn sodium (krō'mō-lĭn)
Crookes' dark space [Sir William Crookes, Brit. physicist, 1832–1919]
Crookes' tube
cross [L. crux]
crossbirth
cross bite
crossbreeding
cross-bridges
cross-dress
crossed
crossed reflexes
cross education
cross-eye
cross-fertilization
crossing over
crossmatching
crossover
Crotalus (krŏt'ă-lŭs) [Gr. krotalon, rattle]
crotamiton (krō″tă-mī'tŏn)
crotaphion (krō-tăf'ē-ŏn) [Gr. krotaphos, the temple]
crotonism (krō'tŏn-ĭzm)
croton oil (krō'tŏn) [Gr. kroton, castor oil plant seed]
croup (croop)
   c., catarrhal
   c., diphtheritic
   c., membranous
   c., spasmodic
croupous (kroo'pŭs)
Crouzon's disease (kroo-zŏnz') [Octave Crouzon, Fr. neurologist, 1874–1938]
crowing (krō'ĭng)
crown [L. corona, wreath]
   c., anatomic
   c., clinical
crowning [L. corona, wreath]
crownwork
CRP   C-reactive protein
CRT   cathode-ray tube
CRTT   certified respiratory therapy technician

crucial (kroo'shăl) [L. crucialis]
cruciate (kroo'shē-āt)
crucible (kroo'sĭ-b'l) [L. crucibulum]
cruciform (kroo'sĭ-form) [L. crux, cross, + forma, shape]
crude (krood) [L. crudus, raw]
crura (kroo'ră) [L., legs]
   c. cerebelli
   c. cerebri
   c. of diaphragm
   c. of the fornix
crural (kroo'răl) [L. cruralis]
crural arch
crural hernia
crural nerve
crural palsies
crus (krŭs) [L.]
   c. cerebri
crush syndrome
crust [L. crusta]
crusta [L.]
crutch [AS. crycc]
Crutchfield tongs [W. Gayle Crutchfield, U.S. surgeon, b. 1900]
crutch paralysis
Cruveilhier-Baumgarten syndrome (kroo-văl-yā'bŏm'găr-tĕn) [Jean Cruveilhier, Fr. pathologist, 1791–1874; P. Clemens von Baumgarten, Ger. pathologist, 1848–1928]
cry (krī)
   c., cephalic
   c., epileptic
   c., hydrocephalic
   c., night
cryalgesia (krī-ăl-jē'zē-ă) [Gr. kryos, cold, + algos, pain]
cryanesthesia (krī-ăn-ĕs-thē'zē-ă) [″ + an-, not, + aisthesis, feeling, perception]
cryesthesia (krī-ĕs-thē'zē-ă) [″ + aisthesis, feeling, perception]
crymodynia (krī″mō-dĭn'ē-ă) [Gr. krymos, frost, + odyne, pain]
crymophilic (krī″mō-fĭl'ĭk) [″ + philein, to love]
crymophylactic (krī″mō-fĭ-lăk'tĭk)

[" + *phylaxis,* guard]

crymotherapy (krī″mō-thĕr′ă-pē)
[" + *therapeia,* treatment]

cryoaerotherapy (krī″ō-ĕr-ō-thĕr′ă-
pē) [Gr. *kryos,* cold, + *aer,* air,
+ *therapeia,* treatment]

cryobank (krī′ō-bănk)

cryobiology (krī″ō-bī-ŏl′ō-jē) [" +
bios, life, + *logos,* word, reason]

cryocautery (krī″ō-kaw′tĕr-ē) [" +
kauter, a burner]

cryoextraction (krī″ō-ĕks-trăk′shŭn)

cryofibrinogen (krī″ō-fī-brĭn′ō-jĕn)

cryogen (krī′ō-jĕn) [" + *gennan,* to
produce]

cryogenic (krī″ō-jĕn′ĭk)

cryoglobulin (krī″ō-glŏb′ū-lĭn) [" +
L. *globulus,* globule]

cryoglobulinemia (krī″ō-glŏb″ū-lĭn-
ē′mē-ă) [" + " + Gr. *haima,*
blood]

cryohypophysectomy (krī″ō-hī″pō-
fĭz-ĕk′tō-mē) [Gr. *kryos,* cold, +
hypo, under, beneath, below, +
physis, growth, + *ektome,* exci-
sion]

cryometer (krī-ŏm′ĕ-tĕr) [" + *metron,* measure]

cryophilic (krī″ō-fĭl′ĭk) [" + *philein,*
to love]

cryoprecipitate (krī″ō-prē-sĭp′ĭ-tāt)

cryopreservation

cryoprobe (krī′ō-prōb)

cryoprotectants

cryoprotective (krī″ō-prō-tĕk′tĭv)

cryoprotein (krī″ō-prō′tē-ĭn)

cryospray (krī′ō-sprā)

cryostat (krī′ō-stăt)

cryosurgery (krī″ō-sĕr′jĕr-ē) [" +
ME. *surgerie,* surgery]

cryothalamotomy (krī″ō-thăl″ă-
mŏt′ō-mē) [" + L. *thalamus,* inner
chamber, + Gr. *tome,* a cutting,
slice]

cryotherapy (krī-ō-thĕr′ă-pē) [" +
therapeia, treatment]

cryotolerant (krī″ō-tŏl′ĕr-ănt) [" +
L. *tolerare,* to bear]

crypt (krĭpt) [Gr. *kryptos,* hidden]
c., anal
c., bony
c. of iris
c. of Lieberkühn
c., synoviparous
c., tonsillar

cryptanamnesia (krĭpt″ăn-ăm-nē′zē-
ă) [" + *an-,* not, + *amnesia,*
forgetfulness]

cryptectomy (krĭp-tĕk′tō-mē) [" +
ektome, excision]

cryptesthesia (krĭp-tĕs-thē′zē-ă)
[" + *aisthesis,* feeling, perception]

cryptic (krĭp′tĭk) [Gr. *kryptikos,* hidden]

cryptitis (krĭp-tī′tĭs) [Gr. *kryptos,* hidden,
+ *itis,* inflammation]

cryptocephalus (krĭp″tō-sĕf′ă-lŭs)
[" + *kephale,* head]

cryptococcosis (krĭp″tō-kŏk-ō′sĭs)
[" + *kokkos,* berry, + *osis,*
condition]

Cryptococcus (krĭp″tō-kŏk′ŭs)

cryptodidymus (krĭp-tō-dĭd′ĭ-mŭs)
[" + *didymos,* twin]

cryptogenic (krĭp″tō-jĕn′ĭk) [" +
gennan, to produce]

cryptogenic infection

cryptolith (krĭp′tō-lĭth) [" + *lithos,*
stone]

cryptomenorrhea (krĭp″tō-mĕn″ō-
rē′ă) [" + *men,* month, +
rhein, to flow]

cryptomerorachischisis (krĭp″tō-
mē″rō-ră-kĭs′kĭ-sĭs) [" + *meros,*
part, + *rhachis,* spine, +
schisis, cleavage]

cryptomnesia (krĭp-tŏm-nē′zē-ă)
[" + *mnesis,* memory]

cryptophthalmus (krĭp″tŏf-thăl′mŭs)
[" + *ophthalmos,* eye]

cryptoplasmic (krĭp″tō-plăz′mĭk)
[" + LL. *plasma,* form, mold]

cryptopodia (krĭp″tō-pō′dē-ă) [Gr.
kryptos, hidden, + *pous,* foot]

cryptopyic (krĭp″tō-pī′ĭk) [" +
pyon, pus]

cryptorchid, cryptorchis (krĭpt-

or'kĭd, -or'kĭs) [" + orchis, testis]

cryptorchidectomy (krĭpt"or-kĭ-dĕk'tō-mē) [" + " + ektome, excision]

cryptorchidism, cryptorchism (krĭpt-or'kĭd-ĭzm, -kĭzm) [" + orchis, testis, + -ismos, condition]

cryptorrhea (krĭp-tō-rē'ă) [" + rhein, to flow]

cryptorrhetic, cryptorrheic (krĭp"tō-rĕt'ĭk, -rē'ĭk)

cryptoscope (krĭp'tō-skōp) [" + skopein, to examine]

cryptosporidiosis

Cryptosporidium

cryptotoxic (krĭp"tō-tŏk'sĭk) [" + toxikon, poison]

cryptoxanthin (krĭp"tō-zăn'thĭn)

cry reflex

crystal (krĭs'tăl) [Gr. krystallos, ice]
  c., apatite
  c.'s, Charcot-Leyden
  c.'s, Charcot-Neumann
  c.'s, Charcot-Robin
  c.'s of hemin
  c.'s, spermin

crystallin (krĭs'tăl-ĭn)

crystalline (krĭs'tă-lĭn)

crystalline deposits

crystalline lens

crystallization (krĭs"tă-lĭ-zā'shŭn) [Gr. krystallos, ice]

crystallography (krĭs"tă-lŏg'ră-fē) [" + graphein, to write]

crystalloid [" + eidos, form, shape]

crystalloiditis (krĭs"tăl-oyd-ī'tĭs) [" + " + itis, inflammation]

crystallophobia [Gr. krystallos, ice, + phobos, fear]

crystalluria (krĭs-tă-lū'rē-ă) [" + ouron, urine]

Crystodigin

CS cesarean section

Cs cesium

c-section cesarean section

CSF cerebrospinal fluid

CS gas

C substance

CT computerized tomography

Ctenocephalides (tĕn-ō-sĕf-ăl'ĭ-dēz) [Gr. ktenodes, like a cockle, + kephale, head]

c-terminal

CTZ chemoreceptor trigger zone

Cu [L. cuprum] copper

cubic measure

cubital (kū'bĭ-tăl) [L. cubitum, elbow]

cubital fossa

cubitus (kū'bĭ-tŭs) [L]
  c. valgus
  c. varus

cuboid (kū'boyd) [Gr. kubos, cube, + eidos, form, shape]

cuboid bone

cu. cm. cubic centimeter

cucurbit (kū-kĕr'bĭt) [L. cucurbita, gourd]

cue

cued speech

cuff (kŭf) [ME. cuffe, glove]
  c., attached gingival
  c., gingival

cuffed endotracheal tube

cuffing (kŭf'ĭng)

cuirass (kwē-răs') [Fr. cuirasse, breastplate]

cul-de-sac (kŭl"dĭ-săk') [Fr., bottom of the sack]

culdocentesis (kŭl"dō-sĕn-tē'sĭs) [" + Gr. kentesis, puncture]

culdoscope (kŭl'dō-skōp)

culdoscopy (kŭl-dŏs'kō-pē)

-cule, -cle [L.] Little

Culex (kū'lĕks) [L., gnat]
  C. pipiens
  C. quinquefasciatus

Culicidae (kū-lĭs'ĭ-dē)

culicide (kū'lĭ-sīd) [L. culex, gnat, + caedere, to kill]

culicifuge (kū-lĭs'ĭ-fūj) [L. culex, gnat, + fugere, to flee]

Cullen's sign (kŭl'ĕnz) [Thomas S. Cullen, U.S. gynecologist, 1863–1953]

culmen (kŭl'mĕn) [L., summit]

cult [L. cultus, care]

cultivation (kŭl"tĭ-vā'shŭn) [L. cultivare,

to cultivate]
cultural (kŭl'tū-răl) [L. *cultura*, tillage]
culture (kŭl'tūr)
  c., blood
  c., cell
  c., contaminated
  c., continuous flow
  c., gelatin
  c., hanging block
  c., hanging drop
  c., negative
  c., positive
  c., pure
  c., slant
  c., stab
  c., stock
  c., streak
  c., tissue
  c., type
culture medium
  c.m., defined
culture shock
cu. mm. *cubic millimeter*
cumulative (kū'mŭ-lă-tĭv) [L. *cumulus*, a heap]
cumulative drug action
cumulus (kū'mŭ-lŭs) [L., a little mound]
  c. oophorus
cuneate (kū'nē-āt) [L. *cuneus*, wedge]
cuneate fasciculus
cuneate funiculus
cuneate nucleus
cuneiform (kū-nē'ĭ-form) [" + *forma*, shape]
cuneiform bones
cuneiform cartilage
cuneo- (kū'nē-ō) [L. *cuneus*, wedge]
cuneocuboid (kū"nē-ō-kū'boyd) [" + Gr. *kubos*, cube, + *eidos*, form, shape]
cuneohysterectomy (kū"nē-ō-hĭs"tĕr-ĕk'tō-mē) [" + Gr. *hystera*, womb, + *ektome*, excision]
cuneus (kū'nē-ŭs) [L., wedge]
cuniculus (kū-nĭk'ū-lŭs) [L., an underground passage]
cunnilinguist (kŭn-ĭ-lĭn'gwĭst) [L. *cunnus*, pudenda, + *lingua*, tongue]

cunnilingus (kŭn-ĭ-lĭn'gŭs)
cunnus (kŭn'ŭs) [L.]
cup [LL. *cuppa*, drinking vessel]
  c., favus
  c., glaucomatous
  c., optic
  c., physiologic
cup arthroplasty of hip
Cupid's bow
cupola, cupula (kū'pō-lă,-pū-lă) [L. *cupula*, little tub]
cupping
cupric (kū'prĭk)
cupric sulfate
cuprous (kū'prŭs)
cuprum (kū'prŭm) [L.]
cupruresis (kū"proo-rē'sĭs) [L. *cuprum*, copper, + Gr. *ouresis*, to void urine]
cupulolithiasis (kū"pū-lō-lĭth-ī'ă-sis) [L. dim. of *cupa*, a tub, + Gr. *lithos*, stone, + *-iasis*, state or condition of]
curare (kū-, koo-răr'ē) [phonetic equivalent of Carib Indian name for extracts of plants used as arrow poisons]
curarization (kū"răr-ī-zā'shŭn)
curative (kū'ră-tĭv) [L. *curare*, to take care of]
curd [ME]
cure [L. *cura*, care]
curet, curette (kū-rĕt') [Fr. *curette*, a cleanser]
curettage (kū"rĕ-tăzh') [Fr.]
  c., periapical
  c., suction
  c., uterine
curettement (kū-rĕt'mĕnt) [Fr.]
Curie (kūr'ē, kū-rē') [Marie Curie, Polish-born Fr. chemist, 1867–1934; Pierre Curie, Fr. chemist, 1859–1906]
curie [Marie Curie]
curiegram (kū'rē-grăm) [*curie* + Gr. *gramma*, letter, piece of writing]
curietherapy (kū"rē-thĕr'ă-pē) [" + Gr. *therapeia*, treatment]
curium (kū'rē-ŭm) [Pierre and Marie Curie]

curled
Curling's ulcer (kŭr'lĭngz) [Thomas Curling, Brit. physician, 1811–1888]
currant jelly clot
current [L. currere, to run]
  c., alternating
  c., direct
curriculum (kŭ-rĭk'ū-lŭm) [L.]
Curschmann's spirals (koorsh'mănz) [Heinrich Curschmann, Ger. physician, 1846–1910]
curse (kĕrs)
  c., Ondine's [Ondine, character in Greek mythology]
curvature [L. curvatura, a slope]
  c., angular
curvature of spine
curve [L. curvus]
  c., dye-dilution
  c., learning
  c., normal
  c. of Carus
  c. of Spee
curvi- [L. curvus, curve]
curvilinear
Cushing, Harvey (koosh'ĭng) U.S. surgeon, 1869–1939
  C.'s disease
  C.'s syndrome
cushingoid (koosh'ĭng-oyd)
cushion
cusp (kŭsp) [L. cuspis, point]
cuspid (kŭs'pĭd)
cuspidate (kŭs'pĭ-dāt) [L. cuspidatus]
cuspidor (kŭs'pĭ-dor)
custom
cut
cutaneous (kū-tā'nē-ŭs) [L. cutis, skin]
cutaneous nerves
cutaneous respiration
cutdown (kŭt'down)
cuticle (kū'tĭ-k'l) [L. cuticula, little skin]
  c., acquired
  c., attachment
  c., dental
  c., enamel
cuticula (kū-tĭk'ū-lă) [L.]
  c. dentis

cuticularization (kū-tĭk"ū-lăr-ĭ-zā'shŭn)
cutin (kū'tĭn) [L. cutis, skin]
cutireaction (kū"tĕ-rē-ăk'shŭn)
  c., von Pirquet's
cutis (kū'tĭs) [L.]
  c. anserina
  c. aurantiasis
  c. hyperelastica
  c. laxa
  c. marmorata
  c. pendula
  c. testacea
  c. unctosa
  c. vera
  c. verticis gyrata
cutization (kū-tĭ-zā'shŭn)
cut throat
cuvette (kŭv-ĕt') [Fr. cuve, a tub]
CVA cerebrovascular accident
CVP central venous pressure
cyanemia (sī"ăn-ē'mē-ă) [Gr. kyanos, dark blue, + haima, blood]
cyanephidrosis (sī"ăn-ĕf"ĭ-drō'sĭs) [" + ephidrosis, sweating]
cyanhemoglobin (sī"ăn-hē"mō-glō'bĭn)
cyanhidrosis (sī-ăn-hī-drō'sĭs) [" + hidrosis, sweat]
cyanide (sī'ă-nīd")
cyanide poisoning
cyanmethemoglobin (sī"ăn-mĕt"hē-mō-glō'bĭn)
cyano- [Gr. kyanos, dark blue]
cyanoacrylate adhesives
cyanocobalamin (sī"ăn-ō-kō-băl'ă-mĭn)
cyanoderma (sī"ă-nō-dĕr'mă) [" + derma, skin]
cyanogen (sī-ăn'ō-jĕn) [" + gennan, to produce]
cyanomycosis (sī"ăn-ō-mī-kō'sĭs) [" + mykes, fungus, + osis, condition]
cyanopathy (sī"ăn-ŏp'ă-thē) [" + pathos, disease, suffering]
cyanophil (sī-ăn'ō-fĭl) [" + philein, to love]
cyanophilous (sī-ăn-ŏf'ĭl-ŭs)

cyanopia, cyanopsia (sī-ăn-ō'pē-ă, -ŏp'sē-ă) [" + *opsis*, sight, appearance, vision]

cyanosed

cyanosis (sī-ă-nō'sĭs) [" + *osis*, condition]

   c., congenital
   c., delayed
   c., enterogenous
   c. retinae
   c., tardive

cyanotic (sī-ăn-ŏt'ĭk)

cyanuria (sī"ă-nū'rē-ă)

cybernetics (sī"bĕr-nĕt'ĭks) [Gr. *kybernetes*, helmsman]

cyberphilia (sī"bĕr-fĭl'ē-ă) [" + *philein*, to love]

cyberphobia (sī"bĕr-fō'bē-ă) [" + *phobos*, fear]

cycad (sī'kăd)

cycasin (sī'kă-sĭn)

cyclacillin (sī-klă-sĭl'ĭn)

cyclamate (sī'klă-māt)

cyclandelate (sī-klăn'dĕ-lāt)

cyclarthrosis (sī-klăr-thrō'sĭs) [Gr. *kyklos*, circle, + *arthron*, joint, + *osis*, condition]

cycle (sī'kl) [Gr. *kyklos*, circle]

   c., cardiac
   c., Cori
   c., gastric
   c., genesial
   c., glycolytic
   c., Krebs
   c., life
   c., menstrual

cyclectomy (sī-klĕk'tō-mē) [Gr. *kyklos*, circle, + *ektome*, excision]

cyclic (sī'klĭk)

cyclic AMP

cyclic AMP synthetase

cyclicotomy (sīk"lĭ-kŏt'ō-mē) [" + *tome*, a cutting, slice]

cyclic vomiting

cyclitis (sĭk-lī'tĭs) [" + *itis*, inflammation]

   c., plastic
   c., purulent

   c., serous

cyclizine hydrochloride

cyclo- [Gr. *kyklos*, circle]

cyclobenzaprine hydrochloride (sī"klō-bĕn'ză-prēn)

cycloceratitis (sī"klō-sĕr"ă-tī'tĭs)

cyclochoroiditis (sī"klō-kō"royd-ī'tĭs) [" + *chorioeides*, skinlike, + *itis*, inflammation]

cyclodialysis (sī"klō-dī-ăl'ĭ-sĭs) [" + *dia*, through, + *lysis*, dissolution]

cycloid (sī'kloyd) [" + *eidos*, form, shape]

cyclokeratitis (sī"klō-kĕr-ă-tī'tĭs) [" + *keras*, cornea, + *itis*, inflammation]

cyclomethycaine sulfate (sī"klō-mĕth'ĭ-kān)

Cyclopar

cyclopentamine hydrochloride (sī"klō-pĕn'tă-mēn)

cyclopentolate hydrochloride (sī"klō-pĕn'tō-lāt)

cyclophoria (sī"klō-fō'rē-ă) [" + *phoros*, bearing]

cyclophosphamide (sī"klō-fŏs'fă-mīd)

cyclopia (sī-klō'pē-ă) [Gr. *kyklos*, circle, + *ops*, eye]

cycloplegia (sī"klō-plē'jē-ă) [" + *plege*, a stroke]

cycloplegic (sī"klō-plē'jĭk)

cyclopropane (sī"klō-prō'pān)

cyclops (sī'klŏps)

cycloserine (sī"klō-sĕr'ĕn)

cyclosis (sī-klō'sĭs) [Gr. *kyklosis*, circulation]

cyclosporine (sī'klō-spor-een)

cyclothiazide (sī"klō-thī'ă-zīd)

cyclothymia (sī"klō-thī'mē-ă) [" + *thymos*, mind, spirit]

cyclotomy (sī-klŏt'ō-mē) [" + *tome*, a cutting, slice]

cyclotron (sī'klō-trŏn)

cyclotropia (sī"klō-trō'pē-ă)

cycrimine hydrochloride (sī'krĭ-mīn)

cyesis (sī-ē'sĭs) [Gr. *kyesis*]

cylicotomy (sīl"ĭ-kŏt'ō-mē) [Gr. *kylix*, cup, + *tome*, a cutting, slice]

cylinder (sĭl′ĭn-dĕr) [Gr. *kylindros*]
  c.'s, crossed
  c.'s, urinary
cylindroadenoma (sī-lĭn″drō-ăd″ĕ-nō′mă) [Gr. *kylindros,* cylinder, + *aden,* gland, + *oma,* tumor]
cylindroid (sĭl-ĭn′droyd) [″ + *eidos,* form, shape]
cylindroma (sĭl″ĭn-drō′mă) [″ + *oma,* tumor]
cylindruria (sĭl″ĭn-drū′rē-ă) [″ + *ouron,* urine]
cyllosis (sĭl-ō′sĭs) [Gr. *kyllosis*]
cymbocephalic (sĭm″bō-sĕ-făl′ĭk) [Gr. *kymbe,* boat, + *kephale,* head]
cynanthropy (sĭn-ăn′thrō-pē) [Gr. *kyon,* dog, + *anthropos,* man]
cynic spasm [Gr. *kynikos,* doglike]
cynophobia (sī″nō-fō′bē-ă) [″ + *phobos,* fear]
cypridophobia (sĭp″rĭ-dō-fō′bē-ă) [Gr. *Kypris,* Venus, + *phobos,* fear]
cypriphobia (sĭp-rĭ-fō′bē-ă)
cyproheptadine   hydrochloride (sī″prō-hĕp′tă-dēn)
cyrtometer (sĭr-tŏm′ĕ-tĕr) [Gr. *kyrtos,* bent, + *metron,* measure]
cyrtosis (sĭr-tō′sĭs) [″ + *osis,* condition]
cyst (sĭst) [Gr. *kystis,* bladder, sac]
  c., adventitious
  c., alveolar
  c., apical
  c., blood
  c., blue dome
  c., branchial
  c., cervical
  c., chocolate
  c., colloid
  c., congenital
  c., daughter
  c., dental
  c., dentigerous
  c., dermoid
  c., distention
  c., echinococcus
  c., epidermal

  c., extravasation
  c., exudation
  c., follicular
  c., Gartner's
  c., hydatid
  c., implantation
  c., intraligamentary
  c., involutional
  c., keratin
  c., meibomian
  c., mucoid
  c., mucous
  c., nabothian
  c., odontogenic
  c., ovarian
  c., parasitic
  c., parovarian
  c., pilonidal
  c., porencephalic
  c., proliferative
  c., radicular
  c., retention
  c., sebaceous
  c., seminal
  c., suprasellar
  c., tubo-ovarian
  c., unilocular
  c., vaginal
  c., vitelline
cystadenocarcinoma (sĭs-tăd″ē-nō-kăr″sĭ-nō′mă) [Gr. *kystis,* bladder, + *aden,* gland, + *karkinos,* crab, + *oma,* tumor]
cystadenoma (sĭst″ăd-ĕn-ō′mă) [″ + ″ + *oma,* tumor]
  c., pseudomucinous
  c., serous
cystalgia (sĭs-tăl′jē-ă) [″ + *algos,* pain]
cystathionine (sĭs″tă-thī′ō-nīn)
cystathioninuria (sĭs″tă-thī″ō-nī-nū′rē-ă)
cystauxe (sĭs-tŏk′sē) [″ + *auxe,* increase]
cystectasy (sĭs-tĕk′tă-sē) [″ + *ektasis,* dilatation]
cystectomy (sĭs-tĕk′tō-mē) [″ + *ektome,* excision]

cysteic acid
cysteine hydrochloride (sĭs′tē-ĭn,
sĭs-tē′ĭn)
cystelcosis (sĭs″tĕl-kō′sĭs) [″ + helkosis, ulceration]
cystic (sĭs′tĭk) [Gr. kystis, bladder]
cystic duct
cysticercoid (sĭs″tĭ-sĕr′koyd) [″ +
kerkos, tail, + eidos, form, shape]
cysticercosis (sĭs″tĭ-sĕr-kō′sĭs) [″ +
″ + osis, condition]
cysticercus (sĭs″tĭ-sĕr′kŭs)
c. cellulosae
cystic fibrosis
cysticotomy (sĭs″tĭ-kŏt′ō-mē) [″ +
tome, a cutting, slice]
cystiform (sĭs′tĭ-form) [″ + L.
forma, form]
cystigerous (sĭs-tĭj′ĕr-ŭs) [″ + L.
gerere, to bear]
cystine (sĭs′tēn) [Gr. kystis, bladder]
cystinemia (sĭs″tĭ-nē′mē-ă) [cystine +
Gr. haima, blood]
cystinosis (sĭs′tĭ-nō′sĭs) [″ + Gr.
osis, condition]
cystinuria (sĭs″tĭ-nū′rē-ă) [″ +
ouron, urine]
cystistaxia (sĭs″tĭ-stăk′sē-ă) [Gr. kystis,
bladder, + staxis, dripping]
cystitis (sĭs-tī′tĭs) [″ + itis, inflamma-
tion]
c., interstitial
cystitome (sĭs′tĭ-tōm) [″ + tome, a
cutting, slice]
cystitomy (sĭs-tĭt′ō-mē)
cysto-, cyst- [Gr. kystis, bladder]
cystoadenoma (sĭs″tō-ăd″ĕ-nō′mă) [″
+ aden, gland, + oma, tumor]
cystocarcinoma (sĭs″tō-kăr″sĭ-nō′mă)
[″ + karkinos, ulcer + oma,
tumor]
cystocele (sĭs′tō-sēl) [″ + kele,
tumor, swelling]
cystocolostomy (sĭs″tō-kō-lŏs′tō-mē)
[″ + kolon, colon, + stoma,
mouth, opening]
cystodiaphanoscopy (sĭs″tō-dī″ă-
făn-ŏs′kō-pē) [″ + dia, through,

+ phanein, to shine, + skopein,
to examine]
cystodynia (sĭs″tō-dĭn′ē-ă) [″ +
odyne, pain]
cystoelytroplasty (sĭs″tō-ē-lĭt′rō-plăs-
tē) [″ + elytron, sheath, +
plassein, to form]
cystoepiplocele (sĭs″tō-ē-pĭp′lō-sēl)
[″ + epiploon, omentum, +
kele, tumor, swelling]
cystoepithelioma (sĭs″tō-ĕp″ĭ-thē″lē-
ō′mă) [″ + epi, upon, + thele,
nipple, + oma, tumor]
cystofibroma (sĭs″tō-fī-brō′mă) [″ +
L. fibra, fiber, + Gr. oma, tumor]
cystogastrostomy (sĭs″tō-găs-trŏs′tō-
mē) [″ + gaster, stomach, +
stoma, mouth, opening]
cystogram (sĭs′tō-grăm) [″ +
gramma, letter, piece of writing]
cystography (sĭs-tŏg′ră-fē) [″ +
graphein, to write]
cystoid (sĭs′toyd) [″ + eidos, form,
shape]
cystojejunostomy (sĭs″tō-jē-jū-nŏs′tō-
mē) [″ + L. jejunum, empty, +
Gr. stoma, mouth, opening]
cystolith (sĭs′tō-lĭth) [″ + lithos,
stone]
cystolithectomy (sĭs-tō-lĭ-thĕk′tō-mē)
[″ + lithos, stone, + ektome,
excision]
cystolithiasis (sĭs-tō-lĭ-thī′ă-sĭs) [Gr.
kystis, bladder, + lithos, stone,
+ -iasis, state or condition of]
cystolithic (sĭs″tō-lĭth′ĭk)
cystolutein (sĭs″tō-loo′tē-ĭn) [″ + L.
luteus, yellow]
cystoma (sĭs-tō′mă) [″ + oma,
tumor]
cystometer (sĭs-tŏm′ĕ-tĕr) [″ +
metron, measure]
cystometrography (sĭs″tō-mĕ-
trŏg′ră-fē) [″ + ″ + graphein,
to write]
cystomorphous (sĭs″tō-mor′fŭs) [″ +
morphe, form]
cystopexy (sĭs′tō-pĕk″sē) [″ +

pexis, fixation]

cystoplasty (sĭs′tō-plăs″tē) [″ + *plassein*, to form]

cystoplegia (sĭs″tō-plē′jē-ă) [″ + *plege*, stroke]

cystoproctostomy (sĭs″tō-prŏk-tŏs′tō-mē) [″ + *proktos*, rectum, + *stoma*, mouth, opening]

cystoptosia, cystoptosis (sĭs″tŏp-tō′sē-ă, -sĭs) [″ + *ptosis*, fall, falling]

cystopyelitis (sĭs″tō-pī-ĕ-lī′tĭs) [″ + *pyelos*, pelvis, + *itis*, inflammation]

cystopyelonephritis (sĭs″tō-pī″ĕ-lō-nĕf-rī′tĭs) [″ + ″ + *nephros*, kidney, + *itis*, inflammation]

cystoradiography (sĭs″tō-rā″dē-ŏg′ră-fē) [″ + L. *radius*, ray, + Gr. *graphein*, to write]

cystorectostomy (sĭs″tō-rĕk-tŏs′tō-mē) [″ + L. *rectum*, straight, + Gr. *stoma*, mouth, opening]

cystorrhagia (sĭs″tō-rā′jē-ă) [″ + *rhegnynai*, to burst forth]

cystorrhaphy (sĭst-or′ă-fē) [″ + *rhaphe*, seam]

cystorrhea (sĭs″tō-rē′ă) [″ + *rhein*, to flow]

cystosarcoma (sĭs″tō-săr-kō′mă) [″ + *sarx*, flesh, + *oma*, tumor]

cystoscope (sĭst′ō-skōp) [″ + *skopein*, to examine]

cystoscopy (sĭs-tŏs′kō-pē) [″ + *skopein*, to examine]

cystospasm (sĭs′tō-spăzm) [Gr. *kystis*, bladder, + *spasmos*, a convulsion]

cystostomy (sĭs-tŏs′tō-mē) [″ + *stoma*, mouth, opening]

cystotome (sĭs′tō-tōm) [″ + *tome*, a cutting, slice]

cystotomy (sĭs-tŏt′ō-mē) [″ + *tome*, a cutting, slice]

cystotrachelotomy (sĭs″tō-trā″kĕ-lŏt′ō-mē) [″ + *trachelos*, neck, + *tome*, a cutting, slice]

cystoureteritis (sĭs″tō-ū-rē″tĕr-ī′tĭs) [″ + *oureter*, ureter, + *itis*, inflammation]

cystoureterogram (sĭs″tō-ū-rē′tĕr-ō-grăm) [″ + ″ + *gramma*, letter, piece of writing]

cystourethritis (sĭs″tō-ū″rē-thrī′tĭs) [″ + *ourethra*, urethra, + *itis*, inflammation]

cystourethrocele (sĭs″tō-ū-rē′thrō-sēl) [″ + ″ + *kele*, tumor, swelling]

cystourethrography (sĭs″tō-ū-rē-thrŏg′ră-fē) [″ + ″ + *graphein*, to write]
    c., chain
    c., voiding

cystourethropexy, retropubic

cystourethroscope (sĭs″tō-ū-rē′thrō-skōp) [″ + *ourethra*, urethra, + *skopein*, to examine]

cystovesiculography (sĭs″tō-vĕ-sĭk-ū-lŏg′ră-fē)

cytarabine (sī-tār′ă-bēn)

cytase (sī′tās) [Gr. *kytos*, cell, + *-ase*, enzyme]

-cyte (sīt) [Gr. *kytos*, cell]

cytidine (sī′tĭ-dĭn)

cyto-, cyt- [Gr. *kytos*, cell]

cytoanalyzer (sī″tō-ăn″ă-lī′zĕr)

cytoarchitectonic (sī″tō-ărk″ĭ-tĕk-tŏn′ĭk) [″ + *architektonike*, architecture]

cytobiology (sī″tō-bī-ŏl′ō-jē) [″ + *bios*, life, + *logos*, word, reason]

cytobiotaxis (sī″tō-bī-ō-tăk′sĭs) [″ + ″ + *taxis*, arrangement]

cytoblast (sī′tō-blăst) [″ + *blastos*, germ]

cytocentrum (sī″tō-sĕn′trŭm) [″ + *kentron*, center]

cytocerastic (sī″tō-sē-răs′tĭk) [″ + *kerastos*, mixed]

cytochalasin B (sī″tō-kăl′ă-sĭn)

cytochemism (sī″tō-kĕm′ĭzm) [″ + *chemeia*, chemistry, + *-ismos*, condition]

cytochemistry (sī″tō-kĕm′ĭs-trē)

cytochrome (sī′tō-krōm) [″ + *chroma*, color]

cytochrome oxidase

cytochrome P-450

cytochylema (sī″tō-kī-lē′mă) [Gr. *kytos*, cell, + *chylos*, juice]

cytocidal (sī″tō-sī′dăl) [″ + L. *cida* fr. *caedere*, to kill]

cytocide (sī′tō-sīd)

cytoclasis (sī″tŏk′lă-sīs) [″ + *klasis*, destruction]

cytoclastic [″ + *klasis*, destruction]

cytoclesis (sī″tō-klē′sīs) [″ + *klesis*, a call]

cytodendrite (sī″tō-děn′drīt) [″ + *dendron*, tree]

cytodiagnosis (sī″tō-dī″ăg-nō′sīs) [″ + *dia*, through, + *gignoskein*, to know]

cytodieresis (sī″tō-dī-ěr′ě-sīs) [″ + *diairesis*, division]

cytodistal (sī″tō-dīs′tăl) [″ + *distare*, to be distant]

cytogenesis (sī″tō-jěn′ěs-īs) [″ + *genesis*, generation, birth]

cytogenetics (sī″tō-jě-nět′īks)

cytogenic (sī-tō-jěn′īk) [″ + *gennan*, to produce]

cytogenous (si-tŏj′ěn-ŭs) [″ + *gennan*, to produce]

cytogeny (sī-tŏj′ě-nē) [″ + *genesis*, generation, birth]

cytoglycopenia (sī″tō-glī-kō-pē′nē-ă) [″ + *glykys*, sweet, + *penia*, lack]

cytohistogenesis (sī″tō-hīs″tō-jěn′ě-sīs) [″ + *histos*, web, + *genesis*, generation, birth]

cytohyaloplasm (sī″tō-hī′ăl-ō-plăzm) [″ + *hyalos*, glass, + LL. *plasma*, form, mold]

cytoid (sī′toyd) [″ + *eidos*, form, shape]

cytoinhibition (sī″tō-īn″hī-bīsh′ŭn) [″ + L. *inhibere*, to restrain]

cytokalipenia (sī″tō-kăl-ī-pē′nē-ă) [″ + L. *kalium*, potassium, + Gr. *penia*, lack]

cytokerastic (sī″tō-kě-răs′tīk) [″ + *kerastos*, mixed]

cytokines

cytokinesis (sī″tō-kī-nē′sīs) [″ + *kinesis*, motion]

cytologist

cytology (sī-tŏl′ō-jē) [″ + *logos*, word, reason]

cytolymph (sī′tō-līmf) [″ + L. *lympha*, lymph]

cytolysin (sī-tŏl′ī-sīn) [″ + *lysis*, dissolution]

cytolysis (sī-tŏl′ī-sīs)

cytomegalic inclusion disease

cytomegalovirus (sī″tō-měg″ă-lō-vī′rŭs)

Cytomel

cytometaplasia (sī″tō-mět″ă-plā′zē-ă) [Gr. *kytos*, cell, + *metaplasis*, change]

cytometer (sī-tŏm′ě-ter) [″ + *metron*, measure]
   c., flow

cytometry (sī-tŏm′ě-trē)

cytomicrosome (sī-tō-mī′krō-sōm) [″ + *mikros*, small, + *soma*, body]

cytomitome (sī″tō-mī′tōm) [″ + *mitos*, thread]

cytomorphology (sī″tō-mor-fŏl′ō-jē) [″ + *morphe*, form, + *logos*, word, reason]

cytomorphosis (sī″tō-mor-fō′sīs) [″ + ″ + *osis*, condition]

cyton (sī′tŏn) [Gr. *kytos*, cell]

cytopathic (sī″tō-păth′īk) [″ + *pathos*, disease, suffering]

cytopathogenic effect (sī″tō-păth″ō-jěn′īk) [″ + *pathos*, disease, suffering, + *gennan*, to produce]

cytopathology (sī″tō-păth-ŏl′ō-jē) [″ + ″ + *logos*, word, reason]

cytopenia [″ + *penia*, lack]

cytophagocytosis (sī″tō-făg″ō-sī-tō′sīs) [″ + *phagein*, to eat, + *kytos*, cell, + *osis*, condition]

cytophagous (sī-tŏf′ă-gŭs)

cytophagy (sī-tŏf′ă-jē)

cytophilic (sī-tō-fīl′īk) [″ + *philein*, to love]

cytophotometry (sī″tō-fō-tŏm′ě-trē)

cytophylaxis (sī″tō-fī-lăk′sīs) [″ + *phylaxis*, guard]

cytophyletic (sī"tō-fī-lĕt'ĭk)[" + phyle, tribe]

cytophysics (sī"tō-fĭz'ĭks) [" + physike, (study of) nature]

cytophysiology (sī"tō-fĭz-ē-ŏl'ō-jē) [" + physis, nature, + logos, word, reason]

cytopipette (sī"tō-pī'pĕt)

cytoplasm (sī'tō-plăzm) [" + LL. plasma, form, mold, from Gr. plassein, to mold, spread out]

cytoplast (sī'tō-plăst)

cytoproximal (sī"tō-prŏk'sĭ-măl) [" + L. proximus, nearest]

cytoreticulum (sī"tō-rĕ-tĭk'ū-lŭm) [" + L. reticulum, network]

cytorrhyctes (sī"tō-rĭk'tēz) [" + oryssein, to dig]

Cytosar-U

cytoscopy (sī-tŏs'kō-pē) [" + skopein, to examine]

cytosine (sī'tō-sīn)
c. arabinoside

cytoskeleton (sī"tō-skĕl'ĕ-tŏn)

cytosol (sī'tō-sŏl)

cytosome (sī'tō-sōm) [" + soma, body]

cytospongium (sī"tō-spŭn'jē-ŭm) [" + sphongos, sponge]

cytost (sī'tŏst) [Gr. kytos, cell]

cytostasis (sī-tŏs'tă-sīs) [" + stasis, standing still]

cytostatic (sī"tō-stăt'ĭk) [" + stasis, standing still]

cytostome (sī'tō-stōm) [" + stoma, mouth, opening]

cytotactic (sī"tō-tăk'tĭk)

cytotaxia, cytotaxis (sī-tō-tăk'sē-ă, -sīs) [" + taxis, arrangement]

cytotherapy [" + therapeia, treatment]

cytothesis (sī-tŏth'ē-sīs) [" + thesis, a placing]

cytotoxic (sī"tō-tŏks'ĭk)

cytotoxic agents

cytotoxin (sī"tō-tŏk'sĭn) [" + toxikon, poison]

cytotrophoblast (sī"tō-trō'fō-blăst) [" + trophe, nourishment, + blastos, germ]

cytotropic (sī"tō-trŏp'ĭk, -trōp'ĭk) [" + trope, a turn]

cytotropism (sī-tŏt'rō-pĭzm) [" + trope, a turn, + -ismos, condition]

Cytoxan (sī-tŏk'săn)

cytozoic (sī"tō-zō'ĭk) [" + zoon, animal]

cytozoon (sī-tō-zō'ŏn)

cyturia (sī-tū'rē-ă) [Gr. kytos, cell, + ouron, urine]

Czermak's spaces (chăr'măks) [Johann N. Czermak, Bohemian physician, 1828–1873]

D

δ Delta

D [L.] *da*, give; *date*; *daughter*; *deciduous*; [L.] *detur*, let it be given; *died*; *diopter*; *divorced*; *doctor*; *deuterium*

D-

d *density*; [L.] *dexter* or *dextro*, right; [L.] *dies*, day; *distal*; *dorsal*; *duration*

D/A *digital to analog*

Da *dalton*

daboia, daboya (dă-boy′ă)

dacarbazine (dă-kăr′bă-zēn)

dacnomania (dăk″nō-mā′nē-ă) [Gr. *daknein*, to bite, + *mania*, insanity]

dacryadenalgia (dăk″rē-ăd-ĕn-ăl′jē-ă) [Gr. *dakryon*, tear, + *aden*, gland, + *algos*, pain]

dacryadenitis (dăk″rē-ăd-ĕ-nī′tĭs) [″ + ″ + *itis*, inflammation]

dacryadenoscirrhus (dăk″rē-ăd″ĕn-ō-skĭr′ŭs) [″ + ″ + *skirrhos*, hardening]

dacryagogatresia (dăk″rē-ă-gŏg″ă-trē′sē-ă) [Gr. *dakryon*, tear, + *agogos*, leading, + *a-*, not, + *tresis*, perforate]

dacryagogue (dăk′rē-ă-gŏg)

dacrycystalgia (dăk″rē-sĭs-tăl′jē-ă) [″ + *kystis*, cyst, + *algos*, pain]

dacryelcosis (dăk″rē-ĕl-kō′sĭs) [″ + *helkosis*, ulceration]

dacryoadenalgia (dăk″rē-ō-ăd″ĕn-ăl′jē-ă) [″ + *aden*, gland, + *algos*, pain]

dacryoadenectomy (dăk″rē-ō-ăd″ĕ-nĕk′tō-mē) [″ + ″ + *ektome*, excision]

dacryoadenitis (dăk″rē-ō-ăd″ĕn-ī′tĭs) [″ + ″ + *itis*, inflammation]

dacryoblennorrhea (dăk″rē-ō-blĕn″ō-rē′ă) [″ + *blenna*, mucus, + *rhein*, to flow]

dacryocele (dăk′rē-ō-sēl) [″ + *kele*, tumor, swelling]

dacryocyst (dăk′rē-ō-sĭst) [″ + *kystis*, cyst]

dacryocystalgia (dăk″rē-ō-sĭs-tăl′jē-ă) [″ + ″ + *algos*, pain]

dacryocystectomy (dăk″rē-ō-sĭs-tĕk′tō-mē) [″ + *kystis*, cyst, + *ektome*, excision]

dacryocystitis (dăk″rē-ō-sĭs-tī′tĭs) [″ + ″ + *itis*, inflammation]

dacryocystoblennorrhea (dăk″rē-ō-sĭs″tō-blĕn-ō-rē′ă) [″ + ″ + *blenna*, mucus, + *rhein*, to flow]

dacryocystocele (dăk″rē-ō-sĭs′tō-sēl) [Gr. *dakryon*, tear, + *kystis*, cyst, + *kele*, tumor, swelling]

dacryocystography (dăk″rē-ō-sĭs-tŏg′ră-fē) [″ + ″ + *graphein*, to write]

dacryocystoptosis (dăk″rē-ō-sĭs-tŏp-tō′sĭs) [″ + ″ + *ptosis*, fall, falling]

dacryocystorhinostenosis (dăk″rē-ō-sĭs″tō-rī-nō-stĕ-nō′sĭs) [″ + ″ + *rhis*, nose, + *stenosis*, act of narrowing]

dacryocystorhinostomy (dăk″rē-ō-sĭs″tō-rī-nŏs′tō-mē) [″ + ″ + ″ + *stoma*, mouth, opening]

dacryocystorhinotomy (dăk″rē-ō-sĭs″tō-rī-nŏt′ō-mē) [″ + ″ + ″ + *tome*, a cutting, slice]

dacryocystosyringotomy (dăk″rē-ō-sĭs″tō-sĭr″ĭn-gŏt′ō-mē) [″ + *kystis*, cyst, + *syrinx*, tube, + *tome*, a cutting, slice]

dacryocystotome (dăk″rē-ō-sĭs′tō-tōm) [″ + ″ + *tome*, a cutting,

179

slice]

dacryocystotomy (dăk″rē-ō-sĭs-tŏt′ō-mē)

dacryocyte

dacryogenic

dacryohelcosis (dăk″rē-ō-hĕl-kō′sĭs) [″ + helcosis, ulceration]

dacryohemorrhea (dăk″rē-ō-hĕm″ō-rē′ă) [″ + haima, blood, + rhein, to flow]

dacryolin (dăk′rē-ō-lĭn) [Gr. dakryon, tear]

dacryolith, dacryolite [″ + lithos, stone]

dacryolithiasis (dăk″rē-ō-lĭ-thī′ă-sĭs) [″ + lithiasis, formation of stones]

dacryoma (dăk″rē-ō′mă) [″ + oma, tumor]

dacryon (dăk′rē-ŏn) [Gr. dakryon]

dacryops (dăk′rē-ŏps) [″ + ops, eye]

dacryopyorrhea (dăk″rē-ō-pī″ō-rē′ă) [″ + pyon, pus, + rhein, to flow]

dacryopyosis [″ + pyosis, suppuration]

dacryorrhea (dăk″rē-ō-rē′ă) [″ + rhein, to flow]

dacryosolenitis (dăk″rē-ō-sō-lĕn-ī′tĭs) [″ + solen, duct, + itis, inflammation]

dacryostenosis (dăk″rē-ō-stĕn-ō′sĭs) [″ + stenosis, act of narrowing]

dacryosyrinx (dăk″rē-ō-sĭ′rĭnks) [″ + syrinx, tube]

dactinomycin

dactyl (dăk′tĭl) [Gr. daktylos, finger]

dactyledema (dăk″tĭl-ĕ-dē′mă) [″ + oidema, swelling]

dactylion

dactylitis [″ + itis, inflammation] d., sickle cell

dactylocampsodynia (dăk″tĭl-ō-kămp″sō-dĭn′ē-ă) [″ + kampsis, bend, + odyne, pain]

dactylogram [″ + gramma, letter, piece of writing]

dactylography [″ + graphein, to write]

dactylogryposis (dăk″tĭl-ō-grĭ-pō′sĭs) [″ + gryposis, curve]

dactylology (dăk-tĭl-ŏl′ō-jē) [″ + logos, word, reason]

dactylolysis (dăk″tĭl-lŏl′ĭ-sĭs) [″ + lysis, dissolution]

dactylomegaly (dăk″tĭl-ō-mĕg′ă-lē) [″ + megas, large]

dactyloscopy (dăk″tĭ-lŏs′kō-pē) [″ + skopein, to examine]

dactylospasm (dăk′tĭ-lō-spăzm) [″ + spasmos, a convulsion]

dactylus (dăk′tĭ-lŭs) [Gr. daktylos]

daily living skills

dairy food substitute

Dakin's solution (dā′kĭns) [Henry D. Dakin, U.S. chemist, 1880–1952]

Dale reaction [Sir Henry H. Dale, 1875–1969]

Dalmane

dalton (dawl′tŏn)

Dalton, John [Brit. chemist, 1766–1844]
> D. -Henry law [Joseph Henry, U.S. physicist, 1797–1878]
> D.'s law

dam

damp
> d., after
> d., black
> d., cold
> d., fire
> d., white

damping

danazol (dă′nă-zōl)

dance, Saint Vitus'

dancing disease

dancing mania

D and C dilation and curettage

dander (dăn′dĕr)

dandruff

dandy fever

Dandy-Walker syndrome (dăn′dē-wawk′ĕr) [Walter E. Dandy, U.S. neurosurgeon, 1886–1946; Arthur E. Walker, U.S. surgeon, b. 1907]

Dane particles [David S. Dane, contemporary Brit. virologist]

Danocrine

danthron (dăn'thrŏn)
Dantrium
dantrolene sodium (dăn'trō-lēn)
Danysz phenomenon [Jean Danysz, Polish pathologist, 1860–1928]
dapsone (dăp'sōn)
Daranide
Daraprim
Darbid
Daricon
Darier's disease (dăr-ē-āz') [J. F. Darier, Fr. dermatologist, 1856–1938]
darkroom
Darling's disease (dăr'lĭngz) [Samuel Taylor Darling, U.S. physician, 1872–1925]
dartoid (dăr'toyd) [Gr. dartos, skinned, + eidos, form, shape]
dartos [Gr.]
dartos muscle reflex
dartrous [Gr. dartos, skinned]
Darvon
Darvon-N
darwinian ear [Charles Robert Darwin, Brit. naturalist, 1809–1882]
darwinian tubercle
darwinism (dăr'wĭ-nĭzm)
dasymeter (dăs-ĭm'ĕ-tĕr)
Datril
Datura (dă-tū'ră)
daughter (daw'tĕr)
daunorubicin hydrochloride
Davidsohn's sign [Hermann Davidsohn, Ger. physician, 1842–1911]
dawn phenomenon
day blindness
day-care center
daydream
dB, db decibel
D.C. Doctor of Chiropractic; direct current
DDD pacing
D.D.S. Doctor of Dental Surgery
DDST Denver Developmental Screening Test
DDT
de- [L. de, from]
deacidification [" + acidus, sour, + facere, to make]

deactivation [" + activus, acting]
dead [AS. dead]
deaf [AS. deaf]
deafferentation (dē-ăf"ĕr-ĕn-tā'shŭn)
deaf-mute
deaf-mutism
deafness [AS.]
   d., aviator's
   d., bass
   d., central
   d., cerebral
   d., ceruminous
   d., conduction
   d., cortical
   d., high frequency
   d., nerve
   d., occupational
   d., ototoxic
   d., perceptive
   d., psychic
   d., tone
   d., word
deamidase (dē-ăm'ĭ-dās)
deamidization (dē-ăm"ĭ-dĭ-zā'shŭn)
deaminase
deamination, deaminization
deaquation (dē"ă-kwā'shŭn) [" + aqua, water]
dearterialization (dē"ăr'tēr"ē-ăl-ĭ-zā'shŭn) [" + Gr. arteria, artery]
dearticulation (dē"ăr-tĭk"ū-lā'shŭn)
death [AS. death]
   d., black
   d., brain
   d., crib
   d., fetal
   d., functional
   d., local
   d., molecular
deathbed
deathbed statement
death rate
death rattle
"death with dignity"
debilitant [L. debilis, weak]
debilitate
debility
débouchement (dā-boosh-mŏn') [Fr.]
Debove's membrane (dĕ-bōvz')

[Georges Maurice Debove, Fr. physician, 1845–1920]

débride (dā-brēd') [Fr.]

débridement (dā-brēd-mŏn') [Fr.]
  d., canal or d., root canal
  d., enzymatic
  d., epithelial

debris (dĕ-brē') [Fr., remains]

debrisoquin (dĕb-rĭs'ō-kwĭn)

debt (dĕt)
  d., oxygen

deca-, dec- [Gr. deka]

Decaderm

Decadron

Decadron-LA

Deca-Durabolin

decagram (dĕk'ă"grăm) [" + gramma, a small weight]

decalcification (dē"kăl-sĭ-fĭ-kā'shŭn) [L. de, from, + calx, lime, + facere, to make]

decalcify

decaliter (dĕk'ă-lē"tĕr) [Gr. deka, ten, + Fr. litre, liter]

decalvant (dē-kăl'vănt) [L. decalvare, to make bald]

decameter (dĕk'ă-mē-tĕr) [Gr. deka, ten, + metron, measure]

decannulation (dē-kăn"nū-lā'shŭn)

decanormal (dĕk"ă-nor'măl) [" + L. norma, rule]

decant (dē-kănt') [L. de, from, + NL. -cantare, side]

decantation

decapitation (dē-kăp"ĭ-tā'shŭn) [" + caput, head]

decapsulation [" + capsula, little box]

decarboxylase (dē"kăr-bŏk'sĭ-lās)

decarboxylation, decarboxylization (dē"kăr-bŏks-ĭ-lā'shŭn, -ĭl"ĭ-zā'shŭn)

Decaspray

decavitamin capsules (dĕk"ă-vī'tă-mĭn)

decay (dē-kā') [" + cadere, to fall, die]
  d., radioactive

deceleration (dē-sĕl"ĕ-rā'shŭn)

decerebrate (dē-sĕr'ĕ-brāt) [" + cerebrum, brain]

decerebrate posture

decerebrate rigidity

decerebration (dē-sĕr-ĕ-brā'shŭn)

dechlorination, dechloridation [" + Gr. chloros, green]

decholesterolization (dē"kō-lĕs"tĕr-ŏl-ĭ-zā'shŭn) [" + chole, bile, + stereos, solid]

Decholin

deci- [L. decimus, tenth]

decibel (dĕs'ĭ-bĕl) [L. decimus, tenth, + bel, unit of sound]

decidophobia [decide, + Gr. phobos, fear]

decidua (dē-sĭd'ū-ă) [L. deciduus, falling off]
  d. basalis
  d. capsularis
  d. menstrualis
  d. parietalis
  d. reflexa
  d. serotina
  d. vera

decidual (dē-sĭd'ū-ăl)

deciduation (dē-sĭd"ū-ā'shŭn)

deciduitis (dē-sĭd"ū-ī'tĭs) [" + Gr. itis, inflammation]

deciduoma (dē-sĭd"ū-ō'mă) [" + Gr. oma, tumor]
  d., benign
  d., Loeb's
  d., malignant

deciduomatosis (dē-sĭd"ū-ō-mă-tō'sĭs) [" + Gr. oma, tumor, + osis, condition]

deciduosarcoma [" + Gr. sarx, flesh, + oma, tumor]

deciduous (dē-sĭd'ū-ŭs) [L. deciduus]

deciduous teeth

decigram (dĕs'ĭ-grăm) [L. decimus, tenth, + Gr. gramma, a small weight]

deciliter (dĕs'ĭ-lē-tĕr) [" + Fr. litre]

decimeter (dĕs'ĭ-mē"tĕr) [" + Gr. metron, measure]

decinormal (dĕs"ĭ-nor'măl) [" + norma, rule]

decipara (dĕs"ĭ-păr'ă) [" + parere, to beget, produce]

decision analysis

decision making

decision tree

Declaration of Geneva

Declaration of Hawaii

declination (dĕk"lĭ-nā'shŭn)

declinator (dĕk'lĭn-ā"tor) [L. declinare, to turn aside]

decline (dē-klīn')

declivis cerebelli (dē-klīv'ĭs sĕr-ĕ-bĕl'ī) [L.]

decoction (dē-kŏk'shŭn) [L. de, down, + coquere, to boil]

decollation (dē"kŏl-ā'shŭn) [" + collum, neck]

décollement (dā-kōl-mŏn') [Fr., ungluing]

decoloration (dē-kŭl"or-ā'shŭn)

decompensation [L. de, from, + compensare, to make good again]

decomplementize

decomposition (dē-kŏm-pō-zĭsh'ŭn) [" + componere, to put together]
   d., double
   d., hydrolytic
   d., simple

decompress

decompression [" + compressio, a squeezing together]
   d., explosive

decompression illness

decongestant

decontamination

decorticate posture

decortication [" + cortex, bark]
   d., pulmonary
   d., renal

decrement (dĕk'rē-mĕnt) [L. decrementum, decrease]

decrepitate (dē-krĕp'ĭ-tāt) [L. decrepitare, to crackle]

decrepitation

decrepitude (dē-krĕp'ĭ-tūd)

decrudescence (dē-kroo-dĕs'ĕns)

decubation (dē-kū-bā'shŭn) [L. de, down, + cumbere, to lie]

decubital

decubitus (dē-kū'bĭ-tŭs) [L., a lying down]
   d., acute
   d., Andral's
   d., dorsal
   d., lateral
   d., ventral

decubitus projections

decubitus ulcer

decurrent (dē-kŭr'ĕnt) [L. decurrere, to run down]

decussate (dē-kŭs'āt) [L. decussare, to make an X]

decussation
   d. of pyramids
   d., optic

decussorium (dē-kŭs-ō'rē-ŭm)

dedifferentiation

dedolation (dĕd"ō-lā'shŭn)

deduction (dē-dŭk'shŭn)

de-efferented state

deep [AS. deop]

deep reflexes

deer fly

deer fly fever

DEF decayed, extracted, and filled

defatted [" + AS. faelt, to fatten]

defecalgesiophobia (dĕf"ĕ-kăl"jē-sē-ō-fō'bē-ă) [L. defaecare, to remove dregs, + Gr. algesis, sense of pain, + phobos, fear]

defecation (dĕf-ĕ-kā'shŭn) [L. defaecare, to remove dregs]

defecation syncope

defect (dē'fĕkt)
   d., congenital
   d., filling
   d., septal

defective [L. defectus, a failure]

defeminization (dē-fĕm"ĭ-nĭ-zā'shŭn)

defense [L. defendre, to repel]

defense mechanism

defense reflex

defensive

defensive medicine

deferens (dĕf'ĕr-ĕnz) [L. *deferens*, carrying away]
deferent (dĕf'ĕr-ĕnt)
deferentectomy (dĕf-ĕr-ĕn-tĕk'tō-mē) [" + Gr. *ektome*, excision]
deferential (dĕf-ĕr-ĕn'shăl) [L. *deferre*, to bring to]
deferentitis (dĕf"ĕr-ĕn-tī'tĭs) [" + Gr. *itis*, inflammation]
deferoxamine mesylate (dĕ-fĕr-ŏks'ă-mēn)
deferred shock
defervescence [L. *defervescere*, to become calm]
defibrillation
    d., electrical
defibrillator (dē-fĭb"rĭ-lā'tor)
defibrination, defibrinization [L. *de*, from, + *fibra*, fiber]
deficiency (dē-fĭsh'ĕn-sē) [L. *deficere*, to lack]
deficiency disease
deficit (dĕf'ĭ-sĭt)
defined medium
definition [L. *definire*, to limit]
definitive
deflection (dē-flĕk'shŭn)
defloration (dĕf"lō-rā'shŭn) [L. *de*, from, + *flos, flor-*, flower]
deflorescence
defluvium (dē-floo'vē-ŭm) [L.]
    d. capillorum
defluxio (dē-flŭk'sē-ō) [L.]
    d. capillorum
    d. ciliorum
defluxion (dē-flŭk'shŭn)
deformability (dē-form"ă-bĭl'ĭ-tē)
deformation [L. *de*, from, + *forma*, form]
deformity
    d., anterior
    d., gunstock
    d., Madelung's
    d., mutilans
    d., seal fin
    d., silverfork
    d., Sprengel's
    d., Velpeau's

    d., Volkmann's
defundation [" + *fundus*, base]
defurfuration (dē"fĕr-fū-rā'shŭn) [" + *furfur*, bran]
deg *degeneration; degree*
deganglionate (dē-găn'glē-ŏn-āt") [" + Gr. *ganglion*, knot]
degenerate [L. *degenerare*, to fall from one's ancestral quality]
degeneration [L. *degeneratio*]
    d., Abercrombie's
    d., adipose
    d., albuminoid
    d., amyloid
    d., ascending
    d., calcareous
    d., caseous
    d., cloudy swelling
    d., colloid
    d., congenital macular
    d., cystic
    d., descending
    d., fatty
    d., fibroid
    d., gray
    d., hepatolenticular
    d., hyaline
    d., hydropic
    d., lardaceous
    d., lipoidal
    d., macular
    d., mucoid
    d., mucous
    d., myxomatous
    d., Nissl
    d., parenchymatous
    d., pigmentary
    d., polypoid
    d., secondary
    d., senile
    d., spongy
    d., subacute combined, of spinal cord
    d., vitreous
    d., wallerian
    d., Zenker's
degenerative
deglutible (dē-gloo'tĭ-bl) [L. *deglutire*,

to swallow]

deglutition (dē"gloo-tĭsh'ŭn)

deglutitive

degradation (dĕg"rĕ-dā'shŭn) [LL. de-gradare, to go down a step]

degree (dĕ-grē')

degustation (dē"gŭs-tā'shŭn) [L. de-gustatio]

dehiscence (dē-hĭs'ĕns) [L. dehiscere, to gape]

dehumanization (dē-hū"măn-ĭ-zā'shŭn) [L. de, from, + humanus, human]

dehumidifier (dē"hū-mĭd'ĭ-fī"ĕr)

dehydrate [L. de, from, + Gr. hydor, water]

dehydration (dē"hī-drā'shŭn)

dehydroandrosterone (dē-hī"drō-ăn-drō-stēr'ōn, -drŏs'tĕr-ōn)

dehydrocholesterol (dē-hī"drō-kō-lĕs'tĕr-ŏl)

dehydrocholic acid

dehydrocorticosterone (dē-hī"drō-kor-tĭ-kōs'tĕr-ōn)

dehydroepiandrosterone (dē-hī"drō-ĕp"ē-ăn-drŏs'tĕr-ōn)

dehydrogenase (dē-hī-drŏj'ē-nās)

dehydrogenate (dē-hī"drŏj'ĕn-āt)

dehydroisoandrosterone (dē-hī"drō-ī"sō-ăn-drŏs'tĕr-ōn)

deinstitutionalization

deionization (dē-ī"ŏn-ī-zā'shŭn)

Deiters' cells (dī'tĕrz) [Otto F. C. Deiters, Ger. anatomist, 1834–1863]

Deiters' nucleus

Deiters' process

déjà entendu (dā'zhă ŏn-tŏn-doo') [Fr., already heard]

déjà vu (dā'zhă voo) [Fr., already seen]

dejecta (dē-jĕk'tă) [L. dejectio, injection]

dejection, dejecture (dē-jĕk'shŭn, -tūr)

Déjérine, Joseph J. (dā"zhĕr-ēn') [Fr. neurologist, 1849–1917]

   D.'s disease

   D. -Sottas atrophy [Jules Sottas, Fr. neurologist, 1866–1943]

   D.'s syndrome

dekaliter

delacrimation (dē-lăk"rĭ-mā'shŭn) [L. de, from, + lacrima, tear]

delactation (dē"lăk-tā'shŭn) [" + lactare, to suckle]

Delalutin

delamination [" + lamina, plate]

Delatestryl

de-lead (dē-lĕd)

deleterious (dĕl"ĕ-tē'rē-ŭs) [Gr. dele-terios]

deletion (dē-lē'shŭn)

Delhi boil

deligation (dĕl-ĭ-gā'shŭn) [L. deligare, to tie up]

delimitation [L. de, from, + limi-tare, to limit]

delinquent (dē-lĭn'kwĕnt)

deliquesce (dĕl"ĭ-kwĕs') [L. delique-scere, to melt away]

deliquescence (dĕl"ĭ-kwĕs'ĕns)

deliquescent (dĕl"ĭ-kwĕs'ĕnt)

délire de toucher (dā-lēr' dŭ too-shā') [Fr.]

deliriant, delirifacient (dē-lĭr'ē-ănt, dē-lĭr"ĭ-fā'shĭ-ĕnt) [L. delirare, to be de-ranged]

delirium (dē-lĭr'ē-ŭm) [L.]

   d., acute

   d., alcoholic

   d., chronic

   d. constantium

   d. cordis

   d. epilepticum

   d., febrile

   d., lingual

   d. mussitans

   d. of negation

   d. of persecution

   d., partial

   d., toxic

   d., traumatic

   d. tremens

delitescence (dĕl"ĭ-tĕs'ĕns) [L. delite-scens, hiding]

deliver [L. deliberare, to free com-pletely]

delivery

d., abdominal
d., forceps
d., postmortem
d., precipitate
d., premature
d., spontaneous
d., vaginal
dellen (děl'ěn)
delomorphous (děl"ō-mor'fŭs) [Gr. *delos*, evident, + *morphe*, form]
delomorphous cells
delousing (dē-lows'ĭng) [L. *de*, from, + AS. *lus*, louse]
delta
Delta-Cortef
deltacortisone (děl"tă-kor'tĭ-sōn)
delta fornicis (děl'tă for'nĭ-sĭs) [L.]
Deltasone
deltoid [Gr. *delta*, letter d, + *eidos*, form, shape]
deltoid ligament
deltoid muscle
deltoid ridge
delusion (dē-loo'zhŭn) [L. *deludere*, to cheat]
d., depressive
d., expansive
d., fixed
d., fleeting
d., nihilistic
d. of grandeur
d. of negation
d. of persecution
d., reference
d., systematized
d., unsystematized
delusional
demand
d., biological oxygen
demarcation (dē"măr-kā'shŭn) [L. *demarcare*, to limit]
demecarium bromide (děm"ē-kā'rē-ŭm)
demeclocycline hydrochloride (děm"ē-klō-sī'klēn)
dement [L. *demens*, mad]
demented
dementia (dē-měn'shē-ă) [L. *demens*,

mad]
d., alcoholic
d., apoplectic
d., dialysis
d., epileptic
d. paralytica
d., postfebrile
d., presenile
d., primary
d., senile
d., syphilitic
d., toxic
Demerol (děm'ěr-ōl)
demi- [L. *dimidius*, half]
demibain (děm'ĭ-băn) [Fr., half bath]
demic (děm'ĭk)[Gr. *demos*, people]
demilune (děm'ĭ-loon) [L. *dimidius*, half, + *luna*, moon]
demineralization [L. *de*, from, + *minare*, to mine]
demise (dē-mīz') [L. *dimittere*, to dismiss]
demodectic (děm-ō-děk'tĭk)
Demodex [Gr. *demos*, fat, + *dex*, worm]
D. folliculorum
demography (dē-mŏg'ră-fē) [Gr. *demos*, people, + *graphein*, to write]
demorphinization (dē-mor"fĭn-ĭ-zā'shŭn)
demotivate
Demours' membrane (dē-mūrz') [Pierre Demours, Fr. ophthalmologist, 1702–1795]
demucosation (dē"mū-kō-sā'shŭn) [L. *demucosatio*]
demulcent [L. *demulcens*, stroking softly]
Demulen
de Musset's sign
demutization (dē"mū-tĭ-zā'shŭn) [L. *de*, from, + *mutus*, mute]
demyelinate (dē-mī'ě-lĭn-āt) [" + Gr. *myelos*, marrow]
demyelination (dē-mī"ě-lĭ-nā'shŭn)
denarcotize (dē-năr'kō-tīz)
denaturation (dē-nā"chŭr-ā'shŭn)

denatured [" + *natura*, nature]
denatured protein
dendraxon (děn-drăk′sŏn) [Gr. *dendron*, tree, + *axon*, axle]
dendric (děn′drĭk)
Dendrid
dendriform (děn′drĭ-form) [" + L. *forma*, shape]
dendrite (děn′drīt) [Gr. *dendrites*, pert. to a tree]
   d.'s, extracapsular
   d.'s, intracapsular
dendritic
dendritic calculus
dendroid (děn′droyd) [" + *eidos*, form, shape]
dendron (děn′drŏn) [Gr., tree]
dendrophagocytosis (děn″drō-făg-ō-sī-tō′sĭs) [" + *phagein*, to eat, + *kytos*, cell, + *osis*, condition]
denervated [L. *de*, from, + Gr. *neuron*, nerve]
dengue (dăng′gă, -gě) [Sp.]
denial (dē-nī′ăl)
denial and isolation
denidation (děn″ĭ-dā′shŭn) [L. *de*, from, + *nidus*, nest]
dens (děnz) [L.]
   d. bicuspidus
   d. caninus
   d. deciduus
   d. incisivus
   d. molaris
   d. permanens
   d. premolaris
   d. sapientiae
   d. serotinus
densimeter (děn-sĭm′ě-těr) [L. *densus*, thick, + Gr. *metron*, measure]
densitometer (děn″sĭ-tŏm′ě-těr)
densitometry (děn″sĭ-tŏm′ě-trē)
density [L. *densitas*, thickness]
dental
dental arch
dental assistant
dental caries
dental chart
dental consonant

dental curve
dental disk
dental dysfunction
dental engine
dental engineering
dental floss
dental formula
dental geriatrics
dentalgia (děn-tăl′jē-ă) [L. *dens*, tooth, + Gr. *algos*, pain]
dental handpiece
dental hygienist
dental index
dental instruments
dental materials
dental plaque
dental prosthesis
dental pulp
dental sealants
dental tape
dentaphone (děn′tă-fōn) [" + Gr. *phone*, sound]
dentate (děn′tāt) [L. *dentatus*, toothed]
dentes [L.]
dentia (děn′shē-ă) [L.]
   d. praecox
   d. tarda
dentibuccal (děn-tĭ-bŭk′l) [L. *dens*, tooth, + *bucca*, cheek]
denticle (děn′tĭ-kl) [L. *denticulus*, little tooth]
denticulate [L. *denticulatus*, small toothed]
denticulate body
dentification [L. *dens*, tooth, + *facere*, to make]
dentiform [" + *forma*, shape]
dentifrice (děn′tĭ-frĭs) [" + *fricare*, to rub]
dentigerous (děn-tĭj′ěr-ŭs) [" + *gerere*, to bear]
dentilabial (děn-tĭ-lā′bē-ăl) [" + *labium*, lip]
dentilingual (děn-tĭ-lĭn′gwăl) [" + *lingua*, tongue]
dentimeter (děn-tĭm′ě-těr) [" + Gr. *metron*, measure]
dentin (děn′tĭn) [L. *dens*, tooth]

dentinal

dentinification [" + *facere,* to make]

dentinitis [" + Gr. *itis,* inflammation]

dentinoblast (děn'tĭn-ō-blăst) [" + Gr. *blastos,* germ]

dentinoclast (děn'tĭn-ō-clăst) [" + Gr. *clastos,* broken]

dentinogenesis (děn"tĭn-ō-jěn'ě-sĭs) [" + *genesis,* generation, birth]
   d. imperfecta

dentinoid [" + Gr. *eidos,* form, shape]

dentinoma [" + Gr. *oma,* tumor]

dentinosteoid (děn"tĭn-ŏs'tē-ōyd) [" + Gr. *osteon,* bone, + *eidos,* form, shape]

dentinum (děn'tĭ-nŭm)

dentiparous (děn-tĭp'ă-rŭs) [" + *parere,* to beget, produce]

dentist [L. *dens,* tooth]

dentistry
   d., esthetic
   d. for children
   d., forensic
   d., four-handed
   d., geriatric
   d., hospital
   d., operative
   d., prosthodontic
   d., public health

dentition [L. *dentitio*]
   d., diphyodont
   d., heterodont
   d., homodont
   d., mixed
   d., monophyodont
   d., permanent
   d., polyphyodont
   d., primary

dentoalveolar (děn"tō-ăl-vē'ō-lăr) [L. *dens,* tooth, + *alveolus,* small hollow]

dentoalveolitis (děn"to-ăl"vē-ō-lī'tĭs) [" + " + Gr. *itis,* inflammation]

dentofacial (děn"tō-fā'shăl)

dentoid [" + Gr. *eidos,* form, shape]

dentoidin

dentulous (děn'tū-lŭs)

denture (děn'chūr)
   d., full
   d., immediate
   d., partial

denturism

denturist

denucleated (dē-nū'klē-āt"ěd) [L. *de,* from, + *nucleus,* kernel]

denudation [L. *denudare,* to lay bare]

denutrition (dē"nū-trĭsh'ŭn) [L. *de,* from, + *nutrire,* to nourish]

Denver classification

Denver Developmental Screening Test

deodorant (dē-ō'dor-ănt) [" + *odorare,* to perfume]

deodorize (dē-ō'dor-īz) [" + *odor,* odor]

deodorizer (dē-ō'dor-īz-ěr)

deontology (dē"ŏn-tŏl'ō-jē) [Gr. *deonta,* needful, + *logos,* word, reason]

deorsum (dē-or'sŭm) [L.]
   d. vergens

deorsumduction (dē-or"sŭm-dŭk'shŭn) [" + *ducere,* to lead]

deorsumversion (dē-or"sŭm-věr'zhŭn) [" + *vertere,* to turn]

deossification (dē-ŏs"ĭ-fĭ-kā'shŭn) [L. *de,* from, + *os,* bone, + *facere,* to make]

deoxidate [" + Gr. *oxys,* sharp]

deoxidation

deoxidizer (dē-ŏk'sĭ-dī-zěr)

deoxycholic acid (dē-ŏk"sē-kō'lĭk)

deoxycorticosterone (dē-ŏk"sē-kor"tē-kŏs'těr-ōn)

deoxygenation (dē-ŏk"sĭ-jěn-ā'shŭn)

deoxyribonuclease (dē-ŏk"sē-rī"bō-nū'klē-ās)

deoxyribonucleic acid (dē-ŏk"sē-rī"bō-nū-klē'ĭk)

deoxyribonucleoprotein (dē-ŏk"sē-rī"bō-nū"klē-ō-prō'tē-ĭn)

deoxyribonucleoside (dē-ŏk"sē-rī"bō-nū'klē-ō-sīd)

deoxyribose (dē-ŏk"sē-rī'bōs)

depancreatize (dē-păn'krē-ă-tīz)
Department of Health and Human Services
Depen
dependence (dē-pĕn'dĕns) [L. *dependere*, to hang down]
depersonalization disorder
depersonalize
de Pezzer's catheter
dephosphorylation (dē-fŏs"for-ī-lā'shŭn) [" + *phosphorylation*]
depigmentation (dē"pĭg-mĕn-tā'shŭn)
depilate (dĕp'ĭl-āt) [L. *depilare*, to deprive of hair]
depilation (dĕp"ĭl-ā'shŭn)
depilatory
depilatory techniques
deplete (dē-plēt') [L. *depletus*, emptied]
depletion (dē-plē'shŭn)
deplumation (dē"ploo-mā'shŭn) [L. *de*, from, + *pluma*, feather]
depolarization (dē-pō"lăr-ĭ-zā'shŭn) [" + *polus*, pole]
depolymerization (dē-pŏl"ĭ-mĕr-ī-zā'shŭn)
Depo-Medrol
Depo-Provera
deposit (dē-pŏz'ĭt) [L. *depositus*, having put aside]
   d., calcareous
   d., tooth
depot (dē'pō, dĕp'ō) [Fr. *depot*, fr. L. *depositum*]
depravation (dĕp"ră-vā'shŭn) [L. *depravare*, completely destroyed]
depressant [L. *depressus*, pressed down]
   d., cardiac
   d., cerebral
   d., motor
   d., respiratory
   d., secretory
depressed (dē-prĕst')
depression (dē-prĕsh'ŭn) [L. *depressio*, a pressing down]
   d., bipolar
   d., endogenous
   d., situational or reactive
   d., unipolar

depressomotor (dē-prĕs'ō-mō"tor) [" + *motor*, mover]
depressor [L.]
   d., tongue
depressor fibers
depressor nerve
depressor reflex
deprivation (dĕp"rī-vā'shŭn) [L. *de*, from, + *privare*, to remove]
   d., emotional
   d., sensory
   d., sleep, effects of
depth [ME. *depthe*]
depth dose
depth perception
depth psychology
depulization (dē-pūl"ĭ-zā'shŭn) [L. *de*, from, + *pulex*, flea]
depurant (dĕp'ū-rănt) [L. *depurare*, to purify]
depuration
depurative
depurator
de Quervain's disease
deradelphus (dĕr-ă-dĕl'fŭs) [Gr. *dere*, neck, + *adelphos*, brother]
deradenitis (dĕr"ăd-ĕn-ī'tĭs) [" + *aden*, gland, + *itis*, inflammation]
deradenoncus (dĕr"ăd-ĕn-ŏnk'ŭs) [" + *onkos*, bulk, mass]
derangement (dē-rānj'mĕnt) [Fr. *deranger*, unbalance]
Dercum's disease (dĕr'kŭms) [Francis X. Dercum, U.S. neurologist, 1856–1931]
derealization
dereism (dē'rē-ĭzm) [L. *de*, from, + *res*, thing]
dereistic (dē"rē-ĭs'tĭk) [" + *res*, thing]
derencephalus (dĕr"ĕn-sĕf'ă-lŭs) [Gr. *dere*, neck, + *enkephalos*, brain]
derivation (dĕr"ĭ-vā'shŭn) [L. *derivare*, to draw off]
derivative (dē-rĭv'ă-tĭv)
derm, derma [Gr. *derma*, skin]
dermabrasion (dĕrm'ă-brā"zhŭn) [" + L. *abrasio*, wearing away]
Dermacentor (dĕr"mă-sĕn'tor)

D. andersoni
D. variabilis
Dermacort
dermad [Gr. *derma*, skin, + L. *ad*, toward]
dermadrome (dĕr'mă-drōm)
dermal
dermalaxia (dĕr″mă-lăk'sē-ă) [" + *malaxis*, softening]
dermalgia (dĕr-măl'jē-ă) [" + *algos*, pain]
dermamyiasis (dĕr-mă-mī-ī'ă-sĭs) [" + *myia*, fly, + *-iasis*, state or condition of]
dermapostasis (dĕr″mă-pŏs'tă-sĭs) [" + *apostasis*, a falling away]
dermat-, dermato- [Gr. *dermatos*]
dermatalgia (dĕr″mă-tăl'jē-ă) [" + *algos*, pain]
dermatatrophia (dĕrm″ăt-ă-trō'fē-ă) [" + *atrophia*, atrophy]
dermatauxe (dĕr-mă-tŏk'sē) [" + *auxe*, increase]
dermatides
dermatitis (dĕr″mă-tī'tĭs) [Gr. *dermatos*, skin, + *itis*, inflammation]
    d., actinic
    d. aestivalis
    d., allergic
    d., atopic
    d., berlock or d.,berloque
    d. calorica
    d., cercarial
    d., contact
    d., cosmetic
    d., exfoliative
    d. herpetiformis
    d. hiemalis
    d. infectiosa eczematoides
    d. medicamentosa
    d. multiformis
    d. papillaris capillitii
    d., poison ivy
    d., primary
    d., radiation
    d., rhus
    d. seborrheica
    d., stasis

    d. venenata
    d. verrucosa
    d., x-ray
dermatoautoplasty (dĕr″mă-tō-aw'tō-plăs″tē) [Gr. *dermatos*, skin, + *autos*, self, + *plassein*, to form]
Dermatobia (dĕr″mă-tō'bē-ă) [" + *bios*, life]
    D. hominis
dermatobiasis (dĕr″mă-tō-bī'ă-sĭs)
dermatocele (dĕr'mă-tō-sēl″) [" + *kele*, tumor, swelling]
    d. lipomatosa
dermatocelidosis (dĕr″mă-tō-sĕl″ĭ-dō'sĭs) [" + *kelis*, spot, + *osis*, condition]
dermatocellulitis (dĕr″mă-tō-sĕl″ū-lī'tĭs) [" + L. *cellula*, little cell, + Gr. *itis*, inflammation]
dermatoconiosis (dĕr″mă-tō-kō″nē-ō'sĭs) [" + *konia*, dust]
dermatocyst (dĕr'mă-tō-sĭst) [" + *kystis*, cyst]
dermatodynia (dĕr″mă-tō-dĭn'ē-ă) [" + *odyne*, pain]
dermatofibroma [" + L. *fibra*, fiber, + Gr. *oma*, tumor]
dermatofibrosarcoma (dĕr″mă-tō-fī″brō-săr-kō'mă) [" + " + Gr. *sarx*, flesh, + *oma*, tumor]
dermatogen (dĕr-măt'ō-jĕn) [" + *gennan*, to produce]
dermatogenous (dĕr″mă-tŏj'ĕn-ŭs)
dermatoglyphics (dĕr″mă-tō-glĭf'ĭks) [" + *glyphe*, a carving]
dermatographia, dermatography
dermatoheliosis
dermatoheteroplasty (dĕr″mă-tō-hĕt'ĕr-ō-plăs″tē) [" + *heteros*, other, + *plassein*, to mold]
dermatokelidosis (dĕr″mă-tō-kĕl″ĭ-dō'sĭs) [" + *kelidoun*, to stain]
dermatologist (dĕr″mă-tŏl'ō-jĭst) [Gr. *dermatos*, skin, + *logos*, word, reason]
dermatology (dĕr″mă-tŏl'ō-jē)
dermatolysis (dĕr″mă-tŏl'ĭ-sĭs) [" + *lysis*, dissolution]

dermatoma (dĕr″mă-tō′mă) [″ + oma, tumor]

dermatome (dĕr′mă-tōm) [Gr. derma, skin, + tome, a cutting, slice]

dermatomere (dĕr′mă-tō-mēr) [Gr. dermatos, skin, + meros, part]

dermatomucosomyositis (dĕr″mă-tō-mū-kō″sō-mī-ō-sī′tĭs) [″ + L. mucosa, mucous membrane, + Gr. mys, muscle, + itis, inflammation]

dermatomycosis (dĕr″mă-tō-mī-kō′sĭs) [″ + mykes, fungus, + osis, condition]

dermatomyoma [″ + mys, muscle, + oma, tumor]

dermatomyositis (dĕr″mă-tō-mī″ō-sī′tĭs) [″ + ″ + itis, inflammation]

dermatoneurosis [″ + neuron, nerve, + osis, condition]

dermatopathia [″ + pathos, disease, suffering]

dermatopathology [″ + ″ + logos, word, reason]

dermatopathy

dermatophiliasis (dĕr″mă-tō-fĭ-lī′ă-sĭs)

dermatophilosis (dĕr″mă-tō-fĭ-lō′sĭs)

dermatophobia [″ + phobos, fear]

dermatophylaxis (dĕr′mă-tō-fĭ-lăk′sĭs) [″ + phylaxis, guard]

dermatophyte (dĕr′mă-tō-fīt) [″ + phyton, plant]

dermatophytid (dĕr″mă-tŏf′ĭ-tĭd)

dermatophytosis (dĕr″mă-tō-fĭ-tō′sĭs) [″ + phyton, plant, + osis, condition]

dermatoplastic [″ + plassein, to form]

dermatoplasty (dĕr′mă-tō-plăs″tē)

dermatorrhagia (dĕr″mă-tō-rā′jē-ă) [Gr. dermatos, skin, + rhegnynai, to burst forth]

dermatorrhea (dĕr″mă-tō-rē′ă) [″ + rhein, to flow]

dermatosclerosis (dĕr″mă-tō-sklĕr-ō′sĭs) [″ + sklerosis, a hardening]

dermatoscopy (dĕr″mă-tŏs′kō-pē) [″ + skopein, to examine]

dermatosis (dĕr″mă-tō′sĭs) [″ + osis, condition]

   d. papulosa nigra

   d., progressive pigmentary

dermatosome (dĕr′mă-tō-sōm) [″ + soma, body]

dermatotherapy [″ + therapeia, treatment]

dermatotome (dĕr′mă-tō-tōm″) [″ + tome, a cutting, slice]

dermatotropic (dĕr″mă-tō-trŏp′ĭk) [″ + trope, a turning]

dermatoxerasia (dĕr″mă-tō-zē-rā′zē-ă) [″ + xerasia, dryness]

dermatozoon [″ + zoon, animal]

dermatozoonosis (dĕr″mă-tō-zō″ō-nō′sĭs) [″ + ″ + nosos, disease]

dermatrophia (dĕr-mă-trō′fē-ă) [″ + atrophia, atrophy]

dermic (dĕr′mĭk) [Gr. derma, skin]

dermis (dĕr′mĭs) [L.]

dermoblast [Gr. derma, skin, + blastos, germ]

dermographia, **dermography** (dĕr-mō-grăf′ē-ă, -mŏg′ră-fē) [″ + graphein, to write]

dermoid (dĕr′moyd) [″ + eidos, form, shape]

dermoid cyst

dermoidectomy (dĕr″moyd-ĕk′tō-mē) [″ + ″ + ektome, excision]

dermolipoma (dĕr″mō-lĭ-pō′mă)

dermomycosis (dĕr″mō-mī-kō′sĭs) [″ + mykes, fungus, + osis, condition]

dermonosology (dĕr″mō-nō-sŏl′ō-jē) [″ + nosos, disease, + logos, word, reason]

dermopathy (dĕr-mŏp′ă-thē) [″ + pathos, disease, suffering]

dermophlebitis (dĕr″mō-flĕ-bī′tĭs) [″ + phleps, blood vessel, vein, + itis, inflammation]

dermophyte (dĕr′mō-fīt) [″ +

phyton, plant]
dermoskeleton [" + *skeleton*]
dermosynovitis (děr″mō-sǐn-ō-vī′tǐs)
[" + L. *synovia,* joint fluid, +
Gr. *itis,* inflammation]
dermotropic (děr″mō-trŏp′ǐk) [" +
trope, a turning]
dermovascular (děr″mō-vǎs′kū-lǎr)
[" + *vas,* vessel]
derodidymus (děr″ō-dǐd′ǐ-mǔs) [Gr.
dere, neck, + *didymos,* double]
DES *diethylstilbestrol*
desalination
desaturation [L. *de,* from, + *saturare,* to fill]
Desault's apparatus (dě-sōz′) [Pierre
J. Desault, Fr. surgeon, 1744 – 1795]
descemetitis (děs″ě-mě-tī′tǐs)
Descemet's membrane (děs-ě-māz′)
[Jean Descemet, Fr. anatomist, 1732 –
1810]
descemetocele (děs″ě-mět′ō-sēl)
descendens (dě-sěn′děns) [L. *de,* from,
+ *scendere,* to climb]
d. hypoglossi
descensus (dě-sěn′sǔs) [L.]
d. testis
d. uteri
d. ventriculi
DES daughters
desensitization
d., systematic
desensitize [L. *de,* from, + *sentire,* to perceive]
desert fever, desert rheumatism
desexualize (dē-sěks′ū-ǎl-īz) [" +
sexus, sex]
Desferal
desferrioxamine (děs-fěr′ē-ŏks′ǎ-
mēn)
desiccant (děs′ǐ-kǎnt)
desiccate (děs′ǐ-kāt) [L. *desiccare,* to
dry up]
desiccation (děs″ǐ-kǎ′shǔn)
"designer drug"
desipramine hydrochloride
(děs-ǐp′rǎ-mēn)
deslanoside (děs-lǎn′ō-sīd)

desmalgia (děs-mǎl′jē-ǎ) [Gr. *desmos,*
band, + *algos,* pain]
desmectasia, desmectasis
(děs-měk-tā′zē-ǎ, -měk′tǎ-sǐs) [" +
ektasis, dilatation]
desmepithelium (děs-měp-ǐ-thē′lē-ǔm)
[" + *epi,* upon, + *thele,* nip-
ple]
desmitis (děs-mī′tǐs) [" + *itis,* in-
flammation]
desmo- [Gr. *desmos*]
desmocranium (děs″mō-krā′nē-ǔm)
[" + L. *cranium*]
desmocyte (děs′mō-sīt) [" + *kytos,*
cell]
desmocytoma (děs″mō-sī-tō′mǎ)
[" + ″ + *oma,* tumor]
desmodynia [" + *odyne,* pain]
desmoenzyme
desmogenous (děs-mǒj′ě-nǔs) [" +
gennan, to produce]
desmography (děs-mǒg′rǎ-fē) [" +
graphein, to write]
desmoid (děs′moyd) [" + *eidos,*
form, shape]
desmology (děs-mǒl′ō-jē) [" +
logos, word, reason]
desmona [" + *oma,* tumor]
desmoneoplasm (děs″mō-nē′ō-
plǎzm) [" + *neos,* new, + LL.
plasma, form, mold]
desmopathy (děs-mǒp′ǎ-thē) [" +
pathos, disease, suffering]
desmoplasia (děs-mō-plā′zē-ǎ) [" +
Gr. *plassein,* to form]
desmoplastic [" + *plassein,* to
form]
desmopressin acetate
desmopyknosis (děs″mō-pǐk-nō′sǐs)
[" + *pyknosis,* condensation]
desmorrhexis (děs-mō-rěk′sǐs) [" +
rhexis, rupture]
desmosis (děs-mō′sǐs) [" + *osis,*
condition]
desmosome (děs′mō-sōm) [" +
soma, body]
desmotomy (děs-mǒt′ō-mē) [" +
tome, a cutting, slice]

desoximetasone (dĕs-ŏk″sē-mĕt′ă-sōn)

desoxy-
desoxycorticosterone (dĕs-ŏk″sē-kor-tĭ-kŏs′tĕr-ōn)
d. acetate

desoxyribonucleic acid (dĕs″ŏk-sē-rīb″ō-nū′klē-ĭk)

despumation (dĕs″pū-mā′shŭn) [L. de, from, + spuma, froth]

desquamate (dĕs′kwă-māt) [L. desquamare, to remove scales]

desquamation (dĕs″kwă-mā′shŭn)
d., furfuraceous

desquamative (dĕs-kwŏm′ă-tĭv)

DES syndrome

destructive [L. destructus, destroyed]

destructive lesion

desudation (dē-sū-dā′shŭn) [L. de, from, + sudare, to perspire]

desulfhydrase (dē″sŭlf-hī′drās)

desynchronosis (dē-sĭn″krō-nō′sĭs) [″ + Gr. synkhronos, same time]

DET diethyltryptamine

det. [L.] detur, let it be given

detachment [O. Fr. destachier, to unfasten]
d., retinal

detail

detector [L. detectus, uncovered]
d., lie
d., optical
d., radiation

detergent [L. detergere, to cleanse]

deterioration [L. deteriorare, to deteriorate]

determinant (dē-tĕr′mĭ-nănt) [L. determinare, to limit]

determination [L. determinatus, limiting]

determinism (dē-tĕr′mĭn-ĭzm) [″ + Gr. -ismos, condition]

detersive [L. detergere, to cleanse]

det. in dup. [L.] detur in duplo, let twice as much be given

detonation (dĕ″tō-nā′shŭn) [L. detonare, to thunder loudly]

detortion, detorsion (dē-tor′shŭn)

detoxicate (dē-tŏk′sĭ-kāt) [L. de, from, + Gr. toxikon, poison]

detoxification [″ + ″ + L. facere, to make]

detoxify (dē-tŏk′sĭ-fī)

detrition (dē-trĭsh′ŭn) [L. detritus, worn down]

detritus (dĭ-trī′tŭs) [L., worn down]

detruncation (dē″trŭn-kā′shŭn) [L. de, from, + truncus, trunk]

detrusor urinae (dē-trū′sor ū-rī′nē) [L.]

detumescence (dē″tū-mĕs′ĕns) [L. de, down, + tumescere, to swell]

deutencephalon (dūt-ĕn-sĕf′ă-lŏn) [Gr. deuteros, second, + enkephalos, brain]

deuteranomalopia (doo″tĕr-ă-nŏm″ă-lō′pē-ă) [″ + anomalos, irregular, + ops, eye]

deuteranopia, deuteranopsia (dū″tĕr-ăn-ō′pē-ă, -ŏp′sē-ă) [″ + anopia, blindness]

deuterate (dū′tĕr-āt)

deuterium (dū-tē′rē-ŭm) [Gr. deuteros, second]
d. oxide

deutero-, deuter-, deuto- [Gr. deuteros, second]

deuteron (dū′tĕr-ŏn)

deuteropathia, deuteropathy [Gr. deuteros, second, + pathos, disease, suffering]

deuteroplasm [″ + LL. plasma, form, mold]

deutoscolex (dū″tō-skō′lĕks) [″ + skolex, worm]

devasation (dē″văs-ā′shŭn) [L. de, from, + vasa, vessel]

devascularization (dē-văs″kū-lăr-ĭ-zā′shŭn) [″ + vascularis, pert. to a vessel]

developer

development [O. Fr. desveloper, to unwrap]
d., cognitive
d., psychomotor and physical, of infant

developmental

developmental milestones
deviance [L. *deviare*, to turn aside]
deviant
   d., sex
deviant behavior
deviate (dē′vē-āt″) [L. *deviare*, to turn aside]
deviation (dē-vē-ā′shŭn)
   d., axis
   d., conjugate
   d., minimum
   d., standard
device (dĭ-vīs′) [O. Fr. *devis*, contrivance]
   d., intrauterine contraceptive
devil's grip
deviometer (dē″vē-ŏm′ĕ-tĕr) [L. *de*, from, + *via*, way, + Gr. *metron*, measure]
devisceration (dē-vĭs″ĕr-ā′shŭn) [″ + *viscus*, internal organ]
devitalization [″ + *vita*, life]
devolution (dĕv″ō-loo′shŭn) [L. *devolvere*, to roll down]
dew cure
dew point
dexamethasone (dĕk″să-mĕth′ă-sōn)
dexbrompheniramine **maleate** (dĕks″brŏm-fĕn-ĭr′ă-mēn)
dexchlorpheniramine **maleate** (dĕks″klor-fĕn-ĭr′ă-mēn)
dexter (dĕks′tĕr) [L.]
dexterity
dextrad (dĕks′trăd) [L. *dexter*, right, + *ad*, toward]
dextral (dĕks′trăl)
dextrality (dĕks-trăl′ĭ-tē)
dextran (dĕks′trăn) [L. *dexter*, right]
dextrase (dĕks′trās)
dextraural (dĕks-traw′răl) [L. *dexter*, right, + *auris*, ear]
dextriferron (dĕks″trī-fĕr′ŏn)
dextrin (dĕks′trĭn) [L. *dexter*, right]
dextrinuria (dĕks″trĭn-ū′rē-ă) [″ + Gr. *ouron*, urine]
dextro- [L. *dexter*, right]
dextroamphetamine **sulfate** (dĕks″trō-ăm-fĕt′ă-mēn sŭl′fāt)

dextrocardia (dĕks″trō-kăr′dē-ă) [″ + Gr. *kardia*, heart]
dextrocardiogram [″ + ″ + *gramma*, letter, piece of writing]
dextrocular (dĕks-trŏk′ū-lăr) [″ + *oculus*, eye]
dextrocularity (dĕks″trŏk-ū-lăr′ĭ-tē)
dextroduction [″ + *ducere*, to lead]
dextrogastria [″ + Gr. *gaster*, belly]
dextroglucose (dĕks″trō-glū′kōs)
dextrogyre (dĕks′trō-jīr)
dextromanual [″ + *manus*, hand]
dextromethorphan (dĕk″strō-mĕth′or-făn)
dextropedal (dĕks-trŏp′ĕ-dăl) [″ + *pes, ped-*, foot]
dextrophobia [″ + Gr. *phobos*, fear]
dextroposition (dĕks″trō-pō-zĭsh′ŭn)
dextropropoxyphene (dĕk″strō-prō-pŏk′sē-fēn)
dextrorotatory (dĕks″trō-rō′tă-tor-ē) [″ + *rotare*, to turn]
dextrose (dĕks′trōs)
dextrose and sodium chloride injection
dextrosinistral (dĕks″trō-sĭn′ĭs-trăl) [L. *dexter*, right, + *sinister*, left]
dextrosuria (dĕks-trō-sū′rē-ă)
dextrothyroxine sodium (dĕks″trō-thī-rŏk′sĭn)
dextrotropic, **dextrotropous** (dĕks″trō-trŏp′ĭk, -trō′pŭs) [″ + Gr. *tropos*, a turning]
dextroversion [″ + *vertere*, to turn]
dezymotize (dē-zī′mō-tīz) [L. *de*, from, + Gr. *zyme*, leaven]
DFP *diisopropyl fluorophosphate*
dg *decigram*
DHE-45
dhobie itch (dō′bē) [Hindi, laundryboy]
di- [Gr. *dis*, twice, double]
diabetes (dī′ă-bē′tēz) [Gr. *diabetes*, passing through]
   d., bronze

d. insipidus
d. mellitus
d.m., brittle
d.m., chemical
d.m., endocrine
d.m., iatrogenic
d.m., insulin-dependent, Type I
d.m., latent
d.m., non-insulin-dependent, Type II
d., pancreatic
d., phlorizin
d., renal
d., true
diabetic (dĭ-ă-bĕt′ĭk)
diabetic acidosis
diabetic center
diabetic coma
diabetic ear
diabetic neuritis
diabetic tabes
diabetogenic (dĭ″ă-bĕt″ō-jĕn′ĭk)
[″ + gennan, to produce]
diabetogenous (dĭ″ă-bē-tŏj′ĕn-ŭs)
Diabinese
diabrosis (dĭ″ă-brō′sĭs) [Gr., eating
through]
diabrotic (dĭ-ă-brŏt′ĭk)
diacele (dĭ′ă-sēl) [Gr. dia, between,
+ koilia, cavity, belly]
diacetate (dĭ-ăs′ĕ-tāt)
diacetemia (dĭ-ăs″ĕ-tē′mē-ă)
diacetic acid (dĭ″ă-sĕt′ĭk)
diacetonuria, diaceturia (dĭ-ăs″ĕ-tō-
nū′rē-ă, dĭ-ăs″ĕ-tū′rē-ă)
diacetylmorphine (dĭ″ă-sē″tĭl-
mor′fēn)
diacid (dĭ-ăs′ĭd) [Gr. dis, twice, double,
+ L. acidus, soured]
diaclasia (dĭ-ă-klā′zē-ă) [Gr. dia,
through, + klan, to break]
diaclast (dĭ′ă-klăst) [″ + klan, to
break]
diacrinous (dĭ-ăk′rĭn-ŭs) [Gr. diakrinein,
to separate]
diacrisis (dĭ-ăk′rĭ-sĭs) [Gr. diakrisis, sep-
aration]
diacritic, diacritical [Gr. dia, through,
+ krinein, to judge]

diaderm [Gr. dia, through, +
derma, skin]
diadochokinesia (dĭ-ăd″ō-kō-kĭn-
ē′zē-ă) [Gr. diadokos, succeeding,
+ kinesis, motion]
diagnose (dī′ăg-nōs) [Gr. diagignoskein, to discern]
diagnosis (dī″ăg-nō′sĭs)
d., antenatal
d. by exclusion
d., clinical
d., cytological
d., differential
d., medical
d., nursing
d., oral
d., pathological
d., physical
d., radiographic
d., serological
diagnosis related group
diagnostic
**Diagnostic and Statistical Manual
of Mental Disorders (Third
Edition – Revised)**
diagnostician (dī″ăg-nŏs-tĭsh′ŭn) [Gr.
diagignoskein, to discern]
diakinesis (dī″ă-kĭ-nē′sĭs) [Gr. dia,
through, + kinesis, motion]
dial (dī′ăl) [L. dialis, daily, fr. dies, day]
d., astigmatic
dialy- [Gr. dia, through, + lysis,
dissolution]
dialysance (dī″ă-lī′săns)
dialysate (dī-ăl′ĭ-sāt)
dialysis (dī-ăl′ĭ-sĭs) [Gr. dia, through,
+ lysis, dissolution]
d., continuous ambulatory peritoneal
d., peritoneal
d., renal
dialysis acidosis
dialysis dementia
dialysis disequilibrium
dialytic
dialyzable (dĭ-ă-līz′ă-b′l)
dialyze (dī′ă-līz)
dialyzer (dī′ă-līz″ĕr) [Gr. dia, through,
+ lysis, dissolution]

diamagnetic [" + *magnes,* magnet]

diameter (dī-ăm'ĕ-tĕr) [" + *metron,* a measure]

    d., anteroposterior, of pelvic cavity
    d., anteroposterior, of pelvic inlet
    d., anteroposterior, of pelvic outlet
    d., bigonial
    d., biparietal
    d., bitemporal
    d., bitrochanteric
    d., bizygomatic
    d., buccolingual
    d., cervicobregmatic
    d., diagonal conjugate, of pelvis
    d., external conjugate
    d., frontomental
    d., interspinous
    d., labiolingual
    d., mentobregmatic
    d., mesiodistal
    d., obstetric, of pelvic inlet
    d., occipitofrontal
    d., occipitomental
    d. of fetal skull
    d. of pelvis

diamid(e) (dī-ăm'ĭd, -īd) [L. *di,* two, + *amide*]

diamidine (dī-ăm'ĭ-dēn)

diamine (dī-ăm'ĭn, -ēn)

diaminuria (dī-ăm"ĭ-nū'rē-ă)

Diamox

dianoetic (dī"ă-nō-ĕt'ĭk) [Gr. *dia,* through, + *nous,* mind]

diapason (dī"ă-pā'sŭn) [" + *pason,* all]

diapause (dī'ă-pawz) [" + *pausis,* pause]

diapedesis (dī"ă-pĕd-ē'sĭs) [" + *pedan,* to leap]

diaphane (dī'ă-fān) [Gr. *dia,* through, + *phainein,* to appear]

diaphanography

diaphanometer (dī"ă-făn-ŏm'ĕ-tĕr) [" + " + *metron,* measure]

diaphanometry (dī"ă-făn-ŏm'ĕt-rē)

diaphanoscope (dī-ă-făn'ō-skōp) [" + *phainein,* to appear, +

skopein, to examine]

diaphanoscopy (dī"ă-făn-ŏs'kō-pē)

diaphemetric (dī"ă-fĕ-mĕt'rĭk) [" + *haphe,* touch, + *metron,* measure]

diaphorase (dī-ăf'ō-rās)

diaphoresis (dī"ă-fō-rē'sĭs) [" + *pherein,* to carry]

diaphoretic (dī"ă-fō-rĕt'ĭk) [" + *pherein,* to carry]

diaphragm (dī'ă-frăm) [Gr. *diaphragma,* a partition]

    d., Bucky
    d., hernia of
    d., pelvic
    d., urogenital

diaphragmalgia (dī"ă-frăg-măl'jē-ă) [Gr. *diaphragma,* a partition, + *algos,* pain]

diaphragmatic

diaphragmatocele (dī"ă-frăg-măt'ō-sēl) [" + *kele,* tumor, swelling]

diaphragmitis (dī"ă-frăg-mī'tĭs) [" + *itis,* inflammation]

diaphragmodynia [" + *odyne,* pain]

diaphyseal (dī"ă-fīz'ē-ăl)

diaphysectomy [Gr. *diaphysis,* a growing through, + *ektome,* excision]

diaphysis (dī-ăf'ĭ-sĭs)

diaphysitis (dī"ă-fĭ-zī'tĭs) [Gr. *diaphysis,* a growing through, + *itis,* inflammation]

Diapid

diaplexus [Gr. *dia,* through, + L. *plexus,* braid]

diapophysis (dī-ă-pŏf'ĭ-sĭs) [" + *apophysis,* outgrowth]

diarrhea (dī-ă-rē'ă) [" + *rhein,* to flow]

    d., acute
    d., dysenteric
    d., emotional
    d., epidemic, in newborn
    d., fatty
    d., infantile
    d., lienteric
    d., membranous

d., mucous
d., purulent
d., simple
d., summer
d., travelers'
diarthric (dĭ-ăr'thrĭk) [Gr. *dis*, twice, double, + *arthron*, joint]
diarthrosis [Gr., a movable articulation]
diarticular [Gr. *dis*, twice, double, + L. *articulus*, joint]
diascope (dĭ'ă-skōp) [" + *skopein*, to examine]
Diasone Sodium Enterab
diastalsis (dĭ-ă-stăl'sĭs) [" + *stalsis*, contraction]
diastaltic
diastase (dĭ'ăs-tās) [Gr. *diastasis*, a separation]
diastasis (dĭ-ăs'tă-sĭs) [Gr.]
d. recti
diastema (dĭ"ă-stē'mă) [Gr. *diastema*, an interval or space]
diastematocrania (dĭ"ă-stĕm"ă-tō-krā'nē-ă) [" + *kranion*, cranium]
diastematomyelia (dĭ"ă-stĕm"ă-tō-mī-ē'lē-ă) [" + *myelos*, marrow]
diastematopyelia (dĭ"ă-stĕm"ă-tō-pī-ē'lē-ă) [" + *pyelos*, pelvis]
diaster [Gr. *dis*, twice, double, + *aster*, star]
diastole (dĭ-ăs'tō-lē) [Gr. *diastellein*, to expand]
diastolic (dĭ-ăs-tŏl'ĭk)
diastolic pressure
d.p., augmented
diataxia [Gr. *dis*, twice, double, + *ataxia*, lack of order]
diatela, diatele (dĭ-ă-tē'lă, -tēl') [Gr. *dia*, between, + L. *tela*, web]
diaterma [" + *terma*, end]
diathermal (dĭ"ă-thĕr'măl) [" + *therme*, heat]
diathermanous
diathermia [Gr. *dia*, through, + *therme*, heat]
diathermic
diathermy (dĭ'ă-thĕr"mē) [Gr. *dia*,

through, + *therme*, heat]
d., medical
d., short-wave
d., surgical
diathesis (dĭ-ăth'ĕ-sĭs) [Gr. *diatithenai*, to dispose]
diathetic
diatom (dĭ'ă-tŏm) [Gr. *diatemnein*, to cut through]
diatomaceous earth (dĭ"ă-tō-mā'shus)
diatomic
diatrizoate meglumine (dĭ"ă-trī-zō'āt)
diatrizoate sodium
diaxon, diaxone [Gr. *dis*, twice, double, + *axon*, axis]
diazepam (dĭ-ăz'ĕ-păm)
diazo-
diazo reaction
diazotize (dĭ-ăz'ō-tīz)
diazoxide (dĭ-ăz-ŏk'sīd)
dibasic (dĭ-bā'sĭk) [" + *basis*, base]
Dibenzyline
diblastula (dĭ-blăs'tū-lă) [" + *blastos*, sprout]
Dibothriocephalus (dĭ-bŏth"rē-ō-sĕf'ăl-ūs)
dibucaine hydrochloride
DIC *disseminated intravascular coagulation*
dicalcic, dicalcium (dĭ-kăl'sĭk) [" + L. *calx*, lime]
dicalcium phosphate (dĭ-kăl'sē-ūm fŏs'fāt)
dicentric (dĭ-sĕn'trĭk)
dicephalus (dĭ-sĕf'ă-lūs) [" + *kephale*, head]
dichloramine-T (dĭ-klor'ă-mēn)
2,4-dichlorophenoxyacetic acid
dichlorphenamide (dĭ"klor-fĕn'ă-mīd)
dichorionic (dĭ"kō-rē-ŏn'ĭk)
dichotomy, dichotomization (dĭ-kŏt'ō-mē, dĭ-kŏt"ō-mī-zā'shŭn) [Gr. *dicha*, twofold, + *tome*, a cutting, slice]
dichroic (dĭ-krō'ĭk)
dichroic mirror

dichroism (dī'krō-ĭzm) [Gr. *dis*, twice, double, + *chroa*, color]

dichromate (dī-krō'māt)

dichromatic

dichromatism (dī-krō'mă-tĭzm)

dichromatopsia (dī"krō-mă-tŏp'sē-ă) [" + *chroma*, color, + *opsis*, sight, appearance, vision]

dichromic

dichromophil [" + *chroma*, color, + *philein*, to love]

dichromophilism (dī"krō-mŏf'ĭl-ĭzm) [" + " + " + *-ismos*, condition]

Dick method [George F. Dick, 1881 – 1967 and Gladys H. Dick, 1881 – 1963, U.S. physicians]

Dick test

dicloxacillin sodium (dī-klŏks"ă-sĭl'ĭn)

Dicodid

dicoelus (dī-sē'lŭs) [" + *koilos*, hollow]

dicophane (dī'kō-fān)

dicoria (dī-kō'rē-ă) [" + *kore*, pupil]

dicoumarol (dī-koo'mă-rŏl)

dicrotic (dī-krŏt'ĭk) [Gr. *dikrotos*, beating double]

dicrotic notch

dicrotic wave

dicrotism (dī'krŏt-ĭzm) [" + *-ismos*, condition]

dictyoma (dĭk"tē-ō'mă) [Gr. *diktyon*, net, + *oma*, tumor]

dictyosome (dĭk'tē-ō-sōm) [" + *soma*, body]

dicumarol (dī-koo'mă-rŏl)

dicyclic (dī-sī'klĭk)

dicyclomine hydrochloride (dī-sī'klō-mēn)

didactic (dī-dăk'tĭk) [Gr. *didaktikos*]

didactylism (dī-dăk'tĭ-lĭzm) [Gr. *dis*, twice, double, + *daktylos*, finger]

didelphic (dī-dĕl'fĭk) [" + *delphys*, uterus]

didymalgia, didymodynia (dĭd-ī-măl'jē-ă, dĭd"ī-mō-dĭn'ē-ă) [Gr. *didymos*, twin, + *algos*, pain]

didymitis (dĭd-ī-mī'tĭs) [" + *itis*, inflammation]

didymus (dĭd'ī-mŭs) [Gr. *didymos*, twin]

die

diechoscope (dī-ĕk'ō-skōp) [Gr. *dis*, twice, double, + *echo*, echo, + *skopein*, to examine]

diecious (dī-ē'shŭs) [" + *oikos*, house]

dieldrin (dī-ĕl'drĭn)

dielectric [Gr. *dia*, through, + *elektron*, amber]

diembryony (dī-ĕm'brē-ŏn"ē)

diencephalon (dī"ĕn-sĕf'ă-lŏn) [Gr. *dis*, twice, double, + *enkephalos*, brain]

dienestrol (dī"ēn-ĕs'trŏl)

Dientamoeba (dī"ĕn-tă-mē'bă)
    D. fragilis

dieresis (dī-ĕr'ĕ-sĭs) [Gr. *diairesis*, a division]

dieretic

diet [Gr. *diaita*, way of living]
    d., balanced
    d., minimum residue
    d., reduction

dietary (dī'ĕ-tā"rē)

dietary fiber

dietetic (dī-ĕ-tĕt'ĭk)

dietetics [Gr. *diaitetikos*]

diethazine hydrochloride (dī-ĕth'ă-zēn)

diethylcarbamazine **citrate** (dī-ĕth"ĭl-kăr-băm'ă-zēn)

diethylpropion **hydrochloride** (dī-ĕth"ĭl-prō'pē-ŏn)

diethylstilbestrol (dī-ĕth"ĭl-stĭl"bĕs'trŏl)

diethyltoluamide (dī-ĕth"ĭl-tŏl-ū'ă-mīd)

diethyltryptamine (dī-ĕth"ĭl-trĭp'tă-mĭn)

dietitian (dī-ĕ-tĭsh'ăn) [Gr. *diaita*, way of living]

Dietl's crisis (dē't'ls) [Joseph Dietl, Pol. physician, 1804 – 1878]

dietotherapy (dī"ĕ-tō-thĕr'ă-pē)

Dieulafoy's triad (dyū-lă-fwăhz') [Georges Dieulafoy, Fr. physician, 1839 – 1911]

differential (dĭf"ĕr-ĕn'shăl) [L. *differre*, to carry apart]
differential amplifier
differential blood count
differential diagnosis
differentiation
diffraction (dĭ-frăk'shŭn) [L. *diffringere*, to break to pieces]
diffraction grating
diffusate (dĭf'ū-sāt) [L. *dis*, apart, + *fundere*, to pour]
diffuse (dĭ-fūs')
diffusible (dĭ-fūz'ĭ-bl)
diffusion (dĭ-fū'zhŭn) [" + *fundere*, to pour]
digastric (dĭ-găs'trĭk) [Gr. *dis*, twice, double, + *gaster*, belly]
digenesis [" + *genesis*, generation, birth]
Digenetica (dĭ-jĕ-nĕt'ĭ-kă)
digest [L. *dis*, apart, + *gerere*, to carry]
digestant
digestible
digestion [L. *digestio*, a taking apart]
   d., artificial
   d., duodenal
   d., extracellular
   d., gastric
   d., intestinal
   d., intracellular
   d., oral
   d., pancreatic
   d., salivary
   d., secondary
digestive (dĭ-jĕs'tĭv)
digestive juice
digestive system
digit (dĭj'ĭt) [L. *digitus*, finger, toe]
digital (dĭj'ĭ-tăl)
digital amniotome
digital radiography
digital subtraction angiography
digitalis (dĭj"ĭ-tăl'ĭs) [L. *digitus*, finger, toe]
digitalis poisoning
digitalization (dĭj"ĭ-tăl-ĭ-zā'shŭn)
digital reflex

digitate [L. *digitus*, finger, toe]
digitation (dĭj-ĭ-tā'shŭn)
digiti (dĭj'ĭ-tī)
digitiform (dĭj'ĭ-tĭ-form)
digitoxin (dĭj-ĭ-tŏk'sĭn)
digitus [L.]
diglossia (dĭ-glŏs'ē-ă) [Gr. *dis*, twice, double, + *glossa*, tongue]
digoxin (dĭ-jŏk'sĭn)
digoxin immune FAB (ovine) for injection
diglyceride (dĭ-glĭs'ĕr-īd)
dignathus (dĭg-nā'thŭs) [" + *gnathos*, jaw]
dihydric (dĭ-hī'drĭk)
dihydrocodeinone   bitartrate (dĭ-hī"drō-kō'dē-ĭ-nōn)
dihydroergotamine   mesylate (dĭ-hī"drō-ĕr-gŏt'ă-mēn)
dihydrosphingosine
dihydrotachysterol (dĭ-hī"drō-tăk-ĭs'tĕr-ŏl)
dihydrotheelin (dĭ-hī"drō-thē'ĕl-ĭn)
dihydroxyaluminum   aminoacetate (dĭ"hī-drŏk"sē-ă-lū'mĭ-nŭm)
dihydroxyaluminum sodium carbonate
dihydroxycholecalciferol (dĭ"hī-drŏk"sē-kō"lē-kăl-sĭf'ĕ-rŏl)
3,4-dihydroxyphenylalanine (dĭ-hī-drŏk"sē-fĕn"ĭl-ăl'ă-nēn)
dihysteria (dĭ"hĭs-tēr'ē-ă) [Gr. *dis*, twice, double, + *hystera*, womb]
diiodohydroxyquin (dĭ"ĭ-ō"dō-hī-drŏk'sē-kwĭn)
diisopropyl phosphorofluoridate
diktyoma (dĭk-tē-ō'mă) [Gr. *diktyon*, net, + *oma*, tumor]
dilaceration (dĭ"lăs-ĕr-ā'shŭn) [L. *dilacerare*, to tear apart]
Dilantin (dĭ-lăn'tĭn)
dilatant (dĭ-lā'tănt) [L. *dilatare*, to enlarge]
dilatation (dĭl-ă-tā'shŭn)
   d., digital
   d., heart
   d., stomach
dilation

dilation and curettage
dilation and evacuation
dilator (dĭ-lā'tor) [L. *dilatare*, to expand]
    d., Barnes'
    d., Bossi's
    d., Goodell's
    d., gynecologic
    d., Hegar's
    d., tent
    d., vaginal
Dilaudid Hydrochloride
dildo, dildoe
diluent (dĭl'ū-ĕnt) [L. *diluere*, to wash away]
dilution (dĭ-loo'shŭn)
dim
dimenhydrinate (dĭ"mĕn-hī'drĭn-āt)
dimension (dĭ-mĕn'shŭn)
dimer (dī'mĕr)
dimercaprol (dĭ-mĕr-kăp'rōl)
Dimetane
dimethicone (dĭ-mĕth'ĭ-kōn)
dimethindene maleate (dĭ"mĕth-ĭn'dēn)
dimethisterone (dĭ"mĕth-ĭs'tĕr-ōn)
dimethylamine (dĭ-mĕth"ĭl-ăm'ĭn)
p-dimethylaminoazobenzene (dĭ-mĕth"ĭl-ăm"ĭ-nō-ăz"ō-bĕn'zēn)
dimethyl phthalate (dĭ-mĕth"ĭl-thăl'āt)
dimethyl sulfoxide (dĭ-mĕth'ĭl sŭlf-ŏks'ĭd)
dimethyltryptamine (dĭ-mĕth"ĭl-trĭp'tă-mēn)
dimetria (dĭ-mē'trē-ă) [Gr. *dis*, twice, double, + *metra*, uterus]
dimorphous (dĭ-mor'fŭs) [" + *morphe*, form]
dimple sign
dimpling
dineuric (dĭ-nū'rĭk) [" + *neuron*, nerve]
dinical (dĭn'ĭ-kl) [Gr. *dinos*, vertigo]
2,4-dinitrophenol (dĭ-nī"trō-fē'nŏl)
Dinoflagellata (dĭ"nō-flăj"ĕ-lā'tă) [" + *flagellum*, whip]
dinoprost tromethamine (dĭ'nō-prŏst)
dinucleotide (dĭ-nū'klē-ō-tīd)

Dioctophyma (dĭ-ōk"tō-fī'mă)
dioctyl calcium sulfosuccinate (dĭ-ŏk'tĭl)
dioctyl sodium sulfosuccinate
Diodrast (dī'ō-drăst)
Diogenes syndrome [Diogenes, Gr. philosopher, 4th century B.C.]
diopter, dioptre [Gr. *dia*, through, + *optos*, visible]
dioptometer (dī"ŏp-tŏm'ĕ-tĕr) [" + " + *metron*, measure]
dioptometry (dī"ŏp-tŏm'ĕ-trē)
dioptral (dī-ŏp'trăl)
dioptric (dī-ŏp'trĭk)
dioptrics
diovulatory (dī-ŏv'ū-lā-tō"rē)
dioxide (dī-ŏk'sīd) [Gr. *dis*, twice, double, + *oxys*, sharp]
dioxin
dioxybenzone (dī-ŏks"ĭ-bĕn'zōn)
dipeptid(e) (dī-pĕp'tĭd, -tīd) [" + *peptein*, to digest]
dipeptidase (dī-pĕp'tĭ-dās)
diperodon (dī-pĕr'ō-dŏn)
Dipetalonema perstans (dī-pĕt"ă-lō-nē'mă)
diphallus (dī-făl'ŭs) [" + *phallos*, penis]
diphasic (dī-fā'zĭk) [" + *phasis*, appearance]
diphemanil methylsulfate (dī-fē'mă-nĭl)
diphenhydramine hydrochloride (dī"fĕn-hī'dră-mēn hī-drō-klō'rĭd)
diphenoxylate hydrochloride (dī"fĕn-ŏk'sĭ-lāt)
diphenylhydantoin sodium (dī-fĕn"ĭl-hī-dăn'tō-ĭn)
diphenylpyraline hydrochloride (dī-fĕn"ĭl-pī'ră-lēn)
diphonia (dī-fō'nē-ă) [Gr. *dis*, twice, double, + *phone*, voice]
2,3-diphosphoglycerate
diphtheria (dĭf-thē'rē-ă) [Gr. *diphthera*, membrane]
    d., cutaneous
    d., laryngeal
    d., surgical
diphtheria antitoxin

diphtherial

diphtheriaphor (dĭf-thē'rē-ă-for) [Gr. *diphthera*, membrane, + *pherein*, to carry]

diphtheria toxin for Schick test

diphtheria toxoid

diphtheric, diphtheritic (dĭf-thē'rĭk, dĭf-thĕr-ĭt'ĭk)

diphtherin (dĭf'thē-rĭn)

diphtheroid (dĭf'thĕ-royd) [" + *eidos*, form, shape]

diphtherotoxin (dif"thĕr-ō-tŏk'sĭn) [" + *toxikon*, poison]

diphthongia (dĭf-thŏn'jē-ă) [Gr. *dis*, twice, double, + *phtongos*, voice]

Diphyllobothrium (dī-fĭl"ō-bŏth'rē-ŭm) [" + *phyllon*, leaf, + *bothrion*, pit]

    D. cordatum

    D. erinacei

    D. latum

diphyodont (dĭf'ē-ō-dŏnt) [" + *phyein*, to produce, + *odous*, tooth]

diplacusis (dĭp"lă-kū'sĭs) [" + *akousis*, hearing]

diplegia (dĭ-plē'jē-ă) [Gr. *dis*, twice, double, + *plege*, a stroke]

    d., infantile

    d., spastic

diplegic (dĭ-plē'jĭk)

diploalbuminuria (dĭp"lō-ăl-bū"mĭn-ū'rē-ă) [Gr. *diplous*, double, + L. *albumen*, white of egg, + Gr. *ouron*, urine]

diplobacillus [" + L. *bacillus*, a little stick]

diplobacterium [" + *bakterion*, little rod]

diploblastic (dĭp"lō-blăs'tĭk) [" + *blastos*, germ]

diplocardia [" + *kardia*, heart]

diplocephaly (dĭp"lō-sĕf'ă-lē) [" + *kephale*, head]

diplococcemia (dĭp"lō-kŏk-sē'mē-ă) [" + *kokkos*, berry, + *haima*, blood]

diplococci (dĭp"lō-kŏk'sē, -kŏk'ī)

Diplococcus (dĭp-lō-kŏk'ŭs) [" + *kokkus*, berry]

    D. pneumoniae

diplococcus (dĭp"lō-kŏk'ŭs)

diplocoria (dĭp"lō-kō'rē-ă) [" + *kore*, pupil]

diploë (dĭp'lō-ē) [Gr. *diploe*, fold]

diploetic, diploic

diplogenesis [Gr. *diplous*, double, + *genesis*, generation, birth]

diploid (dĭp'loyd) [" + *eidos*, form, shape]

diplokaryon (dĭp"lō-kăr'ē-ŏn) [" + *karyon*, nucleus]

diplomellituria (dĭp"lō-mĕl"ĭ-tūr'ē-ă) [" + *meli*, honey, + *ouron*, urine]

diplomyelia (dĭp"lō-mī-ē'lē-ă) [" + *myelos*, marrow]

diploneural [" + *neuron*, nerve]

diplopagus (dĭp-lŏp'ă-gŭs) [" + *pagos*, a thing fixed]

diplophonia (dĭp-lō-fō'nē-ă) [" + *phone*, voice]

diplopia (dĭp-lō'pē-ă) [" + *ope*, sight]

    d., binocular

    d., crossed

    d., direct

    d., heteronymous

    d., monocular

    d., uncrossed

    d., unocular

    d., vertical

diplopiometer (dĭp-lō"pē-ŏm'ĕ-tĕr) [Gr. *diplous*, double, + *ope*, sight, + *metron*, measure]

diploscope [" + *skopein*, to examine]

diplosomatia, diplosomia (dĭp"lō-sō-mā'shē-ă, dĭp"lō-sō'mē-ă) [" + *soma*, body]

diplotene (dĭp'lō-tēn)

dipole (dī'pōl)

dipping

Diprosone

diprosopus (dĭp-rō-sōp'ŭs) [Gr. *dis*, twice, double, + *prosopon*, face]

dipsesis (dĭp-sē'sĭs) [Gr., a thirst]

dipsogen (dĭp'sō-jĕn)

dipsomania (dĭp"sō-mā'nē-ă) [Gr.

dispa, thirst, + *mania,* madness]

dipsophobia (dĭp-sō-fō'bē-ă) [" + *phobos,* fear]

dipsosis (dĭp-sō'sĭs) [" + *osis,* condition]

dipsotherapy (dĭp"sō-thĕr'ă-pē) [" + *therapeia,* treatment]

dipstick (dĭp'stĭk)

Diptera (dĭp'tĕr-ă) [Gr. *dipteros,* having two wings]

dipterous (dĭp'tĕr-ŭs)

dipygus (dī-pī'gŭs) [Gr. *dis,* twice, double, + *pyge,* rump]

dipylidiasis (dĭp"ĭ-lĭ-dī'ă-sĭs)

Dipylidium (dĭp"ĭ-lĭd'ē-ŭm) [Gr. *dipylos,* having two entrances]
    D. caninum

direct [L. *diregere,* to direct]

direct current

directionality

direct light reflex

director

direct reflex

dirigomotor (dĭr"ĭ-gō-mō'tor) [L. *dirigere,* to direct, + *motor,* mover]

Dirofilaria (dī"rō-fī-lā'rē-ă)
    D. immitis

dis- [L. *dis;* Gr. *dis*]

disability (dĭs"ă-bĭl'ĭ-tē)
    d., developmental

disaccharidase (dī-săk'ă-rĭ-dās)

disaccharide (dī-săk'ĭ-rĭd) [Gr. *dis,* twice, double, + *sakkharon,* sugar]

disarticulation [L. *dis,* apart, + *articulus,* joint]

disassimilation [" + *ad,* to, + *similare,* to make like]

disaster [" + L. *astrum,* star, ill-starred]

disc [Gr. *diskos,* quoit]

discharge (dĭs-chărj', dĭs'chărj) [ME. *dischargen,* to discharge]
    d., cerebrocortical
    d., convective
    d., disruptive
    d., lochial

discharge abstract

discharging

discharging lesion

dischronation [L. *dis,* apart, + Gr. *chronos,* time]

discission (dĭs-sĭzh'ŭn) [" + *scindere,* to cut]

discitis (dĭs-kī'tĭs) [Gr. *diskos,* quoit, + *itis,* inflammation]

disclosing agent

discoblastic [" + *blastos,* germ]

discoblastula (dĭs"kō-blăs'tū-lă)

discogenic (dĭs"kō-jĕn'ĭk) [" + *gennan,* to produce]

discography (dĭs-kŏg'ră-fē)

discoid

disconnection syndromes

discoplacenta [Gr. *diskos,* quoit, + *plakous,* a flat cake]

discordance (dĭs-kor'dăns)

discrete (dĭs-krēt') [L. *discretus,* separated]

discrimination [L. *discriminare,* to divide]
    d., one-point
    d., tonal
    d., two-point

discus [Gr. *diskos,* quoit]
    d. articularis
    d. proligerus

disdiaclast (dĭs-dī'ă-klăst) [Gr. *dis,* twice, double, + *diaklan,* to break through]

disdiadochokinesia (dĭs-dī"ă-dō"kō-kĭ-nē'zē-ă) [L. *dis,* apart, + Gr. *diadochos,* succeeding, + *kinesis,* motion]

disease (dĭ-zēz') [Fr. *des,* from, + *aise,* ease]
    d., acute
    d., anticipated
    d., autoimmune
    d., chronic
    d., chronic granulomatous
    d., collagen
    d., communicable
    d., complicating
    d., congenital
    d., constitutional

d., contagious
d., cystine storage
d., deficiency
d., degenerative
d., degenerative joint
d., demyelinating
d., endemic
d., epidemic
d., epizootic
d., extrapyramidal
d., familial
d., focal
d., functional
d., glycogen storage
d., heavy chain
d., hemolytic, of the newborn
d., hemorrhagic, of the newborn
d., hereditary
d., hookworm
d., hypokinetic
d., iatrogenic
d., idiopathic
d., infectious
d., intercurrent
d., iron storage
d., malignant
d., Mediterranean
d., metabolic
d., motor neuron
d., occupational
d., organic
d., pandemic
d., parasitic
d., periodontal
d., psychosomatic
d., secondary
d., self-limited
d., sporadic
d., storage
d., subacute
d., systemic
d., thyrotoxic heart
d., venereal
disengagement [Fr.]
disequilibrium (dĭs-ē″kwĭ-lĭb′rē-ŭm) [L. dis, apart, + aequus, equal, + libra, balance]
dish, Petri

disinfect (dĭs-ĭn-fĕkt′) [″ + inficere, to corrupt]
disinfectant
disinfection
d., concurrent
d. of blankets and woolens
d. of excreta
d. of field of operation
d., terminal
disinfestation (dĭs″ĭn-fĕs-tā′shŭn) [L. dis, apart, + infestare, to strike at]
disinhibition (dĭs″ĭn-hĭ-bĭsh′ŭn)
disinsected
disinsertion
disintegration [″ + integer, entire]
disjoint
disjunction (dĭs-jŭnk′shŭn)
disk [Gr. diskos, a disk]
d., anisotropic
d., articular
d., Bowman's
d., choked
d., dental
d., embryonic
d., epiphyseal
d., germinal
d., herniated intervertebral
d., intervertebral
d., M
d., Merkel's
d., optic
d., proligerous
d., Q
d., slipped
d., tactile
d., Z
diskectomy (dĭs-kĕk′tō-mē)
diskiform (dĭs′kĭ-form)
diskitis (dĭsk-ī′tĭs) [Gr. diskos, disk, + itis, inflammation]
dislocation [L. dis, apart, + locare, to place]
d., closed
d., complete
d., complicated
d., compound
d., congenital

d., consecutive
d., divergent
d., habitual
d., incomplete
d., metacarpophalangeal joint
d., Monteggia's
d., Nélaton's
d., old
d., partial
d., pathologic
d., primitive
d., recent
d., simple
d., slipped
d., subastragalar
d., traumatic
dismember
dismutase (dĭs-mū′tās)
d., superoxide
disocclude
disodium edetate (dĭ-sō′dē-ŭm)
disomus (dĭ-sō′mŭs) [Gr. *dis*, twice, double, + *soma*, body]
disopyramide phosphate (dĭ-sō-pĕr′ă-mīd)
disorder
d., character
disorganization [L. *dis*, apart, + Gr. *organon*, a unified organ]
disorientation (dĭs″ō-rē-ĕn-tā′shŭn) [″ + *oriens*, arising]
disparate points (dĭs′păr-ăt, dĭs-păr′ăt) [L. *disparare*, to separate]
dispensary [L. *dispensare*, to give out]
dispensatory (dĭs-pĕn′să-tō-rē) [L. *dispensatorium*]
dispense (dĭs-pĕns′)
dispersate (dĭs′pŭr-sāt)
disperse (dĭs-pĕrs′) [L. *dis*, apart, + *spargere*, to scatter]
dispersion (dĭs-pĕr′zhŭn)
d., coarse
d., colloidal
d., medium
d., molecular
dispersoid
dispersonalization (dĭs-pĕr″sŏn-ăl-ĭ-zā′shŭn)

dispireme (dī-spī′rēm) [Gr. *dis*, twice, double, + *speirema*, coil]
displacement [Fr. *deplacer*, to lay aside]
disposition [L. *disponere*, to arrange]
disproportion (dĭs″prō-por′shŭn)
d., cephalopelvic
dissect (dĭ-sĕkt′, dī-sĕkt′) [L. *dissecare*, to cut up]
dissection (dĭ-, dĭ-sĕk′shŭn)
disseminated [L. *dis*, apart, + *seminare*, to sow]
disseminated intravascular coagulation
dissipation (dĭs-ĭ-pā′shŭn) [L. *dissipare*, to scatter]
dissociation (dĭs-sō″sē-ā′shŭn) [L. *dis*, apart, + *sociatio*, union]
d., atrioventricular
d., microbic
d. of personality
d., psychological
dissolution [L. *dissolvere*, to dissolve]
dissolve (dĭ-zŏlv′) [L. *dissolvere*, to dissolve]
dissolvent (dĭ-zŏl′vĕnt)
dissolving
dissonance (dĭs′ō-năns)
d., cognitive
distad (dĭs′tăd) [L. *distare*, to be distant]
distal (dĭs′tăl) [L. *distare*, to be distant]
distance
d., focal
d., focal-film
d., interocclusal
d., interocular
d., source-skin
d., source-to-image receptor
d., target-skin
distemper (dĭs-tĕm′pĕr)
distend [L. *distendere*, to stretch out]
distensibility (dĭs-tĕn″sĭ-bĭl′ĭ-tē)
distention
distichiasis (dĭs″tĭ-kī′ă-sīs) [Gr. *distichia*, a double row]
distill (dĭs-tĭl′) [L. *destillare*, to drop from]
distillate (dĭs′tĭl-āt, dĭs-tĭl′āt)
distillation

d., destructive
d., dry
d., fractional
distobuccal (dĭs"tō-bŭk'ăl) [L. *distare*, to be distant, + *bucca*, cheek]
distocclusion (dĭs"tō-kloo'zhŭn)
distogingival (dĭs"tō-jĭn'jĭ-văl) [" + *gingiva*, gum]
distolabial (dĭs"tō-lā'bē-ăl) [" + *labialis*, lips]
distolingual (dĭs"tō-lĭng'gwăl) [" + *lingua*, tongue]
Distoma, Distomum (dĭs'tō-mă, -mŭm) [Gr. *dis*, twice, double, + *stoma*, mouth, opening]
distome
distomia (dĭ-stō'mē-ă) [" + *stoma*, mouth, opening]
distomiasis (dĭs"tō-mī'ă-sĭs)
disto-occlusal (dĭs"tō-ŏ-kloo'zăl)
distortion [L. *distortio*, twist, writhe]
distractibility
distraction (dĭs-trăk'shŭn) [L. *dis*, apart, + *tractio*, a drawing]
distraught (dĭs-trawt') [L. *distrahere*, to perplex]
distress (dĭs-trĕs') [L. *distringere*, to draw apart]
d., fetal
distribution [L. *dis*, apart, + *tribuere*, to allot]
districhiasis (dĭs-trĭk-ī'ă-sĭs) [Gr. *dis*, twice, double, + *thrix*, hair]
distrix (dĭs'trĭks)
disturbance
d., emotional
disulfate (dī-sŭl'fāt)
disulfiram (dī-sŭl'fĭ-răm)
disulfiram poisoning
dithiazanine iodide (dī"thī-ăz'ă-nēn)
Dittrich's plugs (dĭt'rĭks) [Franz Dittrich, Ger. pathologist, 1815–1859]
diurese (dī"ū-rēs')
diuresis (dī"ū-rē'sĭs) [Gr. *diourein*, to urinate]
diuretic (dī"ū-rĕt'ĭk)
Diuril (dī'ū-rĭl)
diurnal [L. *dies*, day]

divagation (dĭ-vă-gā'shŭn) [L. *divagari*, to wander about]
divalent (dī-vā'lĕnt)
divergence (dĭ-vĕr'jĕns) [L. *divergere*, to turn aside]
divergent
diver's paralysis
diverticula (dī"vĕr-tĭk'ū-lă) [L. *devertere*, to turn aside]
diverticulectomy (dī"vĕr-tĭk"ū-lĕk'tō-mē) [" + Gr. *ektome*, excision]
diverticulitis (dī"vĕr-tĭk"ū-lī'tĭs) [" + Gr. *itis*, inflammation]
d., acute
d., chronic
diverticulosis (dī"vĕr-tĭk"ū-lō'sĭs) [" + Gr. *osis*, condition]
diverticulum (dī"vĕr-tĭk'ū-lŭm) [L. *devertere*, to turn aside]
d., false
d., Meckel's
d. of colon
d. of duodenum
d. of jejunum
d. of stomach
d., true
d., Zenker's
diving reflex
division (dĭ-vĭzh'ŭn) [L. *dividere*, to divide]
divulsion (dĭ-vŭl'shŭn) [L. *dis*, apart, + *vellere*, to pluck]
divulsor (dĭ-vŭl'sor) [L. *dis*, apart, + *vellere*, to pluck]
d., pterygium
d., tendon
Dix, Dorothea Lynde [Massachusetts schoolteacher, 1802–1887]
dizygotic twins (dī"zī-gŏt'ĭk) [Gr. *dis*, twice, double, + *zygon*, yoke]
dizziness [AS. *dysig*, foolish]
dl *deciliter*
D.M.D. *Doctor of Dental Medicine*
DMF index
DMSO *dimethyl sulfoxide*
DMT *dimethyltryptamine*
DNA *deoxyribonucleic acid*
DNA probe

DNR *do not resuscitate*
D.O. *Doctor of Osteopathy*
DOA *dead on arrival*
Dobell's solution (dō'bĕlz) [Horace B. Dobell, Brit. physician, 1828 – 1917]
Dobie's globule (dō'bēz) [William M. Dobie, Brit. physician, 1828 – 1915]
Doca Acetate
doctor [L. *docere*, to teach]
d., barefoot
doctrine (dŏk'trĭn)
docusate calcium (dŏk'ū-sāt)
docusate sodium
dog bite
Döhle's bodies (dē'lēz) [Paul Döhle, Ger. pathologist, 1855 – 1928]
dol
Dolene
dolichocephalic (dŏl″ĭ-kō-sĭ-făl'ĭk) [Gr. *dolichos*, long, + *kephale*, head]
dolichocolon (dŏl″ĭ-kō-kō'lŏn) [″ + *kolon*, colon]
dolichofacial (dŏl″ĭ-kō-fā'shăl)
dolichohieric (dŏl″ĭ-kō-hī-ĕr'ĭk) [″ + *hieron*, sacred]
dolichomorphic (dŏl″ĭ-kō-mor'fĭk) [″ + *morphe*, form]
dolichopellic, dolichopelvic (dŏl″ĭ-kō-pĕl'ĭk, -pĕl'vĭk) [″ + *pyelos*, an oblong trough]
dolichosigmoid (dŏl″ĭ-kō-sĭg'moyd) [″ + *sigmoeides*, sigmoid]
dolichuranic (dŏl″ĭk-ū-răn'ĭk) [″ + *ouranos*, palate]
Dolophine Hydrochloride
dolor (dō'lor) [L.]
dolorific (dō″lor-ĭf'ĭk) [L. *dolor*, pain]
dolorimeter (dō″lor-ĭm'ĭ-tĕr) [″ + Gr. *metron*, measure]
dolorogenic [″ + Gr. *gennan*, to produce]
domatophobia (dō-măt-ō-fō'bē-ă) [Gr. *doma*, house, + *phobos*, fear]
domiciliary (dŏm″ĭ-sĭl'ē-ār″ē) [L. *domus*, house]
dominance [L. *dominans*, ruling]
d., ocular

dominant
Donath-Landsteiner phenomenon (dō'năth-lănd'stī-nĕr) [Julius Donath, Austrian physician, 1870 – 1950; Karl Landsteiner, Austrian-born U.S. physician, 1868 – 1943]
donee (dō-nē') [L. *donare*, to give]
Don Juan [After the legendary, promiscuous, Sp. nobleman, Don Juan de Tenerio]
Donnan's equilibrium (dŏn'ănz) [Frederick G. Donnan, Brit. chemist, 1870 – 1956]
donor
d., universal
donor card
Donovan body [Charles Donovan, Ir. physician, 1863 – 1951]
Donovania granulomatis (dŏn-ō-vā'nē-ă)
dopa
dopamine hydrochloride (dō'pă-mēn)
dopaminergic (dō″pă-mēn-ĕr'jĭk)
dopa-oxidase (dō″pă-ŏk'sĭ-dās)
Dopar
doping
d., blood
Doppler effect (dŏp'lĕr) [Johann Christian Doppler, Austrian scientist, 1803 – 1853]
doraphobia (dō″ră-fō'bē-ă) [Gr. *dora*, hide, + *phobos*, fear]
Dorello's canal [Primo Dorello, It. anatomist, 1872 – 1963]
Dorendorf's sign [Hans Dorendorf, Ger. physician, b. 1866]
dornase (dor'nās)
d., pancreatic
dorsa [L.]
dorsabdominal [L. *dorsum*, back, + *abdomen*, belly]
dorsad [″ + *ad*, toward]
dorsal [L. *dorsum*, back]
dorsal cord stimulation
dorsal elevated position
dorsalgia (dōr-săl'jē-ă) [″ + Gr. *algos*, pain]

dorsal inertia posture
dorsalis (dor-sā'lĭs) [L.]
dorsal nerves
dorsal recumbent position
dorsal reflex
dorsal rigid posture
dorsal slit
dorsi-, dorso-, dors- [L.]
dorsiduct [L. *dorsum*, back, + *du-cere*, to lead]
dorsiduction
dorsiflect (dor'sĭ-flĕkt) [" + *flec-tere*, to bend]
dorsiflexion
dorsimesal (dor"sĭ-mĕs'ăl)
dorsimeson (dor-sĭ-mĕs'ŏn) [" + Gr. *meson*, middle]
dorsispinal (dor"sĭ-spī'năl) [" + *spina*, thorn]
dorsocephalad (dor"sō-sĕf'ă-lăd) [" + Gr. *kephale*, head, + L. *ad*, toward]
dorsodynia (dor"sō-dĭn'ē-ă) [" + Gr. *odyne*, pain]
dorsolateral (dor"sō-lăt'ĕr-ăl)
dorsoplantar (dor"sō-plăn'tăr) [" + *planta*, sole of the foot]
dorsosacral [" + *sacrum*, sacred bone]
dorsosacral position
dorsoventral (dor"sō-vĕn'trăl)
dorsum [L.]
dosage [Gr. *dosis*, a giving]
 d. calculation for children
dose (dōs) [Gr. *dosis*, a giving]
 d., absorbed
 d., air
 d., bolus
 d., booster
 d., cumulative
 d., curative
 d., divided
 d., erythema
 d., fatal
 d., infective
 d., maintenance
 d., maximum
 d., maximum permissible

 d., median curative
 d., median infective
 d., median lethal
 d., minimum
 d., primary
 d., skin
 d., therapeutic
 d., threshold
 d., tissue tolerance
 d., toxic
dose response curve
dosimeter (dō-sĭm'ĭ-tĕr) [" + *me-tron*, measure]
dosimetric (dō"sĭ-mĕt'rĭk)
dosimetry (dō-sĭm'ĕt-rē) [" + *me-tron*, measure]
dot
 d., Trantas [Alexios Trantas, Gr. ophthalmologist, 1867–1960]
dotage [ME. *doten*, to be silly]
double (dŭb'l) [L. *duplus*, twofold]
double-blind technique
double-contrast examination
double personality
double touch
double uterus
double vision
douche (doosh) [Fr.]
 d., air
 d., alternating
 d., astringent
 d., circular
 d., cleansing
 d., deodorizing
 d., high
 d., jet
 d., low
 d., medicated
 d., neutral
 d., perineal
 d., Scotch
 d., vaginal
Douglas' cul-de-sac, pouch, space [James Douglas, Scot. anatomist, 1675–1742]
Douglas' fold
douglasitis (dŭg-lăs-ī'tĭs)
dowel [ME. *dowle*, peg]

down
Down syndrome [J. Langdon Down, Brit. physician, 1828 – 1896]
doxapram hydrochloride (dŏk'să-prăm)
Doxinate
doxorubicin **hydrochloride** (dŏk"sō-rū'bĭ-sĭn)
doxycycline (dŏk"sē-sī'klēn)
doxylamine succinate (dŏk-sĭl'ă-mēn)
Doyère's eminence (dwă-yărz') [Louis Doyère, Fr. physiologist, 1811 – 1863]
D.P. *Doctor of Pharmacy*
D.P.H. *Diploma in Public Health*
D.P.M. *Doctor of Podiatric Medicine*
D.P.T.
DR *reaction of degeneration*
Dr *Doctor*
dr *drachm; dram*
drachm (drăm) [Gr. *drachme*, a Gr. unit of weight]
dracontiasis (drăk"ŏn-tī'ă-sĭs) [Gr. *drakontion*, little dragon]
dracunculiasis (dră-kŭng"kū-lī'ă-sĭs)
dracunculosis (dră-kŭng"kū-lō'sĭs)
Dracunculus (dră-kŭng'kū-lŭs)
    D. medinensis
draft, draught
drag
drain (drān) [AS. *dreahnian*, to draw off]
    d., capillary
    d., cigarette
    d., Mikulicz's
    d., nonabsorbable
    d., Penrose
drainage (drān'ĭj)
    d., capillary
    d., closed
    d., closed sterile
    d., funnel
    d., negative pressure
    d., open
    d., postural
    d., suction
    d., tidal
drainage tube

drained weight
dram [Gr. *drachme*]
    d., fluid
Dramamine (drăm'ă-mēn)
dramatism [Gr. *drama*, acting + *-ismos*, condition]
drapetomania (drăp"ĕt-ō-mā'nē-ă) [Gr. *drapetes*, runaway, + *mania*, madness]
drastic [Gr. *drastikos*, effective]
draught (drăft) [ME. *draught*, a pulling]
Draw-a-Person test
drawer sign
draw sheet
dream [AS. *dream*, joy]
drench
drepanocyte (drĕp'ă-nō-sīt) [Gr. *drepane*, sickle, + *kytos*, cell]
drepanocytemia (drĕp"ă-nō-sī-tē'mē-ă) [" + " + *haima*, blood]
drepanocytic (drĕp"ă-nō-sīt'ĭk)
dressing [O. Fr. *dresser*, to prepare]
    d., absorbent
    d., antiseptic
    d., clear transparent covering
    d., dry
    d., fixed
    d., hot moist
    d., nonadherent
    d., occlusive
    d., pressure
    d., protective
    d., transparent synthetic
    d., universal
    d., water
dressing stick
DRG *diagnosis related group*
drift
    d., genetic
    d., mesial
drill
Drinker respirator [Philip Drinker, U.S. engineer in industrial hygiene, 1894 – 1972]
drip [ME. *drippen*, to drip]
    d., intravenous
    d., Murphy

d., nasal
d., postnasal
drive (drīv) [AS. *drifan*]
drive controls
Drolban
dromomania (drō"mō-mā'nē-ă) [Gr. *dromos*, a running, + *mania*, madness]
dromostanolone propionate (drō"mō-stăn'ō-lōn)
dromotropic [" + *tropikos*, a turning]
dronabinol
drop [AS. *dropa*]
d., culture
d.'s, ear
d.'s, eye-
d., foot
d., hanging
d.'s, nose
d., wrist
droperidol (drō-pĕr'ĭ-dŏl)
droplet
droplet infection
dropper
d., medicine
dropsy (drŏp'sē) [Gr. *hydor*, water]
Drosophila (drō-sŏf'ĭ-lă)
D. melanogaster
drowning [ME. *dr(o)unen*, to drown]
drownproofing
drowsiness
d., day-time
Dr.P.H. *Doctor of Public Health*
drug [O. Fr. *drogue*, chemical material]
d.'s, look-alike
drug abuse
drug action
drug addiction
drug administration
drug dependence
drug eruption
drug-fast
drug fever
druggist (drŭg'ĭst)
drug handling
drug interaction
drug overdose

drug rashes
drug reaction
drug receptors
drum
drunkenness [AS. *drinean*, to drink]
drusen (droo'zĕn) [Ger. *Druse*, weathered ore]
dry eye
dry ice
dry measure
dry mouth
Drysdale's corpuscles (drīz'dălz) [Thomas M. Drysdale, U.S. gynecologist, 1831 – 1904]
DTIC-Dome
dt's *delirium tremens*
dualism (dū'ă-lĭzm) [L. *duo*, two, + Gr. *-ismos*, condition]
dual personality
duazomycin (dū-ăz"ō-mī'sĭn)
Dubini's disease (dū-bē'nēz) [Angelo Dubini, It. physician, 1813 – 1902]
Dubin-Johnson syndrome [Isadore Dubin, U.S. pathologist, b. 1913; F.B. Johnson, contemporary U.S. physician]
duboisine (dū-bŏy'sēn)
Dubowitz tool or score [Lilly and Victor Dubowitz, contemporary physicians]
Duchenne, Guillaume B. A. (dū-shĕn') [Fr. neurologist, 1806 – 1875]
D.'s disease
D.'s muscular dystrophy
D.'s paralysis
Duchenne-Aran disease (dū-shĕn'ăr-ăn') [Duchenne; F.A. Aran, Fr. physician, 1817 – 1861]
Duchenne-Erb paralysis (dū-shĕn'ayrb) [Duchenne; W. H. Erb, Ger. internist, 1840 – 1921]
Ducrey's bacillus (dū-krāz') [Augusto Ducrey, It. dermatologist, 1860 – 1940]
duct [L. *ducere*, to lead]
d., accessory pancreatic
d., alveolar
d., Bartholin's
d.'s, biliary

d., cochlear
d., common bile
d., cystic
d., efferent
d., ejaculatory
d., endolymphatic
d., excretory
d., Gartner's
d.'s, hepatic
d., interlobular
d., lacrimal
d.'s, lactiferous
d., Leydig's
d., lymphatic
d., lymphatic, left
d., lymphatic, right
d.'s, mammary
d., mesonephric
d., metanephric
d.'s, milk
d.'s, müllerian
d., nasolacrimal
d.'s of Rivinus
d. of Santorini
d. of the epoophoron
d. of Wirsung
d., omphalomesenteric
d., pancreatic
d.'s, papillary
d., paramesonephric
d.'s, paraurethral
d., parotid
d.'s, prostatic
d.'s, salivary
d.'s, secretory
d., segmental
d.'s, semicircular
d.,'s seminal
d.'s, Skene's
d., spermatic
d., Stensen's
d., striated
d.'s, sublingual
d., submandibular
d.'s, tear
d., testicular
d., thoracic
d., umbilical

d., utriculosaccular
d., vitelline
d., Wharton's
d., wolffian

ductile (dŭk'tĭl) [L. *ductilis*, fr. *ducere*, to lead]

ductless [L. *ducere*, to lead, + AS. *loessa*, less]

ductless glands

ductule (dŭk'tūl)
    d., aberrant

ductulus (dŭk'tū-lŭs)

ductus (dŭk'tŭs)
    d. arteriosus
    d. arteriosus, patent
    d. choledochus
    d. cochlearis
    d. deferens
    d. epoophori longitudinalis
    d. hemithoracicus
    d. hepaticus
    d. hepaticus dexter
    d. hepaticus sinister
    d. prostatici
    d. reuniens
    d., utriculosaccularis
    d. venosus

Duffy system

duipara (doo-ĭp'ă-ră) [L. *duo*, two, + *parere*, to beget, produce]

Duke method

dulcite (dŭl'sĭt) [L. *dulcis*, sweet]

Dulcolax

dull [ME. *dul*]

dullness

dumb [AS.]

dumbness

dumping

dumping syndrome

duodenal (dū-ō-dē'năl, dū-ŏd'ĕ-năl) [L. *duodeni*, twelve]

duodenal bulb

duodenal delay

duodenal ulcer

duodenectasis (dū"ō-dĕn-ĕk'tă-sĭs) [" + Gr. *ektasis*, expansion]

duodenectomy (dū"ō-dĕn-ĕk'tō-mē) [" + Gr. *ektome*, excision]

duodenitis (dū″ŏd-ĕ-nī′tĭs) [″ +
Gr. *itis*, inflammation]
duodenocholecystostomy
(dū″ō-dē″nō-kō-lĭ-sĭs-tŏs′tō-mē) [″ +
Gr. *chole*, bile, + *kystis*, bladder,
+ *stoma*, mouth, opening]
duodenocholedochotomy
(dū″ō-dē″nō-kō-lĕd-ō-kŏt′ō-mē) [″ +
Gr. *choledochos*, bile duct, +
tome, a cutting, slice]
duodenocystostomy (dū″ō-dē″nō-
sĭs-tŏs′tō-mē)
duodenoenterostomy (dū″ō-dē″nō-
ĕn″tĕr-ŏs′tō-mē) [″ + Gr. *enteron*,
intestine, + *stoma*, mouth, open-
ing]
duodenogram (dū-ŏd′ĕ-nō-grăm)
[″ + Gr. *gramma*, letter, piece of
writing]
duodenography (dū″ō-dĕ-nŏg′-ră-fē)
[″ + Gr. *graphein*, to write]
    d., hypotonic
duodenohepatic (dū-ŏd″ĕ-nō″hĕ-
păt′ĭk) [″ + Gr. *hepatos*, liver]
duodenoileostomy (dū″ō-dē″nō-ĭl″ē-
ŏs′tō-mē)
duodenojejunostomy (dū″ō-dē″nō-
jĕ-joo-nŏs′tō-mē) [″ + *jejunum*,
empty, + Gr. *stoma*, mouth, open-
ing]
duodenorrhaphy (dū″ō-dĕ-nor′ă-fē)
[″ + Gr. *rhaphe*, seam]
duodenoscopy (dū″ŏd-ĕ-nŏs′kō-pē)
[″ + Gr. *skopein*, to examine]
duodenostomy (dū″ŏd-ĕ-nŏs′tō-mē)
[″ + Gr. *stoma*, mouth, opening]
duodenotomy (dū″ŏd-ĕ-nŏt′ō-mē)
[″ + Gr. *tome*, a cutting, slice]
duodenum (dū″ō-dē′nŭm, dū-ŏd′ĕ-
nŭm) [L. *duodeni*, twelve]
duplication, duplicature [L. *duplicare*, to double]
duplicitas (dū-plĭs′ĭ-tăs)
dupp (dŭp)
Dupuytren, Baron G. (dū-pwē-trăn′)
[Fr. surgeon, 1777 – 1835]
    D.'s contracture
    D.'s fracture

dura (dū′ră) [L. *durus*, hard]
Durabolin
Duracillin
dural (dū′răl) [L. *durus*, hard]
dura mater [L., hard mother]
duramatral
Durand-Nicolas-Favre disease
duraplasty [″ + Gr. *plassein*, to
form]
Duraquin
duration
durematoma (dū″rĕm-ă-tō′mă) [″ +
Gr. *haima*, blood, + *oma*, tumor]
duritis (dū-rī′tĭs) [″ + Gr. *itis*, inflam-
mation]
duroarachnitis (dū″rō-ăr″ăk-nī′tĭs)
[″ + Gr. *arachne*, spider, +
itis, inflammation]
Duroziez′ murmur (dū-rō″zē-āz′)
[Paul Louis Duroziez, Fr. physician,
1826 – 1897]
dust
    d., blood
    d., ear
    d., house
dust cells
dusting powder
    d.p., absorbable
Duverney's fracture (dū-vĕr-nāz′)
[Joseph G. Duverney, Fr. anatomist,
1648 – 1730]
Duverney's gland
Duvoid
D.V.M. Doctor of Veterinary Medicine
dwarf [AS. *dweorg*, dwarf]
    d., achondroplastic
    d., asexual
    d., hypophyseal
    d., infantile
    d., Levi-Lorain
    d., micromelic
    d., ovarian
    d., phocomelic
    d., physiologic
    d., pituitary
    d., primordial
    d., rachitic
    d., renal

d., thanatophoric
dwarfism
Dy dysprosium
dyad [Gr. duas, pair]
dyadic
Dycill
Dyclone
dyclonine hydrochloride (dī'klō-nēn)
dye
dying
dynamia (dī-năm'ē-ă) [Gr. dynamis, power]
dynamic (dī-năm'ĭk)
dynamics
d., group
d., population
dynamic splint
dynamogenesis (dī"nă-mō-jĕn'ĕ-sĭs) [" + genesis, generation, birth]
dynamogenic [" + gennan, to produce]
dynamograph (dī-năm'ō-grăf) [" + graphein, to write]
dynamometer (dī"nă-mŏm'ĕ-tĕr) [" + metron, measure]
dynamoneure (dī-năm'ō-nūr) [" + neuron, nerve]
dynamoscope (dī-năm'ō-skōp) [" + skopein, to examine]
dynamoscopy (dī-năm-ŏs'kō-pē)
Dynapen
dyne (dīn) [Gr. dynamis, power]
dyphylline (dī-fĭl'ĭn)
Dyrenium
dys- [Gr.]
dysacousia, dysacusis, dysacousma (dĭs"ă-koo'zē-ă, -koo'sĭs, -kooz'mă) [Gr. dys, bad, difficult, painful, disordered, + akousis, hearing]
dysadrenalism (dĭs"ăd-rē'năl-ĭzm)
dysantigraphia (dĭs"ăn-tĭ-grăf'ē-ă) [" + anti, against, + graphein, to write]
dysaphia (dĭs-ă'fē-ă) [" + haphe, touch]
dysarthria (dĭs-ăr'thrē-ă) [" + arthroun, to utter distinctly]

dysarthrosis [" + arthrosis, joint]
dysautonomia (dĭs"aw-tō-nō'mē-ă) [" + autonomia, freedom to use own laws]
dysbarism (dĭs'băr-ĭzm) [" + barys, heavy, + -ismos, condition]
dysbasia (dĭs-bā'zē-ă) [" + basis, a step]
dysboulia (dĭs-bū'lē-ă) [" + boulē, will]
dyscalculia (dĭs"kăl-kū'lē-ă) [" + L. calculare, to compute]
dyscephaly (dĭs-sĕf'ă-lē)
dyschezia (dĭs-kē'zē-ă) [" + chezein, to defecate]
dyschiria (dĭs-kī'rē-ă) [" + cheir, hand]
dyschondroplasia (dĭs"kŏn-drō-plā'zē-ă) [" + chondros, cartilage, + plassein, to form]
dyschroa, dyschroia (dĭs-krō'ă, dĭs-kroy'ă) [" + chroia, complexion]
dyschromatopsia (dĭs"krō-mă-tŏp'sē-ă) [" + chroma, color, + opsis, sight, appearance, vision]
dyschromia
dyschronism (dĭs-krō'nĭzm) [" + chronos, time]
dyscinesia (dĭs-sī-nē'zē-ă)
dyscoria (dĭs-kō'rē-ă) [" + kore, pupil]
dyscrasia (dĭs-krā'zē-ă) [Gr. dyskrasia, bad temperament]
dyscrasic (dĭs-krā'sĭk)
dyscrinism (dĭs-krī'nĭzm) [Gr. dys, bad, difficult, painful, disordered, + krinein, to secrete, + -ismos, condition]
dysdiadochokinesia (dĭs"dī-ăd"ō-kō-kī-nē'sē-ă) [" + diadochos, succeeding, + kinesis, motion]
dysembryoplasia (dĭs-ĕm"brē-ō-plā'sē-ă) [" + embryon, to swell inside, + plassein, to form]
dysemia [" + haima, blood]
dysenteric (dĭs"ĕn-tĕr'ĭk)
dysentery (dĭs'ĕn-tĕr"ē) [" + enteron, intestine]

d., amebic
d., bacillary
d., balantidial
d., malignant
d., viral

dyserethesia (dĭs"ĕr-ē-thē'zē-ă) [" + erethizein, to irritate]

dysergasia (dĭs"ĕr-gă'zē-ă) [" + ergon, work]

dysergastic (dĭs-ĕr-găs'tĭk)

dysergia (dĭs-ĕr'jē-ă) [" + ergon, work]

dysesthesia (dĭs"ĕs-thē'zē-ă) [" + esthesia, sensation]
d., auditory
d. pedis

dysfunction (dĭs-fŭnk'shŭn) [" + L. functio, a performance]

dysgalactia [" + gala, milk]

dysgammaglobulinemia

dysgenesis (dĭs-jĕn'ĕ-sĭs) [" + genesis, generation, birth]
d., gonadal

dysgenic [" + gennan, to produce]

dysgenitalism [" + L. genitalis, to beget, + Gr. -ismos, condition]

dysgerminoma (dĭs"jĕr-mĭn-ō'mă) [" + L. germen, a sprout, + Gr. oma, tumor]

dysgeusia (dĭs-gū'zē-ă) [" + geusis, taste]

dysglandular [" + L. glans, acorn]

dysglobulinemia (dĭs-glŏb"ū-lĭn-ē'mē-ă) [" + L. globulus, globule, + Gr. haima, blood]

dysgnathia (dĭs-nā'thē-ă) [" + gnathos, jaw]

dysgnosia (dĭs-nō'sē-ă) [Gr. dysgnosia, difficulty of knowing]

dysgonesis (dĭs"gō-nē'sĭs) [Gr. dys, bad, difficult, painful, disordered, + gone, seed]

dysgonic

dysgraphia (dĭs-grăf'ē-ă) [" + graphein, to write]

dyshematopoiesia (dĭs-hĕm"ă-tō-poy-ē'sē-ă) [" + haima, blood, + poiein, to make]

dyshidria (dĭs-hĭd'rē-ă) [" + hidros, sweat]

dyshidrosis (dĭs-hī-drō'sĭs) [" + " + osis, condition]

dysidrosis (dĭs-ī-drō'sĭs)

dyskaryosis (dĭs-kăr"ē-ō'sĭs)

dyskeratosis (dĭs"kĕr-ă-tō'sĭs) [" + keras, horn, + osis, condition]

dyskinesia (dĭs"kĭ-nē'sē-ă) [" + kinesis, motion]
d. algera
d., biliary
d. intermittens
d., tardive
d., uterine

dyskinetic

dyslalia (dĭs-lā'lē-ă) [" + lalia, chatter, prattle]

dyslexia (dĭs-lĕk'sē-ă) [" + lexis, diction]

dyslochia (dĭs-lō'kē-ă)[" + lochia, lochia]

dyslogia (dĭs-lō'jē-ă) [" + logos, word, reason]

dysmasesis (dĭs"mă-sē'sĭs) [" + masesis, mastication]

dysmaturity

dysmegalopsia [" + megas, big, + opsis, sight, appearance, vision]

dysmelia (dĭs-mē'lē-ă) [" + melos, limb]

dysmenorrhea (dĭs"mĕn-ō-rē'ă) [" + men, month, + rhein, to flow]
d., congestive
d., inflammatory
d., membranous
d., primary
d., secondary
d., spasmodic

dysmetria (dĭs-mē'trē-ă) [Gr. dys, bad, difficult, painful, disordered, + metron, measure]

dysmetropsia [" + " + opsis, sight, appearance, vision]

dysmimia (dĭs-mĭm'ē-ă) [" +

mimos, imitation]

dysmnesia (dĭs-nē′zē-ă) [″ + *mneme*, memory]

dysmorphophobia (dĭs″mor-fō-fō′bē-ă) [″ + *morphe*, formed, + *phobos*, fear]

dysmorphosis (dĭs″mor-fō′sĭs) [″ + *osis*, condition]

dysmyotonia (dĭs″mī-ō-tō′nē-ă) [″ + *mys*, muscle, + *tonos*, act of stretching, tension, tone]

dysodontiasis (dĭs″ō-dŏn-tī′ă-sĭs) [″ + *odous*, tooth, + *-iasis*, state or condition of]

dysomnias (dĭs-ōm′nē-ăz) [″ + L. *somnus*, sleep]

dysontogenesis (dĭs″ŏn-tō-jĕn′ĕ-sĭs) [″ + *ontos*, being, + *genesis*, generation, birth]

dysontogenetic

dysopia, dysopsia (dĭs-ō′pē-ă, ŏp′sē-ă) [″ + *opsis*, sight, appearance, vision]

dysorexia (dĭs″ō-rĕk′sē-ă) [″ + *orexis*, appetite]

dysosmia (dĭs-ŏz′mē-ă) [″ + *osme*, smell]

dysostosis (dĭs″ŏs-tō′sĭs) [″ + *osteon*, bone, + *osis*, condition]
  d., cleidocranial
  d., craniocerebral
  d., mandibulofacial

dysoxia (dĭs-ŏk′sē-ă)

dysoxidizable [″ + L. *oxidum*, oxide]

dyspancreatism [″ + *pankreas*, pancreas, + *-ismos*, condition]

dyspareunia (dĭs″pă-rū′nē-ă) [″ + *pareunos*, lying beside]

dyspepsia (dĭs-pĕp′sē-ă) [″ + *peptein*, to digest]
  d., acid
  d., alcoholic
  d., biliary
  d., cardiac
  d., gastric
  d., gastrointestinal
  d., hepatic

  d., hysterical

dyspeptic (dĭs-pĕp′tĭk)

dyspermasia [″ + *sperma*, seed]

dyspermatism

dyspermia

dysphagia (dĭs-fā′jē-ă) [″ + *phagein*, to eat]
  d. constricta
  d. lusoria
  d. paralytica
  d., spastica

dysphagy (dĭs′fă-jē)

dysphasia (dĭs-fā′zē-ă) [″ + *phasis*, utterance]

dysphemia (dĭs-fē′mē-ă) [″ + *pheme*, speech]

dysphonia (dĭs-fō′nē-ă) [″ + *phone*, voice]
  d. clericorum
  d. puberum
  d., spasmodic

dysphoria (dĭs-fō′rē-ă) [″ + *pherein*, to bear]

dysphrasia (dĭs-frā′zē-ă) [Gr. *dys*, bad, difficult, painful, disordered, + *phrasis*, diction]

dysphylaxia (dĭs-fĭ-lăk′sē-ă) [″ + *phylaxis*, guard]

dyspigmentation (dĭs″pĭg-mĕn-tā′shŭn)

dyspituitarism (dĭs″pī-tū′ĭ-tăr-ĭzm) [″ + L. *pituita*, mucus, + Gr. *-ismos*, condition]

dysplasia [″ + *plassein*, to form]
  d., anhidrotic
  d., cervical
  d., chondroectodermal
  d., hereditary ectodermal
  d., monostotic fibrous
  d., polyostotic fibrous

dyspnea (dĭsp-nē′ă, dĭsp′nē-ă) [″ + *pnoē*, breathing]
  d., cardiac
  d., expiratory
  d., inspiratory

dyspneic (dĭsp-nē′ĭk)

dyspraxia (dĭs-prăk′sē-ă) [″ + *prassein*, achieve]

dysprosium (dĭs-prō'sē-ŭm)
dysprosody
dysraphia, dysraphism (dĭs-rā'fē-ă, -fĭzm) [" + rhaphe, seam]
   d., spinal
dysrhythmia (dĭs-rĭth'mē-ă) [" + rhythmos, rhythm]
dysstasia [" + stasis, standing still]
dysstatic
dyssynergia [" + synergia, cooperation]
dystaxia (dĭs-tăk'sē-ă) [" + taxis, arrangement]
dystectia (dĭs-tĕk'shē-ă) [" + L. tectum, roof]
dysteleology (dĭs"tē-lē-ŏl'ō-jē) [" + telos, end, + logos, word, reason]
dysthymia (dĭs-thĭm'ē-ă) [" + thymos, mind, spirit]
dysthyreosis (dĭs"thī-rē-ō'sĭs) [" + thyreos, shield, + osis, condition]
dysthyroidism (dĭs-thī'roy-dĭzm) [" + " + eidos, form, shape, + -ismos, condition]
dystocia (dĭs-tō'sē-ă) [" + tokos, birth]
dystonia (dĭs-tō'nē-ă) [" + tonos, act of stretching, tension, tone]
   d. musculum deformans

dystonic
dystopia (dĭs-tō'pē-ă) [" + topos, place]
   d. canthorum
dystopic (dĭs-tŏp'ĭk)
dystopy (dĭs'tō-pē) [" + topos, place]
dystrophia (dĭs-trō'fē-ă) [" + trephein, to nourish]
dystrophic (dĭs-trŏf'ĭk)
dystrophoneurosis (dĭs-trŏf"ō-nū-rō'sĭs) [" + trephein, to nourish, + neuron, nerve, + osis, condition]
dystrophy (dĭs'trō-fē)
   d., adiposogenital
   d., Landouzy-Déjérine
   d., progressive muscular
   d., pseudohypertrophic muscular
dystrypsia (dĭs-trĭp'sē-ă) [" + tripsis, a rubbing, friction]
dysuria (dĭs-ū'rē-ă) [" + ouron, urine]
dysuriac
dyszooamylia (dĭs-zō"ō-ăm-ĭl'ē-ă) [" + zoon, animal, + amylon, starch]
dyszoospermia (dĭs"zō-ō-spĕrm'ē-ă) [" + " + sperma, seed]

E

E emmetropia; energy; Escherichia; eye
E₁ estrone
E₂ estradiol
E₃ estriol
e electric charge; electron; [L.] ex, from
ea. each
EACA epsilon-aminocaproic acid
ead. [L.] eadem, the same
Eales' disease (ēlz) [Henry Eales, Brit. physician, 1852–1913]
ear [AS. ear]
   e., Blainville's
   e., Cagot
   e., cauliflower
   e., external
   e., foreign bodies in
   e., internal
   e., middle
   e., nerve supply of
   e., pierced
earache
ear bones
eardrops
eardrum (ēr'drŭm)
ear dust
ear oximeter
ear plug
earth
   e., alkaline
   e., diatomaceous
   e., fuller's
earth eating
earwax (ēr'wăks)
eat [AS. etan]
Eaton agent
Eberthella (ā"bĕr-tĕl'ă) [K. J. Eberth, Ger. pathologist, 1835–1926]
Ebner's glands [A. G. Victor von Ebner, Austrian histologist, 1842–1925]
Ebola-Marburg virus disease

216

ebonation (ē"bō-nā'shŭn) [L. e, out, + AS. ban, bone]
Ebstein's anomaly (ĕb'stīnz) [Wilhelm Ebstein, Ger. physician, 1836–1912]
ebullism (ĕb'ū-lĭzm) [L. ebullire, to boil over]
eburnation (ĕb"ŭr-nā'shŭn) [L. eburnus, made of ivory]
eburneous (ē-bŭr'nē-ŭs)
EBV Epstein-Barr virus
ecaudate (ē-kaw'dāt) [L. e, without, + cauda, tail]
ecbolic (ĕk-bŏl'ĭk) [Gr. ekbolikos, throwing out]
ECC emergency cardiac care; external cardiac compression
eccentric (ĕk-sĕn'trĭk) [Gr. ek, out, + kentron, center]
eccentro-osteochondrodysplasia (ĕk-sĕn"trō-ŏs"tē-ō-kŏn"drō-dĭs-plā'zhē-ă) [Gr. ekkentros, from the center, + osteon, bone, + chondros, cartilage, + dys, bad, difficult, painful, disordered, + plassein, to form]
eccentropiesis (ĕk-sĕn"trō-pī-ē'sĭs) [" + piesis, pressure]
ecchondroma (ĕk-ŏn-drō'mă) [Gr. ek, out, + chondros, cartilage, + oma, tumor]
ecchondrotome (ĕk-ŏn-drō-tōm) [" + " + tome, a cutting, slice]
ecchymoma (ĕk-ĭ-mō'mă) [" + chymos, juice, + oma, tumor]
ecchymosis (ĕk-ĭ-mō'sĭs) [" + " + osis, condition]
ecchymotic (ĕk-ĭ-mŏt'ĭk) [" + chymos, juice]
eccrine (ĕk'rĭn) [Gr. ekkrinein, to secrete]
eccrine sweat glands

eccritic (ĕk-krĭt′ĭk) [Gr. *ekkritikos*]

eccyclomastopathy (ĕk-sī″klō-măs-tŏp′ă-thē) [Gr. *ek*, out, + *kyklos*, circle, + *mastos*, breast, + *pathos*, disease, suffering]

eccyesis (ĕk″sī-ē′sĭs) [″ + *kyesis*, pregnancy]

ecdemomania (ĕk″dē-mō-mā′nē-ă) [Gr. *ekdemos*, journeying, + *mania*, madness]

ecderon (ĕk′dĕ-rŏn) [Gr. *ek*, out, + *deros*, skin]

ecdysis (ĕk′dĭ-sĭs) [Gr. *ekdysis*, getting out]

ECG, ecg *electrocardiogram*

echeosis (ĕk″ē-ō′sĭs) [Gr. *eche*, loud sound, + *osis*, condition]

echidnase (ĕ-kĭd′nās) [Gr. *echidna*, viper]

echidnin (ĕ-kĭd′nĭn)

Echidnophaga (ĕk″ĭd-nŏf′ă-gă)
   E. gallinacea

echinate (ĕk′ĭ-nāt) [Gr. *echinos*, hedgehog]

echinococcosis (ĕ-kĭ″nō-kŏk-ō′sĭs, ĕk″ĭ-nō-kŏk-ō′sĭs) [″ + *kokkos*, berry, + *osis*, condition]

echinococcotomy (ĕ-kĭ″nō-kŏk-ŏt′ō-mē) [″ + ″ + *tome*, a cutting, slice]

Echinococcus (ĕ-kĭ″nō-kŏk′ŭs)
   E. granulosus
   E. hydatidosus

echinocyte

echinosis (ĕk″ĭ-nō′sĭs) [Gr. *echinos*, hedgehog, + *osis*, condition]

Echinostoma (ĕk″ĭ-nŏs′tō-mă) [″ + *stoma*, mouth, opening]

echinulate (ĕ-kĭn′ū-lāt)

echo (ĕk′ō) [Gr. *ekho*]
   e., amphoric

echoacousia

echocardiogram (ĕk″ō-kăr′dē-ō-grăm″)

echocardiography (ĕk″ō-kăr″dē-ŏg′ră-fē)

echoencephalogram (ĕk″ō-ĕn-sĕf′ă-lō-grăm″)

echogram (ĕk′ō-grăm)

echography (ĕk-ŏg′ră-fē) [″ + *graphein*, to write]

echokinesia (ĕk″ō-kĭn-ē′sē-ă) [″ + *kinesis*, motion]

echolalia (ĕk-ō-lā′lē-ă) [″ + *lalia*, chatter, prattle]

echolocation

echomimia (ĕk″ō-mĭm′ē-ă) [″ + *mimesis*, imitation]

echomotism (ĕk″ō-mō′tĭzm) [″ + L. *motus*, moving]

echopathy (ĕ-kŏp′ă-thē) [″ + *pathos*, disease, suffering]

echophotony (ĕk″ō-fŏt′ō-nē) [″ + *phos*, light, + *tonos*, act of stretching, tension, tone]

echophrasia (ĕk″ō-frā′sē-ă) [″ + *phrasis*, diction]

echopraxia (ĕk″ō-prăk′sē-ă) [″ + *prassein*, to perform]

echo sign

echothiophate iodide (ĕk″ō-thī′ō-fāt)

ECHO virus

Eck's fistula (ĕks) [N. V. Eck, Russian physiologist, 1847 – 1908]

eclabium (ĕk-lā′bē-ŭm) [Gr. *ek*, out, + L. *labium*, lip]

eclampsia (ĕ-klămp′sē-ă) [″ + *lampein*, to shine]

eclamptic

eclamptogenic (ĕk-lămp″tō-jĕn′ĭk) [Gr. *ek*, out, + *lampein*, to shine, + *gennan*, to produce]

eclectic (ĕk-lĕk′tĭk) [Gr. *eklektikos*, selecting]

eclecticism (ĕk-lĕk′tĭ-sĭzm) [″ + *-ismos*, condition]

ecmnesia (ĕk-nē′zē-ă) [Gr. *ek*, out, + *mnesis*, memory]

ECMO *extracorporeal membrane oxygenator*

ecocide (ĕk″ō-sīd′) [Gr. *oikos*, house, + L. *caedere*, to kill]

E. coli *Escherichia coli*

ecologic fallacy

ecology (ē-kŏl′ō-jē) [Gr. *oikos*, house, + *logos*, word, reason]

Economo's disease [Constantin von Economo, Austrian neurologist, 1876–1931]

écorché (ā"kor-shā') [Fr.]

ecosphere (ĕk'ō-sfēr") [Gr. oikos, house, + L. sphera, ball]

ecostate (ē-kŏs'tāt) [L. e, without, + costa, rib]

ecosystem (ĕk'ō-sĭs"tĕm)

Ecotrin

écouvillonage (ā-koo"vē-yō-nŏzh') [Fr. ecouvillon, a stiff brush or swab]

ecphoria (ĕk-for'ē-ă) [Gr. ek, out of, + pherein, to bear]

écrasement (ā-krăz-mŏn') [Fr.]

écraseur (ā-kră-zĕr') [Fr., crusher]

ecstasy (ĕk'stă-sē) [Gr. ekstasis, a standing out]

ecstrophy (ĕk'strō-fē) [Gr. ekstrophe, a turning out]

ECT electroconvulsive therapy

ectad [Gr. ektos, out of, + L. ad, toward]

ectal

ectasia, ectasis (ĕk-tā'sē-ă, ĕk'tă-sĭs) [Gr. ek, out, + teinein, to stretch]
  e., hypostatic
  e. iridis
  e. ventriculi paradoxa

ectatic

ectental [Gr. ektos, out of, + entos, within]

ectental line

ectethmoid (ĕk-tĕth'moyd) [" + ethmos, sieve, + eidos, form, shape]

ecthyma (ĕk-thī'mă) [Gr. ek, out, + thyein, to rush]

ectiris (ĕk-tī-rĭs) [Gr. ektos, out of, + iris, bend, turn]

ecto- [Gr. ekto-, outside]

ectoantigen (ĕk"tō-ăn'tĭ-gĕn) [" + anti, against, + gennan, to produce]

ectoblast (ĕk'tō-blăst) [" + blastos, germ]

ectocardia (ĕk'tō-kăr'dē-ă) [" + kardia, heart]

ectocervical (ĕk"tō-sĕr'vĭ-kăl)

ectocervix (ĕk"tō-sĕr'vĭks)

ectochoroidea (ĕk"tō-kō-roy'dē-ă) [" + khorioeides, choroid]

ectocinerea (ĕk"tō-sĭn-ē'rē-ă) [" + L. cinereus, ashen]

ectocolostomy (ĕk"tō-kŏ-lŏs'tō-mē) [" + kolon, colon, + stoma, mouth, opening]

ectocondyle (ĕk"tō-kŏn'dĭl) [" + kondylos, knuckle]

ectocornea (ĕk-tō-kor'nē-ă) [" + L. corneus, horny]

ectocuneiform (ĕk-tō-kū'nē-ĭ-form) [" + L. cuneus, wedge, + forma, form]

ectocytic (ĕk"tō-sī'tĭk) [" + kytos, cell]

ectodactylism (ĕk"tō-dăk'tĭl-ĭzm) [" + daktylos, finger, + -ismos, condition]

ectoderm (ĕk'tō-dĕrm) [Gr. ektos, out of, + derma, skin]

ectodermal

ectodermatosis,   ectodermosis (ĕk"tō-dĕr"mă-tō'sĭs,   -dĕr-mō'sĭs) [" + derma, skin, + osis, condition]
  e. erosiva pluriorificialis

ectodermic

ectodermoidal (ĕk"tō-dĕr-moyd'ăl) [Gr. ektos, out of, + derma, skin, + eidos, form, shape]

ectoentad (ĕk"tō-ĕn'tăd) [" + entos, within]

ectoenzyme (ĕk"tō-ĕn'zīm) [" + en-, in, + zyme, leaven]

ectogenous (ĕk-tŏj'ĕ-nŭs) [" + gennan, to produce]

ectoglia (ĕk-tŏg'lē-ă) [" + glia, glue]

ectoglobular (ĕk"tō-glŏb'ū-lăr) [" + L. globulus, globule]

ectogony (ĕk-tŏg'ō-nē) [" + gone, seed]

ectolecithal (ĕk"tō-lĕs'ĭ-thăl) [" + lekithos, yolk]

ectomere (ĕk'tō-mēr) [" + meros, part]

ectomesoblast (ĕk"tō-mĕs'ō-blăst)

[" + *mesos*, middle, + *blastos*, germ]

ectomorph (ĕk'tō-morf) [" + *morphe*, form]

-ectomy (ĕk'tō-mē) [Gr. *ektome*, excision]

ectonuclear (ĕk-tō-nū'klē-ăr) [Gr. *ektos*, out of, + L. *nucleus*, kernel]

ectopagus (ĕk-tŏp'ă-gŭs) [" + *pagos*, something fixed]

ectoparasite (ĕk"tō-păr'ă-sīt") [" + Gr. *parasitos*, parasite]

ectoperitonitis (ĕk"tō-pĕr"ĭ-tō-nī'tĭs) [" + *peritonaion*, stretched around or over, + *itis*, inflammation]

ectophyte (ĕk'tō-fīt) [" + *phyton*, plant]

ectopia (ĕk-tō'pē-ă) [Gr. *ektopos*, displaced]

   e. cordis

   e. lentis

   e. pupillae congenita

   e. renis

   e. testis

   e. vesicae

   e., visceral

ectopic (ĕk-tŏp'ĭk)

ectopic beat, complex

ectopic pregnancy

ectopic rhythm

ectopic secretion (ĕk-tŏp'ĭk)

ectoplasm [Gr. *ektos*, out of, + LL. *plasma*, form, mold]

ectoplasmic

ectoplast (ĕk'tō-plăst) [" + *plastikos*, formed]

ectoplastic

ectopotomy (ĕk-tō-pŏt'ō-mē) [Gr. *ektopos*, displaced, + *tome*, a cutting, slice]

ectopterygoid (ĕk"tō-tĕr'ĭ-goyd) [Gr. *ektos*, out of, + *pteryx*, wing, + *eidos*, form, shape]

ectopy (ĕk'tō-pē) [Gr. *ektopos*, displaced]

ectoretina (ĕk"tō-rĕt'ĭ-nă) [Gr. *ektos*, out of, + L. *rete*, net]

ectostosis (ĕk-tŏs-tō'sĭs) [" + *osteon*, bone, + *osis*, condition]

ectothrix (ĕk'tō-thrĭks) [" + *thrix*, hair]

Ectotrichophyton (ĕk"ō-trī-kŏf'ĭ-tŏn) [" + *thrix*, hair, + *phyton*, plant]

ectozoon (ĕk-tō-zō'ŏn) [" + *zoon*, animal]

ectro- [Gr. *ektrosis*, miscarriage]

ectrodactylism (ĕk"trō-dăk'tĭl-īzm) [" + *daktylos*, finger, + *-ismos*, condition]

ectrogeny (ĕk-trŏj'ĕ-nē) [" + *gennan*, to produce]

ectromelia (ĕk"trō-mē'lē-ă) [" + *melos*, limb]

ectromelus (ĕk-trŏm'ĕ-lŭs) [" + *melos*, limb]

ectropic (ĕk-trō'pĭk) [Gr. *ek*, out, + *trope*, turning]

ectropion (ĕk-trō'pē-ŏn)

ectropionize

ectrosyndactyly (ĕk"trō-sĭn-dăk'tĭ-lē) [" + *syn*, together, + *dactylos*, finger]

eczema (ĕk'zĕ-mă) [Gr. *ekzein*, to boil out]

   e., erythematous

   e. fissum

   e. herpeticum

   e. hypertrophicum

   e., lichenoid

   e. marginatum

   e., nummular

   e., pustular

   e., seborrheic

   e. vaccinatum

eczematous (ĕk-zĕm'ă-tŭs)

ED *effective dose; erythema dose*

E.D. *Emergency Department*

ED$_{50}$ *median effective dose*

EDC *expected date of confinement*

Edecrin

edema (ĕ-dē'mă) [Gr. *oidema*, swelling]

   e., acute circumscribed

   e., angioneurotic

   e., blue

   e., brain

   e. bullosum vesicae

   e., cardiac

e., cerebral
e., dependent
e., high-altitude
e., inflammatory
e., laryngeal
e., malignant
e. neonatorum
e. of glottis
e., pitting
e., pulmonary
e., purulent
e., salt

edematogenic (ĕ-dĕm"ă-tō-jĕn'ĭk)
edematous (ĕ-dĕm'ăt-ŭs) [Gr. *oidema*, swelling]
edentia (ē-dĕn'shē-ă) [L. *e*, without, + *dens*, tooth]
edentulous (ē-dĕnt'ū-lŭs)
edetate calcium disodium (ĕd'ē-tāt)
edge

e., bevel
e., chamber
e., cutting
e., denture
e., incisal

edible (ĕd'ĭ-bl) [L. *edere*, to eat]
edrophonium chloride (ĕd"rō-fō'nē-ŭm)
edrophonium test
EDTA ethylenediaminetetraacetic acid
eduction (ē-dŭk'shŭn) [L. *e*, out, + *ducere*, to lead]
edulcorant (ē-dŭl'kō-rănt) [" + *dulcorare*, to sweeten]
edulcorate (ē-dŭl'kō-rāt)
EEE eastern equine encephalitis
EEG electroencephalogram
EENT eyes, ears, nose, and throat
EFA essential fatty acids
E-Ferol
effacement (ĕ-fās'mĕnt)
effect (ĕ-fĕkt') [L. *effectus*, to accomplish]

e., additive
e., Bainbridge
e., cumulative

effectiveness (ĕ-fĕk'tĭv-nĕs)
effector

effector organ
effeminate
effemination (ĕ-fĕm"ĭ-nā'shŭn) [L. *effeminare*, to make feminine]
efferent [L. *efferens*, to bring out]
efferent nerves
effervesce (ĕf"ĕr-vĕs') [L. *effervescere*, to boil up]
effervescence (ĕf-ĕr-vĕs'ĕns)
effervescent
effleurage (ĕf-loor-ăzh') [Fr. *effleurer*, to touch lightly]
efflorescence (ĕf-flor-ĕs'ĕns) [L. *efflorescere*, to bloom]
efflorescent
effluent (ĕf'loo-ĕnt) [L. *effluere*, to flow out]
effluvium (ĕf-loo'vē-ŭm)
effort syndrome
effuse (ĕ-fūs') [L. *effusio*, pour out]
effusion (ĕ-fū'zhŭn)

e., pericardial
e., pleural

Efudex
egersis (ē-gĕr'sĭs) [Gr., a waking]
egesta (ē-jĕs'tă) [L. *egere*, to cast forth]
egg [AS. *aeg*]
eglandulous (ē-glănd'ū-lŭs) [L. *e*, out, + *glandula*, glandule]
ego (ē'gō, ĕg'ō) [L. *ego*, I]
egocentric (ē"gō-sĕn'trĭk) [L. *ego*, I, + Gr. *kentron*, center]
ego-dystonic (ē"gō-dĭs-tŏn'ĭk) [" + Gr. *dys*, bad, difficult, painful, disordered, + *tonos*, act of stretching, tension, tone]
egoism (ē'gō-ĭzm)
egomania (ē"gō-mā'nē-ă) [" + Gr. *mania*, madness]
egophony (ē-gŏf'ō-nē) [Gr. *aix*, goat, + *phone*, voice]
ego strength
ego-syntonic (ē"gō-sĭn-tŏn'ĭk) [" + Gr. *syn*, together, + *tonos*, act of stretching, tension, tone]
egotism (ē'gō-tĭzm)
egotropic (ē"gō-trŏp'ĭk) [L. *ego*, I, + Gr. *tropos*, a turning]

Ehlers-Danlos syndrome (ā'lĕrz-dăn'lŏs) [E. Ehlers, Danish dermatologist, 1863 – 1937; H. A. Danlos, Fr. dermatologist, 1844 – 1912]

Ehrenritter's ganglion (ār'ĕn-rĭt"ĕrs) [Johann Ehrenritter, late eighteenth century Austrian anatomist]

Ehrlich's side-chain theory (ār'lĭks) [Paul Ehrlich, Ger. bacteriologist, 1854 – 1915]

eicosa-

eicosanoids

eidetic (ī-dĕt'ĭk) [Gr. eidos, form, shape]

eidoptometry (ī-dŏp-tŏm'ĕ-trē) [Gr. eidos, form, shape, + optein, to see, + metron, measure]

eighth cranial nerve

Eikenella corrodens (ī"kĕn-ĕl'ă)

eikonometry (ī"kō-nŏm'ĕ-trē) [Gr. eikon, image, + metron, measure]

eiloid (ī'loyd) [Gr. eilein, to coil, + eidos, form, shape]

Eimeria (ī-mē'rē-ă)
E. hominis

einsteinium (īn-stīn'ē-ŭm) [Albert Einstein, German-born U.S. physicist, 1879 – 1955]

Eisenmenger's complex [Victor Eisenmenger, Ger. physician, 1864 – 1932]

eisodic (ī-sŏd'ĭk) [Gr. eis, into, + hodos, way]

ejaculatio (ē-jăk"ū-lā'shē-ō) [L.]
e. praecox

ejaculation (ē-jăk"ū-lā'shŭn) [L. ejaculari, to throw out]
e., retrograde

ejaculatory

ejaculatory duct

ejecta (ē-jĕk'tă) [L. ejectus, thrown out, ejected]

ejection (ē-jĕk'shŭn)
e., ventricular

ejection fraction

EKG elektrokardiogramm

ekphorize (ĕk'fō-rīz) [Gr. ek, out, + phorein, to bear]

elaboration (ē-lăb"ō-rā'shŭn)

elaiopathy (ē"lā-ŏp'ă-thē) [Gr. elaion, oil, + pathos, disease, suffering]

elastase (ē-lăs'tās)

elastic (ē-lăs'tĭk) [NL. elasticus, expansive, impulsive]
e., intermaxillary
e., intramaxillary
e., vertical

elastic bandage

elastic cartilage

elasticity (ē"lăs-tĭs'ĭ-tē)

elastic skin

elastic stocking

elastic tissue

elastin (ē-lăs'tĭn)

elastinase (ē-lăs'tĭn-ās)

elastofibroma (ē-lăs"tō-fī-brō'mă) [" + L. fibra, fiber, + Gr. oma, tumor]

elastoid (ē-lăs'toyd) [" + eidos, form, shape]

elastoma (ē"lăs-tō'mă) [" + oma, tumor]

elastomer (ē-lăs'tō-mĕr) [" + meros, a part]

elastometer (ē"lăs-tŏm'ĕ-tĕr) [" + metron, measure]

elastometry

elastorrhexis (ē-lăs"tō-rĕk'sĭs) [" + rhexis, rupture]

elastose (ē-lăs'tōs)

elastosis (ē"lăs-tō'sĭs) [" + osis, condition]

elation (ē-lā'shŭn) [L. elatus, borne out of]

Elavil

elbow (ĕl'bō) [AS. eln, forearm, + boga, bend]
e., tennis

elbow conformer

elbow jerk

elbow joint

elbow reflex

elbow unit

Eldecort

elective therapy

Electra complex [Gr. Elektra, Agamemnon's daughter, who helped assassinate her mother because of love for her father, whom the former had slain]

electric, -al [Gr. *elektron*, amber]

electricity

  e., frictional
  e., galvanic
  e., induced
  e., magnetic
  e., negative
  e., positive
  e., static

electric light baker

electric shock

electrify [Gr. *elektron*, amber, + L. *facere*, to make]

electrization

electro-, electr- [Gr. *elektron*, amber]

electroaffinity (ē-lĕk"trō-ă-fĭn'ĭ-tē)

electroanalgesia (ē-lĕk"trō-ăn"ăl-jē'zē-ă) [" + *analgesia*, want of feeling]

electroanalysis (ē-lĕk"trō-ă-năl'ĭ-sĭs)

electroanesthesia (ē-lĕk"trō-ăn"ĕs-thē'zē-ă) [" + *an-*, not, + *aisthesis*, feeling, perception]

electrobiology (ē-lĕk"trō-bī-ŏl'ō-jē) [" + *bios*, life, + *logos*, word, reason]

electrobioscopy (ē-lĕk"trō-bī-ŏs'kō-pē) [" + *bios*, life, + *skopein*, to examine]

electrocardiogram (ē-lĕk"trō-kăr'dē-ō-grăm") [" + *kardia*, heart, + *gramma*, letter, piece of writing]

electrocardiograph (ē-lĕk"trō-kăr'dē-ō-grăf) [" + " + *graphein*, to write]

electrocardiography

electrocardiophonograph (ē-lĕk"trō-kăr"dē-ō-fō'nō-grăf) [Gr. *elektron*, amber, + *kardia*, heart, + *phone*, sound, + *graphein*, to write]

electrocatalysis (ē-lĕk"trō-kă-tăl'ĭ-sĭs) [" + *katalyein*, to dissolve]

electrocautery (ē-lĕk"trō-kaw'tĕr-ē) [" + *kauterion*, branding iron]

electrochemistry [" + *chemeia*, chemistry]

electrochemy (ē-lĕk'trō-kĕm-ē)

electrocision (ē-lĕk'trō-sĭzh'ŭn) [" + L. *caedare*, to cut]

electrocoagulation (ē-lĕk"trō-kō-ăg"ū-lā'shŭn) [" + L. *coagulare*, to thicken]

electrocochleography (ē-lĕk"trō-kŏk-lē-ŏg'ră-fē)

electrocontractility (ē-lĕk"trō-kŏn-trăk-tĭl'ĭ-tē) [" + L. *contrahere*, to contract]

electroconvulsive therapy (ē-lĕk"trō-kŏn-vŭl'sĭv)

electrocorticography (ē-lĕk"trō-kor"tĭ-kŏg'ră-fē)

electrocryptectomy (ē-lĕk"trō-krĭp-tĕk'tō-mē) [" + *kryptos*, concealed, + *ektome*, excision]

electrocution (ē-lĕk"trō-kū'shŭn) [" + L. *acutus*, sharpened]

electrode (ē-lĕk'trōd) [" + *hodos*, a way]

  e., active
  e., calomel
  e., depolarizing
  e., dispersive
  e., gas-sending
  e., glass
  e., hydrogen
  e., immobilized enzyme
  e., indifferent
  e., internal reference
  e., ion-selective
  e., multiple point
  e., negative
  e., point
  e., positive
  e., spark-ball
  e., subcutaneous
  e., surface
  e., therapeutic

electrodermal (ē-lĕk"trō-dĕr'măl)

electrodesiccation (ē-lĕk"trō-dĕs"ĭ-kā'shŭn) [Gr. *elektron*, amber, + L. *desiccare*, to dry up]

electrodiagnosis

electrodialysis (ē-lěk″trō-dī-ăl′ĭ-sĭs) [″ + dia, through, + lysis, dissolution]

electrodynamometer (ē-lěk″trō-dī″nă-mŏm′ě-těr) [″ + dynamis, power, + metron, measure]

electroejaculation

electroencephalogram (ē-lěk″trō-ěn-sěf′ă-lō-grăm) [″ + enkephalos, brain, + gramma, letter, piece of writing]

electroencephalograph (ē-lěk-trō-ěn-sěf′ă-lō-grăf) [″ + ″ + graphein, to write]

electroencephalography

electrogoniometer (ē-lěk″trō-gō″ně-ŏm′ě-těr)

electrograph

electrohemostasis (ē-lěk″trō-hě-mŏs′tă-sĭs) [Gr. elektron, amber, + haima, blood, + stasis, standing still]

electrohysterography (ē-lěk″trō-hĭs″těr-ŏg′ră-fē) [″ + hystera, womb, + graphein, to write]

electrology [″ + logos, word, reason]

electrolysis (ē″lěk-trŏl′ĭ-sĭs) [″ + lysis, dissolution]

electrolyte (ē-lěk′trō-līt) [″ + lytos, soluble]
e., amphoteric

electrolytic (ē-lěk″trō-lĭt′ĭk)

electrolytic conduction

electromagnet [″ + magnes, magnet]

electromagnetic

electromagnetic induction

electromagnetic spectrum

electromagnetism

electromassage [″ + Fr. masser, to massage]

electrometer (ē-lěk-trŏm′ě-těr) [″ + metron, measure]

electromotive [″ + L. motor, mover]

electromotive force

electromyogram (ē-lěk″trō-mī′ō-grăm) [Gr. elektron, amber, + mys, muscle, + gramma, letter, piece of writing]

electromyography (ē-lěk″trō-mī-ŏg′ră-fē) [″ + ″ + graphein, to write]

electron [Gr. elektron, amber]

electronarcosis (ē-lěk″trō-năr-kō′sĭs)

electron-dense

electronegative [″ + L. negare, to deny]

electroneurolysis (ē-lěk″trō-nū-rŏl′ĭ-sĭs)

electronic

electronics

electronic voice

electronization [Gr. elektron, amber]

electron microscope

electron volt

electronystagmography (ē-lěk″trō-nĭs″tăg-mŏg′ră-fē) [″ + nystagmos, drowsiness, + graphein, to write]

electro-oculogram (ē-lěk″trō-ŏk′ū-lō-grăm″)

electropathology (ē-lěk″trō-pă-thŏl′ō-jē) [″ + pathos, disease, suffering, + logos, word, reason]

electrophoresis (ē-lěk″trō-for-ē′sĭs) [″ + phoresis, bearing]

electrophorus (ē-lěk″trŏf′ō-rŭs) [″ + phorein, to bear]

electrophrenic (ē-lěk″trō-frěn′ĭk)

electrophrenic respiration

electrophysiology (ē-lěk″trō-fĭz″ē-ŏl′ō-gē) [″ + physis, nature, + logos, word, reason]

electropositive [″ + L. positivus, to put, place]

electropuncture [″ + L. punctura, prick]

electroradiometer (ē-lěk″trō-rā-dē-ŏm′ě-těr) [″ + L. radius, ray, + Gr. metron, measure]

electroresection (ē-lěk″trō-rē-sěk′shŭn)

electroretinogram (ē-lěk″trō-rět′ĭ-nō-grăm)

electroscission (ē-lĕk"trō-sĭ'zhŭn) [" + L. *scindere*, to cut]

electroscope (ē-lĕk'trō-skōp) [" + *skopein*, to examine]

electroshock

electroshock therapy

electrosleep

electrostatic [Gr. *elektron*, amber, + *statikos*, causing to stand]

electrostatic generator

electrostatic unit

electrostimulation (ē-lĕk"trō-stĭm"ū-lā'shŭn)

electrosurgery (ē-lĕk"trō-sŭr'jē-rē) [" + L. *chirurgia*, surgery]

electrosynthesis (ē-lĕk"trō-sĭn'thē-sĭs)

electrotaxis (ē-lĕk"trō-tăk'sĭs) [" + *taxis*, arrangement]

electrothanasia (ē-lĕk"trō-thă-nā'zē-ă) [" + *thanatos*, death]

electrotherapeutics (ē-lĕk"trō-thĕr-ă-pū'tĭks) [" + *therapeutike*, treatment]

electrotherapist (ē-lĕk"trō-thĕr'ă-pĭst) [" + *therapeia*, treatment]

electrotherapy

electrothermotherapy (ē-lĕk"trō-thĕr"mō-thĕr'ă-pē) [" + " + *therapeia*, treatment]

electrotome (ē-lĕk'trō-tōm) [" + *tome*, a cutting, slice]

electrotonic (ē-lĕk"trō-tŏn'ĭk) [" + *tonos*, act of stretching, tension, tone]

electrotonus (ē-lĕk-trŏt'ō-nŭs)

electrotropism (ē-lĕk-trŏt'rō-pĭzm) [" + *trope*, a turning, + *-ismos*, condition]

electrovalence (ē-lĕk"trō-vā'lĕns)

electroversion (ē-lĕk"trō-vĕr'zhŭn)

electuary (ē-lĕk'tū-ă-rē) [Gr. *ekleikhein*, to lick up]

eleidin (ē-lē'ĭ-dĭn) [Gr. *elaion*, oil]

element [L. *elementum*, a rudiment]
   e.'s, trace

eleoma (ĕl"ē-ō'mă) [Gr. *elaion*, oil, + *oma*, tumor]

eleopathy (ĕl"ē-ŏp'ă-thē) [" + *pathos*, disease, suffering]

eleoptene (ĕl-ē-ŏp'tēn) [" + *ptenos*, fleeting]

eleosaccharum (ĕl"ē-ō-săk'ă-rŭm) [" + *sakcharon*, sugar]

eleotherapy (ĕl"ē-ō-thĕr'ă-pē) [Gr. *elaion*, oil, + *therapeia*, treatment]

elephantiasis (ĕl"ĕ-făn-tī'ă-sĭs) [Gr. *elephas*, elephant, + *-iasis*, state or condition of]
   e., scrotal

elevation (ĕl"ĕ-vā'shŭn)
   e.'s, tactile

elevator [L. *elevare*, to raise up, lighten]
   e., periosteal

eleventh cranial nerve

eliminant (ē-lĭm'ĭ-nănt) [L. *e*, out, + *limen*, threshold]

eliminate (ē-lĭm'ĭ-nāt)

elimination

elimination diet

elinguation (ē"lĭn-gwā'shŭn) [" + *lingua*, tongue]

ELISA *enzyme-linked immunoabsorbent assay*

elixir (ē-lĭk'sĕr) [L. from Arabic *al-iksir*]

Elixophyllin

ellipsis (ē-lĭp'sĭs) [Gr. *elleipsis*, condition of falling short, defect]

ellipsoid (ē-lĭp'soyd)

elliptocyte (ē-lĭp'tō-sīt)

elliptocytosis (ē-lĭp"tō-sī-tō'sĭs)
   e., hereditary

Ellis-van Creveld syndrome

elongation (ē"lŏng-gā'shŭn)

elope

eluate (ĕl'ū-āt)

eluent (ē-lū'ĕnt)

elution (ē-lū'shŭn) [L. *e*, out, + *luere*, to wash]

elutriation (ē-lū-trē-ā'shŭn) [L. *elutriare*, to cleanse]

emaciate (ē-mā'sē-āt) [L. *emaciare*, to make thin]

emaciated

emaciation

emaculation (ĕm-ăk"ū-lā'shŭn) [L. *emaculare*, to remove spots]

emailloid (ā-mī'loyd) [Fr. *email*,

enamel, + Gr. *eidos,* form, shape]
emanation [L. *e,* out, + *manare,*
to flow]
  e., actinium
  e., radium
  e., thorium
emasculation (ē-măs"kū-lā'shŭn) [L.
emasculare, to castrate]
embalming (ĕm-bäm'ĭng) [L. *im-,* on,
+ *balsamum,* balsam]
embarrass (ĕm-băr'ăs)
Embden-Meyerhof pathway [G.
G. Embden, Ger. chemist, 1874–
1933; O. Meyerhof, Ger. biochemist,
1884–1951]
embedding [" + AS. *bedd,* to
bed]
embolalia, embololalia (ĕm"bō-
lā'lē-ă, ĕm"bō-lō-lā'lē-ă) [Gr. *embolos,*
stopper, + *lalia,* chatter, prattle]
embole (ĕm'bō-lē) [Gr. *emballein,* to
throw in]
embolectomy (ĕm"bō-lĕk'tō-mē)
[" + *ektome,* excision]
embolic
emboliform [" + L. *forma,* form]
embolism (ĕm'bō-lĭzm) [NL. *embolismus,* intercalary, + *-ismos,* con-
dition]
  e., air
  e., fat
  e., pulmonary
  e., pyemic
embolophrasia (ĕm"bō-lō-frā'zē-ă)
[" + *phrasis,* diction]
embolus (ĕm'bō-lŭs) [Gr. *embolos,*
stopper]
  e., air
  e., amniotic fluid
  e., coronary
  e., pulmonary
emboly (ĕm'bō-lē) [Gr. *emballein,* to
throw in]
embolysis (ĕm-bŏl'ĭ-sĭs)
embrace reflex
embrasure (ĕm-brā'zhŭr) [Fr. *em-
braser,* to widen an opening]
  e., buccal

  e., labial
  e., lingual
  e., occlusal
embrocation (ĕm"brō-kā'shŭn) [Gr.
embroche, lotion]
embryectomy (ĕm"brē-ĕk'tō-mē) [Gr.
embryon, to swell inside, + *ektome,* excision]
embryo (ĕm'brē-ō) [Gr. *embryon,* to
swell inside]
embryocardia (ĕm"brē-ō-kăr'dē-ă)
[" + *kardia,* heart]
embryocidal (ĕm"brē-ō-sī'dal) [Gr.
embryon, to swell inside, + L. *cida*
fr. *caedere,* to kill]
embryoctony (ĕm"brē-ŏk'tō-nē)
[" + *kteinein,* to kill]
embryogenetic, **embryogenic**
[" + *gennan,* to produce]
embryogeny (ĕm"brē-ŏj'ĕ-nē)
embryography [" + *graphein,* to
write]
embryology [" + *logos,* word,
reason]
embryoma (ĕm-brē-ō'mă) [" +
oma, tumor]
embryonal (ĕm'brē-ō-năl)
embryonic (ĕm"brē-ŏn'ĭk) [Gr. *embryon,* to swell inside]
embryonization
embryonoid (ĕm'brē-ō-noyd) [" +
eidos, form, shape]
embryopathy (ĕm"brē-ŏp'ă-thē)
[" + *pathos,* disease, suffering]
embryoplastic [" + *plassein,* to
form]
embryoscopy
embryotocia (ĕm"brē-ō-tō'sē-ă)
[" + *tokos,* birth]
embryotome (ĕm'brē-ō-tōm") [" +
tome, a cutting, slice]
embryotomy (ĕm"brē-ŏt'ō-mē)
embryotoxon (ĕm"brē-ō-tŏks'ŏn)
[" + *toxon,* bow]
embryo transfer
embryotroph (ĕm'brē-ō-trōf) [" +
trophe, nourishment]
embryotrophy (ĕm"brē-ŏt'rō-fē)

embryulcia (ĕm"brē-ŭl'sē-ă) [" + elkein, to draw]

embryulcus (ĕm"brē-ŭl'kŭs) [Gr. embryoulkos, forceps]

emedullate (ē-mĕd'ū-lāt) [L. e, out, + medulla, marrow]

emergency [L. emergere, to raise up]

emergency cardiac care

emergency medical technician

emergency readiness

Emergency Room

emergent [L. emergere, to raise up]

emesis (ĕm'ĕ-sĭs) [Gr. emein, to vomit]
    e., gastric
    e. gravidarum
    e., irritation
    e., nervous
    e., reflex

emesis basin

emetic (ē-mĕt'ĭk) [Gr. emein, to vomit]
    e., direct
    e., indirect

emetine (ĕm'ĕ-tēn) [Gr. emein, to vomit]
    e. bismuth iodide
    e. hydrochloride

emetism [" + -ismos, condition]

emetocathartic (ĕm"ĕ-tō-kă-thăr'tĭk) [" + kathartikos, purging]

emetology (ĕm"ĕ-tŏl'ō-jē) [" + logos, word, reason]

E.M.F. electromotive force; erythrocyte maturation factor

EMG electromyogram

emigration [L. e, out, + migrare, to move]

eminence [" + minere, to hang on]
    e., arcuate
    e., articular, of the temporal bone
    e., auditory
    e., bicipital
    e., blastodermic
    e., canine
    e., collateral
    e., frontal
    e., germinal
    e., hypothenar
    e., iliopectineal
    e., intercondyloid

    e., mamillary
    e., median
    e., nasal
    e., occipital
    e. of Doyère
    e., olivary
    e., parietal
    e.'s, portal
    e., pyramidal
    e., thenar

eminentia (ĕm"ĭn-ĕn'shē-ă) [L.]

emiocytosis (ē"mē-ō-sī-tō'sĭs) [L. emitto, to send forth, + Gr. kytos, cell, + osis, condition]

emissary (ĕm'ĭ-să-rē) [L. e, out, + mittere, to send]

emissary veins

emissio (ē-mĭs'sē-ō) [L.] discharge; emission

emission (ē-mĭsh'ŭn) [L. e, out, + mittere, to send]
    e., nocturnal
    e., thermionic

emmenagogue (ĕm-ĕn'ă-gŏg) [Gr. emmena, menses, + agogos, leading]
    e., direct
    e., indirect

emmenia (ĕ-mē'nē-ă) [Gr. emmena]

emmenic

emmeniopathy (ĕ-mē"nē-ŏp'ă-thē) [Gr. emmena, menses, + pathos, disease, suffering]

emmenology (ĕm"ĕn-ŏl'ō-jē) [" + logos, word, reason]

emmetrope (ĕm'ĕ-trōp) [Gr. emmetros, in measure, + opsis, sight, appearance, vision]

emmetropia (ĕm"ĕ-trō'pē-ă)

emmetropic

Emmet's operation [Thomas A. Emmet, U.S. gynecologist, 1828–1919]

emollient (ē-mŏl'yĕnt) [L. e, out, + mollire, to soften]

emotion (ē-mō'shŭn) [L. emovere, to stir up]

emotional [L. emovere, to stir up]

emotional need
emotivity (ē"mō-tĭv'ĭ-tē)
empasm, empasma (ĕm'păzm, ĕm-păs'mă) [Gr. *en*, in, + *passein*, to sprinkle]
empathic [" + *pathos*, disease, suffering]
empathy (ĕm'pă-thē)
emperipolesis (ĕm-pĕr"ĭ-pō-lē'sĭs) [Gr. *en*, into, + *peripolesis*, a going about]
emperor of pruritus
emphractic (ĕm-frăk'tĭk) [Gr. *emphraxis*, an obstruction]
emphraxis (ĕm-frăk'sĭs) [Gr.]
emphysatherapy (ĕm"fĭz-ă-thĕr'ă-pē) [Gr. *emphysan*, to inflate, + *therapeia*, treatment]
emphysema (ĕm"fĭ-sē'mă) [Gr. *emphysan*, to inflate]
emphysematous (ĕm"fĭ-sĕm'ă-tŭs)
empiric (ĕm-pĭr'ĭk) [Gr. *empeirikos*, skilled, experienced]
empirical (ĕm-pĭr'ĭk-ăl)
empiricism (ĕm-pĭr'ĭs-ĭzm) [Gr. *empeirikos*, skilled, experienced, + *-ismos*, condition]
Empirin
emplastic (ĕm-plăs'tĭk) [Gr. *emplastikos*, clogging]
emplastrum [L.]
emprosthotonos (ĕm"prŏs-thŏt'ō-nŏs) [Gr. *emprosthen*, forward, + *tonos*, act of stretching, tension, tone]
empty follicle syndrome
empty-sella syndrome
emptysis (ĕmp'tĭ-sĭs) [Gr., a spitting]
empyema (ĕm"pī-ē'mă) [Gr.]
  e., interlobular
  e. necessitatis
  e., pulsating
empyesis (ĕm"pī-ē'sĭs) [Gr., suppuration]
empyocele (ĕm'pī-ō-sēl) [Gr. *empyein*, to suppurate, + *kele*, tumor, swelling]
empyreuma (ĕm"pī-roo'mă) [Gr., a live coal]

EMS *emergency medical service*
EMT *emergency medical technician*
emulsification (ē-mŭl"sĭ-fĭ-kă'shŭn) [L. *emulsio*, emulsion, + *facere*, to make]
emulsifier
emulsify (ē-mŭl'sĭ-fĭ)
emulsion [L. *emulsio*]
emulsoid (ē-mŭl'soyd) [" + Gr. *eidos*, form, shape]
emunctory (ē-mŭnk'tō-rē) [L. *emungere*, to cleanse]
E.N.A. *extractable nuclear antigen*
enamel (ĕn-ăm'ĕl) [O. Fr. *esmail*, enamel]
  e., aprismatic
  e., cervical
  e., gnarled
  e. hypoplasia
  e., mottled
enamel organ
enamelum
enanthem, enanthema (ĕn-ăn'thĕm, -ăn-thē'mă) [Gr. *en*, in, + *anthema*, blossoming]
enanthematous (ĕn"ăn-thĕm'ă-tŭs)
enanthesis (ĕn"ăn-thē'sĭs) [Gr. *en*, in, + *anthein*, to bloom]
enanthrope (ĕn-ăn'thrōp) [" + *anthropos*, man]
enantiobiosis (ĕn-ăn"tē-ō-bī-ō'sĭs) [Gr. *enantios*, opposite, + *bios*, life]
enantiomorph (ĕn-ăn'tē-ō-morf")
enantiopathy (ĕn-ăn"tē-ŏp'ă-thē) [" + *pathos*, disease, suffering]
enarthritis (ĕn"ăr-thrī'tĭs) [Gr. *en*, in, + *arthron*, joint, + *itis*, inflammation]
enarthrosis (ĕn"ăr-thrō'sĭs) [" + *arthron*, joint, + *osis*, condition]
en bloc (ĕn blŏk) [Fr., as a whole]
encanthis (ĕn-kăn'thĭs) [Gr. *en*, in, + *kanthos*, corner of the eye]
encapsulation [" + *capsula*, a little box]
encatarrhaphy (ĕn"kăt-ăr'ă-fē) [Gr. *enkatarrhaptein*, to sew in]

enceinte (ŏn-sănt') [Fr.] pregnant
encephalalgia (ĕn-sĕf″ăl-ăl'jē-ă) [Gr. enkephalos, brain, + algos, pain]
encephalatrophy (ĕn-sĕf″ă-lăt'rō-fē) [″ + a-, not, + trophe, nourishment]
encephalic (ĕn″sĕf-ăl'ĭk) [Gr. enkephalos, brain]
encephalitis (ĕn-sĕf″ă-lī'tĭs) [″ + itis, inflammation]
    e., acute disseminated
    e., cortical
    e., epidemic
    e., equine
    e., equine, eastern
    e., equine, western
    e., hemorrhagic
    e., herpes
    e. hyperplastica
    e., infantile
    e., Japanese (B type)
    e., lead
    e. lethargica
    e., meningo-
    e. neonatorum
    e. periaxialis
    e., postinfection
    e., postvaccinal
    e., purulent
    e., Russian spring-summer
    e., St. Louis
    e., toxic
encephalocele (ĕn-sĕf'ă-lō-sēl) [Gr. enkephalos, brain, + kele, tumor, swelling]
encephalocystocele (ĕn-sĕf″ă-lō-sĭs'tō-sēl) [″ + kystis, sac, + kele, tumor, swelling]
encephalogram (ĕn-sĕf'ă-lō-grăm) [″ + gramma, letter, piece of writing]
encephalography (ĕn-sĕf″ă-lŏg'ră-fē) [″ + graphein, to write]
encephaloid (ĕn-sĕf'ă-loyd) [″ + eidos, form, shape]
encephalolith (ĕn-sĕf'ă-lō-lĭth) [″ + lithos, stone]
encephaloma (ĕn-sĕf″ă-lō-mă) [″ + oma, tumor]

encephalomalacia (ĕn-sĕf″ă-lō-mă-lā'sē-ă) [″ + malakia, softening]
encephalomeningitis (ĕn-sĕf″ă-lō-mĕn″ĭn-jī'tĭs) [″ + meninx, membrane, + itis, inflammation]
encephalomeningocele (ĕn-sĕf″ă-lō-mĕ-nĭng'gŏ-sēl) [″ + ″ + kele, tumor, swelling]
encephalomere (ĕn-sĕf'ă-lō-mēr″) [″ + meros, part]
encephalometer (ĕn-sĕf″ă-lŏm'ĕ-tĕr) [″ + metron, measure]
encephalomyelitis (ĕn-sĕf″ă-lō-mī-ĕl-ī'tĭs) [″ + myelos, marrow, + itis, inflammation]
    e., acute disseminated
    e., benign myalgic
    e., equine
    e., postinfectious
    e., postvaccinal
encephalomyeloneuropathy (ĕn-sĕf″ă-lō-mī″ĕ-lō-nū-rŏp'ă-thē)
encephalomyelopathy (ĕn-sĕf″ă-lō-mī″ĕl-ŏp'ă-thē) [″ + ″ + pathos, disease, suffering]
encephalomyeloradiculitis (ĕn-sĕf″ă-lō-mī″ĕ-lō-ră-dĭk″ū-lī'tĭs)
encephalomyocarditis (ĕn-sĕf″ă-lō-mī″ō-kăr-dī'tĭs)
encephalon (ĕn-sĕf'ă-lŏn) [Gr. enkephalos, brain]
encephalopathy (ĕn-sĕf″ă-lŏp'ă-thē) [″ + pathos, disease, suffering]
    e., hepatic
encephalopuncture (ĕn-sĕf″ă-lō-punk'tūr) [″ + L. punctura, prick]
encephalopyosis (ĕn-sĕf″ă-lō-pī-ō'sĭs) [″ + pyosis, suppuration]
encephalorrhagia (ĕn-sĕf″ă-lō-ră'jē-ă) [″ + rhegnynai, to burst forth]
encephalosclerosis (ĕn-sĕf″ă-lō-sklĕ-rō'sĭs) [″ + sklerosis, a hardening]
encephalosis [″ + osis, condition]
encephalospinal [″ + L. spina, thorn, spine]
encephalotome (ĕn-sĕf'ă-lō-tŏm) [Gr. enkephalos, brain, + tome, a cutting, slice]
encephalotomy (ĕn-sĕf″ă-lŏt'ō-mē)

enchondroma (ĕn″kŏn-drō′mă) [Gr. en, in, + chondros, cartilage, + oma, tumor]

enchondrosarcoma (ĕn-kŏn″drō-săr-kō′mă) [″ + ″ + sarx, flesh, + oma, tumor]

enchondrosis (ĕn-kŏn-drō′sĭs) [″ + ″ + osis, condition]

enclave (ĕn′klāv) [Fr. enclaver, to enclose]

enclitic (ĕn-klĭt′ĭk) [Gr. enklinein, to lean on]

encolpitis (ĕn-kŏl-pī′tĭs) [Gr. en, in, + kolpos, vagina, + itis, inflammation]

encopresis (ĕn-kō-prē′sĭs) [″ + kopros, excrement]

encranial [″ + kranion, cranium]

encyesis (ĕn″sĭ-ē′sĭs) [″ + kyesis, pregnancy]

encysted (ĕn-sĭst′ĕd) [″ + kystis, bladder, pouch]

end [AS. ende]

endadelphos (ĕnd″ă-dĕl′fŏs) [Gr. endon, within, + adelphos, brother]

Endamoeba (ĕn″dă-mē′bă)

endangeitis, endangiitis (ĕnd″ăn-jē-ī′tĭs) [Gr. endon, within, + angeion, vessel, + itis, inflammation]

endangium (ĕn-dăn′jē-ŭm) [″ + angeion, vessel]

endaortitis (ĕnd″ā-or-tī′tĭs) [″ + aorte, aorta, + itis, inflammation]

endarterectomy (ĕnd″ăr-tĕr-ĕk′tō-mē)

endarterial (ĕnd″ăr-tē′rē-ăl) [″ + arteria, artery]

endarteritis, endoarteritis (ĕnd-ăr-tĕr-ī′tĭs) [″ + ″ + itis, inflammation]

    e., acute

    e., chronic

    e. deformans

    e. obliterans

    e., syphilitic

end artery

endbrain

end-bud

end-bulb

    e. of Krause

endemic [Gr. en, in, + demos, people]

endemoepidemic (ĕn-dĕm″ō-ĕp-ĭ-dĕm′ĭk) [″ + ″ + epi, on, among, + demos, people]

endergonic (ĕnd″ĕr-gŏn′ĭk) [Gr. endon, within, + ergon, work]

endermatic, endermic [Gr. endon, within, + derma, skin]

endermosis [″ + ″ + osis, condition]

end-feet

ending

endoaneurysmorrhaphy (ĕn″dō-ăn″ū-rĭs-mor′ăf-ē) [Gr. endon, within, + aneurysma, aneurysm, + rhaphe, seam]

endoangiitis (ĕn″dō-ăn-jē-ī′tĭs) [″ + angeion, vessel, + itis, inflammation]

endoantitoxin (ĕn″dō-ăn-tē-tŏk′sĭn) [″ + anti, against, + toxikon, poison]

endoappendicitis (ĕn″dō-ă-pĕn″dĭ-sī′tĭs) [″ + L. appendere, to hang, + Gr. itis, inflammation]

endoauscultation (ĕn″dō-aws″kŭl-tā′shŭn) [″ + L. auscultare, to listen to]

endobiotic (ĕn″dō-bī-ŏt′ĭk) [″ + bios, life]

endoblast (ĕn′dō-blăst) [″ + blastos, germ]

endobronchitis (ĕn″dō-brŏng-kī′tĭs)

endocardiac, endocardial [″ + kardia, heart]

endocarditis (ĕn″dō-kar-dī′tĭs) [″ + ″ + itis, inflammation]

    e., acute bacterial

    e., atypical verrucous

    e., bacterial

    e., chronic

    e., infective

    e., Libman-Sacks

    e., malignant

    e., mural

    e., rheumatic

e., subacute bacterial
e., syphilitic
e., tuberculous
e., ulcerative
e., valvular
e., vegetative
e., verrucous
e. viridans

endocardium [Gr. *endon*, within, + *kardia*, heart]

endocervical (ĕn"dō-sĕr'vĭ-kăl) [" + L. *cervix*, neck]

endocervicitis (ĕn"dō-sĕr"vĭ-sī'tĭs) [" + " + Gr. *itis*, inflammation]

endocervix (ĕn"dō-sĕr'vĭks) [" + L. *cervix*, neck]

endochondral (ĕn"dō-kŏn'drăl) [" + *chondros*, cartilage]

endochorion (ĕn"dō-kō'rē-ŏn) [" + *chorion*, chorion]

endocolitis (ĕn"dō-kō-lī'tĭs) [" + *kolon*, colon, + *itis*, inflammation]

endocolpitis (ĕn"dō-kŏl-pī'tĭs) [" + *kolpos*, vagina, + *itis*, inflammation]

endocorpuscular (ĕn"dō-kor-pŭs'kū-lăr) [" + L. *corpusculum*, small body (corpuscle)]

endocranial (ĕn"dō-krā'nē-ăl) [" + *kranion*, cranium]

endocranitis (ĕn"dō-krā-nī'tĭs) [" + " + *itis*, inflammation]

endocranium (ĕn"dō-krā'nē-ŭm)

endocrinasthenia (ĕn"dō-krĭn"ăs-thē'nē-ă) [Gr. *endon*, within, + *krinein*, to secrete, + *astheneia*, weakness]

endocrine (ĕn'dō-krīn, -krĭn, -krēn) [" + *krinein*, to secrete]

endocrine gland

endocrino- [Gr. *endon*, within, + *krinein*, to secrete]

endocrinology (ĕn"dō-krĭn-ŏl'ō-jē) [" + " + *logos*, word, reason]

endocrinopathic

endocrinopathy (ĕn"dō-krĭn-ŏp'ă-thē) [" + " + *pathos*, disease, suffering]

endocrinotherapy (ĕn"dō-krĭn"ō-thĕr'ă-pē) [" + " + *therapeia*, treatment]

endocyst (ĕn'dō-sĭst) [" + *kystis*, bladder, pouch]

endocystitis (ĕn"dō-sĭs-tī'tĭs) [" + " + *itis*, inflammation]

endocytosis

endoderm (ĕn'dō-dĕrm) [" + *derma*, skin]

endodermal

Endodermophyton (ĕn"dō-dĕr-mŏf'ĭ-tŏn) [" + *derma*, skin, + *phyton*, a growth]

endodiascope (ĕn"dō-dī'ă-skōp) [" + *dia*, through, + *skopein*, to examine]

endodiascopy (ĕn"dō-dī-ăs'kō-pē)

endodontia (ĕn"dō-dŏn'shē-ă) [" + *odous*, tooth]

endodontics (ĕn"dō-dŏn'tĭks)

endodontist

endodontitis (ĕn"dō-dŏn-tī'tĭs) [" + *odous*, tooth, + *itis*, inflammation]

endodontium

endodontologist

endodontology

endoectothrix (ĕn"dō-ĕk'tō-thrĭks) [" + *ektos*, out of, + *thrix*, hair]

endoenteritis (ĕn"dō-ĕn"tĕr-ī'tĭs) [" + *enteron*, intestine, + *itis*, inflammation]

endoenzyme (ĕn"dō-ĕn'zīm) [" + *en*, in, + *zyme*, leaven]

endogamy (ĕn-dŏg'ă-mē) [" + *gamos*, marriage]

endogastric (ĕn"dō-găs'trĭk) [" + *gaster*, belly]

endogastritis (ĕn"dō-găs-trī'tĭs) [" + " + *itis*, inflammation]

endogenic (ĕn"dō-jĕn'ĭk) [" + *gennan*, to produce]

endogenous (ĕn-dŏj'ĕ-nŭs)

endogenous opiate-like substance

endogeny (ĕn-dŏj'ĕ-nē)

endoglobar, endoglobular (ĕn"dō-glōb'ăr, ĕn"dō-glŏb'ū-lăr) [Gr. *endon*, within, + L. *globulus*, a globule]

endognathion (ĕn″dō-năth′ē-ŏn) [Gr. *endon*, within, + *gnathos*, jaw]

endointoxication (ĕn″dō-ĭn-tŏk″sĭ-kā′shŭn) [″ + L. *in*, into, + Gr. *toxikon*, poison]

endolabyrinthitis (ĕn″dō-lăb″ĭ-rĭn-thī′tĭs) [″ + *labyrinthos*, labyrinth, + *itis*, inflammation]

endolaryngeal (ĕn″dō-lă-rĭn′jē-ăl) [″ + *larynx*, larynx]

Endolimax nana (ĕn″dō-lī′măks nă′nă) [″ + *leimax*, meadow]

endolumbar [″ + L. *lumbus*, loin]

endolymph (ĕn′dō-lĭmf) [″ + L. *lympha*, clear fluid]

endolymphatic

endolymphatic duct

endolysin (ĕn-dŏl′ĭ-sĭn) [″ + *lysis*, dissolution]

endolysis

endomastoiditis (ĕn″dō-măs″toy-dī′tĭs) [″ + *mastos*, breast, + *eidos*, form, shape, + *itis*, inflammation]

endometer (ĕn-dŏm′ĕ-tĕr)

endometrectomy (ĕn″dō-mē-trĕk′tō-mē) [″ + *metra*, uterus, + *ektome*, excision]

endometrial (ĕn″dō-mē′trē-ăl) [″ + *metra*, uterus]

endometrial cyst

endometrial dating

endometrial jet washing

endometrioma (ĕn″dō-mē″trē-ō′mă) [Gr. *endon*, within, + *metra*, uterus, + *oma*, tumor]

endometriosis (ĕn″dō-mē″trē-ō′sĭs) [″ + ″ + *osis*, condition]

  e., direct

  e., implantation

  e., internal

  e., metastatic

  e., peritoneal

  e., primary

  e., transplantation

endometritis (ĕn″dō-mē-trī′tĭs) [″ + ″ + *itis*, inflammation]

  e., cervical

  e., decidual

  e. dissecans

  e., puerperal

endometrium (ĕn-dō-mē′trē-ŭm) [Gr. *endon*, within, + *metra*, uterus]

endometry (ĕn-dŏm′ĕ-trē) [Gr. *endon*, within, + *metron*, measure]

endomorph (ĕn″dō-morf′) [″ + *morphe*, form]

endomyocarditis (ĕn″dō-mī-ō-kăr-dī′tĭs) [″ + *mys*, muscle, + *kardia*, heart, + *itis*, inflammation]

endomysium (ĕn″dō-mīs′ē-ŭm) [″ + *mys*, muscle]

endoneuritis [″ + *neuron*, nerve, + *itis*, inflammation]

endoneurium (ĕn″dō-nū′rē-ŭm)

endonuclease (ĕn″dō-nū′klē-ās)

endoparasite (ĕn″dō-păr′ă-sīt) [″ + *para*, alongside, past, beyond, + *sitos*, food]

endopathy (ĕn″dŏp′ă-thē) [″ + *pathos*, disease, suffering]

endopelvic (ĕn″dō-pĕl′vĭk) [″ + L. *pelvis*, basin]

endopelvic fasciae

endopeptidase (ĕn″dō-pĕp′tĭ-dās)

endopericarditis (ĕn″dō-pĕr″ĭ-kăr-dī′tĭs) [″ + *peri*, around, + *kardia*, heart, + *itis*, inflammation]

endoperimyocarditis (ĕn″dō-pĕr″ĭ-mī″ō-kăr-dī′tĭs) [″ + ″ + *mys*, muscle, + *kardia*, heart, + *itis*, inflammation]

endoperitonitis (ĕn″dō-pĕr″ĭ-tō-nī′tĭs) [″ + *peritonaion*, stretched around or over, + *itis*, inflammation]

endophasia (ĕn″dō-fā′zē-ă) [″ + *phasis*, utterance]

endophlebitis (ĕn″dō-flē-bī′tĭs) [″ + *phleps*, blood vessel, vein, + *itis*, inflammation]

  e. obliterans

  e. portalis

endophthalmitis (ĕn″dŏf-thăl-mī′tĭs) [″ + *ophthalmos*, eye, + *itis*, inflammation]

endoplasm [" + LL. *plasma,* form, mold]

endoplasmic reticulum

end organ

  e., neuromuscular

  e., neurotendinous

  e., sensory

endorhinitis (ĕn″dō-rī-nī′tĭs) [Gr. *endon,* within, + *rhis,* nose, + *itis,* inflammation]

endorphins (ĕn-dor′fĭns, ĕn′dor-fĭns)

endorrhachis (ĕn″dō-rā′kĭs) [" + *rhachis,* spine]

endosalpingitis (ĕn″dō-săl″pĭn-jī′tĭs) [" + *salpinx,* tube, + *itis,* inflammation]

endosalpingoma (ĕn″dō-săl″pĭn-gō′mă)

endosalpinx (ĕn″dō-săl′pĭnks) [" + *salpinx,* tube]

endoscope (ĕn″dō-skōp) [" + *skopein,* to examine]

endoscopy (ĕn-dŏs′kō-pē)

endosepsis (ĕn″dō-sĕp′sĭs) [" + *sepsis,* decay]

endoskeleton [" + *skeleton,* skeleton]

endosmometer (ĕn″dŏs-mŏm′ĕ-tĕr) [" + *osmos,* a thrusting, + *metron,* measure]

endosmosis (ĕn″dŏs-mō′sĭs) [" + " + *osis,* condition]

endosome (ĕn′dō-sōm) [" + L. *soma,* body]

endospore [" + *sporos,* seed]

endosteitis (ĕn″dŏs-tē-ī′tĭs) [" + *osteon,* bone, + *itis,* inflammation]

endosteoma (ĕn-dŏs″tē-ō′mă) [" + " + *oma,* tumor]

endosteum (ĕn-dŏs′tē-ŭm) [" + *osteon,* bone]

endostitis (ĕn″dŏs-tī′tĭs) [" + " + *itis,* inflammation]

endostoma (ĕn-dŏs-tō′mă) [" + " + *oma,* tumor]

endostosis (ĕn″dŏs-tō′sĭs) [" + " + *osis,* condition]

endotendineum (ĕn″dō-tĕn-dĭn′ē-ŭm)

[" + L. *tendo,* tendon]

endothelial (ĕn″dō-thē′lē-ăl) [Gr. *endon,* within, + *thele,* nipple]

endotheliocyte (ĕn″dō-thē′lē-ō-sīt″) [" + " + *kytos,* cell]

endotheliocytosis (ĕn″dō-thē″lē-ō-sī-tō′sĭs) [" + " + " + *osis,* condition]

endotheliolysin (ĕn″dō-thē-lē-ŏl′ĭ-sĭn) [" + *thele,* nipple, + *lysis,* dissolution]

endotheliolytic (ĕn″dō-thē-lē-ō-lĭt′ĭk)

endothelioma (ĕn″dō-thē-lē-ō′mă) [" + *thele,* nipple, + *oma,* tumor]

endotheliomyoma (ĕn″dō-thē″lē-ō-mī-ō′mă) [" + " + *mys,* muscle, + *oma,* tumor]

endotheliomyxoma (ĕn″dō-thē″lē-ō-mĭks-ō′mă) [" + " + *myxa,* mucus, + *oma,* tumor]

endotheliosis (ĕn″dō-thē″lē-ō′sĭs)

endotheliotoxin (ĕn″dō-thē-lē-ō-tŏks′ĭn) [" + " + *toxikon,* poison]

endothelium (ĕn″dō-thē′lē-ŭm) [" + *thele,* nipple]

endothermal, endothermic [Gr. *endon,* within, + *therme,* heat]

endothermy (ĕn′dō-thĕr′mē)

endothrix (ĕn′dō-thrĭks) [" + *thrix,* hair]

endothyropexy (ĕn″dō-thī′rō-pĕks″ē) [" + *thyreos,* shield, + *pexis,* fixation]

endotoscope (ĕn-dō′tō-skōp) [" + *ous,* ear, + *skopein,* to examine]

endotoxemia (ĕn″dō-tŏks-ē′mē-ă)

endotoxicosis (ĕn″dō-tŏk″sĭ-kō′sĭs) [Gr. *endon,* within, + *toxikon,* poison, + *osis,* condition]

endotoxin

endotoxin shock

endotracheal tube, cuffed

endotracheitis (ĕn″dō-trā-kē-ī′tĭs) [" + *tracheia,* trachea, + *itis,* inflammation]

endotrachelitis (ĕn″dō-trā-kĕl-ī′tĭs)

[" + *trachelos*, neck, + *itis*, inflammation]

endovasculitis (ĕn″dō-văs″kū-lī′tĭs) [" + L. *vasculum*, vessel, + Gr. *itis*, inflammation]

endovenous (ĕn″dō-vē′nŭs) [" + L. *vena*, vein]

endplate
    e., motor

end product

end result

Enduron

endyma (ĕn′dĭm-ă) [Gr., a garment]

enema (ĕn′ĕ-mă) [Gr.]
    e., antispasmodic
    e., barium
    e., carminative
    e., cleansing
    e., double-contrast
    e., emollient
    e., high
    e., lubricating
    e., medicinal
    e., nutrient
    e., one-two-three
    e., physiological salt solution
    e., retention
    e., saline
    e., soapsuds

energetics (ĕn″ĕr-jĕt′ĭks)

energy (ĕn′ĕr-jē) [Gr. *energeia*]
    e., conservation of
    e., kinetic
    e., latent
    e., potential
    e., radiant

energy expenditure, basal

enervation [L. *enervatio*]

enflagellation (ĕn″flăj-ĕl-lā′shŭn)

enflurane (ĕn′floo-rān)

ENG *electronystagmography*

engagement

Engelmann's disk [Theodor W. Engelmann, Ger. physiologist, 1843–1909]

engine
    e., dental
    e., high-speed
    e., ultraspeed

englobe [Gr. *en, in*, + L. *globus*, a ball]

engorged (ĕn-gorjd′) [O. Fr. *engorgier*, to obstruct, to devour]

engorgement

engram (ĕn′grăm) [Gr. *engramm*]

enhancement (ĕn-hăns′mĕnt)

enissophobia (ĕn-ĭs″ō-fō′bē-ă) [Gr. *enissein*, to reproach, + *phobos*, fear]

enkatarrhaphy (ĕn″kă-tăr′ăf-ē) [Gr. *enkatarrhaptein*, to sew in]

enkephalins (ĕn-kĕf′ă-lĭns)

enlargement (ĕn-lărj′mĕnt)

enol (ē′nŏl)

enolase (ē′nō-lās)

enology (ē-nŏl′ō-jē) [Gr. *oinos*, wine, + *logos*, word, reason]

enomania (ē″nō-mā′nē-ă) [" + *mania*, madness]

enophthalmos (ĕn″ŏf-thăl′mŭs) [Gr. *en, in*, + *ophthalmos*, eye]

enosimania (ĕn″ŏs-ĭ-mā′nē-ă) [Gr. *enosis*, a quaking, + *mania*, madness]

enostosis (ĕn″ŏs-tō′sĭs) [Gr. *en, in*, + *osteon*, bone, + *osis*, condition]

Enovid, Enovid-E

enriched

ensiform (ĕn′sĭ-form) [L. *ensis*, sword, + *forma*, form]

ensisternum (ĕn″sĭs-tĕr′nŭm) [" + Gr. *sternon*, chest]

enstrophe (ĕn′strō-fē) [Gr. *en, in*, + *strephein*, to turn]

ENT *ear, nose, and throat*

entad (ĕn′tăd) [" + L. *ad*, toward]

ental (ĕn′tăl) [Gr. *entos*, within]

entamebiasis (ĕn″tă-mē-bī′ă-sĭs) [" + *amoibe*, change]

Entamoeba (ĕn″tă-mē′bă)
    E. buccalis
    E. coli
    E. gingivalis
    E. histolytica
    E. kartulisi
    E. tetragena
    E. undulans

enteradenitis (ĕn"tĕr-ăd"ĕ-nī'tĭs) [Gr. *enteron*, intestine, + *aden*, gland, + *itis*, inflammation]

enteral (ĕn'tĕr-ăl) [Gr. *enteron*, intestine]

enteral tube feeding

enteralgia (ĕn"tĕr-ăl'jē-ă) [" + *algos*, pain]

enterectasia (ĕn"tĕr-ĕk-tā'sē-ă) [" + *ektasis*, dilatation]

enterectomy (ĕn"tĕr-ĕk'tō-mē) [" + *ektome*, excision]

enterelcosis (ĕn"tĕr-ĕl-kō'sĭs) [" + *helkosis*, ulceration]

enteric (ĕn-tĕr'ĭk) [Gr. *enteron*, intestine]

enteric-coated

enteric fever

enteritis (ĕn"tĕr-ī'tĭs) [" + *itis*, inflammation]

entero-, enter- [Gr. *enteron*, intestine]

enteroanastomosis (ĕn"tĕr-ō-ăn-ăs"tō-mō'sĭs) [" + *anastomosis*, opening]

enteroantigen (ĕn"tĕr-ō-ăn'tĭ-jĕn) [" + *anti*, against, + *gennan*, to produce]

enteroapokleisis (ĕn"tĕr-ō-ăp"ō-klī'sĭs) [" + *apokleisis*, a shutting out]

Enterobacter
    E. aerogenes

Enterobacteriaceae (ĕn"tĕr-ō-băk-tē"rē-ā'sē-ē)

enterobacteriotherapy (ĕn"tĕr-ō-băk-tē"rē-ō-thĕr'ă-pē) [" + *bakterion*, little rod, + *therapeia*, treatment]

enterobiasis (ĕn"tĕr-ō-bī'ă-sĭs) [Gr. *enteron*, intestine, + *bios*, life]

enterobiliary (ĕn"tĕr-ō-bĭl'ē-ăr-ē) [" + L. *bilis*, bile]

Enterobius (ĕn"tĕr-ō'bē-ŭs) [" + *bios*, life]
    E. vermicularis

enterocele (ĕn'tĕr-ō-sēl) [" + *kele*, tumor, swelling]

enterocentesis (ĕn"tĕr-ō-sĕn-tē'sĭs) [" + *kentesis*, puncture]

enterocholecystostomy (ĕn"tĕr-ō-kō"lē-sĭs-tŏs'tō-mē) [" + *chole*, bile, + *kystis*, bladder, + *stoma*, mouth, opening]

enterocholecystotomy (ĕn"tĕr-ō-kō"lē-sĭs-tŏt'ō-mē) [" + " + " + *tome*, a cutting, slice]

enterocinesia (ĕn"tĕr-ō-sĭn-ē'sē-ă) [" + *kinesis*, motion]

enterocinetic (ĕn"tĕr-ō-sĭn-ĕt'ĭk)

enteroclysis (ĕn"tĕr-ŏk'lĭ-sĭs) [" + *klysis*, a washing]

enterococcus (ĕn"tĕr-ō-kŏk'ŭs)

enterocoele (ĕn'tĕr-ō-sēl) [" + *koilia*, cavity, belly]

enterocolectomy (ĕn"tĕr-ō-kō-lĕk'tō-mē) [" + *kolon*, colon, + *ektome*, excision]

enterocolitis (ĕn"tĕr-ō-kō-lī'tĭs) [" + " + *itis*, inflammation]
    e., neonatal necrotizing

enterocolostomy (ĕn"tĕr-ō-kō-lŏs'tō-mē) [" + " + *stoma*, mouth, opening]

enterocrinin (ĕn"tĕr-ŏk'rĭ-nĭn) [" + *krinein*, to separate]

enterocutaneous (ĕn"tĕr-ō-kū-tā'nē-ŭs)

enterocyst (ĕn'tĕr-ō-sĭst) [Gr. *enteron*, intestine, + *kystis*, bladder]

enterocystocele (ĕn"tĕr-ō-sĭs'tō-sēl) [" + *kele*, tumor, swelling]

enterocystoma (ĕn"tĕr-ō-sĭs-tō'mă) [" + " + *oma*, tumor]

enterocystoplasty (ĕn"tĕr-ō-sĭs'tō-plăs"tē) [" + " + *plastos*, formed]

enterodynia (ĕn"tĕr-ō-dĭn'ē-ă) [" + *odyne*, pain]

enteroenterostomy (ĕn"tĕr-ō-ĕn"tĕr-ŏs'tō-mē) [" + *enteron*, intestine, + *stoma*, mouth, opening]

enteroepiplocele (ĕn"tĕr-ō-ē-pĭp'lō-sēl) [" + *epiploon*, omentum, + *kele*, tumor, swelling]

enterogastritis (ĕn"tĕr-ō-găs-trī'tĭs) [" + *gaster*, belly, + *itis*, inflammation]

enterogastrone (ĕn"tĕr-ō-găs'trōn)

enterogenous (ĕn"tĕr-ŏj'ĕ-nŭs) [" +

gennan, to produce]

enterogram [" + *gramma*, letter, piece of writing]

enterography [" + *graphein*, to write]

enterohepatic (ĕn″tĕr-ō-hĕ-păt′ĭk) [" + *hepar*, liver]

enterohepatitis (ĕn″tĕr-ō-hĕp-ă-tī′tĭs) [" + " + *itis*, inflammation]

enterohydrocele (ĕn″tĕr-ō-hī′drō-sēl) [" + *hydor*, water, + *kele*, tumor, swelling]

enteroidea (ĕn″tĕr-oy′dē-ă) [" + *eidos*, form, shape]

enterokinase (ĕn″tĕr-ō-kī′nās) [" + *kinesis*, motion]

enterokinesia

enterolith (ĕn′tĕr-ō-lĭth) [" + *lithos*, stone]

enterolithiasis (ĕn″tĕr-ō-lĭ-thī′ă-sĭs)

enterology [" + *logos*, word, reason]

enterolysis (ĕn″tĕr-ŏl′ĭ-sĭs) [" + *lysis*, dissolution]

enteromegalia, **enteromegaly** (ĕn″tĕr-ō-mĕ-gā′lē-ă, ĕn″tĕr-ō-mĕg′ă-lē) [" + *megas*, large]

Enteromonas hominis (ĕn″tĕr-ŏm′ō-năs hŏm′ĭn-ĭs)

enteromycosis (ĕn″tĕr-ō-mī-kō′sĭs) [" + *mykes*, fungus, + *osis*, condition]

enteromyiasis (ĕn″tĕr-ō-mī-ī′ă-sĭs) [" + *myia*, fly]

enteron (ĕn′tĕr-ŏn) [Gr.]

enteroneuritis (ĕn″tĕr-ō-nū-rī′tĭs) [" + *neuron*, nerve, + *itis*, inflammation]

enteroparesis (ĕn″tĕr-ō-păr′ē-sĭs) [" + *parienai*, let fall]

enteropathogen (ĕn″tĕr-ō-păth′ō-jĕn) [" + *pathos*, disease, suffering, + *gennan*, to produce]

enteropathy (ĕn″tĕr-ŏp′ă-thē) [" + *pathos*, disease, suffering]

enteropeptidase (ĕn″tĕr-ō-pĕp′tĭ-dās)

enteropexy (ĕn′tĕr-ō-pĕks″ē) [" + *pexis*, fixation]

enteroplasty (ĕn′tĕr-ō-plăs″tē) [" + *plassein*, to form]

enteroplegia (ĕn″tĕr-ō-plē′jē-ă) [" + *plege*, stroke]

enteroplex (ĕn′tĕr-ō-plĕks) [" + *plexis*, a weaving]

enteroplexy

enteroproctia (ĕn″tĕr-ō-prŏk′shē-ă) [" + *proktos*, anus]

enteroptosis (ĕn″tĕr-ŏp-tō′sĭs) [" + *ptosis*, fall, falling]

enterorrhaphy (ĕn″tĕr-or′ă-fē) [" + *rhaphe*, seam]

enterorrhexis (ĕn″tĕr-ō-rĕks′ĭs) [" + *rhexis*, rupture]

enteroscope (ĕn′tĕr-ō-skōp″) [" + *skopein*, to examine]

enterosepsis (ĕn″tĕr-ō-sĕp′sĭs) [" + *sepsis*, decay]

enterospasm (ĕn′tĕr-ō-spăzm) [Gr. *enteron*, intestine, + *spasmos*, a convulsion]

enterostasis (ĕn″tĕr-ō-stā′sĭs) [" + *stasis*, standing still]

enterostenosis (ĕn″tĕr-ō-stĕ-nō′sĭs) [" + *stenosis*, act of narrowing]

enterostomal therapist

enterostomy (ĕn″tĕr-ŏs′tō-mē) [" + *stoma*, mouth, opening]

enterotome (ĕn′tĕr-ō-tōm) [" + *tome*, a cutting, slice]

enterotomy (ĕn-tĕr-ŏt′ō-mē)

enterotoxemia (ĕn″tĕr-ō-tŏk-sē′mē-ă)

enterotoxigenic (ĕn″tĕr-ō-tŏk″sĭ-jĕn′ĭk)

enterotoxin (ĕn″tĕr-ō-tŏk′sĭn) [" + *toxikon*, poison]

enterotoxism

enterotropic [" + *trope*, a turning]

enterovirus

enterozoic (ĕn″tĕr-ō-zō′ĭk) [" + *zoon*, animal]

enterozoon (ĕn″tĕr-ō-zō′ŏn)

entheomania (ĕn″thē-ō-mā′nē-ă) [Gr. *entheos*, inspired, + *mania*, madness]

enthesis (ĕn′thĕ-sĭs) [Gr., a putting in]

enthetic (ĕn-thĕt′ĭk)

enthlasis (ĕn'thlă-sĭs) [Gr., dent caused by pressure]

entity (ĕn'tĭ-tē) [L. *ens*, being]

ento- [Gr. *entos*, within]

entoblast (ĕn'tō-blăst) [" + *blastos*, germ]

entocele (ĕn'tō-sēl) [" + *kele*, tumor, swelling]

entochondrostosis (ĕn"tō-kŏn"drŏs-tō'sĭs) [" + *chondros*, cartilage, + *osis*, condition]

entochoroidea (ĕn"tō-kō-roy'dē-ă) [" + *chorioeides*, choroid]

entocineria (ĕn"tō-sĭn-ē'rē-ă) [" + L. *cinereus*, ashen]

entocone (ĕn'tō-kōn) [" + *konos*, cone]

entocornea (ĕn'tō-kor'nē-ă) [" + L. *corneus*, horny]

entocyte (ĕn'tō-sīt) [" + *kytos*, cell]

entoderm (ĕn'tō-dĕrm) [" + *derma*, skin]

entoectad (ĕn"tō-ĕk'tăd) [" + *ektos*, out of, + L. *ad*, toward]

entome (ĕn'tōm) [Gr. *en*, in, + *tome*, a cutting, slice]

entomion (ĕn-tō'mē-ŏn) [Gr. *entome*, notch]

entomology (ĕn"tō-mŏl'ō-jē) [Gr. *entomon*, insect, + *logos*, word, reason]

   e., medical

entophyte (ĕn'tō-fīt) [Gr. *entos*, within, + *phyton*, plant]

entopic [Gr. *en*, in, + *topos*, place]

entoptic (ĕn-tŏp'tĭk) [Gr. *entos*, within, + *optikos*, seeing]

entoptic phenomena

entoretina (ĕn"tō-rĕt'ĭ-nă) [" + L. *rete*, a net]

entotic (ĕn-tō'tĭk, ĕn-tŏt'ĭk) [" + *ous*, ear]

entozoon (ĕn"tō-zō'ŏn) [" + *zoon*, animal]

entrain

entropion (ĕn-trō'pē-ŏn) [Gr. *en*, in, + *trepein*, to turn]

   e., cicatricial

   e., spastic

entropionize (ĕn-trō'pē-ō-nīz)

entropy (ĕn'trō-pē) [Gr. *en*, in, + *trope*, a turning]

enucleate (ē-nū'klē-āt) [L. *enucleare*, to remove the kernel of]

enucleation (ē-nū"klē-ā'shŭn)

enucleator (ē-nū'klē-ā-tor)

enuresis (ĕn"ū-rē'sĭs) [Gr. *enourein*, to void urine]

   e., diurnal

   e., nocturnal

   e., primary

   e., secondary

envelope (ĕn'vĕ-lōp)

   e., nuclear

envenomation (ĕn-vĕn"ō-mā'shŭn)

environment [O. Fr. *en-*, in, + *viron*, circle]

environmental control unit

envy

enzootic (ĕn"zō-ŏt'ĭk) [Gr. *en*, in, + *zoon*, animal]

enzygotic (ĕn"zī-gŏt'ĭk) [Gr. *en*, in, + *zygon*, yoke]

enzygotic twins

enzyme (ĕn'zīm) [" + *zyme*, leaven]

   e., activating

   e.'s, allosteric

   e., amylolytic

   e., autolytic

   e., bacterial

   e.'s, branching

   e., coagulating

   e., deamidizing

   e., debranching

   e., decarboxylating

   e., digestive

   e., extracellular

   e., fermenting

   e., glycolytic

   e., hydrolytic

   e., inhibitory

   e., inorganic

   e., intracellular

   e., inverting

   e., lipolytic

e., mucolytic
e., oxidizing
e., proteolytic
e., redox
e., reducing
e., respiratory
e., splitting
e., steatolytic
e., transferring
e., uricolytic
e., yellow
enzyme induction
enzyme-linked immunoabsorbent assay
enzymology (ĕn″zī-mŏl′ō-jē)
enzymolysis (ĕn-zī-mŏl′ĭ-sĭs) [Gr. en, in, + zyme, leaven, + lysis, dissolution]
enzymopathy (ĕn″zī-mŏp′ă-thē)
enzymopenia (ĕn-zī″mō-pē′nē-ă)
enzymuria (ĕn″zī-mū′rē-ă) [″ + ″ + ouron, urine]
eonism (ē′ō-nĭzm) [Chevalier d'Eon, Fr. political adventurer, 1728–1810]
EOP external occipital protuberance
eosin (ē′ō-sĭn) [Gr. eos, dawn (rose-colored)]
eosinoblast (ē″ō-sĭn′ō-blăst) [″ + blastos, germ]
eosinopenia (ē″ō-sĭn-ō-pē′nē-ă) [″ + penia, lack]
eosinophil (ē″ō-sĭn′ō-fĭl) [″ + philein, to love]
eosinophile (ē″ō-sĭn′ō-fĭl)
eosinophilia (ē″ō-sĭn-ō-fĭl′ē-ă) [Gr. eos, dawn, + philein, to love]
e., urinary
eosinophilic (ē″ō-sĭn-ō-fĭl′ĭk)
eosinophilic leukocytes
eosinophilous (ē″ō-sĭn-ŏf′ĭ-lŭs) [″ + philein, to love]
eosinotactic (ē″ō-sĭn-ō-tăk′tĭk) [″ + taktikos, arranged]
epactal (ē-păk′tăl) [Gr. epaktos, added to]
eparterial (ĕp″ăr-tē′rē-ăl) [Gr. epi, over, upon, + arteria, artery]
epaxial (ĕp-ăk′sē-ăl) [″ + L. axis, axis]
epencephalon (ĕp″ĕn-sĕf′ă-lŏn) [″ + enkephalos, brain]
ependyma (ĕp-ĕn′dĭ-mă) [Gr. ependyma, an upper garment, wrap]
ependymal (ĕp-ĕn′dĭ-măl)
ependymal cells
ependymal layer
ependymitis (ĕp″ĕn-dĭ-mī′tĭs) [″ + itis, inflammation]
ependymoblast (ĕp-ĕn′dĭ-mō-blăst) [″ + blastos, germ]
ependymocyte (ĕp-ĕn′dĭ-mō-sīt) [″ + kytos, cell]
ependymoma (ĕp-ĕn″dĭ-mō′mă) [″ + oma, tumor]
ephebiatrics (ē-fē-bē-ăt′rĭks) [Gr. epi, at, + hebe, youth, + iatrikos, medical]
ephebic (ē-fē′bĭk) [Gr. ephebikos]
ephebology (ĕf-ē-bŏl′ō-jē) [″ + logos, word, reason]
ephedrine (ĕ-fĕd′rĭn, ĕf′ĕ-drēn)
e. hydrochloride
e. sulfate
ephelis (ĕf-ē′lĭs) [Gr. ephelis, freckle]
ephemeral (ĕ-fĕm′ĕr-ăl) [Gr. epi, on, + hemera, day]
ephidrosis (ĕf″ĭ-drō′sĭs) [Gr., a sweating]
e. cruenta
e. tincta
epi-, ep- [Gr.] upon, over, at, in addition to, after
epiandrosterone (ĕp″ē-ăn-drŏs′tĕr-ōn)
epiblast (ĕp′ĭ-blăst) [Gr. epi, upon, + blastos, germ]
epiblastic (ĕp-ĭ-blăs′tĭk)
epiblepharon (ĕp″ĭ-blĕf′ă-rŏn) [″ + Gr. blepharon, eyelid]
epibole, epiboly (ē-pĭb′ō-lē) [Gr. epibole, cover]
epibulbar (ĕp″ĭ-bŭl′băr)
epicanthus [Gr. epi, upon, + kanthos, corner of the eye]
epicardia (ĕp″ĭ-kărd′ē-ă) [″ + kardia, heart]

epicardium

epichordal (ĕp″ĭ-kord′ăl) [″ + *khorde*, cord]

epichorion (ĕp″ĭ-kō′rē-ŏn) [″ + *chorion*]

epicomus (ē-pĭk′ō-mŭs) [″ + *kome*, hair]

epicondylalgia (ĕp″ĭ-kŏn-dĭ-lăl′jē-ă) [″ + *kondylos*, condyle, + *algos*, pain]

epicondyle (ĕp-ĭ-kŏn′dĭl) [″ + *kondylos*, condyle]

epicondylitis (ĕp″ĭ-kŏn″dĭ-lī′tĭs) [″ + ″ + *itis*, inflammation]
e., lateral humeral

epicranium [″ + *kranion*, cranium]

epicranius (ĕp″ĭ-krā′nē-ŭs)

epicrisis (ĕp′ĭ-krī″sĭs) [″ + *krisis*, crisis]

epicritic (ĕp-ĭ-krĭt′ĭk) [Gr. *epikritikos*, judging]

epicystitis [Gr. *epi*, upon, + *kystis*, bladder, + *itis*, inflammation]

epicystotomy (ĕp″ĭ-sĭs-tŏt′ō-mē) [″ + ″ + *tome*, a cutting, slice]

epicyte (ĕp′ĭ-sīt) [″ + *kytos*, cell]

epidemic (ĕp″ĭ-dĕm′ĭk) [″ + *demos*, people]

epidemic viral gastroenteropathy

epidemiologic (ĕp″ĭ-dē-mē-ŏ-lŏj′ĭk) [″ + *demos*, people, + *logos*, word, reason]

epidemiologist (ĕp″ĭ-dē-mē-ŏl′ō-jĭst)

epidemiology (ĕp″ĭ-dē-mē-ŏl′ō-jē)

epidermal, epidermic [″ + *derma*, skin]

epidermatoplasty (ĕp″ĭ-dĕr-măt′ō-plăs-tē) [″ + ″ + *plassein*, to mold]

epidermis (ĕp″ĭ-dĕr′mĭs) [″ + *derma*, skin]

epidermitis (ĕp″ĭ-dĕr-mī′tĭs) [″ + ″ + *itis*, inflammation]

epidermization (ĕp″ĭ-dĕr″mī-zā′shŭn)

epidermodysplasia verruciformis (ĕp″ĭ-dĕr″mō-dĭs-plā′sē-ă)

epidermoid (ĕp″ĭ-dĕr′moyd) [Gr. *epi*, upon, + *derma*, skin, + *eidos*, form, shape]

epidermolysis (ĕp″ĭ-dĕr-mŏl′ĭ-sĭs) [″ + ″ + *lysis*, dissolution]
e. bullosa

epidermoma (ĕp″ĭ-dĕr-mō′mă) [″ + ″ + *oma*, tumor]

epidermomycosis (ĕp-ĭ-dĕr″mō-mī-kō′sĭs) [″ + ″ + *mykes*, fungus, + *osis*, condition]

Epidermophyton (ĕp″ĭ-dĕr-mŏf′ĭ-tŏn) [″ + ″ + *phyton*, plant]
E. floccosum

epidermophytosis (ĕp″ĭ-dĕr-mō-fĭ-tō′sĭs) [″ + ″ + ″ + *osis*, condition]

epidermosis (ĕp″ĭ-dĕr-mō′sĭs) [″ + ″ + *osis*, condition]

epididymectomy (ĕp″ĭ-dĭd″ĭ-mĕk′tō-mē) [″ + *didymos*, testis, + *ektome*, excision]

epididymis (ĕp″ĭ-dĭd′ĭ-mĭs)

epididymitis (ĕp″ĭ-dĭd″ĭ-mī′tĭs) [″ + *didymos*, testis, + *itis*, inflammation]

epididymodeferentectomy (ĕp″ĭ-dĭd″ĭ-mō-dĕf″ĕr-ĕn-tĕk′tō-mē) [″ + ″ + L. *deferens*, carrying away, + Gr. *ektome*, excision]

epididymodeferential (ĕp″ĭ-dĭd″ĭ-mō-dĕf″ĕr-ĕn′shăl)

epididymography (ĕp″ĭ-dĭd″ĭ-mŏg′ră-fē) [″ + ″ + *graphein*, to write]

epididymoorchitis (ĕp″ĭ-dĭd″ĭm-ō-or-kī′tĭs) [″ + *didymos*, testis, + *orchis*, testis, + *itis*, inflammation]

epididymotomy (ĕp″ĭ-dĭd″ĭ-mŏt′ō-mē) [″ + ″ + *tome*, a cutting, slice]

epididymovasostomy (ĕp-ĭ-dĭd″ĭ-mō-văs-ŏs′tō-mē) [″ + ″ + L. *vas*, vessel, + Gr. *stoma*, mouth, opening]

epididymovesiculography (ĕp″ĭ-dĭd″ĭ-mō-vĕ-sĭk″ū-lŏg′ră-fē)

epidural [Gr. *epi*, upon, + L. *durus*, hard]

epidural space

epifascial (ĕp"ĭ-făsh'ē-ăl)
epifolliculitis (ĕp"ĭ-fŏl-lĭk"ū-lī'tĭs) ["
+ L. *folliculus*, follicle, + Gr. *itis*, inflammation]
epigaster [" + *gaster*, belly]
epigastralgia (ĕp"ĭ-găs-trăl'jē-ă)
[" + " + *algos*, pain]
epigastric
epigastric reflex
epigastrium (ĕp"ĭ-găs'trē-ŭm) ["
+ *gaster*, belly]
epigastrocele (ĕp"ĭ-găs'trō-sēl) ["
+ " + *kele*, tumor, swelling]
epigastrorrhaphy (ĕp"ĭ-găs-tror'ă-
fē) [" + " + *rhaphe*, seam]
epigenesis (ĕp"ĭ-jĕn'ĕ-sĭs) [" +
genesis, generation, birth]
epiglottidean (ĕp"ĭ-glŏ-tĭd'ē-ăn)
[" + *glottis*, tongue]
epiglottidectomy (ĕp"ĭ-glŏt"ĭd-ek'tō-
mē) [" + " + *ektome*, excision]
epiglottiditis (ĕp"ĭ-glŏt"tĭd-ī'tĭs) ["
" + *itis*, inflammation]
epiglottis (ĕp"ĭ-glŏt'ĭs) [Gr.]
epiglottitis (ĕp"ĭ-glŏt-ī'tĭs) [" + *itis*,
inflammation]
epihyal (ĕp-ĭ-hī'ăl)
epilate (ĕp'ĭ-lāt) [L. *e*, out, + *pilus*,
hair]
epilating
epilation (ĕp-ĭ-lā'shŭn)
epilatory (ĕ-pĭl'ă-tor-ē)
epilemma (ĕp-ĭ-lĕm'ă) [Gr. *epi*, upon,
+ *lemma*, husk]
epilepsy (ĕp'ĭ-lĕp"sē) [Gr. *epilepsia*, to
seize]
  e., sleep
  e., television
  e., traumatic
epileptic (ĕp"ĭ-lĕp'tĭk) [Gr. *epileptikos*]
epileptiform (ĕp"ĭ-lĕp'tĭ-form) [Gr.
epilepsia, to seize, + L. *forma*,
form]
epileptogenic, **epileptogenous**
(ĕp"ĭ-lĕp-tō-jĕn'ĭk, -tōj'ĕ-nŭs) ["
+ *gennan*, to produce]
epileptoid [" + *eidos*, form,
shape]

epileptology [" + *logos*, word,
reason]
epiloia (ĕp"ĭ-lŏy'ă)
epimandibular (ĕp"ĭ-măn-dĭb'ū-lăr)
[Gr. *epi*, upon, above, + L. *mandibulum*, jaw]
epimer (ĕp'ĭ-mĕr)
epimere (ĕp'ĭ-mĕr) [Gr. *epi*, upon, +
meros, apart]
epimerite (ĕp"ĭ-mĕr'īt) [" + *meros*,
part]
epimorphosis (ĕp"ĭ-mor'fō-sĭs) ["
+ *morphoun*, to give shape, + *osis*,
condition]
epimysium (ĕp"ĭ-mīz'ē-ŭm) ["
+ *mys*, muscle]
epinephrine (ĕp"ĭ-nĕf'rĭn) ["
+ *nephros*, kidney]
  e. bitartrate
epinephrinemia (ĕp"ĭ-nĕf"rĭ-nē'mē-ă)
[" + " + *haima*, blood]
epinephritis (ĕp"ĭ-nĕf-rī'tĭs) [" +
nephros, kidney, + *itis*, inflammation]
epinephroma (ĕp-ĭ-nĕ-frō'mă) ["
" + *oma*, tumor]
epineural (ĕp"ĭ-nū'răl) ["
+ *neuron*, nerve]
epineurium (ĕp"ĭ-nū'rē-ŭm)
epiotic (ĕp"ē-ŏt'ĭk) [" + *ous*, ear]
epiotic center
epipastic (ĕp"ĭ-păs'tĭk) [" + *passein*, to sprinkle]
epipharynx (ĕp"ĭ-făr'ĭnks) ["
+ *pharynx*, throat]
epiphenomenon (ĕp"ĭ-fĕ-nŏm'ĕ-nŏn)
[" + *phainomenon*, phenomenon]
epiphora (ĕ-pĭf'ō-ră) [Gr., downpour]
epiphylaxis (ĕp"ĭ-fĭ-lăks'ĭs) [Gr. *epi*,
upon, + *phylaxis*, guard]
epiphyseal (ĕp"ĭ-fĭz'ē-ăl) ["
+ *physis*, growth]
epiphyseolysis (ĕp"ĭ-fĭz"ē-ŏl'ĭ-sĭs)
[" + " + *lysis*, dissolution]
epiphyseopathy (ĕp"ĭ-fĭz-ē-ŏp'ă-thē)
[" + " + *pathos*, disease, suffering]
epiphysial (ĕp"ĭ-fĭz'ē-ăl)

epiphysis (ĕ-pĭf'ĭ-sĭs) [Gr., a growing upon]

epiphysitis (ĕ-pĭf"ĭ-sī'tĭs) [" + itis, inflammation]

epipial (ĕp"ĭ-pī'ăl) [" + L. pia, tender]

epiplocele (ĕ-pĭp'lō-sēl) [Gr. epiploon, omentum, + kele, tumor, swelling]

epiploenterocele (ĕ-pĭp"lō-ĕn'tĕr-ō-sēl) [" + enteron, intestine, + kele, tumor, swelling]

epiploic (ĕp"ĭ-plō'ĭk) [Gr. epiploon, omentum]

epiploic foramen

epiploitis (ĕ-pĭp"lō-ī'tĭs) [" + itis, inflammation]

epiplomerocele (ĕ-pĭp"lō-mē'rō-sēl) [" + meros, thigh, + kele, tumor, swelling]

epiplomphalocele (ĕ-pĭp"lŏm-făl'ō-sēl) [" + omphalos, navel, + kele, tumor, swelling]

epiploon (ĕ-pĭp'lō-ŏn) [Gr., omentum]

epiplopexy (ĕ-pĭp'lō-pĕks"ē) [" + pexis, fixation]

epiplosarcomphalocele (ĕ-pĭp"lō-săr"kŏm-făl'ō-sēl) [" + sarx, flesh, + omphalos, navel, + kele, tumor, swelling]

epiploscheocele (ĕ-pĭp"lŏs-kē'ō-sēl) [" + oscheon, scrotum, + kele, tumor, swelling]

epipygus (ĕp"ĭ-pī'gŭs) [Gr. epi, upon, + pyge, buttocks]

episclera (ĕp"ĭ-sklē'ră) [" + skleros, hard]

episcleral (ĕp"ĭ-sklē'răl)

episcleritis (ĕp"ĭ-sklē-rī'tĭs) [" + skleros, hard, + itis, inflammation]

episioelytrorrhaphy (ĕ-pĭs"ē-ō-ĕl"ĭ-tror'ă-fē) [" + elytron, vagina, + rhaphe, seam]

episioperineoplasty (ĕ-pĭs"ē-ō-pĕr"ĭ-nē'ō-plăs"tē) [" + perinaion, perineum, + Gr. plassein, to form]

episioperineorrhaphy (ĕ-pĭs"ē-ō-pĕr"ĭ-nē-or'ă-fē) [" + " + rhaphe, seam]

episioplasty (ĕ-pĭs"ē-ō-plăs'tē) [" + plassein, to form]

episiorrhaphy (ĕ-pĭs"ē-or'ă-fē) [" + rhaphe, seam]

episiostenosis (ĕ-pĭs"ē-ō-stĕ-nō'sĭs) [" + stenosis, act of narrowing]

episiotomy (ĕ-pĭs"ē-ŏt'ō-mē) [" + tome, a cutting, slice]

episome (ĕp'ĭ-sōm)

epispadias (ĕp"ĭ-spā'dē-ăs) [Gr. epi, upon, + spadon, a rent]

episplenitis (ĕp"ĭ-splē-nī'tĭs) [" + splen, spleen, + itis, inflammation]

epistasis (ĕ-pĭs'tă-sĭs) [Gr., stoppage]

epistaxis (ĕp"ĭ-stăk'sĭs) [Gr.]

episternal (ĕp"ĭ-stĕr'năl) [Gr. epi, upon, + sternon, chest]

episternum

epistropheus (ĕp"ĭ-strō'fē-ŭs)

epitaxy (ĕp"ĭ-tăk'sē) [Gr. epi-, upon, + taxis, arrangement]

epitendineum (ĕp"ĭ-tĕn-dĭn'ē-ŭm) [" + L. tendere, to stretch]

epitenon (ĕp-ĭ-tĕn'ŏn) [" + tenon, tendon]

epithalamus (ĕp"ĭ-thăl'ă-mŭs) [" + thalamos, chamber]

epithalaxia (ĕp"ĭ-thă-lăk'sē-ă) [" + thele, nipple, + allaxis, exchange]

epithelia [" + thele, nipple]

epithelial (ĕp"ĭ-thē'lē-ăl)

epithelial cancer

epithelial casts

epithelial cells

epithelialization (ĕp"ĭ-thē"lē-ăl-ĭ-zā'shŭn)

epithelial tissue

epitheliitis (ĕp"ĭ-thē"lē-ī'tĭs)

epithelioblastoma (ĕp"ĭ-thē"lē-ō-blăs-tō'mă) [" + thele, nipple, + blastos, germ, + oma, tumor]

epitheliogenic, epitheliogenetic (ĕp"ĭ-thē"lē-ō-jĕn'ĭk, -jĕ-nĕt'ĭk) [" + " + gennan, to produce]

epithelioglandular (ĕp"ĭ-thē"lē-ō-glăn'dū-lăr)

epithelioid (ĕp"ĭ-thē'lē-oyd) [" + " + eidos, form, shape]

epitheliolysin (ĕp″ĭ-thē-lē-ŏl′ĭ-sĭn)
[″ + ″ + lysis, dissolution]
epitheliolysis (ĕp″ĭ-thē-lē-ŏl′ĭ-sĭs)
epithelioma (ĕp″ĭ-thē-lē-ō′mă) [″ +
thele, nipple, + oma, tumor]
  e. adamantinum
  e. adenoides cysticum
  e., basal cell
  e., deep-seated
epitheliomatous (ĕp″ĭ-thē-lē-ō′mă-
tŭs)
epitheliosis (ĕp″ĭ-thē″lē-ō′sĭs) [″ +
thele, nipple, + osis, condition]
epithelium (ĕp″ĭ-thē′lē-ŭm) [″ +
thele, nipple]
  e., attachment
  e., ciliated
  e., columnar
  e., cuboidal
  e., germinal
  e., glandular
  e., laminated
  e., mesenchymal
  e., pavement
  e., pigmented
  e., pseudostratified
  e., reduced enamel
  e., squamous
  e., stratified
  e., sulcular
  e., transitional
epitope (ĕp′ĭ-tōp)
epitrichial layer
epitrichium (ĕp″ĭ-trĭk′ē-ŭm) [Gr. epi,
upon, + trichion, hair]
epitrochlea (ĕp″ĭ-trŏk′lē-ă) [″ +
trochalia, pulley]
epitrochlear (ĕp″ĭ-trŏk′lē-ăr)
epiturbinate (ĕp″ĭ-tĕr′bĭn-āt) [″ +
L. turbo, top]
epitympanum (ĕp″ĭ-tĭm′pă-nŭm)
[″ + tympanon, drum]
epizoic (ĕp″ĭ-zō′ĭk) [″ + zoon, ani-
mal]
epizoicide (ĕp″ĭ-zō′ĭ-sīd) [″ + ″
+ L. caedere, to kill]
epizoon (ĕp″ĭ-zō′ŏn) [″ + zoon,
animal]

epizootic
eponychium (ĕp″ō-nĭk′ē-ŭm) [″ +
onyx, nail]
eponym (ĕp′ō-nĭm) [Gr. eponymos,
named after]
epoophorectomy (ĕp″ō-ŏf-ō-rĕk′tō-
mē) [Gr. epi, upon, + NL. oophoron, ovary, + Gr. ektome, ex-
cision]
epoophoron (ĕp″ō-ŏf′ō-rŏn)
epoxide
epoxy (ĕ-pŏk′sē)
Eprolin
epsilon-aminocaproic acid
epsom salt (ĕp′sŭm)
EPSP excitatory postsynaptic potential
Epstein-Barr virus [M. A. Epstein, Brit.
physician, b. 1921; Y. M. Barr, contemporary Canadian physician]
Epstein's pearls [A. Epstein, Czech.
physician, 1849–1918]
epulis (ĕp-ū′lĭs) [Gr. epoulis, a gumboil]
epuloid (ĕp′ū-loyd) [″ + eidos,
form, shape]
epulosis (ĕp″ū-lō′sĭs) [Gr. epoulosis]
epulotic (ĕp″ū-lŏt′ĭk) [Gr. epoulotikos]
Equanil
equation [L. aequare, to make equal]
equator [L. aequator]
  e. oculi
  e. of cell
  e. of crystalline lens; e. lentis
equatorial
equatorial plate
equi- [L. aequus, equal]
equilibrating (ē-kwĭl′ĭ-brāt-ĭng) [L. ae-
quilibris, in perfect balance]
equilibration
equilibrium [L. aequus, equal, +
libra, balance]
  e., nitrogenous
  e., physiological
equilin (ĕk′wĭl-ĭn) [L. equus, horse]
equine (ē′kwīn) [L. equus, horse]
equinovarus (ē-kwī′nō-vā′rŭs) [L.
equinus, equine, + varus, bent in-
ward]
equipotential (ē″kwĭ-pō-tĕn′shăl) [L.

aequus, equal, + *potentia*, ability]
equivalence (ē-kwĭv'ă-lĕns) [" + *valere*, to be worth]
equivalent (ē-kwĭv'a-lĕnt)
equivalent weight
E.R. external resistance; Emergency Room
Er erbium
eradication
erasion (ē-rā'zhŭn) [L. e, out, + radere, to scrape]
Erben's reflex (ĕrb'ĕnz) [Siegmund Erben, Austrian physician, b. 1863]
erbium (ĕr'bē-ŭm)
Erb's paralysis [Wilhelm H. Erb, Ger. neurologist, 1840–1921]
Erb's point
erectile (ē-rĕk'tĭl) [L. erigere, to erect]
erectile tissue
erection
erector [L. erigere, to erect]
erector spinae reflex
eremophobia (ĕr"ĕm-ō-fō'bē-ă) [Gr. eremos, solitary, + phobos, fear]
erepsin (ē-rĕp'sĭn)
erethism (ĕr'ĕ-thĭzm) [Gr. erethismos, irritation]
   e. mercurialis
erethismic (ĕr"ĕ-thĭz'mĭk)
erethisophrenia (ĕr"ĕ-thĭ-zō-frē'nē-ă) [" + phren, mind]
erethistic (ĕr"ĕ-thĭs'tĭk) [Gr. erethismos, irritation]
erethitic (ĕr"ĕ-thĭt'ĭk)
ereuthrophobia (ĕr"ū-thrō-fō'bē-ă) [Gr. erythros, red, + phobos, fear]
ERG electroretinogram
erg [Gr. ergon, work]
ergasiomania (ĕr-gă"sē-ō-mā'nē-ă) [Gr. ergasia, work, + mania, madness]
ergasiophobia (ĕr-gă"sē-ō-fō'bē-ă) [" + phobos, fear]
ergasthenia (ĕr"găs-thē'nē-ă) [Gr. ergon, work, + astheneia, weakness]
ergastic (ĕr-găs'tĭk) [Gr. ergastikos]
ergastoplasm
ergocalciferol (ĕr-gō-kăl-sĭf'ĕr-ŏl)

ergogenic (ĕr"gō-jĕn'ĭk) [Gr. ergon, work, + gennan, to produce]
ergograph (ĕr'gō-grăf) [" + graphein, to write]
Ergomar
ergometer (ĕr-gŏm'ĕ-tĕr) [" + metron, measure]
   e., bicycle
ergonomics (ĕr"gō-nŏm'ĭks) [" + nomikos, law]
ergonovine maleate (ĕr"gō-nō'vĭn)
ergophobia (ĕr"gō-fō'bē-ă) [" + phobos, fear]
ergophore (ĕr'gō-for) [" + pherein, to bear]
Ergostat
ergostat (ĕr'gō-stăt) [" + statos, standing]
ergosterol (ĕr-gŏs'tĕr-ŏl)
ergot (ĕr'gŏt)
ergotamine (ĕr-gŏt'ă-mēn)
   e. tartrate
ergotherapy (ĕr'gō-thĕr'ă-pē) [" + therapeia, treatment]
ergotism (ĕr'gŏ-tĭzm)
ergot poisoning
ergotrate (ĕr'gō-trāt)
Ergotrate Maleate
ergotropic [Gr. ergon, work, + tropos, a turning]
ergotropy (ĕr-gŏt'rō-pē)
Eristalis (ĕr-ĭs'tă-lĭs)
erode (ē-rōd') [L. erodere]
erogenous (ĕr-ŏj'ĕ-nŭs) [Gr. eros, love, + gennan, to produce]
erogenous zone
erosion (ē-rō'shŭn) [L. erodere, to gnaw away]
   e., dental
   e. of cervix uteri
erosive (ē-rō'sĭv)
erotic (ē-rŏt'ĭk) [Gr. erotikos]
eroticism (ē-rŏt'ĭ-sĭzm) [" + -ismos, condition]
   e., allo-
   e., anal
   e., auto-
   e., oral
erotism (ĕr'ō-tĭzm)

erotogenic (ĕ-rō"tō-jĕn'ĭk) [Gr. eros, love, + gennan, to produce]

erotology (ĕr"ŏ-tŏl'ō-jē) [" + logos, word, reason]

erotomania (ĕ-rō"tō-, ĕ-rŏt"ŏ-mā'nē-ă) [" + mania, madness]

erotopathia (ĕ-rō"tō-, ĕ-rŏt"ō-păth'ē-ă) [" + pathos, disease, suffering]

erotophobia (ĕ-rō"tō-, ĕ-rŏt"ō-fō'bē-ă) [" + phobos, fear]

erratic [L. errare, to wander]

errhine (ĕr'īn) [Gr. en, in, + rhis, nose]

error
  e., type I
  e., type II

erubescence [L. erubescere, to grow red]

eructation (ĕ-rŭk-tā'shŭn) [L. eructare]

eruption (ĕ-rŭp'shŭn) [L. eruptio, a breaking out]
  e., active
  e., creeping
  e., delayed
  e., drug
  e., passive
  e., serum

eruptive

eruptive stage

erysipelas (ĕr"ĭ-sĭp'ĕ-lăs) [Gr. erythros, red, + pella, skin]

erysipelatous (ĕr"ĭ-sĭ-pĕl'ă-tŭs)

erysipeloid (ĕr-ĭ-sĭp'ĕ-loyd) [" + " + eidos, form, shape]

Erysipelothrix rhusiopathiae (ĕr"ĭ-sĭ-pĕl'ŏ-thrĭks) [" + " + thrix, hair]

erysipelotoxin (ĕr"ĭ-sĭp"ĕ-lō-tŏk'sĭn)

erysiphake (ĕr-ĭs'ĭ-fāk)

erythema (ĕr"ĭ-thē'mă) [Gr., redness]
  e. ab igne
  e. annulare
  e. congestivum
  e., diffuse
  e. induratum
  e. infectiosum
  e. intertrigo
  e. marginatum
  e. multiforme

  e. neonatorum
  e. nodosum
  e., punctate
  e. toxicum neonatorum
  e. venenatum

erythematic, erythematous (ĕr"ĭ-thē-măt'ĭk, ĕr"ĭ-thĕm'ă-tŭs) [Gr. erythema, redness]

erythemogenic (ĕr"ĭ-thē"mō-jĕn'ĭk) [" + gennan, to produce]

erythralgia (ĕr"ĭ-thrăl'jē-ă) [" + algos, pain]

erythrasma (ĕr"ĭ-thrăz'mă)

erythredema (ĕ-rĭth"rĕ-dē'mă) [" + oidema, swelling]

erythremia (ĕr"ĭ-thrē'mē-ă) [" + haima, blood]

erythrism (ĕ-rĭth'rĭzm) [" + -ismos, condition]

erythristic (ĕr"ĭ-thrĭs'tĭk)

erythrityl tetranitrate (ĕ-rĭth'rĭ-tĭl)

erythro- [Gr. erythros, red]

erythroblast (ĕ-rĭth'rō-blăst) [" + blastos, germ]

erythroblastemia (ĕ-rĭth"rō-blăs-tē'mē-ă) [" + " + haima, blood]

erythroblastic

erythroblastoma (ĕ-rĭth"rō-blăs-tō'mă) [" + blastos, germ, + oma, tumor]

erythroblastosis (ĕ-rĭth"rō-blăs-tō'sĭs) [" + " + osis, condition]
  e. fetalis

erythrochloropia (ĕ-rĭth"rō-klor-ō'pē-ă) [Gr. erythros, red, + chloros, green, + ops, eye]

erythrochromia (ĕ-rĭth"rō-krō'mē-ă) [" + chroma, color]

Erythrocin Lactobionate-I.V.

erythroclasis (ĕr"ĕ-thrŏk'lă-sĭs)

erythroclastic (ĕ-rĭth-rō-klăs'tĭk) [" + klasis, a breaking]

erythrocyanosis (ĕ-rĭth-rō-sī"ă-nō'sĭs) [" + kyanos, blue, + osis, condition]

erythrocyte (ĕ-rĭth'rō-sīt) [" + kytos, cell]
  e., achromatic

e., basophilic
e., crenated
e., immature
e., orthochromatic
e., polychromatic
erythrocyte sedimentation rate
erythrocythemia (ĕ-rĭth″rō-sī-thē′mē-ă) [Gr. *erythros*, red, + *kytos*, cell, + *haima*, blood]
erythrocytolysin (ĕ-rĭth″rō-sī-tŏl′ĭ-sĭn)
erythrocytolysis (ĕ-rĭth″rō-sī-tŏl′ĭ-sĭs) [″ + ″ + *lysis*, dissolution]
erythrocytometer (ĕ-rĭth″rō-sī-tŏm′ĕ-tĕr) [″ + ″ + *metron*, measure]
erythrocytoopsonin (ĕ-rĭth″rō-sī″tō-ŏp-sō′nĭn) [″ + ″ + *opsonein*, to purchase victuals]
erythrocytopenia (ĕ-rĭth″rō-sī″tō-pē′nē-ă) [″ + ″ + *penia*, lack]
erythrocytopoiesis (ĕ-rĭth″rō-sī″tō-poy-ē′sĭs) [″ + ″ + *poiesis*, making]
erythrocytorrhexis (ĕ-rĭth″rō-sī″tō-rĕk′sĭs) [″ + ″ + *rhexis*, rupture]
erythrocytoschisis (ĕ-rĭth″rō-sī-tŏs′kĭ-sĭs) [″ + ″ + *schisis*, cleavage]
erythrocytosis (ĕ-rĭth″rō-sī-tō′sĭs) [″ + ″ + *osis*, condition]
erythroderma (ĕ-rĭth″rō-dĕr′mă) [″ + *derma*, skin]
e. desquamativum
e. ichthyosiforme congenitum
erythrodermia (ĕ-rĭth″rō-dĕr′mē-ă)
erythrodextrin (ĕ-rĭth″rō-dĕx′trĭn) [″ + L. *dexter*, right]
erythrodontia (ĕ-rĭth″rō-dŏn′shē-ă) [″ + *odous*, tooth]
erythrogenesis (ĕ-rĭth″rō-jĕn′ĕ-sĭs) [″ + *genesis*, generation, birth]
erythroid (ĕr′ĭ-throyd) [″ + *eidos*, form, shape]
erythrokeratodermia (ĕ-rĭth″rō-kĕr″ă-tō-dĕr′mē-ă) [″ + *keras*, horn, + *derma*, skin]
erythrokinetics (ĕ-rĭth″rō-kĭ-nĕt′ĭks) [″ + *kinesis*, motion]
erythroleukemia (ĕ-rĭth″rō-loo-

kē′mē-ă) [Gr. *erythros*, red, + *leukos*, white, + *haima*, blood]
erythroleukosis (ĕ-rĭth″rō-loo-kō′sĭs) [″ + ″ + *osis*, condition]
erythrolysin (ĕr″ĭ-thrŏl′ĭ-sĭn) [″ + *lysis*, dissolution]
erythrolysis
erythromania (ĕ-rĭth″rō-mā′nē-ă) [″ + *mania*, madness]
erythromelalgia (ĕ-rĭth″rō-mĕl-ăl′jē-ă) [″ + *melos*, limb, + *algos*, pain]
erythromelia (ĕ-rĭth″rō-mē′lē-ă) [″ + *melos*, limb]
erythromycin (ĕ-rĭth″rō-mī′sĭn) [″ + *mykes*, fungus]
erythron (ĕr′ĭ-thrŏn) [Gr. *erythros*, red]
erythroneocytosis (ĕ-rĭth″rō-nē″ō-sī-tō′sĭs) [″ + *neos*, new, + *kytos*, cell, + *osis*, condition]
erythronoclastic (ĕ-rĭth″rō-nō-klăs′tĭk) [″ + *klan*, to break]
erythroparasite (ĕ-rĭth″rō-păr′ă-sīt) [″ + *parasitos*, parasite]
erythropathy (ĕr′ĭ-thrŏp′ă-thē) [″ + *pathos*, disease, suffering]
erythropenia (ĕ-rĭth″rō-pē′nē-ă) [″ + *penia*, lack]
erythrophage (ĕ-rĭth′rō-fāj) [″ + *phagein*, to eat]
erythrophagia
erythrophile, erythrophilous (ĕ-rĭth′rō-fĭl, ĕr″ĭ-thrŏf′ĭ-lŭs) [″ + *philein*, to love]
erythrophobia (ĕ-rĭth″rō-fō′bē-ă) [″ + *phobos*, fear]
erythrophose (ĕ-rĭth′rō-fōz) [″ + *phos*, light]
erythrophthisis (ĕ-rĭth″rō-thī′sĭs) [″ + *phthisis*, wasting]
erythropia, erythropsia (ĕr″ĭ-thrō′pē-ă, -thrŏp′sē-ă) [″ + *opsis*, sight, appearance, vision]
erythroplasia (ĕ-rĭth″rō-plā′zē-ă) [″ + *plasis*, molding, forming]
e. of Queyrat
erythropoiesis (ĕ-rĭth″rō-poy-ē′sĭs) [″ + *poiesis*, making]

erythropoietic (ĕ-rĭth″rō-poy-ĕt′ĭk)

erythropoietin (ĕ-rĭth″rō-poy′ĕ-tĭn)

erythroprosopalgia (e-rĭth″rō-prō-sō-păl′jē-ă) [″ + prosopon, face, + algos, pain]

erythropsia (ĕr-ĭ-thrŏp′sē-ă) [″ + opsis, sight, appearance, vision]

erythropsin (ĕ-rĭth-rŏp′sĭn) [″ + opsis, sight, appearance, vision]

erythrorrhexis (ĕ-rĭth″rō-rĕks′ĭs) [″ + rhexis, rupture]

erythrosine sodium

erythrosis (ĕr-ĭ-thrō′sĭs) [″ + osis, condition]

erythrostasis (ĕ-rĭth″rō-stā′sĭs) [″ + stasis, standing still]

erythrotoxin (ĕ-rĭth″rō-tŏk′sĭn) [″ + toxikon, poison]

erythruria (ĕr-ĭ-thrŭ′rē-ă) [″ + ouron, urine]

Es einsteinium

escape [O. Fr. escaper]
    e., vagal
    e., ventricular

escape beat

escape phenomenon

eschar (ĕs′kăr) [Gr. eschara, scab]

escharotic (ĕs-kăr-ŏt′ĭk) [Gr. escharotikos]

escharotomy (ĕs-kăr-ŏt′ō-mē) [Gr. eschara, scab, + tome, a cutting, slice]

Escherichia (ĕsh-ĕr-ĭk′ē-ă)
    E. coli

Escherich's reflex (ĕsh′ĕr-ĭks) [Theodor Escherich, Ger. physician, 1857–1911]

eschrolalia (ĕs-krō-lā′lē-ă) [Gr. aischros, indecent, + lalia, chatter, prattle]

escorcin (ĕs-kor′sĭn)

esculent (ĕs′kū-lĕnt)

escutcheon (ĕs-kŭch′ăn) [L. scutum, a shield]

eserine (ĕs′ĕr-ĭn) [esere, African name for the Calabar bean]

ESF erythropoietic stimulating factor

Esidrix

Eskabarb

Eskalith

Esmarch's bandage (ĕs′mărks) [Johannes F. A. von Esmarch, Ger. surgeon, 1823–1908]

esodic (ē-sŏd′ĭk) [Gr. es, toward, + hodos, way]

esoethmoiditis (ĕs″ō-ĕth″moy-dī′tĭs) [Gr. eso, inward, + ethmos, sieve, + eidos, form, shape, + itis, inflammation]

esogastritis (ĕs″ō-găs-trī′tĭs) [″ + gaster, belly, + itis, inflammation]

esophagalgia (ē-sŏf-ă-găl′jē-ă) [Gr. oisophagos, gullet, + algos, pain]

esophageal (ē-sŏf″ă-jē′ăl)

esophageal web

esophagectasia, esophagectasis (ē-sŏf″ă-jĕk-tā′sē-ă, -jĕk′tă-sĭs) [″ + ektasis, distention]

esophagectomy (ē-sŏf″ă-jĕk′tō-mē) [″ + ektome, excision]

esophagismus (ē-sŏf-ă-jĭs′mŭs) [″ + -ismos, condition]

esophagitis (ē-sŏf-ă-jī′tĭs) [″ + itis, inflammation]

esophagobronchial (ē-sŏf″ă-gō-brŏng′kē-ăl) [″ + bronchos, windpipe]

esophagocele (ē-sŏf′ă-gō-sēl) [″ + kele, tumor, swelling]

esophagodynia (ē-sŏf″ă-gō-dĭn′ē-ă) [Gr. oisophagos, gullet, + odyne, pain]

esophagoenterostomy (ē-sŏf″ă-gō-ĕn-tĕr-ŏs′tō-mē) [″ + enteron, intestine, + stoma, mouth, opening]

esophagogastrectomy (ē-sŏf″ă-gō-găs-trĕk′tō-mē) [″ + gaster, belly, + ektome, excision]

esophagogastroanastomosis (ē-sŏf″ă-gō-găs″trŏ-ă-năs″tō-mō′sĭs) [″ + ″ + anastomosis, opening]

esophagogastroplasty (ē-sŏf′ă-gō-găs′trō-plăs″tē) [″ + ″ + plassein, to form]

esophagogastroscopy (ē-sŏf″ă-gō-găs-trŏs′kō-pē) [″ + ″ + sko-

pein, to examine]

esophagogastrostomy (ē-sŏf"ă-gō-găs-trŏs'tō-mē) [" + " + *stoma*, mouth, opening]

esophagojejunostomy (ĕ-sŏf"ă-gō-jĕ-jū-nŏs'tō-mē) [" + L. *jejunum*, empty, + Gr. *stoma*, mouth, opening]

esophagomalacia (ē-sŏf"ă-gō-mă-lā'sē-ă) [Gr. *oisophagos*, gullet, + *malakia*, softness]

esophagomycosis (ē-sŏf"ă-gō-mī-kō'sĭs) [" + *mykes*, fungus, + *osis*, condition]

esophagomyotomy (ē-sŏf"ă-gō-mī-ŏt'ō-mē) [" + *mys*, muscle, + *tome*, a cutting, slice]

esophagoplasty (ē-sŏf'ă-gō-plăs"tē) [" + *plassein*, to form]

esophagoplication (ē-sŏf"ă-gō-plĭ-kā'shŭn) [" + L. *abplicare*, to fold]

esophagoptosia, esophagoptosis (ē-sŏf"ă-gŏp-tō'sē-ă, -sĭs) [" + *ptosis*, fall, falling]

esophagoscope (ē-sŏf'ă-gō-skōp) [" + *skopein*, to examine]

esophagospasm (ē-sŏf'ă-gō-spăzm") [" + *spasmos*, a convulsion]

esophagostenosis (ē-sŏf"ă-gō-stĕn-ō'sĭs) [" + *stenosis*, act of narrowing]

esophagostomy (ē-sŏf-ă-gŏs'tō-mē) [" + *stoma*, mouth, opening]

esophagotome (ē-sŏf'ă-gō-tōm) [" + *tome*, a cutting, slice]

esophagotomy (ē-sŏf-ă-gŏt'ō-mē)

esophagotracheal (ē-sŏf"ă-gō-trā'kē-ăl)

esophagus (ē-sŏf'ă-gŭs) [Gr. *oisophagos*, gullet]
    e., foreign bodies in

esophoria (ĕs-ō-fō'rē-ă) [Gr. *eso*, inward, + *phorein*, to bear]

esosphenoiditis (ĕs"ō-sfē-noyd-ī'tĭs) [" + *sphen*, wedge, + *eidos*, form, shape, + *itis*, inflammation]

esotropia (ĕs-ō-trō'pē-ă) [" + *tropos*, turning]

ESP *extrasensory perception*

ESR *electron spin resonance*

essence [L. *essentia*, being or quality]

essential [L. *essentialis*]

EST *electroshock therapy*

ester [L. *aether*, ether]

esterase (ĕs'tĕr-ās)

esterification (ĕs-tĕr"ĭ-fĭ-kā'shŭn)

esterize

esthematology (ĕs"thĕm-ă-tŏl'ō-jē) [Gr. *aisthema*, sensation, + *logos*, word, reason]

esthesia (ĕs-thē'zē-ă) [Gr. *aisthesis*, feeling, perception]

esthesiology (ĕs-thē"zē-ŏl'ō-jē) [" + *logos*, word, reason]

esthesiomania (ĕs-thē"zē-ō-mā'nē-ă) [" + *mania*, madness]

esthesiometer, aesthesiometer (ĕs-thē-zē-ŏm'ĕ-tĕr) [" + *metron*, measure]

esthesioneurosis (ĕs-thē"zē-ō-nū-rō'sĭs) [" + *neuron*, nerve, + *osis*, condition]

esthesiophysiology (ĕs-thē"sē-ō-fĭs-ē-ŏl'ō-jē) [" + *physis*, nature, + *logos*, word, reason]

esthesioscopy (ĕs-thē"zē-ŏs'kō-pē) [" + *skopein*, to examine]

estheticokinetic (ĕs-thĕt"ĭ-kō-kĭn-ĕt'ĭk) [" + *kinesis*, motion]

esthetics (ĕs-thĕt'ĭks)

esthiomene (ĕs"thē-ŏm'ĕ-nē) [Gr. *esthiomenos*, eating]

Estinyl

estival (ĕs'tĭ-văl) [L. *aestivus*]

estivoautumnal [" + *autumnalis*, pert. to autumn]

Estrace

estradiol (ĕs-tră-dī'ŏl)
    e. dipropionate

estrin (ĕs'trĭn)

estrinization (ĕs"trĭn-ĭ-zā'shŭn)

estriol (ĕs'trē-ŏl)

estrogen (ĕs'trō-jĕn) [Gr. *oistros*, mad desire, + *gennan*, to produce]
    e.'s, conjugated

estrogenic (ĕs-trō-jĕn'ĭk)

estrone (ĕs′trōn)
estropipate
estrual (ĕs′troo-ăl) [Gr. *oistros*, mad desire]
estruation
estrus, oestrus [Gr. *oistros*, mad desire]
estrus cycle
estuarium (ĕs″tū-ā′rē-ŭm) [L.] Vapor bath
état criblé (ā-tă′ krĕb-lā′) [Fr., sievelike state]
état mamelonné (ā-tă′ mă-mĕl-ŏn-ā′) [Fr., knobby state]
etching (ĕch′ĭng) [Ger. *ätzen*, to feed]
　　e., acid
ethacrynic acid
ethambutol **hydrochloride** (ĕ-thăm′bū-tōl)
Ethamide
ethamivan (ĕth-ăm′ĭ-văn″)
ethanol (ĕth′ă-nŏl)
ethaverine hydrochloride (ĕth″ă-vĕr′ēn)
etchlorvynol (ĕth-klor′vĭ-nŏl)
ethene (ĕth-ēn′)
ether [Gr. *aither*, air]
ether anesthesia
ether asphyxia
ether bed
ethereal (ĕ-thē′rē-ăl) [Gr. *aither*, air]
etherization (ē″thĕr-ĭ-zā′shŭn)
etherize (ē′thĕr-īz)
etheromania (ē″thĕr-ō-mā′nē-ă) [″ + *mania*, madness]
ethics [Gr. *ethos*, moral custom]
　　e., dental
　　e., medical
　　e., nursing
ethinamate (ĕ-thĭn′ă-māt)
ethinyl estradiol (ĕth′ĭ-nĭl)
ethionamide (ĕ-thī″ŏn-ăm′ĭd)
ethionine (ĕ-thī′ō-nĭn)
ethmocarditis (ĕth″mō-kăr-dī′tĭs) [Gr. *ethmos*, sieve, + *kardia*, heart, + *itis*, inflammation]
ethmoid (ĕth′moyd) [″ + *eidos*, form, shape]

ethmoidal
ethmoid bone
ethmoidectomy (ĕth-moy-dĕk′tō-mē) [″ + *eidos*, form, shape, + *ektome*, excision]
ethmoiditis (ĕth″moy-dī′tĭs) [″ + ″ + *itis*, inflammation]
ethmoid sinus
ethnic (ĕth′nĭk) [Gr. *ethnikos*, of a nation]
ethnobiology (ĕth″nō-bī-ŏl′ō-jē) [Gr. *ethnos*, race, + *bios*, life, + *logos*, word, reason]
ethnography (ĕth-nŏg′ră-fē) [″ + *graphein*, to write]
ethnology (ĕth-nŏl′ō-jē) [″ + *logos*, word, reason]
ethology (ē-, ē-thŏl′ō-jē) [Gr. *ethos*, manners, habits, + *logos*, word, reason]
ethopropazine **hydrochloride** (ĕth″ō-prō′pă-zēn)
ethosuximide (ĕth″ō-sŭk′sĭ-mīd)
ethotoin (ĕ-thō′tō-ĭn)
ethoxzolamide (ĕth″ŏks-zōl′ă-mīd)
ethyl (ĕth′ĭl) [Gr. *aither*, air, + *hyle*, matter]
　　e. acetate
　　e. alcohol
　　e. aminobenzoate
　　e. biscoumacetate
　　e. chaulmoograte
　　e. chloride
　　e., vanillin
ethylamine (ĕth″ĭl-ăm′ĭn)
ethylcellulose (ĕth″ĭl-sĕl′ū-lōs)
ethylene (ĕth′ĭl-ēn)
　　e. glycol
　　e. oxide
ethylene anesthesia
ethylenediamine (ĕth″ĭ-lēn-dī′ă-mēn)
ethylenediaminetetraacetic acid
ethylmorphine (ĕth″ĭl-mor′fēn)
ethylnorepinephrine hydrochloride (ĕth″ĭl-nor-ĕp″ĭ-nĕf″rĭn)
ethynodiol diacetate (ĕ-thī″nō-dī′ŏl)
ethynyl (ĕth′ĭ-nĭl)
etiocholanolone (ē″tē-ō-kō-lăn′ō-lōn)
etiologic, etiological (ē″tē-ō-lŏj′ĭk,

-ĭ-kăl) [Gr. *aitia*, cause, + *logos*, word, reason]

etiology (ē"tē-ŏl'ō-jē)

etiotropic (ē"tē-ō-trŏp'ĭk) [Gr. *aita*, cause, + *tropos*, turning]

etretinate

etymology (ĕt"ĭ-mŏl'ō-jē) [L. *etymon*, origin of a word, + *logos*, word, reason]

Eu *europium*

eu- [Gr. *eus*, good]

Eubacteriales (ū"băk-tē-rē-ā'lēz) [Gr. *eus*, good, + *bakterion*, little rod]

Eubacterium (ū"băk-tē'rē-ŭm)

eubiotics (ū"bī-ŏt'ĭks) [" + *bios*, life]

eubolism (ū'bŏl-ĭzm)

eucalyptol (ū"kă-lĭp'tŏl) [" + *kalyptein*, to cover]

eucalyptus oil (ū-kă-lĭp'tŭs)

eucapnia (ū-kăp'nē-ă) [" + *kapnos*, smoke]

eucatropine hydrochloride (ū-kăt'rō-pēn)

euchlorhydria (ū"klor-hī'drē-ă)

eucholia (ū-kō'lē-ă) [" + *chole*, bile]

euchromatin (ū-krō'mă-tĭn) [" + *chroma*, color]

euchylia (ū-kī'lē-ă) [" + *chylos*, juice]

eucrasia (ū-krā'sē-ă) [" + *krasis*, mixture]

eudiaphoresis (ū"dī-ă-fō-rē'sĭs) [" + *dia*, through, + *pherein*, to carry]

eudiometer (ū"dē-ŏm'ĕ-tĕr) [Gr. *eudia*, good weather, + *metron*, measure]

euesthesia (ū-ĕs-thē'sē-ă) [Gr. *eus*, good, + *aisthesis*, feeling, perception]

eugenics (ū-jĕn'ĭks) [" + *gennan*, to produce]

eugenol (ū'jĕn-ŏl)

euglobulin (ū-glŏb'ū-lĭn)

eugonic (ū-gŏn'ĭk) [Gr. *eus*, good, + *gone*, seed]

eukaryon (ū-kăr'ē-ŏn) [" + *kar-*

yon, nucleus]

eukaryote (ū-kăr'ē-ōt)

eukinesia (ū-kĭn-ē'sē-ă) [" + *kinesis*, motion]

Eulenburg's disease (oyl'ĕn-bŭrgz) [Albert Eulenburg, Ger. neurologist, 1840–1917]

Eumycetes (ū"mī-sē'tēz) [" + *mykes*, fungus]

eunoia (ū-noy'ă) [" + *nous*, mind]

eunuch (ū'nŭk) [Gr. *eune*, bed, + *echein*, to guard]

eunuchism (ū'nŭk-ĭzm) [" + " + *-ismos*, condition]
e., pituitary

eunuchoid (ū'nŭ-koyd) [" + " *eidos*, form, shape]

eunuchoidism (ū-'nŭk-oyd-ĭzm) [" + " + " + *-ismos*, condition]

eupancreatism (ū-păn'krē-ă-tĭzm) [Gr. *eus*, good, + *pankreas*, pancreas, + *-ismos*, condition]

eupepsia [" + *pepsis*, digestion]

eupeptic

euphonia (ū-fōn'ē-ă) [" + *phone*, voice]

euphoria (ū-for'ē-ă) [" + *phoros*, bearing]

euplastic (ū-plăs'tĭk) [" + *plastikos*, formed]

euploidy (ū-ploy'dē) [" + *ploos*, fold, + *eidos*, form, shape]

eupnea (ūp-nē'ă) [" + *pnein*, to breathe]

eupraxia (ū-prăks'ē-ă) [" + *prassein*, to do]

eupraxic (ū-prăks'ĭk)

europium (ū-rō'pē-ŭm)

Eurotium (ū-rō'shē-ŭm) [Gr. *euros*, mold]

eury- (ū'rē) [Gr. *eurys*, wide]

eurycephalic (ū"rē-sĕ-făl'ĭk) [" + *kephale*, head]

eustachian (ū-stā'kē-ăn, -shĕn) [Bartolommeo Eustachio, It. anatomist, 1524–1574]

eustachian catheter

eustachianography

eustachian tube

eustachian valve

eustachitis (ū"stă-kī'tĭs)

eusystole (ū-sĭs'tō-lē) [Gr. *eus*, good, + *systellein*, to draw together]

eutectic (ū-tĕk'tĭk) [Gr. *eutektos*]

eutectic mixture

euthanasia (ū-thă-nā'zē-a) [Gr. *eus*, good, + *thanatos*, death]

euthenics (ū-thĕn'ĭks) [Gr. *euthenia*, well-being]

Eutheria

Euthroid

euthyroid (ū-thī'royd)

eutocia (ū-tō'sē-ă) [Gr. *eus*, good, + *tokos*, birth]

Eutonyl

Eutrombicula (ū"trŏm-bĭk'ū-lă)

eutrophication (ū-trŏf"ĭ-kā'shŭn) [Gr. *eutrophein*, to thrive]

ev, eV, EV *electron volt*

evacuant (ē-văk'ū-ănt) [L. *evacuans*, making empty]

evacuate [L. *evacuatio*, emptying]

evacuation (ē-văk"ū-ā'shŭn)

evacuator (ē-văk'ū-ā-tor)

evaginate (ē-văj'ĭ-nāt) [L. *evaginare*, to unsheath]

evagination (ē-văj-ĭ-nā'shŭn)

evaluation

evanescent (ĕv"ă-nĕs'ĕnt) [L. *evanescere*, to vanish]

Evans blue [Herbert M. Evans, U.S. anatomist, 1882–1971]

Evans syndrome [Robert S. Evans, U.S. physician, b. 1912]

evaporation [L. *e*, out, + *vaporare*, to steam]

evenomation (ē-věn"ō-mā'shŭn) [L. *ex*, from, + *venenum*, poison]

eventration (ē"věn-trā'shŭn) [L. *e*, out, + *venter*, belly]

eversion (ē-věr'zhŭn) [" + *vertere*, to turn]

evidement (ā-vēd-mŏn') [Fr., a scooping out]

evidence

evil [AS. *yfel*]

eviration (ē"vī-rā'shŭn) [L. *e*, out, + *vir*, man]

evisceration (ē-vĭs"ĕr-ā'shŭn) [" + *viscera*, viscera]

evisceroneurotomy (ē-vĭs"ĕr-ō-nū-rŏt'ō-mē) [" + " + Gr. *neuron*, nerve, + *tome*, a cutting, slice]

evocation (ĕv"ō-kā'shŭn) [" + *vocare*, to call]

evoked response

evolution (ĕv"ō-lū'shŭn) [L. *e*, out, + *volvere*, to roll]

    e., theory of

evulsion (ē-vŭl'shŭn) [" + *vellere*, to pluck]

Ewing's tumor or sarcoma (ū'ĭngz) [James Ewing, U.S. pathologist, 1866–1943]

ex- [L., Gr. *ex*, out]

exa- 10^{18}

exacerbation (ĕks-ăs"ĕr-bā'shŭn) [" + *acerbus*, harsh]

exaltation [L. *exaltare*, to lift up]

examination [L. *examinare*, to examine]

    e., dental

    e., oral

exangia (ĕks-ăn'jē-ă) [Gr. *ex*, out, + *angeion*, vessel]

exanthem (ĕks-ăn'thĕm) [Gr. *exanthema*, eruption]

    e. subitum

exanthema (ĕks-ăn-thē'mă) [Gr.]

exanthematous (ĕks"ăn-thĕm'ă-tŭs)

exanthrope (ĕks'ăn-thrōp) [Gr. *ex*, out, + *anthropos*, man]

exarticulation (ĕks"ăr-tĭk-ū-lā'shŭn) [L. *ex*, out, + *articulus*, joint]

excavation (ĕks"kă-vā'shŭn) [" + *cavus*, hollow]

    e., atrophic

    e., dental

    e. of optic nerve

    e., rectouterine

excavator (ĕks'kă-vā"tor)

excerebration (ĕk"sĕr-ē-brā'shŭn) [" + *cerebrum*, brain]

exchange transfusion

excipient (ĕk-sĭp'ē-ĕnt) [L. *excipiens*, excepting]

excise (ĕk-sīz') [L. *ex*, out, + *caedere*, to cut]

excision (ĕk-sĭ'zhŭn) [L. *excisio*]

excitability [L. *excitare*, to arouse]
  e., independent
  e., muscle
  e., nerve
  e., reflex

excitant (ĕk-sīt'ănt)

excitation [L. *excitatio*]
  e., direct
  e., indirect

excitation wave

exciting

excitoglandular (ĕk-sīt"ō-glăn'dū-lăr) [L. *excitare*, to arouse, + *glans*, kernel]

excitometabolic (ĕk-sīt"ō-mĕt"ă-bŏl'ĭk) [" + Gr. *metabole*, change]

excitomotor (ĕk-sīt"ō-mō'tor) [" + *motor*, moving]

excitomuscular (ĕk-sīt"ō-mŭs'kū-lăr) [" + Gr. *mys*, muscle]

excitor (ĕk-sī'tor) [L. *excitare*, to arouse]

excitosecretory (ĕk-sīt"ō-sē'krĕ-tor-ē) [" + *secretio*, separation]

excitovascular (ĕk-sī"tō-văs'kū-lăr) [" + *vascularis*, pert. to a vessel]

exclave (ĕks'klāv) [Gr. *ex*, out, + L. *clavis*, key]

exclusion (ĕks-kloo'zhŭn) [L. *exclusio*, fr. *ex*, out, + *claudere*, to shut]

excochleation (ĕks-kŏk-lē-ā'shŭn) [L. *ex*, out, + *cochlea*, spoon]

excoriation (ĕks-kō-rē-ā'shŭn) [" + *corium*, skin]

excrement (ĕks'krĕ-mĕnt) [L. *excrementum*]

excrementitious (ĕks"krĕ-mĕn-tĭsh'ŭs)

excrescence (ĕks-krĕs'ĕns) [L. *ex*, out, + *crescere*, to grow]

excreta (ĕks-krē'tă) [L.]

excrete (ĕks-krēt') [L. *excretus*, sifted out]

excretion (ĕks-krē'shŭn) [L. *excretio*]

excretory (ĕks'krĕ-tō-rē) [L. *excretus*, sifted out]

excursion (ĕks-kŭr'zhŭn) [L. *excursio*]

excurvation (ĕks"kŭr-vā'shŭn) [Gr. *ex*, out, + L. *curvus*, bend]

excystation (ĕk"sĭs-tā'shŭn) [" + *kystis*, cyst]

exencephalia (ĕks"ĕn-sĕf-ā'lē-ă) [" + *enkephalos*, brain]

exenteration (ĕks-ĕn"tĕr-ā'shŭn) [" + *enteron*, intestine]

exercise [L. *exercitus*, having drilled]
  e., active
  e., assistive
  e., blowing
  e., Buerger's postural
  e., Codman's
  e., corrective
  e., crawling
  e., free
  e., isokinetic
  e., isometric
  e., isotonic
  e.'s, Kegel
  e., muscle-setting
  e., passive
  e., range-of-motion
  e., resistive
  e., static
  e., therapeutic

exercise bone

exercise electrocardiogram

exercise-induced asthma

exercise prescription

exercise tolerance test

exeresis (ĕks-ĕr'ĕ-sĭs) [Gr. *exairesis*, taking out]

exergonic (ĕk"sĕr-gŏn'ĭk) [Gr. *ex*, out, + *ergon*, work]

exfetation (ĕks-fē-tā'shŭn) [Gr. *ex*, out, + L. *fetus*, fetus]

exflagellation (ĕks"flăj-ĕ-lā'shŭn) [" + L. *flagellum*, whip]

exfoliation (ĕks"fō-lē-ā'shŭn) [" + L. *folium*, leaf]

exhalation (ĕks"hă-lā'shŭn) [" + L. *halare*, to breathe]

exhaustion [" + L. *haurire*, to drain]

e., heat
exhibit (ĕgs-hĭb'ĭt) [L. exhibere, to display]
exhibitionism [" + Gr. -ismos, condition]
exhibitionist
exhilarant (ĕg-zĭl'ăr-ănt) [L. exhilarare, to gladden]
exhumation (ĕks"hū-mā'shŭn) [L. ex, out, + humus, earth]
exitus (ĕk'sĭ-tŭs) [L., going out]
Ex-Lax
Exna
Exner's nerve (ĕks'nĕrz) [Siegmund Exner, Austrian physiologist, 1846-1926]
Exner's plexus
exo- [Gr. exo, outside]
exobiology (ĕk"sō-bī-ŏl'ō-jē)
exocardia (ĕk"sō-kăr'dē-ă) [" + kardia, heart]
exocardial
exocataphoria (ĕks"ō-kăt-ă-for'ē-ă) [" + kata, down, + phoros, bearing]
exocolitis (ĕks"ō-kō-lī'tĭs) [" + kolon, colon, + itis, inflammation]
exocrine (ĕks'ō-krĭn) [" + krinein, to separate]
exocytosis (ĕks"ō-sī-tō'sĭs) [" + kytos, cell, + osis, condition]
exodeviation (ĕk"sō-dē"vē-ā'shŭn)
exodic (ĕks-ŏd'ĭk) [" + hodos, way]
exodontia (ĕks-ō-dŏn'shē-ă) [" + odous, tooth]
exodontology (ĕks"ō-dŏn-tŏl'ō-jē) [" + " + logos, word, reason]
exoenzyme (ĕk-sō-ĕn'zĭm) [" + en, in, + zyme, leaven]
exoerythrocytic (ĕk"sō-ĕ-rĭth"rō-sī'tĭk) [" + erythros, red, + kytos, cell]
exogamy (ĕks-ŏg'ă-mē) [" + gamos, marriage]
exogastritis (ĕks"ō-găs-trī'tĭs) [" + gaster, belly, + itis, inflammation]
exogenous (ĕks-ŏj'ĕ-nŭs) [" +

gennan, to produce]
exohysteropexy (ĕks"ō-hĭs'tĕr-ō-pĕks"ē) [" + hystera, womb, + pexis, fixation]
exometritis (ĕks-ō-mē-trī'tĭs) [" + metra, womb, + itis, inflammation]
exomphalos (ĕks-ŏm'fă-lŭs) [Gr. ex, out, + omphalos, navel]
exons
exopathic (ĕk"sō-păth'ĭk) [Gr. exo, outside, + pathos, disease, suffering]
exophoria (ĕks"ō-fō'rē-ă) [" + phoros, bearing]
exophthalmia (ĕks"ŏf-thăl'mē-ă) [" + ophthalmos, eye]
e. cachectica
e. fungosa
exophthalmic (ĕks"ŏf-thăl'mĭk)
exophthalmic goiter
exophthalmometer (ĕk"sŏf-thăl-mŏm'ĕ-tĕr)
exophthalmos, exophthalmus (ĕks"ŏf-thăl'mōs, -mŭs)
e., pulsating
exoplasm (ĕk'sō-plăzm) [" + LL. plasma, form, mold]
exoserosis (ĕks"ō-sĕr-ō'sĭs) [" + serum, whey, + Gr. osis, condition]
exoskeleton (ĕk"sō-skĕl'ĕ-tŏn) [" + skeleton, a dried-up body]
exosmosis (ĕks"ŏs-mō'sĭs) [" + osmos, a thrusting, + osis, condition]
exosplenopexy (ĕks"ō-splēn'ō-pĕks-ē) [" + splen, spleen, + pexis, fixation]
exostosis (ĕks"ŏs-tō'sĭs) [" + osteon, bone]
e. bursata
e. cartilaginea
e., dental
e., multiple osteocartilaginous
exoteric (ĕks"ō-tĕr'ĭk) [Gr. exoterikos, outer]
exothermal, exothermic [Gr. exo, outside, + therme, heat]
exothymopexy (ĕks"ō-thī'mō-

pĕks″ē) [″ + *thymos,* thymus gland, + *pexis,* fixation]

exothyropexy (ĕks″ō-thī′rō-pĕks″ē)

exotic (ĕg-zŏt′ĭk) [Gr. *exotikos*]

exotoxin (ĕks″ō-tŏks′ĭn) [Gr. *exo,* outside, + *toxikon,* poison]

exotropia (ĕks″ō-trō′pē-ă) [″ + *tropos,* turning]

expander (ĕk-spăn′dĕr) [L. *expandere,* to spread out]

expansion (ĕks-păn′shŭn) [L. *expandere,* to spread out]

expansive delusion

expectant [Gr. *ex,* out, + L. *spectare,* to watch]

expectation

expected date of confinement

expectorant (ĕk-spĕk′tō-rănt) [Gr. *ex,* out, + L. *pectus,* breast]

expectoration (ĕk-spĕk″tō-rā′shŭn)

expel (ĕks-pĕl′) [L. *expellere*]

experiment [L. *experimentum,* to test]

expiration (ĕks″pī-rā′shŭn) [Gr. *ex,* out, + L. *spirare,* to breathe]
   e., active
   e., passive

expiratory (ĕks-pī′ră-tor″ē)

expiratory center

expire

explant (ĕks-plănt′) [″ + L. *plantare,* to plant]

explode (ĕks-plōd′) [L. *explodere,* fr. *ex,* out, + *plaudere,* to clap the hands]

exploration [L. *explorare,* to search out]

exploratory

explorer
   e., dental

explosive speech

exponent (ĕks′pō-nĕnt)

expose

exposure

express [L. *expressare*]

expression

expressivity

expulsion rate

expulsive [L. *expellere,* to drive out]

exsanguinate (ĕks-săn′gwĭn-āt) [Gr. *ex,* out, + *sanguis,* blood]

exsanguination (ĕk-săn″gwĭn-ā′shŭn)

exsanguine (ĕks-săn′gwĭn)

exsection (ĕk-sĕk′shŭn) [L. *exsectus,* having cut]

Exsel

exsiccant (ĕk-sĭk′ănt) [L. *exsiccare,* to dry out]

exsiccation (ĕk″sĭ-kā′shŭn)

exsiccative (ĕk-sĭk′kă-tĭv)

exsomatize (ĕk-sō′mă-tīz) [Gr. *ex,* out, + *soma,* body]

exsorption (ĕk-sorp′shŭn)

exstrophy (ĕks′trō-fē) [″ + *strephein,* to turn]
   e. of bladder

exsufflation (ĕk″sŭ-flā′shŭn) [″ + *sufflatio,* blown up]

ext. [L. *extractum,* extract]

extemporaneous [LL. *extemporaneus*]

extend (ĕk-stĕnd′) [Gr. *ex,* out, + L. *tendere,* to stretch]

extended care facility

extended family

extender (ĕk-stĕn′dĕr)

extension (ĕks-tĕn′shŭn) [L. *extensio*]
   e., Buck's

extensor [L.]

exterior [L.]

exteriorize

extern(e) (ĕks′tĕrn) [L. *externus,* outside]

external

external fixator

externalia (ĕks″tĕr-nā′lē-ă) [L. *exter,* outside, + *genitalis,* to beget]

externalize (ĕks-tĕr′nă-līz)

exteroceptive (ĕks″tĕr-ō-sĕp′tĭv) [L. *externus,* outside, + *receptus,* having received]

exteroceptor (ĕks″tĕr-ō-sĕp′tor)

exterofective (ĕks″tĕr-ō-fĕk′tĭv) [″ + *facere,* to make]

extima (ĕks′tĭ-mă) [L., outermost]

extinction [L. *exstinctus,* having extinguished]

extinguish (ĕks-tĭng'gwĭsh) [L. *extin-guere,* to render extinct]

extirpation (ĕks-tĭr-pā'shŭn) [L. *extir-pare,* to root out]

extorsion (ĕks-tor'shŭn) [Gr. *ex,* out, + L. *torsio,* twisting]

extra- [L. *extra,* outside]

extra-articular [" + *articulus,* joint]

extra beat

extracapsular (ĕks"tră-kăp'sū-lăr)

extracellular (ĕks"tră-sĕl'ū-lăr)

extracorporeal (ĕks"tră-kor-por'ē-ăl) [" + *corpus,* body]

extracorporeal membrane oxygenator

extracorporeal shock-wave lithotriptor

extracorticospinal (ĕks"tră-kor"tĭ-kō-spī'năl)

extracranial (ĕks"tră-krā'nē-ăl)

extract (ĕks-trăkt', ĕks'trăkt) [L. *extrac-tum*]
　　e., alcoholic
　　e., aqueous
　　e., aromatic fluid
　　e., compound
　　e., ethereal
　　e., fluid
　　e., powdered
　　e., soft
　　e., solid

extraction [L. *extractum,* drawing out]

extractive (ĕks-trăk'tĭv)

extractor
　　e., tissue
　　e., tube

extractum (ĕks-trăk'tŭm) [L., a drawing out]

extracystic (ĕks"tră-sĭs'tĭk) [L. *extra,* outside, + Gr. *kystis,* bladder]

extradural (ĕks-tră-dū'răl) [" + *durus,* hard]

extraembryonic (ĕks"tră-ĕm"brē-ŏn'ĭk) [" + Gr. *embryon,* to swell inside]

extragenital (ĕks"tră-jĕn'ĭ-tăl) [" + *genitalis,* to beget]

extrahepatic (ĕks"tră-hĕ-păt'ĭk) [L. *extra,* outside, + Gr. *hepatos,* liver]

extraligamentous [" + *ligare,* to bind]

extramalleolus (ĕks"tră-măl-lē'ō-lŭs) [" + *malleolus,* little hammer]

extramarginal (ĕks"tră-măr'jĭ-năl) [" + *margo,* margin]

extramarital

extramastoiditis (ĕks"tră-măs"toyd-ī'tĭs) [" + Gr. *mastos,* breast, + *eidos,* form, shape, + *itis,* inflammation]

extramedullary (ĕks"tră-mĕd'ū-lă-rē) [" + *medulla,* marrow]

extramural (ĕks"tră-mū'răl) [" + *murus,* wall]

extraneous (ĕks-trā'nē-ŭs) [L. *ex-traneus,* external]

extranuclear [L. *extra,* outside, + *nucleus,* kernel]

extraocular (ĕks"tră-ŏk'ū-lăr) [" + *oculus,* eye]

extraocular eye muscles

extrapolar [" + *polus,* pole]

extrapyramidal (ĕks"tră-pī-răm'ĭ-dăl)

extrapyramidal syndrome

extrapyramidal system

extrasensory

extrasensory perception

extrasystole (ĕks"tră-sĭs'tō-lē) [" + Gr. *systole,* contraction]
　　e., atrial
　　e., junctional
　　e., nodal
　　e., ventricular

extratubal (ĕks"tră-tū'băl)

extrauterine (ĕks"tră-ū'tĕr-ĭn) [" + *uterus,* womb]

extravaginal (ĕks"tră-văj'ĭ-năl) [" + *vagina,* sheath]

extravasate (ĕks-trăv"ă-sāt) [" + *vas,* vessel]

extravasation (ĕks-trăv"ă-sā'shŭn)

extravascular (ĕks"tră-văs'kū-lăr) [" + *vasculum,* vessel]

extraventricular [" + *ventriculus,*

little belly]
extremital (ĕks-trĕm'ĭ-tăl) [L. *extremus,*
outermost]
extremity
e., lower
e., upper
extrinsic (ĕks-trĭn'sĭk) [LL. *extrinsecus,*
outer]
extrinsic muscles
extrospection (ĕks″trō-spĕk'shŭn) [L.
extra, outside, + *spectare,* to look]
extroversion (ĕks″trō-vĕr'zhŭn) [″ +
vertere, to turn]
extrovert
extrude (ĕks-trūd') [L. *extrudere,* to
squeeze out]
extrusion (ĕks-troo'zhŭn)
extubation (ĕks″tū-bā'shŭn) [Gr. *ex,*
out, + L. *tuba,* tube]
exuberant (ĕg-zū'bĕr-ănt) [L. *exuber-
are,* to be very fruitful]
exudate (ĕks'ū-dāt) [L. *exsudare,* to
sweat out]
exudation (ĕks″ū-dā'shŭn)
exudative (ĕks'ū-dā″tĭv)
exude (ĕg-zūd', ĕk-sūd') [L. *exsudare,*
to sweat out]
exumbilication (ĕks″ŭm-bĭl″ĭ-kā'shŭn)
[Gr. *ex,* out, + L. *umbilicus,* navel]
exuviae (ĕks-ū'vē-ē) [L.]
eye [AS. *eage*]
e., aphakic

e., black
e., crossed
e., dark-adapted
e. deviation
e., dominant
e., dry
e., exciting
e., fixating
e., foreign body in
e., light-adapted
e., pink-
e., squinting
e., sympathizing
eyeball
eye bank
eyebrow
eye contact
eyecup
eyedrops
eye-gaze communicator
eyeglass
eyeground
eyelash
eyelid
e., drooping
e., fused
eyelid closure reflex
eye muscle imbalance
eyepiece (ī'pēs)
eye stones
eyestrain
eyewash

F

F Fahrenheit; field of vision; fluorine; folic acid; formula; function; Fusiformis

F₁

F₂

FA, F.A. fatty acid; filterable agent; first aid; fluorescent antibody

F.A.A.N. Fellow of the American Academy of Nursing

Fab fragment antigen binding

fabella (fă-bĕl'lă) [L., little bean]

fabism (fā'bĭzm) [L. faba, bean, + Gr. -ismos, condition]

fabrication (făb"rĭ-kā'shŭn) [L. fabricatus, having built]

Fabry's disease (fă'brēz) [J. Fabry, Ger. physician, 1860–1930]

F.A.C.D. Fellow of the American College of Dentists

face [L. facies]

    f., moon

facet, facette (făs'ĕt) [Fr. facette, small face]

facetectomy (făs"ĕ-tĕk'tō-mē) [" + Gr. ektome, excision]

facial [L. facialis]

facial bones

facial center

facial nerve

facial paralysis

facial reflex

facial spasm

facies (fā'shē-ēz) [L.]

    f. abdominalis

    f., adenoid

    f. aortica

    f. hepatica

    f. hippocratica

    f. leontina

    f., masklike

    f. mitralis

    f., myopathic

    f., parkinsonian

    f., typhoid

facilitation (fă-sĭl"ĭ-tā'shŭn) [L. facilis, easy]

facing [L. facies, face]

faciobrachial (fā"shē-ō-brā'kē-ăl) [" + Gr. brachion, arm]

faciocephalalgia (fā"shē-ō-sĕf"ă-lăl'jē-ă) [" + Gr. kephale, head, + algos, pain]

faciocervical (fā"shē-ō-sĕr'vĭ-kăl) [" + cervix, neck]

faciolingual (fā"shē-ō-lĭn'gwăl) [" + lingua, tongue]

facioplasty (fā"shē-ō-plăs'tē) [" + Gr. plassein, to form]

facioplegia (fā"shē-ō-plē'jē-ă) [" + Gr. plege, stroke]

facioscapulohumeral (fā"shē-ō-skăp"ū-lō-hū'mĕr-ăl) [" + scapula, shoulder blade, + humerus, shoulder]

F.A.C.O.G. Fellow of the American College of Obstetricians and Gynecologists

F.A.C.P. Fellow of the American College of Physicians

F.A.C.S. Fellow of the American College of Surgeons

F.A.C.S.M. Fellow of the American College of Sports Medicine

factitious (făk-tĭsh'ŭs) [L. facticius, made by art]

factitious disorders

factor [L., maker]

    f., accessory food

    f., antianemic

    f., antihemophilic

    f.'s, coagulation

    f., lethal

    f., milk

    f., proliferation inhibiting

f., Rh
Factorate
facultative (făk'ŭl-tā"tĭv) [L. *facultas*, capability]
faculty
FAD *flavin adenine dinucleotide*
fagopyrism (făg-ō-pīr'ĭzm, -ŏp'ĭ-rĭzm) [L. *fagopyrum*, buckwheat]
Fahrenheit scale (făr'ĕn-hīt") [Gabriel D. Fahrenheit, Ger. physicist, 1686–1736]
failure (fāl'yĕr)
    f., heart
    f., kidney or renal
    f., respiratory
failure to thrive
faint [O. Fr. *faindre*, to feign]
faintness
faith healing
falcate (făl'kāt) [L. *falx*, sickle]
falces (făl'sēz) [L.]
falcial (făl'shăl)
falciform (făl'sĭ-form) [L. *falx*, sickle, + *forma*, form]
falciform ligament
falciform ligament of liver
falciform process
falcular
fallectomy (făl-ĕk'tō-mē)
falling drop
fallopian canal (fă-lō'pē-ăn) [Gabriele Fallopio, It. anatomist, 1523–1562]
fallopian ligament
fallopian tube
Fallot, tetralogy of (făl-ō') [Etienne L. A. Fallot, Fr. physician, 1850–1911]
fallotomy (făl-ŏt'ō-mē)
fallout
false [L. *falsus*]
false-negative (făwls'nĕg'ă-tĭv)
false-positive (făwls'pŏs'ĭ-tĭv)
false ribs
falsification (făwl"sĭ-fĭ-kā'shŭn)
    f., retrospective
falx [L.]
    f. cerebelli
    f. cerebri

f. inguinalis
f. ligmentosa
fames (fā'mēz) [L.]
familial [L. *familia*, family]
familial Mediterranean fever
familial periodic paralysis
family
family planning
family practice
family therapy
Fanconi's syndrome [Guido Fanconi, Swiss pediatrician, 1892–1979]
fang [AS., to plunder]
fango (făn'gō) [Italian, mud]
Fannia (făn'ē-ă)
fantast (făn'tăst) [Gr. *phantasia*, imagination]
fantasy (făn'tă-sē) [Gr. *phantasia*, imagination]
F.A.O.T.A. *Fellow of the American Occupational Therapy Association*
farad (făr'ăd) [Michael Faraday, Brit. physicist, 1791–1867]
faraday (făr'ă-dā)
faradic
faradism
faradization
faradotherapy
farcy (făr'sē) [L. *farcire*, to stuff]
    f., button
farina (fă-rē'nă) [L.]
farinaceous (făr"ĭ-nā'shŭs)
farmer's lung
farpoint
Farre's tubercles (fărz) [John R. Farre, Brit. physician, 1775–1862]
farsighted
farsightedness
fart [Old High Ger. *fezan*, to break wind]
fascia (făsh'ē-ă) [L., a band]
    f., Abernethy's
    f., anal
    f., aponeurotic
    f., Buck's
    f., cervical, deep
    f., cervical, superficial
    f., Cloquet's

f., Colles'
f., cremasteric
f., cribriform
f., crural
f., deep
f., dentate
f., endothoracic
f., extrapleural
f., intercolumnar
f. lata femoris
f., lumbodorsal
f., pectineal
f., pelvic
f., pharyngobasilar
f., plantar
f., Scarpa's
f., superficial
f., thyrolaryngeal
f. transversalis
fasciae (făsh'ē-ē)
fascial (făsh'ē-ăl) [L. *fascia*, a band]
fascial reflex
fasciaplasty (făsh'ē-ă-plăs"tē) [" +
Gr. *plassein*, to form]
fascicle (făs'ĭ-kl) [L. *fasciculus*, little bun-
dle]
fascicular (fă-sĭk'ū-lăr)
fasciculation (fă-sĭk"ū-lă'shŭn)
fasciculus (fă-sĭk'ū-lŭs)
f. cuneatus
f., dorsolateral
f., fundamental
f. gracilis
f., longitudinal, dorsal
f., longitudinal, inferior
f., longitudinal, medial
f., longitudinal, posterior
f., unciform
fasciectomy (făsh"ē-ĕk'tō-mē) [L. *fascia*, band, + Gr. *ektome*, excision]
fasciitis (făs"ē-ī'tĭs)
fasciodesis (făsh"ē-ŏd'ĕ-sĭs) [" +
Gr. *desis*, binding]
Fasciola (fă-sī'ō-lă) [L. *fasciola*, a band]
F. hepatica
fasciola (fă-sī'ō-lă, fă-sē'ō-lă) [L., a
band]
f. cinerea

fasciolar (fă-sē'ō-lăr)
fasciolopsiasis (făs"ē-ō-lŏp-sī'ă-sĭs)
Fasciolopsis buski (făs"ē-ō-lŏp'sĭs)
fascioplasty (făsh'ē-ō-plăs"tē) [" +
Gr. *plassein*, to form]
fasciorrhaphy (făsh-ē-or'ă-fē) [" +
Gr. *rhaphe*, seam]
fasciotomy (făsh-ē-ŏt'ō-mē) [" +
Gr. *tome*, a cutting, slice]
fascitis (fă-sī'tĭs) [" + Gr. *itis*, in-
flammation]
fast [AS. *faest*, fixed; AS. *faestan*, to
hold fast]
f., acid
fastidium (făs-tĭd'ē-ŭm) [L., aversion]
fastigium (făs-tĭj'ē-ŭm) [L., ridge]
fasting [AS. *faestan*, to hold fast]
fastness [AS. *faest*, fixed]
fat [AS. *faett*]
f., neutral
fatal (fāt'l) [L. *fatalis*]
fat emulsion
fatigability (făt"ĭ-gă-bĭl'ĭ-tē)
fatigue (fă-tēg') [L. *fatigare*, to tire]
f., acute
f., chronic
f., muscular
fatty (făt'ē)
fatty acid
f.a., essential
f.a., free
fatty acids, omega 3- (ω3)
fatty casts
fatty change
fatty degeneration
fauces (fŏ'sēz) [L.]
faucial (fŏ'shăl) [L. *fauces*, throat]
faucial reflex
faucitis (fŏ-sī'tĭs) [" + Gr. *itis*, in-
flammation]
fauna (faw'nă) [L. *Faunus*, mythical deity
of herdsmen]
faveolate (fă-vē'ō-lāt) [L. *faveolus*, little
honeycomb]
faveolus (fă-vē'ō-lŭs) [L., little honey-
comb]
favism (fă'vĭzm) [It. *fava*, bean, +
Gr. *-ismos*, condition]

favus (fā'vŭs) [L., honeycomb]
F.D. *fatal dose; focal distance*
F.D.A. *Food and Drug Administration*
Fe [L.] *ferrum,* iron
fear [AS. *faer*]
febricide (fĕb'rĭ-sīd) [L. *febris,* fever,
   + *caedere,* to kill]
febrifacient (fĕb-rĭ-fā'sē-ĕnt) [" +
facere, to make]
febrific (fĕ-brĭf'ĭk)
febrifugal (fĕb-rĭf'ū-găl) [" + *fugare,* to put to flight]
febrifuge (fĕb'rĭ-fūj)
febrile (fē'brĭl, fē'brīl, fĕb'rĭl) [L. *febris,*
fever]
febrile convulsions
febrile state
febriphobia (fĕb"rĭ-fō'bē-ă) [" +
Gr. *phobos,* fear]
febris (fē'brĭs) [L.]
   f. enterica
   f. flava
   f. undulans
fecal (fē'kăl) [L. *faeces,* refuse]
fecalith (fē'kă-lĭth) [" + Gr. *lithos,*
stone]
fecaloid (fē'kă-loyd) [" + Gr.
eidos, form, shape]
fecaloma (fē"kăl-ō'mă) [" + Gr.
oma, tumor]
fecaluria (fē"kăl-ū'rē-ă) [" + Gr.
ouron, urine]
fecal vomit
feces (fē'sēz) [L. *faeces*]
Fechner's law (fĕk'nĕrz) [Gustav T.
Fechner, Ger. philosopher, 1801–
1887]
Fe(C₃H₅O₃)₂
FeCl₂
FeCl₃
FeCO₃
fecula (fĕk'ū-lă) [L. *faecula,* dregs]
feculent (fĕk'ū-lĕnt) [L. *faeculentus*]
fecundate (fē'kŭn-dāt) [L. *fecundare,* to
bear fruit]
fecundation (fē"kŭn-dā'shŭn)
   f., artificial
fecundity (fē-kŭn'dĭ-tē)

feedback
feeder
feeding [AS. *fedan,* to give food to]
   f., artificial
   f., breast
   f., forcible
   f., intravenous
   f., rectal
   f., tube
feeling [AS. *felan,* to feel]
Feen-A-Mint
Feer's disease (fārz) [Emil Feer, Swiss
pediatrician, 1864–1955]
feet [AS. *fet*]
Fehling's solution (fā'lĭngz) [Hermann
von Fehling, Ger. chemist, 1812–
1885]
Feingold diet (fīn'gōld) [Benjamin Feingold, U.S. pediatrician, 1900–1982]
fel (fĕl) [L.]
feline (fē'līn) [L. *feles,* cat]
fellatio (fĕl-ā'shē-ō) [L. *fellare,* to suck]
felon (fĕl'ŏn) [ME. *feloun,* malignant]
feltwork
Felty's syndrome (fĕl'tēz) [A. R. Felty,
U.S. physician, b. 1895]
female [L. *femella,* little woman]
feminine (fĕm'ĭ-nīn)
feminism [L. *femininus*]
feminization
   f., testicular
Feminone
femoral (fĕm'or-ăl) [L. *femoralis*]
femoral artery
femoral reflex
femoral vein
femorocele (fĕm'ō-rō-sēl") [L. *femur,*
thigh, + Gr. *kele,* tumor, swelling]
femorotibial (fĕm"ō-rō-tĭb'ē-ăl) [" +
tibia, shinbone]
femto- [Danish *femten,* fifteen]
femur (fē'mŭr) [L.]
fenestra (fĕn-ĕs'tră) [L., window]
   f. cochleae
   f. rotunda
   f. vestibuli
fenestrated (fĕn'ĕs-trāt"ĕd) [L. *fenestra,* window]

fenestration
fenfluramine hydrochloride (fĕn-floor'ă-mēn)
fenoprofen calcium (fĕn-ō-prō'fĕn)
fentanyl citrate (fĕn'tă-nĭl)
Feosol
Feostat
feral (fĕr'ŭl) [L. *fera*, wild animal]
Fergon
ferment (fĕr-mĕnt', fĕr'mĕnt) [L. *fermentum*]
fermentation
    f., acetic
    f., alcoholic
    f., amylolytic
    f., autolytic
    f., butyric
    f., citric acid
    f., invertin
    f., lactic
    f., oxalic acid
    f., propionic acid
    f., viscous
fermentum (fĕr-mĕn'tŭm) [L.]
fermium (fĕr'mē-ŭm) [Enrico Fermi, 1901–1954]
fern [AS. *fearn*]
fern pattern, ferning
Fero-Gradumet
-ferous [L. *ferre*, to bear]
ferrated (fĕr-āt'ĕd) [L. *ferrum*, iron]
ferri-, ferro- [L. *ferrum*, iron]
ferric
    f. chloride
ferrin
ferritin (fĕr'ĭ-tĭn)
ferrokinetics (fĕr"rō-kĭ-nĕt'ĭks) [" + Gr. *kinesis*, motion]
ferropexia (fĕr-ō-pĕks'ē-ă)
ferroprotein (fĕr"ō-prō'tē-ĭn)
ferrotherapy (fĕr"ō-thĕr'ă-pē) [" + Gr. *therapeia*, treatment]
ferrous (fĕr'ŭs) [L. *ferrum*, iron]
    f. fumarate
    f. gluconate
    f. sulfate
ferruginous (fĕr-ū'jĭ-nŭs) [L. *ferrugo*, iron rust]

ferrule (fĕr'ŭl) [L. *viriola*, little bracelet]
ferrum (fĕr'ŭm) [L., iron]
fertile (fĕr'tĭl) [L. *fertilis*]
fertility (fĕr-tĭl'ĭ-tē)
fertilization [L. *fertilis*, reproductive]
    f., in vitro
fertilizin (fĕr"tĭ-lī'zĭn)
fervescence (fĕr-vĕs'ĕns) [L. *fervescere*, to grow hot]
fester (fĕs'tĕr) [L. *fistula*, ulcer]
festinant (fĕs'tĭ-nănt)
festination (fĕs"tĭ-nā'shŭn) [L. *festinatio*]
festoon (fĕs-toon') [L. *festus*, festal]
fetal (fē'tăl) [L. *fetus*, fetus]
fetal alcohol syndrome
fetal circulation
fetal distress
fetalism (fē'tăl-ĭzm) [" + Gr. *-ismos*, condition]
fetal membranes
feticide (fē'tĭ-sīd) [" + *caedere*, to kill]
fetid (fē'tĭd) [L. *fetidus*, stink]
fetish (fē'tĭsh) [Portug. *feitico*, charm, sorcery]
fetishism (fē'tĭsh-, fĕt'ĭsh-ĭzm) [" + Gr. *-ismos*, condition]
fetochorionic (fē"tō-kor-ē-ŏn'ĭk) [L. *fetus*, fetus, + Gr. *chorion*, membrane]
fetoglobulin (fē"tō-glŏb'ū-lĭn)
fetography (fē-tŏg'ră-fē)
fetology (fē-tŏl'ō-jē) [" + Gr. *logos*, word, reason]
fetometry (fē-tŏm'ĕ-trē) [L. *fetus*, fetus, + Gr. *metron*, measure]
fetoplacental (fē"tō-plă-sĕn'tăl) [" + *placenta*, a flat cake]
fetoprotein (fē"tō-prō'tēn)
fetor (fē'tor) [L.]
    f. ex ore
    f. hepaticus
    f. oris
fetoscope
fetoscopy
fetotoxic (fē"tō-tŏk'sĭk) [L. *fetus*, fetus, + Gr. *toxikon*, poison]

fetus (fē'tŭs) [L.]
  f. amorphus
  f., calcified
  f. in fetu
  f., mummified
  f. papyraceus
  f., parasitic
FEV₁
fever [L. febris]
  f., childbed
  f., continuous
  f., drug
  f., induced
  f., intermittent
  f. of unknown origin
  f., periodic
  f., relapsing
  f., remittent
  f., septic
fever blister
F.F.D. focal film distance
FH₄ 5,6,7,8-tetrahydrofolic acid
fiat (fī'ăt) [L., let there be made]
fiber [L. fibra]
  f., accelerator
  f., afferent
  f., dietary
  f., efferent
  f., inhibitory
  f., medullated
  f., nerve
  f., nonmedullated
  f.'s, Purkinje
  f., unmyelinated
fibercolonoscope (fī″bĕr-kō-lŏn'ō-skōp)
fibergastroscope (fī″bĕr-găs'trō-skōp)
fiberglass
fiber-illuminated (fī'bĕr-ĭl-loo″mĭn-ā″tĕd)
fiberoptic
fiberscope (fī'bĕr-skōp)
fibra (fī'bră) [L.]
fibralbumin (fī″brăl-bū'mĭn) [″ + albumen, white of egg]
fibremia (fī-brē'mē-ă) [″ + Gr. haima, blood]

fibril (fī'brĭl) [L. fibrilla]
  f., muscle
  f., nerve
fibrilla (fĭ-brĭl'ă) [L.]
fibrillar, fibrillary
fibrillated (fī'brĭ-lāt'd) [L. fibrilla, little fiber]
fibrillation (fĭ″brĭl-ā'shŭn)
  f., atrial
  f., ventricular
fibrillogenesis (fĭ-brĭl″ō-jĕn'ĕ-sĭs)
fibrillolysis (fĭ″brĭl-ŏl'ĭ-sĭs) [″ + Gr. lysis, dissolution]
fibrillolytic (fĭ″brĭl-ŏ-lĭt'ĭk)
fibrin (fī'brĭn) [L. fibra, fiber]
  f. foam
fibrinocellular (fī″brĭ-nō-sĕl'ū-lăr)
fibrinogen (fĭ-brĭn'ō-jĕn) [″ + Gr. gennan, to produce]
fibrinogenic, fibrinogenous
fibrinogenolysis (fī″brĭ-nō-jĕ-nŏl'ĭ-sĭs) [″ + ″ + lysis, dissolution]
fibrinogenopenia (fĭ-brĭn″ō-jĕn″ō-pē'nē-ă) [″ + Gr. gennan, to produce, + penia, lack]
fibrinoid (fī'brĭ-noyd) [″ + Gr. eidos, form, shape]
fibrinoid change
fibrinoid material
fibrinokinase (fī″brĭ-nō-kī'nās)
fibrinolysin (fī″brĭn-ŏl'ĭ-sĭn) [L. fibra, fibrin, + Gr. lysis, dissolution]
fibrinolysis (fī″brĭn-ŏl'ĭ-sĭs)
fibrinolytic (fī″brĭn-ō-lĭt'ĭk)
fibrinopenia (fī″brĭn-ō-pē'nē-ă) [″ + Gr. penia, lack]
fibrinopeptide (fī″brĭ-nō-pĕp'tĭd)
fibrinoplastic (fī″brĭn-ō-plăs'tĭk) [″ + Gr. plassein, to form]
fibrinopurulent (fī″brĭ-nō-pū'roo-lĕnt) [″ + purulentus, full of pus]
fibrinoscopy (fĭ-brĭ-nŏs'kō-pē) [″ + Gr. skopein, to examine]
fibrinosis (fĭ-brĭ-nō'sĭs) [″ + Gr. osis, condition]
fibrinous (fī'brĭn-ŭs) [L. fibra, fiber]
fibrinuria (fĭ-brĭn-ū'rē-ă) [″ + Gr. ouron, urine]

fibro- [L. *fibra*]
fibroadenia (fĭ″brō-ă-dē″nē-ă) [″ + Gr. *aden*, gland]
fibroadenoma (fĭ″brō-ăd″ĕ-nō′mă) [″ + ″ + *oma*, tumor]
fibroadipose [″ + *adeps*, fat]
fibroangioma [″ + Gr. *angeion*, vessel, + *oma*, tumor]
fibroareolar (fĭ″brō-ă-rē′ō-lăr) [″ + *areola*, little space]
fibroblast (fĭ′brō-blăst) [″ + Gr. *blastos*, germ]
fibroblastoma (fĭ″brō-blăs-tō′mă) [″ + ″ + *oma*, tumor]
fibrobronchitis (fĭ″brō-brŏn-kī′tĭs) [″ + Gr. *bronchos*, windpipe, + *itis*, inflammation]
fibrocalcific (fĭ″brō-kăl-sĭf′ĭk)
fibrocarcinoma (fĭ″brō-kăr″sĭ-nō′mă) [″ + Gr. *karkinos*, cancer, + *oma*, tumor]
fibrocartilage (fĭ″brō-kăr′tĭ-lĭj) [″ + *cartilago*, gristle]
fibrocellular (fĭ″brō-sĕl′ū-lăr) [″ + *cellula*, little cell]
fibrochondritis (fĭ″brō-kŏn-drī′tĭs) [″ + Gr. *chondros*, cartilage, + *itis*, inflammation]
fibrochondroma (fĭ″brō-kŏn-drō′mă) [″ + ″ + *oma*, tumor]
fibrocyst (fĭ′brō-sĭst) [″ + Gr. *kystis*, cyst]
fibrocystic (fĭ″brō-sĭs′tĭk)
fibrocystic disease of the breast
fibrocystic disease of pancreas
fibrocystoma (fĭ″brō-sĭs-tō′mă) [″ + Gr. *kystis*, cyst, + *oma*, tumor]
fibrocyte (fĭ′brō-sīt) [″ + *kytos*, cell]
fibrodysplasia (fĭ″brō-dĭs-plă′sē-ă) [″ + Gr. *dys*, bad, difficult, painful, disordered, + *plassein*, to form]
fibroelastic (fĭ″brō-ē-lăs′tĭk) [″ + NL. *elasticus*, expansive, impulsive]
fibroelastosis (fĭ″brō-ē″lăs-tō′sĭs)
 f., endocardial
fibroenchondroma (fĭ″brō-ĕn″kŏn-drō′mă) [″ + Gr. *en*, in, +

chondros, cartilage, + *oma*, tumor]
fibroepithelioma (fĭ″brō-ĕp″ĭ-thē″lē-ō′mă) [″ + Gr. *epi*, upon, + *thele*, nipple, + *oma*, tumor]
fibroglia (fĭ-brŏg′lē-ă) [″ + Gr. *glia*, glue]
fibroglioma (fĭ-brō-glī-ō′mă) [″ + Gr. *glia*, glue, + *oma*, tumor]
fibroid (fĭ′broyd) [″ + Gr. *eidos*, form, shape]
 f., interstitial
 f., uterine
fibroidectomy (fĭ-broyd-ĕk′tō-mē) [″ + ″ + *ektome*, excision]
fibrolipoma (fĭ″brō-lĭ-pō′mă) [″ + Gr. *lipos*, fat, + *oma*, tumor]
fibroma (fĭ-brō′mă) [″ + Gr. *oma*, tumor]
 f., intramural
 f. of breast
 f., submucous
 f., subserous
 f., uterine
fibromatosis (fĭ″brō-mă-tō′sĭs) [L. *fibra*, fiber, + Gr. *oma*, tumor, + *osis*, condition]
 f. gingivae
 f., palmar
fibromatous (fĭ-brō′mă-tŭs)
fibromectomy (fĭ″brō-mĕk′tō-mē) [″ + Gr. *oma*, tumor, + *ektome*, excision]
fibromembranous (fĭ″brō-mĕm′bră-nŭs) [″ + *membrana*, web]
fibromuscular (fĭ″brō-mŭs′kū-lăr) [″ + *musculus*, muscle]
fibromyalgia
fibromyitis (fĭ″brō-mī-ī′tĭs) [″ + Gr. *mys*, muscle, + *itis*, inflammation]
fibromyoma (fĭ″brō-mī-ō′mă) [″ + ″ + *oma*, tumor]
fibromyomectomy (fĭ″brō-mī″ō-mĕk′tō-mē) [″ + ″ + *ektome*, excision]
fibromyositis (fĭ″brō-mī″ō-sī′tĭs) [″ + *mys*, muscle, + *itis*, inflammation]
fibromyotomy (fĭ″brō-mī-ŏt′ō-mē)

[" + " + *tome*, a cutting, slice]

fibromyxoma   (fĭ"brō-mĭk-sō'mă)
[" + Gr. *myxa*, mucus, + *oma*, tumor]

fibromyxosarcoma   (fĭ"brō-mĭk"sō-săr-kō'mă) [" + " + *sarkos*, flesh, + *oma*, tumor]

fibroneuroma   (fĭ"brō-nū-rō'mă) [" + Gr. *neuron*, nerve, + *oma*, tumor]

fibro-osteoma   (fĭ"brō-ŏs-tē-ō'mă) [" + Gr. *osteon*, bone, + *oma*, tumor]

fibropapilloma   (fĭ"brō-păp-ĭ-lō'mă) [" + *papilla*, nipple, + Gr. *oma*, tumor]

fibroplasia   (fĭ"brō-plā'sē-ă) [" + Gr. *plasis*, a molding]
   f., retrolental

fibroplastic   (fĭ"brō-plăs'tĭk) [" + Gr. *plassein*, to form]

fibropurulent   (fĭ"brō-pūr'ū-lĕnt) [" + *purulentus*, full of pus]

fibrosarcoma   (fĭ"brō-săr-kō'mă) [L. *fibra*, fiber, + Gr. *sarkos*, flesh, + *oma*, tumor]

fibrose   (fĭ'brōs)

fibroserous   (fĭ"brō-sē'rŭs) [" + *serosus*, serous]

fibrosis   (fĭ-brō'sĭs) [" + Gr. *osis*, condition]
   f., arteriocapillary
   f., diffuse interstitial pulmonary
   f. of lungs
   f., postfibrinosis
   f., proliferative
   f., pulmonary
   f., retroperitoneal
   f. uteri

fibrositis   (fĭ-brō-sī'tĭs) [" + Gr. *itis*, inflammation]

fibrothorax   (fĭ"brō-thō'răks) [" + Gr. *thorax*, chest]

fibrotic   (fĭ-brŏt'ĭk)

fibrous   (fĭ'brŭs) [L. *fibra*, fiber]

fibula   (fĭb'ū-lă) [L., pin]

fibular

fibulocalcaneal   (fĭb"ū-lō-kăl-kā'nē-ăl) [" + *calcaneus*, heel]

ficin   (fī'sĭn) [L. *ficus*, fig]

Fick method   [Adolf Fick, Ger. physician, 1829 – 1901]

F.I.C.S.   *Fellow of the International College of Surgeons*

FID   *flame ionization detector*

field   [AS. *feld*]
   f., auditory
   f., high-power
   f., low-power
   f. of vision

fifth cranial nerve

Fifth disease

fifth ventricle

FIGLU, FIGlu   *formiminoglutamic acid*

FIGLU excretion test

figurate   (fĭg'ū-rāt) [L. *figuratum*, figured]

figure   [L. *figura*]

figure-ground discrimination

fila   (fī'lă) [L. *filum*, thread]

filaceous   (fĭ-lā'shŭs)

filament   [L. *filamentum*]
   f., axial

filamentous

filar   (fī'lăr) [L. *filum*, thread]

Filaria   (fĭl-ā'rē-ă) [L. *filum*, thread]
   F. bancrofti
   F. loa
   F. medinensis
   F. sanguinis hominis

filaria   (fĭl-ā'rē-ă) [L. *filum*, thread]

filarial   (fĭ-lā'rē-ăl)

filariasis   (fĭl-ă-rī'ă-sĭs) [" + Gr. *-iasis*, state or condition of]

filaricidal   (fĭ-lăr"ĭ-sīd'ăl) [" + *cida* fr. *caedere*, to kill]

Filarioidea   (fĭ-lăr"ē-oy'dē-ă)

file   (fīl)

filial generation

filiform   (fĭl'ĭ-form) [" + *forma*, form]

fillet   (fĭl'ĕt) [Fr. *filet*, a band]

filling   (fĭl'ĭng) [AS. *fyllan*, to fill]

film
   f., bite-wing
   f., spot
   f., x-ray

film badge

filopressure (fĭ'lō-prĕ"shūr) [L. *filum*, thread, + *pressura*, pressure]
filovaricosis (fĭ"lō-văr-ĭ-kō'sĭs) [" + *varix*, a dilated vein, + Gr. *osis*, condition]
filter [L. *filtrare*, to strain through]
   f. bed
   f., Berkefeld
   f., infrared
   f., Kitasato's
   f., membrane
   f., Millipore
   f., optical
   f., Pasteur-Chamberland
   f., umbrella
   f., Wood's
filterable [L. *filtrare*, to strain through]
filtrate (fĭl'trāt)
   f., glomerular
filtration (fĭl-trā'shŭn)
filtration of roentgen rays
filtrum [L.]
filum (fī'lŭm) [L.]
   f. coronaria
   f. terminale
fimbria (fĭm'brē-ă) [L., fringe]
   f. ovarica
   f. tubae
fimbriate (fĭm'brē-āt")
fimbriated [L. *fimbria*, fringe]
fimbriocele (fĭm'brē-ō-sēl") [" + Gr. *kele*, tumor, swelling]
fine motor skills
finger [AS.]
   f., baseball
   f., clubbed
   f., dislocation of
   f., hammer
   f., mallet
   f., seal
   f., webbed
finger cot
finger ladder
fingerprint
finger spelling
finger spreader
finger spring
finger-stall

finite
fire [AS. *fyr*]
   f., St. Anthony's
fire emergencies
first aid
first cranial nerves
first-degree A-V block
first intention healing
Fishberg concentration test (fish'bĕrg) [A. M. Fishberg, U.S. physician, b. 1898]
fish poisoning
fishskin disease
fission (fĭsh'ŭn) [L. *fissio*]
fissiparous (fĭ-sĭp'ă-rŭs) [L. *fissus*, cleft, + *parere*, to beget, produce]
fissura (fĭs-ū'ră) [L.]
fissural (fĭsh'ū-răl)
fissure (fĭsh'ūr) [L. *fissura*]
   f., anal
   f., auricular
   f., branchial
   f., Broca's
   f., Burdach's
   f., calcarine
   f., callosomarginal
   f., central
   f., Clevenger's
   f., collateral
   f.'s, Henle's
   f., hippocampal
   f., inferior orbital
   f., interparietal
   f., longitudinal
   f., occipitoparietal
   f. of Bichat
   f. of Sylvius
   f., palpebral
   f., portal
   f., Rolando's
   f., sphenoidal
   f., transverse
   f., umbilical
   f., Wernicke's
   f., zygal
fistula (fĭs'tū-lă) [L., *fistula*, pipe]
   f., anal
   f., arteriovenous

f., biliary
f., blind
f., branchial
f., cervical
f., complete
f., craniosinus
f., enterovaginal
f., fecal
f., gastric
f., horseshoe
f., incomplete
f., metroperitoneal
f., parotid
f., perineovaginal
f., pulmonary arteriovenous, congenital
f., rectovaginal
f., thyroglossal
f., umbilical
f., ureterovaginal
f., vesicouterine
f., vesicovaginal

fistulatome (fĭs'tū-lă-tōm") [" + Gr. *tome*, a cutting, slice]
fistulectomy (fĭs"tū-lĕk'tō-mē) [" + Gr. *ektome*, excision]
fistulization (fĭs"tū-lĭ-zā'shŭn) [L. *fistula*, pipe]
fistuloenterostomy (fĭs"tū-lō-ĕn-tĕr-ŏs'tō-mē) [" + Gr. *enteron*, intestine, + *stoma*, mouth, opening]
fistulous (fĭs'tū-lŭs)
fit (fĭt) [AS. *fitt*]
fitness, biologic
fix
fixation [L. *fixatio*]
f., complement
f., field of
f. of eyes
fixation point
fixative (fĭk'să-tĭv) [L. *fixus*, fastened]
fixed eruption
fixed partial denture
fixing
Fl *fluid*
flaccid (flăk'sĭd) [L. *flaccidus*, flabby]
flaccid paralysis
flagella (flă-jĕl'ă) [L.]

flagellant (flăj'ĕ-lănt) [L. *flagellum*, whip]
flagellate (flăj'ĕ-lāt)
flagellation (flăj"ĕ-lā'shŭn)
flagelliform (flă-jĕl'ĭ-form) [" + *forma*, shape]
flagellum (flă-jĕl'ŭm) [L., whip]
Flagyl
flail chest
flail joint
flames, inhalation of
flange (flănj)
flank [O. Fr. *flanc*]
flap [Dutch *flappen*, to strike]
f., amputation
f., extraction
f., island
f., jump
f., pedicle
f., periodontal
f., skin
f., sliding
f., tube
flare
flash
flashbacks
flash method
flash point
flask [LL. *flasco*]
flatfoot
f., spasmodic
flatness
flatplate
flatulence (flăt'ū-lĕns) [L. *flatulentus*]
flatulent (flăt'ū-lĕnt)
flatus (flā'tŭs) [L., a blowing]
f., vaginal
flatus tube
flatworm
flavedo (flă-vē'dō) [L.]
flavescent (flă-vĕs'ĕnt)
flavin (flā'vĭn)
flavism (flā'vĭzm) [L. *flavus*, yellow, + Gr. *-ismos*, condition]
flavivirus (flā"vē-vī'rŭs)
flavo- [L. *flavus*, yellow]
Flavobacterium
flavone (flā'vōn)

flavoprotein
flavor (flā'vor)
Flaxedil
flaxseed
fl. dr. *fluidram*
flea (flē) [AS. *flea*]
   f., cat
   f., chigger
   f., dog
   f., human
   f., rat
flea bites
flea infestation
fleam (flēm) [Fr. *flieme*]
flecainide acetate
Flechsig's areas (flĕk'zīgz) [Paul E. Flechsig, Ger. neurologist, 1847–1929]
fleece of Stilling
Fleet Bisacodyl
Fleet Enema
Fleet Mineral Oil Enema
Fleming, Sir Alexander (flĕm'ĭng) [Scottish physician, 1881–1955]
flesh [AS. *flaesc*]
   f., examination of animal
   f., goose
   f., proud
Fletcher factor
fletcherism [Horace Fletcher, U.S. dietitian, 1849–1919]
flex [L. *flexus*, bent]
flexibilitas cerea (flĕks"ĭ-bĭl'ĭ-tăs sē'rē-ă) [L.]
flexibility [L. *flexus*, bent]
flexible
flexile (flĕks'ĭl) [L. *flexus*, bent]
flexion (flĕk'shŭn) [L. *flexio*]
flexor (flĕks'or) [L.]
flexura (flĕk-shoo'ră) [L.]
flexure (flĕk'shĕr) [L. *flexura*]
   f., colic, left
   f., colic, right
   f., dorsal
   f., duodenojejunal
   f., hepatic
   f., sigmoid
   f., splenic

flicker
flicker phenomenon
flight of ideas
flint disease
flip-flop
floaters (flō'tĕrs) [AS. *flotian*, float]
floating [AS. *flota*, a raft]
floating kidney
floating ribs
floats
floccillation, floccitation (flŏk"sĭ-lā'shŭn, -tā'shŭn) [L. *floccilatio*]
floccose (flŏk'ōs) [L. *floccosus*, full of wool tufts]
floccular (flŏk'ū-lăr) [L. *flocculus*, little tuft]
flocculation (flŏk"ū-lā'shŭn)
flocculation reaction
flocculence (flŏk'ū-lĕns")
flocculent (flŏk'ū-lĕnt)
flocculus (flŏk'ū-lŭs) [L., little tuft]
flooding (flŭd'ĭng)
Flood's ligament [Valentine Flood, Ir. surgeon, 1800–1847]
floor [AS. *flor*]
floppy-valve syndrome
flora [L. *flos*, flower]
florid [L. *floridus*, blossoming]
Florinef Acetate
Floropryl
floss
   f., dental
flour [L. *flos*, flower]
flow [AS. *flowan*, to flow]
flower [L. *flos*, flower]
flowmeter
flow state
floxuridine (flŏks-ūr'ĭ-dēn)
fl. oz. *fluidounce*
flu (floo)
flucticuli (flŭk-tĭk'ū-lī) [L., little waves]
fluctuant (flŭk'chū-ănt)
fluctuation [L. *fluctuatio*]
flucytosine (flū-sī'tō-sēn")
fludrocortisone (floo"drō-kor'tĭ-sōn)
   f. acetate
fluid [L. *fluidus*]
   f., allantoic

f., amniotic
f., cerebrospinal
f., extracellular
f., extravascular
f., interstitial
f., intracellular
f., intraocular
f., repair
f., seminal
f., serous
f., spinal
f., synovial
fluid balance
fluid diet
fluidextract, fluidextractum [L. *fluidus*, fluid, + *extractum*, extract]
f., aromatic cascara
f., glycyrrhiza
f., ipecac
fluidounce
fluidram
fluid retention
fluke (flook) [AS. *floc*, flatfish]
f., blood
f., intestinal
f., liver
f., lung
flumethasone pivalate (floo-měth'ă-sōn)
flumina pilorum (floo'mĭ-nă pī-lō'rŭm) [L., rivers of hair]
fluocinolone acetonide (floo-ō-sĭn'ō-lŏn)
Fluogen
Fluonid
fluor albus (floo'or ăl'bŭs) [L., white flow]
fluorescein sodium (floo"ō-rĕs'ē-ĭn)
fluorescence (floo"ō-rĕs'ĕnts)
fluorescent (floo-ō-rĕs'ĕnt)
fluorescent antibody
fluorescent screen
fluorescent treponemal antibody-absorption test
Fluorescite
fluoridation (floo"or-ĭ-dā'shŭn)
fluoride (floo'ō-rīd)
f., stannous

fluoride dental treatment
fluoride poisoning
fluorine (floo'ō-rēn, floor'ēn)
Fluor-I-Strip-A.T.
fluoroacetate (floo"or-ō-ăs'ĕ-tāt)
fluoroapatite
fluorocarbon
fluorometer (floo-or-ŏm'ĕ-tĕr)
fluorometholone (floor"ō-měth'ō-lōn)
Fluoroplex
fluoroscope (floo'or-ō-skōp)
fluoroscopy
fluorosis (floo-or-ō'sĭs)
fluorouracil (floor"ō-ŭr'ă-sĭl)
fluoxymesterone (floo-ŏk"sē-mĕs'tĕr-ōn)
fluphenazine enanthate (floo-fĕn'ă-zēn)
fluprednisolone (floo"prĕd-nĭs'ō-lōn)
flurandrenolide (floor"ăn-drĕn'ō-lĭd)
flurazepam hydrochloride (floor-ăz'ĕ-păm)
flurogestone acetate (floor"ō-jĕs'tōn)
flurothyl (floor'ō-thĭl)
fluroxene (floor-ŏks'ēn)
flush [ME. *flusshen*, to fly up]
f., hectic
f., hot
f., malar
flutter [AS. *floterian*, to fly about]
f., atrial
f., diaphragmatic
f., mediastinal
f., ventricular
flutter-fibrillation
flux [L. *fluxus*, a flow]
fly [AS. *fleoge*]
f., black
f., blow
f., bot
f., flesh
f., house
f., sand
f., screwworm
f., Spanish
f., tsetse
f., warble

Fm *fermium*
f.m. [L.] *fiat mistura*, make a mixture
foam (fōm) [AS. *fam*]
foam stability test
focal [L. *focus*, hearth]
focal infection
focal lesion
focal spot
foci (fō'sī) [L.]
focus [L., hearth]
    f., real
    f., virtual
FOD *focus-object distance*
fog
fogging
foil
fold [AS. *fealdan*, to fold]
    f., amniotic
    f., aryepiglottic
    f., circular
    f., costocolic
    f., Douglas'
    f.'s, gastric
    f., genital
    f., gluteal
    f., lacrimal
    f., mesouterine
    f., mucosal
    f., nail
    f., palmate
    f., semilunar, of conjunctiva
    f., transverse, of rectum
    f., ventricular; f., vestibular
    f., vestigial
    f., vocal
folia (fō'lē-ǎ) [L.]
foliaceous (fō-lē-ā'shē-ŭs) [L. *folia*, leaves]
folic acid (fō'lĭk)
folie (fō-lē') [Fr.]
    f. à deux
    f. du doute
    f. du pourquoi
    f. gemellaire
folinic acid
folium (fō'lē-ŭm) [L., leaf]
    f. vermis
follicle [L. *folliculus*, little bag]

f., aggregated
f., atretic
f., dental
f., gastric
f., graafian
f., growing
f., hair
f., lymphatic
f., nabothian
f., ovarian
f., primordial
f., sebaceous
f., solitary
f., thyroid
f., vesicular
follicle-stimulating hormone
follicular
follicular tonsillitis
follicular tumor
folliculitis (fō-lĭk"ū-lī'tĭs) [L. *folliculus*, little bag, + Gr. *itis*, inflammation]
    f. barbae
    f. decalvans
    f., keloidal
folliculoma (fō-lĭk"ū-lō'mǎ) [" + Gr. *oma*, tumor]
folliculose (fō-lĭk'ū-lōs)
folliculosis (fō-lĭk"ū-lō'sĭs) [" + Gr. *osis*, condition]
folliculus (fō-lĭk'ū-lŭs) [L.]
follow-up
Follutein
Folvite
fomentation (fō"mĕn-tā'shŭn) [L. *fomentatio*]
fomes (fō'mēz) [L., tinder]
fomites (fō'mĭ-tēz)
Fontana's spaces (fŏn-tä'nǎz) [Felice Fontana, It. scientist, 1730–1805]
fontanel, fontanelle (fŏn"tǎ-nĕl') [Fr. *fontanelle*, little fountain]
    f., anterior
    f., posterior
fonticulus (fŏn-tĭk'ū-lŭs) [L., little fountain]
food [AS. *foda*]
    f., contamination of
    f., convenience

f., dietetic
f., enriched
f., nutrient substances of
f., textured
food additives
food adulterant
food allergies
Food and Drug Administration
food ball
food chain
food exchange
food poisoning
food requirements
foot [AS. *fot*]
    f., arches of
    f., athlete's
    f., cleft
    f., contracted
    f., flat
    f., immersion
    f., Madura
    f., march
    f., splay
    f., trench
    f., weak
foot and mouth disease
foot board
foot-candle
footdrop
footling presentation
footplate
foot pound
footprint
forage (fō-rŏzh') [Fr., boring]
foramen (for-ā'mĕn) [L.]
    f., apical
    f., condyloid, anterior
    f., condyloid, posterior
    f., epiploic
    f., ethmoidal
    f., external auditory
    f., incisive
    f., infraorbital
    f., internal auditory
    f., interventricular
    f., intervertebral
    f., jugular
    f., Magendie's

f. magnum
f., mandibular
f., mastoid
f., mental
f., obturator
f. of Monro
f. of Vesalius
f. of Winslow
f., olfactory
f., optic
f. ovale
f., palatine
f., palatine (greater and lesser)
f. rotundum
f., sacral, anterior
f., sacral, posterior
f., Scarpa's
f., sciatic, greater
f., sciatic, lesser
f., sphenopalatine
f., spinous
f., supraorbital
f., thebesian
f., transverse
f., vena caval
f., vertebral
f., Weitbrecht's
f., zygomatic-orbital
Forbes' disease [Gilbert B. Forbes, U.S. pediatrician, b. 1915]
force
    f., catabolic
    f., electromotive
    f., G
    f., reserve
    f., unit of
forceps (for'sĕps) [L.]
    f., alligator
    f., artery
    f., bone
    f., capsule
    f., Chamberlen
    f., clamp
    f., dental
    f., dressing
    f., Halsted's
    f., mosquito
    f., needle

f., obstetric
f., rongeur
f., tissue
f., towel
forcipate (for'sĭ-pāt) [L. *forceps*, tongs]
forcipressure [" + *pressura*, pressure]
Fordyce's disease (for'dĭ-sĕs) [John Fordyce, U.S. dermatologist, 1858 – 1925]
Fordyce-Fox disease (for'dĭs-fŏks') [John Fordyce; G. H. Fox, New York dermatologist, 1846 – 1925]
Fordyce's spots
fore- [AS.]
forearm [AS. *fore*, in front, + *arm*, arm]
forebrain [" + *bregen*, brain]
forefinger
forefoot
foregut [" + *gut*, a pouring]
forehead [AS. *forheafod*]
foreign bodies
forelock
f., white
forensic (for-ĕn'sĭk) [L. *forensis*, public]
forensic dentistry
forensic medicine
foreplay
forepleasure [AS. *fore*, in front, + L. *placere*, to please]
foreskin [" + O. Norse *skinn*, skin]
forewaters (for'wăt-ĕrz)
forgetting
fork
f., tuning
form
-form [L. *forma*]
formaldehyde (for-măl'dĕ-hīd)
formaldehyde poisoning
formalin (for'mă-lĭn)
formate (for'māt)
formatio (for-mā'shē-ō) [L.]
f. reticularis
formation
f., reticular
forme fruste (form froost) [Fr., defaced]

formic [L. *formica*, ant]
formic acid
formic aldehyde
formication
formic ether
formiciasis (for"mĭs-ī'ă-sĭs) [L. *formica*, ant, + Gr. *-iasis*, state or condition of]
formilase (for'mĭ-lās)
formiminoglutamic acid
formol (for'mŏl)
form sense
formula [L., a little form]
f., Arneth's
f., chemical
f., dental
f., empirical
f., molecular
f., official
f., spatial or stereochemical
f., structural
formulary [L. *formula*, a little form]
F., National
formyl
fornicate [L. *fornicatus*]; [L. *fornicari*]
fornication
fornices (for'nĭ-sēz) [L.]
fornicolumn [L. *fornix*, arch, + *columna*, column]
fornicommissure (for-nĭ-kŏm'ĭ-sūr) [" + *commissura*, a joining together]
fornix [L., arch]
f. conjunctivae
f. uteri
f. vaginae
Fort Bragg fever [Fort Bragg, North Carolina, a U.S. military base]
fortification spectrum
Foshay's test [Lee Foshay, U.S. physician, 1896 – 1961]
fossa (fŏs'ă) [L.]
f., amygdaloid
f., articular, of mandible
f., articular, of temporal bone
f., axillary
f., canine
f., cerebral

f., Claudius'
f., condylar
f., coronoid
f., cranial
f., digastric
f., epigastric
f., ethmoid
f., glenoid
f., hyaloid
f., hypophyseal
f., iliac
f., incisive
f., infratemporal
f., intercondyloid
f., interpeduncular
f., ischiorectal
f., lacrimal
f., mandibular
f., mastoid
f., nasal
f., navicular
f., olecranon
f. ovalis
f. ovalis cordis
f., ovarian
f., pituitary
f., Rosenmüller's
f., sphenomaxillary
f., sublingual
f., submandibular
f., subpyramidal
f., supraspinous
f. supratonsillaris
f., temporal
fossae (fŏs'ē) [L.]
fossette (fŏ-sĕt') [Fr.]
fossula (fŏs'ū-lă)
Fothergill's disease (fŏth'ĕr-gĭlz) [John Fothergill, Brit. physician, 1712–1780]
foulage (foo-lōzh') [Fr.]
fourchet, fourchette (foor-shĕt') [Fr. *fourchette*, a fork]
fourth cranial nerve
fovea (fō'vē-ă) [L.]
f. capitus
f. centralis retinae
foveate (fō'vē-āt) [L. *foveatus*]
foveation (fō"vē-ā'shŭn)

foveola (fō-vē'ō-lă) [L., little pit]
Fowler's position [George R. Fowler, U.S. surgeon, 1848–1906]
Fowler's solution [Thomas Fowler, Brit. physician, 1736–1801]
Fox-Fordyce disease (fŏks-for'dĭs)
foxglove (fŏks'glŏv)
Fr *francium*
fraction [L. *fractio*, act of breaking]
f. of inspired oxygen
fractional
fractional test meal
fractionation
fracture [L. *fractura*, break]
f., avulsion
f., blow-out
f., closed
f., Colles'
f., comminuted
f., complete
f., complicated
f., compound
f., compression
f., depressed
f., direct
f., dislocation
f., double
f., Duverney's
f., epiphyseal
f., fatigue
f., fissured
f., greenstick
f., hairline
f., hangman's
f., impacted
f., incomplete
f., indirect
f., intrauterine
f., lead pipe
f., LeFort
f., march
f., open
f., overriding
f., pathologic
f., ping-pong
f., Pott's
f., pretrochanteric
f., Smith's
f., spiral

f., spontaneous
f., stellate
f., stress
f., transcervical
f., transverse
fracture dislocation
fragile X syndrome
fragilitas (fră-jĭl'ĭ-tăs) [L.]
  f. crinium
  f. ossium
  f. unguium
fragility
  f., capillary
  f., erythrocyte
  f. of blood
fragment (frăg'mĕnt)
fragment antigen binding
fragmentation [L. fragmentum, detached part]
frambesia (frăm-bē'zē-ă) [Fr. framboise, raspberry]
frambesioma (frăm-bē-zē-ō'mă) [" + Gr. oma, tumor]
frame
  f., Balkan
  f., Bradford [Edward H. Bradford, U.S. orthopedic surgeon, 1848–1926]
  f., quadriplegic standing
  f., Stryker
  f., trial
framework
Franceschetti's syndrome (frăn"chĕs-kĕt'ēz) [Adolph Franceschetti, Swiss ophthalmologist, 1896–1968]
Franciscella tularensis (frăn"sĭ-sĕl'ă too"lă-rĕn'sĭs) [Edward Francis, Tulare County, California]
francium (frăn'sē-ŭm) [Named for France, the country in which it was discovered]
frank
Frankenhäuser's ganglion (frăng'kĕn-hoy"zĕrs) [Ferdinand Frankenhäuser, Ger. gynecologist, 1832–1894]
Frankfort horizontal plane
Franklin glasses [Benjamin Franklin,

U.S. statesman and inventor, 1706–1790]
fraternal twins
fratricide (frăt'rĭ-sīd") [L. fratricidium]
Fraunhofer's lines (frown'hōf-ĕrz) [Joseph von Fraunhofer, Ger. optician, 1787–1826]
F.R.C.P. *Fellow of the Royal College of Physicians*
F.R.C.P.(C.) *Fellow of the Royal College of Physicians of Canada*
F.R.C.S. *Fellow of the Royal College of Surgeons*
F.R.C.S.(C.) *Fellow of the Royal College of Surgeons of Canada*
freckle (frĕk'l) [O. Norse freknur]
  f., Hutchinson's
free association
free base
freebasing
free medical clinics
free radical
freeze-drying
freezing [AS. freosan]
freezing mixtures
freezing point
Freiberg's infraction (frī'bĕrgz) [A. H. Freiberg, U.S. surgeon, 1868–1940]
fremitus (frĕm'ĭ-tŭs) [L.]
  f., tactile
  f., tussive
  f., vocal
frenal (frē'năl) [L. fraenum, bridle]
French scale
frenectomy (frē-nĕk'tō-mē) [" + Gr. ektome, excision]
frenosecretory (frē"nō-sē'krĕ-tor-ē) [L. fraenum, bridle, + secernere, to secrete]
frenotomy (frē-nŏt'ō-mē) [" + Gr. tome, a cutting, slice]
frenuloplasty (frĕn'ū-lō-plăs"tē) [" + Gr. plassein, to form]
frenulum (frĕn'ū-lŭm) [L., a little bridle]
  f. clitoridis
  f. labiorum pudendi
  f. linguae
  f. of ileocecal valve
  f. of the lips, labialis oris

f. of tongue
f. preputii
frenum (frē'nŭm) [L. *fraenum*, bridle]
frenzy (frĕn'zē) [ME. *frenesie*]
frequency [L. *frequens*, often]
fresh frozen plasma
F response
fretum (frē'tŭm) [L.]
Freud, Sigmund (froyd) [Austrian neurologist and psychoanalyst, 1856–1939]
freudian (froy'dē-ăn)
Freund's adjuvant (froynds) [J. Freund, Hungarian-born scientist, 1890–1960]
friable (frī'ă-b'l) [L. *friabilis*]
friction [L. *frictio*]
f., dry
f., moist
frictional electricity
friction rub
f.r., pericardial
Friedländer's bacillus (frēd'lĕn-dĕrz) [Carl F. Friedländer, Ger. physician, 1847–1887]
Friedländer's disease
Friedman's test (frēd'mănz) [Maurice H. Friedman, U.S. physiologist, b. 1903]
Friedreich's ataxia (frēd'rīks) [Nikolaus Friedreich, Ger. neurologist, 1825–1882]
Friedreich's sign
fright [AS. *fryhto*]
f., precordial
fright neuroses
frigid (frĭj'ĭd) [L. *frigidus*]
frigidity (frĭ-jĭd'ĭ-tē)
frigolabile (frĭg"ō-lā'bĭl) [L. *frigor*, cold, + *labilis*, unstable]
frigorific (frĭg"ō-rĭf'ĭk) [L. *frigorificus*]
frigorism [L. *frigor*, cold, + Gr. *-ismos*, condition]
frigostabile (frĭg"ō-stā'bl) [" + *stabilis*, firm]
frigotherapy (frĭg"ō-thĕr'ă-pē) [" + Gr. *therapeia*, treatment]
frit (frĭt) [It. *fritta*, fry]
frog belly

frog face
Fröhlich's syndrome (frā'lĭks) [Alfred Fröhlich, Austrian neurologist, 1871–1953]
Froin's syndrome (frō-ănz') [Georges Froin, Fr. physician, b. 1874]
frolement (frōl-mŏn') [Fr.]
Froment's sign (frō-măz') [Jules Froment, Fr. physician, 1878–1946]
Frommann's lines (frŏm'ănz) [Carl Frommann, Ger. anatomist, 1831–1892]
frons (frŏnz) [L.]
frontad [L. *frons*, front-, brow, + *ad*, toward]
frontal [L. *frontalis*]
frontal bone
frontal lobe
frontal plane
frontal sinuses
fronto- [L. *frons*, brow]
frontomalar (frŏn"tō-mā'lăr) [" + *mala*, cheek]
frontomaxillary (frŏn"tō-măx'ĭ-lār"ē) [" + *maxilla*, jawbone]
frontoparietal (frŏn"tō-pă-rī'ĕ-tăl) [" + *parietalis*, pert. to a wall]
frontotemporal [" + *tempora*, the temples]
front-tap reflex
frost [AS.]
f., uremic
frostbite
frost-itch
frottage (frō-tōzh') [Fr., rubbing]
frotteur (frō-tĕr') [Fr. *frottage*, rubbing]
frozen section
F.R.S. *Fellow of the Royal Society*
fructofuranose (frŭk"tō-fū'ră-nōs)
fructokinase (frŭk"tō-kī'nās)
fructose (frŭk'tōs) [L. *fructus*, fruit]
fructose intolerance
fructosemia (frŭk"tō-sē'mē-ă) [" + Gr. *haima*, blood]
fructoside (frŭk'tō-sīd)
fructosuria (frŭk"tō-sū'rē-ă) [" + Gr. *ouron*, urine]
fruit [L. *fructus*, fruit]
frumentaceous (froo-mĕn-tā'shŭs) [L.

frumentum, grain]
frustration [L. *frustratus,* disappointed]
Fryns syndrome
FSH *follicle-stimulating hormone*
FSH-RF *follicle-stimulating hormone releasing factor*
ft [L.] *fiat* or *fiant,* let there be made; *florentium;* foot
FTA-ABS *fluorescent treponemal antibody-absorption test for syphilis*
5-FU
fuchsin (fook'sĭn)
fucose (fū'kōs)
fucosidosis (fū"kō-sĭ-dō'sĭs)
-fuge [L. *fugare,* to put to flight]
fugitive (fū'jĭ-tĭv) [L. *fugitivus*]
fugue (fūg) [L. *fuga,* flight]
    f., psychogenic
fulgurant (fŭl'gū-rănt) [L. *fulgurans*]
fulgurating [L. *fulgurare,* to lighten]
fulguration (fŭl-gū-rā'shŭn)
fulling [O. Fr. *fauler,* to fill]
full term
fulminant (fool'-, fŭl'mĭ-nănt) [L. *fulminans*]
fulminating
Fulvicin-P/G
Fulvicin-U/F
fumarase (fū'mă-rās)
fumaric acid
fumes [L. *fumus,* smoke]
    f., nitric acid
fumigant (fū'mĭ-gănt) [L. *fumigare,* to make smoke]
fumigation (fū"mĭ-gā'shŭn)
fuming [L. *fumus,* smoke]
function (fŭng'shŭn) [L. *functio,* performance]
functional
functional disease
functional overlay
functional psychosis
functioning tumor
funda (fŭn'dă) [L., sling]
fundal (fŭn'dăl) [L. *fundus,* base]
fundament (fŭn'dă-mĕnt) [L. *fundamentum*]
fundectomy (fŭn-dĕk'tō-mē) [L. *fundus,* base, + Gr. *ektome,* excision]

fundic (fŭn'dĭk)
fundiform (fŭn'dĭ-form) [L. *funda,* sling, + *forma,* shape]
fundoplication (fŭn"dō-plĭ-kā'shŭn)
fundoscopy (fŭn-dŏs'kō-pē) [L. *fundus,* base, + Gr. *skopein,* to examine]
fundus [L., base]
    f. oculi
    f. of bladder
    f. of gallbladder
    f. of stomach
    f. tympani
    f. uteri
funduscope (fŭn'dŭs-skōp) [" + Gr. *skopein,* to examine]
fundusectomy (fŭn"dŭs-ĕk'tō-mē) [" + Gr. *ektome,* excision]
fungal (fŭng'găl)
fungal septicemia
fungate (fŭng'gāt) [L. *fungus,* mushroom]
fungating (fŭn'gāt-ĭng)
fungemia (fŭn-jē'mē-ă) [" + Gr. *haima,* blood]
Fungi (fŭn'jī) [L. *fungus,* mushroom]
fungi
fungicide (fŭn'jĭ-sīd) [L. *fungi,* mushrooms, + *caedere,* to kill]
fungiform (fŭn'jĭ-form) [" + *forma,* shape]
fungiform papillae
fungistasis (fŭn-jĭ-stā'sĭs) [" + Gr. *stasis,* standing still]
fungistat (fŭn'jĭ-stăt) [" + Gr. *statikos,* standing]
fungistatic
fungitoxic (fŭn"jĭ-tŏk'sĭk)
fungoid (fŭn'goyd) [" + Gr. *eidos,* form, shape]
fungosity (fŭn-gŏs'ĭ-tē)
fungous (fŭn'gŭs)
fungus (fŭn'gŭs) [L., mushroom]
funic (fū'nĭk) [L. *funis,* cord]
funicle (fū'nĭ-kl) [L. *funiculus,* little cord]
funic souffle
funicular (fū-nĭk'ū-lăr)
funicular process
funiculitis (fū-nĭk"ū-lī'tĭs) [" + Gr. *itis,* inflammation]

funiculopexy (fū-nĭk'ū-lō-pĕks"ē) [" + Gr. *pexis*, fixation]

funiculus (fū-nĭk'ū-lŭs) [L., little cord]

funiform (fū'nĭ-form) [L. *funis*, cord, + *forma*, shape]

funis (fū'nĭs) [L., cord]

funnel [L. *fundere*, to pour]

funnel breast, funnel chest

funny bone

F.U.O. *fever of unknown origin*

Furacin

Furadantin

furcal [L. *furca*, fork]

furcation (fŭr-kā'shŭn)

furcula (fŭr'kū-lă) [L., little fork]

furfur [L., bran]

furfuraceous (fŭr-fū-rā'shŭs)

furibund (fū'rĭ-bŭnd) [L. *furibundus*]

furor [L., rage]

   f. femininus

furosemide (fū-rō'sĕ-mīd)

furred [O. Fr. *forre*, lining]

furrow [AS. *furh*]

   f., atrioventricular

   f., digital

   f., gluteal

furuncle (fū'rŭng-kl) [L. *furunculus*]

furuncular (fū-rŭng'kū-lăr)

furunculoid (fū-rŭng'kū-loyd) [" + Gr. *eidos*, form, shape]

furunculosis (fū-rŭng"kū-lō'sĭs) [" + Gr. *osis*, condition]

furunculous

furunculus (fū-rŭng'kū-lŭs) [L., a boil]

Fusarium (fū-zā'rē-ŭm) [L. *fusus*, spindle]

fuscin (fŭs'ĭn) [L. *fuscus*, dark brown]

fuse (fūz) [L. *fusus*, poured]

fusible (fū'zĭ-b'l)

fusiform (fū'zĭ-form) [L. *fusus*, spindle, + *forma*, shape]

fusimotor (fū"sĭ-mō'tor)

fusion (fū'shŭn) [L. *fusio*]

   f., diaphyseal-epiphyseal

   f., nuclear

   f., spinal

Fusobacterium

fusocellular [L. *fusus*, spindle, + *cellulus*, little cell]

fusospirochetal (fū"sō-spī-rō-kē'tăl) [" + Gr. *speira*, coil, + *chaite*, hair]

fusospirochetosis (fū"sō-spī"rō-kē-tō'sĭs) [" + " + " + *osis*, condition]

fustigation (fŭs"tĭ-gā'shŭn) [L. *fustigatio*]

fututrix (fū-tū'trĭks)

F wave

FWB *full weight bearing*

G

γ gamma; microgram; immunoglobulin
G newtonian constant of gravitation; giga, 10^9
g force of gravity; gingival; gram; gender
Ga gallium
GABA gamma-aminobutyric acid
gadfly
gadolinium (găd″ō-lĭn′ē-ŭm)
gag
gage (gāj)
gag reflex
gain
   g., secondary
Gaisböck's syndrome (gīs′běks) [Felix Gaisböck, Ger. physician, 1869–1955]
gait (gāt) [ME. gait, passage]
   g., ataxic
   g., cerebellar
   g., double step
   g., drag-to
   g., equine
   g., festinating
   g., gluteal
   g., helicopod
   g., hemiplegic
   g., scissor
   g., spastic
   g., steppage
   g., swing-through
   g., swing-to
   g., tabetic
   g., three-point
   g., two-point
   g., waddling
galact-, galacto- [Gr. gala, milk]
galactacrasia (gă-lăk″tă-krā′zē-ă) [″ + akrasia, bad mixture]
galactagogue (gă-lăk′tă-gŏg) [″ + agogos, leading]

galactan (gă-lăk′tăn)
galactase
galactemia (gă-lăk-tē′mē-ă) [″ + haima, blood]
galactic (gă-lăk′tĭk)
galactidrosis (gă-lăk″tĭ-drō′sĭs) [″ + hidros, sweat]
galactischia (găl″ăk-tĭsk′ē-ă) [″ + ischein, to suppress]
galactoblast (gă-lăk′tō-blăst) [″ + blastos, germ]
galactocele (gă-lăk′tō-sēl) [″ + kele, tumor, swelling]
galactoid
galactokinase (gă-lăk″tō-kī′nās)
galactolipin [″ + lipos, fat]
galactoma (găl-ăk-tō′mă) [″ + oma, tumor]
galactometer [″ + metron, measure]
galactopexic (găl-ăk-tō-pěk′sĭk) [″ + pexis, fixation]
galactopexy (gă-lăk′tō-pěk″sē)
galactophagous (găl″ăk-tŏf′ă-gŭs) [″ + phagein, to eat]
galactophlysis (găl″ăk-tŏf′lĭ-sĭs) [″ + phlysis, eruption]
galactophore (găl-ăk′tō-for) [″ + pherein, to bear]
galactophoritis (găl-ăk″tō-for-ī′tĭs) [″ + ″ + itis, inflammation]
galactophorous (găl″ăk-tŏf′or-ŭs)
galactophthisis (găl″ăk-tŏf′thĭ-sĭs) [″ + phthisis, a wasting]
galactophygous (găl-ăk-tŏf′ĭ-gŭs) [″ + phyge, flight]
galactoplania (gă-lăk″tō-plā′nē-ă) [″ + plane, wandering]
galactopoietic (gă-lăk″tō-poy-ĕt′ĭk) [″ + poiein, to make]
galactopyra (gă-lăk″tō-pī′ră) [″ +

pyr, fire]

galactorrhea (gă-lăk″tō-rē′ă) [″ + *rhein,* to flow]

galactosamine (gă-lăk″tō-săm′ĭn)

galactose (gă-lăk′tōs)

galactosemia (gă-lăk″tō-sē′mē-ă)

galactosidase (gă-lăk″tō-sī′dās)

galactosides (gă-lăk′tō-sīds)

galactosis (găl″ăk-tō′sĭs) [″ + *osis,* condition]

galactostasis (găl″ăk-tŏs′tă-sĭs) [″ + *stasis,* standing still]

galactosuria (găl-ăk″tō-sū′rē-ă) [″ + *ouron,* urine]

galactotherapy (gă-lăk″tō-thĕr′ă-pē) [″ + *therapeia,* treatment]

galactotoxin (gă-lăk″tō-tŏks′ĭn) [″ + *toxikon,* poison]

galactotoxism (gă-lăk″tō-tŏk′sĭzm)

galactotrophy (găl″ăk-tŏt′rō-fē) [″ + *trophe,* nourishment]

galactozymase (gă-lăk″tō-zī′mās) [″ + *zyme,* leaven]

galacturia (găl-ăk-tū′rē-ă) [″ + *ouron,* urine]

galea (gā′lē-ă) [L. *galea,* helmet]
g. aponeurotica

galeanthropy (gă″lē-ăn′thrō-pē) [Gr. *gale,* cat, + *anthropos,* man]

Galeazzi's sign [Riccardo Galeazzi, It. orthopedic surgeon, 1866–1952]

Galen, Claudius [Gr. physician, circa A.D. 129–199]
G.'s veins

galena (gă-lē′nă)

galenic (gă-lĕn′ĭk)

galenicals, galenics (gă-lĕn′ĭ-kăls, -ĭks)

galeophilia (găl″ē-ō-fĭl′ē-ă) [Gr. *gale,* cat, + *philein,* to love]

galeophobia (găl″ē-ō-fō′bē-ă) [″ + *phobos,* fear]

galeropia, galeropsia (găl-ĕr-ō′pē-ă, -ŏp′sē-ă) [Gr. *galeros,* cheerful, + *opsis,* sight, appearance, vision]

gall [AS. *gealla,* sore place]

gallamine triethiodide (găl′ă-mĭn trī″ĕ-thī′ō-dĭd)

gallate (găl′lāt)

gallbladder [AS. *gealla,* sore place, + *blaedre,* bladder]

gall duct [″ + L. *ductus,* a passage]

gallium (găl′ē-ŭm) [L. *Gallia,* Gaul]

gallon [Med. L. *galleta,* jug]

gallop rhythm

gallstone [AS. *gealla,* sore place + *stan,* stone]

Galton's whistle [Sir Francis Galton, Brit. scientist, 1822–1911]

galvanic [Luigi Galvani, It. physiologist, 1737–1798]

galvanic battery

galvanic cell

galvanic current

galvanism

galvanization (găl″văn-ĭ-zā′shŭn)

galvanocautery (găl″vă-nō-kaw′tĕr-ē) [*galvanism* + Gr. *kauterion,* cautery]

galvanocontractility (găl″vă-nō-kŏn″trăk-tĭl′ĭ-tē) [″ + L. *contractus,* drawn together]

galvanofaradization (găl″vă-nō-făr″ă-dĭ-zā′shŭn)

galvanometer (găl″vă-nŏm′ĕ-tĕr) [″ + Gr. *metron,* measure]

galvanopalpation (găl″vă-nō-păl-pā′shŭn) [″ + L. *palpare,* to touch]

galvanopuncture (găl″vă-nō-pŭng′chŭr) [″ + L. *punctura,* prick]

galvanoscope (găl-văn′ō-skōp) [″ + Gr. *skopein,* to examine]

galvanosurgery (găl″vă-nō-sĕr′jĕr-ē) [″ + Gr. *cheir,* hand, + *ergon,* work]

galvanotaxis (găl″vă-nō-tăk′sĭs) [″ + Gr. *taxis,* arrangement]

galvanotherapeutics, galvanotherapy (găl″vă-nō-thĕr″ă-pū′tĭks, -thĕr′ă-pē) [″ + Gr. *therapeia,* treatment]

galvanothermy (găl″văn-ō-thĕrm′ē) [″ + Gr. *therme,* heat]

galvanotonus (găl-văn-ŏt′ō-nŭs) [″ + Gr. *tonos,* act of stretching, tension, tone]

galvanotropism (găl″văn-ŏt′rō-pĭzm) [″ + Gr. *tropos*, a turn]

gamete (găm′ēt) [Gr. *gamein*, to marry]

gamete intrafallopian transfer

gametic (găm-ĕt′ĭk)

gametocide (găm′ĕ-tō-sīd″) [″ + L. *caedere*, to kill]

gametocyte (gă-mē′tō-sīt) [″ + *kytos*, cell]

gametogenesis (găm″ĕt-ō-jĕn′ĕ-sĭs) [″ + *genesis*, generation, birth]

gametogony (găm″ĕ-tŏg′ō-nē)

gametophyte (găm′ĕ-tō-fīt) [″ + *phyton*, plant]

gamic (găm′ĭk) [Gr. *gamein*, to marry]

gamma

gamma benzene hexachloride (găm′ă bĕn′zēn hĕk″să-klor′īd)

gammacism

Gammagee

gamma globulin

Gammar

gamma rays

gammopathy (găm-ŏp′ă-thē)

Gamna's disease

Gamna nodules [Carlo Gamna, It. physician, 1896–1950]

gamo- [Gr. *gamos*, marriage]

gamogenesis (găm″ō-jĕn′ĕ-sĭs) [″ + *genesis*, generation, birth]

gamont (găm′ŏnt) [″ + *on*, being]

gamophobia (găm″ō-fō′bē-ă) [″ + *phobos*, fear]

gampsodactylia (gămp″sō-dăk-tĭl′ē-ă) [Gr. *gampsos*, curved, + *daktylos*, finger]

ganglia (găng′glē-ă)

ganglial (găng′lē-ăl) [Gr. *ganglion*, knot]

gangliated (găng′lē-ă-tĕd)

gangliectomy (găng″glē-ĕk′tō-mē) [″ + *ektome*, excision]

gangliform (găng′lĭ-form) [″ + L. *forma*, shape]

gangliitis (găng″glē-ī′tĭs) [″ + *itis*, inflammation]

ganglioblast (găng″glē-ō-blăst″) [″ + *blastos*, germ]

gangliocyte (găng′glē-ō-sīt″) [″ + *kytos*, cell]

gangliocytoma (găng″glē-ō-sī-tō′mă) [″ + ″ + *oma*, tumor]

ganglioglioma (găng″glē-ō-glī-ō′mă) [″ + *glia*, glue, + *oma*, tumor]

ganglioglioneuroma (găng″glē-ō-glī″ō-nū-rō′mă) [″ + ″ + *neuron*, nerve, + *oma*, tumor]

ganglioma (găng-lē-ō′mă) [″ + *oma*, tumor]

ganglion (găng′lē-ŏn) [Gr.]
  g., abdominal
  g., anterior cerebral
  g., aorticorenal
  g., Arnold's auricular
  g., auricular
  g., autonomic
  g., basal
  g., basal optic
  g., cardiac
  g., carotid
  g., celiac
  g., cephalic
  g., cerebral
  g., cervical
  g., cervicothoracic
  g., cervicouterine
  g., ciliary
  g., coccygeal
  g., collateral
  g., Corti's
  g., dorsal root
  g., false
  g., Frankenhäuser's
  g., gasserian
  g., geniculate
  g., inferior mesenteric
  g., intervertebral
  g., jugular
  g., lateral
  g., lenticular
  g., lumbar
  g., lymphatic
  g., nodose
  g., ophthalmic
  g., otic
  g., parasympathetic

g., petrous
g., pharyngeal
g., phrenic
g., pterygopalatine
g., renal
g., sacral
g., Scarpa's
g., semilunar
g., sensory
g., simple
g., sphenopalatine
g., spinal
g., spiral
g., stellate
g., submandibular
g., superior mesenteric
g., suprarenal
g., sympathetic
g., temporal
g., terminal
g., thoracic
g., trigeminal
g., tympanic
g., vestibular
g., Wrisberg's
g., wrist

ganglionated
ganglionectomy (găng″lē-ō-nĕk′tō-mē) [″ + *ektome*, excision]
ganglioneuroma (găng″lē-ō-nū-rō′mă) [″ + *neuron*, nerve, + *oma*, tumor]
ganglionic (găng-lē-ŏn′ĭk)
ganglionic blockade
ganglionitis (găng″lē-ŏn-ī′tĭs) [″ + *itis*, inflammation]
ganglionostomy (găng″glē-ō-nŏs′tō-mē) [″ + *stoma*, mouth, opening]
ganglioplegia (găng″glē-ō-plē′jē-ă) [″ + *plege*, stroke]
ganglioside (găng′glē-ō-sīd)
gangliosidosis (găng″glē-ō-sī-dō′sĭs)
gangosa (găng-gō′să) [Sp. *gangosa*, muffled voice]
gangrene (găng′grēn) [Gr. *gangraina*, an eating sore]
g., angioneurotic
g., diabetic

g., dry
g., embolic
g., gas
g., humid
g., idiopathic
g., inflammatory
g., moist
g., primary
g., secondary
g., symmetric
g., traumatic

gangrenous
ganoblast (găn′ō-blăst) [Gr. *ganos*, brightness, + *blastos*, cell]
Ganser's syndrome (găn′zĕrz) [Sigbert J. M. Ganser, Ger. psychiatrist, 1853–1931]
Gantanol
Gantrisin
gantry (găn′trē) [Gr. *kanthēlios*, pack ass]
gap [Old Norse *gap*, chasm]
g., auscultatory
Garamycin
Gardnerella vaginalis [Herman Gardner, U.S. physician, d. 1947]
Gardnerella vaginalis vaginitis
Gardner's syndrome [Eldon J. Gardner, U.S. geneticist, b. 1909]
gargarism (găr′găr-ĭzm) [Gr. *gargarisma*]
gargle [Fr. *gargouille*, throat; but may be onomatopoeia for gargle]
gargoylism (găr′goyl-ĭsm)
garlic [AS. *gar*, spear, + *leac*, the leek]
garment, front-opening
Garré's disease (găr-āz′) [Carl Garré, Swiss surgeon, 1858–1928]
Garren gastric bubble [Lloyd and Mary Garren, contemporary U.S. gastroenterologists]
Gartner's duct [Hermann T. Gartner, Danish surgeon and anatomist, 1785–1827]
G.A.S. *general adaptation syndrome*
gas
g., binary

g.'s, blood
g., Clayton
g., coal
g.'s, digestive tract
g., illuminating
g., inert
g., laughing
g., lewisite
g., lung irritant
g., marsh
g., mustard
g., nerve
g., nose irritant
g., sewer
g., suffocating
g., tear
g., toxic
g., vesicant
g., vomiting
g.'s, war
gas bacillus
gas distention
gaseous
gas gangrene
gasoline
gasoline poisoning
gasometric (găs"ō-mĕt'rĭk)
gasometry (găs-ŏm'ĕ-trē)
gasp [Old Norse *geispa*]
gas pains
gasserectomy (găs"ĕr-ĕk'tō-mē)
gaster-, gastero-, gastro- [Gr. *gaster*, belly]
gasteralgia (găs-tĕr-ăl'jē-ă) [" + *algos*, pain]
Gasterophilus (găs"tĕr-ŏf'ĭ-lŭs)
  G. hemorrhoidalis
  G. intestinalis
  G. nasalis
gastorrhagia (găs-tor-ā'jē-ă) [" + *rhegnynai*, to burst forth]
gastralgia (găs-trăl'jē-ă) [" + *algos*, pain]
gastratrophia (găs"tră-trō'fē-ă) [" + *atrophia*, atrophy]
gastrectasia, gastrectasis [" + *ektasis*, dilatation]
gastrectomy (găs-trĕk'tō-mē) [" +

ektome, excision]
gastric (găs'trĭk) [Gr. *gaster*, stomach]
gastric analysis
gastric digestion
gastric glands
gastric inhibitory polypeptide
gastricism (găs'trĭ-sĭzm) [Gr. *gaster*, stomach, + *-ismos*, condition]
gastric juice
gastric lavage
gastric ulcer
gastrin
gastrinoma (găs"trĭn-ō'mă)
gastritis (găs-trī'tĭs) [" + *itis*, inflammation]
  g., acute
  g., atrophic
  g., chronic
  g., giant hypertrophic
  g., toxic
gastro- [Gr. *gaster*, stomach]
gastroanastomosis (găs"trō-ăn-ăs"tō-mō'sĭs) [" + *anastomosis*, outlet]
gastrocamera (găs"trō-kăm'ĕ-ră)
gastrocardiac (găs"trō-kăr'dē-ăk) [" + *kardia*, heart]
gastrocele (găs'trō-sēl) [" + *kele*, tumor, swelling]
gastrocnemius (găs"trŏk-nē'mē-ŭs) [" + *kneme*, leg]
gastrocolic (găs"trō-kŏl'ĭk) [" + *kolon*, colon]
gastrocolic omentum
gastrocolic reflex
gastrocolitis (găs"trō-kō-lī'tĭs) [" + " + *itis*, inflammation]
gastrocoloptosis (găs"trō-kŏl"ŏp-tō'sĭs) [" + " + *ptosis*, fall, falling]
gastrocolostomy (găs"trō-kŏl-ŏs'tō-mē) [" + " + *stoma*, mouth, opening]
gastrocolotomy (găs"trō-kō-lŏt'ō-mē) [" + " + *tome*, a cutting, slice]
gastrocolpotomy (găs"trō-kŏl-pŏt'ō-mē) [" + *kolpos*, vagina, + *tome*, a cutting, slice]

gastrocutaneous (găs"trō-kū-tā'nē-ŭs) [" + cutis, skin]

gastrodialysis (găs"trō-dī-ăl'ĭ-sĭs) [" + dia, through, + lysis, dissolution]

gastrodidymus (găs"trō-dĭd'ĭ-mŭs) [" + didymos, twin]

gastrodisciasis (găs"trō-dĭs-kī'ă-sĭs)

Gastrodiscoides (găs"trō-dĭs-koy'dēz)
G. hominis

gastroduodenal (găs"trō-dū"ō-dĕn'ăl) [Gr. gaster, stomach, + L. duodeni, twelve]

gastroduodenitis (găs"trō-dū-ŏd"ĕn-ī'tĭs) [" + " + Gr. itis, inflammation]

gastroduodenoscopy (găs"trō-dū"ō-dĕnŏs'kō-pē) [" + " + skopein, to examine]

gastroduodenostomy (găs"trō-dū"ō-dĕn-ŏs'tō-mē) [" + " + Gr. stoma, mouth, opening]

gastrodynia (găs"trō-dĭn'ē-ă) [" + odyne, pain]

gastroenteralgia (găs"trō-ĕn"tĕr-ăl'jē-ă) [" + enteron, intestine, + algos, pain]

gastroenteric (găs"trō-ĕn-tĕr'ĭk)

gastroenteritis (găs"trō-ĕn-tĕr-ī'tĭs) [" + enteron, intestine, + itis, inflammation]

gastroenteroanastomosis (găs"trō-ĕn"tĕr-ō-ă-năs"tō-mō'sĭs)

gastroenterocolitis (găs"trō-ĕn"tĕr-ō-kōl-ī'tĭs) [" + " + kolon, colon, + itis, inflammation]

gastroenterocolostomy (găs"trō-ĕn"tĕr-ō-kō-lŏs'tō-mē) [" + " + " + stoma, mouth, opening]

gastroenterology (găs"trō-ĕn"tĕr-ŏl'ō-jē) [" + " + logos, word, reason]

gastroenteropathy (găs"trō-ĕn"tĕr-ŏp'ă-thē)

gastroenteroptosis (găs"trō-ĕn"tĕr-ŏp-tō'sĭs) [" + " + ptosis, fall, falling]

gastroenterostomy (găs"trō-ĕn-tĕr-ŏs'tō-mē) [" + enteron, intestine, + stoma, mouth, opening]

gastroenterotomy (găs"trō-ĕn"tĕr-ŏt'ō-mē) [" + " + tome, a cutting, slice]

gastroepiploic (găs"trō-ĕp"ĭ-plō'ĭk) [" + epiploon, omentum]

gastroesophageal (găs"trō-ĕ-sŏf"ă-jē'ăl) [" + oisophagos, gullet]

gastroesophageal reflux
g.r., chronic

gastroesophagitis (găs"trō-ĕ-sŏf"ă-jī'tĭs) [" + " + itis, inflammation]

gastroesophagostomy (găs"trō-ĕ-sŏf"ă-gŏs'tō-mē) [" + " + tome, a cutting, slice]

gastrofiberscope (găs"trō-fī'bĕr-skōp)

gastrogastrostomy (găs"trō-găs-trŏs'tō-mē) [" + " + stoma, mouth, opening]

gastrogavage (găs"trō-gă-văzh') [" + Fr. gavage, cramming]

gastrogenic (găs"trō-jĕn'ĭk) [" + gennan, to produce]

Gastrografin

gastrohelcosis (găs"trō-hĕl-kō'sĭs) [" + helkos, ulcer]

gastrohepatic [" + hepar, liver]

gastrohepatitis (găs"trō-hĕp-ă-tī'tĭs) [" + " + itis, inflammation]

gastroileac (găs-trō-ĭl'ē-ăk) [" + L. ileum, groin]

gastroileal reflex

gastroileitis (găs"trō-ĭl-ē-ī'tĭs)

gastroileostomy (găs"trō-ĭl-ē-ŏs'tō-mē)

gastrointestinal [" + L. intestinalis, intestine]

gastrointestinal bleeding

gastrointestinal decompression

gastrojejunostomy (găs-trō-jĕ-jū-nŏs'tō-mē) [" + L. jejunum, empty, + Gr. stoma, mouth, opening]

gastrolienal (găs"trō-lī'ĕn-ăl) [" +

L. *lien,* spleen]

gastrolith (găs'trō-lĭth) [" + *lithos,* stone]

gastrolithiasis (găs"trō-lĭth-ī'ă-sĭs)

gastrology (găs-trŏl'ō-jē) [" + *logos,* word, reason]

gastrolysis (găs-trŏl'ĭ-sĭs) [" + *lysis,* dissolution]

gastromalacia (găs-trō-mă-lā'shē-ă) [" + *malakia,* softening]

gastromegaly (găs"trō-měg'ă-lē) [" + *megas,* large]

gastromycosis (găs"trō-mī-kō'sĭs) [" + *mykes,* fungus, + *osis,* condition]

gastromyotomy (găs"trō-mī-ŏt'ō-mē) [" + *mys,* muscle, + *tome,* a cutting, slice]

gastromyxorrhea (găs"trō-mĭks"ō-rē'ă) [" + *myxa,* mucus, + *rhein,* to flow]

gastropancreatitis (găs"trō-păn"krē-ă-tī'tĭs) [" + *pan,* all, + *kreas,* flesh, + *itis,* inflammation]

gastroparalysis (găs"trō-păr-ăl'ĭ-sĭs) [" + *paralyein,* to loosen, disable]

gastropathy (găs-trŏp'ă-thē) [" + *pathos,* disease, suffering]

gastropexy, gastropexis (găs'trō-pěk"sē, -sĭs) [" + *pexis,* fixation]

gastrophrenic (găs"trō-frěn'ĭk) [" + *phren,* diaphragm]

gastroplasty (găs'trō-plăs"tē) [" + *plassein,* to form]

gastroplegia (găs"trō-plē'jē-ă) [" + *plege,* stroke]

gastroplication (găs"trō-plĭ-kā'shŭn) [" + L. *plicare,* to fold]

gastroptosis (găs"trŏp-tō'sĭs) [" + *ptosis,* fall, falling]

gastropulmonary (găs"trō-pŭl'mō-năr-ē) [" + L. *pulmo,* lung]

gastropylorectomy (găs"trō-pī"lor-ěk'tō-mē) [" + *pyloros,* gate-keeper, + *ektome,* excision]

gastropyloric

gastroradiculitis (găs"trō-ră-dĭk"ū-lĭ'tĭs) [" + L. *radix,* root, + Gr.

itis, inflammation]

gastrorrhagia (găs"trō-rā'jē-ă) [" + *rhegnynai,* to burst forth]

gastrorrhaphy (găs-tror'ă-fē) [" + *rhaphe,* seam]

gastrorrhea (găs-trō-rē'ă) [" + *rhein,* to flow]

gastroschisis (găs-trŏs'kĭ-sĭs) [" + *schisis,* cleavage]

gastroscope (găs'trō-skōp) [" + *skopein,* to examine]

gastroscopy (găs-trŏs'kō-pē)

gastrospasm (găs'trō-spăzm) [" + *spasmos,* a convulsion]

gastrosplenic (găs"trō-splěn'ĭk) [" + *splen,* spleen]

gastrostaxis (găs"trō-stăk'sĭs) [" + *staxis,* trickling]

gastrostenosis (găs"trō-stěn-ō'sĭs) [" + *stenosis,* act of narrowing]
  g. cardiaca
  g. pylorica

gastrostogavage (găs-trŏs"tō-gă-văzh') [" + *stoma,* mouth, opening, + Fr. *gaver,* to stuff]

gastrostolavage (găs-trŏs"tō-lă-văzh') [" + Fr. *lavage,* fr. L. *lavare,* to wash]

gastrostoma (găs-trŏs'tō-mă) [" + *stoma,* mouth, opening]

gastrostomy (găs-trŏs'tō-mē)

gastrosuccorrhea (găs"trō-sŭk"or-ē'ă) [" + L. *succus,* juice, + Gr. *rhein,* to flow]

gastrotherapy (găs"trō-thěr'ă-pē) [" + *therapeia,* treatment]

gastrothoracopagus (găs"trō-thō"ră-kŏp'ă-gŭs) [" + *thorax,* chest, + *pagos,* thing fixed]

gastrotome (găs'trō-tōm) [" + *tome,* a cutting, slice]

gastrotomy (găs-trŏt'ō-mē) [" + *tome,* a cutting, slice]

gastrotonometer (găs"trō-tō-nŏm'ě-těr) [" + *tonos,* act of stretching, tension, tone, + *metron,* measure]

gastrotropic (găs"trō-trŏp'ĭk) [" + *tropos,* turning]

gastrotympanites (găs″trō-tǐm″pă-nī′tēz) [″ + *tympanites*, distention]
gastrula (găs′troo-lă) [L., little belly]
gastrulation (găs″troo-lā′shŭn)
Gatch bed [Willis D. Gatch, U.S. surgeon, 1878-1961]
gate
gate theory
gatism (gă′tĭzm) [Fr. *gâter*, to spoil]
Gaucher, Philippe C. E. (gō-shā′) [Fr. physician, 1854-1918]
  G.'s cells
  G.'s disease
gauge (gāj)
Gaultheria Oil
Gault's reflex (gawlts)
gauntlet (gawnt′lĕt) [Fr. *gant*, glove]
gauss (gows) [Johann Carl F. Gauss, Ger. physicist, 1777-1855]
Gauss' sign (gows) [Carl J. Gauss, Ger. gynecologist, 1875-1957]
gauze (gawz) [O. Fr. *gaze*, gauze]
  g., absorbent
  g., antiseptic
  g., aseptic
  g., petrolatum
gavage (gă-văzh′) [Fr. *gaver*, to stuff]
Gavard's muscle (gă-vărz′) [Hyacinthe Gavard, Fr. anatomist, 1753-1802]
gay
Gay's glands [Alexander H. Gay, Russian anatomist, 1842-1907]
Gay-Lussac's law (gā″lŭ-săks′) [Joseph L. Gay-Lussac, Fr. naturalist, 1778-1850]
gaze (gāz)
GB *gallbladder*
Gd *gadolinium*
Ge *germanium*
Gee, Samuel J. (gē) [Brit. physician, 1839-1911]
  G.'s disease
  G.- Thaysen disease
gegenhalten (gā″gĕn-hălt′ĕn) [Ger.]
Geigel's reflex (gī′gĕlz) [Richard Geigel, Ger. physician, 1859-1930]
Geiger counter (gī′gĕr) [Hans Geiger,

Ger. physicist in England, 1882-1945]
gel (jĕl) [L. *gelare*, to congeal]
  g., aluminum hydroxide
gelasmus (jĕ-lăs′mŭs) [Gr. *gelasma*, a laugh]
gelate (jĕl′āt)
gelatin (jĕl′ă-tǐn) [L. *gelatina*, gelatin]
  g., nutrient
gelatinase
gelatin culture
gelatiniferous (jĕl″ăt-ĭn-ĭf′ĕr-ŭs) [″ + *ferre*, to bear]
gelatinize (jĕl-ăt′ĭn-īz) [L. *gelatina*, gelatin]
gelatinoid (jĕl-ăt′ĭn-oyd) [″ + Gr. *eidos*, form, shape]
gelatinolytic (jĕl-ăt″ĭn-ō-lĭt′ĭk) [″ + Gr. *lysis*, dissolution]
gelatinous (jĕl-ăt′ĭn-ŭs)
gelatin sponge, absorbable
gelation (jĕl-ā′shŭn)
Gelfoam
Gellé's test (zhĕl-āz′) [Marie Ernst Gellé, Fr. physician, 1834-1923]
gelose (jĕ′lōs) [L. *gelare*, to congeal]
gelosis (jĕl-ō′sĭs)
gelotherapy (jĕl″ō-thĕr′ă-pē) [Gr. *gelos*, laughter, + *therapeia*, treatment]
gelotripsy (jĕl′ō-trĭp″sē) [L. *gelare*, to congeal, + Gr. *tripsis*, a rubbing, friction]
gemellipara (jĕm″ĕl-lĭp′ă-ră) [L. *gemelli*, twins, + *parere*, to beget, produce]
gemellology (gĕm″ĕl-ŏl′ō-jē) [L. *gemellus*, twin, + Gr. *logos*, word, reason]
gemellus (jĕm-ĕl′ŭs) [L., twin]
gemfibrozil (jĕm-fī′brō-zĭl)
geminate (jĕm′ĭ-nāt) [L. *geminatus*, paired]
gemination (jĕm-ĭ-nā′shŭn)
gemistocyte (jĕm-ĭs′tō-sīt) [Gr. *gemistos*, laden, full, + *kytos*, cell]
gemma (jĕm′mă) [L., bud]
gemmation (jĕm-mā′shŭn) [L. *gem-*

mare, to bud]
gemmule (jĕm'ūl) [L. *gemmula*, little bud]
gena (jē'nă) [L.]
genal (jē'năl)
gender [L. *genus*, kind]
gender identity
   g.i., mistaken
gender role
gender testing
gene (jēn) [Gr. *gennan*, to produce]
   g.'s, allelic
   g.'s, complementary
   g., dominant
   g., histocompatibility
   g., holandric
   g., inhibiting
   g., lethal
   g., modifying
   g., mutant
   g., operator
   g., pleiotropic
   g., recessive
   g., regulator
   g., sex-linked
   g., structural
   g., X-linked
gene amplification
gene map
genera
general adaptation syndrome
generalize [L. *generalis*]
generation (jĕn"ĕr-ā'shŭn) [L. *generare*, to beget]
   g., alternate
   g., asexual
   g., filial
   g., parental
   g., sexual
generative (jĕn'ĕr-ă-tĭv)
generator (gĕn'ĕr-ā"tor)
   g., electric
   g., pulse
   g., x-ray
generic (jĕn-ĕr'ĭk) [L. *genus*, kind]
generic drugs
genesiology (jĕn-ē-zē-ŏl'ō-jē) [Gr. *genesis*, generation, birth, +

logos, word, reason]
genesis (jĕn'ĕ-sĭs)
gene splicing
gene therapy
genetic (jĕn-ĕt'ĭk)
genetic code
genetic counseling
genetic engineering
geneticist (jĕn-ĕt'ĭ-sĭst) [Gr. *gennan*, to produce]
genetics
   g., biochemical
   g., clinical
   g., molecular
genetotrophic (jĕ-nĕt"ō-trōf'ĭk)
genetous (jĕ-nĕt'ŭs)
gene transfer
Geneva Convention
genial (jē'nē-ăl) [Gr. *geneion*, chin]
genic (jĕn'ĭk) [Gr. *gennan*, to produce]
genicular (jĕ-nĭk'ū-lăr)
geniculate (jĕ-nĭk'ū-lāt) [L. *geniculare*, to bend the knee]
geniculate otalgia
geniculocalcarine tract
geniculum (jĕn-ĭk'ū-lŭm) [L. *geniculum*, little knee]
genion (jē'nē-ŏn) [Gr. *geneion*, chin]
genioplasty (jē'nē-ō-plăs"tē) [" + *plassein*, to form]
genital (jĕn'ĭ-tăl) [L. *genitalis*, to beget]
genital herpes
genitalia, genitals (jĕn-ĭ-tāl'ē-ă, jĕn'ĭ-tăls)
   g., ambiguous
   g., female
   g., male
genital warts
genito- [L. *genitivus*, of birth, of generation]
genitocrural (jĕn"ĭ-tō-kroo'răl)
genitofemoral (jĕn"ĭ-tō-fĕm'or-ăl)
genitoplasty (jĕn'ĭ-tō-plăs"tē) [L. *genitalis*, to beget, + Gr. *plassein*, to form]
genitourinary (jĕn"ĭ-tō-ūr'ĭ-năr-ē) [" + Gr. *ouron*, urine]
genitourinary system

genius (jēn′yŭs)
genocide (jĕn″ō-sīd″) [Gr. *genos*, race, + L. *caedere*, to kill]
genodermatosis (jĕn″ō-dĕr-mă-tō′sĭs) [Gr. *gennan*, to produce, + *derma*, skin, + *osis*, condition]
genome (jē′nōm)
Genoptic
genotoxic (jĕn″ō-tŏks′ĭk) [″ + *toxikon*, poison]
genotoxic damage
genotype (jĕn′ō-tīp) [″ + *typos*, type]
gentamicin (jĕn″tă-mī′sĭn)
    g. sulfate
gentian (jĕn′shŭn)
    g. violet
gentianophil(e) (jĕn′shăn-ō-fĭl)
gentianophobic (jĕn″shăn-ō-fō′bĭk)
Gentran 40 and 75
genu (jē′nū) [L.]
    g. extrorsum
    g. introrsum
    g. recurvatum
    g. valgum
    g. varum
genua (jĕn′ū-ă)
genuclast (jĕn′ū-klăst) [″ + Gr. *klan*, to break]
genucubital (jĕn″ū-kū′bĭ-tăl) [″ + *cubitus*, elbow]
genucubital position
genupectoral (jĕn″ū-pĕk′tor-ăl) [″ + *pectus*, breast]
genupectoral position
genus (jē′nŭs) [L. *genus*, kind]
genyplasty (jĕn′ī-plăs″tē) [″ + *plassein*, to form]
geobiology (jē″ō-bī-ŏl′ō-jē) [Gr. *geo*, earth, + *bios*, life, + *logos*, word, reason]
Geocillin
geode (jē′ōd) [Gr. *geodes*, earthlike]
geographic tongue
geomedicine (jē″ō-mĕd′ĭ-sĭn) [Gr. *geo*, earth, + L. *medicina*, medicine]
Geopen
geophagia, geophagism, geo-

phagy (jē-ō-fā′jē-ă, -ŏf′ă-jĭzm, -ŏf′ă-jē) [″ + *phagein*, to eat]
geotaxis (jē″ō-tăk′sĭs) [″ + *taxis*, arrangement]
geotragia (jē″ō-trā′jē-ă) [″ + *trogein*, to chew]
geotrichosis (jē″ō-trī-kō′sĭs)
Geotrichum (jē-ŏt′rī-kŭm)
geotropism (jē″ŏt′rō-pĭzm) [″ + *tropos*, a turning]
gephyrophobia (jē-fī″rō-fō′bē-ă) [Gr. *gephyra*, bridge, + *phobos*, fear]
Gerdy's fibers (zhĕr′dēz) [Pierre N. Gerdy, Fr. physician, 1797 – 1856]
geriatrics (jĕr″ē-ăt′rĭks) [Gr. *geras*, old age, + *iatrike*, medical treatment]
    g., dental
Gerlach's valve (gĕr′lăks) [Joseph von Gerlach, Ger. anatomist, 1820 – 1896]
germ [L. *germen*, sprout, fetus]
    g., dental
    g., hair
    g., wheat
germanium (jĕr-mā′nē-ŭm) [L. *Germania*, Germany]
German measles
germ cell
germ epithelium
germicidal (jĕrm″ĭ-sī′dăl) [L. *germen*, sprout, + *cida* fr. *caedere*, to kill]
germicide (jĕr′mĭ-sīd)
germinal [L. *germen*, sprout]
germinal center
germinal disk
germinal epithelium
germinal vesicle
germination [L. *germinare*, to sprout]
germinoma (jĕr″mĭ-nō′mă)
germ layers
germ plasm
germ theory
geroderma, gerodermia (jĕr-ō-dĕr′mă, -mē-ă) [″ + *derma*, skin]
gerodontology (jĕr″ō-dŏn-tŏl′ō-jē)
geromarasmus (jĕr″ō-măr-ăs′mŭs) [″ + *marasmos*, a wasting]
geromorphism (jĕr″ō-mor′fĭzm) [″ +

morphe, form, + -*ismos*, condition]

gerontal (jĕ-rŏn'tăl) [Gr. *geron*, old man]

gerontology (jĕ-rŏn-tŏl'ō-jē) [" + *logos*, word, reason]

gerontophilia (jĕr"ŏn-tō-fĭl'ē-ă) [" + *philein*, to love]

gerontopia (jĕr"ŏn-tō'pē-ă) [" + *opsis*, sight, appearance, vision]

gerontotherapeutics (jĕr-ŏn"tō-thĕr"ă-pū'tĭks) [" + *therapeia*, treatment]

gerontoxon (jĕ-rŏn-tŏks'ŏn) [" + *toxon*, bow]

Gerota's capsule (gā-rō'tăz) [Dimitru Gerota, Rumanian anatomist, 1867–1939]

gestagen (jĕs'tă-jĕn)

gestalt (gĕs-tawlt') [Ger. *Gestalt*, form]
   g. therapy

gestation (jĕs-tā'shŭn) [L. *gestare*, to bear]
   g., abdominal
   g., cornual
   g., ectopic
   g., interstitial
   g., ovarian
   g., plural
   g., prolonged
   g., secondary
   g., secondary abdominal
   g., tubal
   g., tuboabdominal
   g., tubo-ovarian
   g., uterotubal

gestational assessment

gestation sac

gestation time

gestosis (jĕs-tō'sĭs) [L. *gestare*, to bear, + Gr. *osis*, condition]

gesture

geumaphobia (gū"mă-fō'bē-ă) [Gr. *geuma*, taste, + *phobos*, fear]

GFR glomerular filtration rate

GH growth hormone

Ghon's primary lesion, tubercle (găwnz) [Anton Ghon, Czech. pathologist, 1866–1936]

ghost corpuscle

GH-RH growth hormone-releasing hormones

GI gastrointestinal

Giannuzzi's cells (jăn-noot'sēz) [Guiseppe Giannuzzi, It. anatomist, 1839–1876]

giant [Gr. *gigas*, giant]

giant cell

giant cell tumor

giantism (jī'ăn-tĭzm)

Giardia (jē-ăr'dē-ă) [Alfred Giard, Fr. biologist, 1846–1908]
   G. lamblia

giardiasis (jī"ăr-dī'ă-sĭs)

Gibbon's hydrocele (gĭb'ŏns) [Q. V. Gibbon, U.S. surgeon, 1813–1894]

gibbosity (gĭ-bŏs'ĭ-tē) [LL. *gebbosus*, humped]

gibbous (gĭb'bŭs)

gibbus (gĭb'ŭs) [L. *gibbosus*]

Gibney's boot, bandage (gĭb'nēz) [Virgil P. Gibney, U.S. surgeon, 1847–1927]

Gibson's murmur (gĭb'sŭnz) [George A. Gibson, Scot. physician, 1854–1913]

giddiness [AS. *gydig*, insane]

Giemsa's stain (gēm'zăs) [Gustav Giemsa, Ger. chemist, 1867–1948]

Gifford's reflex (gĭf'fords) [Harold Gifford, U.S. oculist, 1858–1929]

GIFT gamete intrafallopian transfer

giga (jĭg'ă, jī'gă)

gigantism (jī'găn-tĭzm) [Gr. *gigas*, giant, + -*ismos*, condition]
   g., acromegalic
   g., eunuchoid
   g., normal

gigantoblast (jī-găn'tō-blăst) [" + *blastos*, germ]

gigantocyte (jī-găn'tō-sīt) [" + *kytos*, cell]

gigantosoma (jī-găn"tō-sō'mă) [" + *soma*, body]

Gigli's saw (jēl'yēz) [Leonardo Gigli, It. gynecologist, 1863–1908]

Gilbert's syndrome (zhēl-bārz') [Nicolas A. Gilbert, Fr. physician, 1858–1927]

Gilchrist's disease (gĭl′krĭsts) [Thomas C. Gilchrist, U.S. dermatologist, 1862–1927]

Gilles de la Tourette's syndrome [Georges Gilles de la Tourette, Fr. neurologist, 1857–1904]

Gimbernat's ligament (hĭm-bĕr-năts′) [Antonio de Gimbernat, Sp. surgeon, 1734–1790]

gingiva (jĭn-jī′vă, jĭn′jĭ-vă) [L.]
    g., alveolar
    g., attached
    g., free
    g., labial
    g., lingual
    g., marginal

gingival (jĭn′jĭ-văl) [L. gingiva, gum]

gingivalgia (jĭn″jĭ-văl′jē-ă) [″ + Gr. algos, pain]

gingivally (jĭn′jĭ-văl″lē)

gingivectomy (jĭn″jĭ-vĕk′tō-mē) [″ + Gr. ektome, excision]

gingivitis (jĭn-jĭ-vī′tĭs) [″ + Gr. itis, inflammation]
    g., acute necrotizing
    g., expulsive
    g., gravidum
    g., hyperplastic
    g., interstitial
    g., phagedenic
    g., Vincent's

gingivoglossitis (jĭn″jĭ-vō-glŏs-sī′tĭs) [″ + Gr. glossa, tongue, + itis, inflammation]

gingivolabial (jĭn″jĭ-vō-lā′bē-ăl)

gingivoplasty (jĭn′jĭ-vō-plăs″tē) [″ + Gr. plassein, to form]

gingivosis (jĭn″jĭ-vō′sĭs) [″ + Gr. osis, condition]

gingivostomatitis (jĭn″jĭ-vō-stō″mă-tī′tĭs) [″ + Gr. stoma, mouth, opening, + itis, inflammation]
    g., acute necrotizing ulcerative
    g., herpetic

ginglyform (jĭng′lĭ-form) [Gr. ginglymos, hinge, + L. forma, shape]

ginglymoarthrodial (jĭng″lĭ-mō-ăr-thrō′dē-ăl) [″ + arthrodia, gliding joint]

ginglymoid (jĭng′lĭ-moyd) [″ + eidos, form, shape]

ginglymus (jĭng′lĭ-mŭs) [Gr. ginglymos, hinge]

ginseng (jĭn′sĕng) [Chinese jen-shen, man, man image]

Giraldés' organ (hĭr-ăl-dās′) [Joachim A. C. C. Giraldés, Portuguese surgeon in Paris, 1808–1875]

girdle [AS. gyrdel, girdle]
    g., pelvic
    g., shoulder

girdle pain

girdle symptom

Gitaligin

gitalin (jĭt′ă-lĭn)

gitter cell

giving-up

gizzard (gĭz′ărd)

glabella [L. glaber, smooth]

glabrate, glabrous [L. glaber, smooth]

glacial (glā′shăl) [L. glacialis, icy]

gladiate (glā′dē-āt) [L. gladius, sword]

gladiolus (glă-dĭ′ō-lŭs) [L. gladiolus, little sword]

glairy

gland [L. glans, acorn]
    g., absorbent
    g., accessory
    g., acinotubular
    g., acinous
    g., adrenal
    g.'s, aggregate
    g.'s, albuminous
    g., anal
    g., apocrine
    g.'s, areolar
    g.'s, auricular
    g.'s, axillary
    g.'s, Bartholin's
    g.'s, Blandin's
    g.'s, Bowman's
    g.'s, brachial
    g.'s, bronchial

g.'s, Bruch's

g.'s, Brunner's

g.'s, buccal

g., bulbourethral

g.'s, cardiac

g., carotid

g.'s, celiac

g.'s, ceruminous

g.'s, cervical

g.'s, ciliary

g.'s, circumanal

g.'s, Cobelli's

g., coccygeal

g., compound

g., compound tubular

g., conglobate

g., Cowper's

g.'s, cutaneous

g., cytogenic

g., ductless

g.'s, duodenal

g.'s, Ebner's

g., eccrine

g., endocrine

g.'s, female

g.'s, Fraenkel's

g.'s, fundic

g., gastric

g.'s, Gay's

g., genal

g.'s, genital

g.'s, hair

g.'s, haversian

g.'s, hematopoietic

g.'s, hemolymph

g.'s, hepatic

g., holocrine

g.'s, inguinal

g., interscapular

g., interstitial

g.'s, intestinal

g.'s, jugular

g.'s, Krause's

g.'s, labial

g., lacrimal

g.'s, lactiferous

g.'s, Lieberkühn's

g.'s, lingual

g.'s, Littré's

g.'s, lumbar

g., Luschka's

g., lymph; g., lymphatic

g., mammary

g.'s, meibomian

g., merocrine

g., Méry's

g., mixed

g.'s, Moll's

g.'s, Montgomery's

g.'s, Morgagni's

g.'s, muciparous

g.'s, nabothian

g.'s, odoriferous

g.'s of Zies

g.'s, olfactory

g.'s, oxyntic

g.'s, palatine

g.'s, palpebral

g.'s, parathyroid

g.'s, paraurethral

g., parotid

g., peptic

g.'s, Peyer's

g., pineal

g., pituitary

g.'s, preputial

g., prostate

g.'s, pyloric

g., racemose

g., Rivinus

g., saccular

g., salivary

g., sebaceous

g., sentinel

g., seromucous

g.'s, serous

g., sex

g.'s, Skene's

g.'s, solitary

g., sublingual

g., submandibular

g.'s, sudoriferous

g., suprarenal

g.'s, sweat

g.'s, synovial

g., target

g.'s, tarsal
g., thymus
g., thyroid
g.'s, tracheal
g., tubular
g.'s, Tyson's
g., unicellular
g.'s, urethral
g.'s, vaginal
g.'s, vestibular
g.'s, vulvovaginal
g.'s, Waldeyer's
g.'s, Weber's
g., Zuckerkandl's
glanders (glăn'dĕrz)
glandilemma (glăn"dĭ-lĕm'ă) [L. *glans*, acorn, + Gr. *lemma*, sheath]
glandula (glăn'dū-lă)
glandular [L.,*glandula*, little acorn]
glandular therapy
glandule (glăn'dūl)
glans [L. *glans*, acorn]
g. clitoridis
g. penis
Glanzmann's thrombasthenia (glănz'mănz) [Edward Glanzmann, Swiss pediatrician, 1887–1959]
glare [ME. *glaren*, to gleam]
glaserian artery (glă-sē'rē-ăn) [Johann Heinrich Glaser, Swiss anatomist, 1629–1675]
glaserian fissure
Glasgow Coma Scale
glass [AS. *glaes*]
g., leaded
g., photochromic
g., polarized
g., safety
g., tempered
g., ultraviolet transmitting
g., watch
glasses [AS. *glaes*, glass]
g., bifocal
g., safety
g., sun-
g., trifocal
glassy
Glauber's salt (glō'bĕrz) [Johann Ru-

dolf Glauber, Ger. physician, 1604–1668]
glaucoma (glaw-kō'mă) [Gr. *glaukoma*, fr. *glaukos*, gleaming, gray]
g., absolutum
g., chronic
g., congenital
g., infantile
g., juvenile
g., narrow angle
g., open angle
g., simplex
glaucomatous (glaw-kō'mă-tŭs)
GLC *gas-liquid chromatography*
gleet (glēt)
Glénard's disease (glā-nărz') [Frantz Glénard, Fr. physician, 1848–1920]
glenohumeral (glē"nō-hū'mĕr-ăl) [Gr. *glene*, socket, + L. *humerus*, humerus]
glenohumeral ligaments
glenoid (glē'noyd) [" + *eidos*, form, shape]
glenoid cavity
glenoid fossa
glenoid lip
glia (glī'ă) [Gr. *glia*, glue]
glia cells
gliacyte (glī'ă-sīt) [" + *kytos*, cell]
gliadin (glī'ă-dĭn)
glial (glī'ăl)
gliarase (glī'ă-rās) [Gr. *glia*, glue]
glide
g., mandibular
glioblastoma (glī"ō-blăs-tō'mă) [" + *blastos*, germ, + *oma*, tumor]
g. multiforme
gliocyte (glī'ō-sīt) [" + *kytos*, cell]
gliocytoma (glī-ō-sī-tō'mă) [" + " + *oma*, tumor]
gliogenous (glī-ŏj'ĕ-nŭs) [" + *gennan*, to produce]
glioma (glī-ō'mă) [" + *oma*, tumor]
g. retinae
gliomatosis (glī"ō-mă-tō'sīs) [" + " + *osis*, condition]
gliomatous (glī-ō'mă-tŭs)
gliomyoma (glī"ō-mī-ō'mă) [" +

mys, muscle, + *oma*, tumor]

glioneuroma (glī″ō-nū-rō′mă) [″ + *neuron*, nerve, + *oma*, tumor]

gliosarcoma [″ + *sarx*, flesh, + *oma*, tumor]

gliosis (glī-ō′sĭs) [″ + *osis*, condition]

gliosome (glī′ō-sōm) [″ + *soma*, body]

gliotoxin (glī″ō-tŏk′sĭn)

Glisson, Francis (glĭs′ŭn) [Brit. physician and anatomist, 1597–1677]
G.'s capsule
G.'s disease

glissonian cirrhosis

glissonitis

globi (glō′bī) [L.]

globin (glō′bĭn) [L. *globus*, globe]

globoid (glō′boyd) [″ + Gr. *eidos*, form, shape]

globular (glŏb′ū-lăr) [L. *globus*, a globe]

globule (glŏb′ūl) [L. *globulus*, globule]

globulin (glŏb′ū-lĭn) [L. *globulus*, globule]
g., Ac
g., antihemophilic
g., antilymphocyte
g., gamma
g., immune
g., Rh₀(D) immune
g., serum
g., varicella-zoster immune

globulinuria (glŏb″ū-lĭn-ū′rē-ă) [L. *globulus*, globule, + Gr. *ouron*, urine]

globulose (glŏb′ū-lōs) [L. *globulus*, globule]

globus [L.]
g. hystericus
g. major
g. minor
g. pallidus

glomangioma (glō-măn″jē-ō′mă) [L. *glomus*, a ball, + Gr. *angeion*, vessel, + *oma*, tumor]

glomectomy (glō-mĕk′tō-mē)

glomerate (glŏm′ĕr-āt) [L. *glomerare*, to wind into a ball]

glomerular (glō-mĕr′ū-lăr) [L. *glomerulus*, little ball]

glomerular disease

glomeruli (glō-mĕr′ū-lī) [L. *glomerulus*, little ball]

glomerulitis (glō-mĕr″ū-lī′tĭs) [″ + Gr. *itis*, inflammation]

glomerulonephritis (glō-mĕr″ū-lō-nĕ-frī′tĭs) [″ + Gr. *nephros*, kidney, + *itis*, inflammation]

glomerulopathy (glō-mĕr″ū-lŏp′ă-thē)

glomerulosclerosis (glō-mĕr″ū-lō-sklē-rō′sĭs)
g., diabetic
g., intercapillary

glomerulus (glō-mĕr′ū-lŭs) [L.]
g., olfactory

glomoid (glō′moyd)

glomus (glō′mŭs) [L., a ball]
g. caroticum
g. choroideum
g. coccygeum

glossa [Gr. *glossa*, tongue]

glossal

glossalgia (glŏs-săl′jē-ă) [″ + *algos*, pain]

glossectomy (glŏs-ĕk′tō-mē) [″ + *ektome*, excision]

Glossina (glŏs-sī′nă)

glossitis (glŏs-sī′tĭs) [″ + *itis*, inflammation]
g., acute
g. areata exfoliativa
g. desiccans
g., median rhomboid
g., Moeller's
g. parasitica

glosso- [Gr. *glossa*, tongue]

glossocele (glŏs′sō-sēl) [″ + *kele*, tumor, swelling]

glossodynamometer (glŏs″sō-dī″nă-mŏm′ĕ-tĕr) [″ + *dynamis*, power, + *metron*, measure]

glossodynia (glŏs″ō-dĭn′ē-ă) [″ + *odyne*, pain]
g. exfoliativa

glossoepiglottic (glŏs″ō-ĕp-ĭ-glŏt′ĭk)

[" + *epi*, upon, + *glottis*, tongue]

glossoepiglottidean (glŏs"ō-ĕp-ĭ-glŏ-tĭd'ē-ăn)

glossoepiglottidean folds

glossoepiglottidean ligament

glossograph (glŏs'ō-grăf) [" + *graphein*, to write]

glossohyal (glŏs"ō-hī'ăl) [" + *hyoeides*, U-shaped]

glossokinesthetic (glŏs"ō-kĭn"ĕs-thĕt'ĭk) [" + *kinesis*, motion, + *aisthetikos*, perceptive]

glossolabial (glŏs"ō-lā'bē-ăl) [" ⋅ + L. *labium*, lip]

glossolalia (glŏs"ō-lā'lē-ă) [" + *lalia*, chatter, prattle]

glossology (glŏ-sŏl'ō-jē) [" + *logos*, word, reason]

glossolysis (glŏ-sŏl'ĭ-sĭs) [" + *lysis*, dissolution]

glossopalatine (glŏs"ō-păl'ă-tīn)

glossopathy (glŏs-sŏp'ă-thē) [" + *pathos*, disease, suffering]

glossopharyngeal (glŏs"ō-fă-rĭn'jē-ăl) [" + *pharynx*, throat]

glossopharyngeal nerve

glossophytia (glŏs"ō-fī'tē-ă) [Gr. *glossa*, tongue, + *phyton*, plant]

glossoplasty (glŏs'ō-plăs"tē) [" + *plassein*, to form]

glossoplegia (glŏs"ō-plē'jē-ă) [" + *plege*, stroke]

glossoptosis (glŏs"ŏp-tō'sĭs) [" + *ptosis*, fall, falling]

glossopyrosis (glŏs"ō-pī-rō'sĭs) [" + *pyrosis*, a burning]

glossorrhaphy (glŏ-sor'ă-fē) [" + *rhaphe*, seam]

glossoscopy (glŏ-sŏs'kō-pē) [" + *skopein*, to examine]

glossospasm (glŏs'ō-spăzm) [" + *spasmos*, a convulsion]

glossotomy (glŏ-sŏt'ō-mē) [" + *tome*, a cutting, slice]

glossotrichia (glŏs"ō-trĭk'ē-ă) [" + *thrix*, hair]

glossy

glossy skin

glottic [Gr. *glottis*, tongue]

glottis (glŏt'ĭs) [Gr. *glottis*, tongue]
   g., edema of

glottitis (glŏ-tī'tĭs) [" + *itis*, inflammation]

glottology (glŏ-tŏl'ō-jē) [" + *logos*, word, reason]

glucagon (gloo'kă-gŏn)

glucagonoma (glŭ"kă-gŏn-ō'mă)

gluciphore (gloo'sĭ-for)

glucocerebroside (gloo"kō-sĕr'ĕ-brō-sīd")

glucocorticoid (gloo"kō-kort'ĭ-koyd) [Gr. *gleukos*, sweet (new wine), + L. *cortex*, cortex, + Gr. *eidos*, form, shape]

glucofuranose (gloo"kō-fū'ră-nōs)

glucogenesis (gloo"kō-jĕn'ĕ-sĭs)

glucohemia (gloo"kō-hē'mē-ă) [" + *haima*, blood]

glucokinase (gloo"kō-kī'nās)

glucokinetic (gloo"kō-kī-nĕt'ĭk)

Glucometer

gluconeogenesis (gloo"kō-nē"ō-jĕn'ĕ-sĭs) [" + *neos*, new, + *genesis*, generation, birth]

glucopenia (gloo"kō-pē'nē-ă) [" + Gr. *penia*, lack]

glucophore (gloo'kō-for) [" + *phorein*, to carry]

glucoprotein (gloo"kō-prō'tē-ĭn)

glucopyranose (gloo"kō-pī'ră-nōs)

glucosamine (gloo"kō-săm'ēn)

glucose (gloo'kōs) [Gr. *gleukos*, sweet (new wine)]
   g., blood level of
   g., liquid

glucose-6-phosphate dehydrogenase

glucose polymer

glucose tolerance test

glucosidase (gloo-kō'sĭ-dās)

glucoside (gloo'kō-sīd)

glucosin (gloo'kō-sīn)

glucosulfone sodium (gloo"kō-sŭl'fōn)

glucosuria (gloo"kō-sū'rē-ă) [" +

ouron, urine]
glucuronic acid
β-glucuronidase (gloo″kū-rŏn′ĭ-dās)
glucuronide (gloo-kū′rŏn-īd)
glue ear
glue-sniffing
Gluge's corpuscles (gloo′gēz) [Gottlieb Gluge, Ger. pathologist, 1812–1898]
glutamate (gloo′tă-māt)
glutamic acid (gloo-tăm′ĭk) [L. *gluten,* glue, + *ammonium*]
glutamic-oxaloacetic transaminase
glutamic-pyruvic transaminase
glutaminase (gloo-tăm′ĭ-nās)
glutamine (gloo′tă-mīn, -mēn″)
γ-glutamyl transpeptidase
glutaral (gloo′tă-răl)
glutaraldehyde (gloo″tă-răl′dĕ-hīd)
glutathione (gloo-tă-thī′ōn) [″ + Gr. *theion,* sulfur]
   g., reduced
gluteal (gloo′tē-ăl) [Gr. *gloutos,* buttock]
gluteal fold
gluteal reflex
glutelin (gloo′tĕ-lĭn) [L. *gluten,* glue]
gluten [L., glue]
gluten-free diet
gluten-induced enteropathy
glutethimide (gloo-tĕth′ĭ-mīd)
glutin
glutinous (gloo′tĭn-ŭs) [L. *glutinosus,* glue]
glutitis [Gr. *gloutos,* buttock, + *itis,* inflammation]
glycase (glī′kās) [Gr. *glykys,* sweet]
glycemia (glī-sē′mē-ă) [″ + *haima,* blood]
DL-glyceraldehyde (glĭs″ĕr-ăl′dĕ-hīd)
glyceride (glĭs′ĕr-īd) [Gr. *glykys,* sweet]
glycerin (glĭs′ĕr-ĭn)
glycerite (glĭs′ĕr-īt) [L. *glyceritum*]
glycerol (glĭs′ĕr-ŏl) [Gr. *glykys,* sweet]
glyceryl (glĭs′ĕr-ĭl)
   g. monostearate
   g. triacetate
   g. trinitrate

glycine (glī′sēn, -sĭn) [Gr. *glykys,* sweet]
glyco-, glyc- (glī-kō) [Gr. *glykys,* sweet]
glycobiarsol (glī″kō-bī-ăr′sŏl)
glycocalyx (glī″kō-kăl′ĭks)
glycocholate (glī″kō-kōl′āt)
glycocholic acid
glycocin
glycoclastic (glī″kō-klăs′tĭk) [″ + *klan,* to break]
glycocoll (glī′kō-kŏl) [″ + *kolla,* glue]
glycogen (glī′kō-jĕn) [″ + *gennan,* to produce]
glycogenase (glī-kō′jĕn-ās)
glycogenesis (glī″kō-jĕn′ĕ-sĭs) [″ + *genesis,* generation, birth]
glycogenetic
glycogenic
glycogenolysis (glī″kō-jĕn-ŏl′ĭ-sĭs) [″ + *gennan,* to produce, + *lysis,* dissolution]
glycogenolytic (glī″kō-jĕn″ŏ-lĭt′ĭk) [″ + ″ + *lysis,* dissolution]
glycogenosis (glī″kō-jĕn-ō′sĭs) [″ + ″ + *osis,* condition]
glycogen storage disease
   g.s.d., phosphorylase b kinase deficiency
   g.s.d. type Ia
   g.s.d. type Ib
   g.s.d. type II
   g.s.d. type III
   g.s.d. type IV
   g.s.d. type V
   g.s.d. type VI
   g.s.d. type VII
glycogeusia (glī″kō-jū′sē-ă) [Gr. *glykys,* sweet, + *geusis,* taste]
glycohemia (glī″kō-hē′mē-ă) [″ + *haima,* blood]
glycol (glī′kŏl, -kŏl) [″ + *alcohol*]
glycolipid(e) (glī″kō-lĭp′ĭd) [″ + *lipos,* fat]
glycolysis (glī-kŏl′ĭ-sĭs) [″ + *lysis,* dissolution]
glycolytic
glycolytic enzyme
glycometabolic (glī″kō-mĕt-ă-bŏl′ĭk)

[" + *metabole,* change]

glycometabolism (glī"kō-mĕ-tăb'ŏ-lĭzm)

glyconeogenesis (glī"kō-nē"ŏ-jĕn'ē-sĭs) [" + *neos,* new, + *genesis,* generation, birth]

glyconucleoprotein (glī"kō-nū"klē-ŏ-prō'tē-ĭn) [" + L. *nucleus,* kernel, + Gr. *protos,* first]

glycopenia (glī-kō-pē'nē-ă) [" + *penia,* lack]

glycopexic (glī"kō-pĕks'ĭk) [" + *pexis,* fixation]

glycopexis (glī"kō-pĕk'sĭs)

glycophorin (glī"kō-fō'rĭn)

glycopolyuria (glī"kō-pŏl"ē-ū'rē-ă) [" + *polys,* much, + *ouron,* urine]

glycoprival, glycoprivous (glī"kō-prī'văl, -vŭs) [" + L. *privus,* deprived of]

glycoprotein (glī"kō-prō'tē-ĭn) [" + *protos,* first]

glycoptyalism (glī"kō-tī'ăl-ĭzm) [" + *ptyalon,* saliva, + *-ismos,* condition]

glycopyrrolate (glī"kō-pīr'rō-lāt)

glycorrhachia (glī-kō-rā'kē-ă) [" + *rhachis,* spine]

glycorrhea (glī"kō-rē'ă) [" + *rhein,* to flow]

glycosecretory (glī"kō-sē-krē'tō-rē) [" + L. *secretus,* separate]

glycosemia (glī-kō-sē'mē-ă) [" + *haima,* blood]

glycosialia (glī"kō-sī-ăl'ē-ă) [" + *sialon,* saliva]

glycosialorrhea (glī"kō-sī"ăl-ō-rē'ă) [" + " + *rhein,* to flow]

glycoside

glycosphingolipids (glī"kō-sfĭng"ō-lĭp'ĭds)

glycostatic (glī"kō-stăt'ĭk) [Gr. *glykys,* sweet, + *statikos,* standing]

glycosuria (glī"kō-sū'rē-ă) [" + *ouron,* urine]

   g., alimentary

   g., diabetic

   g., emotional

   g., phloridzin

   g., pituitary

   g., renal

glycosyl (glī'kō-sĭl)

glycosylated hemoglobin

glycotropic (glī"kō-trŏp'ĭk) [" + *tropos,* a turning]

glycuresis (glī"kŭ-rē'sĭs) [" + *ouresis,* urination]

glycuronuria (glī-kŭ"rō-nū'rē-ă)

glycylglycine (glĭs"ĭl-glĭs'ĭn)

glycyltryptophan (glĭs"ĭl-trĭp'tō-făn)

glycyrrhiza (glĭs-ĭ-rī'ză) [" + *rhiza,* root]

glyoxalase (glē-ōk'să-lās)

glyoxylic acid

Glysennid

gm *gram*

GML *glabellomeatal line*

gnashing

gnat (năt)

   g., buffalo

gnathalgia (năth-ăl'jē-ă) [Gr. *gnathos,* jaw, + *algos,* pain]

gnathic (năth'ĭk) [Gr. *gnathos,* jaw

gnathion (năth'ē-ŏn)

gnathitis (năth-ī'tĭs) [" + *itis,* inflammation]

gnatho- (năth'ō) [Gr. *gnathos,* jaw]

gnathocephalus (năth"ō-sĕf'ă-lŭs) [" + *kephale,* head]

gnathodynamometer (năth"ō-dī"nă-mŏm'ĕ-tĕr) [" + *dynamis,* power, + *metron,* measure]

gnathodynia (năth"ō-dĭn'ē-ă) [" + *odyne,* pain]

gnathoplasty (năth'ō-plăs"tē) [" + *plassein,* to form]

gnathoschisis (năth-ŏs'kĭ-sĭs) [" + *schizein,* to split]

Gnathostoma (năth-ŏs'tō-mă) [" + *stoma,* mouth, opening]

gnathostomiasis (năth"ō-stō-mī'ă-sĭs)

gnosia (nō'sē-ă) [Gr. *gnosis,* knowledge]

gnotobiotics (nō"tō-bī-ŏt'ĭks) [Gr. *gnotos,* known, + *bios,* life]

GnRH *gonadotropin-releasing hormone*

goat's milk

goblet cell
goggle-eyed
goiter (goy′tĕr) [L. *guttur*, throat]
   g., aberrant
   g., acute
   g., adenomatous
   g., colloid
   g., congenital
   g., cystic
   g., diffuse
   g., diver
   g., endemic
   g., exophthalmic
   g., fibrous
   g., follicular
   g., hyperplastic
   g., intrathoracic
   g., lingual
   g., nodular
   g., parenchymatous
   g., perivascular
   g., retrovascular
   g., simple
   g., substernal
   g., suffocative
   g., toxic
   g., vascular
goitrogens (goy′trō-jĕns) [L. *guttur*, throat, + *gennan*, to produce]
gold
   g. alloy
   g. alloy, dental casting
   G. Au 198 Injection
   g. sodium thiomalate
goldbeater's skin
Goldblatt kidney [Harry Goldblatt, U.S. physician, 1891 – 1977]
gold standard
Golgi apparatus (gŏl′jē) [Camillo Golgi, It. histologist, 1844 – 1926]
Golgi's cells
Golgi's corpuscle
Goll's tract (gŏlz) [Friedrich Goll, Swiss anatomist, 1829 – 1904]
Golytely
gomphosis (gŏm-fō′sĭs) [Gr., bolting together]
gonad (gō′năd, gŏn′ăd) [Gr. *gonos*, offspring, procreation]

gonadal (gō′năd-ăl)
gonadal dysgenesis
gonadectomy (gŏn-ă-dĕk′tō-mē) [Gr. *gonos*, offspring, procreation, + *ektome*, excision]
gonadial (gō-năd′ē-ăl)
gonadopathy (gŏn″ă-dŏp′ă-thē) [″ + *pathos*, disease, suffering]
gonadotherapy (gŏn″ă-dō-thĕr′ă-pē) [″ + *therapeia*, treatment]
gonadotrope (gō-năd′ō-trōp) [″ + *trope*, turning]
gonadotrophic (gŏn″ă-dō-trŏf′ĭk) [″ + *trophe*, nourishment]
gonadotrophic hormones
gonadotropin (gŏn″ă-dō-trō′pĭn)
   g.'s, anterior pituitary
   g., chorionic
gonadotropin-releasing hormone
gonaduct (gŏn′ă-dŭkt) [″ + L. *ductus*, canal]
gonalgia (gō-năl′jē-ă) [Gr. *gony*, knee, + *algos*, pain]
gonangiectomy (gŏn″ăn-jē-ĕk′tō-mē) [Gr. *gone*, seed, + *angeion*, vessel, + *ektome*, excision]
gonarthritis (gŏn″ăr-thrī′tĭs) [Gr. *gony*, knee, + *arthron*, joint, + *itis*, inflammation]
gonarthromeningitis (gŏn-ăr″thrō-mĕn-ĭn-jī′tĭs) [″ + ″ + *meninx*, membrane, + *itis*, inflammation]
gonarthrotomy (gŏn″ăr-thrŏt′ō-mē) [″ + ″ + *tome*, a cutting, slice]
gonatocele (gŏn-ăt′ō-sēl) [″ + *kele*, tumor, swelling]
gonecyst, gonecystis (gŏn′ē-sĭst, gŏn-ē-sĭs′tĭs) [Gr. *gone*, seed, + *kystis*, a bladder]
gonecystitis (gŏn″ē-sĭs-tī′tĭs) [″ + ″ + *itis*, inflammation]
gonecystolith (gŏn″ē-sĭs′tō-lĭth) [″ + ″ + *lithos*, stone]
Gongylonema (gŏn″jĭ-lō-nē′mă) [Gr. *gongylos*, round, + *nema*, thread]
goniometer (gō″nē-ŏm′ĕ-ter) [Gr. *gonia*, angle, + *metron*, measure]
   g., finger
gonion (gō′nē-ŏn) [Gr. *gonia*, angle]

goniopuncture (gō″nē-ō-pŭnk′tūr)
gonioscope (gō′nē-ō-skōp) [″ +
skopein, to examine]
goniosynechia (gō′nē-ō-sĭ-nĕk′ē-ă)
goniotomy (gō″nē-ŏt′ō-mē) [″ +
tome, a cutting, slice]
gono-, gon- (gŏn′ō) [Gr. gonos, offspring, procreation]
gonocide (gŏn′ō-sīd) [″ + L. caedere, to kill]
gonococcal (gŏn″ō-kŏk′ăl) [″ +
kokkos, berry]
gonococcemia (gŏn″ō-kŏk-sē′mē-ă)
[″ + ″ + haima, blood]
gonococci (gŏn″ō-kŏk′sī)
gonococcic (gŏn″ō-kŏk′sĭk) [″ +
kokkos, berry]
gonococcic smears
gonococcide (gŏn″ō-kŏk′sīd) [″ +
″ + L. caedere, to kill]
gonococcocide (gŏn″ō-kŏk′ō-sīd)
gonococcus (gŏn″ō-kŏk′ŭs) [Gr. gonos,
offspring, procreation, + kokkos,
berry]
gonocyte (gŏn′ō-sīt) [″ + kytos,
cell]
gonohemia (gŏn″ō-hē′mē-ă) [″ +
haima, blood]
gonophore (gŏn′ō-for) [″ + phorein, to carry]
gonorrhea (gŏn″ō-rē′ă) [″ +
rhein, to flow]
gonorrheal
gonorrheal arthritis
Gonyaulax catanella (gŏn″ē-
aw′lăks)
gonycampsis (gŏn″ĭ-kămp′sĭs) [Gr.
gony, knee, + kampsis, bending]
gonycrotesis (gŏn″ĭ-krō-tē′sĭs) [″ +
krotesis, knocking]
gonyectyposis (gŏn″ē-ĕk-tĭ-pō′sĭs)
[″ + ektyposis, modeling in relief]
gonyocele (gŏn′ē-ō-sēl) [″ + kele,
tumor, swelling]
gonyoncus (gŏn″ē-ŏn′kŭs) [″ +
onkos, bulk, mass]
Goodell's sign [William Goodell, U.S.
gynecologist, 1829–1894]

Goodpasture's syndrome [E. W.
Goodpasture, U.S. pathologist,
1886–1960]
Good Samaritan Law
goose flesh
Gordon's reflex [Alfred Gordon, U.S.
neurologist, 1874–1953]
gorget (gor′jĕt) [Fr. gorge, throat, because of shape of instrument]
Gossypium (gŏ-sĭp′ē-ŭm) [L.]
gossypol
GOT glutamic-oxaloacetic transaminase
gouge (gowj)
goundou (goon′doo)
gout (gowt) [L. gutta, drop]
   g., abarticular
   g., chronic
   g., tophaceous
gouty
gouty diathesis
Gowers' sign [Sir William R. Gowers,
Brit. neurologist, 1845–1915]
Gowers' tract (gow′ĕrz)
G.P. general practitioner
G-6-PD glucose-6-phosphate dehydrogenase
GPT glutamic-pyruvic transaminase
gr grain
graafian follicle (grăf′ē-ăn) [Regnier
de Graaf, Dutch physician and anatomist, 1641–1673]
gracile (grăs′ĭl) [L. gracilis, slender]
gracile nucleus
gracilis (grăs′ĭ-lĭs) [L., slender]
gradatim (gră-dă′tĭm) [L.]
Gradenigo's syndrome (gră-dĕn-
ē′gōz) [Giuseppe Gradenigo, It. physician, 1859–1926]
gradient (grā′dē-ĕnt)
   g., axial
graduate (grăd′ū-āt, -ăt) [L. gradus, a
step]
graduated
graduated tenotomy
Graefe's sign (grā′fēz) [Albrecht von
Graefe, Ger. ophthalmologist, 1828–
1870]
graft (grăft) [L. graphium, stylus]

g., allograft, allogeneic
g., autodermic
g., autogenous
g., autologous
g., avascular
g., bone
g., cable
g., cadaver
g., delayed
g., dermal
g., fascia
g., fascicular
g., free
g., full-thickness
g., heterodermic
g., heteroplastic
g., homologous
g., isologous
g., lamellar
g., nerve
g., Ollier-Thiersch
g., omental
g., ovarian
g., pedicle
g., periosteum
g., pinch
g., postmortem
g., rope
g., sieve
g., skin
g.'s, split-skin
g., sponge
g., thick-split
g., Thiersch's
g.'s, Wolfe's
g., zooplastic
grafting
graft-versus-host reaction
Graham's law (grā'ǎmz) [Thomas Graham, Brit. chemist, 1805–1869]
grain [L. *granum*]
gram
gram-equivalent
gramicidin (grăm"ĭ-sī'dĭn)
grammeter
Gram's method [Hans C. J. Gram, Danish physician, 1853–1938]
gram molecule

gram-negative
gram-positive
Grancher's disease (grän-shăz') [Jacques J. Grancher, Fr. physician, 1843–1907]
Grancher's sign
grandiose (grän'dē-ōs)
grandiosity
grand mal (grän măl) [Fr., great evil]
granular [L. *granulum*, little grain]
granular cast
granulatio (grän"ū-lā'shē-ō) [L.]
granulation
g., arachnoidal
g., exuberant
granule (grän'ūl) [L. *granulum*, little grain]
g.'s, acidophil
g., agminated
g., albuminous
g., Altmann's
g., amphophil
g., azurophil
g., basal
g.'s, basophil
g., beta
g.'s, chromatin
g., chromophil
g.'s, cone
g.'s, delta
g., eosinophil
g., epsilon
g., glycogen
g.'s, hyperchromatin
g.'s, iodophil
g.'s, juxtaglomerular
g., Kölliker's interstitial
g.'s, metachromatic
g.'s, Much's
g., neutrophil
g., Nissl
g.'s, pigment
g., Plehn's
g., protein
g., rod
g., Schüffner's
g.'s, secretory
g., seminal

g.'s, thread
g.'s, zymogen
granulitis (grăn-ū-lī'tĭs) [L. *granulum*, little grain, + Gr. *itis*, inflammation]
granuloadipose (grăn"ū-lō-ăd'ĭ-pōs)
granuloblast (grăn'ū-lō-blăst) [" + Gr. *blastos*, germ]
granulocyte (grăn'ū-lō-sīt") [" + Gr. *kytos*, cell]
granulocytopenia (grăn"ū-lō-sī"tō-pē'nē-ă) [" + " + *penia*, lack]
granulocytopoiesis (grăn"ū-lō-sī"tō-poy-ē'sĭs) [" + " + *poiein*, to form]
granulocytosis (grăn"ū-lō-sī-tō'sĭs) [" + " + *osis*, condition]
granuloma [" + Gr. *oma*, tumor]
    g. annulare
    g., apical
    g., benign, of thyroid
    g., coccidioidal
    g., dental
    g., eosinophilic
    g. fissuratum
    g., foreign body
    g. fungoides
    g., infectious
    g. inguinale
    g. iridis
    g., lipoid
    g., lipophagic
    g., Majocchi's
    g., malignant
    g., paracoccidioidal
    g. pyogenicum
    g., swimming pool
    g. telangiectaticum
    g.'s, trichophytic
granulomatosis (grăn"ū-lō"mă-tō'sĭs) [L. *granulum*, little grain, + Gr. *oma*, tumor, + *osis*, condition]
    g. siderotica
    g., Wegener's
granulomatous (grăn"ū-lŏm'ă-tŭs)
granulopenia (grăn"ū-lō-pē'nē-ă) [" + Gr. *penia*, lack]
granuloplasm (grăn'ū-lō-plăzm)
granuloplastic (grăn"ū-lō-plăs'tĭk) [" + Gr. *plassein*, to form]

granulopoiesis (grăn"ū-lō-poy-ē'sĭs) [" + Gr. *poiein*, to make]
granulopotent (grăn"ū-lō-pō'tĕnt) [" + *potentia*, power]
granulosa (grăn"ū-lō'să)
granulosa cell tumor
granulosa-theca cell tumor
granulose (grăn'ū-lōs)
granulosis (grăn"ū-lō'sĭs) [" + Gr. *osis*, condition]
    g. rubra nasi
granum (grā'nŭm) [L.]
grape
grape sugar
graph (grăf)
-graph [Gr. *graphos*, written]
graphesthesia (grăf"ĕs-thē'zē-ă) [" + *aisthesis*, feeling, perception]
graphite (grăf'īt) [Gr. *graphein*, to write]
grapho- [Gr. *graphein*, to write]
graphology (grăf-ŏl'ō-jē) [" + *logos*, word, reason]
graphomotor (grăf"ō-mō'tor) [" + L. *motor*, mover]
graphophobia (grăf"ō-fō'bē-ă) [" + *phobos*, fear]
graphorrhea (grăf"ō-rē'ă) [" + *rhein*, to flow]
graphospasm (grăf'ō-spăzm) [" + *spasmos*, a convulsion]
GRAS List *generally recognized as safe*
grasp
grass
grating
grattage (gră-tăzh') [Fr., a scraping]
grave [L. *gravis*, heavy]
gravel [Fr. *gravelle*, coarse sand]
Graves' disease [Robert J. Graves, Irish physician, 1797 – 1853]
grave wax
gravid (grăv'ĭd) [L. *gravida*, pregnant]
gravida (grăv'ĭ-dă) [L.]
gravidism [" + Gr. *-ismos*, condition]
graviditas (gră-vĭd'ĭ-tăs)
gravidity (gră-vĭd'ĭ-tē) [L. *gravida*, pregnant]
gravidocardiac (grăv"ĭd-ō-kăr'dē-ăk)

[" + Gr. *kardia*, heart]
gravimetric (grăv"ĭ-mĕt'rĭk) [L. *gravis*, heavy, + Gr. *metron*, measure]
gravistatic (grăv"ĭ-stăt'ĭk) [" + Gr. *statikos*, causing to stand]
gravitation [L. *gravitas*, weight]
gravity
    g., specific
Gravlee jet washer
gray
gray matter
gray syndrome of the newborn
green
    g., brilliant
    g., indocyanine
    g., malachite
green blindness
Greenfield's disease [J. Godwin Greenfield, Brit. neuropathologist, 1884–1958]
green soap
green soap tincture
greenstick fracture
green vitriol
greffotome (grĕf'ō-tōm) [Fr. *greffe*, graft, + Gr. *tome*, a cutting, slice]
grenz rays [Ger. *Grenze*, boundary]
grid
    g., Fixott-Everett
grief reaction
griffe des orteils (grĕf dāz or-tā') [Fr.]
Grifulvin V
grinder (grīn'dĕr) [AS. *grindan*, to gnash]
grinders' disease
grinding
    g., selective
grip, grippe (grĭp) [Fr. *gripper*, to seize]
gripes (grīps) [AS. *gripan*, to grasp]
griping
Grisactin
griseofulvin
Gris-PEG
gristle (grĭs'ĕl) [AS.]
grits
grocers' itch
groin [AS. *grynde*, abyss]
grommet (grŏm'ĭt)

groove [MD. *groeve*, ditch]
    g., bicipital
    g., branchial
    g., carotid
    g., costal
    g., costovertebral
    g., Harrison's
    g., infraorbital
    g., intertubercular
    g., labial
    g., lacrimal
    g., laryngotracheal
    g., malleolar
    g., medullary
    g.'s, meningeal
    g., musculospiral
    g., mylohyoid
    g., nasolacrimal
    g., nasopalatine
    g., neural
    g., obturator
    g., olfactory
    g., palatine
    g., peroneal
    g., pharyngeal
    g., primitive
    g., pterygopalatine
    g., radial
    g., rhombic
    g., sagittal
    g., sigmoid
    g., subcostal
    g., tympanic
    g., urethral
    g., vertebral
    g., visceral
gross (grōs) [L. *grossus*, thick]
gross anatomy
gross lesion
gross motor skills
ground
ground bundle
ground itch
ground substance
group [It. *gruppo*, knot]
    g., alcohol
    g., azo
    g., coli-aerogenes
    g., colon-typhoid-dysentery

g., peptide
g., prosthetic
g., saccharide
group dynamics
grouping
g., blood
grouping serum
group therapy
group transfer
growing pains
growth [AS. *growan*, to grow]
growth hormone
g.h., human synthetic
gruel [L. *grutum*, meal]
grumose, grumous (groo'mōs,-mŭs) [L. *grumus*, heap]
Grünfelder's reflex (groon'fĕld-ĕrs)
gryposis (grĭ-pō'sĭs) [G. *gryposis*, a crooking]
GSR *galvanic skin response*
G-suit
gt [L.] *gutta*, a drop
gtt [L.] *guttae*, drops
GU *genitourinary*
guaiac (gwī'ăk) [NL. *Guaiacum*]
guaiacol (gwī'ă-kōl)
guaifenesin (gwī-fĕn'ĕ-sĭn)
guanase (gwăn'ās) [Sp. *guano*, from Quechua *huanu*, dung]
guanethidine (gwăn-ĕth'ĭ-dēn)
g., sulfate
guanidine (gwăn'ĭ-dēn)
guanidinemia (gwăn"ĭd-ĕn-ē'mē-ă) [*guanidine* + Gr. *haima*, blood]
guanidoacetic acid
guanine (gwă'nēn)
guanosine (gwăn'ō-sĭn)
gubernaculum (gū"bĕr-năk'ū-lŭm) [L., helm]
g. dentis
g. testis
Gubler's line (goob'lĕrz) [Adolphe Gubler, Fr. physician, 1821–1879]
Gubler's paralysis
Gubler's tumor
Gudden's inferior commissure (gŭd'ĕnz) [Bernard A. von Gudden, Ger. neurologist, 1824–1886]

Gudden's law
guidance
guide
guide dog
guidewire
Guillain-Barré syndrome [G. Guillain, Fr. neurologist, 1876–1961; J. A. Barré, Fr. neurologist, b. 1880]
guillotine (gĭl'ō-tēn) [Fr. instrument for beheading]
guilt (gĭlt)
guinea pig (gĭn'ē pĭg)
guinea worm
Gull's disease [Sir William W. Gull, Brit. physician, 1816–1890]
gullet [L. *gula*, throat]
Gullstrand's slit lamp (gŭl'străndz) [Allvar Gullstrand, Swedish ophthalmologist, 1862–1920]
gum
gumboil
gumma (gŭm'mă) [L. *gummi*, gum]
gummatous (gŭm'ă-tŭs)
gummose (gŭm'ōs)
gummy [L. *gummi*, gum]
Gunn's dots (gŭnz) [Robert M. Gunn, Brit. ophthalmologist, 1850–1909]
gunshot wound
gunstock deformity
Günther's disease [Hans Günther, Ger. physician, 1884–1956]
gurney (gĕr'nē)
gustation (gŭs-tā'shŭn) [L. *gustare*, to taste]
gustatory (gŭs'tă-tō-rē)
gustatory sweating
gustometry (gŭs-tŏm'ĕ-trē) [" + Gr. *metron*, measure]
gut [AS.]
gutta [L., a drop]
gutta-percha (gŭt"ă-pĕr'chă)
guttate [L. *gutta*, drop]
guttatim (gŭt-tā'tĭm) [L.]
guttering (gŭt'ĕr-ĭng)
guttur (gŭt'ŭr) [L. *gutter*, throat]
guttural (gŭt'ŭ-răl)
gutturotetany (gŭt"ŭr-ō-tĕt'ă-nē) [" + Gr. *tetanos*, rigid, stretched]

Guyon's sign (gē-yŏnz') [Felix J. C. Guyon, Fr. surgeon, 1831 – 1920]

Gwathmey's method (gwăth'mēz) [James T. Gwathmey, U.S. surgeon, 1863 – 1944]

Gy gray

gymnastics [Gr. gymnastikos, pert. to nakedness]
    g., ocular
    g., Swedish

gymnophobia (jĭm-nō-fō'bē-ă) [Gr. gymnos, naked, + phobos, fear]

gynander (jī-năn'dĕr, jī-, gī-) [Gr. gyne, woman, + aner, andros, man]

gynandrism (jī-năn'drĭzm)

gynandroid (jī-năn'droyd, jī-, gī-) [" + " + eidos, form, shape]

gynatresia (jī-nă-trē'zē-ă , jī-, gī-) [" + a-, not, + tresis, perforation]

gynecic (jī-nē'sĭk, jī-, gī-) [Gr. gyne, woman]

gyneco-, gyno- [Gr.]

gynecogenic (jĭn"ĕ-kō-jĕn'ĭk) [" + gennan, to produce]

gynecoid (jĭn'ĕ-koyd) [" + eidos, form, shape]

gynecologic, gynecological (gī"nĕ-kō-lŏj'ĭk, jī"-, jĭn"ĕ-; -ĭ-kăl) [" + logos, word, reason]

gynecologic operative procedures

gynecologist (gī"nĕ-kŏl'ō-jĭst, jī"-, jĭn"ĕ-)

gynecology (gī"nĕ-kŏl'ō-jē, jī"-, jĭn"ĕ-) [" + logos, word, reason]

gynecomania (jī"nĕ-kō-mā'nē-ă, gī"-, jĭn"ĕ-) [" + mania, madness]

gynecomastia (jī"nĕ-kō-măs'tē-ă, gī"-, jĭn"ĕ-) [" + mastos, breast]

gynecopathy (jī-nĕ-kŏp'ă-thē, gī"-, jĭn"ĕ-) [" + pathos, disease, suffering]

gynecophonus (jī"nĕ-kŏf'ŏn-ŭs, gī"-, jĭn"ĕ-) [" + phone, voice]

Gyne-Lotrimin

gynephobia (jī"nĕ-fō'bē-ă, gī"-, jĭn"ĕ-) [" + phobos, fear]

Gynergen

gynesic (gī-nē'sĭk, jī-, jĭn-ē'-) [Gr. gyne, woman]

gyniatrics (jī"nē-ăt'rĭks , gī"-, jĭn"ē-) [" + iatrikos, medical treatment]

gynopathic [" + pathos, disease, suffering]

gynoplastics [" + plassein, to form]

gynoplasty

gypsum (jĭp'sŭm) [L.; G. gypsos, chalk]

gyrate (jī'rāt) [Gr. gyros, circle]

gyration (jī-rā'shŭn)

gyre (jīr) [Gr. gyros, circle]

gyrectomy (jī-rĕk'tō-mē) [" + ektome, excision]

gyrencephalic (jī-rĕn-sĕ-făl'ĭk) [" + enkephale, head]

gyri (jī'rī)

gyri breves insulae

gyro- [Gr.]

gyrochrome (jī'rō-krōm) [" + chroma, color]

gyroma (jī-rō'mă) [" + oma, tumor]

gyrometer (jī-rŏm'ĕ-ter) [" + metron, measure]

gyrose (jī'rōs)

gyrospasm (jī'rō-spăzm) [" + spasmos, a convulsion]

gyrous (jī'rŭs) [Gr. gyros, circle]

gyrus (jī'rŭs)
    g., angular
    g., annectent
    g., anterior central
    g., Broca's
    g., callosal
    g. cerebelli
    g., cingulate
    g., dentate
    g. fornicatus
    g., frontal, inferior
    g., frontal, middle
    g., frontal, superior
    g., fusiform
    g., Heschl's
    g., hippocampal
    g., infracalcarine
    g., lingual
    g. longus insulae

g., marginal
g., middle temporal
g., occipital
g., occipitotemporal
g., orbital
g., paracentral
g., parahippocampal
g., paraterminal
g., parietal
g., postcentral
g., precentral

g., profundi cerebri
g. rectus
g., Retzius
g., subcallosal
g., subcollateral
g., supracallosal
g., supracallosus
g., supramarginal
g., temporal
g. transitivus
g., uncinate

H

H *hydrogen*

H, h [L.] *haustus,* a draft of medicine; *height; henry; hora* or *hour; horizontal; hypermetropia*

h *hecto*

h Planck's constant

H⁺ *hydrogen ion*

[H⁺] *hydrogen ion concentration*

¹H *protium*

²H *deuterium*

Haab's reflex (hŏbz) [Otto Haab, Swiss ophthalmologist, 1850–1931]

HaAg *hepatitis A antigen*

habena (hă-bē′nă) [L., rein]

habenal, habenar [L. *habena,* rein]

habenula (hă-bĕn′ū-lă) [L., little rein, strap]
   h. urethralis

habenular

habenular commissure

habenular trigone

habilitation (hă-bĭl″ĭ-tā′shŭn)

habit [L. *habere, habitus,* to have, hold]
   h., chorea
   h., masticatory
   h., spasm

habit training

habituation

habitus [L., habit]

hachement (hăsh-mŏn′) [Fr., chopping]

hacking cough

haem

haem-

Haemadipsa (hē″mă-dĭp′să) [Gr. *haima,* blood + *dipsa,* thirst]
   H. ceylonica

Haemagogus (hē″mă-gŏg′ŭs) [″ + *agogos,* leading]

Haemaphysalis (hĕm″ă-fĭs′ă-lĭs) [″ + *physallis,* bubble]

Haemophilus (hē-mŏf′ĭl-ŭs) [″ +

philein, to love]

Haemosporidia (hē″mō-spō-rĭd′ē-ă)

hafnium (hăf′nē-ŭm)

Hagedorn needle (hă′gĕ-dorn) [Werner Hagedorn, Ger. surgeon, 1831–1894]

Hailey-Hailey disease [W. H. Hailey, 1898–1967; H. E. Hailey, b. 1909, U.S. dermatologists]

hair [AS. *haer*]
   h., auditory
   h., bamboo
   h., beaded
   h., burrowing
   h., gustatory
   h., ingrown
   h., kinky
   h., lanugo
   h., moniliform
   h., pubic
   h., sensory
   h., tactile
   h., taste
   h., terminal
   h., twisted

hair analysis

hairball

hair bulb

hair cell

hair follicle

hair papilla

hair transplantation

hairy tongue

halation (hăl-ā′shŭn) [Gr. *alos,* a halo]

halazone (hăl′ă-zōn)

halcinonide (hăl-sĭn′ō-nīd)

Haldol

Haldrone

half-life

half-value layer

half-value thickness

halfway house
halibut liver oil
halide (hăl′īd)
halisteresis (hă-lĭs″tĕr-ē′sĭs) [Gr. *hals*, salt, + *steresis*, deprivation]
halisteretic
halitosis (hăl-ĭ-tō′sĭs) [L. *halitus*, breath, + Gr. *osis*, condition]
halitus (hăl′ĭ-tŭs)
Haller's anastomotic circle (hăl′ĕrz) [Albrecht von Haller, Swiss physiologist, 1708 – 1777]
Hallervorden-Spatz disease or syndrome [Julius Hallervorden, 1882 – 1965, H. Spatz, 1888 – 1969, Ger. neurologists]
hallex (hăl′ĕks) [L.]
hallucination (hă-loo-sĭ-nā′shŭn) [L. *hallucinari*, to wander in mind]
  h., auditory
  h., extracampine
  h., gustatory
  h., haptic
  h., hypnagogic
  h., kinetic
  h., microptic
  h., motor
  h., olfactory
  h., somatic
  h., tactile
  h., visual
hallucinogen (hă-loo′sĭ-nō-jĕn) [″ + Gr. *gennan*, to produce]
hallucinogenesis (hă-lū″sĭ-nō-jĕn′ĕ-sĭs)
hallucinosis (hă-loo″sĭn-ō′sĭs) [″ + Gr. *osis*, condition]
  h., acute alcoholic
hallus
hallux (hăl′ŭks) [L.]
  h. dolorosus
  h. flexus
  h. malleus
  h. rigidus
  h. valgus
  h. varus
halmatogenesis (hăl″mă-tō-jĕn′ĕ-sĭs) [Gr. *halma*, jump, + *genesis*, gen-

eration, birth]
halo [Gr. *halos*, a halo]
  h., Fick's
  h., glaucomatous
  h., senile peripapillary
halodermia (hăl″ō-dĕr′mē-ă)
Halog
halogen (hăl′ō-jĕn) [Gr. *hals*, salt, + *gennan*, to produce]
haloid (hăl′oyd) [″ + *eidos*, form, shape]
haloid salt
halometer (hă-lŏm′ĕ-tĕr) [Gr. *halos*, a halo, + *metron*, measure]
haloperidol (hă″lō-pĕr′ĭ-dŏl)
halophilic (hăl″ō-fĭl′ĭk) [″ + *philein*, to love]
halosteresis (hă-lŏs″tĕr-ē′sĭs) [Gr. *hals*, salt, + *steresis*, privation]
halo symptom
Halotestin
halothane (hăl′ō-thān)
Halsted's operation (hăl′stĕdz) [William Stewart Halsted, U.S. surgeon, 1852 – 1922]
Halsted's suture
ham [AS. *haum*, haunch]
hamartia (hăm-ăr′shē-ă) [Gr., defect]
hamartoma (hăm-ăr-tō′mă) [Gr. *hamartia*, defect, + *oma*, tumor]
  h., multiple
hamartomatosis (hăm″ăr-tō-mă-tō′sĭs) [″ + ″ + *osis*, condition]
hamate (hăm′āt)
hamate bone
hamatum (hă-mā′tŭm) [L. *hamatus*, hooked]
Hamman, Louis (hăm′ăn) [U.S. physician, 1877 – 1946]
  H.'s disease
  H.-Rich syndrome [Arnold Rich, U.S. pathologist, 1893 – 1968]
hammer
  h., dental
  h., percussion
  h., reflex
hammer finger
hammertoe

hamster

hamstring [AS. *haum,* haunch]
    h.'s, inner
    h., outer

hamstrings

Ham test

hamular (hăm'ū-lăr) [L. *hamulus,* a small hook]

hamulus (hăm'ū-lŭs) [L., a small hook]
    h. cochleae
    h. lacrimalis
    h. pterygoideus

hand [AS.]
    h., ape
    h., claw
    h., cleft
    h., drop
    h., functional position of
    h., lobster-claw
    h., obstetrician's
    h., opera-glass
    h., resting position of
    h., writing

H and E *hematoxylin* and *eosin*

handedness

hand-foot-and-mouth disease

handicap

handpiece (hănd'pēs)
    h., air-bearing turbine
    h., contra-angle
    h., high-speed

Hand-Schüller-Christian disease (hănd-shĭl'ĕr-krĭs'chăn) [Alfred Hand, Jr., U.S. pediatrician, 1868–1949; Arthur Schüller, Austrian neurologist, b. 1874; Henry A. Christian, U.S. pathologist, 1876–1951]

handsock

hanging drop culture

hangman's fracture

hangnail [AS. *ang-,* tight, painful, + *naegel,* nail]

hangover

Hanot's disease (ă-nōz') [Victor C. Hanot, Fr. physician, 1844–1896]

Hansen's bacillus [Gerhard H. A. Hansen, Norwegian physician, 1841–1912]

Hansen's disease

hapalonychia (hăp"ăl-ō-nĭk'ē-ă) [Gr. *hapalos,* soft, + *onyx,* nail]

haphalgesia (hăf"ăl-jē'zē-ă) [Gr. *haphe,* touch, + *algesis,* sense of pain]

haphephobia (hăf"ē-fō'bē-ă) [" + *phobos,* fear]

haplodont (hăp'lō-dŏnt) [" + *odous,* tooth]

haploid [Gr. *haploos,* simple, + *eidos,* form, shape]

haploidy (hăp'loy-dē)

haplopia (hăp-lō'pē-ă) [" + *ops,* vision]

hapten(e) (hăp'tĕn, -tēn) [Gr. *haptein,* to seize]

haptic (hăp'tĭk) [Gr. *haptein,* to touch]

haptics

haptin (hăp'tĭn)

haptoglobin (hăp"tō-glō'bĭn)

haptometer (hăp-tŏm'ĕ-tĕr) [" + *metron,* measure]

haptophil(e) (hăp'tō-fĭl, -fīl) [Gr. *haptein,* to touch, + *philein,* to love]

haptophore (hăp'tō-for) [" + *pherein,* to bring]

haptophoric, haptophorous

hardening [AS. *heardian,* to harden]

hardening of the arteries

hardness
    h. of a gas tube

hardness number

harelip [AS. *hara,* hare, + *lippa,* lip]

harelip suture

harlequin fetus

harmony (hăr'mō-nē)
    h., functional occlusal
    h., occlusal

harness

harpoon (hăr-poon') [Gr. *harpazein,* to seize]

Harris-Benedict equations [James A. Harris, U.S. scientist, b. 1880; Francis G. Benedict, U.S. chemist, physiologist, 1870–1957]

Harrison's groove [Edwin Harrison,

Brit. physician, 1779–1847]
Hartmann's solution [Alexis F. Hartmann, U.S. pediatrician, 1849–1931]
Hartnup disease [*Hartnup*, the family name of the first reported case]
harvest
Harvey, William (hăr'vē) [Brit. physician, 1578–1657]
Hashimoto's struma [Hakura Hashimoto, Japanese surgeon, 1881–1934]
hashish (hăsh'ĭsh) [Arabic, hemp, dried grass]
Hasner's valve or fold [Joseph R. Hasner, Prague ophthalmologist, 1819–1892]
Hassall's corpuscles [Arthur H. Hassall, Brit. chemist and physician, 1817–1894]
Hatchcock's sign
haunch (hawnsh) [Fr. *hanche*]
haustra (haws'trӑ) [L. *haurire*, to draw, drink]
    h. coli
haustral (haw'strӑl)
haustration (haws-trā'shŭn)
haustrum (haw'strŭm) [L. *haurire*, to draw, drink]
haustus (haws'tŭs) [L., a drink]
HAV *hepatitis A virus*
Haverhill fever (hā'vĕr-ĭl) [Haverhill, Mass., U.S., where the initial epidemic occurred]
haversian canal (hă-vĕr'shăn) [Clopton Havers, Brit. physician and anatomist, 1650–1702]
haversian canaliculi
haversian gland
haversian system
hay fever
Hayflick limit [Leonard Hayflick, U.S. microbiologist, b. 1928]
Haygarth's deformities [John Haygarth, Brit. physician, 1740–1827]
hazardous material
hazmat
HB *hepatitis B*
Hb *hemoglobin*

HB Ag *hepatitis B antigen*
Hbg *hemoglobin*
HBV *hepatitis B virus*
HC Cream
HCG *human chorionic gonadotrophin*
HCl *hydrochloric acid*
H.D. *hearing distance*
h.d. [L.] *hora decubitus*, the hour of going to bed
H. disease *Hartnup disease*
HDL *high-density lipoprotein*
He *helium*
head [AS. *heafod*]
    h., after-coming
    h., articular
    h., nerve
headache [AS. *heafod*, head, + *acan*, to ache]
    h., cluster
    h., exertional
    h., histamine
    h., postlumbar puncture
    h., tension
    h., thundering
headgut
head injury
head trauma
heal (hēl) [AS. *hael*, whole]
healer
healing
health (hĕlth) [AS. *haelth*, wholeness]
    h., bill of
    h., board of
    h., department of
    h., industrial
    h., public
health certificate
health education
healthful
health hazard
Health Maintenance Organization
health risk appraisal
healthy
hearing [AS. *hieran*]
    h., after-
hearing aid
hearing distance
hearing hallucinations

heart (härt) [AS. *heorte*]
  h., abdominal
  h., armored
  h., artificial
  h., beriberi
  h., boatshaped
  h., bony
  h., cervical
  h., conduction system of
  h., dilatation of
  h., fatty degeneration of
  h., fatty infiltration of
  h., fibroid
  h., hypertrophy of
  h., irritable
  h., left
  h., palpitation of
  h., right
heart attack
heartbeat
heart block
  h.b., atrioventricular
  h.b., bundle branch
  h.b., complete or third-degree
  h.b., congenital
  h.b., first-degree
  h.b., interventricular
  h.b., partial or second-degree
  h.b., sinoatrial
heartburn
heart disease
  h.d., ischemic
  h.d., risk factors
heart failure
  h.f., backward
  h.f., congestive
  h.f., forward
  h.f., high output
  h.f., left-sided
  h.f., left ventricular
  h.f., low output
  h.f., right-sided
  h.f., right ventricular
heart-lung machine
heart murmur
heart pump, nuclear-powered
heart rate
heart reflex

heart sounds
heart test
heart transplantation
heart valve, prosthetic
heat [AS. *haetu*]
  h., acclimatization to
  h., application of
  h., conductive
  h., convective
  h., conversive
  h., diathermy
  h., dry
  h., initial
  h., latent
  h., latent, of fusion
  h., latent, of vaporization
  h., luminous
  h., mechanical equivalent of
  h., moist
  h., molecular
  h., prickly
  h., radiant
  h., sensible
  h., specific
heat cramps
heat exhaustion
heat gun
heat labile
heatstroke
heat unit
heaves (hēvs)
heavy chain disease
hebephrenia (hē″bĕ-frē′nē-ă) [Gr. *hebe*, youth, + *phren*, mind]
hebephrenic (hē″bĕ-frĕn′ĭk)
Heberden's disease (hē′bĕr-dĕnz) [William Heberden, Brit. physician, 1710–1801]
Heberden's nodes
hebetic (hē-bĕt′ĭk) [Gr. *hebetikos*, youthful]
hebosteotomy (hē-bŏs″tē-ŏt′ō-mē) [Gr. *hebe*, youth, + *osteon*, bone, + *tome*, a cutting, slice]
hebotomy (hē-bŏt′ō-mē)
hecateromeric,   **hecatomeric** (hĕk″ă-tĕr″ ō-mĕr′ĭk, hĕk″ă-tō-mĕr′ĭk) [Gr. *hekateros*, each of two, +

meros, part]
hecto- [Gr. *hekaton*, hundred]
hectogram [" + *gramma*, a small weight]
hectoliter (hĕk'tō-lē"tĕr) [" + *litra*, a pound]
hectometer (hĕk-tōm'ĕ-tĕr) [" + *metron*, measure]
hedonism (hēd'ŏn-īzm) [Gr. *hedone*, pleasure, + *-ismos*, condition]
hedrocele (hĕd'rō-sēl) [Gr. *hedra*, anus, + *kele*, tumor, swelling]
heel [AS. *huela*, heel]
 h., Thomas [H. O. Thomas, Brit. orthopedist, 1834 – 1891]
heel bone
heel puncture
HEENT head, eyes, ears, nose, throat
Heerfordt's disease (hār'forts) [C. F. Heerfordt, Danish ophthalmologist, b. 1871]
Hegar's sign (hā'gărz) [Alfred Hegar, Ger. gynecologist, 1830 – 1914]
Heidenhain's demilunes (hī'dĕn-hīnz) [Rudolph P. Heidenhain, Ger. physiologist, 1834 – 1897]
height (hīt) [AS. *hiehthu*]
Heimlich maneuver (hīm'lĭk) [H. J. Heimlich, U.S. physician, b. 1920]
Heimlich sign
Heineke-Mikulicz pyloroplasty (hī'nĕ-kĕ-mĭk'ū-lĭch) [Walter Hermann Heineke, Ger. surgeon, 1834 – 1901; Johann von Mikulicz-Radecki, Polish surgeon, 1850 – 1905]
Heinz bodies [Robert Heinz, Ger. pathologist, 1865 – 1924]
Heinz body anemia
Heister, spiral valve of (hī'stĕr) [Lorenz Heister, Ger. anatomist, 1683 – 1758]
HeLa cells (hē'lă)
helcoid (hĕl'koyd) [Gr. *helkos*, ulcer, + *eidos*, form, shape]
helcology (hĕl-kŏl'ō-jē) [" + *logos*, word, reason]
helcoma (hĕl-kō'mă) [" + *oma*, tumor]

helcoplasty (hĕl'kō-plăs-tē) [" + *plassein*, to form]
helcosis (hĕl-kō'sĭs) [" + *osis*, condition]
helianthine (hē-lē-ăn'thĭn)
helical (hĕl'ĭ-kăl)
helicine (hĕl'ĭ-sĭn) [Gr. *helix*, coil]
helicine arteries
helicoid (hĕl'ĭ-koyd) [" + *eidos*, form, shape]
helicopodia (hĕl"ĭ-kō-pō'dē-ă) [" + *pous*, foot]
helicotrema (hĕl"ĭ-kō-trē'mă) [" + *trema*, a hole]
heliophobia (hē"lē-ō-fō'bē-ă) [Gr. *helios*, sun, + *phobos*, fear]
heliosis (hē"lē-ō'sĭs) [" + *osis*, condition]
heliotaxis (hē-lē-ō-tăk'sĭs) [" + *taxis*, arrangement]
 h., negative
 h., positive
heliotherapy (hē"lē-ō-thĕr'ă-pē) [" + *therapeia*, treatment]
heliotropism (hē"lē-ŏt'rō-pĭzm) [" + *trepein*, to turn, + *-ismos*, condition]
helium (hē'lē-ŭm) [Gr. *helios*, sun]
helix (hē'lĭks) [Gr., coil]
 h., Watson-Crick
Heller's test [Johann F. Heller, Austrian pathologist, 1813 – 1871]
Hellin's law [Dyonizy Hellin, Polish pathologist, 1867 – 1935]
helminth [Gr. *helmins*, worm]
helminthagogue (hĕl-mĭnth'ă-gŏg) [" + *agogos*, leading]
helminthemesis (hĕl-mĭn-thĕm'ĕ-sĭs) [" + *emesis*, vomiting]
helminthiasis (hĕl-mĭn-thī'ă-sĭs) [" + *-iasis*, state or condition of]
helminthic (hĕl-mĭn'thĭk)
helminthicide (hĕl-mĭn'thĭ-sīd) [" + L. *caedere*, to kill]
helminthoid (hĕl-mĭn'thoyd) [" + *eidos*, form, shape]
helminthology (hĕl"mĭn-thŏl'ō-jē) [" + *logos*, word, reason]

helminthoma (hĕl"mĭn-thō'mă) [" + oma, tumor]

helminthophobia (hĕl-mĭn"thŏ-fō'bē-ă) [" + phobos, fear]

heloma (hē-lō'mă) [Gr. helos, nail, + oma, tumor]

helotomy (hē-lŏt'ō-mē) [" + tome, a cutting, slice]

helplessness

Helweg's bundle (hĕl'vĕgz) [Hans K. S. Helweg, Danish physician, 1847–1901]

hema- (hē'mă, hĕm'-ă) [Gr. haima, blood]

hemachrosis (hē"mă-, hĕm"ă-krō'sĭs) [" + chrosis, coloring]

hemacytometer (hē"mă-, hĕm"ă-sī-tŏm'ĭ-tĕr) [" + kytos, cell, + metron, measure]

hemacytozoon (hē"mă-, hĕm"ă-sī-tō-zō'ŏn) [" + " + zoon, animal]

hemad (hē'măd) [Gr. haima, blood, + L. ad, toward]

hemadostenosis (hē"mă-, hĕm"ă-dō-stĕn-ō'sĭs) [" + stenosis, act of narrowing]

hemadsorption (hĕm"ăd-sorp'shŭn)

hemadynamometer (hē"mă-, hĕm"ă-dī" nă-mŏm'ĭ-ter) [" + dynamis, power, + metron, measure]

hemafecia (hē"mă-, hĕm-ă-fē'sē-ă) [" + L. faeces, refuse]

hemagglutination (hĕm"ă-gloo-tĭ-nā'shŭn) [" + L. agglutinare, to paste to]

hemagglutination inhibition

hemagglutinin (hĕm"ă-gloo'tĭ-nĭn)
  h., cold
  h., warm

hemagogue (hē"mă-, hĕm'ă-gŏg) [" + agogos, leading]

hemal (hē'măl)

hemal arch

hemal gland

hemal node

hemanalysis (hē"măn-, hĕm"ăn-ăl'ĭ-sĭs) [Gr. haima, blood + analyein, to dissolve]

hemangiectasis (hē"măn-, hĕm"ăn-jē-ĕk'tă-sĭs) [" + angeion, vessel, + ektasis, dilatation]

hemangioblast (hē-măn'jē-ō-blăst) [" + " + blastos, germ]

hemangioblastoma (hē-măn"jē-ō-blăs-tō'mă) [" + " + " + oma, tumor]

hemangioendothelioblastoma (hē-măn"jē-ō-ĕn"dō-thē"lē-ō-blăs-tō'mă) [" + " + " + endon, within, + thele, nipple, + blastos, germ, + oma, tumor]

hemangioendothelioma (hē"măn-jē-ō-ĕn"dō-thē-lē-ō'mă) [" + " + " + " + oma, tumor]

hemangiofibroma (hē-măn"jē-ō-fĭ-brō'mă) [" + " + L. fibra, fiber, + Gr. oma, tumor]

hemangioma (hē-măn"jē-ō'mă) [" + angeion, vessel, + oma, tumor]

hemangiomatosis (hē-măn"jē-ō-mă-tō'sĭs) [" + " + " + osis, condition]

hemangiopericytoma (hē-măn"jē-ō-pĕr"ē-sī-tō'mă)

hemangiosarcoma (hē-măn"jē-ō-săr-kō'mă) [" + " + sarkos, flesh, + oma, tumor]

hemaphein (hĕm"ă-fē'ĭn) [" + phaios, dusky, gray]

hemapoiesis (hĕm"ă-poy-ē'sĭs) [" + poiesis, formation]

hemapoietic (hĕm-ă-poy-ĕt'ĭk) [" + poiein, to form]

hemapophysis (hĕm-ă-pŏf'ĭ-sĭs) [" + apo, from, + physis, growth]

hemarthros, hemarthrosis (hĕm-ăr'thrōs, hĕm-ăr-thrō'sĭs) [" + arthron, joint]

hematapostema (hĕm"ăt-ă-pŏs-tē'mă) [Gr. haimatos, blood, + apostema, abscess]

hematein (hĕm"ă-tē'ĭn)

hematemesis (hĕm-ăt-ĕm'ĕ-sĭs) [" + emesis, vomiting]

hematencephalon (hĕm"ăt-ĕn-sĕf'ă-lŏn) [" + enkephalos, brain]

hematherapy (hĕm″ă-thĕr′ă-pē) [Gr. *haima*, blood, + *therapeia*, treatment]

hemathermal (hĕm″ă-, hē″mă-thĕr′măl) [" + *therme*, heat]

hemathermous (hĕm″ă-thĕr′mŭs)

hemathidrosis, hematidrosis (hē-măt″hĭ-drō′sĭs) [Gr. *haimatos*, blood, + *hidros*, sweat, + *osis*, condition]

hematic (hē-măt′ĭk)

hematimeter (hĕm-ă-tĭm′ĕ -tĕr) [" + *metron*, measure]

hematin (hĕm′ă-tĭn)

hematinemia (hē-mă-, hĕm-ă-tĭn-ē′mē-ă)

hematinic (hē-mă-, hĕm-ă-tĭn′ĭk) [Gr. *haima*, blood]

hematinuria (hē″mă-tĭn-ū′rē-ă)

hemato- (hē′mă-tō, hĕm′ă-tō) [Gr. *haimatos*, blood]

hematobilia (hĕm″ă-tō-bĭl′ē-ă) [" + L. *bilis*, bile]

hematobium (hē′mă-, hĕm′ă-tō′bē-ŭm) [" + *bios*, life]

hematoblast (hē′mă-, hĕm′ă-tō-blăst) [" + *blastos*, germ]

hematocele (hē′mă-, hĕm′ă-tō-sēl) [" + *kele*, tumor, swelling]

   h., parametric
   h., pudendal

hematocelia (hĕm″ă-tō-sē′lē-ă) [" + *koilia*, cavity, belly]

hematocephalus (hē′mă-, hĕm″ă-tō-sĕf′ă-lŭs) [" + *kephale*, head]

hematochezia (hĕm″ă-tō-kē′zē-ă) [" + *chezein*, to go to stool]

hematochromatosis (hĕm″ă-tō-krō″mă-tō′sĭs) [" + *chroma*, color, + *osis*, condition]

hematochyluria (hē′mă-, hĕm″ă-tō-kī-lū′rē-ă) [" + *chylos*, juice, + *ouron*, urine]

hematocolpometra (hē″mă-, hĕm″ă-tō-kŏl″pō-mē′tră) [" + *kolpos*, vagina, + *metra*, uterus]

hematocolpos (hē′mă-, hĕm″ă-tō-kŏl′pŏs)

hematocrit (hē-măt′ō-krĭt) [" + *krinein*, to separate]

hematocyst (hē′mă-, hĕm′ă-tō-sĭst) [Gr. *haimatos*, blood, + *kystis*, a bladder]

hematocyte (hē′mă-, hĕm′ă-tō-sīt) [" + *kytos*, cell]

hematocytoblast (hĕm″ă-tō-sī′tō-blăst) [" + " + *blastos*, germ]

hematocytolysis (hē″mă-, hĕm″ă-tō-sī-tŏl′ĭ-sĭs) [" + " + *lysis*, dissolution]

hematocytometer (hē″mă-, hĕm″ă-tō-sī-tŏm′ĕ-ter) [" + " + *metron*, measure]

hematocytozoon (hē″mă-, hĕm″ă-tō-sī-tō-zō′ŏn) [" + " + *zoon*, animal]

hematocyturia (hē″mă-, hĕm″ă-tō-sī-tū′rē-ă) [" + " + *ouron*, urine]

hematogenesis (hē″mă-, hĕm″ă-tō-jĕn′ĕ-sĭs) [" + *genesis*, generation, birth]

hematogenic, hematogenous (hē″mă-, hĕm″ă-tō-jĕn′ĭk, -tŏj′ĕ-nŭs) [" + *gennan*, to produce]

hematohidrosis (hē″mă-, hĕm″ă-tō-hī-drō′sĭs) [" + *hidros*, sweat, + *osis*, condition]

hematoid (hē′mă-, hĕm′ă-toyd) [" + *eidos*, form, shape]

hematoidin (hē′mă-, hĕm-ă-toy′dĭn)

hematokolpos

hematologist (hē″mă-, hĕm″ă-tŏl′ō-jĭst) [" + *logos*, word, reason]

hematology (hē″mă-, hĕm″ă-tŏl′ō-jē)

hematolymphangioma (hē″mă-, hĕm″ă-tō-lĭmf-ăn″jē-ō′mă) [" + L. *lympha*, lymph, + Gr. *angeion*, vessel, + *oma*, tumor]

hematolysis (hē″mă-, hĕm-ă-tŏl′ĭ-sĭs) [" + *lysis*, dissolution]

hematolytic (hĕm-ă-tō-lĭt′ĭk)

hematoma (hē″mă-, hĕm-ă-tō′mă) [Gr. *haimatos*, blood, + *oma*, tumor]

   h. auris
   h., epidural
   h., intracerebral
   h., pelvic

h., subarachnoid
h., subdural
h., vulvar

hematomediastinum (hē"mă-, hĕm"ă-tō-mē"dē-ă-stī'nŭm) [" + L. *mediastinus*, in the middle]

hematometer (hē-mă-tŏm'ĕ-tĕr) [" + *metron*, measure]

hematometra (hē"mă-, hĕm"ă-tō-mē'trä) [" + *metra*, uterus]

hematometry (hĕm"ă-tŏm'ĕ-trē) [" + *metron*, measure]

hematomphalocele (hē"mă-, hĕm"ăt-ŏm-făl'ō-sēl) [" + *omphalos*, navel, + *kele*, tumor, swelling]

hematomyelia (hē"mă-, hĕm"ă-tō-mī-ē'lē-ă) [" + *myelos*, marrow]

hematomyelitis (hē"mă-, hĕm"ă-tō-mī"ĕl-ī'tĭs) [" + " + *itis*, inflammation]

hematomyelopore (hē"măt-, hĕm"ăt-ō-mī'ĕl-ō-por) [" + " + *poros*, passage]

hematonephrosis (hē"mă-, hĕm"ă-tō-nĕ-frō'sĭs) [" + *nephros*, kidney, + *osis*, condition]

hematopathology [" + *pathos*, disease, suffering, + *logos*, word, reason]

hematopericardium (hē"mă-, hĕm"ă-tō-pĕr"ĭ-kăr'dē-ŭm) [" + *peri*, around, + *kardia*, heart]

hematoperitoneum (hē"mă-, hĕm"ă-tō-pĕr"ĭ-tō-nē'ŭm) [" + *peritonaion*, stretched around or over]

hematopexin (hĕm"ă-tō-pĕk'sĭn) [" + *pexis*, fixation]

hematophage (hĕm'ă-tō-fāj) [" + *phagein*, to eat]

hematophagia (hĕm"ă-tō-fā'jē-ă)

hematophagous (hĕm-ă-tŏf'ă-gŭs)

hematophilia (hĕm"ă-tō-fĭl"ē-ă) [" + *philein*, to love]

hematophobia (hē"mă-, hĕm"ă-tō-fō'bē-ă) [" + *phobos*, fear]

hematophyte (hē'mă-, hĕm'ă-tō-fīt) [" + *phyton*, plant]

hematoplastic [" + *plassein*, to form]

hematopoiesis (hē"mă-, hĕm"ă-tō-poy-ē'sĭs) [Gr. *haimatos*, blood, + *poiesis*, formation]
h., extramedullary

hematopoietic (hē"mă-, hĕm"ă-tō-poy-ĕt'ĭk)

hematopoietic system

hematoporphyrin (hē"mă-, hĕm"ă-tō-por'fĭ-rĭn) [" + *porphyra*, purple]

hematoporphyrinuria (hē"mă-, hĕm"ă-tō-por"fĭ-rĭn-ū'rē-ă)[" + " + *ouron*, urine]

hematorrhachis (hĕm-ă-tor'ă-kĭs) [" + *rhachis*, spine]

hematorrhea (hĕm"ă-tō-rē'ă) [" + *rhein*, to flow]

hematosalpinx (hē"mă-, hĕm"ă-tō-săl'pĭnks) [" + *salpinx*, tube]

hematoscheocele (hĕm-ă-tŏs'kē-ō-sēl) [" + *oscheon*, scrotum, + *kele*, tumor, swelling]

hematoscope (hē'mă-, hĕm'ă-tō-skōp) [" + *skopein*, to examine]

hematoscopy (hē"mă-, hĕm-ă-tŏs'kō-pē)

hematose (hē'mă-, hĕm'ă-tōs) [" + *osis*, condition]

hematosepsis (hĕm"ă-tō-sĕp'sĭs) [" + *sepsis*, decay]

hematospectroscope (hĕm"ă-tō-spĕk'trō-skōp) [" + L. *spectrum*, image, + Gr. *skopein*, to examine]

hematospectroscopy (hĕm"ă-tō-spĕk-trŏs'kō-pē)

hematospermatocele (hĕm"ă-tō-spĕr-măt'ō-sēl) [" + *sperma*, seed, + *kele*, tumor, swelling]

hematospermia (hĕm"ă-tō-spĕr'mē-ă)
h. spuria
h. vera

hematostatic (hĕm"ă-tō-stăt'ĭk) [Gr. *haimatos*, blood, + *stasis*, standing still]

hermatosteon (hĕm-ă-tŏs'tē-ŏn) [" + *osteon*, bone]

hematothermal (hĕm"ă-tō-thĕr'măl)

["   +   *therme*, heat]

hematothorax   (hĕm″ă-tō-thō′răks)
["   +   *thorax*, chest]

hematotoxic (hĕm″ă-tō-tŏk′sĭk) ["   +   *toxikon*, poison]

hematotrachelos   (hĕm″ă-tō-tră-kē′lōs) ["   +   *trachelos*, neck]

hematotropic   (hĕm″ă-tō-trŏp′ĭk) ["   +   *tropos*, a turning]

hematotympanum   (hĕm″ă-tō-tĭm′păn-ŭm) ["   +   *tympanon*, drum]

hematoxylin (hĕm″ă-tŏk′sĭ-lĭn)

hematozoon   (hē″mă-,   hĕm″ă-tō-zō′ŏn) ["   +   *zoon*, animal]

hematozymosis (hē″mă-, hĕm″ă-tō-zĭ-mō′sĭs) ["   +   *zymosis*, fermentation]

hematuria   (hē″mă-,   hĕm″ă-tū′rē-ă) ["   +   *ouron*, urine]
   h., renal
   h., urethral
   h., vesical

heme (hēm)

hemeralopia (hĕm″ĕr-ăl-ō′pē-ă) [Gr. *hemera*, day,   +   *alaos*, blind,   +   *ops*, eye]

hemi- (hĕm′ē) [Gr.]

hemiacephalus   (hĕm″ē-ă-sĕf′ă-lŭs) ["   +   *a-*, not,   +   *kephale*, head]

hemiachromatopsia   (hĕm″ē-ă-krō-mă-tŏp′sē-ă) ["   +   "   +   *chroma*, color,   +   *opsis*, sight, appearance, vision]

hemiageusia   (hĕm″ē-ă-gū′zē-ă) ["   +   "   +   *geusis*, taste]

hemialbumin (hĕm″ē-ăl-bū′mĭn) ["   +   L. *albumen*, white of egg]

hemialbumose (hĕm″ē-ăl′bū-mōs)

hemialbumosuria (hĕm″ē-ăl-bū″mō-sū′rē-ă) ["   +   "   +   Gr. *ouron*, urine]

hemialgia   (hĕm-ē-ăl′jē-ă) ["   +   *algos*, pain]

hemiamaurosis   (hĕm″ē-ăm″ŏ-rō′sĭs) ["   +   *amaurosis*, darkness]

hemiamblyopia   (hĕm″ē-ăm″blē-ō′pē-ă) ["   +   *amblys*, dim,   +   *ops*, sight]

hemiamyosthenia (hĕm″ē-ă″mī-ŏs-thē′nē-ă) [Gr. *hemi-*, half,   +   *a-*, not,   +   *mys*, muscle,   +   *sthenos*, strength]

hemianacusia (hĕm″ē-ăn″ă-kū′zē-ă) ["   +   *an-*, not,   +   *akousis*, hearing]

hemianalgesia (hĕm″ē-ăn-ăl-jē′zē-ă) ["   +   "   +   *algos*, pain]

hemianencephaly   (hĕm″ē-ăn″ĕn-sĕf′ă-lē) ["   +   *an-*, not,   +   *enkephalos*, brain]

hemianesthesia   (hĕm″ē-ăn-ĕs-thē′zē-ă) ["   +   "   +   *aisthesis*, feeling, perception]

hemianopia, hemianopsia (hĕm″ē-ă-nŏ′pē-ă , -nŏp′sē-ă) ["   +   *an-*, not,   +   *ops*, eye]
   h., altitudinal
   h., binasal
   h., bitemporal
   h., complete
   h., crossed
   h., heteronymous
   h., homonymous
   h., incomplete
   h., quadrant
   h., unilateral

hemianosmia   (hĕm″ē-ăn-ŏs′mē-ă) [Gr. *hemi-*, half,   +   *an-*, not,   +   *osme*, smell]

hemiapraxia   (hĕm″ē-ă-prăks′ē-ă) ["   +   *a-*, not,   +   *prassein*, to do]

hemiarthroplasty of the hip

hemiarthrosis   (hĕm″ē-ăr-thrō′sĭs) ["   +   *arthron*, joint,   +   *osis*, condition]

hemiasynergia   (hĕm″ē-ă″sĭn-ĕr′jē-ă) ["   +   *a-*, not,   +   *syn*, with,   +   *ergon*, work]

hemiataxia (hĕm″ē-ă-tăks′ē-ă) ["   +   *ataxia*, lack of order]

hemiathetosis   (hĕm″ē-ăth″ē-tō′sĭs) ["   +   *athetos*, without fixed position,   +   *osis*, condition]

hemiatrophy (hĕm-ē-ăt′rō-fē) ["   +

atrophia, atrophy]

hemiballism (hĕm-ē-băl'ĭzm) [" + *balismos*, jumping]

hemiblock (hĕm'ĭ-blŏk)

hemic (hē'mĭk, hĕm'ĭk) [Gr. *haima*, blood]

hemicanities (hĕm"ē-kăn-ĭsh'ĭ-ēz) [Gr. *hemi-*, half, + L. *canities*, gray hair]

hemicardia (hĕm-ē-kăr'dē-ă) [" + *kardia*, heart]

hemicastration (hĕm"ē-kăs-trā'shŭn) [" + L. *castrare*, to prune]

hemicellulose (hĕm-ē-sĕl'ū-lōs)

hemicentrum (hĕm-ē-sĕn'trŭm) [" + *kentron*, center]

hemicephalia (hĕm"ē-sĕ-fā'lē-ă) [" + *kephale*, head]

hemicephalus (hĕm"ē-sĕf'ă-lus)

hemicerebrum (hĕm"ē-sĕr'ĕ-brŭm) [" + L. *cerebrum*, brain]

hemichorea (hĕm-ē-kō-rē'ă) [" + *choreia*, dance]

hemichromatopsia (hĕm"ē-krō-mă-tŏp'sē-ă) [" + *chroma*, color, + *opsis*, sight, appearance, vision]

hemicolectomy (hĕm"ē-kō-lĕk'tō-mē) [" + *kolon*, colon, + *ektome*, excision]

hemicorporectomy (hĕm"ē-kor"pō-rĕk'tō-mē) [" + L. *corpus*, body, + Gr. *ektome*, excision]

hemicrania (hĕm-ē-krā'nē-ă) [" + *kranion*, skull]

hemicraniectomy (hĕm"ē-krā-nē-ĕk'tō-mē) [" + " + *ektome*, excision]

hemicraniosis (hĕm"ē-krā-nē-ō'sĭs) [" + " + *osis*, condition]

hemidesmosome

hemidiaphoresis (hĕm"ē-dī'ă-for-ē'sĭs) [" + *dia*, through, + *pherein*, to carry]

hemidiaphragm (hĕm"ē-dī'ă-frăm) [" + " + *phragma*, wall]

hemidrosis (hĕm"ĭ-drō'sĭs) [" + *hidrosis*, sweating; Gr. *haima*, blood, + *hidrosis*, sweating]

hemidysergia (hĕm"ē-dĭs-ĕr'jē-ă) [Gr.

hemi-, half, + *dys*, bad, difficult, painful, disordered, + *ergon*, work]

hemidysesthesia (hĕm"ē-dĭs-ĕs-thē'zē-ă) [" + " + *aisthesis*, feeling, perception]

hemidystrophy (hĕm"ē-dis'trō-fē) [" + " + *trophe*, nourishment]

hemiectromelia (hĕm"ē-ĕk-trō-mē'lē-ă) [" + *ektro*, abortion, + *melos*, limb]

hemiepilepsy (hĕm"ē-ĕp'ĭ-lĕp-sē) [" + *epilepsia*, to seize]

hemifacial (hĕm"ē-fā'shăl) [" + L. *facies*, face]

hemigastrectomy (hĕm"ē-găs-trĕk'tō-mē) [" + *gaster*, belly, + *ektome*, excision]

hemigeusia (hĕm-ē-gū'sē-ă) [" + *geusis*, taste]

hemiglossal (hĕm"ē-glŏs'săl) [" + *glossa*, tongue]

hemiglossectomy (hĕm"ē-glŏs-sĕk'tō-mē) [" + " + *ektome*, excision]

hemiglossitis [" + " + *itis*, inflammation]

hemignathia (hĕm"ē-năth'ē-ă) [" + *gnathos*, jaw]

hemihepatectomy (hĕm"ē-hĕp'ă-tĕk'tō-mē) [" + *hepatos*, liver, + *ektome*, excision]

hemihidrosis (hĕm"ē-hī-drō'sĭs) [" + *hidros*, sweat, + *osis*, condition]

hemihypalgesia (hĕm"ē-hī"păl-jē'zē-ă) [" + *hypo*, under, beneath, below, + *algesis*, sense of pain]

hemihyperesthesia (hĕm"ē-hī-pĕr-ĕs-thē'zē-ă) [" + *hyper*, over, above, excessive, + *aisthesis*, feeling, perception]

hemihyperidrosis (hĕm"ē-hī-pĕr-ĭ-drō'sĭs) [" + " + *hydrosis*, sweating]

hemihyperplasia (hĕm"ē-hī"pĕr-plā'zē-ă) [" + " + *plassein*, to form]

hemihypertonia (hĕm"ē-hī"pĕr-tō'nē-ă) [" + " + *tonos*, act of stretching, tension, tone]

hemihypertrophy (hĕm″ē-hī-pĕr′trō-fē) [" + " + *trophe*, nourishment]

hemihypesthesia, hemihypoesthesia (hĕm″ē-hī″pĕs-thē′zē-ă, -pō-ĕs-thē′zē-a) [Gr. *hemi*-, half, + *hypo*, under, beneath, below, + *aisthesis*, feeling, perception]

hemihypoplasia (hĕm″ē-hī″pō-plā′zē-ă) [" + " + *plassein*, to form]

hemihypotonia (hĕm″ē-hī-pō-tō′nē-ă) [" + " + *tonos*, act of stretching, tension, tone]

hemikaryon (hĕm″ē-kăr′ē-ŏn) [" + *karyon*, nucleus]

hemilaminectomy (hĕm″ē-lăm″ĭ-nĕk′tō-mē) [" + L. *lamina*, thin plate, + Gr. *ektome*, excision]

hemilaryngectomy (hĕm″ē-lăr″in-jĕk′tō-mē) [" + *larynx*, larynx, + *ektome*, excision]

hemilateral [" + L. *latus*, side]

hemilesion (hĕm″ē-lē′zhŭn) [" + L. *laesio*, a wound]

hemilingual (hĕm″ē-lĭng′gwăl) [" + L. *lingua*, tongue]

hemimacroglossia (hĕm″ē-măk″rō-glŏs′ē-ă) [" + *makros*, large, + *glossa*, tongue]

hemimandibulectomy (hĕm″ē-măn-dĭb-ū-lĕk′tō-mē) [" + L. *mandibula*, lower jawbone, + Gr. *ektome*, excision]

hemimelus (hĕm″ĭ-mē′lŭs) [" + *melos*, limb]

hemin (hē′mĭn) [Gr. *haima*, blood]

heminephrectomy (hĕm″ē-nĕ-frĕk′tō-mē) [Gr. *hemi*-, half, + *nephros*, kidney, + *ektome*, excision]

hemineurasthenia (hĕm″ē-nū-răs-thē′nē-ă) [" + *neuron*, nerve, + *astheneia*, weakness]

hemiopalgia (hĕm″ē-ŏp-ăl′jē-ă) [" + *ops*, eye, + *algos*, pain]

hemiopia (hĕm-ē-ō′pē-ă) [" + *ops*, eye]

hemiopic (hĕm-ē-ŏp′ĭk) [" + *ops*, eye]

hemipagus (hĕm-ĭp′ă-gŭs) [" + *pagos*, a thing fixed]

hemiparalysis [" + *paralyein*, to loosen, disable]

hemiparaplegia (hĕm″ē-păr-ă-plē′jē-ă) [" + " + *plege*, stroke]

hemiparesis (hĕm″ē-păr′ē-sĭs, hĕm-ē-păr-ē′sĭs) [" + *parienai*, let fall]

hemiparesthesia (hĕm″ē-păr-ĕs-thē′zē-ă) [" + *para*, alongside, past, beyond, + *aisthesis*, feeling, perception]

hemipelvectomy (hĕm″ē-pĕl″vĕk′tō-mē) [" + L. *pelvis*, basin, + Gr. *ektome*, excision]

hemiplegia (hĕm-ē-plē′jē-ă) [" + *plege*, a stroke]
   h., capsular
   h., cerebral
   h., facial
   h., spastic
   h., spinal

hemiplegic (hĕm-ē-plē′ĭk)

Hemiptera (hĕm-ĭp′tĕr-ă) [Gr. *hemi*-, half, + *pteron*, wing]

hemipyocyanin (hĕm″ē-pī″ō-sī′ă-nĭn)

hemirachischisis (hĕm″ē-ră-kĭs′kĭ-sĭs) [" + *rhachis*, spine, + *schisis*, cleavage]

hemisacralization (hĕm″ē-sā″krăl-ī-zā′shŭn)

hemisection (hĕm″ē-sĕk′shŭn) [" + L. *sectio*, a cutting]

hemisomus (hĕm″ē-sō′mŭs) [" + *soma*, body]

hemispasm (hĕm′ē-spăzm) [" + *spasmos*, a convulsion]

hemisphere (hĕm′ĭ-sfēr) [" + *sphaira*, sphere]
   h., dominant

hemispheric specialization

hemistrumectomy (hĕm″ē-stroo-mĕk′tō-mē) [" + L. *struma*, goiter, + Gr. *ektome*, excision]

hemisyndrome (hĕm″ē-sĭn′drōm)
[″ + *syndrome*, a running with]
hemithermoanesthesia (hĕm″ē-
thĕr″mō-ăn″ĕs-thē′zē-ă) [Gr. *hemi-*,
half, + *therme*, heat, + *an-*,
not, + *aisthesis*, feeling, percep-
tion]
hemithorax (hĕm″ē-thō′răks) [″ +
thorax, chest]
hemithyroidectomy (hĕm″ē-
thī″royd-ĕk′tō-mē) [″ + *thyreos*,
shield, + *eidos*, form, shape, +
ektome, excision]
hemitomias (hĕm″ĭ-tō′mē-ăs) [Gr. *hemitomias*, half a eunuch]
hemitremor (hĕm″ē-trĕm′or)
hemivertebra (hĕm″ē-vĕr′tĕ-bră)
hemizygosity (hĕm″ē-zī-gŏs′ĭ-tē)
[″ + *zygotos*, yoked]
hemlock [AS. *hemleac*]
hemlock poisoning
hemoagglutination (hē″mō-ă-
gloo″tĭ-nā′shŭn) [Gr. *haima*, blood,
+ L. *agglutinans*, gluing]
hemoagglutinin (hē″mō-ă-gloo′tĭ-nĭn)
hemobilia (hē″mō-bĭl′ē-ă)
hemobilinuria (hē″mō-bĭl-ĭn-ū′rē-ă)
[″ + L. *bilis*, bile, + Gr. *ouron*,
urine]
hemoblast (hē′mō-blăst) [″ +
blastos, germ]
hemochorial (hē″mō-kor′ē-ăl) [″ +
chorion, envelope]
hemochromatosis (hē″mō-krō″mă-
tō′sĭs) [″ + *chroma*, color, +
osis, condition]
    h., exogenous
hemochrome (hē′mō-krōm)
hemochromogen (hē″mō-krō′mō-jĕn)
[″ + *chroma*, color, + *gennan*, to produce]
hemochromometer (hē″mō-krō-
mŏm′ē-tĕr) [″ + ″ + *metron*,
measure]
hemochromoprotein (hē″mō-
krō″mō-prō′tē-ĭn)
hemoclasia (hē″mō-klā′sē-ă) [″ +
klasis, a breaking]

hemoclasis (hē-mŏk′lă-sĭs)
hemoclastic (hē″mō-klăs′tĭk)
hemoconcentration
hemoconia (hē″mō-kō′nē-ă) [Gr.
haima, blood, + *konis*, dust]
hemoconiosis (hē″mō-kō″nē-ō′sĭs)
[″ + ″ + *osis*, condition]
hemocryoscopy (hē″mō-krī-ŏs′kō-pē)
[″ + *kryos*, cold, + *skopein*, to
examine]
hemocrystallin (hē″mō-krĭs′tăl-lĭn)
hemocuprein (hē″mō-kū′prē-ĭn)
hemocyanin (hē″mō-sī′ă-nĭn) [″ +
kyanos, blue]
hemocyte (hē′mō-sīt) [″ + *kytos*,
cell]
hemocytoblast (hē″mō-sī′tō-blăst)
[″ + ″ + *blastos*, germ]
hemocytoblastoma (hē″mō-sī″tō-
blăs-tō′mă) [″ + ″ + ″ +
oma, tumor]
hemocytogenesis (hē″mō-sī″tō-jĕn′ĕ-
sĭs) [″ + *kytos*, cell, + *genesis*,
generation, birth]
hemocytology (hē″mō-sī-tŏl′ō-jē)
[″ + ″ + *logos*, word, reason]
hemocytolysis (hē″mō-sī-tŏl′ĭ-sĭs)
[″ + ″ + *lysis*, dissolution]
hemocytometer (hē″mō-sī-tŏm′ē-tĕr)
[″ + ″ + *metron*, measure]
hemocytophagia
hemocytopoiesis (hē″mō-sī″tō-poy-
ē′sĭs) [″ + *kytos*, cell +
poiesis, formation]
hemocytotripsis (hē″mō-sī″tō-trĭp′sĭs)
[″ + ″ + *tribein*, to rub]
hemocytozoon (hē″mō-sī″tō-zō′ŏn)
[″ + ″ + *zoon*, animal]
hemodiagnosis (hē″mō-dī″ăg-nō′sĭs)
[″ + *dia*, through, + *gnosis*,
knowledge]
hemodialysis (hē″mō-, hĕm″ō-dī-ăl′ĭ-
sĭs) [″ + ″ + *lysis*, dissolution]
hemodialyzer (hē″mō-dī′ă-līz″ĕr)
hemodiastase (hē″mō-dī′ăs-tās)
[″ + *diastasis*, separation]
hemodilution (hē″mō-dī-lū′shŭn)
hemodynamics (hē″mō-dī-năm′ĭks)

[Gr. *haima*, blood, + *dynamis*, power]

hemodynamometer (hē"mō-dī"nă-mŏm'ĕ-ter) [" + " + *metron*, measure]

hemoendothelial (hē"mō-ĕn-dō-thē'lē-ăl)

Hemofil

hemofiltration (hē"mō-fĭl-trā'shŭn)

hemoflagellate (hē"mō-flăj'ĕ-lāt") [" + L. *flagellum*, whip]

hemofuscin (hē"mō-fū'sĭn) [" + L. *fuscus*, brown]

hemogenesis (hē"mō-jĕn'ĕ-sĭs) [" + *genesis*, generation, birth]

hemogenic (hē"mō-jĕn'ĭk) [" + *gennan*, to produce]

hemoglobin (hē"mō-, hĕm"ō-glō'bĭn) [" + L. *globus*, globe]
  h. A_{1c}
  h., fetal
  h., glycosylated

hemoglobinemia (hē"mō-glō-bĭn-ē'mē-ă) [Gr. *haima*, blood, + L. *globus*, globe, + Gr. *haima*, blood]

hemoglobinocholia (hē"mō-glō"bĭn-ō-kō' lē-ă) [" + " + Gr. *chole*, bile]

hemoglobinolysis (hē"mō-glō-bĭn-ŏl'ĭ-sĭs) [" + " + Gr. *lysis*, dissolution]

hemoglobinometer (hē"mō-glō-bĭn-ŏm'ĕ-ter) [" + " + Gr. *metron*, measure]

hemoglobinopathies (hē"mō-glō"bĭ-nŏp'ă-thēz)

hemoglobinopepsia (hē"mō-glō"bĭn-ō-pĕp'sē-ă) [" + L. *globus*, globe, + Gr. *pepsis*, digestion]

hemoglobinophilic (hē"mō-glō-bĭn-ō-fĭl'ĭk) [" + " + Gr. *philein*, to love]

hemoglobinous (hē"mō-glō'bĭ-nŭs)

hemoglobinuria (hē"mō-glō-bĭn-ū'rē-ă) [" + L. *globus*, globe, + Gr. *ouron*, urine]
  h., cold
  h., epidemic

  h., intermittent
  h., malarial
  h., march
  h., paroxysmal
  h., toxic

hemoglobinuric (hē"mō-glō"bĭ-nū'rĭk)

hemogram [Gr. *haima*, blood, + *gramma*, letter, piece of writing]

hemoid (hē'moyd) [" + *eidos*, form, shape]

hemokinesis (hē"mō-kĭ-nē'sĭs) [" + *kinesis*, motion]

hemokonia (hē-mō-kō'nē-ă) [" + *konis*, dust]

hemokoniosis (hē"mō-kō-nē-ō'sĭs) [" + " + *osis*, condition]

hemolith (hē'mō-lĭth) [" + *lithos*, stone]

hemolymph (hē'mō-lĭmf") [" + L. *lympha*, lymph]

hemolymphangioma (hē"mō-lĭm-făn"jē-ō'mă)

hemolysate (hē-mŏl'ĭ-sāt)

hemolysin (hē-mŏl'ĭ-sĭn) [" + *lysis*, dissolution]

hemolysis (hē-mŏl'ĭ-sĭs) [" + *lysis*, dissolution]

hemolytic (hē"mō-lĭt'ĭk)

hemolytic anemia

hemolytic disease of the newborn

hemolytic jaundice

hemolytic uremic syndrome

hemolytopoietic (hē-mŏl"ĭ-tō-poy-ĕt'ĭk) [Gr. *haima*, blood, + *lysis*, dissolution, + *poiein*, to form]

hemolyze (hē'mō-līz)

hemomediastinum (hē"mō-mē"dē-ă-stī'nŭm) [" + L. *mediastinus*, in the middle]

hemometra (hē"mō-mē'tră) [" + *metra*, uterus]

hemonephrosis (hē"mō-nĕ-frō'sĭs) [" + *nephros*, kidney, + *osis*, condition]

hemopathic (hē"mō-păth'ĭk) [" + *pathos*, disease, suffering]

hemopathology (hē"mō-pă-thŏl'ō-jē) [" + " + *logos*, word, reason]

hemopathy (hē-mŏp'ă-thē)

hemoperfusion

hemopericardium (hē″mō-pĕr″ĭ-kăr′dē-ŭm) [″ + *peri*, around, + *kardia*, heart]

hemoperitoneum (hē″mō-pĕr″ĭ-tō-nē′ŭm) [″ + *peritonaion*, stretched around or over]

hemopexin (hē″mō-pĕks′ĭn) [″ + *pexis*, fixation]

hemophage (hē′mō-fāj) [″ + *phagein*, to eat]

hemophagocyte (hē″mō-făg′ō-sīt) [″ + ″ + *kytos*, cell]

hemophagocytosis (hē″mō-făg″ō-sī-tō′sĭs) [″ + ″ + ″ + *osis*, condition]

hemophil (hē′mō-fĭl) [″ + *philein*, to love]

hemophilia (hē″mō-, hĕm″ō-fĭl′ē-ă) [″ + *philein*, to love]
   h., vascular

hemophilia A

hemophilia B

hemophiliac (hē″mō-fĭl′ē-ăk)

hemophilic (hē″mō-fĭl′ĭk)

Hemophilus (hē-mŏf′ĭl-ŭs) [″ + *philein*, to love]
   H. aegyptius
   H. ducreyi
   H. influenzae
   H. pertussis
   H. vaginalis

hemophobia (hē″mō-fō′bē-ă) [Gr. *haima*, blood, + *phobos*, fear]

hemophoric (hē″mō-for′ĭk) [″ + *phoros*, bearing]

hemophthalmia, hemophthalmus (hē″mŏf-thăl′mē-ă, hē″mŏf-thăl′mŭs) [″ + *ophthalmos*, eye]

hemopleura (hē″mō-ploo′ră)

hemopneumopericardium (hē″mō-nū″mō-pĕr″ĭ-kăr′dē-ŭm) [″ + *pneuma*, air, + *peri*, around, + *kardia*, heart]

hemopneumothorax (hē″mō-nū-mō-thō′răks) [″ + ″ + *thorax*, chest]

hemopoiesis (hē″mō-poy-ē′sĭs) [″ + *poiesis*, formation]

hemoprecipitin (hē″mō-prē-sĭp′ĭ-tĭn)

hemoprotein (hē″mō-prō′tē-ĭn)

hemopsonin (hē″mŏp-sō′nĭn) [″ + *opsonein*, to purchase victuals]

hemoptysis (hē-mŏp′tĭ-sĭs) [″ + *ptyein*, to spit]
   h., endemic
   h., parasitic

hemorrhage (hĕm′ĕ-rĭj) [″ + *rhegnynai*, to burst forth]
   h., accidental
   h., antepartum
   h., arterial
   h., capillary
   h., carotid artery
   h., cerebral
   h., concealed
   h., fibrinolytic
   h., internal
   h., intracranial
   h., lung
   h. of knee
   h., petechial
   h., postmenopausal
   h., postpartum
   h., primary
   h., secondary
   h., stomach
   h., thigh
   h., typhoid
   h., unavoidable
   h., uterine
   h., venous
   h., vicarious

hemorrhagenic (hĕm″ō-ră-jĕn′ĭk) [″ + *rhegnynai*, to burst forth, + *gennan*, to form]

hemorrhagic (hĕm-ō-răj′ĭk)

hemorrhagic disease of the newborn

hemorrhagic fevers

hemorrhagic nephrosonephritis

hemorrhagiparous (hĕm″ō-răj-ĭp′ă-rŭs) [″ + *rhegnynai*, to burst forth, + L. *parere*, to beget, produce]

hemorrhoid (hĕm′ō-royd) [Gr. *haimorrhois*]
   h., external
   h., internal

h., prolapsed
h., strangulated
hemorrhoidal (hĕm-ō-roy'dăl)
hemorrhoidectomy (hĕm"ō-royd-ĕk'tō-mē) [Gr. *haimorrhois*, vein liable to bleed, + *ektome*, excision]
hemosalpinx (hē"mō-săl'pĭnks) [Gr. *haima*, blood, + *salpinx*, tube]
hemosiderin (hē"mō-sĭd'ĕr-ĭn) [" + *sideros*, iron]
hemosiderosis (hē"mō-sĭd-ĕr-ō'sĭs) [" + " + *osis*, condition]
hemospasia (hē"mō-spā'zē-ă) [" + *spaein*, to draw]
hemospermia (hē"mō-spĕr'mē-ă) [" + *sperma*, seed]
Hemosporida (hē-mō-spor-ĭ'dē-ă) [" + *sporos*, seed]
hemostasis, hemostasia (hē-mŏs'tă-sĭs, hē"mō-stā'zē-ă) [" + *stasis*, standing still]
hemostat (hē'mō-stăt) [" + *statikos*, standing]
hemostatic (hē"mō-stăt'ĭk)
hemostyptic (hē-mō-stĭp'tĭk) [" + *styptikos*, astringent]
hemotherapeutics (hē"mō-thĕr"ă-pū'tĭks) [" + *therapeutike*, medical practice]
hemotherapy (hē"mō-thĕr'ă-pē) [" + *therapeia*, treatment]
hemothorax (hē"mō-thō'răks) [" + *thorax*, chest]
hemothymia (hē"mō-thī'mē-ă) [" + *thymos*, mind, spirit]
hemotoxin (hē"mō-tŏks'ĭn) [" + *toxikon*, poison]
hemotrophe (hē'mō-trōf)]" + *trophe*, nourishment]
hemotrophic (hē-mō-trōf'ĭk) [" + *trophe*, nourishment]
hemotrophic nutrition
hemotropic (hē-mō-trŏp'ĭk) [" + *tropos*, turning]
hemotympanum (hē"mō-tĭm'pă-nŭm) [" + *tympanon*, drum]
hemozoin (hē"mō-zō'ĭn)
hemozoon (hē"mō-zō'ŏn)

Henderson-Hasselbalch equation [L.J. Henderson, U.S. biochemist, 1878 – 1942; K. A. Hasselbalch, Danish physician, 1874 – 1962]
Henle, Friedrich G. J. (hĕn'lē) [Ger. anatomist, 1809 – 1885]
  H.'s ampulla
  H.'s fissure
  H.'s layer
  H.'s ligament
  H.'s loop
  H.'s membrane
  H.'s sheath
  H.'s tubules
Henoch-Schönlein purpura (hĕn'ōk-shăn'lĭn) [Edouard H. Henoch, Ger. pediatrician, 1820 – 1910; Johann L. Schönlein, Ger. physician, 1793 – 1864]
henry (hĕn'rē) [Joseph Henry, U.S. physicist, 1797 – 1878]
Henry's law (hĕn'rēz) [William Henry, Brit. chemist, 1774 – 1836]
Hensen's cells (hĕn'sĕns) [Victor Hensen, Ger. anatomist and physiologist, 1835 – 1924]
Hensen's disk
Hensen's stripe
hepar (hē'păr) [Gr. *hepatos*, liver]
heparinize (hĕp'ĕr-ĭ-nīz)
heparin lock flush solution
heparin sodium (hĕp'ă-rĭn)
hepatalgia (hĕp"ă-tăl'jē-ă) [Gr. *hepatos*, liver, + *algos*, pain]
hepatalgic (hĕp"ă-tăl'jĭk)
hepatatrophia (hĕp"ăt-ă-trō'fē-ă) [" + *atrophia*, atrophy]
hepatauxe (hĕp"ăt-awk'sē) [" + *auxe*, increase]
hepatectomize (hĕp"ă-tĕk'tō-mīz) [" + *ektome*, excision]
hepatectomy (hĕp"ă-tĕk'tō-mē) [" + *ektome*, excision]
hepatic (hē-păt'ĭk) [Gr. *hepatikos*]
hepatic amebiasis
hepatic coma
hepatic duct
hepatic encephalopathy

hepatic flexure
hepatic lobes
hepaticoduodenostomy (hĕ-păt″ĭ-kō-dū″ō-dĕ-nŏs′tō-mē) [″ + L. *duodeni*, duodenum, + Gr. *stoma*, mouth, opening]
hepaticoenterostomy (hĕ-păt″ĭ-kō-ĕn-tĕr-ŏs′tō-mē) [″ + *enteron*, intestine, + *stoma*, mouth, opening]
hepaticogastrostomy (hĕ-păt″ĭ-kō-găs-trŏs′tō-mē) [″ + *gaster*, stomach, + *stoma*, mouth, opening]
hepaticojejunostomy (hĕ-păt′ĭ-kō-jē″jū-nŏs′tō-mē) [″ + L. *jejunum*, empty, + Gr. *stoma*, mouth, opening]
hepaticolithotomy (hĕ-păt″ĭ-kō-lĭ-thŏt′ō-mē)
hepaticolithotripsy (hĕ-păt″ĭ-kō-lĭth′ō-trĭp-sē) [″ + *lithos*, stone, + *tripsis*, a rubbing, friction]
hepaticostomy (hĕ-păt″ĭ-kŏs′tō-mē) [″ + *stoma*, mouth, opening]
hepaticotomy (hĕ-păt″ĭ-kŏt′ō-mē) [″ + *tome*, a cutting, slice]
hepatic veins
hepatic zones
hepatitis (hĕp″ă-tī′tĭs) [″ + *itis*, inflammation]
　h. A
　h., acute anicteric
　h., acute viral
　h., amebic
　h. B
　h., chronic
　h., delta agent
　h., fulminant
　h., infectious
　h., non-A, non-B
　h., serum
　h., toxic or drug-induced
　h., viral
hepatitis-associated antigen
hepatitis B immune globulin
hepatitis B surface antigen
hepatitis B virus vaccine inactivated
hepatization (hĕp″ă-tĭ-zā′shŭn)
hepato- [Gr. *hepatikos*]

hepatoblastoma (hĕp″ă-tō-blăs-tō′mă) [″ + *blastos*, germ, + *oma*, tumor]
hepatocarcinogen
hepatocarcinoma (hĕp″ă-tō-kăr″sĭn-ō′mă) [″ + *karkinos*, crab, + *oma*, tumor]
hepatocele (hĕp′ă-tō-sēl) [″ + *kele*, tumor, swelling]
hepatocellular (hĕp″ă-tō-sĕl′ū-lăr)
hepatocholangiocystoduodenostomy (hĕp″ă-tō-kō-lăn″jē-ō-sĭs″tō-dū″ō-dĕ-nŏs′tō-mē) [″ + *chole*, bile, + *angeion*, vessel, + *kystis*, bladder, + L. *duodenum*, duodenum, + Gr. *stoma*, mouth, opening]
hepatocholangioduodenostomy (hĕp″ă-tō-kō-lăn″jē-ō-dū-ō-dĕ-nŏs′tō-mē) [″ + ″ + ″ + L. *duodenum*, duodenum, + Gr. *stoma*, mouth, opening]
hepatocholangioenterostomy (hĕp″ă-tō-kō-lăn″jē-ō-ĕn″tĕr-ŏs′tō-mē) [″ + ″ + ″ + *enteron*, intestine, + *stoma*, mouth, opening]
hepatocholangiogastrostomy (hĕp″ă-tō-kō-lăn″jē-ō-găs-trŏs′tō-mē) [″ + ″ + ″ + *gaster*, belly, + *stoma*, mouth, opening]
hepatocholangiostomy (hĕp″ă-tō-kō-lăn-jē-ŏs′tō-mē) [″ + ″ + ″ + *stoma*, mouth, opening]
hepatocholangitis (hĕp″ă-tō-kō-lăn-jī′tĭs) [″ + ″ + ″ + *itis*, inflammation]
hepatocirrhosis (hĕp″ă-tō-sĭ-rō′sĭs) [″ + *kirrhos*, tawny, + *osis*, condition]
hepatocolic (hĕp″ă-tō-kŏl′ĭk) [″ + *kolon*, colon]
hepatocuprein (hĕp″ă-tō-koo′prĭn)
hepatocystic (hĕp″ă-tō-sĭs′tĭk) [″ + *kystis*, bladder]
hepatocyte (hĕp′ă-tō-sīt)
hepatoduodenostomy (hĕp″ă-tō-dū″ō-dĕ-nŏs′tō-mē) [″ + L. *duode-*

num, duodenum, + Gr. *stoma,*
mouth, opening]
hepatodynia   (hĕp"ă-tō-dĭn'ē-ă)
[" + *odyne,* pain]
hepatoenteric   (hĕp"ă-tō-ĕn-tĕr'ĭk)
[" + *enteron,* intestine]
hepatogastric (hĕp"ă-tō-găs'trĭk) [Gr.
hepatikos, liver, + *gaster,* belly]
hepatogenic (hĕp"ă-tō-jĕn'ĭk) [" +
gennan, to produce]
hepatogenous (hĕp"ă-tŏj'ĕ-nŭs)
hepatogram (hĕp'ă-tō-grăm") [" +
gramma, letter, piece of writing]
hepatography   (hĕp"ă-tŏg'ră-fē)
[" + *graphein,* to write]
hepatohemia   (hĕp"ă-tō-hē'mē-ă)
[" + *haima,* blood]
hepatoid [" + *eidos,* form, shape]
hepatojugular (hĕp"ă-tō-jŭg'ū-lăr)
hepatojugular reflex
hepatolenticular   (hĕp"ă-tō-lĕn-tĭk'ū-
lăr) [" + L. *lenticula,* lentil, lens]
hepatolenticular degeneration
hepatolienography   (hĕp"ă-tō-lī"ĕ-
nŏg'ră-fē) [" + L. *lien,* spleen, +
Gr. *graphein,* to write]
hepatolienomegaly   (hĕp"ă-tō-lī"ĕ-
nō-mĕg'ă-lē) [" + " + *megas,*
large]
hepatolith   (hĕp'ă-tō-lĭth)   ["   +
lithos, stone]
hepatolithectomy (hĕp"ă-tō-lĭ-thĕk'-
tō-mē) [" + *lithos,* stone, +
ektome, excision]
hepatolithiasis (hĕp"ă-tō-lĭ-thī'ă-sĭs)
[" + " + *-iasis,* state or condition of]
hepatologist (hĕp"ă-tŏl'ō-jĭst) [" +
logos, word, reason]
hepatology (hĕp"ă-tŏl'ō-jē) [" +
logos, word, reason]
hepatolysin (hĕp"ă-tŏl'ĭ-sĭn) [" +
lysis, dissolution]
hepatolysis (hĕp"ă-tŏl'ĭ-sĭs)
hepatolytic (hĕp"ă-tō-lĭt'ĭk)
hepatoma   (hĕp"ă-tō'mă)   ["   +
oma, tumor]
hepatomalacia (hĕp"ă-tō-mă-lā'sē-ă)

[" + *malakia,* softening]
hepatomegaly (hĕp"ă-tō-mĕg'ă-lē)
[" + *megas,* large]
hepatomelanosis (hĕp"ă-tō-mĕl"ă-
nō'sĭs) [" + *melas,* black, +
osis, condition]
hepatomphalocele (hĕp"ă-tŏm'fă-lō-
sēl") [Gr. *hepatikos,* liver, + *omphalos,* navel, + *kele,* tumor,
swelling]
hepatonecrosis (hĕp"ă-tō-nĕ-krō'sĭs)
[" + *nekrosis,* state of death]
hepatonephric   (hĕp"ă-tō-nĕf'rĭk)
[" + *nephros,* kidney]
hepatonephritis (hĕp"ă-tō-nĕ-frī'tĭs)
[" + " + *itis,* inflammation]
hepatonephromegaly (hĕp"ă-tō-
nĕf"rō-mĕg'ă-lē) [" + " +
megas, large]
  h. glycogenica
hepatopathy (hĕp-ĕ-tŏp'ă-thē) [" +
pathos, disease, suffering]
hepatoperitonitis (hĕp"ă-tō-pĕr"ĭ-tō-
nī'tĭs) [" + *peritonaion,* stretched
around or over, + *itis,* inflamma-
tion]
hepatopexy (hĕp'ă-tō-pĕks"ē) [" +
pexis, fixation]
hepatophage (hĕp'ă-tō-fāj) [" +
phagein, to eat]
hepatopleural   (hĕp"ă-tō-ploo'răl)
[" + *pleura,* side]
hepatopneumonic (hĕp"ă-tō-nū-
mŏn'ĭk) [" + *pneumonikos,* of the
lungs]
hepatoportogram (hĕp"ă-tō-por'tō-
grăm)
hepatoptosia, hepatoptosis (hĕp"
ă-tŏp-tō'sē-ă, -tō'sĭs) [" + *ptosis,*
fall, falling]
hepatopulmonary (hĕp"ă-tō-pŭl'mō-
năr"ē) [" + L. *pulmo,* lung]
hepatorenal (hĕp"ă-tō-rē'năl) [" +
L. *renalis,* kidney]
hepatorrhaphy   (hĕp-ă-tor'ă-fē)
[" + *rhaphe,* seam]
hepatorrhexis   (hĕp"ă-tō-rĕks'-ĭs)
[" + *rhexis,* rupture]

hepatoscan (hĕp'ă-tō-skăn)

hepatoscopy [" + *skopein*, to examine]

hepatosis (hĕp"ă-tō'sĭs) [" + *osis*, condition]

hepatosplenitis (hĕp"ă-tō-splĕ-nī'tĭs) [" + *splen*, spleen, + *itis*, inflammation]

hepatosplenography (hĕp"ă-tō-splĕ-nŏg'ră-fē) [" + " + *graphein*, to write]

hepatosplenomegaly (hĕp"ă-tō-splē"nō-mĕg'ă-lē) [" + " + *megas*, large]

hepatosplenopathy (hĕp"ă-tō-splĕ-nŏp'ă-thē) [" + " + *pathos*, disease, suffering]

hepatostomy (hĕp"ă-tŏs'tō-mē) [" + *stoma*, mouth, opening]

hepatotherapy (hĕp"ă-tō-thĕr'ă-pē) [" + *therapeia*, treatment]

hepatotomy (hĕp"ă-tŏt'ō-mē) [" + *tome*, a cutting, slice]

hepatotoxemia (hĕp"ă-tō-tŏks-ē'mē-ă) [" + *toxikon*, poison, + *haima*, blood]

hepatotoxic

hepatotoxin (hĕp"ă-tō-tŏk'sĭn)

heptachromic (hĕp"tă-krō'mĭk) [Gr. *hepta*, seven, + *chroma*, color]

heptapeptide (hĕp'tă-pĕp'tĭd) [" + *peptein*, to digest]

heptaploidy (hĕp'tă-ploy"dē) [" + *ploos*, fold]

heptose (hĕp'tōs)

heptosuria (hĕp"tō-sū'rē-ă) [" + *ouron*, urine]

herb (ĕrb) [L. *herba*, grass]

herbivorous (hĕr-bĭv'ō-rŭs) [" + *vorare*, to eat]

herd [AS. *heord*]

hereditary (hĕ-rĕd'ĭ-tĕr-ē) [L. *hereditarius*, an heir]

heredity (hĕ-rĕd'ĭ-tē) [L. *hereditas*, heir]

heredo- [L. *hereditas*, heir]

heredoataxia (hĕr"ĕ-dō-ă-tăks'ē-ă) [" + Gr. *ataxia*, lack of order]

heredodegeneration (hĕr"ĕ-dō-dē-jĕn"ĕr-ā'shŭn)

heredofamilial (hĕr"ĕ-dō-fă-mĭl'ē-ăl)

heredoimmunity (hĕr"ĕ-dō-ĭ-mū'nĭ-tē)

Hering, Karl Ewald K. (hĕr'ĭng) [Ger. physiologist, 1834–1918]
   H.-Breuer reflex [Josef Breuer, Ger. physician, 1842–1925]
   H.'s theory

Hering's nerves [Heinrich Ewald Hering, Austrian physician, 1866–1948]

heritable

heritage

hermaphrodism (hĕr-măf'rō-dĭzm)

hermaphrodite (hĕr-măf'rō-dīt) [Gr. *Hermaphroditos*, son of Hermes and Aphrodite, who was man and woman combined]

hermaphroditism (hĕr-măf'rō-dīt-ĭzm)
   h., bilateral
   h., complex
   h., dimidiate
   h., false
   h., lateral
   h., spurious
   h., transverse
   h., true
   h., unilateral

hermetic (hĕr-mĕt'ĭk) [L. *hermeticus*]

hernia (hĕr'nē-ă) [L., rupture]
   h., abdominal
   h., acquired
   h., bladder
   h., cerebral
   h., Cloquet's
   h., complete
   h., concealed
   h., congenital
   h., crural
   h., cystic
   h., direct
   h., diverticular
   h., encysted
   h., epigastric
   h., fascial
   h., fatty
   h., femoral
   h., funicular

h., hiatal
h., Holthouse's
h., incarcerated
h., incisional
h., incomplete
h., indirect
h., inguinal
h., inguinocrural
h., internal
h., interstitial
h., irreducible
h., labial
h., lateral
h., lumbar
h., medial
h., mesocolic
h., nuckian
h., oblique
h., obturator
h. of diaphragm
h., omental
h., ovarian
h., phrenic
h., posterior vaginal
h., properitoneal
h., reducible
h., retroperitoneal
h., Richter's
h., scrotal
h., sliding
h., strangulated
h., umbilical
h., uterine
h., vaginal
h., vaginolabial
h., ventral
hernial (hĕr′nē-ăl) [L. hernia, rupture]
hernial sac
herniated
herniated disk
herniation (hĕr-nē-ā′shŭn)
 h. of nucleus pulposus
 h., tonsillar
 h., transtentorial
hernioenterotomy (hĕr″nē-ō-ĕn″tĕr-ŏt′ō-mē) [″ + Gr. enteron, intestine, + tome, a cutting, slice]
herniography (hĕr″nē-ŏg′ră-fē)

[″ + Gr. graphein, to write]
hernioid (hĕr′nē-oyd) [″ + Gr. eidos, form, shape]
herniolaparotomy (hĕr″nē-ō-lăp″ă-rŏt′ō-mē) [″ + Gr. lapara, loin, + tome, a cutting, slice]
herniology (hĕr″nē-ŏl′ō-jē) [″ + Gr. logos, word, reason]
hernioplasty (hĕr′nē-ō-plăs″tē) [″ + Gr. plassein, to form]
herniopuncture (hĕr″nē-ō-pŭnk′chŭr) [″ + punctura, prick]
herniorrhaphy (hĕr-nē-or′ă-fē) [″ + Gr. rhaphe, seam]
herniotomy (hĕr-nē-ŏt′ō-mē) [″ + Gr. tome, a cutting, slice]
heroin (hĕr′ō-ĭn)
heroin toxicity
heroinism (hĕr′ō-ĭn-ĭzm) [heroin + Gr. -ismos, condition]
herpangina (hĕrp-ăn-jī′nă, hĕrp-ăn′jĭ-nă) [Gr. herpes, creeping skin disease, + L. angina, a choking]
herpes (hĕr′pēz) [Gr. herpes, creeping skin disease]
 h. corneae
 herpesviruses
 herpesvirus simiae encephalomyelitis
 h. facialis
 h. febrilis
 h. genitalis
 h. labialis
 h. menstrualis
 h., ocular
 h. praeputialis
 h. progenitalis
 h. simplex
 h., traumatic
 h. zoster
 h. zoster ophthalmicus
herpetic (hĕr-pĕt′ĭk) [Gr. herpes, creeping skin disease]
herpetic neuralgia
herpetic sore throat
herpetiform (hĕr-pĕt′ĭ-form) [″ + L. forma, form]
herpetism (hĕr′pĕ-tĭzm) [″ + -ismos, condition]

Herplex Liquifilm
Herring bodies [Percy T. Herring, Brit. physiologist, 1872–1967]
Herring track
hersage (ār-săzh') [Fr., a harrowing]
Herter's infantilism [Christian A. Herter, U.S. physician, 1865–1910]
Hertig-Rock embryos [Arthur T. Hertig, U.S. pathologist, b. 1904; John Rock, U.S. gynecologist, b. 1890]
Hertig-Rock ovum
Hertwig's root sheath [Wilhelm A.O. Hertwig, Ger. physiologist, 1849–1922]
hertz [Heinrich R. Hertz, Ger. physicist, 1857–1894]
hesperidin (hĕs-pĕr'ĭ-dĭn)
Hesselbach's hernia (hĕs'ĕl-bŏks) [Franz K. Hesselbach, Ger. surgeon, 1759–1816]
Hesselbach's triangle
hetacillin (hĕt"ă-sĭl'ĭn)
heteradelphia (hĕt"ĕr-ă-dĕl'fē-ă) [Gr. heteros, other, + adelphos, brother]
heteradenia (hĕt"ĕr-ă-dē'nē-ă) [" + aden, gland]
heteradenic (hĕt"ĕr-ă-dĕn'ĭk)
heteradenoma (hĕt"ĕr-ăd-ĕ-nō'mă) [" + aden, gland, + oma, tumor]
heterecious (hĕt"ĕr-ē'shŭs) [" + oikos, house]
heterecism (hĕt"ĕr-ē'sĭzm)
heteresthesia (hĕt"ĕr-ĕs-thē'zē-ă) [" + aisthesis, feeling, perception]
hetero-, heter- [Gr. heteros, other]
heteroagglutination (hĕt"ĕr-ō-ă-gloo"tĭ-nă'shŭn)
heteroagglutinin (hĕt"ĕr-ō-ă-glū'tĭ-nĭn)
heteroalbumose (hĕt"ĕr-ō-ăl'bū-mōs) [" + L. albumen, white of egg]
heteroantibody (hĕt"ĕr-ō-ăn'tĭ-bŏd'ē)
heteroantigen (hĕt"ĕr-ō-ăn'tĭ-jĕn)
heteroautoplasty (hĕt"ĕr-ō-aw'tō-plăs-tē) [" + autos, self, +

plassein, to form]
heteroblastic (hĕt"ĕr-ō-blăs'tĭk) [" + blastos, germ]
heterocellular (hĕt"ĕr-ō-sĕl'ū-lăr)
heterocephalus (hĕt"ĕr-ō-sĕf'ă-lŭs) [" + kephale, head]
heterochiral (hĕt"ĕr-ō-kī'răl) [" + cheir, hand]
heterochromatin (hĕt"ĕr-ō-krō'mă-tĭn) [" + chroma, color]
heterochromatosis (hĕt"ĕr-ō-krō-mă-tō'sĭs) [" + " + osis, condition]
heterochromia (hĕt"ĕr-ō-krō'mē-ă)
    h. iridis
heterochromosome (hĕt"ĕr-ō-krō'mō-sōm)
heterochromous (hĕt"ĕr-ō-krō'mŭs) [" + chroma, color]
heterochronia (hĕt"ĕr-ō-krō'nē-ă) [" + chronos, time]
heterochronic (hĕt"ĕr-ō-krŏn'ĭk)
heterochthonous (hĕt"ĕr-ŏk'thō-nŭs) [Gr. heteros, other, + chthon, a particular land or country]
heterocinesia (hĕt"ĕr-ō-sĭ-nē'zē-ă) [" + kinesis, motion]
heterocladic (hĕt"ĕr-ō-klăd'ĭk) [" + klados, branch]
heterocrisis (hĕt"ĕr-ŏk'rĭ-sĭs) [" + krisis, division]
heterocyclic (hĕt"ĕr-ō-sĭk'lĭk) [" + kyklos, circle]
heterodermic (hĕt"ĕr-ō-dĕr'mĭk) [" + derma, skin]
heterodont (hĕt"ĕr-ō-dŏnt) [" + odous, tooth]
heterodromus (hĕt"ĕr-ŏd'rō-mŭs) [" + dromos, running]
heteroecious
heteroecism
heteroerotism (hĕt"ĕr-ō-ĕr'ŏ-tĭzm) [" + eros, love, + -ismos, condition]
heterogametic (hĕt"ĕr-ō-gă-mĕt'ĭk) [" + gamos, marriage]
heterogamy (hĕt"ĕr-ŏg'ă-mē)
heterogeneity (hĕt"ĕr-ō-jĕ-nē'ĭ-tē)

heterogeneous (hĕt″ĕr-ō-jē′nē-ŭs)
[″ + *genos*, type]
heterogeneous vaccine
heterogenesis (hĕt″ĕ-rō-jĕn′ĕ-sĭs)
[″ + *genesis*, generation, birth]
heterogenetic (hĕt″ĕ-rō-jĕ-nĕt′ĭk)
heterogeusia (hĕt″ĕr-ō-gū′sē-ă)
[″ + *geusis*, taste]
heterograft (hĕt′ĕ-rō-grăft) [″ +
L. *graphium*, stylus]
heterography (hĕt″ĕr-ŏg′ră-fē) [″ +
graphein, to write]
heterohemagglutination (hĕt″ĕr-ō-
hĕm″ă-gloo″tĭ-nā′shŭn)
heterohemagglutinin (hĕt″ĕr-ō-
hĕm″ă-gloo′tĭ-nĭn)
heterohemolysin (hĕt″ĕr-ō-hē-mŏl′ĭ-
sĭn)
heteroimmunity (hĕt″ĕr-ō-ĭm-mū′nĭ-tē)
heteroinfection (hĕt″ĕr-ō-ĭn-fĕk′shŭn)
[Gr. *heteros*, other, + L. *in*, in, +
facere, to make]
heteroinoculation (hĕt″ĕr-ō-ĭn-ŏk″ū-
lā′shŭn) [″ + ″ + *oculus*, bud]
heterokeratoplasty (hĕt″ĕr-ō-kĕr′ă-
tō-plăs″tē) [″ + *keras*, horn, +
plassein, to form]
heterolalia (hĕt″ĕr-ō-lā′lē-ă) [″ +
lalia, chatter, prattle]
heterolateral (hĕt″ĕr-ō-lăt′ĕr-ăl)
[″ + L. *latus*, side]
heteroliteral (hĕt″ĕr-ō-lĭt′ĕr-ăl)
heterologous (hĕt″ĕr-ŏl′ō-gŭs) [″ +
logos, word, reason]
heterology (hĕt″ĕr-ŏl′ō-jē)
heterolysin (hĕt″ĕr-ŏl′ĭ-sĭn) [″ +
lysis, dissolution]
heterolysis (hĕt″ĕr-ŏl′ĭ-sĭs)
heteromeric (hĕt″ĕr-ō-mĕr′ĭk) [″ +
meros, a part]
heterometaplasia (hĕt″ĕr-ō-mĕt″ă-
plā′zē-ă) [″ + *meta*, beyond, +
plassein, to form]
heterometropia (hĕt″ĕr-ō-mĕ-
trō′pē-ă)
heteromorphosis (hĕt″ĕr-ō-mor-
fō′sĭs) [″ + *morphe*, form, +
osis, condition]

heteromorphous (hĕt″ĕr-ō-mor′fŭs)
[″ + *morphe*, form]
heteronomous (hĕt″ĕr-ŏn′ō-mŭs)
[″ + *nomos*, law]
heteronymous (hĕt″ĕr-ŏn′ĭ-mŭs)
[″ + *onyma*, name]
hetero-osteoplasty (hĕt″ĕr-ō-ŏs″tē-
ō-plăs″tē) [″ + *osteon*, bone, +
plassein, to form]
heteropathy (hĕt″ĕr-ŏp′ă-thē) [″ +
pathos, disease, suffering]
heterophany (hĕt″ĕr-ŏf′ă-nē) [″ +
phainein, to appear]
heterophasia (hĕt″ĕr-ō-fā′zē-ă)
[″ + *phasis*, utterance]
heterophemia, **heterophemy**
(hĕt″ĕr-ō-fē′mē-ă,   hĕt-ĕr-ŏf′ĕ-mē)
[″ + *pheme*, speech]
heterophil(e) (hĕt′ĕr-ō-fĭl, -fĭl) [″ +
philein, to love]
heterophilic (hĕt″ĕr-ō-fĭl′ĭk) [Gr. *heteros*, other, + *philein*, to love]
heterophonia (hĕt″ĕr-ō-fō′nē-ă)
[″ + *phone*, voice]
heterophoralgia (hĕt″ĕr-ō-for-ăl′jē-
ă) [″ + *phoros*, bearing, +
algos, pain]
heterophoria (hĕt″ĕ-rō-for′ē-ă) [″ +
phoros, bearing]
heterophthalmos (hĕt″ĕr-ŏf-thăl′mŏs)
[″ + *ophthalmos*, eye]
Heterophyes (hĕt″ĕr-ŏf′ĭ-ēz) [″ +
phye, stature]
    H. heterophyes
heterophyiasis (hĕt″ĕr-ō-fī-ī′ă-sĭs)
[″ + ″ + *-iasis*, state or condition of]
Heterophyidae
heteroplasia (hĕt″ĕr-ō-plā′zē-ă)
[″ + *plassein*, to mold]
heteroplastic (hĕt″ĕr-ō-plăs′tĭk)
heteroploid (hĕt′ĕr-ō-ployd) [″ +
ploos, fold]
heteroprosopus (hĕt″ĕr-ō-prō′sō-pŭs)
[″ + *prosopon*, face]
heteropsia (hĕt″ĕr-ŏp′sē-ă) [″ +
opsis, sight, appearance, vision]
heteroptics (hĕt″ĕr-ŏp′tĭks)

heteropyknosis (hĕt″ĕr-ō-pĭk-nō′sĭs) [″ + pyknos, dense, + osis, condition]

heteroscopy (hĕt″ĕr-ŏs′kō-pē) [″ + skopein, to examine]

heteroserotherapy (hĕt″ĕr-ō-sē″rō-thĕr′ă-pē) [″ + L. serum, whey, + Gr. therapeia, treatment]

heterosexual (hĕt″ĕr-ō-sĕk′shū-ăl) [″ + L. sexus, sex]

heterosexuality (hĕt″ĕr-ō-sĕk″shū-ăl′ĭ-tē)

heterosis (hĕt-ĕr-ō′sĭs) [Gr., alteration]

heterosmia (hĕt″ĕr-ŏs′mē-ă) [Gr. heteros, other, + osme, odor]

heterotaxia (hĕt″ĕr-ō-tăk′sē-ă) [″ + taxis, arrangement]

heterotherm (hĕt″ĕr-ō-thĕrm″)

heterothermy (hĕt′ĕr-ō-thĕr″mē) [″ + therme, heat]

heterotopia (hĕt″ĕr-ō-tō′pē-ă) [″ + topos, place]

heterotopic (hĕt″ĕr-ō-tŏp′ĭk)

heterotopy (hĕt″ĕr-ŏt′ō-pē) [″ + topos, place]

heterotoxin (hĕt″ĕr-ō-tŏk′sĭn) [″ + toxikon, poison]

heterotransplant (hĕt″ĕr-ō-trăns′plănt) [″ + L. trans, across, + plantare, to plant]

heterotrichosis (hĕt″ĕr-ō-trī-kō′sĭs) [″ + trichosis, growth of hair]

heterotroph (hĕt′ĕr-ō-trōf) [″ + trophe, food]

heterotropia (hĕt″ĕr-ō-trō′pē-ă) [″ + tropos, a turning]

heterotypic (hĕt″ĕr-ō-tĭp′ĭk)

heterovaccine (hĕt″ĕr-ō-văk′sēn) [″ + L. vaccinus, pert. to a cow]

heteroxanthine (hĕt″ĕr-ō-zăn′thĭn) [″ + xanthos, yellow]

heteroxenous (hĕt″ĕr-ŏk′sē-nŭs) [″ + xenos, stranger]

heterozygosis (hĕt″ĕr-ō-zī-gō′sĭs) [″ + zygone, yoke, pair, + osis, condition]

heterozygote (hĕt″ĕr-ō-zī′gōt)

heterozygous (hĕt″ĕr-ō-zī′gŭs)

hettocyrtosis (hĕt″ō-sĭr-tō′sĭs) [Gr. hetton, less, + kyrtosis, curvature]

Heubner, Johann Otto L. (hoyb′nĕr) [Ger. pediatrician, 1843–1926]
  H.'s disease
  H.-Herter disease [Christian A. Herter, U.S. pathologist, 1865–1910]

heuristic (hū-rĭs′tĭk) [Gr. heuriskein, to find out, discover]

heurteloup (hĕr′tĕl-oop) [Charles Louis Stanislaus Baron Heurteloup, Fr. surgeon, 1793–1864]

H.E.W. U.S. Department of Health, Education, and Welfare

hex (hĕks) [Ger. Hexe, witch, sorceress]

hex-, hexa- [Gr. hex, six]

hexabasic [Gr. hex, six, + basis, base]

hexachlorophene (hĕks″ă-klō′rō-fēn)

hexachromic [″ + chroma, color]

hexad (hĕk′săd)

hexadactylism (hĕks″ă-dăk′tĭl-ĭzm) [″ + daktylos, finger, + -ismos, condition]

hexadecimal (hĕks″ă-dĕs′ĭ-mŭl) [″ + L. decimus, tenth]

hexafluorenium bromide (hĕk″să-flŭr-ĕn′ē-ŭm)

hexamethonium (hĕks″ă-mĕ-thō′nē-ŭm)

hexaploidy (hĕk′să-ploy″dē) [″ + ploos, fold]

Hexapoda (hĕks-ăp′ō-dă) [″ + pous, foot]

hexatomic (hĕks″ă-tŏm′ĭk) [″ + atomos, indivisible]

hexavaccine (hĕks″ă-văk′sēn) [″ + L. vaccinus, pert. to a cow]

hexavalent (hĕks″ă-vā′lĕnt) [″ + L. valere, to have power]

hexavitamin capsules or tablets

hexestrol (hĕk-sĕs′trōl)

hexing

hexobarbital (hĕk″sō-băr′bĭ-tăl)

hexokinase (hĕks″ō-kī′nās) [″ + kinein, to move, + -ase, enzyme]

hexone (hĕk′sōn) [Gr. hex, six]

hexonic (hĕk-sŏn′ĭk)
hexosamine (hĕk′sōs-ăm‴ĭn)
hexose (hĕk′sōs)
hexosephosphate (hĕks″ōs-fŏs′fāt) [″ + phosphoros, phosphorus]
hexylcaine hydrochloride (hĕk′sĭl-kān)
hexylresorcinol (hĕks″ĭl-rĕ-sor′sĭ-nŏl)
Hey's ligament (hāz) [William Hey, Brit. surgeon, 1736–1819]
HF Hageman factor; high frequency
Hf hafnium
Hg [L.] hydrargyrum, mercury
Hgb hemoglobin
HgCl₂ mercuric chloride; corrosive sublimate
Hg₂Cl₂ mercurous chloride; calomel
HGF human growth factor; hyperglycemic-glycogenolytic factor
HgI₂ mercuric iodide
HgO mercuric oxide
HgS mercuric sulfide
HgSO₄ mercuric sulfate
5-HIAA 5 hydroxyindoleacetic acid
hiatal hernia
hiatus (hī-ā′tŭs) [L., an opening]
    h. aorticus
    h. canalis facialis
    h. esophageus
    h. fallopii
    h. maxillaris
    h., sacral
    h. semilunaris
hibernation (hī″bĕr-nā′shŭn) [L. hiberna, winter]
    h., artificial
hibernoma (hī″bĕr-nō′mă)
Hibiclens
hiccough, hiccup (hĭk′ŭp) [probably of imitative origin]
Hicks sign [John Braxton Hicks, Brit. gynecologist, 1825–1897]
hidebound disease [AS. hyd, a skin, + bindan, to tie up]
hidradenitis (hī-drăd-ĕ-nī′tĭs) [Gr. hidros, sweat, + aden, gland, + itis, inflammation]
hidradenoma (hī″drăd-ĕ-nō′mă)

[″ + ″ + oma, tumor]
hidrocystoma (hī″drō-sĭs-tō′mă) [″ + kystis, cyst, + oma, tumor]
hidropoiesis (hī″drō-poy-ē′sĭs) [″ + poiesis, formation]
hidropoietic (hī″drō-poy-ĕt′ĭk)
hidrorrhea (hī-drō-rē′ă) [″ + rhein, to flow]
hidrosadenitis (hī″drōs-ăd″ĕ-nī′tĭs) [″ + aden, gland + itis, inflammation]
hidroschesis (hī-drŏs′kĕ-sĭs) [″ + schesis, a holding]
hidrosis (hī-drō′-sĭs) [″ + osis, condition]
hidrotic (hī-drŏt′ĭk)
hieralgia (hī-ĕr-ăl′jē-ă) [Gr. hieron, sacrum, + algos, pain]
hierarchy (hī′răr-kē)
hierolisthesis (hī″ĕr-ō-lĭs-thē′sĭs) [″ + olisthanein, to slip]
hierophobia (hī″ĕr-ō-fō′bē-ă) [Gr. hieros, sacred, + phobos, fear]
high, runners'
high blood pressure
high-calorie diet
high-cellulose diet
Highmore, antrum of (hī′mor) [Nathaniel Highmore, Brit. surgeon, 1613–1685]
Highmore's body
high-residue diet
hila (hī′lă) [L.]
hilar (hī′lăr)
hilitis (hī″lī′tĭs) [L. hilus, a trifle, + Gr. itis, inflammation]
hillock (hĭl′ŏk) [ME. hilloc]
    h., anal
    h., axon
    h., seminal
Hill sign [Leonard E. Hill, Brit. physiologist, b. 1866]
Hilton's law [John Hilton, Brit. surgeon, 1804–1878]
Hilton's line
Hilton's muscle
Hilton's sac

hilum (hī'lŭm) [L.]
hilus (hī'lŭs) [L., a trifle]
himantosis (hī"măn-tō'sĭs) [Gr. *himantosis*, a long strap]
hindbrain (hīnd'brān) [AS. *hindan*, behind, + *bragen*, brain]
hindfoot (hīnd'foot)
hindgut (hīnd'gŭt)
hind-kidney (hīnd-kĭd'nē)
Hines and Brown test [Edgar H. Hines, Jr., U.S. physician, b. 1906; George Brown, U.S. physician, 1885–1935]
hinge joint
Hinton's test [William A. Hinton, U.S. bacteriologist, 1883–1959]
hip [AS. *hype*]
  h., congenital dislocation of
  h., dislocation of
  h., dislocation of, backward
  h., dislocation of, downward
  h., dislocation of, forward
  h., snapping
  h., total replacement of
hip joint
hip-joint disease
Hippel's disease, von Hippel-Lindau disease (hĭp'ĕlz, vŏn hĭp'ĕl-lĭn'dow) [Eugen von Hippel, Ger. ophthalmologist, 1867–1939; Arvid Lindau, Swedish pathologist, 1892–1958]
hippocampal (hĭp"ō-kăm'păl) [Gr. *hippokampos*, seahorse]
hippocampal commissure
hippocampal fissure
hippocampal formation
hippocampus major
  h., digitations of
hippocampus minor
Hippocrates (hĭ-pŏk'rŭ-tēz) [5th and 4th centuries B.C.]
hippocratic facies
Hippocratic oath
hippurase (hĭp'ū-rās)
hippuria (hĭ-pū'rē-ŭ) [Gr. *hippos*, horse, + *ouron*, urine]
hippuric acid

hippuricase (hĭ-pūr'ĭ-kās)
hippus (hĭp'ŭs) [Gr. *hippos*, horse]
  h., respiratory
hirci (hĭr'sī) [L., goats]
hircismus (hĭr-sĭs'mŭs)
hircus (hĭr'kŭs) [L., goat]
Hirschberg's reflex (hĭrsh'bĕrgz) [Leonard Keene Hirschberg, U.S. neurologist, b. 1877]
Hirschsprung's disease (hĭrsh'sprŭngz) [Harold Hirschsprung, Dan. physician, 1830–1916]
hirsute (hŭr'sūt) [L. *hirsutus*, shaggy]
hirsuties (hŭr-sū'shē-ēz)
hirsutism (hŭr'sūt-ĭzm)
hirudicide (hĭ-rū'dĭ-sīd) [L. *hirudo*, a leech, + *caedere*, to kill]
hirudin (hĭ-rū'dĭn)
Hirudinea (hĭr"ū-dĭn'ē-ă)
hirudiniasis (hĭr"ū-dĭn-ī'ă-sĭs)
  h., internal
Hirudo (hĭ-roo'dō) [L., leech]
His, Jr., Wilhelm (hĭs) [Ger. physician, 1863–1934]
  H., bundle of
  H.-Werner disease [Heinrich Werner, Ger. physician, 1874–1946]
Hispanic
histaffine (hĭs'tă-fēn) [Gr. *histos*, tissue, + L. *affinis*, having affinity for]
histaminase (hĭs-tăm'ĭ-nās)
histamine (hĭs'tă-mĭn, -mēn)
  h. phosphate
histamine blocking agents
histamine headache
histaminemia (hĭs-tăm"ĭ-nē'mē-ă) [*histamine* + Gr. *haima*, blood]
histaminia (hĭs"tă-mĭn'ē-ă)
histase (hĭs'tās) [Gr. *histos*, tissue]
histenzyme (hĭst-ĕn'zīm) [" + *en*, in, + *zyme*, leaven]
histidase
histidine (hĭs'tĭ-dĭn, -dēn)
histidinemia (hĭs"tĭ-dĭ-nē'mē-ă)
histidinuria (hĭs"tĭ-dĭ-nū'rē-ă)
histioblast (hĭs'tē-ō-blăst")
histiocyte (hĭs'tē-ō-sīt") [Gr. *histion*, lit-

tle web, + *kytos,* cell]

histiocytoma (hĭs″tē-ō-sī-tō′mă) [″ + ″ + *oma,* tumor]

histiocytosis (hĭs″tē-ō-sī-tō′sĭs) [″ + ″ + *osis,* condition]

  h., lipid

  h. X

histiogenic (hĭs-tē-ō-jĕn′ĭk) [″ + *gennan,* to form]

histioid (hĭs′tē-oyd) [″ + *eidos,* form, shape]

histioirritative (hĭs″tē-ō-ĭr′ĭ-tā′tĭv) [″ + L. *irritare,* to excite]

histioma (hĭs″tē-ō′mă) [″ + *oma,* tumor]

histionic (hĭs″tē-ŏn′ĭk)

histo- [Gr. *histos,* web, tissue]

histoblast (hĭs′tō-blăst) [″ + *blastos,* germ]

histochemistry (hĭs″tō-kĕm′ĭs-trē)

histochromatosis (hĭs″tō-krō″mă-tō′sĭs) [″ + *chroma,* color, + *osis,* condition]

histoclastic (hĭs″tō-klăs′tĭk) [″ + *klastos,* breaking]

histocompatibility (hĭs″tō-kŏm-păt″ĭ-bĭl′ĭ-tē)

histocompatibility antigens

histocompatibility genes

histocyte (hĭs′tō-sīt) [″ + *kytos,* cell]

histodiagnosis (hĭs″tō-dī″ăg-nō′sĭs) [″ + *dia,* through, + *gnosis,* knowledge]

histodialysis (hĭs″tō-dī-ăl′ĭ-sĭs) [″ + *dia,* through, + *lysis,* dissolution]

histodifferentiation (hĭs″tō-dĭf″ĕr-ĕn″shē-ă′shŭn)

histogenesis (hĭs-tō-jĕn′ĕ-sĭs) [″ + *genesis,* generation, birth]

histogenetic (hĭs″tō-jĕ-nĕt′ĭk)

histogenous (hĭs-tŏj′ĕ-nŭs)

histogram (hĭs′tō-gram) [L. *historia,* observation, + Gr. *gramma,* letter, piece of writing]

histography [Gr. *histos,* tissue, + *graphein,* to write]

histohematin (hĭs″tō-hĕm′ă-tĭn) [″ + *haima,* blood]

histohematogenous (hĭs″tō-hĕm″ă-tŏj′ĕ-nŭs) [″ + ″ + *gennan,* to form]

histoid (hĭs′toyd) [″ + *eidos,* form, shape]

histokinesis (hĭs-tō-kĭ-nē′sĭs) [″ + *kinesis,* motion]

histological (hĭs″tō-lŏj′ĭ-kăl) [″ + *logos,* word, reason]

histologist (hĭs-tŏl′ō-jĭst)

histology (hĭs-tŏl′ō-jē)

  h., normal

  h., pathologic

histolysis (hĭs-tŏl′ĭ-sĭs) [″ + *lysis,* dissolution]

histolytic (hĭs″tō-lĭt′ĭk)

histoma (hĭs-tō′mă) [″ + *oma,* tumor]

histone (hĭs′tōn, -tŏn) [Gr. *histos,* web, tissue]

histonomy (hĭs-tŏn′ō-mē) [″ + *nomos,* law]

histonuria (hĭs-tŏn-ū′rē-ă) [″ + *ouros,* urine]

histopathology (hĭs″tō-pă-thŏl′ō-jē) [″ + *pathos,* disease, suffering, + *logos,* word, reason]

histophysiology (hĭs″tō-fĭz″ē-ŏl′ō-jē) [″ + *physis,* nature, + *logos,* word, reason]

Histoplasma (hĭs″tō-plăz′mă) [″ + LL. *plasma,* form, mold]

  H. capsulatum

histoplasmin (hĭs″tō-plăz′mĭn)

histoplasmosis (hĭs″tō-plăz-mō′sĭs) [″ + ″ + Gr. *osis,* condition]

historetention (hĭs″tō-rē-tĕn′shŭn) [Gr. *histos,* web, tissue, + L. *re,* back, + *tenere,* to hold]

history (hĭs′tō-rē) [Gr. *historia,* inquiry]

  h., dental

  h., family

  h., medical

histotherapy (hĭs″tō-thĕr′ă-pē) [Gr. *histos,* web, tissue, + *therapeia,* treatment]

histothrombin (hĭs″tō-thrŏm′bĭn) [″ + *thrombos,* a clot]

histotome (hĭs'tō-tōm) [" + *tome,* a cutting, slice]

histotomy (hĭs-tŏt'ō-mē) [" + *tome,* a cutting, slice]

histotoxic (hĭs"tō-tŏk'sĭk) [" + *toxikon,* poison]

histotribe (hĭs'tō-trīb) [" + *tribein,* to crush]

histotroph (hĭs'tō-trōf) [" + *trophe,* nourishment]

histotrophic (hĭs-tō-trŏf'ĭk)

histotropic (hĭs"tō-trŏp'ĭk) [" + *trope,* a turning]

histozoic (hĭs"tō-zō'ĭk) [" + *zoe,* life]

histozyme (hĭs'tō-zīm) [" + *zyme,* leaven]

histrionic (hĭs"trē-ŏn'ĭk) [L. *histrio,* an actor]

histrionic mania

histrionic personality disorder

HIV *human immunodeficiency virus*

hives (hīvz) [of uncertain origin]

Hl *hectoliter; latent hyperopia*

HLA *human leukocyte antigen*

Hm *manifest hyperopia*

HMD *hyaline membrane disease*

HMG *human menopausal gonadotrophin*

HMO *Health Maintenance Organization*

HMS Liquifilm Ophthalmic

HNO₂ *nitrous acid*

HNO₃ *nitric acid*

Ho *holmium*

H₂O *water*

H₂O₂ *hydrogen peroxide*

hoarseness [AS. *has,* harsh]

hobnail liver

Hochsinger's sign (hōk'zĭng-ĕrz) [Karl Hochsinger, Austrian pediatrician, b. 1860]

Hodara's disease (hō-dăr'ăz) [Menahem Hodara, Turkish physician, died 1926]

Hodgkin's disease (hŏj'kĭns) [Thomas Hodgkin, Brit. physician, 1798–1866]

Hodgson's disease (hŏj'sŏnz) [Joseph Hodgson, Brit. physician, 1788–1869]

hodoneuromere (hō"dō-nū'rō-mēr) [Gr. *hodos,* path, + *neuron,* nerve, + *meros,* part]

hof [Ger., court]

Hofbauer cell (hŏf'bow-ĕr) [J. Isfred Isidore Hofbauer, U.S. gynecologist, 1878–1961]

Hoffmann's reflex or sign [Johann Hoffmann, Ger. physician, 1857–1919]

hol-, holo- [Gr. *holos,* entire]

holandric (hŏl-ăn'drĭk) [" + *aner,* man]

holarthritis (hŏl"ăr-thrī'tĭs) [" + *arthron,* joint, + *itis,* inflammation]

Holden's line (hōl'dĕnz) [Luther Holden, Brit. anatomist, 1815–1905]

holergastic (hŏl"ĕr-găs'tĭk)

holism (hōl'ĭzm)

holistic (hō-lĭs'tĭk)

holistic medicine

Hollenhorst plaques or bodies [R. W. Hollenhorst, U.S. ophthalmologist, b. 1913]

hollow (hŏl'ō)

　　h., Sebileau's [Pierre Sebileau, Fr. anatomist, 1860–1953]

hollow-back

Holmgren's test (hōlm'grĕnz) [Alarik F. Holmgren, Swedish physiologist, 1831–1897]

holmium (hŏl'mē-ŭm)

holoacardius (hŏl"ō-ă-kăr'dē-ŭs) [Gr. *holos,* entire, + *a-,* not, + *kardia,* heart]

holoblastic ova (hŏl"ō-blăs'tĭk) [" + *blastos,* germ]

holocrine (hŏl'ō-krĭn) [" + *krinein,* to secrete]

holodiastolic (hŏl"ō-dī"ă-stŏl'ĭk) [" + *diastellein,* to expand]

holoendemic (hŏl"ō-ĕn-dĕm'ĭk) [" + *en,* in, + *demos,* people]

holoenzyme (hŏl"ō-ĕn'zīm) [" + *en,* in, + *zyme,* leaven]

holography (hŏl-ŏg'ră-fē) [" +

graphein, to write]

hologynic (hŏl″ō-jĭn′ĭk) [″ + *gyne*, woman]

holomastigote (hŏl″ō-măs′tĭ-gōt) [″ + *mastix*, lash]

holophytic (hŏl″ō-fĭt′ĭk) [″ + *phyton*, plant]

holoprosencephaly (hŏl″ō-prŏs″ĕn-sĕf′ă-lē) [″ + *proso*, before, + *enkephalos*, brain]

holorachischisis (hŏl″ō-ră-kĭs′kĭ-sĭs) [″ + *rhachis*, spine, + *schisis*, cleavage]

holosystolic (hŏl″ō-sĭs-tŏl′ĭk) [″ + *systellein*, to draw together]

holotetanus, holotonia (hŏl-ō-tĕt′ă-nŭs, hŏl″ō-tō′nē-ah) [″ + *tetanos*, rigid, stretched; ″ + *tonos*, act of stretching, tension, tone]

holotonic (hŏl″ō-tŏn′ĭk)

holotrichous (hōl-ŏt′rĭ-kŭs) [″ + *thrix*, hair]

holozoic (hŏl″ō-zō′ĭk) [″ + *zoion*, animal]

Holter monitor

Holthouse's hernia (hŏlt′howz-ĕs) [Carsten Holthouse, Brit. surgeon, 1810–1901]

homalocephalus (hŏm″ă-lō-sĕf′ă-lŭs) [Gr. *homalos*, level, + *kephale*, head]

Homans' sign (hō′mănz) [John Homans, U.S. surgeon, 1877–1954]

homatropine hydrobromide (hō-măt′rō-pēn)

homatropine methylbromide

homaxial (hō-măk′sē-ăl) [Gr. *homos*, same, + L. *axis*, axis]

home assessment

home health care

homeo- [Gr. *homoios*, like, similar]

homeomorphous (hō″mē-ō-mor′fŭs) [″ + *morphe*, form]

homeo-osteoplasty (hō″mē-ō-ŏs′tē-ō-plăs″tē) [″ + *osteon*, bone, + *plassein*, to form]

homeopathic (hō″mē-ō-păth′ĭk) [″ + *pathos*, disease, suffering]

homeopathist (hō-mē-ŏp′ă-thĭst)

homeopathy (hō-mē-ŏp′ă-thē) [Gr. *homoios*, like, + *pathos*, disease, suffering]

homeoplasia (hō″mē-ō-plā′zē-ă) [″ + *plassein*, to form]

homeoplastic (hō″mē-ō-plăs′tĭk)

homeostasis (hō″mē-ō-stā′sĭs) [″ + *stasis*, standing still]

homeostatic (hō″mē-ō-stăt′ĭk)

homeotherapy (hō″mē-ō-thĕr′ă-pē) [″ + *therapeia*, treatment]

homeothermal (hō″mē-ō-thĕr′măl) [″ + *therme*, heat]

homeotransplant (hō″mē-ō-trăns′plănt) [″ + L. *trans*, across, + *plantare*, to plant]

homeotransplantation (hō″mē-ō-trăns″plăn-tā′shŭn)

homeotypical (hō″mē-ō-tĭp′ĭ-kăl) [″ + *typos*, type]

homesickness [AS. *ham*, home, + *seoc*, ill]

homicide (hŏm′ĭ-sīd) [L. *homo*, man, + *caedere*, to kill]

hominid (hŏm′ĭ-nĭd) [″ + *eidos*, form, shape]

Homo (hō′mō) [L., man]

homo- [Gr. *homos*, same]

homoblastic (hō″mō-blăs′tĭk) [″ + *blastos*, germ]

homocentric (hō″mō-sĕn′trĭk) [″ + *kentron*, center]

homochronous (hō-mōk-rō′nŭs) [″ + *chronos*, time]

homocladic (hō″mō-klăd′ĭk) [″ + *klados*, branch]

homocysteine (hō″mō-sĭs-tē′ĭn)

homocystine (hō″mō-sĭs′tĭn)

homocystinuria (hō″mō-sĭs-tĭn-ū′rē-ă)

homocytotropic (hō″mō-sī″tō-trŏp′ĭk) [″ + *kytos*, cell, + *tropos*, a turning]

homodromous (hō-mŏd′rō-mŭs) [″ + *dromos*, running]

homoerotic (hō″mō-ĕ-rŏt′ĭk)

homogametic (hō″mō-gă-mĕt′ĭk) [″ + *gamos*, marriage]

homogenate (hō-mŏj'ĕ-nāt)
homogeneous (hō"mŏ-jē'nē-ŭs)
[" + *genos*, kind]
homogenesis (hō-mō-jĕn'ĕ-sĭs) [" + *genesis*, generation, birth]
homogenize (hō-mŏj'ĕ-nīz)
homogentisic acid
homogentisuria (hō"mō-jĕn"tĭ-sū'rē-ă)
homoglandular (hō"mō-glăn'dū-lăr) [" + L. *glandula*, a little acorn]
homograft (hō'mō-grăft)
homoiopodal (hō"moy-ŏp'ō-dăl) [Gr. *homoios*, like, + *pous*, pod-, foot]
homoiotherm (hō-moy'ō-thĕrm) [" + *therme*, heat]
homokeratoplasty (hō"mō-ker'ă-tō-plăs"tē)
homolateral [Gr. *homos*, same, + L. *latus*, side]
homologous (hō-mŏl'ō-gŭs) [" + *logos*, word, reason]
homologous organs
homologous series
homologous tissues
homologous vaccine
homologue (hŏm'ō-lŏg)
homology (hō-mŏl'ō-jē) [" + *logos*, word, reason]
homolysin (hō-mŏl'ĭ-sĭn) [" + *lysis*, dissolution]
homonomous (hō-mŏn'ō-mŭs) [" + *nomos*, law]
homonymous (hō-mŏn'ĭ-mŭs) [" + *onyma*, name]
homonymous diplopia
homophil (hō-mō-fĭl) [" + *philein*, to love]
homophile (hō-mō-fĭl')
homophobia
homoplastic (hō"mō-plăs'tĭk) [" + *plassein*, to form]
homoplasty (hō'mō-plăs"tē)
Homo sapiens (hō'mō sā'pē-ĕnz) [L. *homo*, man, + *sapiens*, wise, sapient]
homosexual (hōmō-sĕks'ū-ăl) [Gr. *homos*, same, + L. *sexus*, sex]
homosexuality (hōmō-sĕks"ū-ăl'ĭ-tē)

homostimulant (hōmō-stĭm'ū-lănt) [" + L. *stimulare*, to arouse]
Homo-Tet
homothallic (hōmō-thăl'ĭk)
homotherm (hō'mō-thĕrm) [" + *therme*, heat]
homothermal (hōmō-thĕr'măl)
homotonic (hōmō-tŏn'ĭk) [" + *tonos*, act of stretching, tension, tone]
homotopic (hōmō-tŏp'ĭk) [" + *topos*, place]
homotype (hō'mō-tīp) [" + *typos*, type]
homotypic (hō'mō-tīp'ĭk)
homozygosis (hōmō-zī-gō'sĭs) [" + *zygon*, yoke, pair, + *osis*, condition]
homozygote (hōmō-zī'gōt)
homozygous (hōmō-zī-'gŭs)
homunculus (hō-mŭn'kū-lŭs) [L. diminutive of *homo*, man]
honey [AS. *hunig*]
hook [AS. *hok*, an angle]
hookworm
hookworm disease
hopelessness
hordeolum (hor-dē'ō-lŭm) [L., barleycorn]
   h. internum
horizontal [L. *horizontalis*]
horizontal position
hormesis (hor-mē'sĭs) [Gr. *hormesis*, rapid motion]
hormion (hor'mē-ŏn) [Gr., little chain]
hormonagogue (hor-mŏn'ă-gŏg) [Gr. *hormon*, urging on, + *agogos*, leading]
hormonal (hor-mō'năl)
hormone (hor'mōn) [Gr. *hormon*, urging on]
   h., adaptive
   h., adrenocortical
   h., adrenocorticotropic
   h.'s, adrenomedullary
   h., androgenic
   h.'s, anterior pituitary
   h., antidiuretic
   h., calcitonin

h., corpus luteum
h., cortical
h., ectopic
h., estrogenic
h., follicle
h., follicle-stimulating
h., follicle-stimulating, releasing hormone
h., gastric
h., gonadotropic
h., gonadotropin-releasing
h., growth, human growth
h., human placental lactogen
h., inhibitory
h., interstitial cell-stimulating
h., intestinal
h., lactogenic
h., lipolytic
h., luteal
h., luteinizing
h., luteinizing, releasing hormone
h., luteotropic
h., melanocyte-stimulating
h., ovarian
h., pancreatic
h., parathyroid
h.'s, placental
h., posterior pituitary
h., progestational
h., progesterone
h., prolactin
h., releasing
h.'s, sex
h., somatotrophic
h., somatrophin releasing
h., testicular
h., thyroid
h., thyrotropic

hormonic (hor-mŏn'ĭk) [Gr. *hormon*, urging on]
hormonogenesis (hor"mō-nō-jĕn'ĕ-sĭs) [" + *genesis*, generation, birth]
hormonogenic (hor"mō-nō-jĕn'ĭk) [" + *gennan*, to produce]
hormonology (hor"mō-nŏl'ō-jē) [" + *logos*, word, reason]
hormonopoiesis (hor"mō-nō-poy-ē'sĭs) [" + *poiesis*, formation]

hormonopoietic (hor"mō-nō-poy-ĕt'ĭk)
hormonotherapy (hor"mō-nō-thĕr'ă-pē)
hormonotropic (hor"mō-nō-trŏp'ĭk)
horn
h., anterior, of spinal cord
h., cicatricial
h., cutaneous
h., dorsal
h. of Ammon
h., posterior
h., sebaceous
h., ventral
h., warty

Horner's syndrome (hor'nĕrz) [Johann F. Horner, Swiss ophthalmologist, 1831–1886]
hornet sting
horny
horopter (hō-rŏp'tĕr) [Gr. *horos*, limit, + *opter*, observer]
horripilation (hor"ĭ-pĭ-lā'shŭn) [L. *horrere*, to bristle, + *pilus*, hair]
horsepower
horseshoe fistula
horseshoe kidney
hospice (hŏs'pĭs)
hospital [L. *hospitalis*, pert. to a guest]
h., base
h., camp
h., evacuation
h., field

hospitalism [L. *hospitalis*, pert. to a guest, + Gr. *-ismos*, condition]
hospitalization
host [L. *hospes*, a stranger]
h., accidental
h., alternate
h., definitive
h., final
h., immunocompromised
h., intermediate
h. of predilection
h., primary
h., reservoir
h., secondary
h., transfer

hostility (hŏ-stĭl'ĭ-tē)
hot [AS. *hat, hot*]
hot flashes
hotline
Hottentot apron [Hottentot, southern African population]
hottentotism (hŏt'ĕn-tŏt-ĭsm) [*Hottentot* + Gr. *-ismos*, condition]
hot water bag
hourglass contraction
hourglass stomach
housefly
housemaid's knee
house physician
house staff
house surgeon
Houston's muscle (hūs'tŏns) [John Houston, Irish surgeon, 1802 – 1845]
Houston's valves
Howell-Jolly bodies [William H. Howell, U.S. physiologist, 1860 – 1945; Justin Jolly, Fr. histologist, 1870 – 1953]
Howship's lacunae [John Howship, Brit. surgeon, 1781 – 1841]
Howship's symptom
Hp *haptoglobin*
H.P. Acthar Gel
HPG *human pituitary gonadotropin*
HPL *human placental lactogen*
HPLC *high pressure* or *high performance liquid chromatography*
HPO₃ *metaphosphoric acid*
H₃PO₂ *hypophosphorous acid*
H₃PO₃ *phosphorous acid*
H₃PO₄ *orthophosphoric acid*
H₄P₂O₆ *hypophosphoric acid*
hr *hour*
H reflex [after Hoffmann who described it in 1918]
H.S. *house surgeon*
h.s. [L.] *hora somni, at bedtime*
H₂S *hydrogen sulfide*
HSA *human serum albumin*
H₂SO₃ *sulfurous acid*
H₂SO₄ *sulfuric acid*
H-substance
5-HT *5-hydroxytryptamine*

Ht *total hypermetropia*
ht *height*
Hubbard tank
Huguier's canal (ū-gē-āz') [Pierre C. Huguier, Fr. surgeon, 1804 – 1873]
Huhner test (hoon'ĕr) [Max Huhner, U.S. urologist, 1873 – 1947]
hum
  h., venous
human [L. *humanus*, human]
human bite
human growth hormone, synthetic
human immunodeficiency virus
human insulin
human placental lactogen
Humatin
humectant (hū-mĕk'tănt) [L. *humectus*, moist]
humeral (hū'mĕr-ăl) [L. *humerus*, upper arm]
humeroradial (hū"mĕr-ō-rā'dē-ăl) [" + *radius*, wheel spoke, ray]
humeroscapular (hū"mĕr-ō-skăp'ū-lăr) [" + *scapula*, shoulder blade]
humeroulnar (hū"mĕr-ō-ŭl'năr) [" + *ulna*, elbow]
humerus (hū'mĕr-ŭs) [L., upper arm]
  h., fracture of
humid [L. *humidus*, moist]
humid gangrene
humidifier (hū-mĭd'ĭ-fī"ĕr)
humidity [L. *humiditas*]
  h., relative
humor (hū'mor) [L. *humor*, fluid]
  h., aqueous
  h., crystalline
  h., vitreous
humoral (hū'mor-ăl) [L. *humor*, fluid]
humpback (hŭmp'băk)
Humulin
hunchback (hŭnch'băk)
hunger [AS. *hungur*]
  h., air
hunger contractions
hunger cure
Hunner's ulcer (hŭn'ĕrz) [Guy LeRoy Hunner, U.S. surgeon, 1868 – 1957]
Hunter's canal [John Hunter, Scot.

anatomist and surgeon, 1728 – 1793]

Hunter's disease [C. H. Hunter, contemporary Canadian physician]

hunterian chancre

Huntington chorea or disease [G. Huntington, U.S. physician, 1850 – 1916]

Hunt's neuralgia or syndrome [James R. Hunt, U.S. neurologist, 1872 – 1937]

Hurler's syndrome (hoor'lĕrz) [Gertrud Hurler, Austrian pediatrician]

Hürthle cells (hĕr'tĕl) [Karl Hürthle, Ger. histologist, 1860 – 1945]

Hürthle cell tumor

Huschke's auditory teeth (hoosh'kĕz) [Emil Huschke, Ger. anatomist, 1797 – 1858]

    H.'s canal

    H.'s foramen

    H.'s valve

Hutchinson, Sir Jonathan [Brit. surgeon, 1828 – 1913]

    H.-Gilford disease [Hastings Gilford, Brit. physician, 1861 – 1941]

    H.'s patch

    H.'s pupil

    H.'s teeth

    H.'s triad

Hu-Tet

Huxley's layer (hŭks'lēz) [Thomas H. Huxley, Brit. physiologist and naturalist, 1825 – 1895]

hyalin (hī'ă-lĭn) [Gr. hyalos, glass]

hyaline (hī'ă-lĭn)

hyaline bodies

hyaline cartilage

hyaline casts

hyaline membrane disease

hyalinization (hī"ă-lĭn"ĭ-zā'shŭn)

hyalinosis (hī"ă-lĭn-ō'sĭs) [Gr. hyalos, glass, + osis, condition]

hyalinuria (hī"ă-lĭn-ū'rē-ă) [" + ouron, urine]

hyalitis (hī-ă-lī'tĭs) [" + itis, inflammation]

    h., asteroid

    h. punctata

    h. suppurativa

hyalo- [Gr. hyalos, glass]

hyaloenchondroma (hī"ă-lō-ĕn"kŏn-drō'mă) [" + en, in, + chondros, cartilage, + oma, tumor]

hyalogen (hī-ăl'ō-jĕn) [" + gennan, to produce]

hyaloid (hī'ă-loyd) [" + eidos, form, shape]

hyaloid artery

hyaloid canal

hyaloiditis (hī"ă-loyd-ī'tĭs) [" + eidos, form, shape, + itis, inflammation]

hyaloid membrane

hyalomere (hī'ă-lō-mēr") [" + meros, part]

hyalomucoid (hī"ă-lō-mū'koyd) [" + L. mucus, mucus, + Gr. eidos, form, shape]

hyalonyxis (hī"ă-lō-nĭk'sĭs) [" + nyxis, puncture]

hyalophagia, hyalophagy (hī"ă-lō-fā'jē-ă, hī"ă-lŏf'ă-jē) [" + phagein, to eat]

hyalophobia (hī"ă-lō-fō'bē-ă) [" + phobos, fear]

hyaloplasm (hī'ă-lō-plăzm) [" + LL. plasma, form, mold]

hyaloserositis (hī"ă-lō-sē"rō-sī'tĭs) [" + L. serum, whey, + Gr. itis, inflammation]

    h., progressive multiple

hyalosis (hī"ă-lō'sĭs) [" + osis, condition]

    h., asteroid

hyalosome (hī-ăl'ō-sōm) [" + soma, body]

hyalotome (hī-ăl'ō-tōm) [Gr. hyalos, glass]

hyaluronic acid

hyaluronidase (hī"ă-lūr-ŏn'ĭ-dās)

Hyazyme

hybrid (hī'brĭd) [L. hybrida, mongrel]

hybridization (hī'brĭd-ī-zā'shŭn)

hybridoma (hī"brĭ-dō'mă)

hydantoin (hī-dăn'tō-ĭn)

hydatid (hī'dă-tĭd) [Gr. hydatis, watery vesicle]

    h., sessile

h., stalked
hydatid disease
hydatid fremitus
hydatidiform (hī″dă-tĭd′ĭ-form) [″ +
L. *forma,* shape]
hydatid mole
hydatidocele (hī″dă-tĭd′ō-sēl) [″ +
kele, tumor, swelling]
hydatid of Morgagni
hydatidoma (hī″dă-tĭd-ō′mă) [″ +
oma, tumor]
hydatidosis (hī″dă-tĭd-ō′sĭs) [Gr. *hydatis,* watery vesicle, + *osis,* con-
dition]
hydatidostomy (hī″dă-tĭ-dŏs′tō-mē)
[″ + *stoma,* mouth, opening]
hydatiform (hī-dăt′ĭ-form) [″ + L.
forma, form]
hydatism (hī′dă-tĭzm) [″ + *-ismos,*
condition]
hydradenitis (hī″drăd-ĕn-ī′tĭs) [Gr.
hydros, sweat, + *aden,* gland,
+ *itis,* inflammation]
hydradenoma (hī″drăd-ĕ-nō′mă)
[″ + ″ + *oma,* tumor]
hydraeroperitoneum (hī-drā″ĕr-ō-
pĕr″ĭ-tō-nē′ŭm) [Gr. *hydor,* water, +
aer, air + *peritonaion,* stretched
around or over]
hydragogue (hī′dră-gŏg) [″ +
agogos, leading]
hydralazine hydrochloride (hī-
drăl′ă-zēn)
Hydralyn
hydramnion, hydramnios (hī-
drăm′nē-ŏn, -ŏs) [″ + *amnion,* a
caul on a lamb]
hydranencephaly (hī″drăn-ĕn-sĕf′ă-
lē) [″ + *an-,* not, + *enkephalos,* brain]
hydrargyria (hī″drăr-jĭr′ē-ă) [″ +
argyros, silver]
hydrarthrosis (hī″drăr-thrō′sĭs) [″ +
arthron, joint, + *osis,* condition]
h., intermittent
hydrase (hī′drās)
hydrate (hī′drāt)
hydrated (hī′dră-tĕd) [L. *hydratus*]

hydration (hī-drā′shŭn)
hydraulics (hī-draw′lĭks) [Gr. *hydor,*
water, + *aulos,* pipe]
hydrazine (hī′dră-zĭn)
Hydrea
hydremia (hī-drē′mē-ă) [Gr. *hydor,*
water, + *haima,* blood]
hydrencephalocele (hī″drĕn-sĕf′ă-lō-
sēl) [″ + *enkephalos,* brain, +
kele, tumor, swelling]
hydrencephalomeningocele (hī″
drĕn-sĕf″ă-lō-mĕ-nĭng′gō-sēl) [″ +
″ + *meninx,* membrane, +
kele, tumor, swelling]
hydrencephalus (hī″drĕn-sĕf′ă-lŭs)
hydrepigastrium (hī″drĕp-ĭ-găs′trē-
ŭm) [″ + *epi,* upon, + *gaster,*
belly]
hydriatric (hī-drē-ăt′rĭk) [″ + *iatrikos,* healing]
hydriatrics (hī-drē-ăt′rĭks)
hydriatrist (hī-drī′ă-trĭst)
hydride (hī′drīd)
hydrion (hī-drī′ŏn)
hydro- [Gr. *hydor,* water]
hydroa (hĭd-rō′ă)
hydroappendix (hī″drō-ă-pĕn′dĭks)
[″ + L. *appendere,* to hang upon]
hydrobilirubin (hī″drō-bĭl″ĭ-roo′bĭn)
[″ + L. *bilis,* bile, + *ruber,* red]
hydrobromate (hī″drō-brō′māt)
[″ + *bromos,* stench]
hydrocalycosis (hī″drō-kăl″ĭ-kō′sĭs)
[″ + *kalyx,* cup of a flower, +
osis, condition]
hydrocarbon (hī″drō-kăr′bŏn) [″ +
L. *carbo,* coal]
h., alicyclic
h., aliphatic
h., aromatic
h., cyclic
h., saturated
h., unsaturated
hydrocele (hī′drō-sēl) [″ + *kele,*
tumor, swelling]
h., acute
h., cervical
h., chronic

h., congenital
h., encysted
h. feminae
h. hernialis
h., infantile
h. muliebris
h., spermatic
h. spinalis
hydrocelectomy (hī"drō-sē-lĕk'tō-mē) [" + " + ektome, excision]
hydrocephalic [" + kephale, head]
hydrocephalocele (hī"drō-sĕf'ă-lō-sēl) [" + " + kele, tumor, swelling]
hydrocephaloid (hī"drō-sĕf'ă-loyd) [" + " + eidos, form, shape]
hydrocephaloid disease
hydrocephalus (hī-drō-sĕf'ă-lŭs) [" + kephale, head]
h., communicating
h., congenital
h., external
h., internal
h., noncommunicating
h., normal pressure
h., secondary
hydrochlorate (hī"drō-klō'rāt) [Gr. hydor, water, + chloros, green]
hydrochloric acid
hydrochloride (hī"drō-klō'rīd)
hydrochlorothiazide (hī"drō-klō"rō-thī'ă-zīd)
hydrocholecystis (hī"drō-kō"lĭ-sĭs'tĭs) [" + chole, bile, + kystis, bladder]
hydrocholeresis (hī"drō-kō"lĕr-ē'sĭs) [" + " + hairesis, a taking]
hydrocholeretic (hī"drō-kō"lĕr-rĕt'ĭk)
hydrocirsocele (hī"drō-sĭr'sō-sēl) [" + kirsos, varix, + kele, tumor, swelling]
hydrocodone bitartrate (hī"drō-kō'dōn)
hydrocolloid (hī"drō-kŏl'loyd) [" + kollodes, glutinous]
hydrocolpos (hī"drō-kŏl'pŏs) [" + kolpos, vagina]

hydroconion (hī"drō-kō'nē-ŏn) [" + konis, dust]
hydrocortisone (hī"drō-kor'tĭ-sōn)
h. acetate
hydrocyanic acid
hydrocyst (hī'drō-sĭst) [Gr. hydor, water, + kystis, bladder]
hydrocystoma [" + " + oma, tumor]
hydrodiascope (hī"drō-dī'ă-skōp) [" + dia, through, + skopein, to examine]
hydrodictiotomy (hī"drō-dĭk"tē-ŏt'ō-mē) [" + diktyon, retina, + tome, a cutting, slice]
HydroDIURIL
hydroencephalocele (hī"drō-ĕn-sĕf'ă-lō-sēl) [" + enkephalos, brain, + kele, tumor, swelling]
hydroflumethiazide (hī"drō-floo"mĕ-thī'ă-zīd)
hydrogel (hī'drō-jĕl) [" + L. gelare, to congeal]
hydrogen [" + gennan, to produce]
hydrogen acceptor
hydrogenase (hī'drō-jĕn-ās)
hydrogenate (hī'drō-jĕn-āt")
hydrogenation (hī"drō-jĕn-ā'shŭn)
hydrogen cyanide
hydrogen dioxide
hydrogen donor
hydrogen iodide
hydrogen ion
hydrogen ion concentration
hydrogen ion scale
hydrogen peroxide
h. p., solution of
hydrogen sulfide
hydroglossa (hī"drō-glŏs'ă) [Gr. hydor, water, + glossa, tongue]
hydrogymnasium (hī"drō-jĭm-nā'zē-ŭm) [" + gymnazein, to train naked]
hydrogymnastics (hī"drō-jĭm-năs'tĭks)
hydrohematonephrosis (hī"drō-hĕm"ă-tō-nĕf-rō'sĭs) [" + haima, blood, + nephros, kidney, +

osis, condition]

hydrohymenitis (hī″drō-hī″mĕn-ī′tĭs)
[″ + *hymen*, membrane, +
itis, inflammation]

hydrokinetics (hī″drō-kī-nĕt′ĭks) [″ +
kinesis, motion]

hydrolabile (hī″drō-lā′bĭl)

hydrolase (hī′drō-lās)

hydrology (hī-drŏl′ō-jē) [″ +
logos, word, reason]

hydrolysate (hī-drŏl′ĭ-sāt)
h., protein

hydrolysis (hī-drŏl′ĭ-sĭs) [″ + *lysis*,
dissolution]

hydrolytic (hī-drō-lĭt′ĭk)

hydrolyze (hī′drō-līz)

hydroma (hī-drō′mă) [Gr. *hydor*,
water, + *oma*, tumor]

hydromeiosis (hī″drō-mī-ō′sĭs) [″ +
meiosis, dimunition]

hydromeningitis (hī″drō-mĕn″ĭn-jī′tĭs)
[″ + *meninx*, membrane, +
itis, inflammation]

hydromeningocele (hī″drō-mĕn-
ĭn′gō-sēl) [″ + ″ + *kele*, tumor,
swelling]

hydrometer (hī-drŏm′ĕ-tĕr) [″ +
metron, measure]

hydrometra (hī″drō-mē′tră) [″ +
metra, uterus]

hydrometrocolpos (hī″drō-mē″trō-
kŏl′pŏs) [″ + *metra*, uterus, +
kolpos, vagina]

hydromicrocephaly (hī″drō-mī″krō-
sĕf′ă-lē) [″ + *mikros*, small, +
kephale, head]

hydromorphone hydrochloride
(hī″drō-mor′fōn)

Hydromox

hydromphalus (hī-drŏm′fă-lŭs) [″ +
omphalos, navel]

hydromyelia (hī″drō-mī-ē′lē-ă) [″ +
myelos, marrow]

hydromyelocele (hī″drō-mī-ĕl′ō-sēl)
[″ + ″ + *kele*, tumor, swelling]

hydromyelomeningocele (hī″drō-
mī″ē-lō-mē-nĭng′gō-sēl) [″ +
myelos, marrow, + *meninx*, mem-

brane, + *kele*, tumor, swelling]

hydromyoma (hī″drō-mī-ō′mă) [″ +
mys, muscle, + *oma*, tumor]

hydronephrosis (hī″drō-nĕf-rō′sĭs)
[″ + *nephros*, kidney, + *osis*,
condition]

hydroparasalpinx (hī″drō-păr″ă-
săl′pĭnks) [Gr. *hydor*, water, +
para, alongside, past, beyond, +
salpinx, tube]

hydroparotitis (hī″drō-păr″ō-tī′tĭs)
[″ + ″ + *ous*, ear, + *itis*,
inflammation]

hydropathic (hī″drō-păth′ĭk) [″ +
pathos, disease, suffering]

hydropathy (hī-drŏp′ă-thē)

hydropenia (hī″drō-pē′nē-ă) [″ +
penia, lack]

hydropericarditis [″ + *peri*,
around, + *kardia*, heart, +
itis, inflammation]

hydropericardium (hī″drō-pĕr″ĭ-kăr′
dē-ŭm)

hydroperinephrosis (hī″drō-pĕr″ĭ-
nē-frō′sĭs) [″ + *peri*, around, +
nephros, kidney, + *osis*, condition]

hydroperion (hī″drō-pĕr′ē-ŏn) [″ +
″ + *oon*, egg]

hydroperitoneum (hī″drō-pĕr″ĭ-tō-
nē′ŭm) [″ + *peritonaion*, stretched
around or over]

hydropexis (hī″drō-pĕk′sĭs) [″ +
pexis, fixation]

hydrophilia (hī-drō-fĭl′ē-ă) [″ +
philein, to love]

hydrophilic lyophilic colloid

hydrophilic ointment

hydrophilism (hī-drŏf′ĭ-lĭzm) [″ + ″
+ *-ismos*, condition]

hydrophilous (hī-drŏf′ĭ-lŭs)

hydrophobia (hī-drō-fō′bē-ă) [Gr.
hydor, water, + *phobos*, fear]

hydrophobophobia (hī″drō-fō″bō-
fō′bē-ă) [″ + ″ + *phobos*,
fear]

hydrophthalmos (hī″drŏf-thăl′mŏs)
[″ + *ophthalmos*, eye]

hydrophysometra (hī″drō-fī″sō-

mē'trȧ) [" + *physa*, air, +
metra, uterus]

hydropic (hī-drŏp'ĭk) [Gr. *hydropikos*]

hydropneumatosis (hī″drō-nū″mȧ-tō'sĭs) [" + *pneumatosis*, inflation]

hydropneumopericardium (hī″drō-nū″mō-pĕr-ĭ-kăr'dē-ŭm) [" + " + *peri*, around, + *kardia*, heart]

hydropneumoperitoneum (hī″drō-nū″mō-pĕr″ĭ-tō-nē'ŭm) [" + " + *peritonaion*, stretched around or over]

hydropneumothorax (hī″drō-nū″mō-thō'răks) [" + " + *thorax*, chest]

hydrops, hydropsy (hī'drŏps, hī-drŏp'sē) [Gr.]
- h. abdominis
- h., endolymphatic
- h. fetalis
- h. folliculi
- h. gravidarum
- h., labyrinthine
- h. tubae
- h. tubae profluens

hydropyonephrosis (hī″drō-pī″ō-nĕf-rō'sĭs) [Gr. *hydor*, water, + *pyon*, pus, + *nephros*, kidney, + *osis*, condition]

hydroquinone (hī″drō-kwĭn'ōn)

hydrorheostat (hī″drō-rē'ō-stăt) [" + *rheos*, current, + *histanai*, to place]

hydrorrhachis (hī-dror'ȧ-kĭs) [" + *rhachis*, spine]

hydrorrhachitis (hī-dror-ȧ-kī'tĭs) [" + " + *itis*, inflammation]

hydrorrhea (hī″drō-rē'ȧ) [" + *rhein*, to flow]
- h. gravidarum

hydrosalpinx (hī″drō-săl'pĭnks) [" + *salpinx*, tube]
- h., intermittent

hydrosarcocele (hī″drō-săr'kō-sēl) [" + *sarx*, flesh, + *kele*, tumor, swelling]

hydroscheocele (hī-drŏs'kē-ō-sēl″) [" + *oscheon*, scrotum, + *kele*, tumor, swelling]

hydrosis (hī-drō'sĭs)

hydrosol (hī'drō-sŏl)

hydrosphygmograph (hī″drō-sfĭg'mō-grăf) [" + *sphygmos*, pulse, + *graphein*, to write]

hydrostat (hī'drō-stăt) [" + *statikos*, standing]

hydrostatic (hī″drō-stăt'ĭk) [" + *statikos*, standing]

hydrostatic densitometry

hydrostatics (hī″drō-stăt'ĭks)

hydrostatic test

hydrostatic weighing

hydrosudotherapy (hī″drō-soo″dō-thĕr'ȧ-pē) [" + L. *sudor*, sweat, + Gr. *therapeia*, treatment]

hydrosulfuric acid

hydrosyringomyelia (hī″drō-sīr-ĭng″ō-mī-ē'lē-ȧ) [" + *syrinx*, tube, + *myelos*, marrow]

hydrotaxis (hī″drō-tăk'sĭs) [" + *taxis*, arrangement]

hydrotherapeutics (hī″drō-thĕr″ȧ-pū'tĭks) [Gr. *hydor*, water, + *therapeia*, treatment]

hydrotherapist (hī″drō-thĕr'ȧ-pĭst)

hydrotherapy (hī-drō-thĕr'ȧ-pē) [" + *therapeia*, treatment]

hydrothermic (hī″drō-thĕr'mĭk)

hydrothionammonemia (hī″drō-thī″ō-năm″ō-nē'mē-ȧ) [" + *theion*, sulfur, + *ammoniakos*, of Amen, from near whose temple it came, + *haima*, blood]

hydrothionemia (hī″drō-thī″ō-nē'mē-ȧ) [" + " + *haima*, blood]

hydrothionuria (hī″drō-thī″ō-nū'rē-ȧ) [" + " + *ouron*, urine]

hydrothorax (hī″drō-thō'răks) [" + *thorax*, chest]

hydrotis (hī-drō'tĭs) [" + *ous*, ear]

hydrotomy (hī-drŏt'ō-mē) [" + *tome*, a cutting, slice]

hydrotropism (hī-drŏt-rō'pĭzm) [" + *trope*, a turning]

hydrotympanum (hī″drō-tĭm'pȧ-nŭm) [" + *tympanon*, drum]

hydroureter (hī″drō-ū-rē'tĕr) [" +

oureter, ureter]
hydrous (hī′drŭs)
hydrovarium (hī″drō-vā′rē-ŭm) [″ +
NL. *ovarium*, ovary]
hydroxide (hī-drŏk′sīd) [″ + *oxys*,
sour]
hydroxocobalamin (hī-drŏk″sō-kō-
băl′ă-mĭn)
hydroxy acids (hī-drŏk′sē)
**hydroxyamphetamine hydrobro-
mide** (hī-drŏk″sē-ăm-fĕt′ă-mēn hī″
drō-brō′mīd)
hydroxyapatite (hī-drŏk″sē-ăp′ă-tīt)
hydroxybenzene (hī-drŏk″sē-bĕn′
zēn)
hydroxybutyric acid
hydroxybutyric dehydrogenase
hydroxychloroquine sulfate (hī-
drŏk″sē-klō′rō-kwīn)
25-hydroxycholecalciferol (hī-
drŏk″sēkō″lē-kăl-sīf′ĕ-rŏl)
17-hydroxycorticosterone (hī-
drŏk″sē-kor″tĭ-kō-stĕr′ōn)
hydroxydione sodium succinate
(hī-drŏk″sē-dī′ōn)
hydroxyl
hydroxylase (hī-drŏk′sī-lās)
hydroxylysine (hī″drŏk-sĭl′ĭ-sīn)
hydroxyprogesterone caproate
(hī-drŏk″sē-prō-jĕs′tĕr-ōn)
hydroxyproline (hī-drŏk″sē-prō′lĭn)
hydroxypropyl methycellulose
hydroxystilbamidine isethionate
(hī-drŏk″sē-stĭl-băm′ĭ-dēn)
5-hydroxytryptamine (hī-drŏk″sē-
trĭp′tă-mēn)
hydroxyurea (hī-drŏk″sē-ū-rē′ă)
hydroxyzine hydrochloride (hī-
drŏk′sī-zēn)
hydruria (hī-droo′rē-ă) [Gr. *hydor*,
water, + *ouron*, urine]
hygiene (hī′jēn) [Gr. *hygieinos*, health-
ful]
　h., community
　h., dental
　h., industrial
　h., mental
　h., oral

hygienic (hī″jē-ĕn′ĭk)
hygienics
hygienist (hī-jē′nĭst, hī′jē-ĕn-ĭst)
　h., dental
hygienization (hī″jē-ĕn-ī-zā′shŭn)
hygric (hī′grĭk) [Gr. *hygros*, moisture]
hygroblepharic (hī″grō-blĕ-făr′ĭk)
[″ + *blepharon*, eyelid]
hygroma (hī-grō′mă) [″ + *oma*,
tumor]
　h., cystic
hygrometer (hī-grŏm′ĕ-tĕr) [″ +
metron, measure]
hygroscopic (hī-grō-skŏp′ĭk) [″ +
skopein, to examine]
hygroscopy (hī-grŏs′kō-pē)
hygrostomia (hī-grō-stō′mē-ă) [″ +
stoma, mouth, opening]
Hygroton
hyl-, hylo- [Gr. *hyle*, matter]
hyla (hī′lă)
hyloma (hī-lō′mă) [Gr. *hyle*, matter,
+ *oma*, tumor]
hymen (hī′mĕn) [Gr.]
　h., annular
　h. biforis
　h., cribriform
　h. denticulatus
　h., fenestrated
　h., imperforate
　h., lunar
　h., ruptured
　h., septate
　h., unruptured
hymenal (hī′mĕn-ăl)
hymenectomy (hī″mĕn-ĕk′tō-mē)
[″ + *ektome*, excision]
hymenitis (hī-mĕn-ī′tĭs) [″ + *itis*, in-
flammation]
Hymenolepis (hī″mĕ-nŏl′ĕ-pĭs)[″ +
lepis, rind]
　H. nana
hymenology (hī′mĕn-ŏl′ō-jē) [″ +
logos, word, reason]
Hymenoptera (hī″mĕn-ŏp′tur-ă) [Gr.
hymenopteros, membrane-winged]
hymenorrhaphy (hī″mĕn-or′ă-fē)
[″ + *rhaphe*, seam]

hymenotome (hī-mĕn'ō-tōm) [" + *tome*, a cutting, slice]
hymenotomy (hī"mĕn-ŏt'ō-mē)
hyo- [Gr. *hyoeides*, U-shaped]
hyobasioglossus (hī"ō-bā"sē-ō-glŏs'ŭs) [" + *basis*, base, + *glossa*, tongue]
hyoepiglottic, hyoepiglottidean (hī"ō-ĕp"ĭ-glŏt'ĭk, hī"ō-ĕp"ĭ-glŏt-ĭd'ē-ăn) [" + *epi*, upon, *glottis*, tongue]
hyoglossal (hī"ō-glŏs'ăl) [" + *glossa*, tongue]
hyoglossus (hī"ō-glŏs'ŭs)
hyoid (hī'oyd) [Gr. *hyoeides*, U-shaped]
hyoid arch
hyoid bone
hyopharyngeus (hī"ō-făr-ĭn'jē-ŭs) [" + *pharynx*, throat]
hyoscine hydrobromide
hyoscyamus (hī"ō-sī'ă-mŭs) [Gr. *hys*, a pig, + *kyamos*, bean]
hyoscyamus poisoning
hypacousia, hypacusia, hypacusis (hī"pă-koo'sē-ă, -kū'sē-ă, -sĭs) [Gr. *hypo*, under, beneath, below, + *akousis*, hearing]
hypalbuminosis (hī"păl-bū-mĭn-ō'sĭs) [" + L. *albumen*, white of egg, + Gr. *osis*, condition]
hypalgesia (hī-păl-jē'zē-ă) [" + *algesis*, sense of pain]
hypalgia (hī-păl'jē-ă) [" + *algos*, pain]
hypamnios (hī-păm'nē-ŏs) [" + *amnion*, caul of a lamb]
hypaphrodisia (hī-păf"rō-dĭz'ē-ă) [Gr. *hypo*, under, beneath, below, + *aphrodisia*, sexual pleasure]
hypaxial (hī-păks'ē-ăl) [" + *axon*, axle]
hyper- [Gr. *hyper*, over, above, excessive]
Hyperab
hyperacid (hī"pĕr-ăs'ĭd) [" + L. *acidus*, sour]
hyperacidaminuria (hī"pĕr-ăs"ĭd-ăm-ĭn-ū'rē-ă) [" + " + *amine* + Gr. *ouron*, urine]

hyperacidity (hī"pĕr-ă-sĭd'ĭ-tē) [" + L. *acidus*, sour]
hyperactive child syndrome
hyperactivity
hyperacuity (hī"pĕr-ă-kū'ĭ-tē) [Gr. *hyper*, over, above, excessive, + L. *acuitas*, sharpness]
hyperacusis (hī"pĕr-ă-kū'sĭs) [" + *akousis*, hearing]
hyperacute (hī"pĕr-ă-kūt')
hyperadenosis (hī"pĕr-ăd"ĭ-nō'sĭs) [" + *aden*, gland, + *osis*, condition]
hyperadiposis, hyperadiposity (hī"pĕr-ăd"ĭ-pō'sĭs, -pŏs'ĭ-tē) [" + L. *adeps*, fat, + Gr. *osis*, condition]
hyperadrenalism (hī"pĕr-ă-drē'năl-ĭzm)
hyperadrenocorticalism (hī"pĕr-ă-drē"nō-kor'tĭ-kăl-ĭzm)
hyperalbuminemia (hī"pĕr-ăl-bū"mĭ-nē'mē-ă) [" + L. *albumen*, white of egg, + Gr. *haima*, blood]
hyperaldosteronism (hī"pĕr-ăl"dō-stĕr'ōn-ĭzm)
hyperalgesia (hī"pĕr-ăl-jē'zē-ă) [" + *algesis*, sense of pain]
hyperalgia (hī-pĕr-ăl'jē-ă) [" + *algos*, pain]
hyperalimentation (hī"pĕr-ăl"ĭ-mĕn-tā'shŭn)
hyperalkalinity (hī"pĕr-ăl-kă-lĭn'ĭ-tē)
hyperaminoacidemia (hī"pĕr-ăm"ĭ-nō-ăs"ĭ-dē'mē-ă)
hyperammonemia (hī"pĕr-ăm"mō-nē'mē-ă)
  h., congenital
hyperamylasemia (hī"pĕr-ăm"ĭl-ăs-ē'mē-ă)
hyperanacinesia, hyperanacinesis (hī"pĕr-ăn"ă-sĭn-ē'zē-ă, -sĭs)
hyperanakinesis (hī"pĕr-ăn"ă-kĭ-nē'sĭs) [" + *anakinesis*, exercise]
hyperaphia (hī"pĕr-ă'fē-ă) [" + *haphe*, touch]
hyperaphic (hī-pĕr-ăf'ĭk)
hyperazotemia (hī"pĕr-ăz"ō-tē'mē-ă) [" + L. *azotum*, nitrogen, +

Gr. *haima*, blood]

hyperazoturia (hī″pĕr-ăz″ō-tū′rē-ă)
[″ + ″ + Gr. *ouron*, urine]

hyperbaric chamber

hyperbaric oxygen

hyperbaric oxygen therapy

hyperbarism (hī″pĕr-băr′ĭzm)

hyperbetalipoproteinemia (hī″pĕr-
bā″tă-lĭp″ō-prō″tē-ĭn-ē′mē-ă)

hyperbilirubinemia (hī″pĕr-bĭl″ĭ-roo-
bĭn-ē′mē-ă) [Gr. *hyper*, over, above,
excessive, + L. *bilis*, bile, +
ruber, red, + Gr. *haima*, blood]

hyperbrachycephaly (hī″pĕr-brăk″
ē-sĕf′ă-lē) [″ + *brachys*, short,
+ *kephale*, head]

hyperbulia (hī″pĕr-bū′lē-ă) [″ +
boule, will]

hypercalcemia (hī″pĕr-kăl-sē′mē-ă)
[″ + L. *calx*, lime, + Gr.
haima, blood]
   h., idiopathic

hypercalciuria (hī″pĕr-kăl″sē-ū′rē-ă)
[″ + ″ + Gr. *ouron*, urine]

hypercapnia (hī″pĕr-kăp′nē-ă) [″ +
kapnos, smoke]

hypercarbia

hypercatharsis (hī″pĕr-kă-thăr′sĭs)
[″ + *katharsis*, to cleanse, purify]

hypercellularity (hī″pĕr-sĕl″ū-lăr′ĭ-tē)

hypercementosis (hī″pĕr-sē″mĕn-
tō′sĭs) [″ + L. *cementum*, cement,
+ Gr. *osis*, condition]

hyperchloremia (hī″pĕr-klō-rē′mē-ă)
[″ + *chloros*, green, + *haima*,
blood]

hyperchlorhydria (hī″pĕr-klor-hī′drē-
ă) [″ + ″ + *hydor*, water]

hyperchloridation (hī″pĕr-klō″rĭ-
dā′shŭn)

hypercholesterolemia (hī″pĕr-kō-
lĕs″tĕr-ŏl-ē′mē-ă) [″ + *chole*, bile,
+ *stereos*, solid, + *haima*,
blood]
   h., familial

hypercholesterolia (hī″pĕr-kō-lĕs″
tĕr-ō′lē-ă) [″ + ″ + *stereos*,
solid]

hypercholia (hī″pĕr-kō′lē-ă) [″ +
chole, bile]

hyperchromasia (hī″pĕr-krō-mā′zē-ă)
[Gr. *hyper*, over, above, excessive,
+ *chroma*, color]

hyperchromatic (hī″pĕr-krō-măt′ĭk)
[″ + *chroma*, color]

hyperchromatic cell

hyperchromatism (hī″pĕr-krō′mă-
tĭzm) [″ + ″ + *-ismos*, condi-
tion]

hyperchromatopsia (hī″pĕr-krō″mă-
tŏp′sē-ă) [″ + ″ + *opsis*, sight,
appearance, vision]

hyperchromatosis (hī″pĕr-krō″mă-
tō′sĭs) [″ + *chroma*, color, +
osis, condition]

hyperchromia (hī″pĕr-krō′mē-ă)

hyperchromic (hī-pĕr-krō′mĭk)

hyperchylia (hī″pĕr-kī′lē-ă) [Gr. *hyper*,
over, above, excessive, + *chylos*,
juice]

hyperchylomicronemia (hī″pĕr-kī″
lō-mī″krō-nē′mē-ă)

hypercoagulability (hīpĕr-kō-ăg″ū-
lă-bĭl′ĭ-tē)

hypercorticism (hī″pĕr-kor′tĭ-sĭzm)

hypercrinism (hī″pĕr-krī′nĭsm) [″ +
krinein, to separate, + *-ismos*,
condition]

hypercryalgesia (hī″pĕr-krī″ăl-jē′zē-
ă) [″ + *kryos*, cold, + *algesis*,
sense of pain]

hypercryesthesia (hī″pĕr-krī″ĕs-
thē′zē-ă) [″ + ″ + *aisthesis*,
feeling, perception]

hypercupremia (hī″pĕr-kū-prē′mē-ă)

hypercyanosis (hī″pĕr-sī″ă-nō′sĭs)
[″ + *kyanos*, dark blue, +
osis, condition]

hypercyanotic (hī″pĕr-sī″ă-nŏt′ĭk)

hypercyesis (hī″pĕr-sī-ē′sĭs) [″ +
kyesis, gestation]

hypercythemia (hī″pĕr-sī-thē′mē-ă)
[″ + *kytos*, cell, + *haima*,
blood]

hypercytosis (hī″pĕr-sī-tō′sĭs) [″ +
″ + *osis*, condition]

hyperdactylia (hī"pĕr-dăk-tĭl'ē-ă) [Gr. *hyper*, over, above, excessive, + *daktylos*, finger]

hyperdicrotic (hī"pĕr-dĭ-krŏt'ĭk) [" + *dikrotos*, beating double]

hyperdistention (hī"pĕr-dĭs-tĕn'shŭn) [" + L. *distendere*, to stretch out]

hyperdontia (hī"pĕr-dŏn'shē-ă)

hyperdynamia (hī"pĕr-dī-nă'mē-ă) [" + *dynamis*, force]
  h. uteri

hypereccrisia, hypereccrisis (hī"pĕr-ĕk-krīs'ē-ă, -ĕk'krī-sĭs) [" + *ekkrisis*, excretion]

hypereccritic (hī-pĕr-ĕk-krīt'ĭk)

hyperemesis (hī"pĕr-ĕm'ĕ-sĭs) [" + *emesis*, vomiting]
  h. gravidarum
  h. lactentium

hyperemia (hī"pĕr-ē'mē-ă) [" + *haima*, blood]
  h., active
  h., arterial
  h., Bier's
  h., constriction
  h., leptomeningeal
  h., passive
  h., reactive
  h., venous

hyperemization (hī"pĕr-ē"mĭ-zā'shŭn)

hyperemotivity (hī"pĕr-ē"mō-tĭv'ĭ-tē) [Gr. *hyper*, over, above, excessive, + L. *emovere*, to disturb]

hypereosinophilic syndrome

hypereosinophilia (hī"pĕr-ē"ō-sĭn-ō-fĭl'ē-ă) [" + *eos*, dawn, + *philein*, to love]

hyperepinephrinemia (hī"pĕr-ĕp"ĭ-nĕf"rĭ-nē'mē-ă) [" + " + *nephros*, kidney, + *haima*, blood]

hyperequilibrium (hī"pĕr-ē"kwī-lĭb'rē-ŭm) [" + L. *aequus*, equal, + *libra*, balance]

hypererethism (hī"pĕr-ĕr'ĭ-thĭzm) [" + *erethisma*, stimulation]

hyperergasia (hī"pĕr-ĕr-gā'sē-ă) [" + *ergasia*, work]

hyperergia (hī"pĕr-ĕr'jē-ă)

hyperergy (hī'pĕr-ĕr"jē) [" + *ergon*, energy]

hyperesophoria (hī"pĕr-ĕs"ō-fō'rē-ă) [" + *eso*, inward, + *phorein*, to bear]

hyperesthesia (hī"pĕr-ĕs-thē'zē-ă) [" + *aisthesis*, feeling, perception]
  h., acoustic
  h., cerebral
  h., gustatory
  h., muscular
  h., optic
  h. sexualis
  h., tactile

hyperesthetic (hī"pĕr-ĕs-thĕt'ĭk)

hyperexophoria (hī"pĕr-ĕks"ō-fō'rē-ă) [" + *exo*, outward, + *phorein*, to bear]

hyperexplexia

hyperextension (hī"pĕr-ĕks-tĕn'shŭn) [" + L. *extendere*, to stretch out]

hyperferremia (hī"pĕr-fĕr-rē'mē-ă)

hyperfibrinogenemia (hī"pĕr-fī-brĭn"ō-jĕ-nē'mē-ă)

hyperflexion (hī"pĕr-flĕk'shŭn)

hyperfunction [Gr. *hyper*, over, above, excessive, + L. *functio*, performance]

hypergalactia (hī-pĕr-găl-ăk'shē-ă) [" + *gala*, milk]

hypergammaglobulinemia (hī"pĕr-găm"ă-glŏb"ū-lĭ-nē'mē-ă)

hypergamy (hī-pĕr'gă-mē) [" + *gamos*, marriage]

hypergasia (hĭp-ĕr-gā'sē-ă)

hypergenesis (hī"pĕr-jĕn'ĕ-sĭs) [" + *genesis*, generation, birth]

hypergenitalism (hī"pĕr-jĕn'ĭt-ăl-ĭzm) [" + L. *genitalis*, to beget]

hypergeusesthesia, hypergeusia (hī"pĕr-gūs-ĕs-thē'sē-ă, -gū'sē-ă) [" + *geusis*, taste + *aisthesis*, feeling, perception]

hypergia (hī-pĕr'jē-ă)

hyperglandular (hī"pĕr-glăn'dū-lăr) [" + L. *glandula*, a little acorn]

hyperglobulinemia (hī"pĕr-glŏb"ū-lĭn-ē'mē-ă) [" + L. *globulus*, a globule, + Gr. *haima*, blood]

hyperglycemia (hī″pĕr-glī-sē′mē-ă)
[″ + *glykys*, sweet, + *haima*,
blood]

hyperglyceridemia (hī″pĕr-glĭs″ĕr-ĭ-
dē′mē-ă)

hyperglycinemia (hī″pĕr-glī″sĭ-
nē′mē-ă)

hyperglycogenolysis (hī″pĕr-glī″kō-
jĕn-ŏl′ĭ-sĭs) [″ + ″ + *gennan*,
to form, + *lysis*, dissolution]

hyperglycoplasmia (hīpĕr-glī″kō-
plăz′mē-ă) [″ + ″ + LL.
plasma, form, mold]

hyperglycorrhachia (hī″pĕr-glī″kō-
rā′kē-ă) [″ + *glykys*, sweet, +
rhachis, spine]

hyperglycosemia (hī″pĕr-glī-kō-
sē′mē-ă) [″ + ″ + *haima*,
blood]

hyperglycosuria (hī″pĕr-glī″kō-sū′rē-
ă) [″ + ″ + *ouron*, urine]

hypergnosia (hī″pĕr-nō′sē-ă) [″ +
gnosis, knowledge]

hypergonadism (hī″pĕr-gō′năd-ĭzm)
[″ + *gone*, seed, + *-ismos*,
condition]

hyperguanidinemia (hī″pĕr-gwăn″ĭ-
dĭn-ē′mē-ă) [″ + Sp. *guano*, dung,
+ *haima*, blood]

hyperhedonia, hyperhedonism
(hī″pĕr-hē-dŏ′nē-ă, -hē′dŏn-ĭzm) [Gr.
hyper, over, above, excessive, +
hedone, pleasure, + *-ismos*, con-
dition]

Hyper-Hep

hyperhidrosis (hī″pĕr-hī-drō′sĭs)
[″ + *hidros*, sweat, + *osis*,
condition]

hyperhydration (hī″pĕr-hī-drā′shŭn)

hyperimmune (hī″pĕr-ĭm-mūn′)

hyperinflation (hī″pĕr-ĭn-flā′shŭn)

hyperinosemia (hī″pĕr-ī″nō-sē′mē-ă)
[″ + *inos*, fiber, + *haima*,
blood]

hyperinosis (hī″pĕr-ĭ-nō′sĭs) [″ +
inos, fiber, + *osis*, condition]

hyperinsulinism (hī″pĕr-ĭn′sū-lĭn-ĭzm)

[″ + L. *insula*, island, + Gr.
-ismos, condition]

hyperinvolution (hī″pĕr-ĭn″vō-lū′shŭn)
[″ + L. *involvere*, to enwrap]
h. uteri

hyperirritability (hī″pĕr-ĭr″ĭ-tă-bĭl′ĭ-tē)

hyperisotonic [″ + *isos*, equal,
+ *tonos*, act of stretching, tension,
tone]

hyperkalemia, hyperkaliemia (hī″
pĕr-kă-lē′mē-ă, -kăl″ē-ē′mē-ă)
[″ + L. *kalium*, potassium, +
Gr. *haima*, blood]

hyperkeratinization (hī″pĕr-kĕr″ă-
tĭn″ĭ-zā′shŭn) [″ + *keras*, horn]

hyperkeratomycosis (hī″pĕr-kĕr″ă-
tō-mī-kō′sĭs) [″ + ″ + *mykes*,
fungus, + *osis*, condition]

hyperkeratosis [″ + ″ +
osis, condition]
h. congenitalis
h., epidermolytic

hyperketonemia (hī″pĕr-kē″tō-
nē′mē-ă)

hyperketonuria (hī″pĕr-kē-tō-nūr′ē-ă)

hyperketosis (hī″pĕr-kē-tō′sĭs)

hyperkinesia, hyperkinesis (hī″pĕr-
kī-nē′zē-ă, -nē′sĭs) [Gr. *hyper*, over,
above, excessive, + *kinesis*, mo-
tion]

hyperlactation (hī″pĕr-lăk-tā′shŭn)
[″ + L. *lactare*, to suckle]

hyperlipemia (hī″pĕr-lĭp-ē′mē-ă)
[″ + *lipos*, fat, + *haima*,
blood]

hyperlipoproteinemia (hī″pĕr-lĭp″ō-
prō′tē-ĭn-ē′mē-ă)

hyperliposis (hī″pĕr-lĭ-pō′sĭs) [″ +
lipos, fat, + *osis*, condition]

hyperlithuria (hī″pĕr-lĭth-ū′rē-ă) [″ +
lithos, stone, + *ouron*, urine]

hypermastia (hī″pĕr-măs′tē-ă) [″ +
mastos, breast]

hypermature (hī″pĕr-mă-tūr′) [″ +
L. *maturus*, ripe]

hypermature cataract

hypermegasoma (hī″pĕr-mĕg″ă-
sō′mă) [″ + *megas*, large, +

soma, body]
hypermelanoses
hypermenorrhea (hī″pĕr-mĕn″ō-rē′ă)
[" + *men,* month, + *rhein,* to
flow]
hypermetabolic state (hī″pĕr-mĕt″ă-
bŏl′ĭk)
hypermetabolism (hī″pĕr-mĕ-tăb′ō-
lĭzm)
  h., extrathyroidal
hypermetaplasia (hī″pĕr-mĕt″ă-
plă′sē-ă) [" + *meta-,* after, +
plassein, to form]
hypermetria (hī″pĕr-mē′trē-ă) [Gr.
hyper, over, above, excessive, +
metron, measure]
hypermetrope (hī″pĕr-mĕt′rōp)
[" + " + *ops,* eye]
hypermetropia (hī″pĕr-mē-trō′pē-ă)
hypermetropic (hī″pĕr-mē-trŏp′ĭk)
hypermimia (hī″pĕr-mĭm′ē-ă) [" +
mimesis, imitation]
hypermnesia (hī″pĕrm-nē′zē-ă)
[" + *mneme,* memory]
hypermobility (hī″pĕr-mō-bĭl′ĭ-tē)
hypermorph (hī′pĕr-morf) [" +
morphe, form]
hypermotility (hī″pĕr-mō-tĭl′ĭ-tē)
[" + L. *motio,* motion]
hypermyatrophy (hī″pĕr-mī-ăt′rō-fē)
[" + *mys,* muscle, + *atrophia,*
atrophy]
hypermyesthesia (hī″pĕr-mī″ĕs-
thē′sē-ă) [" + " + *aisthesis,*
feeling, perception]
hypermyotonia (hī″pĕr-mī″ō-tō′nē-ă)
[" + " + *tonos,* act of stretching, tension, tone]
hypermyotrophy (hī″pĕr-mī-ŏt′rō-fē)
[" + " + *trophe,* nourishment]
hypernatremia (hī″pĕr-nă-trē′mē-ă)
[" + L. *natron,* sodium, + Gr.
haima, blood]
hyperneocytosis (hī″pĕr-nē″ō-sī-
tō′sĭs) [" + *neos,* new, +
kytos, cell, + *osis,* condition]
hypernephroma (hī″pĕr-nĕ-frō′mă)
[" + *nephros,* kidney, + *oma,*
tumor]

hyperneurotization (hī″pĕr-nū-rŏt″ĭ-
ză′shŭn) [" + *neuron,* nerve]
hypernitremia (hī″pĕr-nī-trē′mē-ă)
[" + *nitron,* niter, + *haima,*
blood]
hypernormal (hī″pĕr-nor′măl) [" +
L. *norma,* rule]
hypernormocytosis (hī″pĕr-nor″mō-
sī-tō′sĭs) [" + " + Gr. *kytos,*
cell, + *osis,* condition]
hypernutrition (hī″pĕr-nū-trĭsh′ŭn)
[" + L. *nutrire,* to nourish]
hyperonychia (hī″pĕr-ō-nĭk′ē-ă)
[" + *onyx,* nail]
hyperope (hī′pĕr-ōp) [" + *ops,*
eye]
hyperopia (hī″pĕr-ō′pē-ă) [" +
ops, eye]
  h., absolute
  h., axial
  h., facultative
  h., latent
  h., manifest
  h., relative
  h., total
hyperorchidism (hī″pĕr-or′kĭd-ĭzm)
[Gr. *hyper,* over, above, excessive,
+ *orchis,* testicle, + *-ismos,* con-
dition]
hyperorexia (hī″pĕr-ō-rĕks′ē-ă)
[" + *orexis,* appetite]
hyperorthocytosis (hī″pĕr-or″thō-sī-
tō′sĭs) [" + *orthos,* straight, +
kytos, cell, + *osis,* condition]
hyperosmia (hī″pĕr-ŏz′mē-ă) [" +
osme, smell]
**hyperosmolar hyperglycemic non-
ketotic coma**
hyperosmolarity (hī″pĕr-ŏz″mō-
lăr′ĭ-tē)
hyperostosis (hī″pĕr-ŏs-tō′sĭs) [" +
osteon, bone, + *osis,* condition]
  h., frontal internal
  h., infantile cortical
  h., Morgagni′s
hyperovaria [Gr. *hyper,* over, above,
excessive, + NL. *ovarium,* ovary]
hyperoxaluria (hī″pĕr-ŏk″să-lū′rē-ă)
  h., enteric

h., primary
hyperoxemia (hī″pĕr-ŏk-sē′mē-ă)
[″ + oxys, sharp, + haima,
blood]
hyperoxia (hī″pĕr-ŏk′sē-ă)
hyperpancreatism (hī″pĕr-păn′krē-
ă-tĭzm) [″ + pankreas, pancreas,
+ -ismos, condition]
hyperparasitism (hī″pĕr-păr′ă-
sī″tĭzm)
hyperparathyroidism (hī″pĕr-păr″ă-
thī′roy-dĭzm) [″ + para, alongside,
past, beyond, + thyreos, shield,
+ eidos, form, shape, + -ismos,
condition]
hyperpathia [″ + pathos, disease, suffering]
hyperpepsia (hī″pĕr-pĕp′sē-ă) [″ +
pepsis, digestion]
hyperpepsinia (hī″pĕr-pĕp-sĭn′ē-ă)
[″ + pepsis, digestion]
hyperperistalsis (hī″pĕr-pĕr″ĭ-stăl′sĭs)
[″ + peri, around, + stalsis,
contraction]
hyperphalangism (hī″pĕr-făl-ăn′jĭzm)
[″ + phalanx, line of battle, +
-ismos, condition]
hyperphasia (hī″pĕr-fā′zē-ă) [″ +
phasis, utterance]
hyperphenylalaninemia
(hī″pĕr-fĕn″ĭl-ăl″ă-nĭ-nē′mē-ă)
hyperphonia (hī″pĕr-fō′nē-ă) [″ +
phone, voice]
hyperphoria (hī″pĕr-fō′rē-ă) [″ +
phorein, to bear]
hyperphosphatasemia (hī″pĕr-
fŏs″fă-tă-sē′mē-ă)
hyperphosphatemia (hī″pĕr-fŏs″fă-
tē′mē-ă) [″ + L. phosphas, phosphate, + Gr. haima, blood]
hyperphosphaturia (hī″pĕr-fŏs-fă-
tū′rē-ă) [″ + ″ + Gr. ouron,
urine]
hyperphospheremia (hī″pĕr-fŏs-fĕr-
ē′mē-ă) [″ + ″ + Gr. haima,
blood]
hyperphrenia (hī″pĕr-frē′nē-ă) [Gr.
hyper, over, above, excessive, +
phren, mind]

hyperpiesia, hyperpiesis (hī″pĕr-pī-
ē′zē-ă, -pī′ĕ-sīs) [″ + piesis, pres-
sure]
hyperpietic (hī″pĕr-pī-ĕt′ĭk)
hyperpigmentation (hī″pĕr-pĭg″mĕn-
tā′shŭn)
hyperpituitarism (hī″pĕr-pĭ-tū′ĭ-tăr-
ĭsm) [″ + L. pituita, mucus, +
Gr. -ismos, condition]
hyperplasia (hī″pĕr-plā′zē-ă) [″ +
plassein, to form]
h., fibrous
h., lipoid
hyperplastic (hī″pĕr-plăs′tĭk)
hyperploidy (hī″pĕr-ploy′dē)
hyperpnea (hī″pĕrp′nē-ă) [″ +
pnoia, breath]
hyperpotassemia (hī″pĕr-pŏt″ă-
sē′mē-ă)
hyperpragic (hī″pĕr-prăj′ĭk) [″ +
praxis, action]
hyperpraxia (hī″pĕr-prăk′sē-ă)
hyperprolactinemia (hī″pĕr-prō-
lăk″tĭn-ē′mē-ă)
hyperprolinemia (hī″pĕr-prō″lĭ-
nē′mē-ă)
hyperproteinemia (hī″pĕr-prō″tē-ĭn-
ē′mē-ă) [″ + protos, first, +
haima, blood]
hyperproteinuria (hī″pĕr-prō″tē-ĭn-
ū′rē-ă) [″ + ″ + ouron, urine]
hyperpselaphesia (hī″pĕrp-sĕl″ă-
fē′zē-ă) [Gr. hyper, over, above, excessive, + pselaphesis, touch]
hyperptyalism (hī″pĕr-tī′ăl-ĭzm) [″ +
ptyalon, spittle]
hyperpyretic (hī″pĕr-pī-rĕt′ĭk)
hyperpyrexia (hī″pĕr-pī-rĕks′ē-ă)
[″ + pyressein, to be feverish]
h., malignant
hyperpyrexial (hī″pĕr-pī-rĕk′sē-ăl)
hyperreactive (hī″pĕr-rē-ăk′tĭv)
hyperreflexia (hī″pĕr-rē-flĕk′sē-ă)
[″ + L. reflexus, to bend, turn]
hyperresonance (hī″pĕr-rĕz′ō-năns)
[″ + L. resonare, to resound]
hypersalemia (hī″pĕr-săl-ē′mē-ă)
hypersalivation (hī″pĕr-săl″ĭ-vā′shŭn)
[″ + L. salivatio, salivation]

hypersecretion (hī″pĕr-sē-krē′shŭn) [″ + L. secretio, separation]
hypersensibility (hī″pĕr-sĕn″sī-bĭl′ĭ-tē) [″ + L. sensibilitas, sensibility]
hypersensitiveness (hī″pĕr-sĕn′sī-tĭv-nĕs) [″ + L. sensitivus, sensitive]
hypersensitivity (hī″pĕr-sĕn″sī-tĭv′ĭ-tē)
hypersensitization (hī″pĕr-sĕn″sī-tī-zā′shŭn)
hypersialosis (hī″pĕr-sī″ă-lō′sĭs)
hypersomnia (hī″pĕr-sŏm′nē-ă) [″ + L. somnus, sleep]
hypersplenism (hī″pĕr-splĕn′ĭzm)
hypersthenia (hī″pĕr-sthē′nē-ă) [Gr. hyper, over, above, excessive, + sthenos, strength]
hypersthenic (hī″pĕr-sthĕn′ĭk)
hypersthenuria (hī″pĕr-sthĕn-ū′rē-ă) [″ + sthenos, strength, + ouron, urine]
hypersusceptibility (hī″pĕr-sŭ-sĕp″tĭ-bĭl′ĭ-tē) [″ + L. suscipere, to take up, + -bilis, able]
hypersystole (hī″pĕr-sĭs′tō-lē) [″ + systole, contraction]
hypersystolic (hī″pĕr-sĭs-tŏl′ĭk)
hypertelorism (hī″pĕr-tĕl′or-ĭzm) [″ + telouros, distant]
hypertensinogen (hī″pĕr-tĕn-sĭn′ō-jĕn)
hypertension [″ + L. tensio, tension]
   h., benign
   h., essential
   h., Goldblatt
   h., malignant
   h., portal
   h., primary
   h., renal
hypertensive (hī″pĕr-tĕn′sĭv)
Hyper-Tet
hyperthecosis (hī″pĕr-thē-kō′sĭs)
hyperthelia (hī″pĕr-thē′lē-ă) [Gr. hyper, over, above, excessive, + thele, nipple]
hyperthermalgesia (hī″pĕr-thĕrm″ăl-jē′zē-ă) [″ + therme, heat, + algesis, sense of pain]

hyperthermia (hī″pĕr-thĕr′mē-ă) [″ + therme, heat]
   h., malignant
hyperthermoesthesia (hī″pĕr-thĕrm″ō-ĕs-thē′zē-ă) [″ + ″ + aisthesis, feeling, perception]
hyperthrombinemia (hī″pĕr-thrŏm″bĭn-ē′mē-ă) [″ + thrombos, clot, + haima, blood]
hyperthymia (hī″pĕr-thī′mē-ă) [″ + thymos, mind, spirit]
hyperthyroidism (hī″pĕr-thī′royd-ĭzm) [″ + thyreos, shield, + eidos, form, shape, + -ismos, condition]
hyperthyrosis (hī″pĕr-thī-rō′sĭs)
hyperthyroxinemia (hī″pĕr-thī-rŏk″sī-nē′mē-ă)
hypertonia (hī″pĕr-tō′nē-ă) [″ + tonos, act of stretching, tension, tone]
hypertonic (hī″pĕr-tŏn′ĭk)
hypertonicity (hī″pĕr-tŏn-ĭ′sĭ-tē)
hypertonus (hī″pĕr-tō′nŭs)
hypertoxicity (hī″pĕr-tŏk-sĭs′ĭ-tē) [″ + toxikon, poison]
hypertrichiasis (hī″pĕr-trĭk-ī′ă-sĭs) [″ + thrix, hair, + -iasis, state or condition of]
hypertrichophobia (hī″pĕr-trĭk″ō-fō′bē-ă) [″ + ″ + phobos, fear]
hypertrichophrydia (hī″pĕr-trĭk″ō-frĭd′ē-ă) [″ + ″ + ophrys, eyebrow]
hypertrichosis (hī″pĕr-trī-kō′sĭs) [″ + ″ + osis, condition]
hypertriglyceridemia (hī″pĕr-trī-glĭs″ĕr-ĭ-dē′mē-ă)
hypertrophia (hī″pĕr-trō′fē-ă) [Gr. hyper, over, above, excessive, + trophe, nourishment]
hypertrophic (hī″pĕr-trŏf′ĭk) [″ + trophe, nourishment]
hypertrophy (hī-pĕr′trŏ-fē) [″ + trophe, nourishment]
   h., adaptive
   h., benign prostatic
   h., cardiac
   h., compensatory

h., concentric
h., eccentric
h., false
h., Marie's
h., numerical
h., physiological
h., pseudomuscular
h., simple
h., true
h., ventricular
h., vicarious

hypertropia [Gr. hyper, over, above, excessive, + tropos, turning]

hyperuricemia (hī″pĕr-ū″rĭs-ē′mē-ă) [″ + ouron, urine, + haima, blood]

hyperuricuria (hī″pĕr-ū″rĭk-ū′rē-ă) [″ + ″ + ouron, urine]

hypervalinemia (hī″pĕr-văl″ĭn-ē′mē-ă)

hypervascular (hī″pĕr-văs′kū-lăr) [″ + L. vasculus, vessel]

hyperventilation (hī″pĕr-vĕn″tĭ-lā′shŭn)[″ + L. ventilatio, ventilation]

hyperviscosity (hī″pĕr-vĭs-kŏs′ĭ-tē) [″ + L. viscosus, gummy]

hypervitaminosis (hī″pĕr-vī″tă-mĭn-ō′sĭs) [″ + L. vita, life, + amine + Gr. osis, condition]

hypervolemia (hī″per-vŏl-ē′mē-ă) [″ + L. volumen, volume, + Gr. haima, blood]

hypesthesia (hī″pĕs-thē′zē-ă) [Gr. hypo, under, beneath, below, + aisthesis, feeling, perception]

hypha (hī′fă) [Gr. hyphe, web]

hyphedonia (hĭp″hĕ-dō′nē-ă) [Gr. hypo, under, beneath, below, + hedone, pleasure]

hyphema (hī-fē′mă) [Gr. hyphaimos, suffused with blood]

hyphidrosis (hĭp-hĭd-rō′sĭs) [Gr. hypo, under, beneath, below, + hidros, sweat]

Hyphomycetes (hī″fŏ-mī-sē′tēz) [Gr. hyphe, web, + mykes, fungus]

hypinosis (hĭp″ĭn-ō′sĭs) [Gr. hypo, under, beneath, below, + inos, fiber, + osis, condition]

hypnagogic (hĭp-nă-gŏj′ĭk) [Gr. hypnos, sleep, + agogos, leading]

hypnagogic state

hypnagogue (hĭp′nă-gŏg)

hypnalgia (hĭp-năl′jē-ă) [″ + algos, pain]

hypnic (hĭp′nĭk) [Gr. hypnos, sleep]

hypnoanalysis (hĭp″nō-ă-năl′ĭ-sĭs) [″ + analyein, to dissolve]

hypnoanesthesia (hĭp″nō-ăn″ĕs-thē′zē-ă)

hypnodontics (hĭp″nō-dŏn′tĭks)

hypnogenetic (hĭp″nō-jĕ-nĕt′ĭk) [″ + gennan, to produce]

hypnoidal (hĭp-noy′dăl) [″ + eidos, form, shape]

hypnoidization (hĭp″noy-dĭ-zā′shŭn) [″ + eidos, form, shape]

hypnolepsy (hĭp′nō-lĕp″sē) [″ + lepsis, seizure]

hypnology (hĭp-nŏl′ō-jē) [″ + logos, word, reason]

hypnonarcoanalysis (hĭp″nō-năr″kō-ă-năl′ĭ-sĭs)

hypnonarcosis (hĭp″nō-năr-kō′sĭs)

hypnophobia (hĭp″nō-fō′bē-ă) [″ + phobos, fear]

hypnopompic (hĭp″nō-pŏm′pĭk) [″ + pompe, procession]

hypnosis (hĭp-nō′sĭs) [″ + osis, condition]

hypnosophy (hĭp-nŏs′ō-fē) [″ + sophia, wisdom]

hypnotherapy (hĭp″nō-thĕr′ă-pē) [″ + therapeia, treatment]

hypnotic (hĭp-nŏt′ĭk) [Gr. hypnos, sleep]

hypnotics (hĭp-nŏt′ĭks) [Gr. hypnos, sleep]

hypnotism (hĭp′nō-tĭzm) [″ + -ismos, condition]

hypnotist (hĭp′nō-tĭst) [Gr. hypnos, sleep]

hypnotize (hĭp′nō-tīz)

hypnotoxin (hĭp″nō-tŏk′sĭn)

hypo, hypo-, hyp- (hī′pō) [Gr. hypo, under, beneath, below]

hypoacidity (hī″pō-ă-sĭd′ĭ-tē) [″ + L. *acidus*, sour]

hypoacusis (hī″pō-ă-kū′sĭs) [″ + *akousis*, hearing]

hypoadenia (hī″pō-ă-dē′nē-ă) [″ + *aden*, gland]

hypoadrenalism (hī″pō-ăd-rē′năl-ĭzm) [″ + L. *ad*, to, + *renalis*, pert. to kidney, + Gr. *-ismos*, condition]

hypoadrenocorticism (hī″pō-ă-drē″ nō-kor′tĭ-sĭzm)

hypoaffectivity (hī″pō-ăf′fĕk-tĭv′ĭ-tē)

hypoalbuminemia (hīpō-ăl-bū″mĭn-ē′ mē-ă)

hypoaldosteronism (hī″pō-ăl″dŏ-stĕr′ŏn-ĭzm)

hypoalimentation [″ + L. *alimentum*, nourishment]

hypoallergenic [″ + *allos*, other, + *ergon*, work]

hypoazoturia (hī″pō-ăz-ō-tū′rē-ă) [″ + L. *azotum*, nitrogen, + Gr. *ouron*, urine]

hypobaric (hī″pō-băr′ĭk) [″ + *baros*, weight]

hypobaropathy (hī″pō-băr-ŏp′ă-thē) [″ + ″ + *pathos*, disease, suffering]

hypoblast (hī′pō-blăst) [″ + *blastos*, germ]

hypoblastic (hī-pō-blăs′tĭk)

hypobulia (hī″pō-bū′lē-ă) [″ + *boule*, will]

hypocalcemia (hī″pō-kăl-sē′mē-ă) [″ + L. *calx*, lime, + Gr. *haima*, blood]

hypocalciuria (hī″pō-kăl″sē-ū′rē-ă)

hypocapnia (hī″pō-kăp′nē-ă) [Gr. *hypo*, under, beneath, below, + *kapnos*, smoke]

hypocarbia (hī″pō-kăr′bē-ă)

hypocellularity (hī″pō-sĕl″ū-lăr′ĭ-tē)

hypochloremia (hī″pō-klō-rē′mē-ă) [″ + *chloros*, green, + *haima*, blood]

hypochlorhydria (hī″pō-klor-hī′drē-ă) [″ + ″ + *hydor*, water]

hypochlorite salts

hypochlorite salts poisoning

hypochlorization (hī″pō-klō″rī-zā′shŭn)

hypochlorous acid

hypochloruria (hī″pō-klor-ū′rē-ă) [″ + *chloros*, green, + *ouron*, urine]

hypocholesteremia (hī″pō-kō-lĕs-tĕr-ē′mē-ă) [″ + *chole*, bile, + *stereos*, solid, + *haima*, blood]

hypochondria (hī″pō-kŏn′drē-ă) [″ + *chondros*, cartilage]

hypochondriac (hī″pō-kŏn′drē-ăk)

hypochondriac region

hypochondriacal (hī″pō-kŏn-drī′ă-kăl) [″ + *chondros*, cartilage]

hypochondrial reflex (hī″pō-kŏn′drē-ăl)

hypochondriasis (hī″pō-kŏn-drī′ă-sĭs) [″ + *chondros*, cartilage, + *-iasis*, state or condition of]

hypochondrium (hī″pō-kŏn′drē-ŭm)

hypochromasia (hī″pō-krō-mā′sē-ă) [″ + *chroma*, color]

hypochromatism (hī″pō-krō′mă-tĭzm) [″ + *chroma*, color]

hypochromatosis (hī″pō-krō-mă-tō′sĭs) [″ + ″ + *osis*, condition]

hypochromia (hī″pō-krō′mē-ă)

hypochromic (hī″pō-krōm′ĭk)

hypochylia (hī″pō-kī′lē-ă) [Gr. *hypo*, under, beneath, below, + *chylos*, juice]

hypocinesia (hī″pō-sĭn-ē′zē-ă) [″ + *kinesis*, motion]

hypocomplementemia (hī″pō-kŏm″ plĕ-mĕn-tē′mē-ă)

hypocondylar (hī″pō-kŏn′dĭ-lăr) [″ + *kondylos*, condyle]

hypocone (hī″pō-kōn) [″ + *konos*, cone]

hypoconid (hī″pō-kō′nĭd)

hypocorticism (hī″pō-kor′tĭ-sĭzm)

hypocrinism (hī″pō-krī′nĭzm) [″ + *krinein*, to separate, + *-ismos*, condition]

hypocupremia (hī″pō-kū-prē′mē-ă)

hypocyclosis (hī″pō-sī-klō′sĭs) [″ + *kyklos*, circle]

h., ciliary
h., lenticular
hypocystotomy (hī″pō-sĭs-tŏt′ō-mē)
[″ + *kystis,* a bladder, + *tome,* a cutting, slice]
hypocythemia (hī″pō-sī-thē′mē-ă)
[″ + *kytos,* cell, + *haima,* blood]
hypodactylia (hī″pō-dăk-tĭl′ē-ă)
[″ + *daktylos,* finger]
Hypoderma (hī″pō-dĕr′mă) [″ + *derma,* skin]
hypodermatoclysis (hī″pō-dĕr-mă-tŏk′lĭ-sĭs)
hypodermatomy (hī″pō-dĕr-măt′ō-mē) [″ + *derma,* skin, + *tome,* a cutting, slice]
hypodermiasis (hī″pō-dĕr-mī′ă-sĭs)
[″ + ″ + *-iasis,* state or condition of]
hypodermic (hī″pō-dĕr′mĭk) [″ + *derma,* skin]
h., intracutaneous
h., intramuscular
h., intraspinal
h., intravenous
h., subcutaneous
hypodermoclysis (hī″pō-dĕr-mŏk′lĭ-sĭs) [Gr. *hypo,* under, beneath, below, + *derma,* skin, + *klysis,* a washing]
hypodipsia (hī″pō-dĭp′sē-ă) [″ + *dipsa,* thirst]
hypodontia (hī″pō-dŏn′shē-ă)
hypodynamia (hī″pō-dĭ-nă′mē-ă)
[″ + *dynamis,* power]
hypoeccrisia (hī″pō-ĕk-krĭs′ē-ă) [″ + *ek,* out, + *krisis,* separation]
hypoeccritic (hī″pō-ĕk-krĭt′ĭk)
hypoendocrinism (hī″pō-ĕn-dŏk′rĭ-nĭzm) [″ + *endon,* within, + *krinein,* to separate, + *-ismos,* condition]
hypoendocrisia (hī″pō-ĕn″dō-krĭz′ē-ă)
hypoeosinophilia (hī″pō-ē″ō-sĭn″ō-fĭl′ē-ă) [Gr. *hypo,* under, beneath, below, + *eos,* dawn, + *philein,* to love]

hypoepinephria (hī″pō-ĕp″ĭ-nĕf′rē-ă)
[″ + *epi,* upon, + *nephros,* kidney]
hypoergasia (hī″pō-ĕr-gă′sē-ă)
[″ + *ergon,* work]
hypoergia (hī″pō-ĕr′jē-ă)
hypoergic (hī″pō-ĕr′jĭk)
hypoergy (hī″pō-ĕr′jē) [″ + *ergon,* work]
hypoesophoria (hī″pō-ĕs″ō-fō′rē-ă)
[″ + *eso,* inward, + *phorein,* to bear]
hypoesthesia (hī″pō-ĕs-thē′zē-ă)
[″ + *aisthesis,* feeling, perception]
hypoexophoria (hī″pō-ĕks-ō-fō′rē-ă)
[″ + *exo,* outward, + *phorein,* to bear]
hypoferremia (hī″pō-fĕ-rē′mē-ă)
hypofibrinogenemia (hī″pō-fī-brĭn″ō-jĕ-nē′mē-ă)
hypofunction (hī″pō-fŭnk′shŭn)
hypogalactia (hī″pō-gă-lăk′tē-ă)
[″ + *gala,* milk]
hypogammaglobulinemia (hī″pō-găm″ă-glŏb″ū-lĭ-nē′mē-ă)
h., acquired
h., congenital
hypogastric (hī″pō-găs′trĭk) [″ + *gaster,* belly]
hypogastric artery
hypogastric plexus
hypogastric region
hypogastrium (hī″pō-găs′trē-ŭm)
hypogenesis (hī″pō-jĕn′ĕ-sĭs) [Gr. *hypo,* under, beneath, below, + *genesis,* generation, birth]
hypogenitalism (hī″pō-jĕn′ĭ-tăl-ĭzm)
[″ + L. *genitalis,* to beget, + Gr. *-ismos,* condition]
hypogeusia (hī″pō-gū′sē-ă) [″ + *geusis,* taste]
h., idiopathic
hypoglossal (hī″pō-glŏs′ăl) [″ + *glossa,* tongue]
hypoglossal alternating hemiplegia
hypoglossal nerve
hypoglottis (hī″pō-glŏt′ĭs)
hypoglycemia (hī″pō-glī-sē′mē-ă)

[" + *glykys*, sweet, + *haima*, blood]

hypoglycemic (hī″pō-glī-sē′mĭk)

hypoglycemic agents, oral

hypoglycemic shock

hypoglycogenolysis (hī″pō-glī″kō-jĕn-ŏl′ĭ-sĭs) [Gr. *hypo*, under, beneath, below, + *glykys*, sweet, + *gennan*, to produce, + *lysis*, dissolution]

hypoglycorrhachia (hī″pō-glī″kō-rā′kē-ă) [" + " + *rhachis*, spine]

hypognathous (hī-pŏg′nă-thŭs) [" + *gnathos*, jaw]

hypogonadism (hī″pō-gō′năd-ĭzm) [" + *gone*, semen, + *-ismos*, condition]

hypogonadotropic (hī″pō-gŏn″ă-dō-trōp′ĭk)

hypohepatia (hī″pō-hĕ-pă′tē-ă) [" + *hepar*, liver]

hypohidrosis (hī″pō-hī-drō′sĭs) [" + *hidros*, sweat, + *osis*, condition]

hypohyloma (hī″pō-hī-lō′mă) [" + *hyle*, matter, + *oma*, tumor]

hypoinsulinism [" + L. *insula*, island, + Gr. *-ismos*, condition]

hypoisotonic (hī″pō-ī″sō-tŏn′ĭk) [" + *isos*, equal, + *tonos*, act of stretching, tension, tone]

hypokalemia (hī″pō-kă-lē′mē-ă) [" + Mod. L. *kalium*, potash, + Gr. *haima*, blood]

hypokalemic (hī″pō-kă-lē′mĭk)

hypokinesia (hī″pō-kī-nē′zē-ă) [" + *kinesis*, motion]

hypokinetic (hī″pō-kī-nĕt′ĭk)

hypolemmal (hī″pō-lĕm′ăl) [" + *lemma*, sheath]

hypoleydigism (hī″pō-lī′dĭg-ĭzm)

hypolipidemic (hī″pō-lĭp″ĭ-dē′mĭk)

hypoliposis (hī″pō-lĭ-pō′sĭs) [" + *lipos*, fat, + *osis*, condition]

hypologia (hī-pō-lō′jē-ă) [" + *logos*, word, reason]

hypolymphemia (hī″pō-lĭm-fē′mē-ă) [" + L. *lympha*, lymph, + Gr. *haima*, blood]

hypomagnesemia (hī″pō-măg″nĕ-sē′mē-ă)

hypomania (hī″pō-mā′nē-ă) [" + *mania*, madness]

hypomastia (hī-pō-măs′tē-ă) [" + *mastos*, breast]

hypomazia (hī″pō-mā′zē-ă) [" + *mazos*, breast]

hypomelanoses

hypomenorrhea (hī″pō-mĕn-ō-rē′ă) [" + *men*, month, + *rhein*, to flow]

hypomere (hī′pō-mēr) [" + *meros*, part]

hypometabolism (hī″pō-mĕ-tăb′ō-lĭzm) [" + *metabole*, change, + *-ismos*, condition]

hypometria (hī″pō-mē′trē-ă) [" + *metron*, measure]

hypometropia (hī″pō-mĕ-trōp′ē-ă) [" + " + *ops*, eye]

hypomnesia, hypomnesis (hī″pŏm-nē′zē-ă, -nē′sĭs) [" + *mnesis*, memory]

hypomorph (hī′pō-morf) [" + *morphe*, form]

hypomotility (hī″pō-mō-tĭl′ĭ-tē) [" + L. *motus*, moved]

hypomyotonia (hī″pō-mī″ō-tō′nē-ă) [" + *mys*, muscle, + *tonos*, act of stretching, tension, tone]

hypomyxia (hī″pō-mĭks′ē-ă) [" + *myxa*, mucus]

hyponanosoma (hī″pō-năn-ō-sō′mă) [" + *nanos*, dwarf, + *soma*, body]

hyponatremia (hī″pō-nă-trē′mē-ă) [" + L. *natron*, sodium, + Gr. *haima*, blood]

hyponeocytosis (hī″pō-nē″ō-sī-tō′sĭs) [" + *neos*, new, + *kytos*, cell, + *osis*, condition]

hyponoia (hī″pō-noy′ă) [" + *nous*, mind]

hyponychium (hī-pō-nĭk′ē-ŭm) [Gr. *hypo*, under, beneath, below, + *onyx*, nail]

hyponychon (hī-pŏn′ĭ-kŏn) [" + *onyx*, nail]

hypo-orthocytosis (hī″pō-or″thō-sī-tō′sĭs) [″ + *orthos,* straight, + *kytos,* cell, + *osis,* condition]

hypopallesthesia (hī″pō-păl″ĕs-thē′zē-ă) [″ + *pallein,* to shake, + *aisthesis,* feeling, perception]

hypopancreatism (hī″pō-păn′krē-ă-tĭzm) [″ + *pankreas,* pancreas, + *-ismos,* condition]

hypoparathyreosis (hī″pō-păr-ă-thī-rē-ō′sĭs) [″ + *para,* alongside, past, beyond, + *thyreos,* shield, + *osis,* condition]

hypoparathyroidism (hī″pō-păr-ă-thī′royd-ĭzm) [″ + ″ + ″ + *eidos,* form, shape, + *-ismos,* condition]

hypopepsia (hī″pō-pĕp′sē-ă) [″ + *pepsis,* digestion]

hypopepsinia (hī″pō-pĕp-sĭn′ē-ă)

hypoperistalsis (hī″pō-pĕr″ĭ-stăl′sĭs)

hypophalangism (hī″pō-fă-lăn′jĭzm)

hypopharynx (hī″pō-făr′ĭnks) [″ + *pharynx,* throat]

hypophonesis (hī″pō-fō-nē′sĭs) [″ + *phone,* voice]

hypophonia (hī″pō-fō′nē-ă)

hypophoria (hī″pō-fō′rē-ă) [″ + *phorein,* to bear]

hypophosphatasia (hī″pō-fŏs″fă-tā′zē-ă)

hypophosphatemia (hī″pō-fŏs″fă-tē′mē-ă) [″ + L. *phosphas,* phosphate, + Gr. *haima,* blood]

hypophosphaturia (hī″pō-fŏs″fă-tū′rē-ă) [″ + ″ + Gr. *ouron,* urine]

hypophrenia (hī″pō-frē′nē-ă) [″ + *phren,* mind]

hypophrenic (hī″pō-frĕn′ĭk) [″ + *phren,* diaphragm, mind]

hypophyseal (hī″pō-fĭz′ē-ăl) [″ + *physis,* growth]

hypophysectomy (hī-pŏf″ĭ-sĕk′tō-mē) [″ + ″ + *ektome,* excision]

hypophyseoportal (hī″pō-fĭz″ē-ō-por′tăl)

hypophyseoprivic (hī″pō-fĭz″ē-ō-prĭv′ĭk)

hypophysis (hī-pŏf′ĭ-sĭs) [Gr., an undergrowth]
  h. cerebri
  h. sicca

hypophysitis (hī-pŏf″ĭ-sī′tĭs) [Gr. *hypo,* under, beneath, below, + *physis,* growth, + *itis,* inflammation]

hypopiesis (hī″pō-pī-ē′sĭs) [″ + *piesis,* pressure]

hypopigmentation (hī″pō-pĭg″mĕn-tā′shŭn)

hypopinealism (hī″pō-pĭn′ē-ăl-ĭzm) [″ + L. *pineus,* of the pine, + Gr. *-ismos,* condition]

hypopituitarism (hī″pō-pĭ-tū′ĭ-tă-rĭzm) [″ + L. *pituita,* mucus, + Gr. *-ismos,* condition]

hypoplasia (hī″pō-plā′zē-ă) [″ + *plasis,* formation]

hypopnea (hī″pŏp-nē′ă) [″ + *pnoia,* breath]

hypoporosis (hī″pō-pō-rō′sĭs) [″ + *poros,* passage, + *osis,* condition]

hypoposia (hī″pō-pō′zē-ă) [″ + *posis,* drinking]

hypopotassemia (hī″pō-pō″tăs-sē′mē-ă) [″ + *potassium* + Gr. *haima,* blood]

hypopraxia (hī″pō-prăk′sē-ă) [″ + *praxis,* action]

hypoproteinemia (hī″pō-prō″tē-ĭn-ē′mē-ă) [″ + *protos,* first, + *haima,* blood]

hypoproteinosis (hī″pō-prō″tē-ĭ-nō′sĭs)

hypoprothrombinemia (hī″pō-prō-thrŏm″bĭn-ē′mē-ă) [″ + L. *pro,* for, + Gr. *thrombos,* clot, + *haima,* blood]

hypopselaphesia (hī″pŏp-sĕl-ă-fē′zē-ă) [″ + *pselaphesis,* touch]

hypoptyalism (hī″pō-tī′ăl-ĭzm) [″ + *ptyalon,* saliva, + *-ismos,* condition]

hypopyon (hī-pō′pē-ŏn) [″ + *pyon,* pus]

hyporeactive (hī″pō-rē-ăk′tĭv)

hyporeflexia [″ + L. *reflexus,* to bend, turn]

hyposalemia (hī″pō-săl-ē′mē-ă) [″ + L. *sal*, salt, + Gr. *haima*, blood]
hyposalivation (hī″pō-săl″ĭ-vā′shŭn)
hyposarca (hī″pō-săr′kă) [″ + *sarx*, flesh]
hyposcleral (hī″pō-sklē′răl)
hyposecretion (hī″pō-sē-krē′shŭn)
hyposensitive (hī″pō-sĕn′sĭ-tĭv) [″ + L. *sentire*, to feel]
hyposensitization (hī″pō-sĕn″sĭ-tĭ-zā′shŭn)
hyposialadenitis (hī″pō-sī″ăl-ăd-ē-nī′tĭs) [Gr. *hypo*, under, beneath, below, + *sialon*, saliva, + *aden*, gland, + *itis*, inflammation]
hyposmia (hī-pŏz′mē-ă) [″ + *osme*, smell]
hyposmolarity (hī-pŏz″mō-lăr′ĭ-tē)
hyposomnia (hī″pō-sŏm′nē-ă)
hypospadia, hypospadias (hī″pō-spā′dē-ă, -ăs) [″ + *span*, to draw]
hyposphresia (hī″pŏs-frē′sē-ă) [″ + *osphresis*, smell]
hypostasis (hī″pŏs′tă-sĭs) [″ + *stasis*, standing still]
hypostatic (hī″pō-stăt′ĭk) [″ + *statikos*, standing]
hypostatic pneumonia
hyposteatolysis (hī″pō-stē-ă-tŏl′ĭ-sĭs) [″ + *stear*, fat, + *lysis*, dissolution]
hyposthenia (hī″pŏs-thē′nē-ă) [″ + *sthenos*, strength]
hypostheniant (hī″pŏs-thē′nē-ănt)
hyposthenic (hī-pŏs-thĕn′ĭk)
hyposthenuria (hī″pŏs-thĕn-ū′rē-ă) [″ + *sthenos*, strength, + *ouron*, urine]
   h., tubular
hypostomia (hī″pō-stō′mē-ă) [″ + *stoma*, mouth, opening]
hypostosis (hĭp″ŏs-tō′sĭs) [″ + *osteon*, bone, + *osis*, condition]
hypostypsis (hī″pō-stĭp′sĭs) [″ + *stypsis*, a contracting]
hypostyptic (hī″pō-stĭp′tĭk)
hyposynergia (hī″pō-sĭn-ĕr′jē-ă)

[″ + *syn*, together, + *ergon*, work]
hypotaxia (hī″pō-tăks′ē-ă) [″ + *taxis*, arrangement]
hypotelorism (hī″pō-tĕl′ō-rĭzm) [″ + *telouros*, distant]
hypotension [″ + L. *tensio*, tension]
   h., orthostatic
hypotensive
hypothalamus (hī″pō-thăl′ă-mŭs) [″ + *thalamos*, chamber]
hypothenar (hī-pōth′ē-năr) [″ + *thenar*, palm]
hypothenar eminence
hypothermal (hī″pō-thĕr′măl) [″ + *therme*, heat]
hypothermia (hī″pō-thĕr′mē-ă)
hypothermia blanket
hypothesis (hī-pŏth′ē-sĭs) [″ + *thesis*, a placing]
hypothrombinemia (hī″pō-thrŏm-bĭn-ē′mē-ă) [″ + *thrombos*, clot, + *haima*, blood]
hypothymia (hī″pō-thī′mē-ă) [″ + *thymos*, mind, spirit]
hypothymism (hī″pō-thī′mĭzm) [″ + *thymos*, thymus gland, + *-ismos*, condition]
hypothyroid (hī″pō-thī′royd) [″ + *thyreos*, shield, + *eidos*, form, shape]
hypothyroidism (hī″pō-thī′royd-ĭzm)
hypotonia (hī″pō-tō′nē-ă) [″ + *tonos*, act of stretching, tension, tone]
hypotonic (hī-pō-tŏn′ĭk)
hypotoxicity (hī″pō-tŏks-ĭs′ĭ-tē) [″ + *toxikon*, poison]
hypotrichosis (hī″pō-trī-kō′sĭs) [″ + *thrix*, hair, + *osis*, condition]
hypotrophy (hī-pŏt′rŏ-fē) [″ + *trophe*, nourishment]
hypotropia (hī″pō-trō′pē-ă) [″ + *trope*, a turning]
hypotympanotomy (hī″pō-tĭm″pă-nŏt′ō-mē)
hypotympanum (hī″pō-tĭm′pă-nŭm)
hypouricuria (hī″pō-ū-rĭ-kū′rē-ă)

[" + *ouron*, urine, + *ouron*, urine]

hypourocrinia (hī″po-ūr″ō-krīn′ē-ă) [" + " + *krinein*, to separate]

hypovaria (hī″pō-vā′rē-ă) [" + NL. *ovarium*, ovary]

hypovenosity (hī″pō-vĕn-ŏs′ĭ-tē) [" + L. *venosus*, pert. to a vein]

hypoventilation (hī″pō-vĕn″tĭ-lā′shŭn) [" + L. *ventilatio*, ventilation]

hypovitaminosis (hī″pō-vī″tă-mĭn-ō′sĭs) [" + L. *vita*, life, + *amine* + Gr. *osis*, condition]

hypovolemia (hī″pō-vō-lē′mē-ă) [" + L. *volumen*, volume]

hypovolia (hī″pō-vō′lē-ă)

hypoxanthine (hī″pō-zăn′thĭn, -thēn) [" + *xanthos*, yellow]

hypoxemia (hī-pŏks-ē′mē-ă) [" + *oxygen* + *haima*, blood]

hypoxia (hī″pŏks′ē-ă)

hypoxic lap swimming

HypRho-D

hypsarrhythmia (hĭp″săr-ĭth′mē-ă) [Gr. *hypsi*, high, + *a-*, not, + *rhythmos*, rhythm]

hypsibrachycephalic (hĭp″sē-brăk″ē-sĕ-făl′ĭk) [Gr. *hypsi*, high, + *brachys*, broad, + *kephale*, head]

hypsicephalic (hĭp″sē-sĕ-făl′ĭk) [" + *kephale*, head]

hypsicephaly (hĭp-sē-sĕf′ă-lē)

hypsiconchous (hĭp″sē-kŏng′kŭs) [" + *konche*, shell]

hypsiloid (hĭp′sĭ-loyd) [Gr. *upsilon*, U or Y, + *eidos*, form, shape]

hypsiloid ligament

hypsistenocephalic (hĭp″sē-stĕn″ō-sĕ-făl′ĭk) [" + *stenos*, narrow, + *kephale*, head]

hypsocephalous (hĭp″sō-sĕf′ă-lŭs) [Gr. *hypsos*, height, + *kephale*, head]

hypsokinesis (hĭp″sō-kĭ-nē′sĭs) [" + *kinesis*, motion]

hypsophobia (hĭp″sō-fō′bē-ă) [" + *phobos*, fear]

hypurgia (hī-pŭr′jē-ă) [Gr. *hypourgia*, help]

hysteralgia (hĭs-tĕr-ăl′jē-ă) [Gr. *hystera*, womb, + *algos*, pain]

hysteratresia (hĭs″tĕr-ă-trē′zē-ă) [" + *a-*, not, + *tresis*, perforation]

hysterectomy (hĭs-tĕr-ĕk′tō-mē) [" + *ektome*, excision]
  h., abdominal
  h., cesarean
  h., Porro
  h., radical
  h., subtotal
  h., supracervical
  h., supravaginal
  h., total
  h., vaginal

hysteresis (hĭs″tĕr-ē′sĭs) [Gr., a coming too late]

hystereurynter (hĭs″tĕr-ū-rĭn′tĕr) [Gr. *hystera*, womb, + *eurynein*, to stretch]

hysteria (hĭs-tĕ′rē-ă) [Gr. *hystera*, womb]
  h., anxiety
  h., major
  h., mass
  h., minor

hysteriac (hĭs-tĕr′ē-ăk) [Gr. *hystera*, womb]

hysteric, hysterical

hysteric ataxia

hysteric chorea

hystericoneuralgic (hĭs-tĕr″ĭk-ō-nū-răl′jĭk) [" + *neuron*, nerve, + *algos*, pain]

hysteritis (hĭs-tĕr-ī′tĭs) [" + *itis*, inflammation]

hystero-, hyster- [Gr. *hystera*, womb]

hysterobubonocele (hĭs″tĕr-ō-bū-bŏn′ō-sēl) [" + *boubon*, groin, + *kele*, tumor, swelling]

hysterocele (hĭs′tĕr-ō-sēl) [" + *kele*, tumor, swelling]

hysterocleisis (hĭs″tĕr-ō-klī′sĭs) [" + *kleisis*, closure]

hysterocystocleisis (hĭs″tĕr-ō-sĭs″tō-klī′sĭs) [" + *kystis*, a bladder, +

kleisis, closure]

hysterodynia   (hĭs″tĕr-ō-dĭn′ē-ă)
[″ + *odyne,* pain]

hysterogastrorrhaphy   (hĭs″tĕr-ō-
găs-tror′ă-fē) [″ + *gaster,* belly,
+ *rhaphe,* seam]

hysterogenic (hĭs″tĕr-ō-jĕn′ĭk) [″ +
gennan, to produce]

hysterogram (hĭs′tĕr-ō-grăm)

hysterography   (hĭs″tĕ-rŏg′ră-fē)
[″ + *graphein,* to write]

hysteroid (hĭs′tĕr-oyd) [″ + *eidos,*
form, shape]

hysterolaparotomy (hĭs″tĕr-ō-lăp″ă-
rŏt′ō-mē) [″ + *lapara,* flank, +
tome, a cutting, slice]

hysterolith (hĭs′tĕr-ō-lĭth) [″ +
lithos, stone]

hysterology (hĭs-tĕr-ŏl′ō-jē) [″ +
logos, word, reason]

hysterolysis (hĭs″tĕr-ŏl′ĭ-sĭs) [″ +
lysis, dissolution]

hysteromania   (hĭs″tĕr-ō-mā′nē-ă)
[″ + *mania,* madness]

hysterometer (hĭs″tĕ-rŏm′ĕ-tĕr) [″ +
metron, measure]

hysterometry (hĭs″tĕ-rŏm′ĕ-trē)

hysteromyoma   (hĭs″tĕr-ō-mī-ō′mă)
[Gr. *hystera,* womb, + *mys,* muscle, + *oma,* tumor]

hysteromyomectomy   (hĭs″tĕr-ō-
mī″ō-mĕk′tō-mē) [″ + ″ + *ektome,* excision]

hysteromyotomy (hĭs″tĕr-ō-mī-ŏt′ō-
mē) [″ + ″ + *tome,* a cutting,
slice]

hystero-oophorectomy   (hĭs″tĕr-ō-
ō″ō-for-ĕk′tō-mē) [″ + NL. oo-
phoron, ovary, + Gr. *ektome,* ex-
cision]

hysteropathy (hĭs″tĕr-ŏp′ă-thē) [″ +
pathos, disease, suffering]

hysteropexy (hĭs′tĕr-ō-pĕk″sē) [″ +
pexis, fixation]

hysteropia (hĭs″tĕr-ō′pē-ă) [″ +
ops, eye]

hysteropsychosis (hĭs″tĕr-ō-sī-kō′sĭs)
[″ + *psyche,* mind, + *osis,*

condition]

hysteroptosia,   hysteroptosis
(hĭs″tĕr-ŏp-tō′sē-ă, -sĭs) [″ + *ptosis,*
fall, falling]

hysterorrhaphy   (hĭs-tĕr-or′ă-fē)
[″ + *rhaphe,* seam]

hysterorrhexis   (hĭs″tĕr-ō-rĕk′sĭs)
[″ + *rhexis,* rupture]

hysterosalpingectomy   (hĭs″tĕr-ō-
săl″pĭn-jĕk′tō-mē) [″ + *salpinx,*
tube, + *ektome,* excision]

hysterosalpingography   (hĭs″tĕr-ō-
săl″pĭn-gŏg′ră-fē) [″ + ″ +
graphein, to write]

hysterosalpingo-oophorectomy
(hĭs″tĕr-ō-săl-pĭng″gō-ō″ō-for-ĕk′tō-
mē) [″ + ″ + NL. *oophoron,*
ovary, + Gr. *ektome,* excision]

hysterosalpingostomy   (hĭs″tĕr-ō-
săl″pĭng-ŏs′tō-mē) [″ + ″ +
stoma, mouth, opening]

hysteroscope (hĭs′tĕr-ō-skōp) [″ +
skopein, to examine]

hysteroscopy (hĭs″tĕr-ŏs′kō-pē)

hysterospasm (hĭs′tĕr-ō-spăzm″) [Gr.
hystera, womb, + *spasmos,* a con-
vulsion]

hysterostomatocleisis   (hĭs″tĕr-ō-
stō″mă-tō-klī′sĭs) [″ + *stoma,*
mouth, opening, + *kleisis,* closure]

hysterostomatomy (hĭs″tĕr-ō-stō-
măt′ō-mē) [″ + ″ + *tome,* a
cutting, slice]

hysterotome (hĭs′tĕr-ō-tōm) [″ +
tome, a cutting, slice]

hysterotomy (hĭs-tĕr-ŏt′ō-mē)

hysterotrachelectomy   (hĭs″tĕr-ō-
trā″kĕl-ĕk′tō-mē) [″ + *trachelos,*
neck, + *ektome,* excision]

hysterotracheloplasty   (hĭs″tĕr-ō-
trā′kĕl-lō-plăs″tē) [″ + ″ +
plassein, to form]

hysterotrachelorrhaphy   (hĭs″tĕr-ō-
trā″kĕl-or′ă-fē) [″ + ″ +
rhaphe, seam]

hysterotrachelotomy   (hĭs″tĕr-ō-
trā″kĕl-ŏt′ō-mē) [″ + ″ +
tome, a cutting, slice]

hysterotraumatic (hĭs″tĕr-ō-traw-mǎt′ĭk) [″ + *trauma*, wound]

hysterotubography (hĭs″tĕr-ō-tū-bŏg′rǎ-fē)

hysterovagino-enterocele (hĭs″tĕr-ō-vǎj″ĭn-ō-ĕn′tĕr-ō-sēl) [″ + L. va-gina, sheath, + Gr. *enteron*, intestine, + *kele*, tumor, swelling]

Hytakerol

Hz *hertz*

HZV *herpes zoster virus*

I

I *iodine; quantity of electricity expressed in amperes*

¹³¹I *radioactive iodine*

¹³²I *radioactive iodine*

i *optically inactive*

-ia *condition*

IABC *intra-aortic balloon counterpulsation*

IABP *intra-aortic balloon pump*

I and O *intake and output*

ianthinopsia (ī-ăn″thī-nŏp′sē-ă) [Gr. *ianthinos*, violet colored, + *opsis*, sight, appearance, vision]

-iasis [Gr., same as; the state or condition of]

iatraliptics (ī″ă-tră-lĭp′tĭks) [Gr. *iatreia*, cure, + *aleiphein*, to anoint]

iatric (ī-ăt′rĭk) [Gr. *iatrikos*, medical]

iatro- [Gr. *iatros*, physician]

iatrochemistry (ī-ăt″rō-kĕm′ĭs-trē) [″ + *chemeia*, chemistry]

iatrogenic disorder (ī″ăt-rō-jĕn′ĭk) [″ + *gennan*, to produce]

iatrogeny (ī″ă-trŏj′ĕ-nē)

iatrology (ī″ă-trŏl′ō-jē) [″ + *logos*, word, reason]

iatrotechniques (ī-ăt″rō-tĕk-nēks′) [″ + *techne*, art]

I band *isotropic light band*

IBC *iron-binding capacity*

ibuprofen

IBW *ideal body weight*

IC *inspiratory capacity*

ICD *intrauterine contraceptive device; International Classification of Diseases*

ice (īs) [AS. *is*]
    i., dry

ice bag

iceberg phenomenon

Iceland disease

Iceland moss

ice treatment

ichnogram (ĭk′nō-grăm) [Gr. *ichnos*, footstep, + *gramma*, letter, piece of writing]

ichor (ī′kor) [Gr. *ichor*, serum]

ichoremia (ī″kor-ē′mē-ă) [″ + *haima*, blood]

ichorous (ī′kor-ŭs) [Gr. *ichor*, serum]

ichthammol (ĭk′thă-mŏl)

ichthyism, ichthyismus (ĭk′thē-īzm, ĭk″thē-īz′mŭs) [Gr. *ichthys*, fish, + *-ismos*, condition]

ichthyo- [Gr. *ichthys*, fish]

ichthyoacanthotoxism (ĭk″thē-ō-ă-kăn″thō-tŏk′sĭzm) [″ + *akantha*, thorn, + *toxikon*, poison, + *-ismos*, condition]

ichthyohemotoxin (ĭk″thē-ō-hē″mō-tŏk′sĭn) [″ + *haima*, blood, + *toxikon*, poison]

ichthyoid (ĭk′thē-oyd) [″ + *eidos*, form, shape]

ichthyology (ĭk″thē-ŏl′ō-jē) [″ + *logos*, word, reason]

ichthyootoxin (ĭk″thē-ō″ō-tŏk′sĭn) [″ + *oon*, egg, + *toxikon*, poison]

ichthyophagous (ĭk″thē-ŏf′ă-gŭs) [″ + *phagein*, to eat]

ichthyophobia (ĭk-thē-ō-fō′bē-ă) [″ + *phobos*, fear]

ichthyosarcotoxin (ĭk″thē-ō-săr″kō-tŏk′sĭn) [″ + *sarx*, flesh, + *toxikon*, poison]

ichthyosis (ĭk″thē-ō′sĭs) [″ + *osis*, condition]
    i. congenita
    i. fetalis
    i. hystrix
    i., lamellar, of newborn
    i. vulgaris

ichthyotic (ĭk″thē-ŏt′ĭk) [Gr. *ichthys*, fish]
ichthyotoxicology (ĭk″thē-ō-tŏk″sĭ-kŏl′ō-jē) [″ + *toxikon*, poison, + *logos*, word, reason]
ichthyotoxin (ĭk″thē-ō-tŏk′sĭn) [″ + *toxikon*, poison]
icing
ICN *International Council of Nurses*
iconolagny (ī-kŏn″ō-lăg′nē) [Gr. *eikon*, image, + *lagneia*, lewdness]
icosa- (ī-kō′să) [Gr. *eikosi*, twenty]
ICS *intercostal space*
I.C.S. *International College of Surgeons*
ICSH *interstitial cell-stimulating hormone*
ictal (ĭk′tăl) [L. *ictus*, a blow or stroke]
icteric (ĭk-tĕr′ĭk) [Gr. *ikteros*, jaundice]
icteritious (ĭk-tĕr-ĭsh′ŭs)
icteroanemia (ĭk″tĕr-ō-ă-nē′mē-ă) [″ + *an-*, not, + *haima*, blood]
icterogenic, icterogenous (ĭk″tĕr-ō-jĕn′ĭk, -ŏj′ĕn-ŭs) [″ + *gennan*, to produce]
icterohematuric (ĭk″tĕr-ō-hēm″ă-tū′rĭk) [″ + *haima*, blood, + *ouron*, urine]
icterohemoglobinuria (ĭk″tĕr-ō-hē″mō-glō″bĭ-nū′rē-ă) [″ + *haima*, blood, + L. *globus*, globe, + Gr. *ouron*, urine]
icterohepatitis (ĭk″tĕr-ō-hĕp-ă-tī′tĭs) [″ + *hepar*, liver, + *itis*, inflammation]
icteroid (ĭk′tĕr-oyd) [″ + *eidos*, form, shape]
icterus (ĭk′tĕr-ŭs) [Gr. *ikteros*, jaundice]
   i. gravis neonatorum
   i., hemolytic
   i. neonatorum
   i., nonobstructive
   i., obstructive
ictus [L., stroke]
   i. cordis
   i. epilepticus
   i. sanguinis
   i. solis
ICU *intensive care unit*
ID *identification; infective dose; inside di-*

ameter; intradermal
ID₅₀
id [L. *id*, it; later translators of Freud's writings believed that the word *es* should have been translated to *it* and not to id]
id. L. *idem*, the same
-id [Gr. *eidos*, form, shape]
IDDM *insulin-dependent diabetes mellitus*
idea [Gr., form]
   i., autochthonous
   i., compulsive
   i., dominant
   i., fixed
   i.'s, flight of
   i. of reference
ideal [L. *idea*, model]
ideation (ī-dē-ā′shŭn)
idée fixe (ē-dā′ fĕks′) [Fr.]
identical [L. *identicus*, the same]
identification [″ + *facere*, to make]
   i., dental
identification, palm and sole system of
identity (ī-dĕn′tĭ-tē)
   i., ego
   i., gender
ideo- [Gr. *idea*, form]
ideogenous, ideogenetic (ĭd-ē-ŏj′ĕn-ŭs, -ō-jē-nĕt′ĭk) [″ + *gennan*, to produce]
ideology (ĭdē-ŏl′ō-jē) [″ + *logos*, word, reason]
ideomotion (ī″dē-ō-mō′shŭn) [″ + L. *motus*, moving]
ideomotor (ī″dē-ō-mō′tor)
ideomuscular (ī″dē-ō-mŭs′kū-lăr) [″ + L. *musculus*, muscle]
ideophrenic (ĭd″ē-ō-frĕn′ĭk) [″ + *phrenitikos*, insane]
ideoplastia (ĭd-ē-ō-plăs′tē-ă) [″ + *plassein*, to form]
ideovascular (ĭd″ē-ō-văs′kū-lăr)
idio- [Gr. *idios*, own]
idiochromosome (ĭd″ē-ō-krō′mō-sōm) [″ + *chroma*, color, + *soma*,

body]

idiocrasy (ĭd″ē-ŏk′ră-sē) [″ + krasis, temperament]

idiocratic (ĭd″ē-ō-krăt′ĭk)

idiocy [Gr. idiotes, ignorant person]
   i., complete
   i., cretinoid
   i., epileptic
   i., genetous
   i., hemiplegic
   i., hydrocephalic
   i., intrasocial
   i., microcephalic
   i., paralytic
   i., paraplegic
   i., sensorial
   i., traumatic

idiogamist (ĭd″ē-ŏg′ă-mĭst) [Gr. idios, own, + gamos, marriage]

idiogenesis (ĭd″ē-ō-jĕn′ĕ-sĭs) [″ + genesis, generation, birth]

idioglossia (ĭd″ē-ō-glŏs′ē-ă) [″ + glossa, tongue]

idiogram (ĭd′ē-ō-grăm″) [″ + gramma, letter, piece of writing]

idioisolysin (ĭd″ē-ō-ī-sŏl′ĭ-sĭn) [″ + isos, equal, + lysis, dissolution]

idiolalia (ĭd″ē-ō-lā′lē-ă) [″ + lalia, chatter, prattle]

idiolysin (ĭd″ē-ŏl′ĭ-sĭn) [″ + lysis, dissolution]

idiometritis (ĭd″ē-ō-mĕ-trī′tĭs) [″ + metra, uterus, + itis, inflammation]

idiomiasma (ĭd″ē-ō-mī-ăz′mă) [″ + miasma, stain]

idiomuscular (ĭd″ē-ō-mŭs′kū-lăr) [″ + L. musculus, a muscle]

idiomuscular contraction

idiopathic (ĭd″ē-ō-păth′ĭk) [″ + pathos, disease, suffering]

idiopathic pulmonary fibrosis

idiopathy (ĭd-ē-ŏp′ă-thē)

idiophrenic (ĭd″ē-ō-frĕn′ĭk) [″ + phren, mind]

idiopsychologic (ĭd″ē-ō-sī″kō-lŏj′ĭk) [″ + psyche, mind, + logos, word, reason]

idioreflex (ĭd″ē-ō-rē′flĕks) [″ + L.

reflexus, to bend, turn]

idiospasm (ĭd′ē-ō-spăzm) [″ + spasmos, a convulsion]

idiosyncrasy (ĭd″ē-ō-sĭn′kră-sē) [″ + syn, together, + krasis, mixture]

idiosyncrasy of effect

idiosyncrasy to a drug

idiosyncratic (ĭd″ē-ō-sĭn-krăt′ĭk)

idiot [Gr. idiotes, ignorant person]

idiotic

idiotrophic (ĭd″ē-ō-trŏf′ĭk) [Gr. idios, own, + trophe, nourishment]

idiotropic (ĭd″ē-ō-trŏp′ĭk) [″ + trope, a turning]

idiotropic type

idiot-savant (ēd-jō′să-vănt) [Fr., learned idiot]

idiotype

idiotypic (ĭd″ē-ō-tĭp′ĭk) [Gr. idios, own, + typos, type]

idiovariation (ĭd″ē-ō-văr″ē-ā′shŭn) [″ + L. variare, to vary]

idioventricular (ĭd″ē-ō-vĕn-trĭk′ū-lăr) [″ + L. ventriculus, little belly]

idoxuridine (ī-dŏks-ūr′ĭ-dēn)

IDU 5-iodo-2′deoxyuridine; idoxuridine

IgA *immunoglobulin gamma A*

IgD *immunoglobulin gamma D*

IgE *immunoglobulin gamma E*

IgG *immunoglobulin gamma G*

IgM *immunoglobulin gamma M*

ignatia (ĭg-nā′shē-ă) [L.]

igniextirpation (ĭg″nē-ĕks″tĭr-pā′shŭn) [L. ignis, fire, + exstirpare, to root out]

ignioperation (ĭg″nē-ŏp″ĕr-ā′shŭn) [″ + operatio, a working]

ignipuncture (ĭg″nē-pŭnk′chūr) [″ + punctura, prick]

ignis (ĭg′nĭs) [L., fire]
   i. infernalis
   i. sacer
   i. Sancti Antonii

I.H. *infectious hepatitis*

ILD *interstitial lung disorders*

ilea

ileac (ĭl′ē-ăk)

ileal (ĭl′ē-ăl)

ileal bypass

ileal conduit

ileectomy (ĭl″ē-ĕk′tō-mē) [L. *ileum*, ileum, + Gr. *ektome*, excision]

ileitis (ĭl″ē-ī′tĭs) [″ + Gr. *itis*, inflammation]
   i., regional

ileo- (ĭl″ē-ō) [L. *ileum*]

ileocecal (ĭl″ē-ō-sē′kăl) [″ + *caecus*, blind]

ileocecal valve

ileocecostomy (ĭl″ē-ō-sē-kŏs′tō-mē) [″ + ″ + Gr. *stoma*, mouth, opening]

ileocecum (ĭl″ē-ō-sē′kŭm)

ileocolic (ĭl″ē-ō-kŏl′ĭk) [″ + Gr. *kolon*, colon]

ileocolitis (ĭl″ē-ō-kō-lī′tĭs) [″ + ″ + *itis*, inflammation]

ileocolostomy (ĭl″ē-ō-kō-lŏs′tō-mē) [″ + ″ + *stoma*, mouth, opening]

ileocolotomy (ĭl″ē-ō-kō-lŏt′ō-mē) [″ + ″ + *tome*, a cutting, slice]

ileocystoplasty (ĭl″ē-ō-sĭst′ō-plăs″tē) [″ + Gr. *kystis*, bladder, + *plassein*, to form]

ileocystostomy (ĭl″ē-ō-sĭs-tŏs′tō-mē) [″ + ″ + *stoma*, mouth, opening]

ileoileostomy (ĭl″ē-ō-ĭl″ē-ŏs′tō-mē) [″ + *ileum*, small intestine, + Gr. *stoma*, mouth, opening]

ileoproctostomy (ĭl″ē-ō-prŏk-tŏs′tō-mē) [″ + Gr. *proktos*, rectum, + *stoma*, mouth, opening]

ileorectal (ĭl″ē-ō-rĕk′tăl) [″ + *rectum*, rectum]

ileorectostomy (ĭl″ē-ō-rĕk-tŏs′tō-mē) [″ + ″ + Gr. *stoma*, mouth, opening]

ileorrhaphy (ĭl″ē-or′ă-fē) [″ + Gr. *rhaphe*, seam]

ileosigmoidostomy (ĭl″ē-ō-sĭg″moyd-ŏs′tō-mē) [″ + Gr. *sigma*, letter S, + *eidos*, form, shape, + *stoma*, mouth, opening]

ileostomy (ĭl′ē-ŏs′tō-mē) [″ + Gr. *stoma*, mouth, opening]
   i., urinary

ileotomy (ĭl″ē-ŏt′ō-mē) [″ + Gr. *tome*, a cutting, slice]

ileotransversostomy (ĭl″ē-ō-trăns″vĕr-sŏs′tō-mē) [″ + *transversus*, crosswise, + Gr. *stoma*, mouth, opening]

ileum (ĭl″ē-ŭm) [L., ileum]
   i., duplex

ileus (ĭl′ē-ŭs) [Gr. *eileos*, a twisting]
   i., adynamic
   i., dynamic
   i., mechanical
   i., meconium
   i. paralyticus
   i., postoperative
   i., spastic
   i. subparta

ilia

iliac [L. *iliacus*, pert. to ilium]

iliac crest

iliac fascia

iliac fossa

iliac region

iliac roll

iliac spine

ilio- [L. *ilium*, flank]

iliococcygeal (ĭl″ē-ō-kŏk-sĭj′ē-ăl) [″ + Gr. *kokkyx*, coccyx]

iliocolotomy (ĭl″ē-ō-kō-lŏt′ō-mē) [″ + Gr. *kolon*, colon, + *tome*, a cutting, slice]

iliocostal (ĭl″ē-ō-kŏs′tăl) [″ + *costa*, rib]

iliofemoral (ĭl″ē-ō-fĕm′or-ăl) [″ + *femoralis*, pert. to femur]

iliohypogastric (ĭl″ē-ō-hī″pō-găs′trĭk) [″ + Gr. *hypo*, under, beneath, below, + *gaster*, stomach]

ilioinguinal (ĭl″ē-ō-ĭn′gwĭ-năl) [″ + *inguinalis*, pert. to groin]

iliolumbar (ĭl″ē-ō-lŭm′bar) [″ + *lumbus*, loin]

iliopagus (ĭl″ē-ŏp′ă-gŭs) [″ + Gr. *pagos*, thing fixed]

iliopectineal (ĭl″ē-ō-pĕk-tĭn′ē-ăl) [L. *ilium*, flank, + *pecten*, a comb]

iliopelvic (ĭl″ē-ō-pĕl′vĭk) [″ + pelvis, basin]

iliopsoas (ĭl″ē-ō-sō′ăs) [″ + Gr. psoa, loin]

iliopsoas abscess

iliosacral (ĭl″ē-ō-sā′krăl) [″ + sacralis, pert. to sacrum]

iliosciatic (ĭl″ē-ō-sī-ăt′ĭk) [″ + sciaticus, pert. to the ischium]

iliospinal (ĭl″ē-ō-spī′năl) [″ + spinalis, pert. to the spine]

iliothoracopagus (ĭl″ē-ō-thō″ră-kōp′ă-gŭs) [″ + Gr. thorax, chest, + pagos, thing fixed]

iliotibial (ĭl″ē-ō-tĭb′ē-ăl) [″ + tibialis, pert. to tibia]

iliotibial band

ilioxiphopagus (ĭl″ē-ō-zī-fŏp′ă-gŭs) [″ + Gr. xiphos, sword, + eidos, form, shape, + pagos, thing fixed]

ilium (ĭl′ē-ŭm) [L., groin, flank]

ill (ĭl) [Old Norse illr, bad]

illaqueation (ĭl″ăk-wē-ā′shŭn) [L. illa queare, to ensnare]

illegitimate

illinition (ĭl-ĭ-nĭsh′ŭn) [L. illinire, to smear]

illness (ĭl′nĭs) [Old Norse illr, bad, + AS. -ness, state of]
    i., catastrophic

illuminating gas

illumination (ĭl-lū-mĭn-ā′shŭn) [L. illuminare, to light up]
    i., axial
    i., central
    i., dark-field
    i., direct
    i., focal
    i., oblique
    i., through
    i., transmitted light

illuminism

illusion [L. illusio]
    i., optical

illusional

Ilosone

Ilotycin

Ilozyme

I.M. intramuscular(ly)

I.M.A. Industrial Medical Association

ima (ī′mă) [L., lowest]

image (ĭm′ĭj) [L. imago, likeness]
    i., body
    i., direct
    i., double
    i., false
    i., inverted
    i., latent
    i., mirror
    i., radiographic
    i., real
    i., true
    i., virtual

image intensifier

imagery (ĭm′ĭj-rē) [L. imago, likeness]
    i., auditory
    i., smell
    i., tactile
    i., taste
    i., visual

imagination [L. imago, likeness]

imaging

imago (ĭ-mā′gō) [L., likeness]

Imavate

imbalance [L. in-, not, + bilanx, two scales]
    i., autonomic
    i., sympathetic
    i., vasomotor

imbecile (ĭm′bĕ-sĭl) [L. imbecillus, feeble]

imbecility

imbed [L. in, in, (put) into, + AS. bedd, bed]

imbibition (ĭm″bĭ-bĭsh′ŭn) [″ + bibere, to drink]

imbricate, imbricated (ĭm′brĭ-kāt, -ĕd) [L. imbricare, to tile]

imbrication (ĭm″brĭ-kā′shŭn) [L. imbricare, to tile]

Imferon

imidazole (ĭm″ĭd-ăz′ōl″)

imide (ĭm′ĭd)

imipramine hydrochloride (ĭ-mĭp′ră-mēn)

immature (ĭm″mă-tūr′) [L. in-, not, + maturus, ripe]

immediate [″ + mediare, to be in middle]

immedicable (ĭ-mĕd′ĭ-kă-b′l) [L. *immedicabilis*]

immersion (ĭm-ĕr′shŭn) [L. *in*, into, + *mergere*, to dip]
   i., homogeneous

immersion foot

immersion lens, oil

immiscible (ĭ-mĭs′ĭ-bl) [L. *in-*, not, + *miscere*, to mix]

immobilization [" + *mobilis*, movable]

immune (ĭm-ūn′) [L. *immunis*, safe]

immune body

immune reaction

immune response

immunifacient (ĭ-mū″nĭ-fā′shĕnt) [" + *facere*, to make]

immunity [L. *immunitas*]
   i., acquired
   i., active
   i., cell-mediated
   i., congenital
   i., herd
   i., local
   i., natural
   i., passive

immunization [L. *immunitas*, immunity]
   i., deliberate
   i., natural

immunizing unit

immunoassay (ĭm″ū-nō-ăs′sā) [L. *immunis*, safe, + O. Fr. *assai*, trial]

immunobiology (ĭm″ū-nō-bī-ŏl′ō-jē) [" + Gr. *bios*, life, + *logos*, word, reason]

immunochemistry (ĭm″ū-nō-kĕm′ĭs-trē) [" + Gr. *chemeia*, chemistry]

immunochemotherapy (ĭm″ū-nō-kē′mō-thĕr″ă-pē) [" + " + *therapeia*, treatment]

immunocompetence (ĭm″ū-nō-kŏm′pĕ-tĕns)

immunocompromised

immunoconglutinin (ĭm″ū-nō-kŏn-gloo′tĭ-nĭn) [" + *conglutinare*, to glue together]

immunodeficiency (ĭm″ū-nō-dĕ-fĭsh′ĕn-sē)

immunodiagnosis (ĭm″ū-nō-dī″ăg-nō′sĭs)

immunodiffusion (ĭm″ū-nō-dĭ-fū′zhŭn)

immunoelectrophoresis (ĭ-mū″nō-ē-lĕk″trō-fō-rē′sĭs)

immunofluorescence (ĭm″ū-nō-floo″ō-rĕs′ĕns)

immunofluorescent method

immunogen (ĭ-mū-nō-jĕn) [" + Gr. *gennan*, to produce]

immunogenetics (ĭm″ū-nō-jĕ-nĕt′ĭks) [" + Gr. *gennan*, to produce]

immunogenic (ĭm″ū-nō-jĕn′ĭk)

immunogenicity (ĭm″ū-nō-jĕ-nĭs′ĭ-tē)

immunoglobulin (ĭm″ū-nō-glŏb′ū-lĭn)
   i. A
   i. D
   i. E
   i. G
   i. M

immunohematology (ĭ-mū-nō-hēm″ă-tŏl′ō-jē) [L. *immunis*, safe, + Gr. *haima*, blood, + *logos*, word, reason]

immunologic (ĭm″ū-nō-lŏj′ĭk) [" + Gr. *logos*, word, reason]

immunologic diseases

immunologist (ĭm″ū-nŏl′ō-jĭst)

immunology (ĭm″ū-nŏl′ō-jē) [" + Gr. *logos*, word, reason]

immunopathology (ĭm″ū-nō-pă-thŏl′ō-jē)

immunoprecipitation (ĭm″ū-nō-prē-sĭp″ĭ-tā′shŭn)

immunoproliferative (ĭm″ū-nō-prō-lĭf′ĕr-ă-tĭv)

immunoprotein (ĭm″ū-nō-prō′tē-ĭn) [" + Gr. *protos*, first]

immunoreactant (ĭ-mū″nō-rē-ăk′tănt)

immunoreaction (ĭ-mū″nō-rē-ăk′shŭn)

immunoselection (ĭm″ū-nō-sē-lĕk′shŭn)

immunostimulant (ĭm″ū-nō-stĭm′ū-lănt)

immunosuppression (ĭm″ū-nō-sū-prĕsh′ŭn)

immunosuppressive (ĭm″ū-nō-sū-prĕs′ĭv)

immunosuppressive agent

immunosurgery (ĭ-mū″nō-sĕr′jĕr-ē)

immunosurveillance (ĭm″ū-nō-sĕrvā'lĕns)

immunotherapy (ĭm"ū-nō-thĕr'ă-pē) [" + Gr. *therapeia*, treatment]

immunotoxin (ĭm"ū-nō-tŏk'sĭn) [" + Gr. *toxikon*, poison]

immunotransfusion (ĭ-mū"nō-trăns-fū'zhŭn) [" + *trans*, across, + *fusus*, poured]

impacted [L. *impactus*, pressed on]

impaction (ĭm-pǎk'shŭn) [L. *impactio*, a pressing together]

impairment

impalpable (ĭm-pǎl'pǎ-bl) [L. *in-*, not, + *palpare*, to touch]

impar (ĭm'pǎr) [L., unequal]

imparidigitate (ĭm-pǎr"ĭ-dĭj'ĭ-tāt) [" + *digitus*, finger, toe]

impatent (ĭm-pǎ'tĕnt) [" + *patere*, to be open]

impedance (ĭm-pē'dǎns) [L. *impedire*, to hinder]

   i., acoustic

imperative [L. *imperativus*, commanding]

imperception [L. *in-*, not, + *percipere*, to perceive]

imperforate (ĭm-pĕr'fō-rāt) [" + *per*, through, + *forare*, to bore]

imperforate hymen

imperforation [L. *imperforatus*, not open]

imperious acts

impermeable [L. *in-*, not, + *permeare*, to pass through]

impervious [L. *impervius*]

impetiginous (ĭm"pĕ-tĭj'ĭ-nŭs) [L. *impetiginosus*]

impetigo (ĭm-pĕ-tī'gō, -tē'gō) [L.]

   i. contagiosa

   i. herpetiformis

implant (ĭm-plǎnt'; ĭm'plǎnt) [L. *in-*, into, + *plantare*, to plant]

   i., brain

   i., dental

   i., tooth

implantation (ĭm"plǎn-tā'shŭn) [" + *plantare*, to plant]

   i., hypodermic

   i., teratic

implosion

implosion flooding

imponderable [L. *in-*, not, + *pondus*, weight]

impostors, medical

impotence, impotency [" + *potentia*, power]

   i., anatomic

   i., atonic

   i., functional

   i., organic

   i., psychic

   i., symptomatic

   i., vasculogenic

impotent (ĭm'pō-tĕnt)

impotentia (ĭm"pō-tĕn'shē-ă) [L.]

impregnate (ĭm-prĕg'nāt) [L. *impregnare*, to make pregnant]

impregnated

impregnated carbon

impregnation (ĭm"prĕg-nā'shŭn) [L. *impregnare*, to make pregnant]

   i., artificial

impressio (ĭm-prĕs'sē-ō) [L., impression]

   i. cardiaca hepatis

   i. colica

   impressiones digitatae

   i. duodenalis

   i. gastrica

   i. renalis

impression [L. *impressio*]

   i., digitate

   i., final

impression materials

impression tray

imprinting

impulse (ĭm'pŭls) [L. *impulsus*]

   i., cardiac

   i., ectopic

   i., enteroceptive

   i., excitatory

   i., exteroceptive

   i., inhibitory

   i., nervous

   i., proprioceptive

impulsion

IMV *intermittent mandatory ventilation*

In *indium*
in- [L. *in*, into; L. *in-*, not]
inaction (ĭn-ăk′shŭn) [L. *in-*, not, + *actio*, act]
inactivate [″ + *activus*, acting]
inactivation
inactivation of complement
inadequacy (ĭn-ăd′ĕ-kwă-sē) [″ + *adaequare*, to be equal]
inanimate [″ + *animatus*, alive]
inanition (ĭn″ă-nĭsh′ŭn) [L. *inanis*, empty]
inapparent
inappetence (ĭn-ăp′ĕ-tĕns) [″ + *appetere*, to long for]
Inapsine
inarticulate [″ + *articulus*, joined]
in articulo mortis (ĭn ăr-tĭk′ū-lō mor′tĭs) [L.]
inassimilable (ĭn″ă-sĭm′ĭ-lă-bl) [″ + *assimilis*, to make similar]
inborn
inbreeding [″ + AS. *bredan*, to cherish]
incandescent [L. *incandescere*, to glow]
incaparina
incarcerated [L. *incarcerare*]
incarceration
incarial bone (ĭn-kā′rē-ăl)
incarnatio (ĭn″kăr-nā′shē-ō)
   i. unguis
incasement
incentive spirometry
inception [L. *inceptio*, taking in, beginning]
incest (ĭn′sĕst) [L. *incestus*, unchaste, incest]
incidence [L. *incidens*, falling upon]
incident
incineration (ĭn-sĭn″ĕr-ā′shŭn) [L. *in*, into, + *cineres*, ashes]
incipient (ĭn-sĭp′ē-ĕnt) [L. *incipere*, to begin]
incisal (ĭn-sī′zăl)
incise (ĭn-sīz′) [L. *incisus*]
incised (ĭn-sīzd′)
incision (ĭn-sĭzh′ŭn) [L. *incisio*]
incisive (ĭn-sī′sĭv) [L. *incisivus*]

incisive bone
incisor (ĭn-sī′zor) [L., a cutter]
   i.'s, central
   i., prostatic
incisura (ĭn-sī-sū′ră) [L.]
   i. angularis gastrica
incisure (ĭn-sīz′ūr) [L. *incisura*, a cutting into]
   i. of Rivinus
   i.'s of Schmidt-Lanterman
incitant (in-sīt′ănt) [L. *incitare*, to set in motion]
inclination [L. *inclinere*, to slope]
inclinometer (ĭn″klĭ-nŏm′ĕ-ter) [″ + Gr. *metron*, measure]
inclusion [L. *inclusus*, enclosed]
   i., cell
   i., dental
   i., fetal
inclusion blennorrhea
inclusion bodies
inclusion conjunctivitis
incoagulability (ĭn″kō-ăg″ū-lă-bĭl′ĭ-tē) [L. *in-*, not, + *coagulare*, to congeal]
incoercible (ĭn″kō-ĕr′sĭ-bl) [L. *in-*, not, + *coercere*, to restrain]
incoherence (ĭn″kō-hēr′ĕns) [″ + *cohairens*, adhering]
incoherent (ĭn″kō-hē′rĕnt)
incombustible [″ + *combustus*, burned]
incompatibility [L. *incompatibilis*]
   i., physiological
incompatible
incompetence, incompetency [L. *in-*, not, + *competere*, to be suitable]
   i., aortic
   i., ileocecal
   i., mental
   i., muscular
   i., pyloric
   i., relative
   i., valvular
incompetent
incompetent palatal syndrome
incompressible [″ + *compressus*,

pressed together]
incontinence [" + *continere,* to stop]
  i., active
  i., anal
  i., giggle
  i., intermittent
  i. of milk
  i. of urine
  i., overflow
  i., paralytic
  i., passive
  i., urinary stress
incoordinate [L. *in-,* not, + *coordinare,* to arrange]
incoordination (ĭn″kō-or″dĭ-nā′shŭn)
incorporation [L. *in,* into, + *corporare,* to form into a body]
increment (ĭn′krĕ-mĕnt) [L. *incrementum*]
incretogenous (ĭn″krē-tŏj′ĕ-nŭs) [L. *in,* into, + *secernere,* to secrete, + Gr. *gennan,* to produce]
incrustation [L. *in,* on, + *crusta,* shell, crust]
incubation (ĭn″kū-bā′shŭn) [L. *incubare,* to lie on]
incubator
incubus (ĭn′kū-bŭs) [L. *incubare,* to lie upon]
incudal (ĭng′kū-dăl) [L. *incus,* anvil]
incudectomy (ĭng″kū-dĕk′tō-mē) [" + Gr. *ektome,* excision]
incudiform (ĭn-kū′dĭ-form) [" + *forma,* shape]
incudomalleal (ĭng″kū-dō-măl′ē-ăl) [" + *malleus,* a hammer]
incudostapedial (ĭn″kū-dō-stă-pē′dē-ăl) [" + *stapes,* a stirrup]
incurable [L. *in-,* not, + *curare,* to care for]
incurvation (ĭn″kŭr-vā′shŭn) [L. *incurvare,* to bend in]
incus (ĭng′kŭs) [L., anvil]
  i., lenticular process of
incyclophoria (ĭn-sī″klō-for′ē-ă) [L. *in-,* not, + Gr. *kyklos,* circle, + *phoros,* bearing]

incyclotropia (ĭn-sī″klō-trō′pē-ă) [" + " + *tropos,* turning]
in d. [L.] *in dies,* daily
indagation (ĭn″dă-gā′shŭn) [L. *indagatus,* searching]
indecision
indentation [L. *in,* in, + *dens,* tooth]
independent living
independent living skills
index (ĭn′dĕks) [L., an indicator]
  i., alveolar
  i., cardiac
  i., cephalic
  i., cerebral
  i., DMF
  i., leukopenic
  i., opsonic
  i., oral hygiene
  i., pelvic
  i., periodontal (Ramfjord)
  i., phagocytic
  i., refractive
  i., therapeutic
  i., thoracic
  i., vital
index case
indican (ĭn′dĭ-kăn)
indicanemia (ĭn″dĭ-kăn-ē′mē-ă) [*indican* + Gr. *haima,* blood]
indicant (ĭn′dĭ-kănt)
indicanuria (ĭn″dĭ-kăn-ū′rē-ă) [" + Gr. *ouron,* urine]
indication [L. *indicare,* to show]
  i., causal
  i., symptomatic
indicator [L. *indicare,* to show]
indifferent [L. *in-,* not, + *differre,* to differ]
indigenous (ĭn-dĭj′ĕn-ŭs) [L. *indigenus,* born in]
indigestible (ĭn″dĭ-jĕs′tĭ-bl) [L. *in-,* not, + *digerere,* to separate]
indigestion [" + *digerere,* to separate]
indigitation (ĭn-dĭj″ĭ-tā′shŭn) [L. *in,* in, + *digitus,* finger, toe]
indigo

Indigo Carmine
indigotindisulfonate sodium (ĭn″dĭ-gō″tĭn-dĭ-sŭl′fō-nāt)
indigouria (ĭn″dĭ-gō-ū′rē-ă) [Gr. *indikon*, Indian dye, + *ouron*, urine]
indisposition [L. *in-*, not, + *dispositus*, arranged]
indium (ĭn′dē-ŭm) [L. *indicum*, indigo]
indium chlorides in 113m injection
individuation (ĭn″dĭ-vĭd″ū-ā′shŭn)
Indocin
indocyanine green
indolaceturia (ĭn″dō-lăs″ē-tū′rē-ă) [*indole* + L. *acetum*, vinegar, + Gr. *ouron*, urine]
indole (ĭn′dōl)
indolent (ĭn′dō-lĕnt) [LL. *indolens*, painless]
indolent ulcer
indologenous (ĭn″dō-lŏj′ĕn-ŭs) [*indole* + Gr. *gennan*, to produce]
indoluria (ĭn″dōl-ū′rē-ă) [″ + Gr. *ouron*, urine]
indomethacin (ĭn″dō-mĕth′ă-sĭn)
indoxyl (ĭn-dŏk′sĭl) [Gr. *indikon*, indigo, + *oxys*, sharp]
indoxylemia (ĭn-dŏk″sĭl-ē′mē-ă) [″ + ″ + *haima*, blood]
indoxyluria (ĭn″dŏk-sĭl-ū′rē-ă) [″ + ″ + *ouron*, urine]
induced (ĭn-dūsd′) [L. *inducere*, to lead in]
inducer (ĭn-dūs′ĕr)
inductance
induction (ĭn-dŭk′shŭn) [L. *inductio*, leading in]
inductor (ĭn-dŭk′tĕr)
inductorium (ĭn″dŭk-tō′rē-ŭm)
inductotherm (ĭn-dŭk′tō-thĕrm) [L. *inducere*, to lead in, + Gr. *therme*, heat]
inductothermy
indulin (ĭn′dū-lĭn)
indulinophil(e) (ĭn″dū-lĭn′ō-fĭl, -fīl)
indurate (ĭn′dū-rāt) [L. *in*, in, + *durus*, hard]
indurated
induration

i., black
i., brown
i., cyanotic
i., granular
i., gray
i., red
indurative (ĭn′dūr-ā″tĭv)
indusium (ĭn-dū′zē-ŭm) [L., tunic]
i. griseum
inebriant (ĭn-ē′brē-ănt) [L. *inebrius*, drunken]
inebriate
inebriation (ĭn-ē″brē-ā′shŭn)
inelastic [L. *in-*, not, + NL. *elasticus*, expansive, impulsive]
inert (ĭn-ĕrt′) [L. *iners*, unskilled, idle]
inertia (ĭn-ĕr′shē-ă) [L., inactivity]
i., uterine
in extremis (ĭn ĕks-trē′mĭs) [L.]
infant [L. *infans*]
i., development of
i., post-term
i., preterm
i., respiration of
i., temperature of
i., term
infanticide (ĭn-făn′tĭ-sīd) [LL. *infanticidium*]
infantile (ĭn′făn-tĭl) [Fr. *infantilis*]
infantilism (ĭn-făn′tĭl-ĭzm, ĭn′făn-tĭl-ĭzm″) [″ + Gr. *-ismos*, condition]
i., angioplastic
i., Brissaud's
i., cachectic
i., celiac
i., dysthyroidal
i., hepatic
i., hypophyseal
i., idiopathic
i., intestinal
i., myxedematous
i., pituitary
i., renal
i., sex
i., symptomatic
i., universal
infant stimulation
infarct [L. *infarctus*]

i., anemic
i., bland
i., calcareous
i., cicatrized
i., hemorrhagic
i., infected
i., pale
i., red
i., septic
i., uric acid
i., white
infarction
i., cardiac
i., cerebral
i., evolution of
i., extension of
i., myocardial
i., pulmonary
infect [ME. infecten]
infection (ĭn-fĕk'shŭn)
i., acute
i., airborne
i., apical
i., chronic
i., concurrent
i., contagious
i., cross
i., droplet
i., dustborne
i., endogenous
i., exogenous
i., fungus
i., local
i., low-grade
i., metastatic
i., mixed
i., opportunistic
i., protozoal
i., pyogenic
i., secondary
i., simple
i., subacute
i., subclinical
i., systemic
i., terminal
i., waterborne
infectious (ĭn-fĕk'shŭs) [ME. infecten, infect]

infectious disease
infectious mononucleosis
infecundity (ĭn-fē-kŭn'dĭ-tē) [L. infecunditas, sterility]
inferior (ĭn-fē'rē-or) [L. inferus, below]
inferiority complex
infertility
i., secondary
infest [L. infestare, to attack]
infestation
infibulation (ĭn-fĭb-ū-lā'shŭn) [L. in, in, + fibula, clasp]
infiltrate (ĭn-fĭl'trāt, ĭn'fĭl-trāt) [" + filtrare, to strain through]
infiltration (ĭn"fĭl-trā'shŭn)
i., adipose
i., amyloid
i., anesthesia
i., calcareous
i., cellular
i., fatty
i., glycogenic
i., lymphocytic
i., pigmentary
i., purulent
i., serous
i., urinous
i., waxy
infinite distance
infinity
infirm [L. infirmis]
infirmary [L. infirmarium]
infirmity
Inflamase
inflammation [L. inflammare, to flame within]
i., acute
i., adhesive
i., bacterial
i., catarrhal
i., chronic
i., exudative
i., fibrinous
i., granulomatous
i., hemorrhagic
i., hyperplastic
i., interstitial
i., parenchymatous

i., productive
i., proliferative
i., pseudomembranous
i., purulent
i., reactive
i., serous
i., specific
i., subacute
i., suppurative
i., toxic
i., traumatic
i., ulcerative
inflammatory [L. *inflammare*, to flame within]
inflammatory response
inflation (ĭn-flā'shŭn) [L. *in*, into, + *flare*, to blow]
inflator (ĭn-flā'tor)
inflection (ĭn"flĕk'shŭn) [" + *flectere*, to bend]
influenza (ĭn"flū-ĕn'ză) [It., influence]
i., Asian
influenzal (ĭn"flū-ĕn'zăl) [It. *influenza*, influence]
influenza virus vaccine
infolding
informed consent
infra- [L. *infra*, below, underneath]
infra-axillary (ĭn"fră-ăks'ĭl-ă-rē) [" + *axilla*, little axis]
infrabulge (ĭn'fră-bŭlj)
infraclavicular (ĭn"fră-klă-vĭk'ū-lăr) [" + *clavicula*, little key]
infracortical (ĭn"fră-kor'tĭ-kăl) [" + *cortex*, rind]
infracostal (ĭn"fră-kŏs'tăl) [" + *costa*, rib]
infracotyloid (ĭn"fră-kŏt'ĭ-loyd) [" + Gr. *kotyloeides*, cup shaped]
infraction (ĭn-frăk'shŭn) [L. *infractus*, to destroy]
infradentale
infradiaphragmatic (ĭn"fră-dī"ă-frăg-măt'ĭk)
infraglenoid (ĭn"fră-glē'noyd) [L. *infra*, below, underneath, + Gr. *glene*, cavity, + *eidos*, form, shape]
infraglottic (ĭn"fră-glŏt'ĭk) [" + Gr.

glottis, tongue]
infrahyoid (ĭn"fră-hī'oyd) [" + Gr. *hyoeides*, U-shaped]
inframammary [" + *mamma*, breast]
inframandibular (ĭn"fră-măn-dĭb'ū-lăr) [" + *mandibula*, lower jawbone]
inframarginal [" + *margo*, a margin]
inframaxillary [" + *maxilla*, jawbone]
infranuclear (ĭn"fră-nū'klē-ăr) [" + *nucleus*, kernel]
infraocclusion [" + *occlusio*, a shutting up]
infraorbital (ĭn-fră-or'bĭ-tăl) [" + *orbita*, track]
infrapatellar (ĭn"fră-pă-tĕl'ăr) [" + *patella*, a small pan]
infrapsychic (ĭn"fră-sī'kĭk) [" + Gr. *psyche*, mind]
infrapubic [" + *pubes*, hair on genitals]
infrared rays
infrascapular [" + *scapula*, shoulder blade]
infrasonic (ĭn"fră-sŏn'ĭk) [L. *infra*, below, underneath, + *sonus*, sound]
infraspinous [" + *spina*, thorn]
infrasternal [" + Gr. *sternon*, chest]
infratemporal (ĭn"fră-tĕm'pō-răl) [" + *temporalis*, pert. to the temple]
infratonsillar (ĭn"fră-tŏn'sĭ-lăr) [" + *tonsilla*, almond]
infratrochlear (ĭn"fră-trŏk'lē-ăr) [" + *trochlea*, pulley]
infraumbilical (ĭn"fră-ŭm-bĭl'ĭ-kăl) [" + *umbilicus*, a pit]
infraversion (ĭn"fră-vĕr'zhŭn) [" + *versio*, a turning]
infriction [L. *in*, into, + *frictio*, rubbing]
infundibulectomy (ĭn"fŭn-dĭb"ū-lĕk'tō-mē) [L. *infundibulum*, funnel, +

Gr. *ektome*, excision]
infundibuliform   (ĭn″fŭn-dĭb′ū-lĭ-form)
["   +   *forma*, form]
   i. fascia
infundibulopelvic   (ĭn″fŭn-dĭb″ū-lō-
pĕl′vĭk) ["   +   *pelvis*, basin]
infundibulum   (ĭn″fŭn-dĭb′ū-lŭm) [L.]
   i., ethmoidal
   i. of hypothalamus
   i. of the uterine tube
infusible   [L. *in-*, not,   +   *fusio*, fusion; L. *in*, into,   +   *fundere*, to pour]
infusion   (ĭn-fū′zhŭn) [L. *infusio*]
   i., continuous
   i., intravenous
   i., subcutaneous
infusodecoction   (ĭn-fū″sō-dē-kŏk′
shŭn) ["   +   *de*, down,   +
coquere, to boil]
Infusoria   (ĭn-fū-sō′rē-ă)
infusum   (ĭn-fū′sŭm) [L., infusion]
ingesta   (ĭn-jĕs′tă) [L. *in*, into,   +
gerere, to carry]
ingestant   (ĭn-jĕs′tănt) ["   +   *gerere*,
to carry]
ingestion
Ingrassia's apophyses   (ĭn-gră′sē-ăs)
[Giovanni Filippo Ingrassia, It. anatomist, 1510–1580]
ingravescent   (ĭn″grăv-ĕs′ĕnt) ["   +
gravesci, to grow heavy]
ingredient   (ĭn-grē′dē-ĕnt) [L. *ingredi*, to
enter]
ingrowing   [L. *in*, into,   +   AS. *growan*, to grow]
ingrown nail
inguen   (ĭn′gwĕn) [L.]
inguinal   (ĭng′gwĭ-năl) [L. *inguinalis*, pert.
to the groin]
inguinal canal
inguinal glands
inguinal hernia
inguinal ligament
inguinal reflex
inguinal region
inguinal ring
inguinocrural   (ĭng″gwĭ-nō-kroo′răl) [L.
inguen, groin,   +   *cruralis*, pert. to

the leg]
inguinodynia   (ĭn″gwĭ-nō-dĭn′ē-ă)
["   +   Gr. *odyne*, pain]
inguinolabial   (ĭng″gwĭ-nō-lā′bē-ăl)
["   +   *labialis*, pert. to the lips]
inguinoscrotal   (ĭng″gwĭ-nō-skrō′tăl)
["   +   *scrotum*, a bag]
INH   isoniazid
inhalant   [L. *inhalare*, to inhale]
inhalation   (ĭn″hă-lā′shŭn) [L. *inhalatio*]
inhalation therapy
inhale   (ĭn-hāl′) [L. *inhalare*]
inhaler
inherent   (ĭn-hĕr′ĕnt) [L. *inhaerens*, to in-
here]
inherent cauterization
inheritance   (ĭn-hĕr′ĭ-tăns) [L. *inheredi-
tare*, to inherit]
   i., maternal
inherited
inhibin   (ĭn-hĭb′ĭn)
inhibited sexual excitement
inhibition   (ĭn″hĭ-bĭsh′ŭn) [L. *inhibere*, to
restrain]
   i., competitive
   i., contact
   i., noncompetitive
   i., psychic
   i., selective
inhibitor
inhibitory   (ĭn-hĭb′ĭ-tō-rē)
inhibitory nerve
inhibitrope   (ĭn-hĭb′ĭ-trōp) ["   +   Gr.
tropos, a turning]
inhomogeneity   (ĭn-hō″mō-jĕ-nē′ĭ-tē)
[L. *in-*, not,   +   Gr. *homos*, same,
   +   *genos*, kind]
iniac, inial   (ĭn″ē-ăk, -ăl) [Gr. *inion*, back
of the head]
iniencephalus   (ĭn′ē-ĕn-sĕf′ă-lŭs)
["   +   *enkephalos*, brain]
inion   (ĭn′ē-ŏn) [Gr.]
iniopagus   (ĭn″ē-ŏp′ă-gŭs) ["   +
pagos, thing fixed]
iniops   (ĭn′ē-ŏps) ["   +   *ops*, eye]
initial   (ĭn-ĭsh′ăl) [L. *initium*, beginning]
initis   (ĭn-ī′tĭs) [Gr. *inos*, fiber,   +   *itis*,
inflammation]

inject [L. *injicere*, to throw in]
injected [L. *injectus*, thrown in]
injection (ĭn-jĕk'shŭn)
  i., epidural
  i., fractional
  i., hypodermic
  i., intra-alveolar
  i., intracardial
  i., intracutaneous
  i., intralingual
  i., intramuscular
  i., intraosseous
  i., intraperitoneal
  i., intravenous
  i., jet
  i., rectal
  i., sclerosing
  i., spinal
  i., subcutaneous
  i., vaginal
  i., Z-track
injectors
  i.'s, pressure
injury [L. *injurius*, unjust]
  i., egg-white
  i., internal
  i., steering wheel
ink poisoning
inlay (ĭn'lā) [L. *in*, in, + AS. *lecgan*, to lay]
inlet
  i. of pelvis
INN *International Nonproprietary Names*
innate (ĭn-nāt') [" + *natus*, born]
innervate (ĭn-nĕr'vāt, ĭn'ĕr-vāt) [" + *nervus*, nerve]
innervation (ĭn"ĕr-vā'shŭn)
  i., collateral
  i., double
  i., reciprocal
innidiation (ĭ-nĭd"ē-ā'shŭn) [" + *nidus*, nest]
innocent (ĭn'ō-sĕnt) [L. *innocens*]
innocuous (ĭ-nŏk'ū-ŭs) [L. *innocuus*]
innominate (ĭ-nŏm'ĭ-nāt) [L. *innominatus*, unnamed]
innominate artery

innominate bone
innominate veins
innoxious (ĭ-nŏk'shŭs) [L. *in*, not, + *noxius*, harmful]
inochondritis (ĭn"ō-kŏn-drī'tĭs) [Gr. *inos*, fiber, + *chondros*, cartilage, + *itis*, inflammation]
inochondroma (ĭn"ō-kŏn-drō'mă) [" + " + *oma*, tumor]
inoculability (ĭn-ŏk"ū-lă-bĭl'ĭ-tē) [" + *oculus*, bud]
inoculable
inoculate
inoculation (ĭn-ŏk"ū-lā'shŭn)
  i., animal
inoculum (ĭn-ŏk'ū-lŭm) [L.]
inocyst (ĭn'ō-sĭst) [Gr. *inos*, fiber, + *kystis*, a bladder]
inocyte (ĭn'ō-sīt) [" + *kytos*, cell]
inogenesis (ĭn"ō-jĕn'ĕ-sĭs) [" + *genesis*, generation, birth]
inogenous (ĭn-ŏj'ĭ-nŭs) [" + *gennan*, to produce]
inoglia (ĭn-ŏg'lē-ă) [" + *glia*, glue]
inohymenitis (ĭn"ō-hī"mĕn-ī'tĭs) [" + *hymen*, membrane, + *itis*, inflammation]
inolith (ĭn'ō-lĭth) [" + *lithos*, stone]
inomyositis (ĭn"ō-mī"ō-sī'tĭs) [" + *mys*, muscle, + *itis*, inflammation]
inomyxoma (ĭn"ō-mĭk-sō'mă) [" + *myxa*, mucus, + *oma*, tumor]
inoneuroma (ĭn"ō-nū-rō'mă) [" + *neuron*, nerve, + *oma*, tumor]
inoperable [L. *in-*, not, + *operari*, to work]
inopexia (ĭn-ō-pĕk'sē-ă) [Gr. *inos*, fiber, + *pexis*, fixation]
inorganic [L. *in-*, not, + Gr. *organon*, an organ]
inorganic acid
inorganic chemistry
inorganic compound
inosclerosis (ĭn"ō-sklĕ-rō'sĭs) [Gr. *inos*, fiber, + *skleros*, hard]
inoscopy [" + *skopein*, to examine]
inosculating [L. *in*, in, + *osculum*,

little mouth]

inosculation (ĭn-ŏs"kū-lā'shŭn)

inose (ĭn'ōs)

inosemia (ĭn-ō-sē'mē-ă) [Gr. *inos*, fiber, + *haima*, blood]

inosinic acid [" + L. *acidus*, sour]

inosite (ĭn'ō-sīt)

inositis (ĭn"ō-sī'tĭs) [" + *itis*, inflammation]

inositol (ĭn-ŏs'ĭ-tŏl)

inosituria (ĭn"ō-sĭ-tū'rē-ă) [*inositol* + Gr. *ouron*, urine]

inosuria (ĭn-ō-sū'rē-ă) [Gr. *inos*, fiber, + *ouron*, urine; *inositol* + Gr. *ouron*, urine]

inotropic (ĭn"ō-trŏp'ĭk) [Gr. *inos*, fiber, + *trepein*, to influence]

inpatient

inquest [L. *in*, into, + *quaerere*, to seek]

insalivation [" + *saliva*, spittle]

insalubrious (ĭn-săl-ū'brē-ŭs) [L. *in*, not, + *salus*, health]

insane (ĭn-sān') [" + *sanus*, sound]

insanitary

insanity [L. *insanitas*, insanity]

insatiable (ĭn-sā'shē-ă-bl) [L. *insatiabilis*]

inscriptio (ĭn-skrĭp'shē-ō) [L.]
    i. tendinea

inscription (ĭn-skrĭp'shŭn) [L. *in*, upon, + *scribere*, to write]

insect [L. *insectum*]

Insecta

insect bites and stings

insecticide (ĭn-sĕk'tĭ-sīd) [L. *insectum*, insect, + *caedere*, to kill]

insectifuge (ĭn-sĕk'tĭ-fūj) [" + *fugare*, to put to flight]

Insectivora (ĭn"sĕk-tĭv'ō-ră) [" + *vorare*, to devour]

insectivore (ĭn-sĕk'tĭ-vor)

insect repellents

insecurity

insemination (ĭn-sĕm"ĭn-ā'shŭn) [L. *in*, into, + *semen*, seed]
    i., artificial
    i., heterologous artificial
    i., homologous artificial

insenescence (ĭn"sĕ-nĕs'ĕns) [" + *senescens*, growing old]

insensible [L. *in*-, not, + *sensibilis*, appreciable]

insertion [L. *in*, into, + *serere*, to join]
    i., velamentous

insheathed (ĭn-shēthd') [" + AS. *sceath*, sheath]

insidious (ĭn-sĭd'ē-ŭs) [L. *insidiosus*, cunning]

insight

insipid (ĭn-sĭp'ĭd) [LL. *insipidus*]

in situ (ĭn sī'tū, sĭt'ū) [L.]

insolation (ĭn"sō-lā'shŭn) [L. *insolare*, to expose to the sun]

insoluble (ĭn-sŏl'ū-bl) [L. *insolubilis*]

insomnia (ĭn-sŏm'nē-ă) [L. *insomnis*]

insomniac (ĭn-sŏm'nē-ăk)

insorption (ĭn-sorp'shŭn) [L. *in*, into, + *sorbere*, to suck in]

inspect [L. *inspectare*, to examine]

inspection

inspectionism (ĭn-spĕk'shŭn-ĭzm)

inspersion (ĭn-spĕr'zhŭn) [L. *in*, upon, + *spargere*, to sprinkle]

inspiration (ĭn"spĭr-ā'shŭn) [L. *in*, in, + *spirare*, to breathe]
    i., crowing
    i., external
    i., forcible
    i., full
    i., internal

inspirator (ĭn'spī-rā"tor)

inspiratory (ĭn-spīr'ă-tor"ē)

inspirometer (ĭn"spī-rŏm'ē-tĕr) [" + " + Gr. *metron*, measure]

inspissate (ĭn-spĭs'āt) [L. *inspissatus*, thickened]

inspissated (ĭn-spĭs'ā-tĕd)

inspissation (ĭn-spĭ-sā'shŭn)

instep

instillation (ĭn"stĭl-ā'shŭn) [L. *in*, into, + *stillare*, to drop]

instillator

instinct (ĭn'stĭngkt) [L. *instinctus*, instigation]

i., death
i., herd
instinctive
institutional review board
instruction
   i., dental hygiene
instrument (ĭn'stroo-mĕnt) [L. *instrumentum*, tool]
   i., dental
instrumental
instrumental activities of daily living
instrumentarium (ĭn'stroo-mĕn-tā'rē-ŭm)
instrumentation
insufficiency (ĭn"sŭ-fĭsh'ĕn-sē) [L. *in-*, not, + *sufficiens*, sufficient]
   i., adrenal
   i., aortic
   i., cardiac
   i., coronary
   i., gastric
   i., hepatic
   i., ileocecal
   i., mitral
   i., muscular
   i. of ocular muscles
   i., pulmonary valvular
   i., renal
   i., respiratory
   i., thyroid
   i., valvular
   i., venous
insufflate [L. *insufflare*, to blow into]
insufflation
   i., perirenal
   i., tubal
insufflator (ĭn'sŭ-flā"tor)
insula (ĭn'sū-lă) [L.]
insular (ĭn'sū-lăr) [L. *insula*, island]
insulation [L. *insulare*, to make into an island]
insulator
insulin [L. *insula*, island]
   i., human
   i., NPH
   i., single component or monocomponent

i. suspension, isophane
i. suspension, protamine zinc
i., synthetic
i. zinc suspension, extended
i. zinc suspension, prompt
insulinase (ĭn'sū-lĭn-ās)
insulinemia (ĭn-sū-lĭn-ē'mē-ă) [L. *insula*, island, + Gr. *haima*, blood]
insulin lipodystrophy
insulinogenesis (ĭn"sū-lĭn-ō-jĕn'ĕ-sĭs) [" + Gr. *genesis*, generation, birth]
insulinogenic (ĭn"sū-lĭn"ō-jĕn'ĭk) [" + Gr. *gennan*, to produce]
insulinoid (ĭn'sū-lĭn-oyd) [" + Gr. *eidos*, form, shape]
insulinoma (ĭn"sū-lĭn-ō'mă) [" + Gr. *oma*, tumor]
insulin pump
insulin shock
insulitis (ĭn"sū-lī'tĭs) [" + Gr. *itis*, inflammation]
insuloma (ĭn"sū-lō'mă) [" + Gr. *oma*, tumor]
insulopathic (ĭn"sū-lō-păth'ĭk) [" + Gr. *pathos*, disease, suffering]
insultus (ĭn-sŭl'tŭs) [L.]
insusceptibility (ĭn"sŭ-sĕp"tĭ-bĭl'ĭ-tē) [L. *in*, not, + *suscipere*, to take up]
intake (ĭn-tāk')
   i. and output
Intal
integration (ĭn"tĕ-grā'shŭn) [L. *integrare*, to make whole]
   i., primary
   i., secondary
integrator (ĭn'tĕ-grā"tor)
integument (ĭn-tĕg'ū-mĕnt) [L. *integumentum*, a covering]
integumentary (ĭn-tĕg-ū-mĕn'tă-rē)
integumentary system
intellect [L. *intelligere*, to understand]
intellectual
intellectualization (ĭn"tĕ-lĕk"chū-ăl-ĭ-zā'shŭn)
intelligence [L. *intelligere*, to understand]
   i., artificial
intelligence quotient

intelligence test
intemperance [L. *in,* not, + *temperare,* to moderate]
intensifying [L. *intensus,* intense, + *facere,* to make]
intensifying screen
intensimeter (ĭn″tĕn-sĭm′ĭ-tĕr) [″ + Gr. *metron,* measure]
intensity (ĭn-tĕn′sĭ-tē)
intensive (ĭn-tĕn′sĭv)
intention (ĭn-tĕn′shŭn) [″ + *tendere,* to stretch]
   i., first
   i., second
   i., third
intention tremor
interacinar (ĭn″tĕr-ăs′ĭ-năr) [L. *inter,* between, + *acinus,* grape]
interalveolar (ĭn″tĕr-ăl-vē′ō-lăr) [″ + *alveolus,* little tub]
interarticular [″ + *articulus,* joint]
interarytenoid (ĭn″tĕr-ăr″ē-tē′noyd) [″ + Gr. *arytaina,* ladle, + *eidos,* form, shape]
interatrial (ĭn″tĕr-ā′trē-ăl) [″ + *atrium,* hall]
interauricular (ĭn″tĕr-aw-rĭk′ū-lăr) [″ + *auricula,* little ear]
interbrain [″ + AS. *braegen,* brain]
intercadence (ĭn″tĕr-kā′dĕns) [″ + *cadere,* to fall, die]
intercalary (ĭn-tĕr′kă-lĕr″ē) [″ + *calare,* to call]
intercalated (ĭn-tĕr′kăl-āt-ĕd)
intercalated ducts
intercanalicular (ĭn″tĕr-kăn″ă-lĭk′ū-lăr) [″ + *canalicularis,* pert. to a canaliculus]
intercapillary (ĭn″tĕr-kăp′ĭ-lăr-ē) [″ + *capillaris,* hairlike]
intercarotic (ĭn″tĕr-kă-rŏt′ĭk) [L. *inter,* between, + Gr. *karos,* deep sleep]
intercarpal (ĭn″tĕr-kăr′păl) [″ + Gr. *karpalis,* pert. to the carpus]
intercartilaginous (ĭn″tĕr-kăr″tĭ-lăj′ĭ-nŭs) [″ + *cartilago,* cartilage]

intercavernous (ĭn″tĕr-kăv′ĕr-nŭs) [″ + L. *caverna,* a hollow]
intercellular (ĭn″tĕr-sĕl′ū-lăr) [″ + *cella,* compartment]
intercerebral (ĭn″tĕr-sĕr′ĕ-brăl) [″ + *cerebrum,* brain]
interchange
interchondral (ĭn″tĕr-kŏn′drăl) [″ + Gr. *chondros,* cartilage]
intercilium (ĭn″tĕr-sĭl′ē-ŭm) [″ + *cilium,* eyelash]
interclavicular (ĭn″tĕr-klă-vĭk′ū-lăr) [″ + *clavicula,* clavicle]
intercoccygeal (ĭn″tĕr-kŏk-sĭj′ē-ăl) [″ + Gr. *kokkyx,* coccyx]
intercolumnar (ĭn″tĕr-kō-lŭm′năr) [″ + *columna,* column]
intercolumnar fascia
intercolumnar fibers
intercondylar, intercondyloid, intercondylous [″ + Gr. *kondylos,* knuckle]
intercostal [″ + *costa,* rib]
intercostal muscles, external
intercostal muscles, internal
intercostobrachial (ĭn″tĕr-kŏs″tō-brā′kē-ăl) [″ + ″ + *brachium,* arm]
intercostohumeral (ĭn″tĕr-kŏs-tō-hū′mĕr-ăl) [″ + ″ + *humerus,* upper arm]
intercourse [L. *intercursus,* running between]
   i., sexual
intercricothyrotomy (ĭn″tĕr-krī″kō-thī-rŏt′ō-mē) [L. *inter,* between, + Gr. *krikos,* ring, + *thyreos,* shield, + *tome,* a cutting, slice]
intercristal (ĭn″tĕr-krĭs′tăl) [″ + *crista,* crest]
intercrural (ĭn″tĕr-krū′răl) [″ + *crus,* limb]
intercurrent [″ + *currere,* to run]
intercusping [″ + *cuspis,* point]
interdent
interdental [″ + *dens,* tooth]
interdentium (ĭn″tĕr-dĕn′shē-ŭm)
interdigitation [″ + *digitus,*

finger, toe]
interest checklist
interface
interfascicular (ĭn″tĕr-făs-ĭk′ū-lăr)
[″ + *fasciculus*, bundle]
interfemoral [″ + *femoralis*, pert.
to the thigh]
interference [″ + *ferire*, to strike
interference of impulses
interferometer (ĭn″tĕr-fĕr-ŏm′ĕ-tĕr)
interferon (ĭn-tĕr-fĕr′ŏn)
interfibrillar, interfibrillary (ĭn″tĕr-
fĭb′rĭ-lăr, -rī-lăr″ē) [″ + *fibrilla*, a
small fiber]
interfilamentous (ĭn″tĕr-fĭl″ă-mĕn′tŭs)
[″ + *filamentum*, filament]
interfilar (ĭn-tĕr-fī′lăr) [″ + *filum*,
thread]
interfilar mass
interganglionic [″ + *ganglion*, a
swelling]
intergemmal (ĭn″tĕr-jĕm′ăl) [″ +
gemma, bud]
interglobular [″ + *globulus*, glo-
bule]
interglobular dentin
interglobular spaces
intergluteal (ĭn″tĕr-gloo′tē-ăl) [″ +
Gr. *gloutos*, buttock]
intergonial
intergyral (ĭn″tĕr-jī′răl) [″ + Gr.
gyros, circle]
interhemicerebral (ĭn″tĕr-hĕm″ĭ-
sĕr′ĕ-brăl) [″ + Gr. *hemi*, half, +
L. *cerebrum*, brain]
interictal (ĭn″tĕr-ĭk′tăl) [″ + *ictus*, a
blow]
interior [L. *internus*, within]
interischiadic (ĭn″tĕr-ĭs″kē-ăd′ĭk) [L.
inter, between, + Gr. *ischion*, hip]
interkinesis (ĭn″tĕr-kī-nē′sĭs) [″ +
Gr. *kinesis*, motion]
interlabial
interlamellar (ĭn″tĕr-lă-mĕl′ăr) [″ +
lamella, layer]
interleukin-1
interleukin-2
interlobar (ĭn″tĕr-lō′băr) [″ +

lobus, lobe]
interlobitis (ĭn″tĕr-lō-bī′tĭs) [″ + ″
+ Gr. *itis*, inflammation]
interlobular (ĭn″tĕr-lŏb′ū-lăr) [″ +
lobulus, lobule]
interlobular emphysema
intermalleolar (ĭn″tĕr-mă-lē′ō-lăr)
[″ + *malleolus*, little hammer]
intermammary (ĭn″tĕr-măm′ă-rē)
[″ + *mamma*, breast]
intermamillary (ĭn″tĕr-măm′ĭ-lăr″ē)
[″ + *mammilla*, nipple]
intermarriage [″ + *maritare*, to
marry]
intermaxillary [″ + *maxilla*, jaw-
bone]
intermediary (ĭn″tĕr-mē′dē-ăr-ē)
[″ + *medius*, middle]
intermediary metabolism
intermediate (ĭn″tĕr-mē′dē-ĭt) [″ +
medius, middle]
intermedin (ĭn″tĕr-mē′dĭn)
intermediolateral [″ + ″ +
latus, side]
intermedius (ĭn″tĕr-mē′dē-ŭs) [″ +
medius, middle]
intermembranous (ĭn″tĕr-mĕm′bră-
nŭs) [″ + *membrana*, membrane]
intermeningeal (ĭn″tĕr-mĕn-ĭn′jē-ăl)
[″ + *meninx*, membrane]
intermenstrual (ĭn″tĕr-mĕn′stroo-ăl)
[″ + Gr. *men*, month]
intermetacarpal (ĭn″tĕr-mĕt″ă-
kăr′păl) [″ + Gr. *meta*, beyond,
+ *karpos*, wrist]
intermission [″ + *mittere*, to send]
intermittence [″ + *mittere*, to
send]
intermittent (ĭn″tĕr-mĭt′ĕnt)
intermittent fever
**intermittent positive-pressure
breathing**
intermittent pulse
intermural (ĭn″tĕr-mū′răl) [L. *inter*, between, + *murus*, wall]
intermuscular [″ + *musculus*, mus-
cle]
intern (ĭn′tĕrn) [L. *internus*, within]

internal [L. *internus,* within]
internal bleeding
internal ear
internal injury
internalization (ĭn-tĕr″năl-ĭ-zā′shŭn)
internal medicine
internal secretion
internarial (ĭn″tĕr-nā′rē-ăl) [L. *inter,* between, + *nares,* nostrils]
internasal (ĭn″tĕr-nā′zăl) [″ + *nasus,* nose]
internatal (ĭn″tĕr-nā′tăl) [″ + *nates,* buttocks]
International Classification of Diseases
International Symbol of Access
International System of Units
international unit
interneuron (ĭn″tĕr-nū′rŏn) [L. *inter,* between, + Gr. *neuron,* nerve]
internist
internode [″ + *nodus,* knot]
internship (ĭn′tĕrn-shĭp)
internuclear (ĭn″tĕr-nū′klē-ăr) [″ + *nucleus,* a kernel]
internuncial (ĭn″tĕr-nŭn′shē-ăl) [″ + *nuncius,* messenger]
internuncial neuron
internus (ĭn-tĕr′nŭs) [L., within]
interocclusal (ĭn″tĕr-ŏ-kloo′zăl) [L. *inter,* between, + *occlusio,* a shutting up]
interoceptive [L. *internus,* within, + *capere,* to take]
interoceptor (ĭn″tĕr-ō-sĕp′tor)
　i., general
　i., special
interofective (ĭn″tĕr-ō-fĕk′tĭv) [″ + *afficere,* to influence]
interoinferior (ĭn″tĕr-ō-ĭn-fē′rē-or) [″ + *inferus,* below]
interolivary [L. *inter,* between, + *oliva,* olive]
interorbital [″ + *orbita,* orbit]
interosseous [″ + *os,* bone]
interpalpebral (ĭn″tĕr-păl′pĕ-brăl) [″ + *palpebra,* eyelid]
interparietal (ĭn″tĕr-pă-rī′ĕ-tăl) [″ + *paries,* wall]
interparietal bone
interparietal suture
interparoxysmal (ĭn″tĕr-păr″ŏk-sĭz′măl) [″ + Gr. *paroxysmos,* spasm]
interpeduncular (ĭn″tĕr-pĕ-dŭnk′ū-lăr) [L. *inter,* between, + *pedunculus,* peduncle]
interpersonal
interphalangeal (ĭn″tĕr-fă-lăn′jē-ăl) [″ + Gr. *phalanx,* line of battle]
interphase
interpolar (ĭn″tĕr-pō′lăr) [″ + *polus,* pole]
interpolar path
interpolation (ĭn-tĕr″pō-lā′shŭn)
interposed (ĭn′tĕr-pōzd)
interposition (ĭn″tĕr-pō-zĭsh′ŭn)
interpretation
interproximal [″ + *proximus,* next]
interproximal space
interpubic (ĭn-tĕr-pū′bĭk) [″ + *pubes,* pubes]
interpupillary [″ + *pupilla,* pupil]
interpupillary distance
interradicular
interradicular bone
interradicular fibers
interrenal (ĭn″tĕr-rē′năl) [L. *inter,* between, + *ren,* kidney]
interscapilium (ĭn″tĕr-skă-pĭl′ē-ŭm) [″ + *scapula,* shoulder blade]
interscapular
interscapular reflex
interscapulum (ĭn-tĕr-skăp′ū-lŭm)
intersection
intersegmental (ĭn″tĕr-sĕg-mĕn′tăl) [″ + *segmentum,* a portion]
interseptal (ĭn″tĕr-sĕp′tăl) [″ + *saeptum,* a partition]
intersex (ĭn′tĕr-sĕks)
　i., female
　i., male
　i., true
intersexuality (ĭn″tĕr-sĕks″ū-ăl′ĭ-tē)
interspace

interspinal (ĭn-tĕr-spī′năl) [″ + spinalis, pert. to the spine]
interstice (ĭn-tĕr′stĭs) [L. interstitium]
interstitial (ĭn″tĕr-stĭsh′ăl)
interstitial cells of testes
interstitial cell-stimulating hormone
interstitial cystitis
interstitial fluid
interstitial lung disorders
interstitial tissue
interstitium (ĭn″tĕr-stĭsh′ē-ŭm) [L.]
intersystole (ĭn″tĕr-sĭs′tō-lē) [L. inter, between, + Gr. systole, contraction]
intertarsal (ĭn″tĕr-tăr′săl) [″ + Gr. tarsos, flat of the foot, flat surface, edge of eyelid]
intertransverse (ĭn″tĕr-trăns-vĕrs′) [″ + transversus, turned across]
intertriginous (ĭn″tĕr-trĭj′ĭ-nŭs)
intertrigo (ĭn″tĕr-trī′gō) [″ + terere, to rub]
intertrochanteric (ĭn″tĕr-trō″kăn-tĕr′ĭk) [″ + Gr. trochanter, trochanter]
intertrochanteric line
intertubular (ĭn″tĕr-tū′bū-lăr) [″ + tubulus, tubule]
interureteral, interureteric (ĭn″tĕr-ū-rē′tĕr-ăl, ĭn″tĕr-ū″rē-tĕr′ĭk) [″ + Gr. oureter, ureter]
intervaginal (ĭn″tĕr-văj′ĭ-năl) [″ + vagina, sheath]
interval [″ + vallum, a breastwork]
  i., atriocarotid
  i., A-V
  i., cardioarterial
  i., focal
  i., isometric
  i., lucid
  i., passive
  i., postsphygmic
  i., P-R
  i., presphygmic
  i., Q-R
  i., QRS
  i., QRST

  i., Q-T
intervalvular (ĭn″tĕr-văl′vū-lăr) [L. inter, between, + valva, leaf of a folding door]
intervascular [″ + vasculum, a vessel]
intervention (ĭn″tĕr-vĕn′shŭn)
  i., crisis
  i., nursing
interventricular [″ + ventriculum, a small cavity]
intervertebral [″ + vertebra, joint]
intervertebral disk
intervillous (ĭn″tĕr-vĭl′ŭs) [″ + villus, tuft]
intestinal [L. intestinum, intestine]
intestinal bypass surgery
intestinal flora
intestinal gases
intestinal juice
intestinal obstruction
intestinal perforation
intestinal putrefaction
intestinal reflex
intestinal tubes
intestine (ĭn-tĕs′tĭn) [L. intestinum]
  i., large
  i., small
intestinum (ĭn″tĕs-tī′nŭm) [L.]
  i. crassum
  i. rectum
  i. tenue
intima (ĭn′tĭ-mă) [L.]
intimal (ĭn′tĭ-măl)
intimitis (ĭn″tĭ-mī′tĭs) [L. intima, innermost, + Gr. itis, inflammation]
intolerance [L. in-, not, + tolerare, to bear]
intorsion (ĭn-tor′shŭn) [L. in, toward, + torsio, twisting]
intoxicant (ĭn-tŏks′ĭ-kănt)
intoxication [L. in, in, + Gr. toxikon, poison]
  i., water
intra-abdominal [L. intra, within, + abdomen, belly]
intra-acinous (ĭn-tră-ăs′ĭ-nŭs) [″ +

acinus, grape]

intra-aortic balloon counterpulsation

intra-arterial [" + Gr. *arteria,* artery]

intra-articular (ĭn″tră-ăr-tĭk′ū-lăr) [" + *articulus,* little joint]

intra-atrial (ĭn″tră-ā′trē-ăl) [" + Gr. *atrion,* hall]

intrabronchial (ĭn″tră-brŏng′kē-ăl) [" + Gr. *bronchos,* windpipe]

intrabuccal (ĭn″tră-bŭk′ăl) [" + *bucca,* cheek]

intracanalicular (ĭn″tră-kăn″ă-lĭk′ū-lăr) [" + *canalicularis,* pert. to a canaliculus]

intracapsular [" + *capsula,* little box]

intracapsular fracture

intracardiac

intracarpal (ĭn″tră-kăr′păl) [" + Gr. *karpalis,* pert. to the carpus]

intracartilaginous (ĭn″tră-kăr″tĭ-lăj′ĭn-ŭs) [" + *cartilago,* gristle]

intracellular (ĭn″tră-sĕl′ū-lăr) [" + *cellula,* cell]

intracerebellar (ĭn″tră-sĕr″ĕ-bĕl′ăr) [" + *cerebellum,* little brain]

intracerebral (ĭn″tră-sĕr′ĕ-brăl) [" + *cerebrum,* brain]

intracervical (ĭn″tră-sĕr′vĭ-kăl) [" + *cervicalis,* pert. to the neck]

intracisternal (ĭn″tră-sĭs-tĕr′năl) [" + *cisterna,* box, chest]

intracostal (ĭn″tră-kŏs′tăl) [" + *costa,* rib]

intracranial [" + Gr. *kranion,* skull]

intractable (ĭn-trăk′tă-b′l)

intracutaneous [" + *cutis,* skin]

intracutaneous injection

intracutaneous reaction

intracystic [" + Gr. *kystis,* bladder]

intrad (ĭn′trăd)

intradermal [" + Gr. *derma,* skin]

intradermal reaction (ĭn″tră-dĕr″măl rē-ăk′shŭn) [" + " + L. *re,*

back, + *agere,* to do]

intraduct (ĭn′tră-dŭkt) [" + *ductus,* a canal]

intraduodenal (ĭn″tră-dū″ō-dē′năl) [" + *duodeni,* twelve]

intradural (ĭn-tră-dū′răl) [" + *durus,* hard]

intraepidermal (ĭn″tră-ĕp″ĭ-dĕr′măl) [L. *intra,* within, + Gr. *epi,* upon, + *derma,* skin]

intraepithelial (ĭn″tră-ĕp″ĭ-thē′lē-ăl) [" + " + *thele,* nipple]

intrafebrile [" + *febris,* fever]

intrafilar (ĭn-tră-fī′lăr) [" + *filum,* thread]

intragastric [" + Gr. *gaster,* belly]

intragastric balloon

intragemmal (ĭn″tră-jĕm′ăl) [" + *gemma,* bud]

intraglandular [" + *glans,* acorn]

intragyral (ĭn″tră-jī′răl) [" + Gr. *gyros,* circle]

intrahepatic (ĭn″tră-hĕ-păt′ĭk) [" + Gr. *hepatikos,* pert. to the liver]

intraintestinal [" + *intestinum,* intestine]

intralaryngeal (ĭn″tră-lă-rĭn′jē-ăl) [" + Gr. *larynx,* larynx]

intralesional (ĭn″tră-lē′zhŭn-ăl) [" + *laesio,* a wound]

intraligamentary [" + *ligamentum,* a binding]

intraligamentous

intralingual

intralobar (ĭn″tră-lō′băr) [" + *lobus,* a lobe]

intralobular (ĭn″tră-lŏb′ū-lăr) [" + *lobulus,* a lobule]

intralocular (ĭn″tră-lŏk′ū-lăr) [" + *loculus,* a cavity]

intralumbar [" + *lumbus,* loin]

intraluminal (ĭn″tră-lū′mĭ-năl) [" + *lumen,* light]

intramastoiditis (ĭn″tră-măs″tŏyd-ī′tĭs) [" + Gr. *mastos,* breast, + *eidos,* form, shape, + *itis,* inflammation]

intramedullary (ĭn″tră-mĕd′ū-lăr″ē)

[" + *medullaris*, marrow]
intramural [" + *murus*, a wall]
intramuscular [" + *musculus*, a muscle]
intramuscular injection
intranasal [" + *nasus*, nose]
intraocular [" + *oculus*, eye]
intraoperative (ĭn″tră-ŏp′ĕr-ă″tĭv) [L. *intra*, within, + *operativus*, working]
intraoral [" + *oralis*, pert. to the mouth]
intraorbital [" + *orbita*, mark of a wheel]
intraosseous (ĭn″tră-ŏs′ē-ŭs) [" + *os*, bone]
intraovarian (ĭn″tră-ō-vā′rē-ăn)[" + NL. *ovarium*, ovary]
intraparietal (ĭn″tră-pă-rī′ē-tăl) [" + *paries*, wall]
intrapartum (ĭn″tră-păr′tŭm) [" + *partus*, birth]
intrapelvic (ĭn″tră-pĕl′vĭk) [" + *pelvis*, basin]
intraperitoneal [" + Gr. *peritonaion*, stretched around or over]
intraplacental (ĭn″tră-plă-sĕn′tăl) [" + *placenta*, a flat cake]
intrapleural [" + Gr. *pleura*, rib]
intrapontine (ĭn″tră-pŏn′tēn) [" + *pons*, bridge]
intrapsychic, intrapsychical (ĭn″tră-sī′kĭk, -kĭ-kăl) [" + Gr. *psyche*, mind]
intrapulmonary [" + *pulmo*, lung]
intrapyretic (ĭn″tră-pī-rĕt′ĭk) [" + Gr. *pyretos*, fever]
intrarectal (ĭn″tră-rĕk′tăl) [" + *rectum*, straight]
intrarenal (ĭn″tră-rē′năl) [" + *renalis*, pert. to the kidney]
intraretinal (ĭn″tră-rĕt′ĭ-năl) [" + *retina*, retina]
intrascrotal (ĭn″tră-skrō′tăl) [" + *scrotum*, a bag]
intraspinal [L. *intra*, within, + *spina*, thorn]

intrathecal (ĭn″tră-thē′kăl) [" + Gr. *theke*, sheath]
intrathoracic (ĭn″tră-thō-răs′ĭk) [" + Gr. *thorax*, chest]
intratracheal (ĭn″tră-trāk′ē-ăl) [" + Gr. *tracheia*, trachea]
intratracheal anesthesia
intratubal [" + *tubus*, hollow tube]
intratympanic (ĭn″tră-tĭm-păn′ĭk) [" + Gr. *tympanon*, drum]
intrauterine (ĭn″tră-ū′tĕr-ĭn) [" + *uterus*, womb]
intrauterine contraceptive device
intravasation (ĭn-trăv″ă-zā′shŭn) [" + *vas*, vessel]
intravascular
intravenous (ĭn-tră-vē′nŭs) [" + *vena*, vein]
intravenous feeding
intravenous infusion
intravenous infusion pump
intravenous injection
intravenous medication
intravenous treatment
intraventricular [L. *intra*, within, + *ventriculus*, ventricle]
intravesical (ĭn″tră-vĕs′ĭ-kăl) [" + *vesica*, bladder]
intravital [" + *vita*, life]
intravital stain
intra vitam (ĭn′tră vī′tăm) [L.] During life
intravitelline (ĭn″tră-vī-tĕl′ĭn) [" + *vitellus*, yoke]
intravitreous (ĭn″tră-vĭt′rē-ŭs) [" + *vitreus*, glassy]
intrinsic [L. *intrinsicus*, on the inside]
intrinsic factor
intrinsic muscles
introducer [L. *intro*, into, + *ducere*, to lead]
introflexion (ĭn″trō-flĕk′shŭn) [" + *flexus*, bent]
introitus (ĭn-trō′ĭ-tŭs) [L.]
    i. canalis sacralis
    i. laryngis
    i. vaginae
introjection [" + *jacere*, to throw]
intromission (ĭn″trō-mĭsh′ŭn) [" +

mittere, to send]
intromittent (ĭn-trō-mĭt′ĕnt)
introns
Intropin
introspection [″ + *spicere,* to look]
introsusception (ĭn″trō-sŭ-sĕp′shŭn) [″ + *suscipere,* to receive]
introversion (ĭn″trō-vĕr′shŭn) [″ + *versio,* a turning]
introvert
intubate (ĭn′tū-bāt) [L. *in,* into, + *tuba,* a tube]
intubation (ĭn″tū-bā′shŭn)
intubator
intuition
intumesce (ĭn-tū-mĕs′) [L. *intumescere*]
intumescence
intumescent (ĭn-tū-mĕs′ĕnt)
intussusception (ĭn″tŭ-sŭ-sĕp′shŭn) [L. *intus,* within, + *suscipere,* to receive]
intussusceptum (ĭn″tŭ-sŭ-sĕp′tŭm) [L.]
intussuscipiens (ĭn″tŭ-sŭ-sĭp′ē-ĕns) [L.]
Inuit [Eskimo]
inulase (ĭn′ū-lās)
inulin
inunction (ĭn-ŭngk′shŭn) [L. *in,* into, + *unguere,* to anoint]
inustion (ĭn-ŭs′chŭn) [″ + *urere,* to burn]
in utero (ĭn ū′tĕr-ō) [L.]
in vacuo (ĭn văk′ū-ō) [L.]
invaginate (ĭn-văj′ĭn-āt) [L. *invaginatio*]
invaginated
invagination
invalid [L. *in-,* not, + *validus,* strong]
invasion [L. *in,* into, + *vadere,* to go]
invasive
invasive procedure
invermination [″ + *vermis,* worm]
inverse-square law
Inversine
inversion (ĭn-vĕr′zhŭn) [L. *inversio,* to turn inward]
   i., uterine

invert (ĭn-vĕrt′)
invertase (ĭn-vĕr′tās)
invertebrate [L. *in-,* not, + *vertebratus,* vertebrate]
invertin (ĭn-vĕr′tĭn)
invertor (ĭn-vĕr′tor)
invert sugar
investing [L. *in,* into, + *vestire,* to clothe]
investment
inveterate [″ + *vetus,* old]
inviscation (ĭn″vĭs-kā′shŭn) [L. *in,* among, + *viscum,* slime]
in vitro (ĭn vē′trō) [L., in glass]
in vivo (ĭn vē′vō) [L., in the living body]
involucre, involucrum (ĭn′vō-lū″kĕr, ĭn″vō-lū′krŭm) [″ + *volvere,* to wrap]
involuntary [L. *in-,* not, + *voluntas,* will]
involution (ĭn″vō-lū′shŭn) [″ + *volvere,* to roll]
   i. of uterus
   i., senile
   i., sexual
involutional (ĭn-vō-lū′shŭn-ăl)
involutional melancholia
Io Ionium
iocetamic acid
Iodamoeba (ī″ō-dă-mē′bă)
   I. bütschlii
iodide (ī′ō-dīd)
   i., cesium
iodide I 125 solution, sodium
iodinate (ī-ō′dĭ-nāt)
iodinated I 131 albumin injection
iodine (ī′ō-dĭn, ī′ō-dēn) [Gr. *ioeides,* violet colored]
   i., protein-bound
   i., radioactive
   i., tincture of
iodine poisoning
iodine tincture
iodinophilous (ī″ō-dĭn-ŏf′ĭ-lŭs) [Gr. *ioeides,* violet colored, + *philos,* love]
iodipamide meglumine injection
iodipamide sodium I 131

iodism (ī'ō-dĭzm)
iodize
iodized
iodized salt
5-iodo-2'-deoxyuridine
iododerma (ī-ō"dō-dĕr'mă) [" + derma, skin]
iodoform (ī-ō'dō-form) [Gr. ioeides, violet colored, + L. forma, form]
iodoformism (ī'ō-dō-form"ĭzm) [" + " + Gr. -ismos, condition]
iodoglobulin (ī"ō-dō-glŏb'ū-lĭn) [" + L. globus, globe]
iodohippurate sodium I 131 injection (ī-ō"dō-hĭp'ū-rāt)
iodophilia (ī"ō-dō-fĭl'ē-ă) [" + philein, to love]
   i., extracellular
   i., intracellular
iodophor (ī-ō'dō-for)
iodopyracet (ī-ō"dō-pī'ră-sĕt)
iodoquinol (ī-ō"dō-kwĭn'ŏl)
iodotherapy [Gr. ioeides, violet colored, + therapeia, treatment]
iodum (ī-ō'dŭm) [L.]
IOML infraorbitomeatal line
ion [Gr. ion, going]
   i., dipolar
   i., hydrogen
   i., hydroxyl
Ionamin
ion-exchange resins
ionic [Gr. ion, going]
ionic medication
ionium (ī-ō'nē-ŭm)
ionization
ionization chamber
ionize
ionogen (ī-ŏn'ō-jĕn) [Gr. ion, going, + gennan, to produce]
ionometer [" + metron, measure]
ionophose (ī'ō-nō-fōz) [" + phos, light]
ionotherapy (ī"ŏn-ō-thĕr'ă-pē) [" + therapeia, treatment]
iontophoresis (ī-ŏn"tō-fō-rē'sĭs) [" + phorein, to carry]
iontoquantimeter (ī-ŏn"tō-kwŏn-tĭm'ĕ-ter) [" + L. quantus, how much, + Gr. metron, measure]
iontoradiometer (ī-ŏn"tō-rā"dē-ŏm'ī-tĕr) [" + L. radius, ray, + Gr. metron, measure]
iontotherapy (ī-ŏn"tō-thĕr'ă-pē) [" + therapeia, treatment]
IOP intraocular pressure
iopanoic acid
iophendylate (ī"ō-fĕn'dĭ-lāt)
iophobia (ī"ō-fō'bē-ă) [Gr. ios, poison, + phobos, fear]
iotacism (ī-ō'tă-sĭzm) [Gr. iota, letter i]
iothalamate meglumine injection (ī-ō-thăl'ă-māt)
I.P. intraperitoneal; isoelectric point
ipecac (ĭp'ĕ-kăk)
I.P.L. interpupillary line
ipodate calcium (ī'pō-dāt)
ipodate sodium
IPPB intermittent positive-pressure breathing
IPPV intermittent positive-pressure ventilation
ipratropium bromide
iproniazid (ī"prō-nī'ă-zīd)
ipsi- [L. ipse, same]
ipsilateral (ĭp"sĭ-lăt'ĕr-ăl) [" + latus, side]
IPSP inhibitory postsynaptic potential
IQ intelligence quotient
IR infrared
I.R. internal resistance
Ir iridium
iralgia (ĭr-ăl'jē-ă) [Gr. iris, bend, turn, + algos, pain]
irascible (ĭ-răs'ĭ-bl) [LL. irascibilis]
IRB institutional review board
irid- [Gr. iridos, colored circle]
iridadenosis (ĭr"ĭd-ăd-ĭn-ō'sĭs) [L. iris, bend, turn, + Gr. aden, gland, + osis, condition]
iridal (ī'rĭd-ăl)
iridalgia (ī"rĭd-ăl'jē-ă) [" + algos, pain]
iridauxesis (ĭr"ĭd-ŏk-sē'sĭs) [" + auxesis, increase]
iridectome (ĭr"ĭ-dĕk'tōm) [" +

tome, a cutting, slice]

iridectomesodialysis   (ĭr″ĭ-dĕk″tō-mēs″ō-dī-ăl′ĭ-sĭs) [″ + *ektome,* excision,   +   *mesos,* middle,   + *dia,* through,   +   *lysis,* dissolution]

iridectomize (ĭr″ĭd-ĕk′tō-mīz) [″ + *ektome,* excision]

iridectomy

i., optical

iridectropium   (ĭr-ĭ-dĕk-trō′pē-ŭm) [″ + *ektrope,* a turning aside]

iridemia (ĭr-ĭ-dē′mē-ă) [″ + *haima,* blood]

iridencleisis (ĭr″ĭ-dĕn-klī′sĭs) [″ + *enklein,* to lock in]

iridentropium   (ĭr″ĭ-dĕn-trō′pē-ŭm) [″ + *en,* in,   + *tropein,* to turn]

irideremia (ĭr″ĭd-ĕr-ē′mē-ă) [″ + *eremia,* lack]

irides (ĭr′ĭ-dēz) [Gr.]

iridescence (ĭr″ĭ-dĕs′ĕns) [L. *iridescere,* to gleam like a rainbow]

iridesis (ĭ-rīd′ĕ-sĭs) [″ + *desis,* a binding]

iridic (ĭ-rĭd′ĭk) [Gr. *iris,* bend, turn]

iridis, rubeosis

iridium (ĭ-rĭd′ē-ŭm) [Gr. *iris,* bend, turn]

irido- [Gr. *iridos,* colored circle]

iridoavulsion   (ĭr″ĭ-dō-ăv-ŭl′shŭn) [″ + L. *avulsio,* a pulling away from]

iridocapsulitis   (ĭr″ĭd-ō-kăp-sū-lī′tĭs) [″ + L. *capsula,* little box,   + Gr. *itis,* inflammation]

iridocele (ĭ-rīd′ō-sēl) [″ + *kele,* tumor, swelling]

iridochorioiditis,   iridochoroiditis (ĭr″ĭ-dō-kō″rē-oy-dī′tĭs,   ĭr″ĭ-dō-kō-roy-dī′tĭs) [″ + *chorioeides,* skinlike,   + *itis,* inflammation]

iridocoloboma   (ĭr″ĭd-ō-kŏl″ō-bō′mă) [″ + *koloboma,* mutilation]

iridoconstrictor (ĭr″ĭ-dō-kŏn-strĭk′tor)

iridocyclectomy   (ĭr″ĭ-dō-sī-klĕk′tō-mē) [″ + *kyklos,* circle,   + *ektome,* excision]

iridocyclitis (ĭr″ĭd-ō-sī-klī′tĭs) [″ + ″   + *itis,* inflammation]

i., heterochromic

iridocyclochoroiditis   (ĭr″ĭ-dō-sī″klō-kō″roy-dī′tĭs) [″ + ″   + *chorioeides,* skinlike,   + *itis,* inflammation]

iridocystectomy (ĭr″ĭ-dō-sĭs-tĕk′tō-mē) [″ + *kystis,* bladder,   + *ektome,* excision]

iridodesis (ĭr-ĭ-dŏd′ĕ-sĭs) [″ + *desis,* a binding]

iridodiagnosis [″ + *dia,* through,   + *gnosis,* knowledge]

iridodialysis (ĭr″ĭd-ō-dī-ăl′ĭ-sĭs) [″ + *dia,* through,   + *lysis,* dissolution]

iridodilator [″ + L. *dilatare,* to dilate]

iridodonesis (ĭr″ĭd-ō-dō-nē′sĭs) [″ + *donesis,* tremor]

iridokeratitis (ĭr″ĭ-dō-kĕr″ă-tī′tĭs) [″ + *keras,* horn,   + *itis,* inflammation]

iridokinesis (ĭr″ĭd-ō-kĭn-ē′sĭs) [Gr. *iridos,* colored circle,   + *kinesis,* motion]

iridoleptynsis (ĭr″ĭ-dō-lĕp-tĭn′sĭs) [″ + *leptynsis,* attenuation]

iridology (ĭr″ĭ-dŏl′ō-jē) [″ + *logos,* word, reason]

iridomalacia (ĭr″ĭd-ō-mă-lā′shē-ă) [″ + *malakia,* softness]

iridomedialysis (ĭr″ĭd-ō-mē-dē-ăl′ĭ-sĭs) [″ + L. *medius,* in middle,   + Gr. *dia,* through,   + *lysis,* dissolution]

iridomesodialysis (ĭr″ĭd-ō-mĕs″ō-dī-ăl′ĭ-sĭs) [″ + *mesos,* middle,   + *dia,* through,   + *lysis,* dissolution]

iridomotor [″ + L. *motor,* that which moves]

iridoncus (ĭr-ĭ-dong′kŭs) [″ + *onkos,* bulk, mass]

iridoparalysis [″ + *paralyein,* to loosen, disable]

iridoparelkysis (ĭr″ĭ-dō-păr-ĕl′kĭ-sĭs) [″ + *parelkysis,* protraction]

iridopathy (ĭr″ĭ-dŏp′ă-thē) [″ + *pathos,* disease, suffering]

iridoperiphacitis,   iridoperiphakitis (ĭr″ĭ-dō-pĕr″ĭ-fă-sī′tĭs,   -pĕr″ĭ-fă-kī′tĭs)

[" + *peri*, around, + *phakos*, lens, + *itis*, inflammation]

iridoplegia (ĭr″ĭd-ō-plē′jē-ă) [" + *plege*, stroke]
  i., accommodative
  i., complete
  i., reflex

iridoptosis (ĭr″ĭ-dŏp-tō′sĭs) [" + *ptosis*, fall, falling]

iridopupillary (ĭr″ĭ-dō-pū′pĭ-lĕr″ē) [" + L. *pupilla*, pupil]

iridorrhexis (ĭr″ĭd-ō-rĕk′sĭs) [" + *rhexis*, rupture]

iridoschisis (ĭr″ĭ-dŏs′kĭ-sĭs) [" + *schisis*, cleavage]

iridosclerotomy (ĭr″ĭd-ō-sklē-rŏt′ō-mē) [" + *skleros*, hard, + *tome*, a cutting, slice]

iridosteresis (ĭr″ĭ-dō-stē-rē′sĭs) [" + *steresis*, loss]

iridotasis (ĭr-ĭ-dŏt′ă-sĭs) [" + *tasis*, a stretching]

iridotomy (ĭr-ĭ-dŏt′ō-mē) [" + *tome*, a cutting, slice]

iris [Gr., bend, turn]
  i. bombé
  i., chromatic asymmetry of
  i., piebald

Irish moss

irisopsia (ī″rĭs-ŏp′sē-ă) [Gr. *iris*, bend, turn, + *opsis*, sight, appearance, vision]

iritic (ī-rĭt′ĭk) [Gr. *iris*, bend, turn]

iritis [" + *itis*, inflammation]
  i., plastic
  i., primary
  i., purulent
  i., secondary
  i., serous

iritoectomy (ī″rĭ-tō-ĕk′tō-mē) [" + *ektome*, excision]

iritomy (ī-rĭt′ō-mē) [" + *tome*, a cutting, slice]

iron (ī′ĕrn) [AS. *iren*; L. *ferrum*]

iron dextran injection

iron lung

iron poisoning

iron sorbitex injection

iron storage disease

irotomy (ī-rŏt′ō-mē) [Gr. *iris*, bend, turn, + *tome*, a cutting, slice]

irradiate (ĭ-rā′dē-āt) [L. *in*, into, + *radiare*, to emit rays]

irradiating

irradiation
  i., interstitial
  i. of reflexes

irrational

irreducible (ĭr″rē-dū′sĭ-bl) [L. *in-*, not, + *re*, back, + *ducere*, to lead]

irrelevance [" + *relevans*, raising]

irrespirable (ĭr″rē-spī′ră-bl) [" + *respirare*, to breathe again]

irreversible

irrigate [L. *in*, into, + *rigare*, to carry water]

irrigation
  i., bladder
  i., colonic

irrigator

irritability [L. *irritabilis*, irritable]
  i., muscular
  i., nervous

irritable

irritant

irritant poisons

irritation [L. *irritatio*]
  i., spinal
  i., sympathetic

irritative

ischemia (ĭs-kē′mē-ă) [Gr. *ischein*, to hold back, + *haima*, blood]
  i., intestinal
  i., myocardial

ischesis (ĭs-kē′sĭs)

ischia (ĭs′kē-ă) [L.]

ischiac, ischiadic (ĭs′kē-ăk, ĭs-kē-ăd′ĭk)

ischial (ĭs′kē-ăl) [Gr. *ischion*, hip]

ischialgia (ĭs″kē-ăl′jē-ă) [" + *algos*, pain]

ischiatic (ĭs″kē-ăt′ĭk) [Gr. *ischion*, hip]

ischiatitis (ĭs″kē-ă-tī′tĭs) [" + *itis*, inflammation]

ischidrosis (ĭs″kĭ-drō′sĭs) [Gr. *ischein*, to hold back, + *hidrosis*, sweat]

ischio- [Gr. *ischion*, hip]

ischioanal (ĭs″kē-ō-ā′năl) [″ + L. *anus*, anus]

ischiobulbar (ĭs″kē-ō-bŭl′băr) [″ + L. *bulbus*, bulb]

ischiocapsular (ĭs″kē-ō-kăp′sū-lăr) [″ + L. *capsula*, capsule]

ischiocavernosus (ĭs″kē-ō-kă″vĕr-nō′sŭs) [″ + L. *cavernosus*, cavernous]

ischiocele (ĭs′kē-ō-sēl) [″ + *kele*, tumor, swelling]

ischiococcygeus (ĭs″kē-ō-kŏk-sĭj′ē-ŭs) [″ + *kokkyx*, coccyx]

ischiodynia (ĭs″kē-ō-dĭn′ē-ă) [″ + *odyne*, pain]

ischiofemoral (ĭs″kē-ō-fĕm′or-ăl) [″ + L. *femur*, thigh]

ischiofibular (ĭs″kē-ō-fĭb′ū-lăr) [″ + L. *fibula*, pin]

ischiohebotomy (ĭs″kē-ō-hē-bŏt′ō-mē) [″ + *hebe*, pubes, + *tome*, a cutting, slice]

ischioneuralgia (ĭs″kē-ō-nū-răl′jē-ă) [″ + *neuron*, nerve, + *algos*, pain]

ischionitis (ĭs″kē-ō-nī′tĭs) [″ + *itis*, inflammation]

ischiopubic (ĭs″kē-ō-pū′bĭk) [″ + L. *pubes*, the pubes]

ischiopubiotomy (ĭs″kē-ō-pū″bē-ŏt′ō-mē)

ischiorectal (ĭs″kē-ō-rĕk′tăl) [″ + L. *rectus*, straight]

ischiorectal abscess

ischiosacral (ĭs″kē-ō-sā′krăl) [″ + L. *sacralis*, pert. to the sacrum]

ischiovaginal (ĭs″kē-ō-văj′ĭ-năl) [″ + L. *vagina*, sheath]

ischium (ĭs′kē-ŭm) [Gr. *ischion*, hip]

ischo- (ĭs′kō) [Gr. *ischein*, to hold back]

ischogalactic (ĭs″kō-gă-lăk′tĭk) [″ + *gala*, milk]

ischuretic (ĭs″kū-rĕt′ĭk) [″ + *ouron*, urine]

ischuria (ĭs-kū′rē-ă) [″ + *ouron*, urine]

I.S.C.L.T. *International Society of Clinical Laboratory Technologists*

iseikonia (ĭs″ī-kō′nē-ă) [Gr. *isos*, equal, + *eikon*, image]

isinglass (ī′sĭn-glăs)

island [AS. *igland*, island]
i., blood
i.'s of Calleja
i.'s of Langerhans
i. of Reil
i., pancreatic

islet (ī′lĕt)
i.'s of Calleja
i.'s of Langerhans [Paul Langerhans, Ger. pathologist, 1847 – 1888]
i.'s, Walthard's [Max Walthard, Swiss gynecologist, 1867 – 1933]

Ismelin

I.S.O. *International Standards Organization*

iso- [Gr. *isos*, equal]

isoagglutination (ī″sō-ă-gloo″tĭ-nā′shŭn) [″ + L. *agglutinare*, to glue to]

isoagglutinin (ī″sō-ă-glŭ′tĭn-ĭn) [″ + L. *agglutinare*, to glue to]

isoagglutinogen (ī″sō-ă-ġlū-tĭn′ō-jĕn)

isoanaphylaxis (ī″sō-ăn″ă-fĭ-lăk′sĭs) [″ + *ana*, against, + *phylaxis*, guard]

isoantibody (ī″sō-ăn′tĭ-bŏd″ē)

isoantigen (ī″sō-ăn′tĭ-jĕn) [″ + L. *anti*, against, + *gennan*, to produce]

isobar (ī′sō-băr) [″ + *baros*, weight]

isobaric (ī″sō-băr′ĭk)

isobucaine hydrochloride (ī″sō-bū′kān)

isocaloric (ī″sō-kă-lō′rĭk) [″ + L. *calor*, heat]

isocarboxazid (ī″sō-kăr-bŏk′să-zĭd)

isocellular [″ + L. *cellula*, cell]

isochromatic (ī″sō-krō-măt′ĭk) [″ + *chroma*, color]

isochromatophil(e) (ī″sō-krō-măt′ō-fĭl, -fĭl) [″ + ″ + *philein*, to love]

isochromosome (ī″sō-krō′mō-sōm) [″ + ″ + *soma*, body]

isochronal (ī-sŏk′rō-năl) [" + chronos, time]

isochronia (ī″sō-krō′nē-ă) [Gr. isos, equal, + chronos, time]

isochronous (ī-sŏk′rō-nŭs)

isochroous (ī-sŏk′rō-ŭs) [" + chroa, color]

isocitrate dehydrogenase (ī″sō-cīt′rāt dē″hī-drŏj′ĕn-ās)

isocolloid (ī-sō-kŏl′oyd) [" + kollodes, glutinous]

isocomplement [" + L. complere, to complete]

isocoria (ī″sō-kō′rē-ă) [" + kore, pupil]

isocortex (ī″sō-kor′tĕks) [" + L. cortex, bark]

isocytosis (ī″sō-sī-tō′sīs) [" + kytos, cell, + osis, condition]

isocytotoxin (ī″sō-sī″tō-tŏk′sīn) [" + " + toxikon, poison]

isodactylism (ī-sō-dăk′tīl-īzm) [" + daktylos, finger]

isodiametric (ī″sō-dī-ă-mĕt′rĭk) [" + dia, across, + metron, measure]

isodontic (ī″sō-dŏn′tĭk) [" + odous, tooth]

isodose (ī′sō-dōs)

isodynamic (ī″sō-dī-năm′ĭk) [" + dynamis, power]

isoelectric (ī″sō-ē-lĕk′trĭk) [" + elektron, amber]

isoelectric period

isoenergetic [Gr. isos, equal, + energeia, energy]

isoenzyme (ī″sō-ĕn′zīm) [" + en, in, + zyme, leaven]

isoetharine hydrochloride (ī-sō-ĕth′ă-rēn)

Isofedrol

isoflurophate (ī-sō-floo′rō-fāt)

isogamete (ī″sō-găm′ēt) [" + gamete, wife, gametes, husband]

isogamy (ī-sŏg′ă-mē) [" + gamos, marriage]

isogeneic (ī″sō-jĕn-ē′ĭk)

isogeneric (ī″sō-jĕ-nĕr′ĭk) [" + L. genus, kind]

isogenesis (ī″sō-jĕn′ĕ-sīs) [" + genesis, generation, birth]

isogenic (ī″sō-jĕn′ĭk)

isograft [" + L. graphium, stylus]

isohemagglutination (ī″sō-hĕm″ă-gloo″tī-nā′shŭn) [" + haima, blood, + L. agglutinare, to glue to]

isohemagglutinin (ī″sō-hĕm″ă-glū′tĭn-ĭn) [" + haima, blood, + L. agglutinare, to glue to]

isohemolysin (ī″sō-hē-mŏl′ĭ-sīn) [" + " + lysis, dissolution]

isohemolysis (ī″sō-hē-mŏl′ĭ-sīs)

isohypercytosis (ī″sō-hī″pĕr-sī-tō′sīs) [" + hyper, over, above, excessive, + kytos, cell, + osis, condition]

isohypocytosis (ī″sō-hī″pō-sī-tō′sīs) [" + hypo, under, beneath, below, + kytos, cell, + osis, condition]

isoiconia (ī″sō-ī-kō′nē-ă) [Gr. isos, equal, + eikon, image]

isoiconic (ī″sō-ī-kŏn′ĭk)

isoimmunization [" + L. immunis, safe]

isokinetic exercise

isolate [It. isolato, isolated]

isolation
   i., infectious
   i., protective
   i., reverse

isolation ward

isoleucine (ī″sō-lū′sēn)

isologous (ī-sŏl′ō-gŭs)

isolophobia (ī″sō-lō-fō′bē-ă) [It. isolato, isolated, + Gr. phobos, fear]

isolysin (ī-sŏl′ĭ-sīn) [Gr. isos, equal, + lysis, dissolution]

isolysis (ī-sŏl′ĭ-sīs)

isolytic (ī-sō-lĭt′ĭk)

isomer (ī′sō-mĕr) [Gr. isos, equal, + meros, part]

isomerase (ī-sŏm′ĕr-ās)

isomeric (ī″sō-mĕr′ĭk)

isomerism (ī-sŏm′ĕr-īzm)

isomerization (ī-sŏm″ĕr-ī-zā′shŭn)

isometric [" + metron, measure]

isometric contraction

isometric contraction phase
isometric exercise
isometric muscle
isometropia (ī"sō-mĕ-trō'pē-ă) [" + " + *ops*, eye]
isomorphism (ī-sō-mor'fĭzm) [" + *morphe*, form, + *-ismos*, condition]
isomorphous (ī"sō-mor'fŭs)
isoniazid (ī"sō-nī'ă-zĭd)
isonicotinoylhydrazine (ī"sō-nĭk"ō-tĭn"ō-ĭl-hī'dră-zēn)
isonormocytosis (ī"sō-nor"mō-sī-tō'sĭs) [" + L. *norma*, rule, + Gr. *kytos*, cell, + *osis*, condition]
isopathy (ī-sŏp'ă-thē) [Gr. *isos*, equal, + *pathos*, disease, suffering]
isophoria (ī"sō-fō'rē-ă) [" + *phorein*, to carry]
isopia (ī-sō'pē-ă) [" + *ops*, vision]
isoplastic (ī"sō-plăs'tĭk) [" + *plastos*, formed]
isoprecipitin (ī"sō-prē-sĭp'ĭ-tĭn) [" + L. *praecipitare*, to cast down]
isopropamide iodide (ī"sō-prō'pă-mīd)
isopropanol (ī"sō-prō'pă-nŏl)
isopropyl alcohol
isoproterenol hydrochloride (ī"sō-prō"tĕ-rē'nŏl)
isopters (ī-sŏp'tĕrz) [" + *opter*, observer]
Isopto Atropine
Isopto Carbachol
Isopto Carpine
Isopto Cetamide
Isopto Eserine
Isopto Frin
Isopto Homatropine
Isopto Hyoscine
isopyknosis (ī"sō-pĭk-nō'sĭs) [" + *pyknosis*, condensation]
Isordil
isoserotherapy (ī"sō-sē"rō-thĕr'ă-pē) [" + L. *serum*, whey, + Gr. *therapeia*, treatment]
isoserum (ī"sō-sē'rŭm)
isosexual (ī"sō-sĕks'ū-ăl)
isosmotic (ī"sŏs-mŏt'ĭk) [" + *osmos*, impulsion]

isosorbide dinitrate tablets (ī"sō-sor'bīd)
Isospora (ī-sŏs'pō-ră) [" + *sporos*, seed]
   I. hominis
isospore (ī'sō-spor) [Gr. *isos*, equal, + *sporos*, seed]
isosthenuria (ī"sōs-thĕn-ū'rē-ă) [" + *sthenos*, strength, + *ouron*, urine]
isostimulation [" + L. *stimulare*, to goad]
isotherapy (ī"sō-thĕr'ă-pē) [" + *therapeia*, treatment]
isothermal [" + *therme*, heat]
isothermognosis (ī"sō-thĕrm"ŏg-nō'sĭs) [" + " + *gnosis*, knowledge]
isotherms (ī'sō-thĕrmz)
isotones (ī'sō-tōnz)
isotonia (ī"sō-tō'nē-ă) [" + *tonos*, act of stretching, tension, tone]
isotonic (ī"sō-tŏn'ĭk)
isotonic exercise
isotonicity (ī"sō-tō-nĭs'ĭ-tē)
isotonic solution
isotope (ī'sō-tōp) [" + *topos*, place]
   i., radioactive
isotope cisternography
isotretinoin
isotropic (ī"sō-trŏp'ĭk) [" + *tropos*, a turning]
isotropy (ī-sŏt'rō-pē)
isotypes
isotypical (ī-sō-tĭp'ĭ-kăl) [" + *typos*, mark]
isovalericacidemia (ī"sō-vă-lĕr'ĭk-ăs"ĭ-dē'mē-ă)
isoxsuprine hydrochloride (ī-sŏk'sū-prēn)
isozyme (ī'sō-zīm)
issue (ĭsh'ū) [ME.]
isthmectomy (ĭs-mĕk'tō-mē) [Gr. *isthmos*, isthmus, + *ektome*, excision]
isthmian (ĭs'mē-ăn)
isthmitis (ĭs-mī'tĭs) [" + *itis*, inflammation]
isthmoparalysis (ĭs"mō-pă-răl'ĭ-sĭs)

[" + *paralyein*, to loosen, disable]
isthmoplegia (ĭs"mō-plē'jē-ă) [" +
plege, a stroke]
isthmospasm (ĭs'mō-spăzm") [" +
spasmos, a convulsion]
isthmus (ĭs'mŭs) [L.; Gr. *isthmos*, isthmus]
   i., aortic
   i. faucium
   i. glandulae thyroideae
   i. of eustachian tube
   i. of thyroid
   i. of uterine tube
   i. of uterus
   i., pharyngeal
   i. pharyngonasalis
   i. tubae auditivae
   i. tubae uterinae
   i. uteri
Isuprel Hydrochloride
isuria (ĭ-sū'rē-ă) [Gr. *isos*, equal, +
ouron, urine]
itch [ME. *icchen*]
   i., baker's
   i., barber's
   i., dhobie
   i., grain
   i., grocer's
   i., ground
   i., jock
   i., seven-year
   i., swimmer's
   i., winter
itching
itch mite
iter (ī'tĕr) [L.]
iteral (ī'tĕr-ăl)

iteroparity (ĭt"ĕr-ō-păr'ĭ-tē) [L. *iterare*,
to repeat, + *parere*, to beget,
produce]
ithycyphosis, ithyokyphosis (ĭth"ĭ-
sī-fō'sĭs, ĭth"ē-ō-kĭ-fō'sĭs) [Gr. *ithys*,
straight, + *kyphos*, humped]
ithylordosis (ĭth"ĭ-lor-dō'sĭs) [" +
lordosis, a bending forward]
ITP idiopathic thrombocytopenic pur-
pura
I.U. immunizing unit; international unit
IUCD intrauterine contraceptive device
IUD intrauterine device
I.V. intravenous(ly)
Ivadantin
IVC intravenous cholangiography
IVCD intraventricular conduction defect
ivermectin
IVF in vitro fertilization
I.V.P. intravenous pyelography
I.V. push
I.V.T. intravenous transfusion
I.V.U. intravenous urography
Ivy method (ī'vē) [Andrew C. Ivy, U.S.
physiologist, 1893 – 1978]
ivy poisoning
Ixodes (ĭks-ō'dēz) [Gr. *ixodes*, like bird-
lime]
ixodiasis (ĭks"ō-dī'ă-sĭs)
ixodic (ĭks-ŏd'ĭk)
Ixodidae (ĭks-ŏd'ĭ-dē)
Ixodides (ĭks-ŏd'ĭ-dēz)
Ixodoidea (ĭks"ō-doy'dē-ă)
ixomyelitis (ĭks"ō-mī-ĕ-lī'tĭs) [Gr.
ixodes, like birdlime, + *myelos*,
marrow, + *itis*, inflammation]

J

J *joule*

Jaboulay's amputation (zhǎ"boo-lāz') [Mathieu Jaboulay, Fr. surgeon, 1860–1913]

Jaboulay's button

jacket [O. Fr. *jacquet*, jacket]
j., porcelain
j., Sayre's
j., strait-

jackknife position

jackscrew

jacksonian epilepsy [John Hughlings Jackson, Brit. neurologist, 1835–1911]

Jacob, Arthur [Irish ophthalmologist, 1790–1874]
J.'s membrane
J.'s ulcer

Jacobson, Ludwig [Danish anatomist, 1783–1843]
J.'s cartilage
J.'s nerve
J.'s organ
J.'s sulcus

Jacquemier's sign (zhǎk-mē-āz') [Jean Jacquemier, Fr. obstetrician, 1806–1879]

jactatio (jǎk-tā'shē-ō) [L.]

jactitation (jǎk"tǐ-tā'shǔn) [L. *jactitatio*, tossing]

Jaeger's test types (yā'gěrz) [Edward Jaeger von Jastthal, Austrian ophthalmologist, 1818–1884]

jamais vu (zhǎm'ā voo) [Fr., never seen]

James fibers [T. N. James, U.S. cardiologist and physiologist, b. 1925]

Janeway lesions [E. G. Janeway, U.S. physician, 1841–1911]

janiceps (jǎn'ǐ-sěps) [L. *Janus*, a two-faced god, + *caput*, head]

Janimine

Jansky-Bielschowsky syndrome (jǎn'skē-bē-ǎl-show'skē) [Jan Jansky, Czech physician, 1873–1921; Max Bielschowsky, Ger. neuropathologist, 1869–1940]

jar
j., bell
j., heel

jargon (jǎr'gǔn) [O. Fr., a chattering]

Jarvis' snare [William C. Jarvis, U.S. laryngologist, 1855–1895]

jaundice (jawn'dǐs) [Fr. *jaune*, yellow]
j., acholuric
j., cholestatic
j., congenital
j., hematogenous
j., hemolytic
j., hemorrhagic
j., hepatocanalicular
j., hepatocellular
j., hepatogenous
j., infectious
j., leptospiral
j., malignant
j., nonhemolytic
j., obstructive
j. of newborn
j., parenchymatous
j., physiologic
j., posthepatic
j., regurgitation
j., retention
j., spirochetal
j., toxic

Javelle water (zhǔ-věl') [Javel, a city now part of Paris]

jaw [ME. *iawe*]
j., cleft
j., crackling
j., dislocation of

j., lumpy
j., swelling of
jaw winking
jejunal (jē-jū'năl) [L. *jejunum*, empty]
jejunectomy (jē"jū-něk'tō-mē) [" + Gr. *ektome*, excision]
jejunitis (jē"jū-nī'tĭs) [" + Gr. *itis*, inflammation]
jejunocecostomy (jē-joo"nō-sē-kŏs'tō-mē) [" + *caecum*, blindness, + Gr. *stoma*, mouth, opening]
jejunocolostomy (jē-jū"nō-kōl-ŏs'tō-mē) [" + Gr. *kolon*, colon, + *stoma*, mouth, opening]
jejunoileal (jē-joo"nō-ĭl'ē-ăl) [" + *ileum*, small intestine]
jejunoileitis (jē-jū"nō-ĭl"ē-ī'tĭs) [" + " + Gr. *itis*, inflammation]
jejunoileostomy (jē-jū"nō-ĭl"ē-ŏs'tō-mē) [" + " + Gr. *stoma*, mouth, opening]
jejunojejunostomy (jē-jū"nō-jē"jū-nŏs'tō-mē) [" + *jejunum*, empty, + Gr. *stoma*, mouth, opening]
jejunorrhaphy (jē"joo-nor'ă-fē) [" + Gr. *rhaphe*, seam]
jejunostomy (jē"jū-nŏs'tō-mē) [" + Gr. *stoma*, mouth, opening]
jejunotomy (jē"jū-nŏt'ō-mē) [" + Gr. *tome*, a cutting, slice]
jejunum (jē-jū'nŭm) [L., empty]
j., inflammation of
jelly [L. *gelare*, to freeze]
j., contraceptive
j., mineral
j., petroleum
j., vaginal
j., Wharton's
Jendrassik's maneuver (yĕn-drä'sĭks) [Ernö Jendrassik, Hungarian physician, 1858–1921]
Jenner, Edward [Brit. physician, 1749–1823]
Jenner's stain [Louis Jenner, Brit. physician, 1866–1904]
jerk (jĕrk)
j., Achilles; j., ankle
j., biceps

j., elbow
j., jaw
j., knee
j., tendon
j., triceps surae
jet lag
jigger
jimson weed
jitters (jĭt'ĕrz)
Jobst pressure garment
Jocasta complex (jō-kăs'tă) [Jocasta, mother in the Oedipus complex, who was the wife and mother of Oedipus]
Joffroy's reflex (zhŏf-rwhäz') [Alexis Joffroy, Fr. physician, 1844–1908]
Joffroy's sign
jogger's heel
jogging
joint [L. *junctio*, a joining]
j., amphidiarthrodial
j., arthrodial
j., ball-and-socket
j., biaxial
j., bilocular
j., bleeders'
j., Brodie's
j., Budin's
j., cartilaginous
j., Charcot's
j., Chopart's
j., cochlear
j., compound
j., condyloid
j.'s, craniomandibular
j., diarthrodial
j., dry
j., ellipsoid
j., enarthrodial
j., false
j.'s, fibrous
j., flail
j., ginglymoid
j., gliding
j., hemophilic
j., hinge
j., hip
j., immovable
j.'s, intercarpal

j., irritable
j., knee
j., midcarpal
j., mixed
j., movable
j., multiaxial
j., pivot
j., plane
j., polyaxial
j., receptive
j., rotary
j., saddle
j., simple
j., spheroid
j., spiral
j., sternoclavicular
j.'s, subtalar
j., synarthrodial
j., synovial
j.'s, tarsometatarsal
j.'s, temporomandibular
j., trochoid
j., uniaxial
j., unilocular

joint approximation
joint capsule
joint cavity
joint mice
joint protection
Jones criteria [T.D. Jones, U.S. physician, 1899–1954]
joule (jūl) [James P. Joule, Brit. physicist, 1818–1899]
jugal [L. jugalis, of a yoke]
jugal bone
jugale (jū-gā'lē)
jugal process
jugate (jū'gāt) [L. jugatus, joined]
jugomaxillary (joo″gō-măk'sĭ-lăr″ē)
jugular (jŭg'ū-lăr) [L. jugularis]
jugular foramen
jugular fossa
jugular ganglion
jugular process
jugular veins
jugulate (jŭg'ū-lāt) [L. jugulare, to cut the throat]
jugulation (jŭg″ū-lā'shŭn)

jugulum (jŭg'ū-lŭm) [L.]
jugum (jū'gŭm) [L., a yoke]
j. penis
j. petrosum
juice [L. jus, broth]
j., alimentary
j., gastric
j., intestinal
j., pancreatic
jujitsu, jiujitsu (jū-jĭt'sū) [Japanese]
jumentous (jū-mĕn'tŭs) [L. jumentum, beast of burden]
Jumping Frenchmen of Maine
junction (jŭnk'shŭn) [L. junctio, a joining]
j., amelodentinal
j., cementodentinal
j., cementoenamel
j., dentinocemental
j., dentinoenamel
j., dentogingival
j., interneuronal
j., mucocutaneous
j., mucogingival
j., myoneural
j., sclerocorneal
j., squamocolumnar
j., tight
junctional epithelium
junctura (jŭnk-tū'ră) [L., a joining]
juniper tar (joo'nĭ-pĕr)
junket [L. juncus]
jurisprudence (joor″ĭs-proo'dĕns) [L. juris prudentia, knowledge of law]
j., dental
j., medical
jury-mast (jūr'ē-măst) [L. jurare, to be right, + AS. masc, a stick]
jusculum (jŭs'kū-lŭm) [L.]
Juster's reflex [Emile Juster, 20th century Fr. neurologist]
justo major (jŭs'tō mā'jor) [L.]
justo minor (jŭs'tō mī'nor) [L.]
jute (jūt) [Sanskrit juta, matted hair]
juvenile (jū'vĕ-nīl″) [L. juvenis, young]
juvenile cell
juvenile rheumatoid arthritis
juxta- [L., near]
juxta-articular (jŭks″tă-ăr-tĭk'ū-lăr) ["

+ *articulus,* joint]

juxtaglomerular (jŭks"tă-glō-mĕr'ū-lăr) [" + *glomus,* ball]

juxtaglomerular apparatus

juxtaglomerular cells

juxtangina (jŭks"tăn-jĭ'nă) [" + *angina,* a choking]

juxtaposition (jŭks"tă-pō-zĭ'shŭn) [" + *positio,* place]

juxtapyloric (jŭks"tă-pī-lor'ĭk) [" + Gr. *pyloros,* gatekeeper]

juxtaspinal (jŭks"tă-spī'năl) [" + *spina,* thorn]

K

K [L. *kalium*, potassium]
K, k Gr. letter *kappa; Kelvin temperature scale; kilo*
Ka *cathode*
Kabikinase
Kader's operation (kǎ'dĕrs) [Bronislaw Kader, Polish surgeon, 1863–1937]
kaif (kīf) [Arabic, quiescence]
kainophobia (kī-nō-fō'bē-ǎ) [Gr. *kainos*, new, + *phobos*, fear]
kaiserling (kī'zĕr-lĭng) [Karl Kaiserling, Ger. pathologist, 1869–1942]
kakidrosis (kǎk-ĭ-drō'sĭs) [Gr. *kakos*, bad, + *hidrosis*, sweat]
kakke (kŏk'kā) [Japanese]
kakosmia (kǎk-ŏz'mē-ǎ) [Gr. *kakos*, bad, + *osme*, smell]
kakotrophy (kǎk-ŏt'rō-fē) [" + *trophe*, nourishment]
kala-azar (kǎ'lǎ ǎ-zǎr') [Hindi, black fever]
kaliemia (kā-lē-ē'mē-ǎ) [Arabic, *gali*, potash, + Gr. *haima*, blood]
kaligenous (kā-lĭj'ĕ-nŭs) [" + Gr. *gennan*, to produce]
kalimeter (kǎ-lĭm'ĕ-ter) [" + Gr. *metron*, measure]
kaliopenia (kǎ"lē-ō-pē'nē-ǎ) [L. *kalium*, potassium, + Gr. *penia*, lack]
kalium (kā'lē-ŭm) [L.]
kaliuresis (kǎ"lē-ū-rē'sĭs) [" + Gr. *ouresis*, urination]
kallidin (kǎl'ĭ-dĭn)
kallikrein (kǎl-ĭ-krē'ĭn) [Gr. *kallikreas*, pancreas]
kallikreinogen (kǎl"ĭ-krī'nō-jĕn) [" + *gennan*, to produce]
kanamycin sulfate (kǎn"ǎ-mī'sĭn)
Kanner syndrome [Leo Kanner, Austrian psychiatrist in the U.S., b. 1894]

Kantrex
Kaochlor
kaolin (kā'ō-lĭn) [Fr., from Mandarin Chinese *kao*, high, + *ling*, mountain]
kaolinosis (kā"ō-lĭn-ō'sĭs)
Kaon
Kaon-Cl
Kaopectate
Kaposi, Moritz K. (kǎp'ō-sē") [Hungarian dermatologist, 1837–1902]
    K.'s disease
    K.'s sarcoma
    K.'s varicelliform eruption
Kappadione
karaya gum (kǎr'ā-ǎ)
Karman catheter [Harvey Karman, contemporary U.S. psychologist]
Karnofsky Index (or Scale) [D. A. Karnofsky, 20th century physician]
Kartagener's syndrome (kǎr'tǎ-gǎ"nĕrz) [Manes Kartagener, Swiss physician, 1897–1975]
karyo- [Gr. *karyon*, nucleus]
karyochromatophil (kǎr"ē-ō-krō-māt'ō-fĭl) [" + *chroma*, color, + *philein*, to love]
karyochrome (kǎr'ē-ō-krōm")
karyoclasis (kǎr-ē-ŏk'lǎ-sĭs) [Gr. *karyon*, nucleus, + *klasis*, a breaking]
karyocyte (kǎr'ē-ō-sīt) [" + *kytos*, cell]
karyogamy (kǎr-ē-ŏg'ǎ-mē) [" + *gamos*, marriage]
karyogenesis (kǎr"ē-ō-jĕn'ĕ-sĭs) [" + *genesis*, generation, birth]
karyokinesis (kǎr"ē-ō-kĭn-ē'sĭs) [" + *kinesis*, motion]
karyokinetic (kǎr"ē-ō-kĭ-nĕt'ĭk)
karyoklasis (kǎr"ē-ŏk'lǎ-sĭs) [" + *klasis*, a breaking]
karyolobism (kǎr"ē-ō-lō'bĭzm) [" +

L. *lobus*, lobe, + Gr. *-ismos*, condition]

karyolymph [" + L. *lympha*, lymph]

karyolysis (kăr-ē-ŏl′ĭ-sĭs) [" + *lysis*, dissolution]

karyolytic (kăr-ē-ō-lĭt′ĭk)

karyomegaly (kăr″ē-ō-mĕg′ă-lē) [" + *megas*, large]

karyomere (kăr′ē-ō-mēr″) [" + *meros*, part]

karyomicrosome (kăr″ē-ō-mī′krō-sōm) [" + *mikros*, small, + *soma*, body]

karyomitome (kăr″ē-ŏm′ĭ-tōm) [" + *mitos*, thread]

karyomitosis (kăr″ē-ō-mī-tō′sĭs) [" + *mitos*, thread, + *osis*, condition]

karyomorphism (kăr-ē-ō-mor′fĭzm) [" + *morphe*, form, + *-ismos*, condition]

karyon (kăr′ē-ŏn) [Gr.]

karyophage (kăr′ē-ō-fāj) [" + *phagein*, to eat]

karyopyknosis (kăr″ē-ō-pĭk-nō′sĭs) [" + *pyknos*, thick, + *osis*, condition]

karyorrhexis (kăr″ē-ō-rĕk′sĭs) [" + *rhexis*, rupture]

karyosome (kăr′ē-ō-sōm) [" + *soma*, body]

karyostasis (kăr″ē-ŏs′tă-sĭs) [" + *stasis*, standing still]

karyotheca (kăr″ē-ō-thē′kă) [" + *theke*, sheath]

karyotype (kăr′ē-ō-tīp) [" + *typos*, mark]

karyozoic (kăr″ē-ō-zō′ĭk) [" + *zoon*, animal]

Kasabach-Merritt syndrome [Haig H. Kasabach, U.S. pediatrician, 1898–1943; K. K. Merritt, U.S. physician, b. 1886]

Kashin-Beck disease [N. I. Kashin, Russian physician, 1825–1872; E. V. (Bek) Beck]

kata- [Gr. *kata*, down]

katabolism (kă-tăb′ō-lĭsm) [" +

ballein, to throw, + *-ismos*, condition]

kataplasia (kăt-ă-plā′sē-ă)

katathermometer (kăt″ă-thĕr-mŏm′ĕ-ter) [" + *therme*, heat, + *metron*, measure]

katatonia (kăt-ă-tō′nē-ă) [" + *tonos*, act of stretching, tension, tone]

kathisophobia (kăth″ĭ-sō-fō′bē-ă) [Gr. *kathizein*, to sit down, + *phobos*, fear]

kation (kăt′ē-ŏn) [Gr., descending]

katophoria (kăt″ō-fō′rē-ă)

katotropia (kăt″ō-trō′pē-ă) [Gr. *kata*, down, + *tropos*, a turning]

katzenjammer (kăts′ĕn-yăm′ĕr) [Ger. *katzen*, cats, + *jammer*, distress, misery]

kava [Tongan, bitter]

Kawasaki disease [Tomsaku Kawasaki, contemporary Japanese pediatrician]

Kay Ciel

Kayser-Fleischer ring (kī′zĕr-flī′shĕr) [Bernard Kayser, 1869–1954; Bruno Fleischer, 1848–1904, Ger. physicians]

KBr potassium bromide

kc kilocycle

KC₂H₃O₂ potassium acetate

$KC_2H_3O_2$ potassium acetate

KCl potassium chloride

KClO potassium hypochlorite

KClO₃ potassium chlorate

K₂CO₃ potassium carbonate

k.c.p.s. kilocycles per second

kefir, kefyr (kĕf′ĕr) [Caucasus region of Russia]

Keflex

Keflin

Kegel exercises [A. H. Kegel, contemporary U.S. physician]

Keith's bundle, node (kēths) [Sir Arthur Keith, Brit. anatomist, 1866–1955]

Keith-Flack node [Sir Arthur Keith; Martin William Flack, Brit. physiologist, 1882–1931]

Keith-Wagener-Barker classifica-

tion
kelis (kē′lĭs) [Gr., blemish]
Kell blood group
Kelly's pad [Howard A. Kelly, U.S. surgeon, 1858–1943]
keloid (kē′lŏyd) [Gr. *kele*, tumor, swelling, + *eidos*, form, shape]
  k., acne
keloidosis (kē″loy-dō′sĭs) [″ + ″ + *osis*, condition]
kelotomy (kē-lŏt′ō-mē) [″ + *tome*, a cutting, slice]
kelp
Kelvin scale [William Thompson Kelvin, Brit. physicist, 1824–1907]
Kemadrin
Kempner rice-fruit diet (kĕmp′nĕr) [Walter Kempner, U.S. physician, b. 1903]
Kenacort
Kenalog
Kenny treatment [Sister Elizabeth Kenny, Australian nurse, 1886–1952]
kenophobia (kĕn″ō-fō′bē-ă) [Gr. *kenos*, empty, + *phobos*, fear]
kenotoxin (kē′nō-tŏk-sĭn) [″ + *toxikon*, poison]
Kent's bundles [A. F. S. Kent, Brit. physiologist, 1863–1958]
kerasin (kĕr′ă-sĭn)
keratalgia (kĕr″ă-tăl′jē-ă) [Gr. *keras*, horn, + *algos*, pain]
keratectasia (kĕr″ă-tĕk-tā′sē-ă) [″ + *ektasis*, extension]
keratectomy (kĕr-ă-tĕk′tō-mē) [″ + *ektome*, excision]
keratiasis (kĕr-ă-tī′ă-sĭs) [″ + -*iasis*, state or condition of]
keratic (kĕr-ăt′ĭk)
keratin (kĕr′ă-tĭn)
  k., hard
  k., soft
keratinase (kĕr′ă-tĭ-nās)
keratinization
keratinize (kĕr′ă-tĭn-īz) [Gr. *keras*, horn]
keratinocyte (kĕ-răt′ĭ-nō-sīt) [″ + *kytos*, cell]

keratinous (kĕr-ăt′ĭ-nŭs)
keratitic precipitates
keratitis (kĕr-ă-tī′tĭs) [″ + *itis*, inflammation]
  k., band-shaped
  k. bullosa
  k., deep
  k., dendritic
  k. disciformis
  k., fascicular
  k., herpetic
  k., hypopyon
  k., interstitial
  k., lagophthalmic
  k., mycotic
  k., neuroparalytic
  k., parenchymatous
  k., phlyctenular
  k., punctate
  k., purulent
  k., sclerosing
  k., superficial punctate
  k., trachomatous
  k., traumatic
  k., xerotic
kerato-, kerat- [Gr. *keras*, horn]
keratoacanthoma (kĕr″ă-tō-ăk″ăn-thō′mă) [″ + *akantha*, thorn, + *oma*, tumor]
keratocele (kĕr-ăt′ō-sēl) [″ + *kele*, tumor, swelling]
keratoconjunctivitis (kĕr″ă-tō-kŏn-jŭnk″tĭ-vī′tĭs)
  k., epidemic
  k., flash
  k., phlyctenular
  k. sicca
  k., virus
keratoconus (kĕr-ă-tō-kō′nŭs) [″ + *konos*, cone]
keratocyte (kĕr′ă-tō-sīt)
keratoderma (kĕr″ă-tō-dĕr′mă) [″ + *derma*, skin]
  k. blennorrhagica
  k. climactericum
keratodermatitis (kĕr″ă-tō-dĕr″mă-tī′tĭs) [″ + ″ + *itis*, inflammation]

keratodermia
keratogenous (kĕr-ă-tŏj′ĕ-nŭs) [″ +
gennan, to produce]
keratoglobus (kĕr″ă-tō-glō′bŭs)
[″ + L. globus, circle]
keratohelcosis (kĕr″ă-tō-hĕl-kō′sĭs)
[″ + helkosis, ulceration]
keratohemia (kĕr″ă-tō-hē′mē-ă)
[″ + haima, blood]
keratohyalin
keratoid (kĕr′ă-toyd) [″ + eidos,
form, shape]
keratoiditis (kĕr″ă-toyd-ī′tĭs) [″ +
″ + itis, inflammation]
keratoiritis (kĕr″ă-tō-ī-rī′tĭs) [″ +
iris, bend, turn, + itis, inflammation]
keratoleptynsis (kĕr″ă-tō-lĕp-tin′sĭs)
[″ + leptynein, to make thin]
keratoleukoma (kĕr″ă-tō-lū-kō′mă) [″
+ leukos, white, + oma, tumor]
keratolysis (kĕr-ă-tŏl′ĭ-sĭs) [″ +
lysis, dissolution]
    k., pitted
keratolytic (kĕr″ă-tō-lĭt′ĭk)
keratoma (kĕr″ă-tō′mă) [″ + oma,
tumor]
keratomalacia (kĕr″ă-tō-mă-lā′shē-ă)
[″ + malakia, softness]
keratome (kĕr′ă-tōm) [″ + tome, a
cutting, slice]
keratometer (kĕr-ă-tŏm′ĕ-ter) [″ +
metron, measure]
keratometry (kĕr″ă-tŏm′ĕ-trē) [″ +
metron, measure]
keratomileusis (kĕr″ă-tō-mī-loo′sĭs)
[″ + smileusis, carving]
keratomycosis (kĕr″ă-tō-mī-kō′sĭs)
[″ + mykes, fungus, + osis,
condition]
keratonosis (kĕr″ă-tō-nō′sĭs) [″ +
nosos, disease]
keratonyxis (kĕr″ă-tō-nĭks′ĭs) [″ +
nyssein, to puncture]
keratopathy, band (kĕr″ă-tŏp′ă-thē)
[″ + pathos, disease, suffering]
keratoplasty (kĕr′ă-tō-plăs″tē) [″ +
plassein, to form]
    k., optic

k., refractive
k., tectonic
keratoprotein (kĕr″ă-tō-prō′tē-ĭn)
[″ + protos, first]
keratorrhexis (kĕr″ă-tō-rĕks′ĭs) [″ +
rhexis, rupture]
keratoscleritis (kĕr″ă-tō-sklĕr-ī′tĭs)
[″ + skleros, hard, + itis, in-
flammation]
keratoscope (kĕr′ăt-ō-skōp) [″ +
skopein, to examine]
keratoscopy
keratose (kĕr′ă-tōs) [Gr. keras, horn]
keratosis (kĕr-ă-tō′sĭs) [″ + osis,
condition]
    k., actinic
    k. climactericum
    k. follicularis
    k. nigricans
    k., oral
    k. palmaris et plantaris
    k. pharyngis
    k. pilaris
    k. punctata
    k., seborrheic
    k. senilis
keratotome (kĕr-ăt′ō-tōm) [″ +
tome, a cutting, slice]
keratotomy (kĕr-ă-tŏt′ō-mē)
    k., radial
keraunoneurosis (kĕ-raw″nō-nū-
rō′sĭs) [Gr. keraunos, lightning, +
neuron, nerve, + osis, condition]
keraunophobia (kĕ-raw″nō-fō′bē-ă)
[″ + phobos, fear]
Kerckring's folds (kĕrk′rĭngz) [Theo-
dorus Kerckring, Dutch anatomist,
1640 – 1693]
kerectomy (kē-rĕk′tō-mē) [Gr. keras,
horn, + ektome, excision]
kerion (kē′rē-ŏn) [Gr., honeycomb]
Kerley lines [P. J. Kerley, Brit. radiologist, b. 1900]
kernicterus (kĕr-nĭk′tĕr-ŭs) [Ger.]
Kernig's sign (kĕr′nĭgz) [Vladimir Kernig, Russian physician, 1840 – 1917]
kerosene (kĕr′ō-sēn)
Ketaject

Ketalar
ketamine hydrochloride
keto acid (kē″tō-ăs′ĭd)
ketoacidosis (kē″tō-ă″sĭ-dō′sĭs) [Ger. *keton*, alter. of *azeton*, acetone, + L. *acidus*, sour, + Gr. *osis*, condition]
ketoaciduria (kē″tō-ăs″ĭ-dū′rē-ă) [″ + ″ + Gr. *ouron*, urine]
ketogenesis (kē-tō-jĕn′ĕ-sĭs) [″ + Gr. *genesis*, generation, birth]
ketogenic diet (kē-tō-jĕn′ĭk) [″ + Gr. *gennan*, to produce]
ketohexose (kē″tō-hĕks′ōs) [″ + *hex*, six, + -*ose*]
ketolysis (kē-tŏl′ĭ-sĭs) [″ + Gr. *lysis*, dissolution]
ketolytic
ketone (kē′tōn)
ketone bodies
ketonemia (kē″tō-nē′mē-ă) [″ + Gr. *haima*, blood]
ketone threshold
ketonuria (kē-tō-nū′rē-ă) [″ + Gr. *ouron*, urine]
ketoplasia (kē-tō-plā′sē-ă) [″ + Gr. *plassein*, to form]
ketoplastic [″ + Gr. *plastikos*, formed]
ketose
ketosis (kē-tō′sĭs) [″ + Gr. *osis*, condition]
17-ketosteroid
ketosuria (kē″tō-sū′rē-ă)
ketotic
keV *kiloelectron volts*
Key-Retzius foramina (kē′rĕt′zē-ŭs) [Ernst A. H. Key, Swedish physician, 1832–1901; Magnus G. Retzius, Swedish histologist, 1842–1919]
kg *kilogram*
kg-m *kilogram-meter*
KHCO₃ *potassium bicarbonate*
KHSO₄ *potassium bisulfate*
kHz *kilohertz*
KI *potassium iodide*
kibe (kīb) [Welsh *cibi*, chilblain]
kidney [ME. *kidenei*]

k., amyloid
k., artificial
k., cake
k., contracted
k., cystic
k., embolic contracted
k., fatty
k., flea-bitten
k., floating
k., fused
k., Goldblatt
k., granular
k., horseshoe
k., hypermobile
k., lardaceous
k., lump
k., movable
k., polycystic
k., red contracted
k., sacculated
k., sponge
k., syphilitic
k., wandering
k., waxy
kidney failure
kidney stone
Kienböck's disease (kēn′bĕks) [Robert Kienböck, Austrian physician, 1871–1953]
Kiernan's spaces (kēr′nănz) [Francis Kiernan, Brit. physician, 1800–1874]
Kiesselbach's plexus (kē′sĕl-bŏks) [Wilhelm Kiesselbach, Ger. laryngologist, 1839–1902]
Kilian's pelvis (kĭl′ē-ănz) [Hermann F. Kilian, Ger. gynecologist, 1800–1863]
kilocalorie
kilocycle (kĭl′ō-sī″k′l)
kilogram [Fr. *kilo*, a thousand, + *gramme*, a small weight]
kilogram-meter
kilohertz
kilojoule
kiloliter (kĭl′ō-lē″tĕr) [Fr. *kilolitre*]
kilomegacycles
kilometer [Fr. *kilometre*]
kilopascal (kĭl″ō-păs-kăl′) [″ + Pa-

scal, Fr. scientist]
kilounit (kĭl″ō-ū′nĭt)
kilovolt [Fr. *kilo,* a thousand, + *volt*]
kilovoltage peak
kilowatt
Kimmelstiel-Wilson syndrome [Paul Kimmelstiel, Ger. physician, 1900–1970; Clifford Wilson, Brit. physician, b. 1906]
kinanesthesia (kĭn-ăn-ĕs-thē′zē-ă) [Gr. *kinesis,* motion, + *an-,* not, + *aisthesis,* feeling, perception]
kinase (kĭn′ās)
kinematics [Gr. *kinematos,* movement]
kinematograph (kĭn″ĕ-măt′o-grăf)
kineplastic (kĭn″ĭ-plăs′tĭk) [Gr. *kinein,* to move, + *plastikos,* formed]
kineplasty
kinesalgia (kĭn″ĕ-săl′jē-ă) [Gr. *kinesis,* motion, + *algos,* pain]
kinescope (kĭn′ĕ-skōp) [″ + *skopein,* to examine]
kinesia (kī-nē′sē-ă)
kinesialgia (kĭ-nē″sē-ăl′jē-ă) [″ + *algos,* pain]
kinesiatrics (kĭ-nē″sē-ăt′rĭks) [″ + *iatrikos,* curative]
kinesics (kĭ-nē′sĭks)
kinesimeter (kĭn″ĕ-sĭm′ĕ-tĕr) [″ + *metron,* measure]
kinesiodic (kĭ-nē″sē-ŏd′ĭk) [″ + *hodos,* path]
kinesiology (kĭ-nē″sē-ŏl′ō-jē) [″ + *logos,* word, reason]
kinesioneurosis (kĭ-nē″sē-ō-nū-rō′sĭs) [″ + *neuron,* nerve, + *osis,* condition]
  k., external
  k., vascular
  k., visceral
kinesiotherapy (kĭ-nē″sē-ō-thĕr′ă-pē) [″ + *therapeia,* treatment]
kinesis (kĭn-ē′sĭs) [Gr., motion]
kinesitherapy [″ + *therapeia,* treatment]
kinesodic (kĭn″ĕ-sŏd′ĭk) [″ + *hodos,* path]

kinesthesia (kĭn″ĕs-thē′zē-ă) [″ + *aisthesis,* feeling, perception]
kinesthesiometer (kĭn″ĕs-thē-zē-ŏm′ĕ-tĕr) [″ + ″ + *metron,* measure]
kinesthetic
kinetic (kĭ-nĕt′ĭk) [Gr. *kinesis,* motion]
kinetics
kinetocardiography
kinetosis (kĭn″ĕ-tō′sĭs) [″ + *osis,* condition]
kinetotherapy (kĭ-nĕt″ō-thĕr′ă-pē) [″ + *therapeia,* treatment]
kingdom [AS. *cyningdom*]
kinin (kī′nĭn) [Gr. *kinesis,* motion]
kininases, plasma
kininogen
kink [Low Ger. *kinke,* a twist in rope]
kinky hair disease
kino- (kī′nō) [Gr. *kinein,* to move]
kinocilium (kī″nō-sĭl′ē-ŭm) [″ + L. *cilium,* eyelash]
kinomometer (kī″nō-mŏm′ĕ-tĕr) [″ + *metron,* measure]
kinship (kĭn′shĭp)
kiotome (kī′ō-tōm) [Gr. *kion,* column, + *tome,* a cutting, slice]
kiotomy (kī-ŏt′ō-mē)
Kirschner's wire (kērsh′nĕrz) [Martin Kirschner, Ger. surgeon, 1879–1942]
Kisch's reflex (kĭsh′ĕs) [Bruno Kisch, Ger. physiologist, 1890–1966]
kitasamycin (kĭt″ă-să-mī′sĭn)
kite apparatus
KJ *knee jerk*
KK *knee kick (knee jerk)*
kl *kiloliter*
Klebcil
Klebsiella (klĕb″sē-ĕl′ă) [T. A. Edwin Klebs, Ger. bacteriologist, 1834–1913]
  K. ozaenae
  K. pneumoniae
  K. rhinoscleromatis
Klebs-Loeffler bacillus (klĕbs-lĕf′lĕr) [T. A. Edwin Klebs; Friedrich Loeffler, Ger. bacteriologist, 1852–1915]
klepto- (klĕp′tō) [Gr. *kleptein,* to steal]

kleptolagnia (klĕp"tō-lăg'nē-ă) [" + *lagneia*, lust]
kleptomania (klĕp-tō-mā'nē-ă) [" + *mania*, madness]
kleptomaniac
kleptophobia (klĕp-tō-fō'bē-ă) [" + *phobos*, fear]
Klieg eye (klēg) [after John H. Kliegl, Ger. manufacturer, 1869–1959]
Klinefelter's syndrome (klīn'fĕl-tĕrs) [Harry F. Klinefelter, Jr., U.S. physician, b. 1912]
Klippel's disease (klĭ-pĕlz') [Maurice Klippel, Fr. neurologist, 1858–1942]
Klippel-Feil syndrome [Maurice Klippel; André Feil, Fr. physician, b. 1884]
Klonopin
K-Lor
Klumpke's paralysis (kloomp'kĕz) [Madame A. Dejerine Klumpke, Fr. neurologist, 1859–1927]
Klüver-Bucy syndrome [Heinrich Klüver, U.S. neurologist, b. 1897; Paul C. Bucy, U.S. neurologist, b. 1904]
K-Lyte
km *kilometer*
kMc *kilomegacycle*
KMnO₄ *potassium permanganate*
Knapp's forceps (năps) [Herman J. Knapp, U.S. ophthalmologist, 1832–1911]
kneading (nēd'ĭng) [AS. *cnedan*]
knee [AS. *cneo*]
   k., Brodie's
   k., dislocation of
   k., game
   k., housemaid's
   k., knock-
   k., locked
kneecap
knee-chest position
knee-jerk reflex
knee joint
knee of internal capsule
Kneipp cure (nīp) [Rev. Father Sebastian Kneipp, Ger. priest, 1821–1897]
kneippism (nīp'ĭzm)
knemometry (nē-mŏm'ĕt-rē) [Gr.

kneme, shinbone, + *metron*, measure]
knife (nīf) [AS. *cnif*]
   k., electric
   k., gold
   k., interdental
   k., periodontal
   k., plaster
knismogenic (nĭs"mō-jĕn'ĭk) [Gr. *knismos*, tickling, + *gennan*, to produce]
knitting [AS. *cnyttan*, to make knots]
KNO₃ *potassium nitrate*
knob (nŏb) [ME. *knobbe*]
knock-knee
knot [AS. *cnotta*]
   k., false
   k., granny
   k., Hensen's
   k., primitive
   k., square
   k., surgical
   k., syncytial
   k., true
knuckle (nŭk'ĕl) [Middle Low Ger. *knokel*]
knuckle pads
K.O.C. *cathodal opening contraction*
Koch, Robert (kōk) Ger. bacteriologist, 1843–1910
   K.'s bacillus
   K.'s law
   K.'s phenomenon
   K.'s postulates
Koch, Walter (kōk) Ger. surgeon, b. 1880
   K.'s node
kocherization (kŏk"ĕr-ĭ-zā'shŭn)
Kocher's reflex (kō'kĕrz) [Theodor Kocher, Swiss surgeon, 1841–1917]
Koebner phenomenon [H. Koebner, Ger. dermatologist, 1838–1904]
KOH *potassium hydroxide*
Köhler's disease (kă'lĕrz) [Alban Köhler, Ger. physician, 1874–1947]
Kohlrausch's fold (kōl'rowsh-ĕs) [Otto L. B. Kohlrausch, Ger. physician, 1811–1854]

Kohnstamm's phenomenon (kŏn'stămz) [Oscar Kohnstamm, Ger. physician, 1871–1917]

koilocyte (koy'lō-sīt) [Gr. *koilos*, hollow, + *kytos*, cell]

koilocytotic atypia (koy"lō-sī-tŏt'ĭk ă-tĭp'ē-ă) [" + " + *osis*, condition, + *a-*, not, + *typicalis*, typical]

koilonychia (koy-lō-nĭk'ē-ă) [" + *onyx*, nail]

koilorrhachic (koy"lō-răk'ĭk) [" + *rhachis*, spine]

koilosternia (koy"lō-stĕr'nē-ă) [" + Gr. *sternon*, chest]

kolp- [Gr. *kolpos*, vagina]

kolpitis (kŏl-pī'tĭs) [" + *itis*, inflammation]

kolypeptic (kō"lē-pĕp'tĭk) [Gr. *kolyein*, to hinder, + *pepsis*, digestion]

Konakion

Kondoleon's operation (kŏn-dō'lē-ŏnz) [Emmanuel Kondoleon, Gr. surgeon, 1879–1939]

Kondremul

koniocortex (kō"nē-ō-kor'tĕks) [Gr. *konis*, dust, + L. *cortex*, rind]

koniology [" + *logos*, word, reason]

koniometer (kō-nē-ŏm'ĕ-ter) [" + *metron*, measure]

koniosis (kō-nē-ō'sĭs) [" + *osis*, condition]

Konyne HT

kopf-tetanus [Ger. *Kopf*, head, + *tetanos*, rigid, stretched]

kophemia (kō-fē'mē-ă) [Gr. *kophan*, to become stupid, + *pheme*, speech]

Koplik's spots [Henry Koplik, U.S. pediatrician, 1858–1927]

kopophobia (kŏp"ō-fō'bē-ă) [Gr. *kopos*, fatigue, + *phobos*, fear]

Korányi's sign (kō-răn'yēz) [Friedrich von Korányi, Hung. physician, 1828–1913]

koro (kō'rō)

koronion (kō-rō'nē-ŏn) [Gr. *korone*, crest]

Korotkoff's sounds (kō-rŏt'kŏfs) [Nikolai S. Korotkoff, Russian physician, 1874–1920]

Korsakoff's syndrome (kor'să-kŏfs) [Sergei S. Korsakoff, Russian neurologist, 1854–1900]

kosher (kō'shĕr) [Hebrew *kasher*, proper]

koumiss (koo'mĭs) [Tartar *kumyz*]

Kr *krypton*

Krabbe's disease (krăb'ēz) [Knud H. Krabbe, Danish neurologist, 1885–1961]

Kraepelin's classification (krā'pā-lĭnz) [Emil Kraepelin, Ger. psychiatrist, 1856–1926]

krait (krāt)

kraurosis (krŏ-rō'sĭs) [Gr. *krauros*, dry]
  k. penis
  k. vulvae

Krause, Karl (krowz) Ger. anatomist, 1797–1868
  K.'s glands
  K.'s valve

Krause, Wilhelm (krowz) Ger. anatomist, 1833–1910
  K.'s bulbs; K.'s end bulbs
  K.'s membrane

Krebs cycle [Sir Hans Krebs, Ger. biochemist, 1900–1981]

Krönig's area (krā'nĭgz) [Georg Krönig, Ger. physician, 1856–1911]

Krukenberg's chopsticks [Hermann Krukenberg, Ger. surgeon, 1863–1935]

Krukenberg's tumor (kroo'kĕn-bĕrgz) [Frederick Krukenberg, Ger. pathologist, 1871–1946]

krypton (krĭp'tŏn) [Gr. *kryptos*, hidden]

K₂SO₄ *potassium sulfate*

KUB *kidneys, ureters, bladder*

kubisagari (koo-bĭs"ă-gă'rē) [Japanese, hang-head]

Kufs' disease [H. Kufs, Ger. psychiatrist, 1871–1955]

Kugelberg-Welander disease [E. Kugelberg, b. 1913; L. Welander, b. 1909; Swedish neurologists]

kumiss, kumyss (koo'mĭs) [Tartar *kumyz*]

Kümmell's disease or spondylitis (kĭm'ĕlz) [Hermann Kümmell, Ger. surgeon, 1852–1937]

Kupffer's cells (koop'fĕrz) [Karl W. von Kupffer, Ger. anatomist, 1829–1902]

kuru (koo'roo)

Kussmaul, Adolph (koos'mowl) Ger. physician, 1822–1902
    K.'s breathing
    K.'s disease

kv *kilovolt*

kvp *kilovoltage peak*

kwashiorkor (kwăsh-ē-or'kor) [Ghana, Africa, deposed child, i.e., child that is no longer suckled]

Kwell

Kyasanur Forest disease

kyestein, kiestein (kī-ĕs'tē-ĭn) [Gr. *kyesis*, pregnancy]

kyllosis (kĭl-lō'sĭs) [Gr., crippling]

kymatism [Gr. *kyma*, wave, + *-ismos*, condition]

kymogram (kī'mō-grăm)

kymograph (kī'mō-grăf) [Gr. *kyma*, wave, + *graphein*, to write]

kymography

kymoscope [" + *skopein*, to examine]

kynocephalus (kĭ"nō-sĕf'ă-lŭs) [Gr. *kyon*, dog, + *kephale*, head]

kynurenine (kĭ"nū-rĕn'ĭn) [" + L. *ren*, kidney]

kyogenic (kī"ō-jĕn'ĭk) [Gr. *kyesis*, pregnancy, + *gennan*, to produce]

kypho- [Gr. *kyphos*, a hump]

kyphorachitis (kī"fō-răk-ī'tĭs) [" + *rhachis*, spine, + *itis*, inflammation]

kyphos (kī'fŏs) [Gr., hump]

kyphoscoliosis (kī"fō-skō"lē-ō'sĭs) [" + *skoliosis*, crookedness]

kyphosis (kĭ-fō'sĭs) [Gr., humpback]

kyphotic (kĭ-fŏt'ĭk)

kyrtorrhachic (kĭr"tō-răk'ĭk) [Gr. *kyrtos*, curved, + *rhachis*, spine]

kysthitis (kĭs-thī'tĭs) [Gr. *kysthos*, vagina, + *itis*, inflammation]

kysthoptosis (kĭs-thŏp-tō'sĭs) [" + *ptosis*, fall, falling]

kyto- [Gr. *kytos*, cell]

L

Λ, λ lambda
L, l Lactobacillus; Latin; left; left eye; length; lethal; light sense; liter
L₊ limes tod
L₀ limes nul
LA left atrium
La lanthanum
lab.
Labbé's vein (lăb-āz') [Léon Labbé, Fr. surgeon, 1832–1916]
labeling
la belle indifference [Fr., beautiful indifference]
labia (lā'bē-ă) [L.]
   l. majora
   l. minora
labial (lā'bē-ăl) [L. labialis]
labial glands
labialism (lā'bē-ăl-ĭzm) [" + Gr. -ismos, condition]
LaBID
labile (lā'bĭl) [L. labi, to slip]
   l., heat
lability (lă-bĭl'ĭ-tē)
   l., emotional
labioalveolar (lā"bē-ō-ăl-vē'ō-lăr) [L. labium, lip, + alveolus, little hollow]
labiocervical (lā"bē-ō-sĕr'vĭ-kl) [" + cervix, neck]
labiochorea (lā"bē-ō-kō-rē'ă) [" + Gr. choreia, dance]
labioclination (lā"bē-ō-klĭ-nā'shŭn) [" + Gr. klinein, to slope]
labiodental (lā"bē-ō-dĕn'tăl) [" + dens, tooth]
labiogingival (lā"bē-ō-jĭn'jĭ-văl) [" + gingiva, gum]
labioglossolaryngeal (lā"bē-ō-glŏs"ō-lăr-ĭn'jē-ăl) [" + Gr. glossa, tongue, + larynx, larnyx]
labioglossopharyngeal (lā"bē-ō-glŏs"ō-făr-ĭn'jē-ăl) [" + " + pharynx, throat]
labiograph (lā'bē-ō-grăf) [" + Gr. graphein, to write]
labiomental (lā"bē-ō-mĕn'tăl) [" + mentum, chin]
labiomycosis (lā"bē-ō-mī-kō'sĭs) [" + Gr. mykes, fungus, + osis, condition]
labionasal (lā"bē-ō-nā'zăl) [" + nasus, nose]
labiopalatine (lā"bē-ō-păl'ă-tīn) [" + palatum, palate]
labioplasty (lā'bē-ō-plăs"tē) [" + Gr. plassein, to form]
labiotenaculum (lā"bē-ō-tĕn-ăk'ū-lŭm) [" + tenaculum, a hook]
labioversion (lā"bē-ō-vĕr'zhŭn) [" + versio, a turning]
labium (lā'bē-ŭm) [L.]
   l. cerebri
   l. inferius oris
   l. majus
   l. minus
   l. minus pudendi
   l. oris
   l. superius oris
   l. tympanicum
   l. urethrae
   l. uteri
   l. vestibulare
labor [L., work]
   l., active
   l., arrested
   l., artificial
   l., complicated
   l., dry
   l., false
   l., induction of
   l., instrumental
   l., missed

l., normal
l., precipitate
l., premature
l., spontaneous
l., trial of

laboratory (lăb'ră-tor"ē) [L. *laboratorium*]

Laborde's method (lă-bordz') [Jean B. V. Laborde, Fr. physician, 1830–1903]

labret (lā'brĕt) [L. *labrum*, lip]

labrocyte (lăb'rō-sīt) [Gr. *labros*, greedy, + *kytos*, cell]

labrum (lā'brŭm) [L., lip]

labyrinth (lăb'ĭ-rĭnth) [Gr. *labyrinthos*, maze]
l., bony
l., ethmoidal
l., membranous
l., olfactory
l., osseous

labyrinthectomy (lăb-ĭ-rĭn-thĕk'tō-mē) [" + *ektome*, excision]

labyrinthine (lăb-ĭ-rĭn'thĭn)

labyrinthitis (lăb"ĭ-rĭn-thī'tĭs) [" + *itis*, inflammation]

labyrinthotomy (lăb"ĭ-rĭn-thŏt'ō-mē) [" + *tome*, a cutting, slice]

labyrinthus (lăb"ĭ-rĭn'thŭs) [L., Gr. *labyrinthos*, maze]

lac (lăk) [L.]

lacerable (lăs'ĕr-ă-b'l) [L. *lacerare*, to tear]

lacerate (lăs'ĕr-āt) [L. *lacerare*, to tear]

lacerated

laceration

laceration of cervix

laceration of perineum

lacertus (lă-sĕr'tŭs) [L., lizard]
l. cordis
l. fibrosus

laciniate (lă-sĭn'ē-āt) [L. *lacinia*, fringe]

lacrima (lăk'rĭ-mă) [L.]

lacrimal (lăk'rĭm-ăl) [L. *lacrima*, tear]

lacrimal apparatus

lacrimal bone

lacrimal duct

lacrimal gland

lacrimal reflex

lacrimal sac

lacrimation [L. *lacrima*, tear]
l., test for

lacrimator

lacrimatory (lăk'rĭ-mă-tō"rē)

lacrimonasal (lăk"rĭ-mō-nā'zăl) [" + *nasus*, nose]

lacrimotome (lăk'rĭ-mō-tōm) [" + Gr. *tome*, a cutting, slice]

lacrimotomy (lăk'rĭm-ŏt'ō-mē) [" + Gr. *tome*, a cutting, slice]

lactacid

lactacidemia (lăk-tăs"ĭ-dē'mē-ă) [" + " + Gr. *haima*, blood]

lactaciduria (lăkt-ă-sĭd-ū'rē-ă) [" + " + Gr. *ouron*, urine]

lactagogue (lăk'tă-gŏg) [" + Gr. *agogos*, leading]

lactalbumin [" + *albumen*, coagulated white of egg]

lactam (lăk'tăm)

β-lactamase (bā"tă-lăk'tă-mās)

β-lactamase-resistant antibiotics

lactase [" + *-ase*, enzyme]

lactase deficiency syndrome

lactate (lăk'tāt)

lactate dehydrogenase

lactation (lăk-tā'shŭn) [L. *lactatio*, a sucking]

lacteal (lăk'tē-ăl) [L. *lacteus*, of milk]

lactenin (lăk'tĕn-ĭn)

lactescence (lăk-tĕs'ĕns) [L. *lactescere*, to become milky]

lactic (lăk'tĭk) [L. *lac*, milk]

lactic acid

lactic acid fermentation

lactic acidosis

lactic dehydrogenase

lacticemia (lăk-tĭ-sē'mē-ă) [" + Gr. *haima*, blood]

lactiferous (lăk-tĭf'ĕr-ŭs) [" + *ferre*, to bear]

lactiferous ducts

lactiferous glands

lactification (lăk"tĭ-fĭ-kā'shŭn) [" + *facere*, to make]

lactifuge (lăk'tĭ-fūj) [" + *fugare*, to expel]

lactigenous (lăk-tĭj'ĕn-ŭs) [" + Gr.

gennan, to produce]

lactigerous (lăk-tĭj'ĕr-ŭs) [" + gerere, to carry]

lactinated (lăk'tĭ-nāt"ĕd)

lactivorous (lăk-tĭv'or-ŭs) [" + vorare, to devour]

Lactobacillus (lăk-tō-bă-sĭl'ŭs) [" +
bacillus, little rod]
    L. acidophilus
    L. bulgaricus
    L. casei
    L. helveticus

lactobutyrometer (lăk"tō-bū-tĭ-rŏm'ĕ-
tĕr) [" + Gr. boutyron, butter, +
metron, measure]

lactocele (lăk'tō-sēl) [" + Gr. kele,
tumor, swelling]

lactochrome (lăk'tō-krōm) [" +
Gr. chroma, color]

lactocrit (lăk'tō-krĭt) [" + Gr. krites,
judge]

lactodensimeter (lăk"tō-dĕn-sĭm'ĕ-
tĕr) [" + densus, thick, + Gr.
metron, meter]

lactoflavin (lăk'tō-flā"vĭn) [" +
flavus, yellow]

lactogen (lăk'tō-jĕn) [L. lac, milk, +
Gr. gennan, to produce]

lactogenic [" + Gr. gennan, to
produce]

lactogenic hormone

lactoglobulin (lăk"tō-glŏb'ū-lĭn) [" +
globulus, globule]
    l.'s, immune

lactometer (lăk-tŏm'ĕ-tĕr) [" +
Gr. metron, measure]

lacto-ovovegetarian (lăk"tō-ō"vō-
vĕj"ĕ-tā'rē-ăn)

lactophosphate (lăk"tō-fŏs'fāt) [" +
phosphas, phosphate]

lactoprotein (lăk"tō-prō'tē-ĭn) [" +
Gr. protos, first]

lactorrhea (lăk-tō-rē'ă) [" + Gr.
rhein, to flow]

lactose

lactose intolerance

lactoserum (lăk-tō-sēr'ŭm) [" +
serum, whey]

lactosuria (lăk-tō-sū'rē-ă) [" + Gr.

ouron, urine]

lactotherapy (lăk-tō-thĕr'ă-pē) [" +
Gr. therapeia, treatment]

lactotoxin (lăk"tō-tŏks'ĭn) [" + Gr.
toxikon, poison]

lactovegetarian

lactulose

lacuna (lă-kū'nă) [L., a pit]
    l., absorption
    l., blood
    l., bone
    l., Howship's
    l., intervillous
    l. laterales
    l. magna
    l. of the urethra
    l. pharyngis
    l., trophoblastic
    l. vasorum
    l., venous

lacunae (lă-kū'nē) [L.]

lacunar (lă-kū'năr) [L. lacuna, pit]

lacunar disease

lacunes (lă-kūnz')

lacunula (lă-kū'nū-lă) [L., little pit]

lacunule (lă-kū'nūl) [L. lacunula]

lacus (lā'kŭs) [L., lake]
    l. lacrimalis

LAD left anterior descending

Laënnec's cirrhosis (lā"ĕ-nĕks') [René
T. H. Laënnec, Fr. physician, 1781 –
1826]

Laënnec's pearls

Laënnec's thrombus

Laetrile

Lafora, Gonzalo R. (lă-fō'ră)
    L.'s bodies
    L.'s disease

lag

lageniform (lă-jĕn'ĭ-form) [L. lagena,
flask, + forma, shape]

lagophthalmos, lagophthalmus
(lăg"ŏf-thăl'mōs, -mŭs) [Gr. lagos, hare,
+ ophthalmos, eye]
    l., nocturnal

lag phase

la grippe (lă grĭp') [Fr.]

laity (lā'ĭ-tē) [Gr. laos, the people]

lake [L. lacus]

laked
laking
LAL *limulus amebocyte lysate*
La Leche League
laliatry (lăl-ī'ă-trē) [Gr. *lalia*, chatter, prattle, + *iatria*, therapy]
lallation (lă-lā'shŭn) [L. *lallatio*]
lalognosis (lăl-ŏg-nō'sĭs) [Gr. *lalia*, chatter, prattle, + *gnosis*, understanding]
lalopathology (lăl"ō-pă-thŏl'ō-jē) [" + *pathos*, disease, suffering, + *logos*, word, reason]
lalopathy (lă-lŏp'ă-thē) [" + *pathos*, disease, suffering]
lalophobia (lăl"ō-fō'bē-ă) [" + *phobos*, fear]
laloplegia (lăl-ō-plē'jē-ă) [" + *plege*, a stroke]
lalorrhea (lăl"ō-rē'ă) [" + *rhein*, to flow]
Lamarck's theory (lă-mărks') [Jean Baptiste P. A. Lamarck, Fr. naturalist, 1744–1829]
Lamaze technique or method (lă-măz') [Fernand Lamaze, Fr. obstetrician, 1890–1957]
lambda (lăm'dă) [Gr.]
lambdacism (lăm'dă-sĭzm) [Gr. *lambdakismos*]
lambdoid, lambdoidal (lăm'doyd, lăm-doyd'ăl) [Gr. *lambda*, L, + *eidos*, form, shape]
lambdoid suture
lambert [Johann H. Lambert, Ger. physicist, 1728–1777]
Lamblia intestinalis (lăm'blē-ă) [Wilhelm D. Lambl, Bohemian physician, 1824–1895]
lambliasis (lăm-blī'ă-sĭs)
lame [AS. *lama*]
lamella (lă-mĕl'ă) [L., a little plate]
   l., bone
   l., circumferential
   l., concentric
   l., enamel
   l., ground
   l., haversian

   l., interstitial
   l., medullary
   l., periosteal
   l., triangular
   l., vitreous
lamellar (lă-mĕl'ăr)
lameness
lamina (lăm'ĭ-nă) [L.]
   l., alar
   l., anterior elastic
   l., basal
   l. basalis choroideae
   l. basilaris ductus cochlearis
   l., Bowman's
   l. cartilaginis cricoideae
   l. chorioidcapillaris
   l. cribrosa
   l. cribrosa sclerae
   l., dental
   l. dura
   l., epithelial
   l. fusca sclerae
   l., interpubic fibrocartilaginous
   l., labial
   l., medullary, internal
   l. multiformis
   l. of vertebral arch
   l. papyracea
   l., perpendicular
   l. propria mucosae
   l., pterygoid
   l., rostral
   l. suprachoroidea
   l., terminal
   l., vestibular
   l. vitrea
   l. zonalis
laminae (lăm'ĭ-nē)
laminagram (lăm'ĭ-nă-grăm) [L. *lamina*, thin plate, + Gr. *gramma*, letter, piece of writing]
laminagraph (lăm'ĭ-nă-grăf) [" + Gr. *graphein*, to write]
laminagraphy (lăm"ĭ-năg'ră-fē) [" + Gr. *graphein*, to write]
laminar air flow
Laminaria digitata (lăm-ĭ-năr'ē-ă dĭj-ĭ-tā'tă)

laminarin (lăm"ĭ-nā'rĭn)
laminated (lăm'ĭn-āt"ĕd) [L. *lamina*, thin plate]
lamination (lăm"ĭn-ā'shŭn)
laminectomy (lăm"ĭ-nĕk'tō-mē) [" + Gr. *ektome*, excision]
laminitis (lăm-ĭn-ī'tĭs) [" + Gr. *itis*, inflammation]
laminotomy (lăm"ĭ-nŏt'ō-mē) [" + Gr. *tome*, a cutting, slice]
lamp [Gr. *lampein*, to shine]
　l., Gullstrand's
　l., infrared
　l., slit
　l., sun
　l., ultraviolet
lamprophonia (lăm"prō-fō'nē-ă) [Gr. *lampros*, clear, + *phone*, voice]
lamprophonic (lăm"prō-fŏn'ĭk)
lana (lăn'ă) [L.]
lanatoside C (lăn-ăt'ō-sīd)
lance (lăns) [L. *lancea*]
Lancefield classification (lăns'fēld) [Rebecca Lancefield, U.S. bacteriologist, b. 1895]
lancet (lăn'sĕt) [L. *lancea*, lance]
lancinating (lăn'sĭ-nāt"ĭng) [L. *lancinare*, to tear]
L and A *light and accommodation*
landmark
　l., bony
　l., cephalometric
　l., craniometric
　l., orbital
　l., radiographic
　l., soft tissue
Landouzy-Déjérine atrophy (lăn-dū-zē' dĕ"zhĕ-rēn') [Louis T. J. Landouzy, Fr. physician, 1845–1917; Joseph Jules Déjérine, Fr. neurologist, 1849–1917]
Landry's paralysis (lăn-drēz') [Jean Baptiste O. Landry, Fr. neurologist, 1826–1865]
Landsteiner's classification (lănd'stī-nĕrz) [Karl Landsteiner, Austrian-born U.S. biologist, 1868–1943]
Lane's kinks [Sir W. Arbuthnot Lane,

Brit. surgeon, 1856–1943]
Langerhans' islands (lăng'ĕr-hănz) [Paul Langerhans, Ger. pathologist, 1847–1888]
Langer's lines (lăng'ĕrz) [Carl Ritter von Langer, Austrian anatomist, 1819–1887]
Langer's muscle
Lange's test (lăng'ĕz) [Carl Lange, Ger. physician, b. 1883]
Langhans' layer (lăng'hăns) [Theodor Langhans, Ger. pathologist, 1839–1915]
languor (lăng'gĕr) [L. *languere*, to languish]
laniary (lăn'ē-ā"rē) [L. *laniare*, to tear to pieces]
lanolin (lăn'ō-lĭn) [L. *lana*, wool]
　l., anhydrous
Lanoxin
lanthanum (lăn'thă-nŭm)
lanuginous (lă-nū'jĭn-ŭs)
lanugo (lă-nū'gō) [L. *lana*, wool]
laparectomy (lăp"ă-rĕk'tō-mē) [Gr. *lapara*, flank, + *ektome*, excision]
laparo- [Gr. *lapara*, flank]
laparocele (lăp'ă-rō-sēl) [" + *kele*, tumor, swelling]
laparocholecystotomy (lăp"ăr-ō-kōl"ē-sĭs-tŏt'ō-mē) [" + *chole*, bile, + *kystis*, bladder, + *tome*, a cutting, slice]
laparocolectomy (lăp"ă-rō-kō-lĕk'tō-mē) [" + *kolon*, colon, + *ektome*, excision]
laparocolostomy, laparocolotomy (lăp"ăr-ō-kō-lŏs'tō-mē, lăp"ăr-ō-kō-lŏt'ō-mē) [" + " + *stoma*, mouth, opening]
laparocystectomy (lă"pă-rō-sĭs-tĕk'tō-mē) [" + *kystis*, bladder, + *ektome*, excision]
laparocystidotomy (lăp"ăr-ō-sĭst-ĭ-dŏt'ō-mē) [" + " + *tome*, a cutting, slice]
laparocystotomy (lăp"ăr-ō-sĭs-tŏt'ō-mē)
laparoenterostomy (lăp"ă-rō-

ĕn"tĕr-ŏs'tō-mē) [" + enteron, intestine, + stoma, mouth, opening]

laparoenterotomy (lăp"ăr-ō-ĕn"tĕrŏt'ō-mē) [" + " + tome, a cutting, slice]

laparogastroscopy (lăp"ă-rō-găstrŏs'kō-pē) [" + gaster, belly, + skopein, to examine]

laparogastrostomy (lăp"ăr-ō-găstrŏs'tō-mē) [" + " + stoma, mouth, opening]

laparogastrotomy (lăp"ă-rō-găstrŏt'ō-mē) [" + " + tome, a cutting, slice]

laparohepatotomy (lăp"ăr-ō-hĕp"ătŏt'ō-mē) [" + hepar, liver, + tome, a cutting, slice]

laparohysterectomy (lăp"ăr-ōhĭs"tĕr-ĕk'tō-mē) [" + hystera, womb, + ektome, excision]

laparohystero-oophorectomy (lăp"ăr-ō-hĭs"tĕr-ō-ō"ō-for-ĕk'tō-mē) [" + " + NL. oophoron, ovary, + Gr. ektome, excision]

laparohysteropexy (lăp"ăr-ōhĭs'tĕr-ō-pĕks-ē) [" + " + pexis, fixation]

laparohysterosalpingo-oophorectomy (lăp"ăr-ō-hĭs"tĕr-ō-săl-pīn"gōō"ō-fō-rĕk'tō-mē) [" + hystera, womb, + salpinx, tube, + NL. oophoron, ovary, + Gr. ektome, excision]

laparohysterotomy (lăp"ăr-ōhĭs"tĕr-ŏt'ō-mē) [" + " + tome, a cutting, slice]

laparoileotomy (lăp"ăr-ō-ĭl-ē-ŏt'ō-mē) [" + L. ileum, ileum, + Gr. tome, a cutting, slice]

laparomyitis (lăp"ăr-ō-mī-ī'tĭs) [" + mys, muscle, + itis, inflammation]

laparomyomectomy (lăp"ăr-ō-mī"ōmĕk'tō-mē) [" + " + oma, tumor, + ektome, excision]

laparonephrectomy (lăp"ăr-ō-nĕfrĕk'tō-mē) [" + nephros, kidney, + ektome, excision]

laparorrhaphy (lăp-ă-ror'ă-fē) [" +

rhaphe, seam]

laparosalpingectomy (lăp"ăr-ō-sălpīn-jek'tō-mē) [" + salpinx, tube, + ektome, excision]

laparosalpingo-oophorectomy (lăp"ăr-ōsăl-pīn"gō-ō"ŏf-ō-rĕk'tō-mē) [" + " + NL. oophoron, ovary, + Gr. ektome, excision]

laparosalpingotomy (lăp"ăr-ō-sălpīn-gŏt'ō-mē) [" + " + tome, a cutting, slice]

laparoscope (lăp'ă-rō-skōp") [" + skopein, to examine]

laparoscopy (lăp-ăr-ŏs'kō-pē) [" + skopein, to examine]

laparosplenectomy (lăp"ăr-ō-splĕnĕk'tō-mē) [" + splen, spleen, + ektome, excision]

laparosplenotomy (lăp"ăr-ō-splĕnŏt'ō-mē) [" + " + tome, a cutting, slice]

laparotomy (lăp-ăr-ŏt'ō-mē) [" + tome, a cutting, slice]

laparotrachelotomy (lăp"ăr-ō-trākĕl-ŏt'ō-mē) [" + trachelos, neck, + tome, a cutting, slice]

laparotyphlotomy (lăp"ăr-ō-tĭ-flŏt'ō-mē) [" + typhlon, cecum, + tome, a cutting, slice]

lap board

lapinization (lăp"ĭn-ī-zā'shŭn) [Fr. lapin, rabbit]

lapis (lă'pĭs) [L.]

lard [L. lardum, fat]
l., benzoinated

lardaceous (lăr-dā'shŭs) [L. lardum, fat]

Largon

Larodopa

larva [L., mask]
l. currens
l. migrans, cutaneous
l. migrans, visceral

larval (lăr'văl) [L. larva, mask]

larvate [L. larva, mask]

larvicide [" + caedere, to kill]

larviphagic (lăr"vĭ-fā'jĭk) [" + Gr. phagein, to eat]

laryngalgia (lăr-ĭn-găl'jē-ă) [Gr. lar-

ynx, larynx, + *algos*, pain]
laryngeal (lăr-ĭn'jē-ăl) [Gr. *larynx*, lar-
ynx]
laryngeal reflex
laryngeal vertigo
laryngectomee (lăr"ĭn-jĕk'tō-mē)
[" + *ektome*, excision]
laryngectomy (lăr"ĭn-jĕk'tō-mē) [" +
ektome, excision]
laryngemphraxis (lăr"ĭn-jĕm-frăk'sĭs)
[" + *emphraxis*, an obstruction]
laryngismal (lăr"ĭn-jĭs'măl) [" +
-*ismos*, condition]
laryngismus (lăr"ĭn-jĭs'mŭs) [" +
-*ismos*, condition]
laryngitic (lăr-ĭn-jĭt'ĭk) [Gr. *larynx*, lar-
ynx]
laryngitis (lăr-ĭn-jī'tĭs) [" + *itis*, in-
flammation]
   l., acute catarrhal
   l., atrophic
   l., chronic
   l., croupous
   l., diphtheritic
   l., membranous
   l., syphilitic
   l., tuberculous
laryngo- [Gr. *larynx*, larynx]
laryngocele (lăr-ĭn'gō-sēl) [" +
kele, tumor, swelling]
laryngocentesis (lăr-ĭn"gō-sĕn-tē'sĭs)
[" + *kentesis*, puncture]
laryngoedema
laryngofissure (lăr-ĭng"gō-fĭsh'ŭr)
[" + L. *fissura*, a cleft]
laryngogram (lă-rĭng'gō-grăm) [" +
gramma, letter, piece of writing]
laryngograph (lăr-ĭng'ō-grăf) [" +
graphein, to write]
laryngography (lăr"ĭn-gŏg'ră-fē)
laryngologist (lăr"ĭn-gŏl'ō-jĭst) [" +
logos, word, reason]
laryngology
laryngomalacia (lăr-ĭng"gō-mă-
lā'shē-ă) [" + *malakia*, softness]
laryngometry (lăr"ĭn-gŏm'ĕ-trē)
[" + *metron*, measure]
laryngoparalysis (lăr-ĭn"gō-păr-ăl'ĭ-

sĭs) [" + *paralyein*, to loosen, dis-
able]
laryngopathy (lăr"ĭn-gŏp'ă-thē)
[" + *pathos*, disease, suffering]
laryngophantom (lăr"ĭn-gō-făn"tŏm)
[" + *phantasma*, image]
laryngopharyngeal (lăr-ĭn"gō-făr-
ĭn"jē-ăl) [" + *pharynx*, throat]
laryngopharyngectomy (lăr-ĭn"gō-
făr-ĭn-jĕk'tō-mē) [" + " + *ektome*, excision]
laryngopharyngeus (lă-rĭng"gō-fă-
rĭn'jē-ŭs)
laryngopharyngitis (lăr-ĭn"gō-făr-ĭn-
jī'tĭs) [" + " + *itis*, inflamma-
tion]
laryngopharyngography (lă-rĭng"
gō-fă-rĭn-jŏg'ră-fē) [" + " +
graphein, to write]
laryngopharynx (lăr-ĭn"gō-făr'ĭnks)
[Gr. *larynx*, larynx, + *pharynx*,
throat]
laryngophony (lăr"ĭn-gŏf'ō-nē) [" +
phone, voice]
laryngophthisis (lăr"ĭng-gŏf'thĭ-sĭs)
[" + *phthisis*, a wasting]
laryngoplasty (lăr-ĭn'gō-plăs"tē)
[" + *plassein*, to form]
laryngoplegia (lă-rĭng"gō-plē'jē-ă)
[" + *plege*, stroke]
laryngoptosis (lă-rĭng"gō-tō'sĭs)
[" + *ptosis*, fall, falling]
laryngorhinology (lăr-ĭn"gō-rīn-ŏl'ō-
jē) [" + *rhis*, nose, + *logos*,
word, reason]
laryngorrhagia (lăr"ĭn-gō-rā'jē-ă)
[" + *rhegnynai*, to flow forth]
laryngorrhea (lăr"ĭn-gō-rē'ă) [" +
rhein, to flow]
laryngoscleroma (lăr-ĭn"gō-sklĕ-
rō'mă) [" + *skleros*, hard, +
oma, tumor]
laryngoscope (lăr-ĭn'gō-skōp) [" +
skopein, to examine]
laryngoscopic (lăr"ĭn-gō-skŏp'ĭk)
[" + *skopein*, to examine]
laryngoscopist (lăr"ĭng-gŏs'kō-pĭst)
[" + *skopein*, to examine]

laryngoscopy (lăr"ĭn-gŏs'kō-pē)
   l., direct
   l., indirect
laryngospasm (lăr-ĭn'gō-spăzm)
   [" + spasmos, a convulsion]
laryngostenosis (lăr-ĭng"gō-stĕ-
   nō'sĭs) [" + stenosis, act of narrow-
   ing]
   l., compression
   l., occlusion
laryngostomy (lăr-ĭn-gŏs'tō-mē)
   [" + stoma, mouth, opening]
laryngostroboscope (lăr"ĭn-gō-
   strō'bō-skōp) [" + strobos, whirl,
   + skopein, to view]
laryngotomy (lăr-ĭn-gŏt'ō-mē) [" +
   tome, a cutting, slice]
   l., inferior
   l., median
   l., subhyoid or superior
laryngotracheal (lă-rĭng"gō-trā'kē-ăl)
   [" + tracheia, trachea]
laryngotracheitis (lăr-ĭn"gō-trā-kē-
   ī'tĭs) [" + " + itis, inflammation]
laryngotracheobronchitis (lă-
   rĭng"gō-trā"kē-ō-brŏng-kī'tĭs) [" +
   " + bronchos, windpipe, +
   itis, inflammation]
laryngotracheotomy (lăr-ĭn"gō-trā-
   kē-ŏt'ō-mē) [" + " + tome, a
   cutting, slice]
laryngoxerosis (lăr-ĭn"gō-zĕr-ō'sĭs)
   [" + xeros, dry, + osis, condi-
   tion]
larynx (lăr'ĭnks) [Gr.]
   l., foreign bodies in
Lasan
lascivia (lă-sĭv'ē-ă) [L. lascivire, to be
   wanton]
Lasègue's sign (lă-sĕgz') [Ernest C. Lasègue, Fr. physician, 1816–1883]
laser (lā'zĕr)
laser angioplasty
laser cane
Lasix
Lassa fever [Lassa, city in Africa]
lassitude (lăs'ĭ-tūd) [L. lassitudo, weari-
   ness]

last sacraments
latah (lă'tă)
latency (lā'tĕn-sē) [L. latens, lying hid-
   den]
latency period
latent
latent content
latent heat
latent image
latent period
laterad (lăt'ĕr-ăd) [L. latus, side, +
   ad, toward]
lateral (lăt'ĕr-ăl) [L. lateralis]
lateralis (lăt"ĕr-ā'lĭs) [L.]
laterality (lăt"ĕr-ăl'ĭ-tē)
   l., crossed
   l., dominant
lateral sinus
latericeous, lateritious (lăt"ĕr-ĭsh'ŭs)
   [L. later, brick]
lateroabdominal (lăt"ĕr-ō-ăb-dŏm'ĭ-
   năl) [L. lateralis, pert. to side, +
   abdomen, belly]
laterodeviation (lăt"ĕr-ō-dē"vē-
   ā'shŭn) [" + deviare, to turn aside]
lateroduction (lăt"ĕr-ō-dŭk'shŭn)
   [" + ducere, to lead]
lateroflexion (lăt"ĕr-ō-flĕk'shŭn)
   [" + flexis, bending]
lateroposition (lăt"ĕr-ō-pō-zĭsh'ŭn)
   [" + positio, position]
lateropulsion (lăt"ĕr-ō-pŭl'shŭn) [L. lateralis, pert. to side, + pulsus, driv-
   ing]
laterosemiprone position (lăt"ĕr-ō-
   prōn')
laterotorsion (lăt"ĕr-ō-tor'shŭn) [" +
   torsio, a twisting]
lateroversion (lăt"ĕr-ō-vĕr'shŭn)
   [" + versio, a turning]
latex (lā'tĕks) [L., fluid]
lathyrism (lăth'ĭr-ĭzm) [Gr. lathyros,
   vetch]
lathyrogen (lăth'ĭ-rō-jĕn) [" +
   gennan, to produce]
Latino
latissimus (lă-tĭs'ĭ-mŭs) [L., widest]
latitude

latrine (lă-trēn') [L. *latrina*]
   l., pit
latrodectism (lăt"rō-dĕk'tĭzm) [*Latrodectus* + Gr. *-ismos*, condition]
Latrodectus (lăt"rō-dĕk'tŭs) [L. *latro*, robber, + Gr. *daknein*, biting]
   L. mactans
LATS *long-acting thyroid stimulator*
lattice (lăt'ĭs)
latus (lā'tŭs) [L., broad]
latus, lata, latum (lā'tŭs, lā'tă, lăt'ŭm) [L., broad]
laudable [L. *laudabilis*, praiseworthy]
laudanum (lăw'dăn-ŭm)
laugh (lăf) [ME. *laughen*, to laugh]
   l., sardonic
laughing gas (lăf'ĭng)
laughter, compulsive
laughter reflex (lăf'tĕr)
Laurence-Moon-Biedl syndrome (law'rĕns-moon'bē'dĕl) [John L. Laurence, Brit. ophthalmologist, 1830–1874; Robert C. Moon, U.S. ophthalmologist, 1844–1914; Arthur Biedl, Prague endocrinologist, 1869–1933]
lavage (lă-văzh') [Fr., from L. *lavare*, to wash]
   l., gastric
law [AS. *laga*, law]
   l., all-or-none
   l., Avogadro's
   l., Bell's
   l., biogenetic
   l., Boyle's
   l., Charles'
   l., Courvoisier's
   l., Fechner's
   l., Gay-Lussac's
   l., Graham's
   l., Haeckel's
   l., Hilton's
   l., Hooke's
   l., Koch's
   l., Marey's
   l., Mariotte's
   l.'s, Mendel's
   l., Murphy's
   l., Nysten's

   l. of definite proportions
   l. of the heart
   l. of the intestine
   l. of Magendie
   l. of mass action
   l. of multiple proportions
   l. of reciprocal proportions
   l. of specificity of nervous energy
   l., periodic
   l.'s, Rubner's
   l., Sutton's
   l., Waller's, of degeneration
   l., Weber's
   l., Wolff's
lawrencium (lă-rĕn'sē-ŭm) [Ernest O. Lawrence, U.S. physicist, 1901–1958]
lax (lăks) [L. *laxus*, slack]
laxation (lăk-sā'shŭn) [L. *laxare*, to loosen]
laxative (lăk'să-tĭv) [L. *laxare*, to loosen]
laxative regimen
laxator (lăk-sā'tor) [L. *laxare*, to loosen]
   l. tympani
layer (lā'ĕr) [ME. *leyer*]
   l., ameloblastic
   l., bacillary
   l., basal
   l., blastodermic
   l., choriocapillary
   l., claustral
   l., clear
   l., columnar
   l., compact
   l., cuticular, of epithelium
   l., enamel
   l., ependymal
   l., ganglionic
   l., germ
   l., germinative
   l., granular exterior
   l., granular interior
   l., half-value
   l., Henle's
   l., horny
   l., Huxley's
   l., Langhans'
   l., malpighian

l., mantle
l., molecular
l., nervous
l., odontoblastic
l. of pyramidal cells
l. of rods and cones
l., osteogenetic; l., Ollier's
l., outer nuclear
l., papillary
l., pigment
l., prickle cell
l., Purkinje
l., reticular
l., somatic
l., spinous
l., splanchnic
l., spongy
l., subendocardial
l., subendothelial
l., Tome's granular
l., Weil's basal
l., zonal, of hypothalamus
lazaretto (lăz″ă-rĕt′ō) [It. *lazzaro*, a leper]
lb *pound*
LBBB *left bundle branch block*
LD *lethal dose*
LD$_{50}$ *median lethal dose*
LDH *lactic dehydrogenase*
LDL *low-density lipoprotein*
L-dopa
L.E. *lupus erythematosus*
leachate
leaching (lēch′ĭng) [AS. *leccan*, to wet]
lead (lēd) [AS. *laedan*, to guide]
l., bipolar
l., esophageal
l., limb
l., precordial
l., unipolar
lead (lĕd) Latin *plumbum*
l. acetate
l. monoxide
lead apron
lead colic
lead encephalopathy
lead line
lead pipe contraction

lead poisoning, acute
lead poisoning, chronic
leads (lēdz)
leaf (lĕf) [AS.]
lean (lēn) [AS. *hlaene*, without flesh]
lean body mass
learning, latent
learning curve
learning disability
learning theory
Leber's disease (lā′bĕrz) [Theodor Leber, Ger. ophthalmologist, 1840–1917]
Leber's plexus
Leboyer method (lĕ-boy-yā′) [Frederick Leboyer, contemporary Fr. obstetrician]
Lecat's gulf (lā-kăz′) [Claude N. Lecat, Fr. surgeon, 1700–1768]
L.E. cell *lupus erythematosus* cell
lechery (lĕtch′ĕr-ē) [Fr. *lecher*, to lick]
lecithal (lĕs′ĭ-thăl) [Gr. *lekithos*, egg yolk]
lecithin (lĕs′ĭth-ĭn) [Gr. *lekithos*, egg yolk]
lecithin/sphingomyelin ratio
lecithinase (lĕs′ĭ-thĭn-ās)
l., cobra
lecithoblast (lĕs′ĭ-thō-blăst″) [″ + *blastos*, germ]
lecithoprotein (lĕs″ĭ-thō-prō′tē-ĭn) [″ + *protos*, first]
lectin (lĕk′tĭn) [L. *legere*, to pick and choose]
lectual (lĕkt′ū-ăl) [L. *lectus*, bed]
LED *light-emitting diode*
leech (lētch) [AS. *laece*]
l., artificial
Lee's ganglion (lēz) [Robert Lee, Brit. gynecologist and obstetrician, 1793–1877]
lees
Leeuwenhoek's disease (lū′ĕn-hōks) [Antonj van Leeuwenhoek, Dutch microscopist, 1632–1723]
left
left-handedness
left lateral recumbent position

leg (lĕg) [ME.]
  l., badger
  l., baker
  l., bandy
  l., Barbadoes
  l., bayonet
  l., bird
  l., boomerang
  l., bow-
  l., milk
  l., restless
  l., scissor
  l., white
Legg-Calvé-Perthes   disease
(lĕg′kăl-vā′pĕr′tĕz) [Arthur T. Legg, U.S.
surgeon, 1874–1939; Jacques Calvé,
Fr. orthopedist, 1875–1954; Georg
C. Perthes, Ger. surgeon, 1869–
1927]
Legg's disease (lĕgz) [Arthur T. Legg]
leggings (lĕg′gĭngs) [ME. leg, leg]
Legionnaires' disease [after individuals stricken while attending an American Legion convention in Philadelphia, PA, in 1976]
legitimacy (lĕ-jĭt′ĭ-mă-sē) [L. legitimus, lawful]
legume (lĕ′gūm) [L. legumen, pulse, bean]
legumelin (lĕg-ū′mĕl-ĭn) [L. legumen, pulse, bean]
legumin (lĕ-gū′mĭn)
Leiner's disease (lī′nĕrz) [Karl Leiner, Austrian pediatrician, 1871–1930]
leiodermia (lī″ō-dĕr′mē-ă) [Gr. leios, smooth, + derma, skin]
leiomyofibroma (lī″ō-mī″ō-fī-brō′mă) [″ + mys, muscle, + L. fibra, fiber, + Gr. oma, tumor]
leiomyoma (lī″ō-mī-ō′mă) [″ + ″ + oma, tumor]
  l., epithelioid
  l. uteri
leiomyosarcoma (lī″ō-mī″ō-săr-kō′mă) [″ + ″ + sarx, flesh, + oma, tumor]
leiotrichous (lī-ŏt′rĭ-kŭs) [″ + thrix, hair]

Leishman-Donovan bodies
Leishmania (lēsh-mā′nē-ă) [Sir William B. Leishman, Brit. medical officer, 1865–1926]
  L. braziliensis
  L. donovani
  L. tropica
leishmaniasis (lēsh″mă-nī′ă-sĭs)
  l., American
  l., cutaneous
  l., mucocutaneous
  l., visceral
lema (lē′mă) [Gr. leme]
lemmocyte (lĕm′ō-sīt) [Gr. lemma, husk, + kytos, cell]
lemniscus (lĕm-nĭs′kŭs) [Gr. lemniskos, a ribbon]
lemon [Persian limun, lemon]
lemoparalysis (lē″mō-pă-răl′ĭ-sĭs) [Gr. laimos, gullet, + paralyein, to loosen, disable]
lemostenosis [″ + stenosis, act of narrowing]
length
  l., basialveolar
  l., basinasal
  l., crown-heel
  l., crown-rump
  l., focal
  l., wave
lenitive (lĕn′ĭ-tĭv) [L. lenire, to soothe]
lens (lĕnz) [L. lens, lentil]
  l., achromatic
  l., aplanatic
  l., apochromatic
  l., biconcave
  l., biconvex
  l., bifocal
  l., concave spherical
  l., contact
  l., convexoconcave
  l., convex spherical
  l., corneal contact
  l., crystalline
  l., cylindrical
  l., implanted
  l., omnifocal
  l., orthoscopic

l., soft contact
l., spherical
l., trial
l., trifocal
lentectomy (lĕn-tĕk'tō-mē) [L. *lens*, lentil, + Gr. *ektome*, excision]
lenticonus (lĕn"tĭ-kō'nŭs) [" + *conus*, cone]
lenticular [L. *lenticularis*, lentil]
lenticular fossa
lenticular glands
lenticular nucleus
lenticulostriate (lĕn-tĭk"ū-lō-strī'āt) [" + *striatus*, streaked]
lenticulothalamic
lentiform (lĕnt'ĭ-form) [L. *lens*, lentil, + *forma*, shape]
lentiginosis (lĕn-tĭj"ĭ-nō'sĭs) [L. *lentigo*, freckle, + Gr. *osis*, condition]
lentiginous (lĕn-tĭj'ĭn-ŭs) [L. *lentigo*, freckle]
lentiglobus (lĕn"tĭ-glō'bŭs) [L. *lens*, lentil, + *globus*, sphere]
lentigo (lĕn-tī'gō) [L., freckle]
l. maligna
lentitis (lĕn-tī'tĭs) [L. *lens*, lentil, + Gr. *itis*, inflammation]
leontiasis (lē"ŏn-tī'ă-sĭs) [Gr. *leon*, lion, + *-iasis*, state or condition of]
l. ossea
leotropic (lē-ō-trŏp'ĭk) [Gr. *laios*, left, + *tropos*, a turning]
leper (lĕp'ĕr) [Gr. *lepros*, scaly]
lepidic (lĕ-pĭd'ĭk) [Gr. *lepis*, scale]
lepido- [Gr. *lepis*, scale]
Lepidoptera (lĕp"ĭ-dŏp'tĕr-ă) [" + *pteron*, feather, wing]
lepidosis (lĕp"ĭ-dō'sĭs) [" + *osis*, condition]
lepothrix (lĕp'ō-thrĭks) [" + *thrix*, hair]
lepra (lĕp'ră) [Gr. *lepra*, leprosy]
l. alba
l. Arabum
l. maculosa
leprechaunism (lĕp'rē-kŏn"ĭzm)
leprid (lĕp'rĭd) [Gr. *lepra*, leprosy, + *eidos*, form, shape]

leprology (lĕp-rŏl'ō-jē) [" + *logos*, word, reason]
leproma (lĕp-rō'mă) [" + *oma*, tumor]
lepromatous (lĕp-rō'mă-tŭs)
lepromin (lĕp'rō-mĭn)
lepromin skin test
leprosarium
leprostatic (lĕp"rō-stăt'ĭk) [" + *statikos*, standing]
leprosy (lĕp'rō-sē) [Gr. *lepros*, scaly]
leprotic (lĕp-rŏt'ĭk) [Gr. *lepra*, leprosy]
leprous (lĕp'rŭs)
leptocephalia (lĕp"tō-sĕ-fā'lē-ă) [Gr. *leptos*, slender, + *kephale*, head]
leptocephalus
leptochromatic (lĕp"tō-krō-măt'ĭk) [" + *chromatin*]
leptocyte (lĕp'tō-sīt) [" + *kytos*, cell]
leptocytosis (lĕp"tō-sī-tō'sĭs) [" + " + *osis*, condition]
leptodactyly (lĕp"tō-dăk'tĭ-lē) [" + *daktylos*, finger]
leptomeninges (lĕp"tō-mĕn-ĭn'jēs) [" + *meninx*, membrane]
leptomeningitis (lĕp"tō-mĕn-ĭn-jī'tĭs) [" + " + *itis*, inflammation]
leptomeningopathy (lĕp"tō-mĕn"ĭn-gŏp'ă-thē) [" + " + *pathos*, disease, suffering]
leptomeninx
leptonema (lĕp"tō-nē'mă) [" + *nema*, thread]
leptopellic (lĕp"tō-pĕl'ĭk) [" + *pellis*, basin]
leptophonia (lĕp"tō-fō'nē-ă) [" + *phone*, voice]
leptoprosopia (lĕp"tō-prō-sō'pē-ă) [" + *prosopon*, face]
leptorhine, leptorrhine (lĕp'tor-rīn) [" + *rhis*, nose]
leptoscope (lĕp'tō-skōp) [" + *skopein*, to examine]
leptosome (lĕp'tō-sōm) [" + *soma*, body]
Leptospira (lĕp-tō-spī'ră) [" + *speira*, coil]

L. icterohaemorrhagiae
leptospire (lĕp'tō-spīr)
leptospirosis (lĕp"tō-spī-rō'sĭs) [" + " + osis, condition]
leptospiruria (lĕp"tō-spīr-ū'rē-ă) [" + " + ouron, urine]
leptotene (lĕp'tō-tēn) [" + tainia, ribbon]
leptothricosis (lĕp"tō-thrī-kō'sĭs) [" + thrix, hair]
Leptus autumnalis
leresis (lĕ-rē'sĭs) [Gr.]
Leriche's syndrome (lĕ-rēsh'ĕz) [René Leriche, Fr. surgeon, 1879–1955]
Leri's plenonosteosis (lā'rēz) [André Leri, Fr. physician, 1875–1930]
lesbian (lĕs'bē-ăn) [Gr. lesbios, pert. to island of Lesbos]
lesbianism
Lesch-Nyhan disease [M. Lesch, b. 1939, W. L. Nyhan, b. 1926, U.S. pediatricians]
lesion (lē'zhŭn) [L. laesio, a wound]
  l., degenerative
  l., diffuse
  l., discharging
  l., focal
  l., indiscriminate
  l., initial, of syphilis
  l., irritative
  l., local
  l., peripheral
  l., primary
  l., structural
  l., systemic
  l., toxic
  l., vascular
LET linear energy transfer
lethal [Gr. lethe, oblivion]
lethargic (lĕ-thăr'jĭk) [Gr. lethargos, drowsiness]
lethargy (lĕth'ăr-jē) [Gr. lethargos, drowsiness]
  l., African
  l., hysteric
  l., induced
  l., lucid

lethe (lē'thē) [Gr., oblivion]
lethologica (lĕth-ō-lōj'ĭ-kă) [Gr. lethe, forgetfulness, + logos, word, reason]
Letterer-Siwe disease (lĕt'ĕr-ĕr-sī'wē) [Erich Letterer, Ger. physician, b. 1895; S. August Siwe, Ger. physician, b. 1897]
Leu leucine
leucine (loo'sĭn) [Gr. leukos, white]
leucine aminopeptidase
leucinosis (loo"sĭn-ō'sĭs) [" + osis, condition]
leucinuria (loo"sĭn-ū'rē-ă) [" + ouron, urine]
leucism (loo'sĭzm) [" + -ismos, condition]
leucismus (loo-sĭz'mŭs) [" + -ismos, condition]
leucitis (loo-sī'tĭs) [" + itis, inflammation]
leucovorin calcium (loo"kō-vō'rĭn)
leukapheresis (loo"kă-fĕ-rē'sĭs) [" + aphairesis, removal]
leukemia (loo-kē'mē-ă) [Gr. leukos, white, + haima, blood]
  l., acute granulocytic
  l., acute lymphocytic
  l., acute myelogenous
  l., chronic lymphocytic
  l., chronic myelogenous
  l., hairy cell
leukemic (loo-kēm'ĭk) [" + haima, blood]
leukemid (loo-kē'mĭd)
leukemogenesis (loo-kē"mō-jĕn'ĕ-sĭs) [" + " + genesis, generation, birth]
leukemoid (loo-kē'moyd) [" + " + eidos, form, shape]
Leukeran
leukin (loo'kĭn)
leuko-, leuk- [Gr. leukos, white]
leukoagglutinin (loo"kō-ă-gloo'tĭ-nĭn) [" + L. agglutinans, gluing]
leukoblast (loo'kō-blăst) [" + blastos, germ]
leukoblastosis (loo"kō-blăs-tō'sĭs)

["   +   "   +   *osis*, condition]
leukocidin (loo-kō-sī'dĭn) ["   +   L. *caedere*, to kill]
leukocytal (loo"kō-sī'tăl) ["   +   *kytos*, cell]
leukocyte (loo'kō-sīt) ["   +   *kytos*, cell]
   l., acidophilic
   l., agranular
   l., basophil
   l., eosinophilic
   l., granular
   l., heterophilic
   l., lymphoid
   l., neutrophilic
   l., nongranular
   l., polymorphonuclear
leukocythemia (loo"kō-sī-thē'mē-ă) [Gr. *leukos*, white,   +   *kytos*, cell,   +   *haima*, blood]
leukocytic (loo"kō-sĭt'ĭk) ["   +   *kytos*, cell]
leukocytoblast (loo"kō-sī'tō-blast) ["   +   "   +   *blastos*, germ]
leukocytogenesis (loo"kō-sī'tō-jĕn'ĕ-sĭs) ["   +   *kytos*, cell,   +   *genesis*, generation, birth]
leukocytoid (loo'kō-sī"toyd) ["   +   "   +   *eidos*, form, shape]
leukocytolysin
leukocytolysis (loo"kō-sī-tŏl'ĭ-sĭs) ["   +   *kytos*, cell,   +   *lysis*, dissolution]
leukocytoma (loo"kō-sī-tō'mă) ["   +   "   +   *oma*, tumor]
leukocytopenia (loo"kō-sī"tō-pē'nē-ă) ["   +   "   +   *penia*, lack]
leukocytoplania (loo"kō-sī"tō-plā'nē-ă) ["   +   "   +   *plane*, wandering]
leukocytopoiesis (loo"kō-sī"tō-poy-ē'sĭs) ["   +   "   +   *poiein*, to make]
leukocytosis (loo"kō-sī-tō'sĭs) ["   +   *kytos*, cell,   +   *osis*, condition]
   l., basophilic
   l., mononuclear
   l., pathologic
leukocytotaxis (loo"kō-sī'tō-tăk'sĭs) [Gr. *leukos*, white,   +   *kytos*, cell,   +   *taxis*, arrangement]
leukocytotoxin (loo"kō-sī"tō-tŏk'sĭn) ["   +   "   +   *toxikon*, poison]
leukocyturia (loo"kō-sī-tū'rē-ă) ["   +   "   +   *ouron*, urine]
leukoderma (loo-kō-dĕr'mă) ["   +   *derma*, skin]
   l., syphilitic
leukodiagnosis (loo"kō-dī"ăg-nō'sĭs) ["   +   *dia*, through,   +   *gnosis*, knowledge]
leukodystrophy (lu"kō-dĭs'trō-fē)
   l., metachromatic
leukoedema (loo"kō-ē-dē'mă) ["   +   *oidema*, swelling]
leukoencephalitis (loo"kō-ĕn-sĕf-ă-lī'tĭs) ["   +   *enkephalos*, brain   +   *itis*, inflammation]
leukoerythroblastosis (loo"kō-ĕ-rĭth"rō-blăs-tō'sĭs) ["   +   *erythros*, red,   +   *blastos*, germ,   +   *osis*, condition]
leukokeratosis (loo"kō-kĕr-ă-tō'sĭs) ["   +   *keras*, horn,   +   *osis*, condition]
leukokoria (loo"kō-kō'rē-ă) ["   +   *kore*, pupil]
leukokraurosis (loo"kō-kraw-rō'sĭs) ["   +   *krauros*, dry,   +   *osis*, condition]
leukolymphosarcoma (loo"kō-lĭm"fō-săr-kō'mă) ["   +   L. *lympha*, lymph,   +   Gr. *sarx*, flesh,   +   *oma*, tumor]
leukolysis (loo-kŏl'ĭ-sĭs) ["   +   *lysis*, dissolution]
leukoma (loo-kō'mă) ["   +   *oma*, tumor]
   l. adherens
leukomaine (loo'kō-mān) [Gr. *leukoma*, whiteness]
leukomainemia (loo"kō-mā-nē'mē-ă) ["   +   *haima*, blood]
leukomatous (loo-kō'mă-tŭs) [Gr. *leukos*, white,   +   *oma*, tumor]
leukomyelitis (loo"kō-mī-ĕ-lī'tĭs) ["   +   *myelos*, marrow,   +   *itis*, inflammation]
leukomyelopathy (loo"kō-mī-ĕl-

öp′ă-thē) [″ + ″ + *pathos,*
disease, suffering]
leukonecrosis   (loo″kō-nĕ-krō′sĭs)
[″ + *nekrosis,* state of death]
leukonychia (loo″kō-nĭk′ē-ă) [″ +
onyx, nail]
leukopathia (loo″kō-păth′ē-ă) [″ +
pathos, disease, suffering]
  l. unguium
leukopedesis   (loo″kō-pĕ-dē′sĭs)
[″ + *pedan,* to leap]
leukopenia (loo″kō-pē′nē-ă) [″ +
penia, lack]
leukoplakia   (loo″kō-plă′kē-ă)
[″ + *plax,* plate]
  l. buccalis
  l. lingualis
  l. vulvae
leukoplasia (loo-kō-plă′zē-ă)
leukopoiesis (loo″kō-poy-ē′sĭs) [″ +
poiesis, formation]
leukopoietic (loo″kō-poy-ĕt′ĭk) [″ +
poiein, to make]
leukopsin
leukorrhagia (loo″kō-rā′jē-ă) [″ +
rhegnynai, to burst forth]
leukorrhea   (loo″kō-rē′ă)   [″ +
rhein, to flow]
leukosarcoma (loo″kō-săr-kō′mă) [Gr.
leukos, white, + *sarx,* flesh, +
oma, tumor]
leukosis (loo-kō′sĭs) [″ + *osis,* con-
dition]
leukotactic   (loo″kō-tăk′tĭk)   [″ +
taxis, arrangement]
leukotaxine (loo″kō-tăk′sĭn)
leukotaxis (loo″kō-tăks′ĭs)
leukotomy (loo-kŏt′ō-mē) [″ +
tome, a cutting, slice]
leukotoxic   (loo″kō-tŏks′ĭk)   [″ +
toxikon, poison]
leukotoxin   (loo″kō-tŏk′sĭn)   [″ +
toxikon, poison]
leukotrichia (loo″kō-trĭk′ē-ă) [″ +
thrix, hair]
leukotrienes
leukous (loo′kŭs) [Gr. *leukos,* white]
levallorphan tartrate (lĕv″ăl-lor′făn)
levarterenol bitartrate   (lĕv″ăr-tĕ-

rē′nŏl bī-tăr′trāt)
levator (lē-vā′tor) [L., lifter]
  l. ani
  l. palpebrae superioris
LeVeen shunt [Harry LeVeen, U.S. surgeon, b. 1917]
level of activities
lever (lĕv′ĕr, lē′vĕr) [L. *levare,* to raise]
levigation (lĕv″ĭ-gā′shŭn) [L. *levigare,*
to render smooth]
Levin's tube   (lē-vĭnz′) [Abraham L.
Levin, U.S. physician, 1880–1940]
levitation [L. *levitas,* lightness]
levocardia (lē″vō-kăr′dē-ă) [L. *laevus,*
left, + Gr. *kardia,* heart]
levoclination (lē″vō-klĭ-nā′shŭn) [″ +
clinatus, leaning]
levocycloduction   (lē″vō-sĭ″klō-
dŭk′shŭn) [″ + Gr. *kyklos,* circle,
+ L. *ducere,* to lead]
levodopa
Levo-Dromoran
levoduction (lē″vō-dŭk′shŭn) [L. *laevus,*
left, + *ducere,* to lead]
levography   (lē-vŏg′ră-fē)   [″ +
Gr. *graphein,* to write]
levogyration (lē″vō-jī-rā′shŭn) [″ +
gyrare, to turn]
levogyrous (lē″vō-jī′rŭs) [″ + *gyrare,* to turn]
levonordefrin (lē″vō-nor′dĕ-frĭn)
Levopa
Levophed
levophobia   (lĕv″ō-fō′bē-ă)   [″ +
Gr. *phobos,* fear]
Levoprome
levopropoxyphene   napsylate
(lē″vō-prō-pŏk′sĕ-fēn)
levorotation (lē″vō-rō-tā′shŭn) [″ +
rotare, to turn]
levorotatory (lē″vō-rō′tă-tor-ē)
levorphanol tartrate (lĕv-or′fă-nŏl)
levothyroxine   sodium   (lē″vō-thī-
rŏk′sēn)
levotorsion, levoversion   (lē″vō-
tor′shŭn, lē″vō-vĕr′shŭn) [″ + *torsio,* a twisting]
levulinic acid
levulose (lĕv′ū-lōs) [L. *laevus,* left]

levulosemia (lĕv″ū-lō-sē′mē-ă) [″ + Gr. *haima*, blood]

levulosuria (lĕv″ū-lō-sū′rē-ă) [″ + Gr. *ouron*, urine]

lewisite (lū′ĭ-sīt) [W. L. Lewis, U.S. chemist, 1879–1943]

Lewy bodies [Frederic H. Lewy, Ger. neurologist, 1885–1950]

Leyden jar (lī′dĕn) [Ernest V. von Leyden, Ger. physician, 1832–1910]

Leydig cells (lī′dĭg) [Franz von Leydig, Ger. anatomist, 1821–1908]

L.F.A. left frontoanterior

L-forms [named for *Lister* Institute]

L.F.P. left frontoposterior

L.F.T. left frontotransverse

LH *luteinizing hormone*

Lhermitte's sign (lār′mĭts) [Jacques Jean Lhermitte, Fr. neurologist, 1877–1959]

LHRH *luteinizing hormone releasing hormone*

Li *lithium*

libidinous (lĭ-bĭd′ĭ-nŭs) [L. *libidinosus*, pert. to desire]

libido (lĭ-bī′dō, -bē′dō) [L., desire]

Libman-Sacks disease (lĭb′măn-săks′) [Emanuel Libman, U.S. physician, 1872–1946; Benjamin Sacks, U.S. physician 1896–1939]

Libritabs

Librium

lice

licensure
  l., individual
  l., institutional

licentiate (lī-sĕn′shē-ăt)

lichen (lī′kĕn) [Gr. *leichen*, lichen]
  l., myxedematous
  l. nitidus
  l. pilaris
  l. planopilaris
  l. planus
  l. ruber moniliformis
  l. ruber planus
  l. sclerosus et atrophicus
  l. scrofulosus
  l. simplex chronicus

  l. spinulosus
  l. striatus
  l. tropicus

lichenification (lī-kĕn″ĭ-fĭ-kā′shŭn) [Gr. *leichen*, lichen, + L. *facere*, to make]

lichenin (lī′kĕ-nĭn)

lichenoid (lī′kĕn-oyd) [″ + *eidos*, form, shape]

Lichtheim's syndrome (lĭkt′hīmz) [Ludwig Lichtheim, Ger. physician, 1845–1928]

licorice (lĭk′ĕr-ĭs, -ĕr-ĭsh) [ME.]

lid [ME.]

Lida-Mantle

lidocaine (lī′dō-kān)
  l. hydrochloride

lid reflex

lie, transverse

Lieberkühn crypts (lē′bĕr-kēn) [Johann N. Lieberkühn, Ger. anatomist, 1711–1756]

lie detector

lien (lī′ĕn) [L.]
  l. accessorius
  l. mobilis

lienal (lī-ē′năl) [L. *lien*, spleen]

lienitis (lī″ĕ-nī′tĭs) [″ + Gr. *itis*, inflammation]

lienocele (lī-ē′nō-sēl) [″ + Gr. *kele*, tumor, swelling]

lienography (lī″ē-nŏg′ră-fē) [″ + Gr. *graphein*, to write]

lienomalacia (lī-ē″nō-mă-lā′shē-ă) [″ + Gr. *malakia*, softening]

lienomedullary (lī-ē″nō-mĕd′ū-lăr-ē) [″ + *medulla*, marrow]

lienomyelogenous (lī-ē″nō-mī-ĕl-ŏj′ē-nŭs) [″ + Gr. *myelos*, marrow, + *gennan*, to produce]

lienomyelomalacia (lī-ē″nō-mī″ĕl-ō-mă-lā′shē-ă) [″ + ″ + *malakia*, softening]

lienopancreatic (lī-ē″nō-păn″krē-ăt′ĭk) [″ + Gr. *pankreas*, pancreas]

lienorenal (lī-ē″nō-rē′năl) [″ + *renalis*, pert. to kidney]

lienotoxin (lī-ē″nō-tŏk′sĭn) [″ +

Gr. *toxikon,* poison]
lientery (lī′ĕn-tĕr′ē) [Gr. *leios,* smooth,
  + *enteron,* intestine]
lienunculus (lī″ĕn-ŭng′kū-lŭs)
life (līf) [AS.]
life expectancy
life extension
life sciences
life span
lifestyle
life support
ligament (lĭg′ă-mĕnt) [L. *ligamentum,* a
  band]
  l., accessory
  l., acromioclavicular
  l., alar
  l., annular
  l., apical
  l.'s, arcuate
  l., arterial
  l.'s, auricular
  l., broad, of liver
  l., broad, of uterus
  l.'s, capsular
  l.'s, carpal
  l., caudal
  l., check
  l., conoid
  l., coracoacromial
  l., coracoclavicular
  l., coracohumeral
  l., coronary, of liver
  l., costocolic
  l., costocoracoid
  l.'s, costotransverse
  l., costotransverse, middle
  l.'s, costovertebral
  l., cricopharyngeal
  l., cricothyroid
  l., cricotracheal
  l., cruciate
  l., cruciform
  l., crural
  l., deltoid
  l., dentate
  l., dentoalveolar
  l., falciform, of liver
  l., fundiform, of penis

l., gastrophrenic
l., Gimbernat's
l., gingivodental
l.'s, glenohumeral
l., glenoid
l., Henle's
l., hepaticoduodenal
l., iliofemoral
l., iliolumbar
l., iliopectineal
l., infundibulopelvic
l., inguinal
l., interclavicular
l., interspinal
l., ischiocapsular
l., lacunar
l., lateral occipitoatlantal
l.'s, lateral odontoid
l.'s, lateral, of liver
l.'s, Lisfranc's
l., Lockwood's
l., medial
l.'s, meniscofemoral
l.'s, nephrocolic
l., nuchal
l.'s, palpebral
l., patellar
l., pectineal
l., periodontal
l., Petit's
l., phrenocolic
l., popliteal arcuate
l., Poupart's
l., pterygomandibular
l.'s, pubic arcuate
l., pulmonary
l., rhomboid, of clavicle
l., round, of femur
l., round, of liver
l., round, of uterus
l.'s, sacroiliac
l., sacrospinous
l., sacrotuberous
l., sphenomandibular
l., spiral, of cochlea
l., stylohyoid
l., stylomandibular
l., suprascapular

l., supraspinal
l., suspensory
l., suspensory, of axilla
l., suspensory, of lens
l., suspensory, of ovary
l., suspensory, of penis
l.'s, suspensory, of uterus
l.'s, sutural
l., temporomandibular
l., tendinotrochanteric
l., transverse crural
l., transverse humeral
l., transverse, of atlas
l., transverse, of hip joint
l., transverse, of knee joint
l., trapezoid
l.'s, triangular, of liver
l., umbilical, lateral
l., umbilical, median
l., uterorectosacral
l., uterosacral
l., venous, of liver
l., ventricular, of larynx
l., vesicouterine
l., vestibular
l., vocal
l., Weitbrecht's
l.'s, yellow

ligamenta

ligamentopexis (lĭg″ă-mĕn″tō-pĕks′ĭs) [L. *ligamentum*, band, + Gr. *pexis*, fixation]

ligamentous (lĭg″ă-mĕn′tŭs) [L. *ligamentum*, band]

ligamentum (lĭg″ă-mĕn′tŭm) [L., a band]

ligand (lī′gănd, lĭg′ănd) [L. *ligare*, to bind]

ligase (lī′gās, lĭg′ās)

ligate (lī′gāt)

ligation (lī-gā′shŭn)

ligature (lĭg′ă-chūr) [L. *ligatura*, a binding]

light (līt) [AS. *leohte*, not heavy]

light (līt) [AS. *lihtan*, to shine]
l., axial
l., cold
l., diffused

l., idioretinal; l., intrinsic
l., oblique
l., polarized
l., reflected
l., refracted
l., transmitted
l., white
l., Wood's

light adaptation
light diet
light difference
lightening [AS. *leohte*, not heavy]
light-headed
lightning safety rules
lightning streaks, Moore's
light reflex
light sense
light therapy
light unit
Lignac-Fanconi disease
lignin (lĭg′nĭn)
lignocaine (lĭg′nō-kān)
lignoceric acid
limb (lĭm) [AS. *lim*]
l., anacrotic
l., anterior, of internal capsule
l., ascending, of renal tubule
l., catacrotic
l., descending, of renal tubule
l., pectoral
l., pelvic
l., phantom
l., thoracic

limbic (lĭm′bĭk) [L. *limbus*, border]
limbic system
limbus (lĭm′bŭs) [L., border]
l. alveolaris
l. conjunctivae
l. corneae
l., corneoscleral
l. fossae ovalis
l. lamina spiralis ossae
l. palpebrales, anteriores
l. palpebralis, posterior
l. sphenoidalis

lime (lĭm) [AS. *lim*, glue]
l., chlorinated
l., slaked

l., soda
l., sulfurated
l. water
lime [Fr.]
limen (lī'měn) [L.]
l. nasi
l. of insula
limes nul
limes tod
liminal (lĭm'ĭ-năl) [L. limen, threshold]
limit (lĭm'ĭt)
l., assimilation
l., audibility
l., elastic
l., Hayflick's
l. of flocculation
l. of perception
l., quantum
limitans (lĭm'ĭ-tăns) [L. limitare, to limit]
limitation (lĭm"ĭ-tā'shŭn)
limitation of motion
limosis (lĭ-mō'sĭs) [Gr. limos, hunger]
limotherapy (lĭ"mō-thĕr'ă-pē) [" + therapeia, treatment]
limulus amebocyte lysate test
Lincocin
lincomycin hydrochloride (lĭn"kō-mī'sĭn)
lincture, linctus (lĭnk'tūr, -tŭs) [L. linctus, a licking]
lindane (lĭn'dān)
Lindau's disease (lĭn'dowz) [Arvid Lindau, Swedish pathologist, 1892–1958]
Lindau-von Hippel disease (lĭn'dow-vŏn-hĭp'ĕl) [Arvid Lindau; Eugen von Hippel, Ger. ophthalmologist, 1867–1939]
line (lĭn) [L. linea]
l., abdominal
l., absorption
l., alveolobasilar
l., alveolonasal
l., auriculobregmatic
l.'s, axillary
l., base
l., basiobregmatic
l., Baudelocque's

l.'s, Beau's
l., biauricular
l., blue
l., canthomeatal
l., cement
l., cervical
l.'s, cleavage
l., costoarticular
l., costoclavicular
l., Douglas'
l., epiphyseal
l., gingival
l., glabellomeatal
l.'s, gluteal
l., gum
l., iliopectineal
l., incremental
l., incremental, of Retzius
l., incremental, of von Ebner
l., infraorbitomeatal
l., interauricular
l., intercondylar
l., interpupillary
l., intertrochanteric
l., intertuberal
l.'s, Kerley's
l., lead
l., lip
l., mamillary
l., mammary
l., median
l., mentomeatal
l., milk
l., mucogingival
l., mylohyoid
l., nasobasilar
l., nuchal, superior and inferior
l., oblique, of fibula
l., oblique, of radius
l. of demarcation
l. of fibula, oblique
l. of fixation
l. of ilium, intermediate
l. of mandible, oblique
l.'s of Owen
l., parasternal
l., pectineal
l., popliteal, of femur

l., popliteal, of tibia
l., resting
l., reversal
l., scapular
l., semilunar
l., Shenton's
l., sight
l., sternal
l., sternomastoid
l.'s, supracondylar, medial and lateral
l., supraorbital
l., temporal, of frontal bone
l., umbilicopubic
l., visual
l.'s, Zöllner's
linea (lĭn'ē-ă) [L., line]
l. alba
l. albicantes
l. aspera
l. costoarticularis
l. nigra
l. semilunaris
l. splendens
l. sternalis
l. striae atrophicae
l. terminalis
l. transversae ossis sacri
linear (lĭn'ē-ăr) [L. linea, line]
linear energy transfer
liner (lĭn'ĕr)
l., cavity
l., soft
lingua (lĭng'gwă) [L.]
l. frenata
l. geographica
l. nigra
l. plicata
lingual (lĭng'gwăl) [L. lingua, tongue]
linguiform (lĭng'gwĭ-form) [" + forma, shape]
lingula (lĭng'gū-lă) [L., little tongue]
l. cerebelli
l. of lung
l. of mandible
l. of sphenoid
lingulectomy (lĭng"gū-lĕk'tō-mē) [L. lingula, little tongue, + Gr. ektome,

excision]
linguoclasia (lĭng'gwō-klă'zē-ă) [L. lingua, tongue, + Gr. klasis, destruction]
linguoclination (lĭng'gwō-klī-nā'shŭn) [" + clinatus, leaning]
linguodental
linguodistal (lĭng"gwō-dĭs'tăl) [" + distare, to be distant]
linguogingival (lĭng"gwō-jĭn'jĭ-văl) [" + gingiva, gum]
linguomesial
linguo-occlusal (lĭng"gwō-ŏ-kloo'zăl) [" + occludere, to shut up]
linguopapillitis (lĭng"gwō-păp"ĭ-lĭ'tĭs) [" + papilla, nipple, + Gr. itis, inflammation]
linguopulpal
linguoversion (lĭng"gwō-vĕr'zhŭn) [" + versio, a turning]
liniment [L. linimentum, smearing substance]
l., camphor
l., medicinal soft soap
linimentum (lĭn-ĭ-mĕn'tŭm) [L.]
linitis (lĭn-ī'tĭs) [Gr. linon, flax, + itis, inflammation]
l. plastica
linkage
l., sex
linseed [AS. linsaed]
lint (lĭnt) [L. linteum, made of linen]
lintin (lĭn'tĭn)
liothyronine sodium (lī"ō-thī'rō-nēn)
liotrix tablets (lī'ō-trĭks)
lip [AS. lippa]
l., cleft
l., double
l., glenoid
l., Hapsburg
l.'s, oral
l., tympanic
l., vestibule
lipacidemia (lĭp"ăs-ĭ-dē'mē-ă) [Gr. lipos, fat, + L. acidus, acid, + Gr. haima, blood]
lipaciduria (lĭp"ăs-ĭ-dū'rē-ă) [" + " + Gr. ouron, urine]

liparocele (lĭp'ă-rō-sēl) [" + kele, tumor, swelling]

liparous (lĭp'ă-rŭs) [Gr. lipos, fat]

lipase (lī'pās, lĭ'pās) [" + -ase, enzyme]
  l., pancreatic

lipasuria (lĭp"ăs-ū'rē-ă) [" + " + Gr. ouron, urine]

lipectomy (lĭ-pĕk'tō-mē) [" + ektome, excision]
  l., suction

lipedema (lĭp"ĕ-dē'mă) [" + oidema, swelling]

lipemia (lĭ-pē'mē-ă) [" + haima, blood]
  l., alimentary
  l. retinalis

lipid(e) (lĭp'ĭd, -īd) [Gr. lipos, fat]

lipid histiocytosis

lipidosis

lipiduria (lĭp"ĭ-dū'rē-ă) [" + Gr. ouron, urine]

lipin (lĭp'ĭn) [Gr. lipos, fat]

Lipiodol (lĭp-ī'ō-dŏl) [" + L. oleum, oil]

lipo-, lip- [Gr. lipos, fat]

lipoarthritis (lĭp"ō-ărth-rī'tĭs) [" + arthron, joint, + itis, inflammation]

lipoatrophia, lipoatrophy (lĭ"pō-ă-trō'fē-ă, lĭ"pō-ăt'rō-fē) [" + a-, not, + trophe, nourishment]

lipoblast (lĭp'ō-blăst) [" + blastos, germ]

lipoblastoma (lĭp"ō-blăs-tō'mă) [" + " + oma, tumor]

lipocardiac (lĭp"ō-kăr'dē-ăk) [" + kardia, heart]

lipocatabolic (lĭp"ō-kăt"ă-bŏl'ĭk) [" + katabole, a casting down]

lipocele (lĭp'ō-sēl) [" + kele, tumor, swelling]

lipoceratous (lĭp"ō-sĕr'ă-tŭs) [" + L. cera, wax]

lipocere (lĭp'ō-sēr) [" + L. cera, wax]

lipochondrodystrophy (lĭp"ō-kŏn"drō-dĭs'trō-fē) [" + chondros, cartilage, + dys, bad, difficult,

painful, disordered, + trephein, to nourish]

lipochondroma (lĭp"ō-kŏn-drō'mă) [" + " + oma, tumor]

lipochrome (lĭp'ō-krōm) [" + chroma, color]

lipoclasis (lĭp-ŏk'lă-sĭs) [" + klasis, breaking]

lipoclastic (lĭp-ō-klăs'tĭk)

lipocyte (lĭp'ō-sīt) [" + kytos, cell]

lipodieresis (lĭp"ō-dī-ĕr'ē-sĭs) [" + diairesis, a taking]

lipodystrophy (lĭp"ō-dĭs'trō-fē) [" + dys, bad, difficult, painful, disordered, + trophe, nourishment]
  l., insulin
  l., intestinal
  l., progressive

lipoferous (lĭp-ŏf'ĕr-ŭs) [" + L. ferre, to carry]

lipofibroma (lĭp"ō-fī-brō'mă) [" + L. fibra, fiber, + Gr. oma, tumor]

lipofuscin (lĭp"ō-fŭs'sĭn)

lipofuscinosis (lĭp"ō-fū"sĭn-ō'sĭs) [lipofuscin + Gr. osis, condition]

Lipo Gantrisin

lipogenesis (lĭp"ō-jĕn'ĕ-sĭs) [Gr. lipos, fat, + genesis, generation, birth]

lipogenetic, lipogenic (lĭp"ō-jĕ-nĕt'ĭk, lĭp"ō-jĕn'ĭk)

lipogenous (lĭp-ŏj'ĕ-nŭs)

lipogranuloma (lĭp"ō-grăn-ū-lō'mă) [" + L. granulum, granule, + Gr. oma, tumor]

lipogranulomatosis (lĭp"ō-grăn"ū-lō-mă-tō'sĭs) [" + " + " + osis, condition]

Lipo-Hepin

lipoid (lĭp'oyd) [" + eidos, form, shape]

lipoidemia (lĭp"oy-dē'mē-ă) [" + " + haima, blood]

lipoidosis (lĭp-oy-dō'sĭs) [" + " + osis, condition]
  l., arterial
  l., cerebroside

lipoiduria (lĭp"oy-dū'rē-ă) [" + " + ouron, urine]

lipolipoidosis (lĭp″ō-lĭp″oy-dō′sĭs) [″ + *lipos*, fat, + *eidos*, form, shape, + *osis*, condition]

lipolysis (lĭp-ŏl′ĭ-sĭs) [″ + *lysis*, dissolution]

lipolytic (lĭp-ō-lĭt′ĭk)

lipolytic digestion

lipolytic enzyme

lipoma (lĭ-pō′mă) [Gr. *lipos*, fat, + *oma*, tumor]
   l. arborescens
   l., cystic
   l., diffuse
   l. diffusum renis
   l. durum
   l., hernial
   l., nasal
   l., osseous
   l. telangiectodes

lipomatoid (lĭ-pō′mă-toyd) [″ + ″ + *eidos*, form, shape]

lipomatosis (lĭp″ō-mă-tō′sĭs) [″ + *oma*, tumor + *osis*, condition]
   l. renis

lipomatous (lĭp-ō′mă-tŭs)

lipomeningocele (lĭp″ō-mĕ-nĭng′gō-sēl) [″ + *meninx*, membrane, + *kele*, tumor, swelling]

lipomeria (lĭ″pō-mē′rē-ă) [Gr. *leipein*, to leave, + *meros*, a part]

lipometabolic (lĭp″ō-mĕt″ă-bŏl′ĭk) [″ + *metabole*, change]

lipometabolism (lĭp-ō-mĕ-tăb′ŏl-ĭzm) [″ + ″ + *-ismos*, condition]

lipomyoma (lĭp″ō-mī-ō′mă) [″ + *mys*, muscle, + *oma*, tumor]

lipomyxoma (lĭp″ō-mĭks-ō′mă) [″ + *myxa*, mucus, + *oma*, tumor]

lipopectic (lĭp-ō-pĕk′tĭk) [″ + *pexis*, fixation]

lipopenia (lĭp″ō-pē′nē-ă) [″ + *penia*, lack]

lipopenic (lĭp″ō-pē′nĭk)

lipopeptid, lipopeptide (lĭp″ō-pĕp′tĭd, -tīd)

lipopexia (lĭp″ō-pĕk′sē-ă)

lipophage (lĭp′ō-fāj) [″ + *phagein*, to eat]

lipophagia, granulomatous (lĭp″ō-fă′jē-ă)

lipophagic (lĭp-ō-fă′jĭk)

lipophagy (lĭ-pŏf′ă-jē)

lipophanerosis (lĭp″ō-făn″ĕ-rō′sĭs) [″ + *phaneros*, visible, + *osis*, condition]

lipophil (lĭp′ō-fĭl) [″ + *philein*, to love]

lipophilia (lĭp″ō-fĭl′ē-ă) [″ + *philos*, love]

lipopolysaccharide (lĭp″ō-pŏl″ē-săk′ă-rīd)

lipoproteins
   l., high-density
   l., low-density
   l., very low density

liposarcoma (lĭp″ō-săr-kō′mă) [Gr. *lipos*, fat, + *sarx*, flesh, + *oma*, tumor]

liposis (lĭ-pō′sĭs) [″ + *osis*, condition]

liposoluble (lĭp″ō-sŏl′ū-b′l) [″ + L. *solubilis*, soluble]

liposome (lĭp′ō-sōm) [″ + *soma*, body]

lipostomy (lĭ-pŏs′tō-mē) [Gr. *leipein*, to fail, + *stoma*, mouth, opening]

lipothymia (lĭ″pō-thī′mē-ă) [Gr. *lipothymein*, to faint]

lipotrophy (lĭ-pŏt′rō-fē) [Gr. *lipos*, fat, + *trophe*, nourishment]

lipotropic (lĭp-ō-trŏp′ĭk) [″ + *trope*, a turning]

lipotropic factors

lipotropism, lipotropy (lĭ-pŏt′rō-pĭzm, -pē) [″ + *trope*, a turn, + *-ismos*, condition]

lipovaccine (lĭp″ō-văk′sēn)

lipoxeny (lĭ-pŏks′ĕ-nē) [Gr. *leipein*, to fail, + *xenos*, host]

lipoxidase (lĭ-pŏk′sĭ-dās)

lipoxygenase (lĭ-pŏks′ĭ-jĕ-nās)

Lippes loop (lĭ′pēz) [Jacob Lippes, U.S. obstetrician, b. 1924]

lipping (lĭp′ĭng)

lippitude (lĭp′ĭ-tūd) [L. *lippitudo*, fr. *lippus*, blear-eyed]

lip reading
lip reflex
lipsis (lĭp'sĭs) [Gr. *leipein*, to fail]
  l. animi
lipuria (lĭ-pū'rē-ă) [Gr. *lipos*, fat, + *ouron*, urine]
Liquaemin Sodium
liquefacient (lĭk"wĕ-fā'shĕnt) [L. *liquere*, to be fluid, + *facere*, to make]
liquefaction (lĭk"wĕ-făk'shŭn)
liquescent (lĭk-wĕs'sĕnt) [L. *liquescere*, to become liquid]
liqueur (lĭ-kĕr') [Fr.]
liquid (lĭk'wĭd) [L. *liquere*, to be fluid]
liquid air therapy
liquid crystals
liquid diet
liquid measure
liquor (lĭk'ĕr) [L.]
  l. amnii
  l. folliculi
  l. sanguinis
liquor solutions
Lisfranc's ligament (lĭs-frănks') [Jacques Lisfranc, Fr. surgeon, 1790–1847]
lisping (lĭsp'ĭng) [AS. *wlisp*, lisping]
lissencephalous (lĭs"sĕn-sĕf'ă-lŭs) [Gr. *lissos*, smooth, + *enkephalos*, brain]
lissotrichy (lĭs-sŏt'rĭ-kē) [" + *thrix*, hair]
Lister, Baron Joseph (lĭs'tĕr) [Brit. surgeon, 1827–1912]
listeriosis, listerosis (lĭs-tĕr"ē-ō'sĭs, lĭs"tĕr-ō'sĭs)
lisuride
liter (lē'tĕr) [Fr. *litre*, liter]
lithagogue (lĭth'ă-gŏg) [Gr. *lithos*, stone, + *agogos*, leading]
Lithane
lithecbole (lĭ-thĕk'bō-lē) [" + *ekbole*, expulsion]
lithectasy (lĭth-ĕk'tă-sē) [" + *ektasis*, dilatation]
lithectomy (lĭ-thĕk'tō-mē) [" + *ektome*, excision]

lithemia (lĭth-ē'mē-ă) [" + *haima*, blood]
lithiasis (lĭth-ī'ă-sĭs)
  l. biliaris
  l. nephritica
  l. renalis
lithic acid (lĭth'ĭk)
lithicosis (lĭth"ĭ-kō'sĭs) [Gr. *lithikos*, made of stone]
lithium (lĭth'ē-ŭm) [Gr. *lithos*, stone]
  l. carbonate
litho-, lith- [Gr. *lithos*, stone]
lithocenosis (lĭth"ō-sĕn-ō'sĭs) [" + *kenosis*, evacuation]
lithoclast (lĭth'ō-klăst) [" + *klastos*, broken]
lithoclasty (lĭth'ō-klăs"tē)
lithoclysmia (lĭth-ō-klĭz'mē-ă) [" + *klysma*, a clyster]
lithocystotomy (lĭth"ō-sĭs-tŏt'ō-mē) [" + *kystis*, bladder, + *tome*, a cutting, slice]
lithodialysis (lĭth"ō-dī-ăl'ĭ-sĭs) [" + *dia*, through, + *lysis*, dissolution]
lithogenesis (lĭth"ō-jĕn'ĕ-sĭs) [" + *genesis*, generation, birth]
lithokelyphopedion (lĭth"ō-kĕl"ĭ-fō-pē'dē-ŏn) [" + *kelyphos*, sheath, + *paidion*, child]
lithokelyphos (lĭth"ō-kĕl'ĭ-fŏs) [" + *kelyphos*, sheath]
lithokonion (lĭth"ō-kō'nē-ŏn) [" + *konios*, dusty]
litholabe (lĭth'ō-lāb) [" + *lambanein*, to hold]
litholapaxy (lĭth-ŏl'ă-păks"ē) [Gr. *lithos*, stone, + *lapaxis*, evacuation]
lithology (lĭth-ŏl'ō-jē) [" + *logos*, word, reason]
litholysis (lĭth-ŏl'ĭ-sĭs) [" + *lysis*, dissolution]
lithometer (lĭth-ŏm'ĕ-tĕr) [" + *metron*, measure]
lithometra (lĭth-ō-mē'tră) [" + *metra*, uterus]
lithomyl (lĭth'ō-mĭl) [" + *myle*, mill]
Lithonate

lithonephritis (lĭth"ō-nĕ-frī'tĭs) [" + nephros, kidney, + itis, inflammation]

lithonephrotomy (lĭth"ō-nē-frŏt'ō-mē) [" + nephros, kidney, + tome, a cutting, slice]

lithontriptic (lĭth-ŏn-trĭp'tĭk) [" + tribein, to rub]

lithopedion (lĭth"ō-pē'dē-ŏn) [" + paidion, child]

lithophone (lĭth'ō-fōn) [" + phone, sound]

lithoscope (lĭth'ō-skōp) [" + skopein, to examine]

Lithotabs

lithotome (lĭth'ō-tōm) [" + tome, a cutting, slice]

lithotomy (lĭth-ŏt'ō-mē) [" + tome, a cutting, slice]
  l., bilateral
  l., high
  l., lateral
  l., median
  l., rectal
  l., vaginal

lithotomy position

lithotony (lĭth-ŏt'ō-nē) [Gr. lithos, stone, + teinein, to stretch]

lithotresis (lĭth"ō-trē'sĭs) [" + tresis, boring]

lithotripsy (lĭth'ō-trĭp"sē) [" + tribein, to rub]

lithotriptic (lĭth-ō-trĭp'tĭk)

lithotriptor (lĭth'ō-trĭp"tor) [" + tripsis, a rubbing, friction]

lithotriptoscopy (lĭth"ō-trĭp-tŏs'kō-pē) [" + " + skopein, to examine]

lithotrite (lĭth'ō-trīt) [" + tribein, to rub]

lithotrity (lĭth-ŏt'rĭ-tē)

lithous (lĭth'ŭs) [Gr. lithos, stone]

lithoxiduria (lĭth"ŏks-ĭ-dū'rē-ă) [" + L. oxidum, oxide, + Gr. ouron, urine]

lithuresis (lĭth"ū-rē'sĭs) [" + ouresis, urination]

lithureteria (lĭth"ū-rē-tē'rē-ă) [" + oureter, ureter]

lithuria (lĭth-ū'rē-ă) [" + ouron, urine]

litmus (lĭt'mŭs)

litmus paper

litter (lĭt'tĕr) [O. Fr. litiere, offspring at birth, bed]

Little's disease [William John Little, Brit. physician, 1810–1894]

Littre's glands (lē'trz) [Alexis Littre, Fr. surgeon, 1658–1725]

littritis (lĭt-trī'tĭs)

Litzmann's obliquity [Karl K.T. Litzmann, Ger. gynecologist, 1815–1890]

live birth

livedo (lĭv-ē'dō) [L. livedo, lividness]
  l. reticularis

liver (lĭv'ĕr) [AS. lifer]
  l., abscess of
  l., acute yellow atrophy of
  l., amyloid
  l., biliary cirrhotic
  l., cancer of
  l., cirrhosis of
  l., cysts of
  l., fatty
  l., floating
  l., foamy
  l., hobnail
  l., inflammation of
  l., lardaceous
  l., nutmeg
  l., wandering
  l., waxy

liver extract

liver failure

liver flap

liver fluke, human

liver spots

livid (lĭv'ĭd) [L. lividus, lead-colored]

lividity (lĭ-vĭd'ĭ-tē)

living will

livor (lī'vor) [L., a black-and-blue spot]
  l. mortis

lixiviation (lĭks"ĭv-ē-ā'shŭn) [L. lixivia, lye]

L.L.E. left lower extremity

LLQ left lower quadrant

L.M.A.   *left mentoanterior*
L.M.P.   *left mentoposterior*
L.M.T.   *left mentotransverse*
L.O.A.   *left occipitoanterior*
load
loading, carbohydrate
loading test
loaiasis
Loa loa   (lō′ă) [W. African]
lobar   (lō′băr) [Gr. *lobos*, lobe]
lobar pneumonia
lobate   (lō′bāt) [L. *lobatus*, lobed]
lobe   (lōb) [Gr. *lobos*, lobe]
    l., anterior, of hypophysis
    l., azygos
    l., caudate, of liver
    l., central
    l., flocculonodular
    l., frontal
    l.'s, hepatic
    l., insular
    l.'s, lateral, of prostate
    l.'s, lateral, of thyroid gland
    l., limbic
    l., occipital
    l.'s of cerebrum
    l. of ear
    l.'s of lungs
    l. of mamma
    l.'s of pancreas
    l. of parotid, accessory
    l.'s of prostate
    l., olfactory
    l.'s, orbital
    l., parietal
    l., posterior, of hypophysis
    l., prefrontal
    l., pyramidal, of thyroid
    l., quadrate, of liver
    l., Riedel's
    l., spigelian
    l., temporal
lobectomy   (lō-běk′tō-mē) [Gr. *lobos*,
    lobe,   +   *ektome*, excision]
lobelia   (lō-bē′lē-ă)
lobeline   (lŏb′ĕ-lēn)
lobi
lobitis   (lō-bī′tĭs) [″   +   *itis*, inflamma-
tion]
Loboa loboi
Lobo's disease
lobotomy   (lō-bŏt′ō-mē) [Gr. *lobos*,
    lobe,   +   *tome*, a cutting, slice]
Lobstein's disease   (lŏb′stīnz) [Johann
    F. G. C. M. Lobstein, Ger. surgeon,
    1777–1835]
lobular   (lŏb′ū-lăr) [L. *lobulus*, small lobe]
lobulate, lobulated   (lŏb′ū-lāt, -lāt-ĕd)
lobule   (lŏb′ūl) [L. *lobulus*, small lobe]
    l., central, of cerebellum
    l.'s of epididymis
    l. of kidney
    l. of liver
    l.'s of lung
    l.'s of testis
    l.'s of thymus
    l., paracentral
    l., parietal
    l., primary pulmonary
lobuli
lobulus   (lŏb′ū-lŭs) [L.]
lobus   (lō′bŭs) [L.]
local   (lō′kăl) [L. *locus*, place]
localization   (lō-kăl-ĭ-zā′shŭn)
    l., cerebral
localized   (lō′kăl-īzd)
localizer
locator   (lō′kā-tĕr)
lochia   (lō′kē-ă) [Gr. *lochia*]
    l. alba
    l. cruenta
    l. purulenta
    l. rubra
    l. serosa
lochial   (lō′kē-ăl)
lochiocolpos   (lō″kē-ō-kŏl′pŏs) [Gr. *lochia*, discharge following childbirth,
    +   *kolpos*, vagina]
lochiometra   (lō″kē-ō-mē′tră) [″   +
metra, uterus]
lochiometritis   (lō″kē-ō-mē-trī′tĭs)
    [″   +   ″   +   *itis*, inflammation]
lochiorrhagia   (lō′kē-ō-rā′jē-ă) [″   +
rhegnynai, to break forth]
lochiorrhea   (lō″kē-ō-rē′ă) [″   +
rhein, to flow]

lochioschesis (lō″kē-ŏs′kĕ-sĭs) [″ + *schesis*, retention]

lochometritis (lō″kō-mē-trī′tĭs) [″ + *metra*, uterus, + *itis*, inflammation]

loci [L.]

locked-in syndrome

Locke's solution, Locke-Ringer's solution [Frank S. Locke, Brit. physician, 1871–1949; Sydney Ringer, Brit. physiologist, 1835–1910]

lockjaw

Lockwood's ligament [Charles B. Lockwood, Brit. surgeon, 1856–1914]

loco (lō′kō) [Sp., cracked brain]

locomotion (lō″kō-mō′shŭn) [L. *locus*, place, + *movere*, to move]

locomotor (lō″kō-mō′tor)

locomotor ataxia

locomotorium (lō″kō-mō-tō′rē-ŭm)

locular (lŏk′ū-lăr) [L. *loculus*, a small space]

loculated (lŏk′ū-lāt-ĕd)

loculi (lŏk′ū-lī)

loculus (lŏk′ū-lŭs) [L.]

locum tenens (lō′kŭm tĕn′ĕns) [L. *locus*, place, + *tenere*, to hold]

locus (lō′kŭs) [L. *locus*, a place]
   l. ceruleus
   l. niger

locus of control

Loeffler's bacillus (lĕf′lĕrz) [Friedrich A. J. Loeffler, Ger. bacteriologist, 1852–1915]

Löffler's endocarditis (lĕf′lĕrz) [Wilhelm Löffler, Swiss physician, b. 1887]

logadectomy (lŏg″ă-dĕk′tō-mē) [Gr. *logades*, the whites of the eyes, + *ektome*, excision]

logaditis (lŏg″ă-dī′tĭs) [″ + *itis*, inflammation]

logagnosia (lŏg″ăg-nō′sē-ă) [Gr. *logos*, word, reason, + *a-*, not, + *gnosis*, knowledge]

logagraphia (lŏg-ă-grăf′ē-ă) [″ + ″ + *graphein*, to write]

logamnesia (lŏg-ăm-nē′zē-ă) [″ + *amnesia*, forgetfulness]

logaphasia (lŏg″ă-fā′zē-ă) [″ +

a-, not, + *phasis*, utterance]

logasthenia (lŏg″ăs-thē′nē-ă) [″ + ″ + *sthenos*, strength]

logoklony (lŏg′ō-klŏn-ē) [″ + *klonein*, to agitate]

logokophosis (lŏg″ō-kō-fō′sĭs) [″ + *kophosis*, deafness]

logomania (lŏg-ō-mā′nē-ă) [″ + *mania*, madness]

logoneurosis (lŏg″ō-nū-rō′sĭs) [″ + *neuron*, nerve, + *osis*, condition]

logopathia (lŏg-ō-păth′ē-ă) [″ + *pathos*, disease, suffering]

logopedia (lŏg″ō-pē′dē-ă) [″ + *pais*, child]

logoplegia (lŏg-ō-plē′jē-ă) [″ + *plege*, stroke]

logorrhea (lŏg″ō-rē′ă) [″ + *rhein*, to flow]

logospasm (lŏg′ō-spăzm) [″ + *spasmos*, a convulsion]

-logy [Gr. *logos*, word, reason]

loiasis (lō-ī′sĭs)

loin (loyn) [O. Fr. *loigne*, long part]

lolism

lomustine (lō-mŭs′tēn)

loneliness

Long, Crawford Williamson [U.S. physician, 1815–1878]

long-acting thyroid stimulator

longevity (lŏn-jĕv′ĭ-tē) [L. *longaevus*, aged]

longing

longissimus (lŏn-jĭs′ĭ-mŭs) [L.]

longitudinal (lŏn″jĭ-tū′dĭ-năl) [L. *longitudo*, length]

longsightedness

longus (lŏng′gŭs) [L.]

loop [ME. *loupe*]
   l., cervical
   l., closed
   l., Henle's
   l., Lippes
   l.'s of capillary

loosening of associations

L.O.P. *left occipitoposterior*

lophotrichea (lŏf-ō-trĭk′ē-ă) [Gr. *lophos*, tuft, + *thrix*, hair]

lophotrichous (lŏf-ŏt′rĭ-kŭs)
lordoma (lor-dō′mă) [Gr.]
lordoscoliosis (lor″dō-skō″lē-ō′sĭs)
[Gr. *lordosis*, bending, + *skoliosis*, crookedness]
lordosis (lor-dō′sĭs) [Gr.]
Lorfan
L.O.T. *left occipitotransverse*
lotio (lō′shē-ō) [L.]
   l. alba
lotion (lō′shŭn) [L. *lotio*]
   l., calamine
   l., white
Lotrimin
Lotusate
loudness
Louis-Bar syndrome (loo-wē′băr)
[Denise Louis-Bar, 20th century European physician]
loupe (loop) [Fr.]
louse [AS. *lus*]
   l., body
   l., crab
   l., head
lousiness
lovastatin
love [ME.]
Loven's reflex (lō-vănz′) [Otto K. Loven, Swed. physician, 1835–1904]
lower motor neuron lesion
Lowe's syndrome (lōz) [Charles U. Lowe, U.S. pediatrician, b. 1921]
Lowman balance board [Charles LeRoy Lowman, U.S. orthopedist, b. 1879]
low-protein diet
low-salt diet
lox *liquid oxygen*
loxapine succinate (lŏks′ă-pēn)
loxarthron (lŏks-ăr′thrŏn) [Gr. *loxos*, slanting, + *arthron*, joint]
loxia (lŏks′ē-ă) [Gr., slanting]
Loxosceles (lŏks-ŏs′sĕ-lēz)
loxoscelism (lŏk-sŏs′sĕ-lĭzm)
loxotic (lŏks-ŏt′ĭk) [Gr. *loxos*, slanting]
loxotomy (lŏks-ŏt′ō-mē) [″ + *tome*, a cutting, slice]
lozenge (lŏz′ĕnj) [Fr.]

L-phase variants
L.P.N. *licensed practical nurse*
Lr *lawrencium*
L.R.C.P. *licentiate of the Royal College of Physicians*
L.R.C.S. *licentiate of the Royal College of Surgeons*
LRF *luteinizing hormone releasing factor*
L.S.A. *left sacroanterior*
L.Sc.A. *left scapuloanterior*
L.Sc.P. *left scapuloposterior*
LSD *lysergic acid diethylamide*
L.S.P. *left sacroposterior*
L/S ratio *lecithin/sphingomyelin ratio*
L.S.T. *left sacrotransverse*
LTC *long-term care*
LTH *luteotropic hormone*
Lu *lutetium*
lubb-dupp (lŭb-dŭp′)
lubricant (loo′brĭ-kănt) [L. *lubricans*]
lubricating enema
Lucas-Championnière's disease (lū-kă′shaw″pē-ŏn-ē-ayrz′) [J. M. M. Lucas-Championnière, Fr. surgeon, 1843–1913]
lucid (lū′sĭd) [L. *lucidus*, clear]
lucid interval
lucidity (lū-sĭd′ĭ-tē)
luciferase (loo-sĭf′ĕr-ās)
luciferin (loo-sĭf′ĕr-ĭn)
lucifugal (loo-sĭf′ū-găl) [L. *lux*, light, + *fugere*, to flee from]
lucipetal (loo-sĭp′ĭ-tăl) [″ + *peter*, to seek]
lucotherapy (lū″kō-thĕr′ă-pē) [″ + Gr. *therapeia*, treatment]
Ludwig's angina (lūd′vĭgz) [Wilhelm F. von Ludwig, Ger. surgeon, 1790–1865]
L.U.E. *left upper extremity*
Luer-Lok syringe (lū′ĕr-lŏk′)
lues (lū′ēz) [L.]
luetic (lū-ĕt′ĭk)
Lugol's solution (lū′gŏlz) [Jean G. A. Lugol, Fr. physician, 1786–1851]
lumbago (lŭm-bā′gō) [L. *lumbus*, loin]
lumbar (lŭm′băr) [L. *lumbus*, loin]
lumbarization (lŭm″băr-ĭ-zā′shŭn)

lumbar nerves
lumbar plexus
lumbar puncture
lumbar reflex
lumbar region
lumbar vertebrae
lumbo- [L. *lumbus*, loin]
lumboabdominal (lŭm″bō-ăb-dŏm′ĭ-năl) [″ + *abdomen*, belly]
lumbocolostomy (lŭm″bō-kō-lŏs′tō-mē) [″ + Gr. *kolon*, colon, + *stoma*, mouth, opening]
lumbocolotomy (lŭm″bō-kō-lŏt′ō-mē) [″ + ″ + *tome*, a cutting, slice]
lumbocostal (lŭm″bō-kŏs′tăl) [″ + *costa*, rib]
lumbodynia (lŭm″bō-dĭn′ē-ă) [″ + Gr. *odyne*, pain]
lumboiliac (lŭm″bō-ĭl′ē-ăk) [″ + *iliacus*, pert. to ilium]
lumboinguinal (lŭm″bō-ĭng′gwĭ-năl) [″ + *inguinalis*, pert. to the groin]
lumbosacral
lumbosacral plexus
lumbrical (lŭm′brĭ-kăl) [L. *lumbricus*, earthworm]
lumbrical bar
lumbricalis
lumbricide (lŭm′brĭ-sīd) [″ + *caedere*, to kill]
lumbricoid (lŭm′brĭ-koyd) [″ + Gr. *eidos*, form, shape]
lumbricosis (lŭm″brĭ-kō′sĭs) [″ + Gr. *osis*, condition]
Lumbricus (lŭm-brĭ′kŭs)
lumbricus (lŭm-brĭ′kŭs)
lumbus [L.]
lumen (lū′mĕn) [L., light]
Luminal
luminal (lū′mĭ-năl)
Luminal Sodium
luminescence (loo″mĭ-nĕs′ĕns)
luminiferous (loo″mĭ-nĭf′ĕr-ŭs) [L. *lumen*, light, + *ferre*, to bear]
luminophore (loo′mĭ-nō-for″) [″ + Gr. *phoros*, bearing]
luminous (loo′mĭ-nŭs)
lumirhodopsin (loo″mĭ-rō-dŏp′sĭn)

lumpectomy (lŭm-pĕk′tō-mē) [*lump* + Gr. *ektome*, excision]
lunacy (lū′nă-sē) [L. *luna*, moon]
lunar
lunate
lunatic (lū′nă-tĭk) [L. *luna*, moon]
lunatomalacia (loo-nă″tō-mă-lā′shē-ă)
lung (lŭng) [AS. *lungen*]
    l., blast
    l.'s, compliance of
    l., edema of
    l., iron
lung abscess
lung cancer
lung collapse
    l.c., hypostatic
    l.c., passive
lung fluke
lung hemorrhage
lung inflammation
lungmotor
lung surfactant
lung transplantation
lungworm (lŭng′wĕrm)
lunula (lū′nū-lă) [L., little moon]
    l. of valves of heart
lupiform (lū′pĭ-form) [L. *lupus*, wolf, + *forma*, shape]
lupoid (loo′poyd) [″ + Gr. *eidos*, form, shape]
lupous (lū′pŭs)
lupus (lū′pŭs) [L., wolf]
    l. erythematosus, discoid
    l. erythematosus, systemic
    l. pernio
    l. vulgaris
LUQ *left upper quadrant*
Lust's reflex (lŭsts) [Franz Alexander Lust, Ger. pediatrician, b. 1880]
lusus naturae (loo′sŭs nă-chū′rē)
luteal [L. *luteus*, yellow]
luteal hormone
lutein (lū′tē-ĭn)
lutein cells
luteinic (loo″tē-ĭn′ĭk)
luteinization (lū″tē-ĭn-ĭ-zā′shŭn)
luteinizing hormone

luteinizing hormone releasing hormone

Lutembacher's syndrome (loo'tĕm-băk"ĕrz) [René Lutembacher, Fr. physician, 1884–1916]

luteohormone (loo"tē-ō-hor'mōn)

luteolysin (loo"tē-ō-lǐ'sǐn) [" + Gr. *lysis*, dissolution]

luteoma (lū"tē-ō'mǎ) [L. *luteus*, yellow, + Gr. *oma*, tumor]

luteotropin (loo"tē-ō-trō'pǐn)

lutetium (lū-tē'shē-ŭm)

luteum (lū'tē-ŭm) [L.]
   l., corpus

lutin (lū'tǐn)

Lutz-Splendore-Almeida disease [A. Lutz, Brazilian physician, 1855–1940; A. Splendore, contemp. It. physician; Floriano P. de Almeida, Brazilian physician, b. 1898]

lux (lŭks) [L., light]

luxation (lŭks-ā'shŭn) [L. *luxatio*, dislocation]

luxus (lŭks'ŭs) [L.]

Luys' body (lū-ēz') [Jules B. Luys, Fr. physician, 1828–1898]

LV *left ventricle*

L.V.N. *licensed vocational nurse*

lyase (lǐ'ās)

lycanthropy (lǐ-kǎn'thrō-pē) [Gr. *lykos*, wolf, + *anthropos*, man]

lycopene (lǐ'kō-pēn)

lycopenemia (lǐ"kō-pě-nē'mē-ǎ) [*lycopene* + Gr. *haima*, blood]

lycoperdonosis (lǐ"kō-pěr"dŏn-ō'sǐs) [Gr. *lykos*, wolf, + *perdesthai*, to break wind, + *osis*, condition]

lycopodium (lǐ-kō-pō'dē-ŭm)

lycorexia (lǐ-kō-rěk'sē-ǎ) [Gr. *lykos*, wolf + *orexis*, appetite]

lye (lǐ) [AS. *leag*]

lye poisoning

lying-in

Lyme disease, Lyme arthritis [Lyme, Connecticut, U.S.A., where the disease was originally described]

lymph (lǐmf) [L. *lympha*]
   l., animal

   l., inflammatory
   l., intercellular

lymphadenectasis (lǐm-fǎd"ě-něk'tǎ-sǐs) [L. *lympha*, lymph, + Gr. *aden*, gland, + *ektasis*, dilatation]

lymphadenectomy (lǐm-fǎd"ě-něk'tō-mē) [" + " + *ektome*, excision]

lymphadenia (lǐm"fǎ-dē'nē-ǎ)
   l. ossea

lymphadenitis (lǐm-fǎd"ěn-ī'tǐs) [" + " + *itis*, inflammation]
   l., tuberculous

lymphadenocele (lǐm-fǎd'ě-nō-sēl") [" + " + *kele*, tumor, swelling]

lymphadenogram (lǐm-fǎd'ě-nō-grǎm") [" + " + *gramma*, letter, piece of writing]

lymphadenography (lǐm-fǎd"ě-nŏg'rǎ-fē) [" + " + *graphein*, to write]

lymphadenoid (lǐm-fǎd'ě-noyd) [" + " + *eidos*, form, shape]

lymphadenopathy (lǐm-fǎd"ě-nŏp'ǎ-thē) [" + " + *pathos*, disease, suffering]
   l., dermatopathic

lymphadenosis benigna cutis (lǐm-fǎd"ě-nō'sǐs) [" + " + *osis*, condition]

lymphadenotomy (lǐm-fǎd"ě-nŏt'ō-mē) [" + " + *tome*, a cutting, slice]

lymphadenovarix (lǐm-fǎd"ě-nō-vā'rǐks) [" + " + L. *varix*, a twisted vein]

lymphagogue (lǐmf'ǎ-gŏg) [" + Gr. *agogos*, leading]

lymphangial (lǐm-fǎn'jē-ǎl) [" + Gr. *angeion*, vessel]

lymphangiectasis (lǐm-fǎn"jē-ěk'tǎ-sǐs) [" + " + *ektasis*, dilatation]

lymphangiectomy (lǐm-fǎn"jē-ěk'tō-mē) [" + " + *ektome*, excision]

lymphangiitis (lǐm-fǎn"jē-ī'tǐs) [" + " + *itis*, inflammation]

lymphangioendothelioma (lǐm-fǎn"jē-ō-ěn"dō-thē-lē-ō'mǎ) [" + " + *endon*, within, + *thele*, nipple,

+ *oma*, tumor]

lymphangiofibroma (lĭm-făn"jē-ō-fĭ-brō'mă) [" + Gr. *angeion*, vessel, + L. *fiber*, fiber, + Gr. *oma*, tumor]

lymphangiogram (lĭm-făn'jē-ō-grăm) [" + " + *gramma*, letter, piece of writing]

lymphangiography (lĭm-făn"jē-ŏg'ră-fē) [" + " + *graphein*, to write]

lymphangiology (lĭm-făn"jē-ŏl'ŏ-jē) [" + " + *logos*, word, reason]

lymphangioma (lĭm-făn"jē-ō'mă) [" + " + *oma*, tumor]
   l., cavernous
   l., cystic

lymphangiophlebitis (lĭm-făn"jē-ō-flĕ-bī'tĭs) [" + " + *phleps*, blood vessel, vein, + *itis*, inflammation]

lymphangioplasty (lĭm-făn'jē-ō-plăs"tē) [" + Gr. *angeion*, vessel, + *plassein*, to form]

lymphangiosarcoma (lĭm-făn"jē-ō-săr-kō'mă) [" + " + *sarx*, flesh, + *oma*, tumor]

lymphangiotomy (lĭm-făn"jē-ŏt'ō-mē) [" + " + *tome*, a cutting, slice]

lymphangitis (lĭm"făn-jī'tĭs) [" + Gr. *angeion*, vessel, + *itis*, inflammation]

lymphatic (lĭm-făt'ĭk) [L. *lymphaticus*]
   l., afferent
   l., efferent

lymphatic blockade
lymphatic capillary
lymphatic organ

lymphaticostomy (lĭm-făt"ĭ-kŏs'tō-mē) [L. *lymphaticus*, lymphatic, + Gr. *stoma*, mouth, opening]

lymphatic system
lymphatic vessels

lymphatism (lĭm'fă-tĭzm) [" + Gr. -*ismos*, condition]

lymphatitis (lĭm"fă-tī'tĭs) [" + Gr. *itis*, inflammation]

lymphatology (lĭm"fă-tŏl'ō-jē) [" +
Gr. *logos*, word, reason]

lymphatolysis (lĭm"fă-tŏl'ĭ-sĭs) [" + Gr. *lysis*, dissolution]

lymphatolytic (lĭm"fă-tō-lĭt'ĭk)

lymph cell

lymph channel

lymphectasia (lĭmf"ĕk-tā'zē-ă) [L. *lympha*, lymph, + Gr. *ektasis*, dilatation]

lymphedema (lĭmf-ĕ-dē'mă) [" + Gr. *oidema*, swelling]
   l., congenital

lymphemia (lĭm-fē'mē-ă) [" + Gr. *haima*, blood]

lymphendothelioma (lĭmf"ĕn-dō-thē-lē-ō'mă) [" + Gr. *endon*, within, + *thele*, nipple, + *oma*, tumor]

lymphenteritis (lĭmf"ĕn-tĕr-ī'tĭs) [" + Gr. *enteron*, intestine, + *itis*, inflammation]

lymph follicle

lymphization (lĭm"fī-zā'shŭn)

lymph node

lymphnoditis (lĭmf"nō-dī'tĭs) [" + *nodus*, knot, + Gr. *itis*, inflammation]

lymph nodule

lymphoblast (lĭm'fō-blăst) [" + Gr. *blastos*, germ]

lymphoblastic (lĭm"fō-blăs'tĭk) [" + Gr. *blastos*, germ]

lymphoblastoma (lĭm"fō-blăst-ō'mă) [" + " + *oma*, tumor]

lymphoblastomatosis (lĭm"fō-blăs"tō-mă-tō'sĭs) [" + " + *oma*, tumor, + *osis*, condition]

lymphoblastosis (lĭm"fō-blăs-tō'sĭs) [" + " + *osis*, condition]

lymphocele (lĭm'fō-sēl) [L. *lympha*, lymph, + Gr. *kele*, tumor, swelling]

lymphocyte (lĭm'fō-sīt) [L. *lympha*, lymph, + Gr. *kytos*, cell]
   l., B
   l., T

lymphocythemia (lĭm"fō-sī-thē'mē-ă) [" + Gr. *kytos*, cell, + *haima*, blood]

lymphocytoblast (lĭm"fō-sī'tō-blăst")

[" + " + *blastos*, germ]
lymphocytoma (lĭm"fō-sī-tō'mă)
[" + " + *oma*, tumor]
lymphocytopenia (lĭm"fō-sīt"ō-pē'nē-ă) [" + " + *penia*, lack]
lymphocytopoiesis (lĭm"fō-sīt"ō-poy-ē'sĭs) [" + " + *poiesis*, production]
lymphocytosis (lĭm"fō-sī-tō'sĭs) [" + " + *osis*, condition]
lymphocytotoxin (lĭm"fō-sīt"ō-tŏks'ĭn) [" + " + *toxikon*, poison]
lymphoduct (lĭm'fō-dŭkt) [" + *ducere*, to lead]
lymphoepithelioma (lĭm"fō-ĕp"ĭ-thē-lē-ō'mă) [" + Gr. *epi*, at, + *thele*, nipple, + *oma*, tumor]
lymphogenesis (lĭm"fō-jĕn'ĕ-sĭs) [" + Gr. *genesis*, generation, birth]
lymphogenous (lĭm-fŏj'ĕn-ŭs) [" + Gr. *gennan*, to produce]
lymphoglandula (lĭm"fō-glăn'dū-lă) [" + *glandula*, little gland]
lymphogonia (lĭm"fō-gō'nē-ă) [" + Gr. *gonos*, offspring, procreation]
lymphogram (lĭm'fō-grăm) [" + Gr. *gramma*, letter, piece of writing]
lymphogranuloma inguinale
lymphogranulomatosis (lĭm"fō-grăn-ū-lō"mă-tō'sĭs) [" + *granulum*, granule, + Gr. *oma*, tumor, + *osis*, condition]
lymphogranuloma venereum (lĭm"fō-grăn"ū-lō'mă) [" + " + Gr. *oma*, tumor]
lymphogranuloma venereum antigen
lymphography (lĭm-fŏg'ră-fē) [L. *lympha*, lymph, + Gr. *graphein*, to write]
lymphoid (lĭm'foyd) [" + Gr. *eidos*, form, shape]
lymphoid cells
lymphoidectomy (lĭm"foyd-ĕk'tō-mē) [" + " + *ektome*, excision]
lymphoidocyte (lĭm-foyd'ō-sīt) [" + " + *kytos*, cell]
lymphokines (lĭm'fō-kīnz)

lymphokinesis (lĭm"fō-kī-nē'sĭs) [" + Gr. *kinesis*, motion]
lymphology (lĭm-fŏl'ō-jē) [" + Gr. *logos*, word, reason]
lymphoma (lĭm-fō'mă) [" + Gr. *oma*, tumor]
　l., African
　l., Burkitt's
　l., clasmocytic
　l., giant follicular
　l. granulomatous
　l., lymphoblastic
　l., lymphocytic
　l., malignant, histiocytic
　l., malignant, mixed cell
　l., malignant, poorly differentiated diffuse lymphocytic
　l., malignant, undifferentiated
　l., malignant, well-differentiated diffuse lymphocytic
lymphomatoid (lĭm-fō'mă-toyd) [L. *lympha*, lymph, + Gr. *oma*, tumor, + *eidos*, form, shape]
lymphomatosis (lĭm"fō-mă-tō'sĭs) [" + " + *osis*, condition]
lymphomatous (lĭm-fō'mă-tŭs)
lymphomyxoma (lĭm"fō-mĭk-sō'mă) [" + Gr. *mys*, muscle, + *oma*, tumor]
lymphonodus (lĭm"fō-nō'dŭs) [" + *nodus*, knot]
lymphopathia venereum
lymphopathy (lĭm-fŏp'ă-thē) [" + Gr. *pathos*, disease, suffering]
lymphopenia (lĭm-fō-pē'nē-ă) [" + Gr. *penia*, lack]
lymphoplasty (lĭm'fō-plăs"tē) [" + Gr. *plassein*, to form]
lymphopoiesis (lĭm"fō-poy-ē'sĭs) [" + Gr. *poiesis*, production]
lymphopoietic (lĭm"fō-poy-ĕt'ĭk) [" + Gr. *poiein*, to produce]
lymphoproliferative (lĭm"fō-prō-lĭf'ĕr-ă-tĭv)
lymphoprotease
lymphoreticular (lĭm"fō-rĕ-tĭk'ū-lăr) [" + *reticula*, net]
lymphoreticular disorders

lymphoreticular system

lymphoreticulosis, benign, of inoculation (lĭm″fō-rē-tĭk″ū-lō′sĭs) [″ + ″ + Gr. osis, condition]

lymphorrhagia (lĭm″fō-rā′jē-ă) [″ + Gr. rhegnynai, to burst forth]

lymphorrhea (lĭm″fō-rē′ă) [″ + Gr. rhein, to flow]

lymphorrhoid (lĭm′fō-royd)

lymphosarcoma (lĭm″fō-săr-kō′mă) [″ + Gr. sarx, flesh, + oma, tumor]

lymphosarcomatosis (lĭm″fō-săr″kō-mă-tō′sĭs) [″ + ″ + ″ + osis, condition]

lymphostasis (lĭm″fŏs′tă-sĭs) [″ + Gr. stasis, standing still]

lymphotaxis (lĭm″fō-tăk′sĭs) [″ + Gr. taxis, arrangement]

lymphotome (lĭm′fō-tōm) [″ + Gr. tome, a cutting, slice]

lymphotomy (lĭm-fŏt′ō-mē) [″ + Gr. tome, a cutting, slice]

lymphotoxin (lĭm″fō-tŏk′sĭn) [″ + Gr. toxikon, poison]

lymphotrophy (lĭm-fŏt′rō-fē) [″ + Gr. trophe, nourishment]

lymph sinus

lymph spaces

lymphuria (lĭm-fū′rē-ă) [″ + Gr. ouron, urine]

lymph vascular (lĭmf-văs′kū-lăr) [″ + vasculus, a little vessel]

lynestrenol (lĭn-ĕs′trē-nŏl)

lyo- [Gr. lyein, to dissolve]

lyochrome (lī′ō-krōm) [″ + chroma, color]

lyoenzyme (lī″ō-ĕn′zīm) [″ + en, in, + zyme, leaven]

lyogel (lī′ō-jĕl)

Lyon hypothesis (lī′ŏn) [Mary Lyon, Brit. geneticist, b. 1925]

lyophil(e) (lī′ō-fĭl, -fīl) [″ + philos, love]

lyophilic (lī″ō-fĭl′ĭk)

lyophilization (lī-ŏf″ĭ-lĭ-zā′shŭn)

lyophobe, lyophobic (lī′ō-fōb, lī″ō-fō′bĭk) [Gr. lyein, to dissolve, + phobos, fear]

lyosorption (lī″ō-sorp′shŭn) [″ + sorbere, to suck in]

lyotrope (lī′ō-trōp) [″ + tropos, a turning]

lyotropic (lī″ō-trŏp′ĭk) [″ + tropikos, turning]

lypressin (lī-prĕs′ĭn)

lyra (lī′ră) [L., Gr., lyre]

lysate (lī′sāt)

lyse (līz) [Gr. lysis, dissolution]

lysemia (lī-sē′mē-ă) [″ + haima, blood]

lysergic acid diethylamide

lysimeter (lī-sĭm′ĕ-tĕr) [Gr. lysis, dissolution, + metron, measure]

lysin (lī′sĭn)

lysine (lī′sēn)
  l. acetate
  l. hydrochloride

lysinogen (lī-sĭn′ō-jĕn) [Gr. lysis, dissolution, + gennan, to produce]

lysis (lī′sĭs) [Gr., dissolution]

lysocephalin (lī″sō-sĕf′ă-lĭn)

Lysodren

lysogen (lī′sō-jĕn) [″ + gennan, to produce]

lysogenesis (lī″sō-jĕn′ĕ-sĭs) [″ + genesis, generation, birth]

lysogenic (lī-sō-jĕn′ĭk) [″ + Gr. gennan, to produce]

lysogeny (lī-sŏj′ĕ-nē)

Lysol (lī′sŏl)

Lysol poisoning

lysolecithin (lī″sō-lĕs′ĭ-thĭn)

lysosomal storage diseases

lysosome (lī′sō-sōm)

lysozyme (lī′sō-zīm) [Gr. lysis, dissolution, + zyme, leaven]

lyssa (lĭs′să) [Gr., frenzy]

Lyssavirus

lyssoid (lĭs′oyd) [Gr. lyssa, frenzy, + eidos, form, shape]

lyssophobia (lĭs-ō-fō′bē-ă) [″ + phobos, fear]

lyterian (lī-tēr′ē-ăn) [Gr. lyein, to dissolve]

lytic (lĭt′ĭk)

lyze (līz) [Gr. lysis, dissolution]

M

μ [*mu*, the twelfth letter of the Greek alphabet]; *micro-*

M *master* or *medicine* in professional titles; *mille*, a thousand; *misce*, mix; *molar*

m *meter*, *minim*, *meta-*, *mol*, *mole*

MA mental age

M.A. Master of Arts

ma. milliampere

Maalox

MAC *maximum allowable concentration*

Mace

mace (mās) [L. *macis*]

macerate (măs′ĕr-āt)

maceration (măs-ĕr-ā′shŭn) [L. *macerare*, to make soft]

Mache unit (mä′kĕ) [Heinrich Mache, Austrian physicist, 1876–1954]

machine

Machover test [Karen Alper Machover, U.S. psychologist, b. 1902]

macies (mā′shē-ēz) [L., wasting]

macrencephalia, **macrencephaly** (măk-rĕn″sĕ-fā′lē-ă, -sĕf′ă-lē) [Gr. *makros*, large, + *enkephalos*, brain]

macro-, macr- [Gr. *makros*, large]

macroamylase (măk″rō-ăm′ĭ-lās)

macroamylasemia (măk″rō-ăm″ĭl-ă-sē′mē-ă)

macrobiosis (măk″rō-bī-ō′sĭs) [Gr. *makros*, large, + *biosis*, life]

macrobiota (măk″rō-bī-ō′tă)

macroblepharia (măk″rō-blĕ-fā′rē-ă) [Gr. *makros*, large, + *blepharon*, eyelid]

macrobrachia (măk″rō-brā′kē-ă) [″ + *brachion*, arm]

macrocardius (măk″rō-kăr′dē-ŭs) [″ + *kardia*, heart]

macrocephalia (măk″rō-sĕ-fā′lē-ă)

[″ + *kephale*, head]

macrocephalic

macrocephalous (măk″rō-sĕf′ă-lŭs)

macrocephaly (măk-rō-sĕf′ă-lē)

macrocheilia (măk″rō-kī′lē-ă) [″ + *cheilos*, lip]

macrocheiria (măk-rō-kī′rē-ă) [″ + *cheir*, hand]

macrochemistry

macrocnemia (măk″rōk-nē′mē-ă) [″ + *kneme*, shin]

macrocolon (măk″rō-kō′lŏn) [″ + *kolon*, colon]

macroconidium (măk″rō-kō-nĭd′ē-ŭm)

macrocornea (măk-rō-kor′nē-ă) [″ + L. *cornu*, horn]

macrocyst (măk′rō-sĭst) [″ + *kystis*, bladder]

macrocyte [″ + *kytos*, cell]

macrocythemia, **macrocytosis** (măk″rō-sī-thē′mē-ă, măk″rō-sī-tō′sĭs) [″ + ″ + *haima*, blood]

macrodactylia (măk″rō-dăk-tĭl′ē-ă) [″ + *daktylos*, finger]

Macrodantin

Macrodex

macrodontia (măk″rō-dŏn′shē-ă) [″ + *odous*, tooth]

macroesthesia (măk″rō-ĕs-thē′zē-ă) [Gr. *makros*, large, + *aisthesis*, feeling, perception]

macrofauna (măk″rō-faw′nă)

macroflora (măk″rō-flō′ră)

macrogamete (măk″rō-găm′ĕt) [″ + *gamete*, wife]

macrogametocyte (măk″rō-gă-mē′tō-sīt)

macrogenitosomia praecox (măk″rō-jĕn″ĭ-tō-sō′mē-ă prē′kŏks) [″ + L. *genitalis*, to beget, + Gr. *soma*, body, + L. *praecox*, early]

macrogingivae   (măk″rō-jĭn-jĭ′vē)
[″ + L. *gingiva*, gum]

macroglia   (măk-rŏg′lē-ă) [″ +
glia, glue]

macroglobulin (măk″rō-glŏb′ū-lĭn)

macroglobulinemia   (măk-rō-glŏb″ū-
lĭn-ē′mē-ă)
m., Waldenström's

macroglossia [Gr. *makros*, large, +
glossa, tongue]

macrognathia   (măk-rō-nā′thē-ă)
[″ + *gnathos*, jaw]

macrography (măk-rŏg′ră-fē) [″ +
graphein, to write]

macrogyria [″ + *gyros*, circle]

macrolabia (măk-rō-lā′bē-ă) [″ +
L. *labium*, lip]

macroleukoblast (măk″rō-lū′kō-blăst)
[″ + *leukos*, white, + *blastos*,
germ]

macrolymphocyte (măk″rō-lĭmf′ō-sīt)
[″ + L. *lympha*, lymph, + Gr.
kytos, cell]

macromania (măk″rō-mā′nē-ă) [″ +
mania, madness]

macromastia   (măk-rō-măs′tē-ă)
[″ + *mastos*, breast]

macromelia [″ + *melos*, limb]

macromelus (măk-rŏm′ē-lŭs) [″ +
melos, limb]

macromere   (măk′rō-mēr) [″ +
meros, a part]

macromethod (măk′rō-mĕth″ŏd)

macromolecule (măk″rō-mŏl′ĕ-kūl)

macromonocyte (măk″rō-mŏn′ō-sīt)

macromyeloblast   (măk″rō-mī′ĕ-lō-
blăst) [″ + *myelos*, marrow, +
blastos, germ]

macronormoblast   (măk″rō-nor′mō-
blăst) [″ + L. *norma*, rule, +
Gr. *blastos*, germ]

macronucleus (măk″rō-nū′klē-ŭs)

macronychia (măk″rō-nĭk′ē-ă) [″ +
onyx, nail]

macropathology   (măk″rō-pă-
thŏl′ō-jē)

macrophage,   macrophagus
(măk′rō-făj, măk-rŏf′ă-gŭs) [″ +

phagein, to eat]
m., fixed
m., free

macrophage activating factor

**macrophage migration inhibiting
factor**

macrophagocyte (măk″rō-făg′ō-sīt)

macrophallus (măk″rō-făl′ŭs) [Gr.
makros, large, + *phallos*, penis]

macrophthalmia (măk″rŏf-thăl′mē-ă)
[″ + *ophthalmos*, eye]

macroplasia (măk″rō-plā′zē-ă) [″ +
plasis, forming]

macropodia (măk-rō-pō′dē-ă) [″ +
pous, foot]

macropolycyte   (măk″rō-pŏl′ē-sīt)
[″ + *polys*, many, + *kytos*,
cell]

macropromyelocyte   (măk″rō-prō-
mī′ĕ-lō-sīt)

macroprosopia (măk″rō-prō-sō′pē-ă)
[″ + *prosopon*, face]

macropsia (măk-rŏp′sē-ă) [″ +
opsis, sight, appearance, vision]

macrorhinia (măk-rō-rĭn′ē-ă) [″ +
rhis, nose]

macroscelia (măk-rō-sē′lē-ă) [″ +
skelos, leg]

macroscopic (măk-rō-skŏp′ĭk) [″ +
skopein, to examine]

macroscopy (măk-rŏs′kō-pē)

macrosigmoid (măk″rō-sĭg′moyd)

macrosis (mă-krō′sĭs) [″ + *osis*,
condition]

macrosmatic (măk″rŏs-măt′ĭk) [″ +
osmasthai, to smell]

macrosomatia,   macrosomia
(măk″rō-sō-mā′shē-ă, măk-rō-sō′mē-ă)
[Gr. *makros*, large, + *soma*, body]

macrospore (măk′rō-spor)

macrostereognosis   (măk″rō-stē″rē-
ō-nō′sĭs) [″ + *stereos*, solid, +
gnosis, knowledge]

macrostomia   (măk-rō-stō′mē-ă)
[″ + *stoma*, mouth, opening]

macrostructure (măk′rō-strŭk″tūr)

macrotia (măk-rō′shē-ă) [″ + *ous*,
ear]

macrotome   (măk′rō-tōm) [″ +

tome, a cutting, slice]
macrotooth
macula (măk'ū-lă) [L., spot]
   maculae acusticae
   m. albidae
   m. atrophicae
   m. caeruleae
   m., cerebral
   m. corneae
   m. cribrosa
   m. densa
   m. flava laryngis
   m. folliculi
   m. germinativa
   m. gonorrhoeica
   m. lutea retinae
   m. sacculi
   m. utriculi
macular (măk'ū-lăr) [L. *macula,* spot]
maculate(d) (măk'ū-lāt, -lāt-ĕd)
maculation (măk-ū-lā'shŭn) [L. *macula,* spot]
macule (măk'ūl) [L. *macula,* spot]
maculocerebral (măk″ū-lō-sĕr'ē-brăl) [″ + *cerebrum,* brain]
maculopapular (măk″ū-lō-păp'ū-lăr)
maculopathy (măk″ū-lŏp'ă-thē) [″ + Gr. *pathos,* disease, suffering]
mad
madarosis (măd-ă-rō'sĭs) [Gr. *madaros,* bald]
madder (măd'ĕr)
Madelung's deformity [Otto W. Madelung, Strasbourg surgeon, 1846–1926]
Madelung's disease
madescent (măd-ĕs'ĕnt) [L. *madescere,* to become moist]
madidans (măd'ĭ-dăns) [L. *madidus,* wet]
Madura foot
maduromycosis (măd-ū″rō-mī-kō'sĭs)
mafenide acetate (măf'ĕn-īd)
magaldrate (măg'ăl-drāt)
Magendie's foramen (mă-jĕn'dēz) [François Magendie, Fr. physiologist, 1783–1855]
magenblase syndrome [Ger. *Magen,* stomach, + *Blase,* bubble]

magenstrasse (măg″ĕn-străs'ē) [″ + *strasse,* street]
magenta (mă-jĕn'tă)
maggot
maggot treatment
magic thinking
magistery (măj'ĭs-tĕr″ē) [L. *magister,* master]
magistral (măj'ĭs-trăl)
magma (măg'mă) [Gr.]
magnesia (măg-nē'zē-ă) [magnetic stone found in Magnesia, region of ancient Thessaly]
   m., milk of
magnesia and alumina (tablets)
magnesium [L.]
   m. carbonate
   m. chloride
   m. citrate oral solution
   m. gluconate
   m. hydroxide
   m. oxide
   m. phosphate
   m. salicylate
   m. stearate
   m. sulfate
   m. trisilicate
magnet [Gr. *magnes,* magnet]
   m., horseshoe
magnetic
magnetic field
magnetic lines of force
magnetic resonance imaging
magnetism (măg'nĕ-tĭzm) [Gr. *magnes,* magnet, + *-ismos,* condition]
magnetoelectricity (măg-nē″tō-ē″lĕk-trĭs'ĭ-tē) [″ + *elektron,* amber]
magnetometer (măg″nĕ-tŏm'ĕ-tĕr) [″ + *metron,* measure]
magneton (măg'nĕ-tŏn)
magnetotherapy (măg-nē″tō-thĕr'ă-pē) [″ + *therapeia,* treatment]
magnetropism (măg-nĕt'rō-pĭzm) [″ + *trope,* a turn]
magnification (măg-nĭ-fĭ-kā'shŭn) [L. *magnus,* great, + *facere,* to make]
magnum [L.]
Mahaim fibers [I. Mahaim, contempo-

rary Fr. physician]
maidenhead
maim (măm) [ME. *maymen*, to cripple]
main (măn) [Fr.]
   m. en griffe
mainstreaming
maintainer
   m., space
Majocchi's disease (mă-yŏk′ēz) [Domenico Majocchi, It. physician, 1849–1929]
Majocchi's granuloma
major histocompatibility gene complex
mal (măl) [Fr., from L. *malum*, an evil]
   m. de Cayenne
   m. de mer
   m. perforant
   m. perforant palatin
mala (mā′lă) [L., cheek]
malabsorption syndrome
malacia (mă-lā′shē-ă) [Gr. *malakia*, softening]
malacoma (măl-ă-kō′mă)
malacoplakia (măl″ă-kō-plā′kē-ă) [Gr. *malakos*, soft, + *plax*, plaque]
   m. vesicae
malacosarcosis (măl″ă-kō-săr-kō′sĭs) [″ + *sarx*, flesh, + *osis*, condition]
malacosis (măl-ă-kō′sĭs) [″ + *osis*, condition]
malacosteon (măl-ă-kŏs′tē-ŏn) [″ + *osteon*, bone]
malacotic (măl-ă-kŏt′ĭk)
malacotomy (măl-ă-kŏt′ō-mē) [Gr. *malakos*, soft, + *tome*, a cutting, slice]
malactic (mă-lăk′tĭk) [Gr. *malakos*, soft]
maladie de Roger (măl″ă-dē′) [Henry L. Roger, Fr. physician, 1809–1891]
maladjusted
malady (măl′ă-dē) [Fr. *maladie*, illness, from L. *malum*, an evil]
malaise (mă-lāz′) [Fr.]
malalignment (măl″ă-līn′mĕnt)
malar (mā′lăr) [L. *mala*, cheek]
malar bone

malaria (mă-lā′rē-ă) [It. *malaria*, bad air]
   m., cephalgic
   m., cerebral
   m., estivoautumnal
   m., falciparum
   m., latent
   m., quartan
   m., quotidian
   m., tertian
   m., vivax
malariacidal (mă-lā″rē-ă-sī′dăl) [It. *malaria*, bad air, + L. *cida* fr. *caedere*, to kill]
malarial (mă-lăr′ē-ăl) [It. *malaria*, bad air]
malariology (mă-lăr-ē-ŏl′ō-jē)
malariotherapy (mă-lăr-ē-ō-thĕr′ă-pē)
malarious (mă-lăr′ē-ŭs)
Malassezia (măl″ă-sē′zē-ă) [Louis C. Malassez, Fr. physiologist, 1842–1910]
malassimilation (măl″ă-sĭm-ĭ-lā′shŭn) [L. *malus*, ill, + *assimilatio*, making like]
malate (mā′lāt)
malathion (măl″ă-thī′ŏn)
malaxate (măl′ăk-sāt) [L. *malaxare*, to soften]
malaxation (măl-ăks-ā′shŭn)
maldigestion (măl″dĭ-jĕs′chŭn)
male [O. Fr.]
malemission (măl″ē-mĭsh′ŭn) [L. *malus*, evil, + *e*, out, + *mittere*, to send]
maleruption (măl-ē-rŭp′shŭn)
malformation (măl-for-mā′shŭn) [″ + *formatio*, a shaping]
   m., tooth
malfunction (măl-fŭnk′shŭn)
malic (mā′lĭk, măl′ĭk) [L. *malum*, apple]
malic acid
malice (măl′ĭs) [L. *malus*, bad]
malign (mă-līn′) [ME. *maligne*]
malignancy (mă-lĭg′năn-sē) [L. *malignus*, of bad kind]
malignant (mă-lĭg′nănt)

malinger (mă-lǐng′ĕr) [Fr. *malingre*, weak, sickly]

malingerer (mă-lǐng′gĕr-ĕr)

malinterdigitation (măl″ĭn-tĕr-dĭj″ĭ-tā′shŭn)

malleable (măl′ē-ă-b′l) [L. *mallere*, to hammer]

malleation (măl-lē-ā′shŭn)

malleoincudal (măl″ē-ō-ĭng′kū-dăl) [L. *malleus*, hammer, + *incus*, anvil]

malleolar (măl-ē′ō-lăr) [L. *malleolus*, little hammer]

malleolus (măl-ē′ō-lŭs) [L.]
  m., external
  m., internal

malleotomy (măl″ē-ŏt′ō-mē) [″ + Gr. *tome*, a cutting, slice]

mallet

mallet finger

mallet toe

malleus (măl′ē-ŭs) [L., hammer]

Mallophaga (măl-ŏf′ă-gă) [Gr. *mallos*, wool, + *phagein*, to eat]

Mallory-Weiss syndrome [G. Kenneth Mallory, U.S. pathologist, b. 1900; Soma Weiss, U.S. internist, 1898–1942]

malnutrition (măl″nū-trĭ′shŭn)
  m., protein-energy

malocclusion
  m., classification of

malonylurea (măl″ō-nĭl-ū′rē-ă)

malpighian body (măl-pĭg′ē-ăn) [Marcello Malpighi, It. anatomist, founder of histology, 1628–1694]

malpighian capsule

malpighian layer

malpighian pyramid

malposition (măl-pō-zĭ′shŭn) [L. *malus*, evil, + *positio*, placement]

malpractice [″ + Gr. *praxis*, an action]

malpresentation [″ + *praesentatio*, a presenting]

malrotation (măl″rō-tā′shŭn)

malt [AS. *mealt*]

Malta fever

maltase (mawl′tās) [AS. *mealt*, grain]

malt extract

maltose (mawl′tōs)

maltosuria (mawl″tō-sūr′ē-ă) [″ + Gr. *ouron*, urine]

malt sugar

malturned

malum (mā′lŭm) [L., an evil]
  m. articulorum senilis
  m. coxae senilis
  m. perforans pedis
  m. venereum

malunion [L. *malus*, evil, + *unio*, oneness]

mamanpian (mă-măn″pē-ăn′) [Fr. *maman*, mother, + *pian*, yaw]

mamelon (măm′ĕ-lŏn) [Fr., nipple]

mamill-

mamma (măm′ă) [L., breast]

mammal (măm′ăl)

mammalgia (măm-ăl′jē-ă) [L. *mamma*, breast, + Gr. *algos*, pain]

mammaplasty (măm′ă-plăs″tē) [″ + Gr. *plassein*, to form]

mammary (măm′ă-rē) [L. *mamma*, breast]

mammary glands

mammectomy (măm-měk′tō-mē) [″ + Gr. *ektome*, excision]

mammilla (mă-mĭl′lă) [L., nipple]

mammillary (măm′ĭl-lār-ē) [L. *mammilla*, nipple]

mammillated (măm′mĭl-lā-těd)

mammillation (măm-ĭl-lā′shŭn)

mammilliform (măm-mĭl′ĭ-form) [″ + *forma*, shape]

mammilliplasty (măm-mĭl′ĭ-plăs″tē) [″ + Gr. *plassein*, to form]

mammillitis (măm″mĭl-ī′tĭs) [″ + Gr. *itis*, inflammation]

mammitis (măm-ī′tĭs) [L. *mamma*, breast, + Gr. *itis*, inflammation]

mammogen (măm′ō-jĕn) [″ + Gr. *gennan*, to produce]

mammogram (măm′ō-grăm) [″ + Gr. *gramma*, letter, piece of writing]

mammography (măm-ŏg′ră-fē) [″ + Gr. *graphein*, to write]

mammoplasty (măm′ō-plăs″tē) [″ +

Gr. *plassein*, to form]
  m., augmentation
  m., reduction
mammose (măm′ōs) [L. *mammosus*]
mammotomy (măm-ŏt′ō-mē) [L. *mamma*, breast, + Gr. *tome*, a cutting, slice]
mammotrophic (măm″ō-trŏf′ĭk) [″ + Gr. *trophe*, nourishment]
man [AS. *mann*]
manchette (măn-chĕt′) [Fr., a cuff]
manchineel (măn″kĭ-nēl′) [Sp. *manzanilla*, small apple]
mancinism (măn′sĭn-ĭzm) [L. *mancus*, crippled]
Mandelamine
mandelic acid
mandible (măn′dĭ-bl) [L. *mandibula*, lower jawbone]
mandibula (măn-dĭb′ū-lă) [L.]
mandibular (măn-dĭb′ū-lăr)
mandibular reflex
mandibulopharyngeal (măn-dĭb″ū-lō-fă-rin′jē-ăl) [″ + Gr. *pharynx*, throat]
mandrel, mandril (măn′drĕl)
mandrin (măn′drĭn) [Fr.]
maneuver [Fr. *manoeuvre*, from L. *manu operari*, to work by hand]
  m., Crede's
  m., Heimlich
  m., Leopold's
  m., Mauriceau-Smellie-Veit
  m., Müller's
  m., Munro Kerr
  m., Pinard's
  m., Prague
  m., Scanzoni
  m., Valsalva's
manganese (măn′gă-nēz) [L. *manganesium*]
manganese poisoning
mange (mānj)
mania (mā′nē-ă) [Gr., madness]
  m., puerperal
  m., religious
  m., transitory
  m., unproductive

maniac (mā′nē-ăk)
maniacal (mă-nī′ă-kl)
manic (măn′ĭk)
manic-depressive psychosis
manifest
manifestation
manifest squint
manikin [D. *manneken*, little man]
maniphalanx (măn″ĭ-fā′lănks) [L. *manus*, hand, + Gr. *phalanx*, line of battle]
manipulation [L. *manipulare*, to handle]
manipulative surgery
manna (măn′ă) [L.]
mannans (măn′ănz)
mannerism
mannitol (măn′ĭ-tŏl)
Mannkopf's sign [Emil W. Mannkopf, Ger. physician, 1836–1918]
mannose (măn′ōs)
mannoside (măn′ō-sīd)
mannosidosis (măn″ōs-ĭ-dō′sĭs)
manometer (măn-ŏm′ĕt-ĕr) [Gr. *manos*, thin, + *metron*, measure]
  m., saline
Mansonella (măn″sō-nĕl′ă)
  M. ozzardi
mansonelliasis (măn″sō-nĕl-ī′ă-sĭs) [*Mansonella* + Gr. *-iasis*, state or condition of]
Mansonia (măn-sō′nē-ă)
mantle [AS. *mentel*, a garment]
  m., dentin
Mantoux reaction (măn-tū′) [Charles Mantoux, Fr. physician, 1877–1947]
manual (măn′ū-ăl) [L. *manus*, hand]
manual muscle test
manubrium (mă-nū′brē-ŭm) [L., handle]
  m. sterni
manudynamometer (măn″ū-dī″nă-mŏm′ĕ-tĕr) [L. *manus*, hand, + Gr. *dynamis*, force, + *metron*, measure]
manus (mā′nŭs) [L., hand]
MAO *monoamine oxidase*
map
  m., genetic

m., linkage
maple bark disease
maple syrup urine disease
mapping
marantic (mă-răn'tĭk) [Gr. *marantikos*, wasting away]
marantology (mă"răn-tŏl'ō-jē) [Gr. *marasmos*, a dying away, + *logos*, word, reason]
marasmic (mă-răz'mĭk) [Gr. *marasmos*, a dying away]
marasmoid (mă-răz'moyd) [" + *eidos*, form, shape]
marasmus (măr-ăz'mŭs)
marble bones
Marburg virus disease [Marburg, Germany]
marc (mărk) [Fr.]
Marchiafava-Micheli syndrome (măr"kēă-fă'vă-mē-kā'lē) [Ettore Marchiafava, It. pathologist, 1847–1935; F. Micheli, It. clinician, 1872–1937]
marcid (măr'sĭd) [L. *marcere*, to waste away]
Marcus Gunn pupil [Robert Marcus Gunn, Brit. ophthalmologist, 1850–1909]
Marezine Hydrochloride
Marfan's syndrome [Bernard-Jean Antonin Marfan, Fr. physician, 1858–1942]
margarine
margin [L. *marginalis*, border]
marginal (măr'jĭn-ăl)
margination (măr"jĭ-nā'shŭn)
marginoplasty (mar-jĭn'ō-plăs"tē) [L. *marginalis*, border, + Gr. *plassein*, to mold]
margo (măr'gō) [L.]
   m. acutus
   m. obtusus
Marie's ataxia (mă-rēz') [Pierre Marie, Fr. physician, 1853–1940]
Marie's disease
Marie's sign
marijuana, marihuana (măr"ĭ-wă'nă)
Marinol
mark [AS. *mearc*]

m., birth-
m., port-wine
m., strawberry
marker
   m., fecal
Marplan
marrow [AS. *mearh*]
   m., gelatinous
   m., red
   m., spinal
   m., yellow
marrow aspiration
marrow transplantation
marsh fever
marsh gas
Marsh's test [James Marsh, Brit. chemist, 1789–1846]
marsupialization (măr-sū"pē-ăl-ĭ-zā'shŭn) [L. *marsupium*, pouch]
marsupium (măr-sū'pē-ŭm) [L., pouch]
maschaladenitis (măs"kăl-ăd"ĕ-nī'tĭs) [Gr. *maschale*, armpit, + *aden*, gland, + *itis*, inflammation]
maschaliatry (măs-kăl-ī-ă'trē) [" + *iatreia*, healing]
maschaloncus (măs"kăl-ŏng'kŭs) [" + *onkos*, bulk, mass]
masculation (măs-kū-lā'shŭn) [L. *masculus*, a male]
masculine (măs'kū-lĭn)
masculinization
masculinovoblastoma (măs"kū-lĭn-ō"vō-blăs-tō'mă)
maser microwave amplification by stimulation emission of radiation
mask [Fr. *masque*]
   m., BLB
   m., death
   m., ecchymotic
   m., Hutchinson's
   m., luetic
   m. of pregnancy
   m., Parkinson's
masked
masochism (măs'ō-kĭzm) [Leopold von Sacher-Masoch, Austrian novelist, 1835–1895]
   m., sexual

masochist (măs'ō-kĭst)
mass [L. *massa*]
  m., cell
  m., epithelial
  m., inner cell
  m., intermediate cell
massa [L., mass]
  m. intermedia
massage [Gr. *massein*, to knead]
  m., auditory
  m., cardiac
  m., electrovibratory
  m., general
  m., introductory
  m., local
  m., tremolo
  m., vapor
  m., vibratory
masseter (măs-sē'tĕr) [Gr. *maseter*, chewer]
masseur (mă-soor') [Fr.]
masseuse (mă-sooz') [Fr.]
massive (măs'sĭv) [Fr. *massif*]
massive collapse of the lung
mass number
massotherapy (măs-ō-thĕr'ă-pē) [Gr. *massein*, to knead, + *therapeia*, treatment]
mass psychogenic illness
MAST *military antishock trousers*
mastadenitis (măst-ăd-ĕ-nī'tĭs) [Gr. *mastos*, breast, + *aden*, gland, + *itis*, inflammation]
mastadenoma (măst"ă-dĕ-nō'mă) [" + " + *oma*, tumor]
mastalgia (măst-ăl'jē-ă) [" + *algos*, pain]
mastatrophia, mastatrophy (măst-ă-trō'fē-ă, măst-ăt'rō-fē) [" + *atrophia*, want of nourishment]
mastauxe (măs-tawk'sē) [" + *auxe*, increase]
mast cells [Gr. *masten*, to feed]
mastectomy (măs-tĕk'tō-mē) [Gr. *mastos*, breast, + *ektome*, excision]
Master two-step test [A. M. Master, U.S. physician, 1895–1973]

masthelcosis (măs"thĕl-kō'sĭs) [Gr. *mastos*, breast, + *helkosis*, ulceration]
mastic (măs'tĭk)
mastication (măs-tĭ-kā'shŭn) [L. *masticare*, to chew]
masticatory (măs'tĭk-ă-tō"rē) [L. *masticare*, to chew]
Mastigophora (măs"tĭ-gŏf'ō-ră)
mastigote (măs'tĭ-gōt)
mastitis (măs-tī'tĭs) [Gr. *mastos*, breast, + *itis*, inflammation]
  m., cystic
  m., interstitial
  m., parenchymatous
  m., puerperal
  m., stagnation
mastocarcinoma (măst"ō-kăr-sĭn-ō'mă) [" + *karkinos*, crab, + *oma*, tumor]
mastochondroma (măst"ō-kŏn-drō'mă) [" + *chondros*, cartilage, + *oma*, tumor]
mastocyte (măs'tō-sīt) [Gr. *masten*, to feed, + *kytos*, cell]
mastocytoma (măs"tō-sī-tō'mă) [" + " + *oma*, tumor]
mastocytosis (măs"tō-sī-tō'sĭs) [" + " + *osis*, condition]
mastodynia (măst-ō-dĭn'ē-ă) [Gr. *mastos*, breast, + *odyne*, pain]
mastography [" + *graphein*, to write]
mastoid (măs'toyd) [" + *eidos*, form, shape]
mastoidal (măs-toy'dăl)
mastoidale (măs-toy-dā'lē)
mastoidalgia (măs-toyd-ăl'jē-ă) [Gr. *mastos*, breast, + *eidos*, form, shape, + *algos*, pain]
mastoid antrum
mastoid cells
mastoidectomy [" + " + *ektome*, excision]
mastoideocentesis (măs-toyd"ē-ō-sĕn-tē'sĭs) [" + " + *kentesis*, puncture]
mastoiditis (măs-toyd-ī'tĭs) [" + "

+ *itis,* inflammation]
m., Bezold's
m. externa
m., sclerosing
mastoidotomy (măs-toyd-ŏt'ō-mē)
[" + " + *tome,* a cutting, slice]
mastoid portion of temporal bone
mastoid process
mastology (măs-tŏl'ō-jē) [" +
logos, word, reason]
mastomenia (măs-tō-mē'nē-ă) [" +
menes, menses]
mastoncus (măst-ŏng'kŭs) [" +
onkos, bulk, mass]
masto-occipital (măs"tō-ŏk-sĭp'ĭ-tăl)
mastoparietal (măs"tō-pă-rī'ĕ-tăl)
mastopathy (măs-tŏp'ă-thē) [Gr.
mastos, breast, + *pathos,* disease,
suffering]
mastopexy (măs'tō-pĕks-ē) [" +
pexis, fixation]
mastoplasia (măst-ō-plā'zē-ă) [" +
plassein, to form]
mastoplasty (măs'tō-plăs"tē) [" +
plassein, to form]
mastoptosis (măs"tō-tō'sĭs) [" +
ptosis, fall, falling]
mastorrhagia (măs-tor-ā'jē-ă) [" +
rhegnynai, to burst forth]
mastoscirrhus (măs-tō-skĭr'ŭs) [" +
skirros, hardness]
mastosquamous (măs-tō-skwā'mŭs)
mastostomy (măs-tŏs'tō-mē) [" +
stoma, mouth, opening]
mastotomy (măs-tŏt'ō-mē)
masturbate (măs'tĕr-bāt) [L. *mastur-
bari,* fr. *manus,* hand, + *stuprare,*
to defile]
masturbation (măs"tĕr-bā'shŭn)
match [ME. *macche,* lamp wick]
matching
m., cross
m. of blood
match poisoning
maté (mă-tā') [Sp., vessel for preparing
leaves]
mater (mā'tŭr) [L., mother]
m., dura

m., pia
materia alba (mă-tē'rē-ă ăl'bă) [L.,
white matter]
material
m., base
m., impression
materia medica (mă-tē'rē-ă mĕd'ĭ-kă)
[L., medical matter]
maternal [L. *maternus*]
maternal deprivation syndrome
maternity (mă-tĕr'nĭ-tē)
mating [ME. *mate,* companion]
m., assortative
m., random
matrilineal (mă"trī-lĭn'ē-ăl) [L. *mater,*
mother, + *linea,* line]
matrix (mā'trĭks) [L.]
m. unguis
matrixitis (mā-trĭks-ī'tĭs)
matter
m., gray
m., white
Matulane
maturate (măt'ū-rāt) [L. *maturus,* ripe]
maturation (măt"ū-rā'shŭn)
m., enamel
mature (mă-tūr')
maturity
matutinal (mă-tū'tĭ-năl) [L. *matutinalis,*
morning]
matzoon (măt-zūn') [Armenian]
Maurer's dots (mow'ĕrz) [Georg
Maurer, Ger. physician in Sumatra, b.
1909]
Maxidex
maxilla [L., jawbone]
maxillary (măk'sĭ-lĕr"ē)
maxillary sinus
maxillitis (măks"ĭl-ī'tĭs) [L. *maxilla,* jawbone, + Gr. *itis,* inflammation]
maxillodental (măk-sĭl"ō-dĕn'tăl)
[" + *dens,* tooth]
maxillofacial (măks-ĭl"ō-fā'shăl)
maxillojugal (măk-sĭl"ō-jū'găl)
maxillomandibular (măk-sĭl"ō-măn-
dĭb'ū-lăr) [" + *mandibula,* lower
jawbone]
maxillopalatine (măk-sĭl"ō-păl'ă-tīn)

maxillotomy (măk″sĭ-lŏt′ō-mē) [″ + Gr. *tome*, a cutting, slice]
maxima (măk′sĭ-mă) [L.]
maximal (măks′ĭ-măl) [L. *maximus*, greatest]
maximum (măks′ĭ-mŭm) [L.]
maximum allowable concentration
maximum breathing capacity
maximum permissible dose
Mayo-Robson's point [Arthur Mayo-Robson, Brit. surgeon, 1853–1933]
maze
mazindol
mazopexy (mā′zō-pĕk″sē) [Gr. *mazos*, breast, + *pexis*, fixation]
mazoplasia (mā″zō-plā′zē-ă) [″ + *plassein*, to form]
M.B. *Bachelor of Medicine*
m.b. [L.] *misce bene*, mix well
MBC *maximum breathing capacity*
M.B.D. *minimal brain dysfunction*
μc *microcurie*
M.C. *Master of Surgery; Medical Corps*
Mc *megacurie*
mc *millicurie*
McArdle's disease [B. McArdle, contemporary Brit. pediatrician]
McBurney's incision [Charles McBurney, U.S. surgeon, 1845–1914]
McBurney's point
McBurney's sign
McCarthy's reflex [Daniel J. McCarthy, U.S. neurologist, 1874–1958]
McCormac's reflex
mcg *microgram*
MCH *mean corpuscular hemoglobin*
mc.h. *millicurie hour*
MCHC *mean corpuscular hemoglobin concentration*
μCi *microcurie*
McMurray's sign [Thomas P. McMurray, Brit. orthopedic surgeon, 1887–1949]
M.C.P. *metacarpophalangeal joint*
MCV *mean corpuscular volume*
M.D. [L.] *Medicinae, Doctor*
Md *mendelevium*
MDA *multiple drug resistance*

meal (mēl) [AS. *mael*, measure, meal]
mean [L. *medius*, middle]
　　m., arithmetic
mean corpuscular hemoglobin
mean corpuscular hemoglobin concentration
mean corpuscular volume
measles (mē′zls) [Dutch *maselen*]
　　m., black
　　m., German
　　m., hemorrhagic
measles and mumps virus vaccine, live
measles and rubella virus vaccine, live
measles, mumps, and rubella virus vaccine, live
measles virus vaccine, live
measly (mē′zlē)
measure (mĕ′zhūr) [L. *mensura*, a measuring]
Measurin
meat [AS. *mete*, food]
meatal (mē-ā′tăl) [L. *meatus*, passage]
meatometer (mē-ă-tŏm′ĕt-ĕr) [″ + Gr. *metron*, measure]
meatorrhaphy (mē″ă-tor′ăf-ē) [″ + Gr. *rhaphe*, seam]
meatoscope (mē-ăt′ō-skōp) [″ + Gr. *skopein*, to examine]
meatoscopy (mē-ă-tŏs′kō-pē) [″ + Gr. *skopein*, to examine]
meatotome (mē-ăt′ō-tōm) [″ + Gr. *tome*, a cutting, slice]
meatotomy (mē″ă-tŏt′ō-mē)
meatus (mē-ā′tŭs) [L.]
　　m. acusticus externus
　　m. acusticus internus
　　m., external auditory
　　m., internal auditory
　　m. nasi communis
　　m. nasi inferior
　　m. nasi medius
　　m. nasi superior
　　m. nasopharyngeus
　　m. urinarius
Mebaral
mebendazole (mĕ-bĕn′dă-zōl)
mebutamate (mĕ-bū′tă-māt)

mecamylamine hydrochloride (měk″ă-mĭl′ă-mīn)
mechanical rectifier
mechanics [Gr. *mechane*, machine]
mechanism
    m., countercurrent
    m., defense
    m., Duncan's
mechanocyte (měk′ă-nō-sīt″) [″ + *kytos*, cell]
mechanoreceptor (měk″ă-nō-rē-sĕp′tor)
mechanotherapy (měk″ăn-ō-thĕr′ă-pē) [Gr. *mechane*, machine, + *therapeia*, treatment]
mechlorethamine (měk″lor-ĕth′ă-mēn)
mecism (mē′sĭzm) [Gr. *mekos*, length]
Meckel, Johann Friedrich [the elder] (měk′ĕl) Ger. anatomist, 1724–1774
    M.'s ganglion
    M.'s space
Meckel, Johann Friedrich [the younger] (měk′ĕl) Ger. anatomist, 1781–1833
    M.'s cartilage
    M.'s diverticulum
meckelectomy (měk-ĕl-ĕk′tō-mē)
meclizine hydrochloride (měk′lĭ-zēn)
meclocycline sulfosalicylate
meconium (mē-kō′nē-ŭm) [Gr. *mekonion*, poppy juice]
meconium ileus
mecystasis (mē-sĭs′tă-sĭs)
M.E.D. *minimal effective dose*
medi- [L., middle]
media (mē′dē-ă) [L.]
mediad (mē′dē-ăd) [L. *medium*, middle, + *ad*, toward]
medial [L. *medialis*]
medialis (mē″dē-ā′lĭs) [L.]
median (mē′dē-ăn) [L. *medianus*]
median line
median nerve
median plane
mediastinal (mē″dē-ăs-tī′năl) [L. *mediastinalis*]
mediastinitis (mē″dē-ăs″tī-nī′tĭs) [″ + Gr. *itis*, inflammation]

mediastinography (mē″dē-ăs″tī-nŏg′ră-fē) [″ + Gr. *graphein*, to write]
mediastinopericarditis (mē-dē-ăs″tī-nō-pĕr″ĭ-kăr-dī′tĭs) [″ + Gr. *peri*, around, + *kardia*, heart, + *itis*, inflammation]
mediastinoscopy (mē″dē-ăs″tī-nŏs′kō-pē) [″ + *skopein*, to examine]
mediastinotomy (mē″dē-ăs″tī-nŏt′ō-mē) [″ + *tome*, a cutting, slice]
mediastinum (mē″dē-ăs-tī′nŭm) [L., in the middle]
    m. testis
mediate (mē′dē-āt)
mediation (mē″dē-ā′shŭn)
mediator (mē′dē-ā″tŏr)
medic
medicable (mĕd′ĭ-kă-bl) [L. *medicari*, to heal]
Medicaid
medical (mĕd′ĭ-kăl)
medical assistant
medical audit
medical corpsman
Medic Alert
medical examiner
medical history
medical informatics
medical jurisprudence
medical preparations
medical record
medical record, problem-oriented
medical records librarian
medicament [L. *medicamentum*]
medicamentosus (mĕd″ĭ-kă-mĕn-tō′sŭs)
Medicare
medicate (mĕd′ĭ-kāt) [L. *medicatus*]
medication (mĕd-ĭ-kā′shŭn)
    m., hypodermic
    m., ionic
    m., sublingual
    m., substitutive
medication route
medicinal (mě-dĭ′sĭn-ăl) [L. *medicina*, medicine]
medicinal enema

medicine
 m., aerospace
 m., clinical
 m., community
 m., dental
 m., disaster
 m., emergency
 m., environmental
 m., experimental
 m., family
 m., folk
 m., forensic
 m., group
 m., industrial
 m., internal
 m., legal
 m., nuclear
 m., occupational
 m., patent
 m., physical
 m., preclinical
 m., preventive
 m., proprietary
 m., psychosomatic
 m., socialized
 m., sports
 m., tropical
 m., veterinary
medicine man
medicinerea (mĕd"ĭ-sĭn-ē'rē-a) [L. *medius*, middle, + *cinerea*, ashen]
medicochirurgical (mĕd"ĭ-kō-kī-rŭr'jĭ-kăl) [L. *medicus*, medical, + Gr. *cheir*, hand, + *ergon*, work]
medicolegal (mĕd"ĭ-kō-lē'găl) [" + *legalis*, legal]
medicomechanical (mĕd"ĭ-kō-mĕ-kăn'ĭ-kăl)
medicopsychology (mĕd"ĭ-kō-sī-kŏl'ō-jē)
medicopter
medicornu (mĕd"ĭ-kor'nū) [L. *medius*, middle, + *cornu*, horn]
Medihaler-Epi
Medina worm
medio- [L. *medius*, middle]
mediocarpal (mē"dē-ō-kăr'păl)
mediolateral (mē"dē-ō-lăt'ĕr-ăl)

medionecrosis (mē"dē-ō-nē-krō'sĭs) [" + *nekrosis*, state of death]
mediopontine (mē"dē-ō-pŏn'tĭn) [" + *pons*, bridge]
mediotarsal (mē"dē-ō-tăr'săl)
medisect (mē'dĭ-sĕkt) [" + *secare*, to cut]
Mediterranean anemia
Mediterranean fever, familial
medium (mēd'ē-ŭm)
 m., clearing
 m., contrast
 m., culture
 m., defined
 m., nutrient
 m., radiopaque
 m., refracting
 m., separating
medium-chain triglycerides
medius (mē'dē-ŭs) [L., middle]
MEDLARS Medical Literature Analysis and Retrieval System
MEDLINE MEDLARS on line
medrogestone (mĕd-rō-jĕs'tōn)
Medrol
medroxyprogesterone acetate (mĕd-rŏk"sē-prō-jĕs'tĕr-ōn)
medrysone (mĕd'rĭ-sōn)
medulla (mĕ-dŭl'lă) [L., marrow]
 m., adrenal
 m. nephrica
 m. oblongata
 m. of hair
 m. of kidneys
 m. of ovary
 m. ossium
 m. spinalis
medullary (mĕd'ū-lār-ē) [L. *medullaris*]
medullated (mĕd'ū-lāt"ĕd)
medullated nerve fiber
medullation
medullectomy (mĕd"ū-lĕk'tō-mē) [L. *medulla*, marrow, + Gr. *ektome*, excision]
medullitis (mĕd-ū-lī'tĭs) [" + Gr. *itis*, inflammation]
medullization (mĕd"ū-lĭ-zā'shŭn)
medulloadrenal (mĕ-dŭl"ō-ă-drē'năl)

[" + *ad*, to, + *ren*, kidney]
medulloarthritis (mĕ-dŭl"ō-ăr-thrī'tĭs)
[L. *medulla*, marrow, + Gr.
arthron, joint, + *itis*, inflammation]
medulloblast (mĕ-dŭl'ō-blăst) [" +
Gr. *blastos*, germ]
medulloblastoma (mĕ-dŭl"ō-blăs-
tō'mă) [" + Gr. *blastos*, germ, +
oma, tumor]
medulloepithelioma (mĕ-dŭl"ō-ĕp"ĭ-
thēl-ē-ō'mă) [" + Gr. *epi*, upon,
+ *thele*, nipple, + *oma*, tumor]
Mees lines
mefenamic acid
mega- [Gr. *megas*, large]
megabladder (mĕg"ă-blăd'ĕr) [" +
AS. *blaedre*, bladder]
megabucks (mĕg'ă-bŭks)
megacardia (mĕg"ă-kăr'dē-ă)
Megace
megacephalic (mĕg-ă-sĕf-ăl'ĭk)
megacolon (mĕg-ă-kō'lŏn) [" +
kolon, colon]
　　m., toxic
megacurie (mĕg"ă-kū'rē) [" +
curie]
megadontia (mĕg"ă-dŏn'shē-ă)
[" + *odous, odont-*, tooth]
megadyne (mĕg'ă-dīn)
megaesophagus (mĕg"ă-ē-sŏf'ă-gŭs)
[" + *oisophagos*, gullet]
megahertz (mĕg'ă-hĕrtz)
megakaryoblast (mĕg"ă-kăr'ē-ō-
blăst)
megakaryocyte (mĕg"ă-kăr'ē-ō-sīt")
[" + *karyon*, nucleus, + *kytos*,
cell]
megakaryocytosis (mĕg"ă-kăr"ē-ō-
sī-tō'sĭs) [" + " + " +
osis, condition]
megalencephaly (mĕg"ăl-ĕn-sĕf'ă-lē)
[" + *enkephalos*, brain]
megalgia (mĕg-ăl'jē-ă) [" + *algos*,
pain]
megalo- [Gr. *megas*, large]
megaloblast (mĕg'ă-lō-blăst) [" +
blastos, germ]
megalocardia (mĕg"ă-lō-kăr'dē-ă)

[" + *kardia*, heart]
megalocephalic (mĕg-ă-lō-sĕf-ăl'ĭk)
[" + *kephale*, head]
megalocephaly (mĕg"ă-lō-sĕf'ă-lē)
[" + *kephale*, head]
megalocheiria (mĕg"ă-lō-kī'rē-ă)
[" + *cheir*, hand]
megalocornea (mĕg"ă-lō-kor'nē-ă)
[" + L. *cornu*, horn]
megalocystis (mĕg"ă-lō-sĭs'tĭs) [" +
kystis, bladder]
megalocyte (mĕg'ă-lō-sīt) [" +
kytos, cell]
megalodactylous (mĕg"ă-lō-dăk'tĭl-
ŭs) [" + *daktylos*, finger]
megalodontia (mĕg"ă-lō-dŏn'shē-ă)
[" + *odous*, tooth]
megaloesophagus (mĕg"ă-lō-ē-
sŏf'ă-gŭs) [" + *oisophagos*, gullet]
megalogastria (mĕg"ă-lō-găs'trē-ă)
[" + *gaster*, belly]
megaloglossia (mĕg"ă-lō-glŏs'sē-ă)
[" + *glossa*, tongue]
megalographia (mĕg"ă-lō-grā'fē-ă)
[" + *graphein*, to write]
megalohepatia (mĕg"ă-lō-hĕ-
păt'ē-ă) [" + *hepar*, liver]
megalokaryocyte (mĕg"ă-lō-kăr'ē-
ō-sīt) [" + *karyon*, nucleus, +
kytos, cell]
megalomania (mĕg"ă-lō-mā'nē-ă)
[" + *mania*, madness]
megalomelia (mĕg'ă-lō-mēl'ē-ă)
[" + *melos*, limb]
megalonychosis (mĕg'ă-lō"nĭ-kō'sĭs)
[" + *onyx*, nail]
megalopenis (mĕg'ă-lō-pē'nĭs) [" +
L. *penis*, penis]
megalophthalmus (mĕg"ă-lŏf-
thăl'mŭs) [" + *ophthalmos*, eye]
megalopodia (mĕg"ă-lō-pō'dē-ă)
[" + *pous*, foot]
megalopsia (mĕg"ă-lŏp'sē-ă) [" +
opsis, sight, appearance, vision]
megaloscope (mĕg'ă-lō-skōp") [" +
skopein, to examine]
megalosplenia (mĕg"ă-lō-splēn'ē-ă)
[" + *splen*, spleen]

megalospore (mĕg'ă-lō-spor")
megalosyndactyly (mĕg'ă-lō-sĭn-dăk'tĭl-ē) [" + syn, with, + daktylos, finger]
megaloureter (mĕg"ă-lō-ū-rē'tĕr, -ūr'ĕ-tĕr) [" + oureter, ureter]
megaprosopous (mĕg"ă-prŏs'ō-pŭs) [" + prosopon, face]
megarectum (mĕg-ă-rĕk'tŭm) [" + L. rectum, straight]
megaseme (mĕg'ă-sēm) [" + sema, sign]
megavitamin (mĕg"ă-vī'tă-mĭn)
megavolt (mĕg'ă-vŏlt)
megestrol acetate (mĕ-jĕs'trōl)
meglumine (mĕg'lū-mēn)
    m. antimonate
megohm (mĕg'ōm)
megophthalmos (mĕg-ŏf-thăl-mōs) [" + ophthalmos, eye]
megrim (mē'grĭm)
meibomian cyst (mī-bō'mē-ăn) [Heinrich Meibom, Ger. anatomist, 1638–1700]
meibomian gland
meibomitis (mī-bō"mĭ'tĭs)
meio- [Gr. meioun, diminution]
meiogenic (mī"ō-jĕn'ĭk) [Gr. meiosis, diminution, + gennan, to produce]
meiosis (mī-ō'sĭs) [Gr., diminution]
Meissner's corpuscles (mīs'nĕrz) [Georg Meissner, Ger. histologist, 1829–1905]
Meissner's plexus
mel [L.]
melagra (mĕl-ă'gră) [Gr. melos, limb, + agra, seizure]
melalgia (mĕl-ăl'jē-ă) [" + algos, pain]
melancholia (mĕl-ăn-kō'lē-ă) [Gr. melankholia, sadness]
    m., affective
    m. agitata
    m., climacteric
    m., involutional
    m., panphobic
    m., sexual
    m. simplex

    m. stuporosa
    m., suicidal
melanedema (mĕl-ăn-ĕ-dē'mă) [Gr. melas, black, + oidema, swelling]
melanemia (mĕl-ăn-ē'mē-ă) [" + haima, blood]
melanephidrosis, melanidrosis (mĕl"ăn-ĕf"ĭ-drō'sĭs, mĕl"ăn-ĭd-rō'sĭs) [" + ephidrosis, sweating]
melaniferous (mĕl"ăn-ĭf'ĕr-ŭs) [" + L. ferre, to carry]
melanin [Gr. melas, black]
melanism (mĕl'ăn-ĭzm) [" + -ismos, condition]
melano- [Gr. melas, black]
melanoameloblastoma (mĕl"ă-nō-ă-mĕl"ō-blăs-tō'mă) [" + O. Fr. amel, enamel, + Gr. blastos, germ, + oma, tumor]
melanoblast (mĕl'ăn-ō-blăst", mĕl-ăn'ō-blăst) [" + blastos, germ]
melanoblastoma (mĕl"ă-nō-blăs-tō'mă) [" + " + oma, tumor]
melanocarcinoma (mĕl"ă-nō-kăr-sĭn-ō'mă) [" + karkinos, cancer, + oma, tumor]
melanocyte (mĕl'ăn-ō-sīt, mĕl-ăn'ō-sīt) [" + kytos, cell]
melanocyte-stimulating hormone
melanocytoma (mĕl"ă-nō-sī-tō'mă) [" + kytos, cell, + oma, tumor]
melanoderm (mĕl'ăn-ō-dĕrm) [" + derma, skin]
melanoderma (mĕl"ăn-ō-dĕr'mă)
melanodermatitis (mĕl"ă-nō-dĕr"mă-tī'tĭs) [" + " + itis, inflammation]
melanoepithelioma (mĕl"ăn-ō-ĕp"ĭ-thē-lē-ō'mă) [" + epi, upon, + thele, nipple, + oma, tumor]
melanogen (mĕ-lăn'ō-jĕn) [" + gennan, to produce]
melanogenesis (mĕl"ăn-ō-jĕn'ĕ-sĭs) [" + genesis, generation, birth]
melanoglossia (mĕl"ăn-ō-glŏs'ē-ă) [" + glossa, tongue]
melanoid (mĕl'ă-noyd) [" + eidos, form, shape]

melanoleukoderma (mĕl″ăn-ō-lū″kō-dĕr′mă) [″ + leukos, white, + derma, skin]
  m. colli

melanoma (mĕl″ă-nō′mă) [″ + oma, tumor]

melanomatosis (mĕl″ă-nō″mă-tō′sĭs) [″ + ″ + osis, condition]

melanonychia (mĕl″ă-nō-nĭk′ē-ă) [″ + onyx, nail]

melanopathy (mĕl″ă-nŏp′ă-thē) [″ + pathos, disease, suffering]

melanophage (mĕl′ă-nō-fāj″) [″ + phagein, to eat]

melanophore (mĕl′ăn-ō-for) [″ + phoros, bearing]

melanoplakia (mĕl″ăn-ō-plā′kē-ă) [″ + plax, a flat plain]

melanorrhagia, melanorrhea (mĕl″ăn-ō-rā′jē-ă, mĕl″ăn-ō-rē′ă) [″ + rhegnynai, to burst forth]

melanosarcoma (mĕl″ă-nō-săr-kō′mă) [″ + sarx, flesh, + oma, tumor]

melanoscirrhus (mĕl″ă-nō-skĭr′ŭs) [Gr. melas, black, + skirros, hardness]

melanosis (mĕl-ăn-ō′sĭs) [″ + osis, condition]
  m. lenticularis

melanosome (mĕl′ă-nō-sōm″) [″ + soma, body]

melanotic

melanotrichia linguae (mĕl″ăn-ō-trĭk′ē-ă lĭng′gwē) [″ + thrix, hair, + L. linguae, tongue]

melanotroph (mĕl′ă-nō-trōf″) [″ + trophe, nutrition]

melanuria (mĕl-ăn-ū′rē-ă) [″ + ouron, urine]

melasma (mĕl-ăz′mă) [Gr., a black spot]
  m. gravidarum

melatonin (mel″ă-tō′nĭn)

melena (mĕl′ē-nă, mĕl-ē′nă) [Gr. melaina, black]
  m. neonatorum

melenic (mĕl-ē′nĭk) [Gr. melaina, black]

melicera, meliceris (mĕl-ĭ-sēr′ă, -ĭs)

[Gr. meli, honey, + keros, wax]

melioidosis (mē″lē-oy-dō′sĭs) [Gr. melis, a distemper of asses, + eidos, form, shape, + osis, condition]

melissophobia (mĕ-lĭs″ō-fō′bē-ă) [Gr. melissa, bee, + phobia, fear]

melitagra

melitemia (mĕl-ĭ-tē′mē-ă) [Gr. meli, honey, + haima, blood]

melitensis (mĕl-ĭ-tĕn′sĭs)

melitis (mĕl-ĭ′tĭs) [Gr. melon, cheek, + itis, inflammation]

melitoptyalism (mĕl″ĭ-tō-tī′ăl-ĭzm) [″ + ptyalon, saliva]

melituria (mĕl-ĭ-tū′rē-ă) [″ + ouron, urine]

Mellaril

mellitum (mĕ-lī′tŭm) [L.]

melo-, mel- [Gr. melon, cheek; melos, limb]

melomelus (mē-lŏm′ē-lŭs) [Gr. melos, limb, + melos, limb]

meloncus (mĕl-ŏn′kŭs) [Gr. melon, cheek, + onkos, bulk, mass]

melonoplasty (mĕl′ŏn-ō-plăs″tē) [″ + plassein, to form]

meloplasty (mĕl′ō-plăs-tē) [″ + plassein, to form; Gr. melos, limb, + plassein, to form]

melorheostosis (mĕl″ō-rē″ŏs-tō′sĭs) [Gr. melos, limb, + rhein, to flow, + osteon, bone, + osis, condition]

melosalgia (mĕl″ō-săl′jē-ă) [″ + algos, pain]

meloschisis (mē-lŏs′kĭ-sĭs) [Gr. melon, cheek, + schistos, divided]

melotia (mĕ-lō′shē-ă) [″ + ous, ear]

melphalan (mĕl′fă-lăn)

melting point

member [L. membrum]

membrane (mĕm′brān) [L. membrana]
  m., alveolocapillary
  m., alveodental
  m., arachnoid
  m., atlanto-occipital

m., basement
m., basilar
m., Bowman's
m., Bruch's
m., buccopharyngeal
m., cell
m., choroid
m., costocoracoid
m., cricothyroid
m., croupous
m., decidual
m., Descemet's
m., diphtheritic
m., drum
m., egg
m., elastic
m., enamel
m., false
m., fenestrated
m., fetal
m., fibrous
m., glassy
m., glial cell
m., Henle's elastic
m., homogeneous
m., Huxley's
m., hyaline
m., hyaloid
m., hyoglossal
m., interosseous
m., Krause's
m., laryngeal mucous
m., limiting, external
m., limiting, internal
m., lingual mucous
m., masticatory mucous
m., medullary
m., mucous
m., nasal mucous
m., Nasmyth's
m., nictitating
m., nuclear
m., obturator
m., olfactory
m., oral
m., oronasal
m., otolithic
m., palatal mucous

m., peridental
m., periodontal
m., permeable
m., pharyngeal
m., pharyngeal mucous
m., placental
m., plasma
m., pseudoserous
m., pupillary
m., pyogenic
m., quadrangular
m., Reissner's
m., Ruysch's
m., Scarpa's
m., schneiderian
m., Schwann's
m., selectively permeable
m., semipermeable
m., serous
m., Shrapnell's
m., submucous
m., synovial
m., tectorial
m., thyrohyoid
m., tympanic
m., unit
m., vestibular mucous
m., virginal
m., vitelline
m., vitreous
m., yolk

membranectomy (měm″brăn-něk′tō-mē) [L. *membrana*, membrane, + Gr. *ektome*, excision]

membranella (měm″bră-něl′ă)

membrane potential

membraniform (měm-brā′nĭ-form)

membranocartilaginous (měm″brăn-ō-kăr-tĭ-lăj′ĭ-nŭs)

membranoid (měm′bră-noyd) [L. *membrana*, membrane, + Gr. *eidos*, form, shape]

membranous

membrum muliebre (měm′brŭm mū-lē-ě′brē) [L., female member]

membrum virile (měm′brŭm vĭr-il′ē) [L., male member]

memory [L. *memoria*]

m., anterograde
m., long-term
m., retrograde

menacme (măn-ăk′mē) [Gr. *men,* month, + *akme,* top]

menadiol sodium diphosphate

menadione (měn″ă-dī′ōn)
m. sodium bisulfite

menarchal, menarcheal, menarchial

menarche (měn-ăr′kē) [Gr. *men,* month, + *arche,* beginning]

mendelevium (měn-dě-lē′vē-ŭm)

mendelism (měn′děl-ĭzm)

Mendel's laws [Gregor Johann Mendel, Austrian monk, 1822–1884]

Mendel's reflex [Kurt Mendel, Ger. neurologist, 1874–1946]

Ménétrier's disease (mān″ă-trē-ārz′) [Pierre Ménétrier, Fr. physician, 1859–1935]

menhidrosis, menidrosis (měn-hī-drō′sĭs, měn″ĭ-drō′sĭs) [Gr. *men,* month, + *hidros,* sweat]

Ménière's disease (mān″ē-ārz′) [Prosper Ménière, Fr. physician, 1799–1862]

meningeal (měn-ĭn′jē-ăl)

meningeocortical (mě-nĭn″jē-ō-kor′tĭ-kăl) [Gr. *meninx,* membrane, + L. *corticalis,* pert. to cortex]

meningeorrhaphy (mě-nĭn″jē-or′ă-fē) [″ + *rhaphe,* seam]

meninges (měn-ĭn′jēz) [Gr.]

meningioma (měn-ĭn″jē-ō′mă) [Gr. *meninx,* membrane, + *oma,* tumor]

meningiomatosis (mě-nĭn″jē-ō-mă-tō′sĭs) [″ + ″ + *osis,* condition]

meningism (měn-ĭn′jĭzm) [″ + *-ismos,* condition]

meningismus

meningitic (měn-ĭn-jĭt′ĭk) [Gr. *meninx,* membrane]

meningitis (měn-ĭn-jī′tĭs) [″ + *itis,* inflammation]
m., acute
m., acute aseptic
m., basilar

m., cerebral
m., cerebrospinal
m., listeria
m., pneumococcal
m., serosa circumscripta
m., serous
m., spinal
m., sterile
m., traumatic
m., tuberculous

meningitophobia (měn″ĭn-jĭt″ō-fō′bē-ă) [Gr. *meninx,* membrane, + *phobos,* fear]

meningo- (měn-ĭn′gō) [Gr. *meninx,* membrane]

meningoarteritis (měn-ĭn″gō-ăr″těr-īt′ĭs) [″ + *arteria,* artery, + *itis,* inflammation]

meningocele (měn-ĭn′gō-sēl) [″ + *kele,* tumor, swelling]

meningococcal polysaccharide vaccine group A

meningococcal polysaccharide vaccine group C

meningococcemia (měn-ĭn″gō-kŏk-sē′mē-ă) [″ + *kokkyx,* coccyx, + *haima,* blood]

meningococci (měn-ĭn″gō-kŏk′sī)

meningococcidal (mě-nĭng″gō-kŏk-sī′dăl) [″ + ″ + L. *cida* fr. *caedere,* to kill]

meningococcus (měn-ĭn″gō-kŏk′ŭs)

meningocortical (měn-ĭn″gō-kor′tĭ-kăl)

meningocyte (mě-nĭng′gō-sīt) [″ + *kytos,* cell]

meningoencephalitis (měn-ĭn″gō-ěn-sěf″ă-lī′tĭs) [″ + *enkephalos,* brain, + *itis,* inflammation]
m. due to Naegleria and Acanthamoeba

meningoencephalocele (měn-ĭn″gō-ěn-sěf″ăl-ō-sēl) [″ + ″ + *kele,* tumor, swelling]

meningoencephalomyelitis (měn-ĭn″gō-ěn-sěf″ăl-ō-mī-ěl-ī′tĭs) [″ + ″ + *myelos,* marrow, + *itis,* inflammation]

meningoencephalopathy

(mĕ-nĭng"gō-ĕn-sĕf"ă-lŏp'ă-thē) [" +
" + *pathos*, disease, suffering]
meningomalacia (mĕn-ĭn"gō-mă-lā'shē-ă) [" + *malakia*, softening]
meningomyelitis (mĕn-ĭn"gō-mī"ĕl-ī'tĭs) [" + *myelos*, marrow, + *itis*, inflammation]
meningomyelocele (mĕn-ĭn"gō-mī-ĕl'ō-sēl) [" + " + *kele*, tumor, swelling]
meningomyeloradiculitis (mĕ-nĭng"gō-mī"ĕ-lō-ră-dĭk"ū-lī'tĭs) [" + " + L. *radicula*, radicle, + Gr. *itis*, inflammation]
meningo-osteophlebitis (mĕ-nĭng"gō-ŏs"tē-ō-flĕ-bī'tĭs) [" + *osteon*, bone, + *phleps*, blood vessel, vein, + *itis*, inflammation]
meningopathy (mĕn-ĭn-gŏp'ă-thē) [" + *pathos*, disease, suffering]
meningoradicular (mĕ-nĭng"gō-ră-dĭk'ū-lăr) [" + L. *radicula*, radicle]
meningoradiculitis (mĕ-nĭng"gō-ră-dĭk"ū-lī'tĭs) [" + " + Gr. *itis*, inflammation]
meningorrhachidian (mĕn-ĭn"gō-ră-kĭd'ē-ăn) [" + *rhachis*, spine]
meningorrhagia (mĕn-ĭn"gō-rā'jē-ă) [" + *rhegnynai*, to burst forth]
meningorrhea (mĕn-ĭn"gō-rē'ă) [" + *rhein*, to flow]
meningosis (mĕn"ĭn-gō'sĭs) [" + *osis*, condition]
meningotyphoid (mĕn-ĭn"gō-tī'foyd)
meningovascular (mĕn-ĭn"gō-văs'kū-lăr)
meninguria (mĕn"ĭn-gū'rē-ă) [Gr. *meninx*, membrane, + *ouron*, urine]
meninx (mē'nĭnks) [Gr., membrane]
meniscectomy (mĕn"ĭ-sĕk'tō-mē) [" + *ektome*, excision]
menisci (mĕn-ĭs'ē)
meniscitis (mĕn"ĭ-sī'tĭs) [Gr. *meniskos*, crescent, + *itis*, inflammation]
meniscocyte (mĕn-ĭs'kō-sīt) [" + *kytos*, cell]
meniscocytosis (mĕn-ĭs"kō-sī-tō'sĭs) [" + " + *osis*, condition]

meniscus (mĕn-ĭs'kŭs) [Gr. *meniskos*, crescent]
m. articularis
menometrorrhagia (mĕn"ō-mĕt-rō-rā'jē-ă) [Gr. *men*, month, + *metra*, womb, + *rhegnynai*, to burst forth]
menopause (mĕn'ō-pawz) [" + *pausis*, cessation]
m., artificial
m., male
m., premature
m., surgical
menophania (mĕn-ō-fā'nē-ă) [" + *phainesthai*, to appear]
menoplania (mĕn-ō"plā'nē-ă) [" + *plane*, deviation]
menorrhagia (mĕn"ō-rā'jē-ă) [" + *rhegnynai*, to burst forth]
menorrhalgia (mĕn-ō-răl'jē-ă) [" + *rhein*, to flow, + *algia*, pain]
menorrhea (mĕn"ō-rē'ă)
menostasis (mĕn-ŏs'tă-sĭs) [" + *stasis*, standing still]
menostaxis (mĕn"ō-stăk'sĭs) [" + *staxis*, dripping]
menotropins (mĕn"ō-trō'pĭns)
menoxenia (mĕn-ŏk-sē'nē-ă) [" + *xenos*, strange]
menses (mĕn'sēz) [L., month]
menstrual (mĕn'stroo-ăl) [L. *menstrualis*]
menstrual cycle
menstrual epilepsy
menstrual extraction
menstrual regulation
menstruant (mĕn'stroo-ănt) [L. *menstruare*, to discharge the menses]
menstruate (mĕn'stroo-āt)
menstruation (mĕn-stroo-ā'shŭn) [L. *menstruare*, to discharge the menses]
m., anovulatory
m., retrograde
m., suppressed
m., vicarious
menstruous (mĕn'stroo-ŭs)
menstruum (mĕn'stroo-ŭm) [L. *menstruus*, menstrual fluid]
mensual (mĕn'sū-ăl) [L. *mensis*, month]

mensuration (mĕn-sū-rā'shŭn) [L. mensuratio]

mentagrophyton (mĕn"tă-grŏf'ĭ-tŏn) [L. mentagra, sycosis, + Gr. phyton, plant]

mental [L. mens, mind; mentum, chin]

mental age

mental deficiency

mental disorder

mental fog

mental health

mental hygiene

mental illness

mentality

Mental Measurements Yearbook

mental retardation

mental status

mentation (mĕn-tā'shŭn)

Mentha [L.]

M. piperita

M. pulegium

M. viridis

menthol

menton (mĕn'tŏn) [L. mentum, chin]

mentulagra (mĕn"tū-lăg'ră) [L. mentula, penis, + Gr. agra, seizure]

mentulate (mĕn'tū-lāt) [L. mentula, penis]

mentulomania (mĕn"tū-lō-mā'nē-ă) [" + Gr. mania, madness]

mentum [L.]

mepacrine hydrochloride (mĕp'ă-krĭn)

mepazine (mĕp'ă-zēn)

mepenzolate bromide (mĕ-pĕn'zō-lāt)

meperidine hydrochloride (mĕ-pĕr'ĭ-dēn)

mephenesin (mĕ-fĕn'ĕ-sĭn)

mephentermine sulfate (mĕ-fĕn'tĕr-mēn)

mephenytoin (mĕ-fĕn'ĭ-tō-ĭn)

mephitic [L. mephiticus, mephitis, foul exhalation]

mephobarbital (mĕf"ō-băr'bĭ-tăl)

Mephyton

mepivacaine hydrochloride (mĕ-pĭv'ă-kān)

meprednisone (mĕ-prĕd'nĭ-sōn)

meprobamate (mĕ-prō'bă-māt)

Meprospan

meprylcaine hydrochloride (mĕp'rĭl-kăn)

mEq milliequivalent

meralgia (mĕr-ăl'jē-ă) [Gr. meros, thigh, + algos, pain]

m. paresthetica

merbromin (mĕr-brō'mĭn)

mercaptan (mĕr-kăp'tăn)

mercaptomerin sodium injection (mĕr-kăp"tō-mĕr'ĭn)

mercaptopurine (mĕr-kăp"tō-pū'rēn)

Mercier's bar (mĕr-sē-āz') [Louis A. Mercier, Fr. urologist, 1811 – 1882]

mercurial (mĕr-kū'rē-ăl) [L. mercurialis]

mercurial diuretics

mercurialism (mĕr-kū'rē-ăl-ĭzm) [L. mercurius, mercury, + Gr. -ismos, condition]

mercurialized (mĕr-kū'rē-ăl-īzd)

mercurial palsy

mercurial rash

mercuric (mĕr-kū'rĭk)

m. chloride

m. oxide, yellow

mercuric chloride poisoning

Mercurochrome

mercurous (mĕr-kū'rŭs, mĕr'kū-rŭs)

m. chloride

mercurous chloride poisoning

mercury (mĕr'kū-rē) [L. mercurius]

m., ammoniated

m. bichloride

m. chloride, mild

mercury poisoning

mercy (mĕr'sē) [L. merces, reward]

meridian (mĕ-rĭd'ē-ăn)

m. of eye

merinthophobia (mĕr-ĭn"thō-fō'bē-ă) [Gr. merinthos, a cord, + phobia, fear]

merispore (mĕr'ĭ-spor) [Gr. meros, a part, + sporos, seed]

meristic (mĕr-ĭs'tĭk) [Gr. meristikos, fit for dividing]

mero- [Gr. meros, a part]

meroacrania (mĕr"ō-ă-krā'nē-ă) [" + *a-*, not, + *kranion*, skull]

meroblastic (mĕr-ō-blăst'ĭk) [" + *blastos*, germ]

merocele (mĕr'ō-sēl) [" + *kele*, tumor, swelling]

merocoxalgia (mĕr"ō-kŏk-săl'jē-ă) [" + L. *coxa*, hip, + Gr. *algos*, pain]

merocrine (mĕr'ō-krĭn) [" + *krinein*, to separate]

merodiastolic (mĕr"ō-dī-ă-stŏl'ĭk)

meroergasia (mĕr"ō-ĕr-gă'zē-ă) [Gr. *meros*, a part, + *ergasia*, work]

merogenesis (mĕr"ō-jĕn'ĕ-sĭs) [" + *genesis*, generation, birth]

merogony (mĕ-rŏg'ō-nē) [" + *gonos*, offspring, procreation]

meromelia (mĕr"ō-mē'lē-ă) [" + *melos*, limb]

meromicrosomia (mĕr"ō-mī"krō-sō'mē-ă) [" + *mikros*, small, + *soma*, body]

meromyosin (mĕr"ō-mī'ō-sĭn)

meronecrosis (mĕr"ō-nĕk-rō'sĭs) [" + *nekrosis*, state of death]

meropia (mĕr-ō'pē-ă) [" + *ops*, vision]

merorrhachischisis (mĕ"rō-ră-kĭs'kĭ-sĭs) [" + *rhachis*, spine, + *schisis*, cleavage]

merosmia (mĕr-ŏs'mē-ă) [" + *osme*, odor]

merosystolic (mĕr"ō-sĭs-tŏl'ĭk) [" + *systole*, a contraction]

merotomy (mĕr-ŏt'ō-mē) [" + *tome*, a cutting, slice]

merozoite (mĕr"ō-zō'ĭt) [" + *zoon*, animal]

merozygote (mĕr"ō-zī'gōt) [" + *zygotos*, yoked together]

Merthiolate

Meruvax

mesad (mē'săd) [Gr. *mesos*, middle, + L. *ad*, toward]

mesal (mē'săl)

mesangium (mĕs-ăn'jē-ŭm)

Mesantoin

mesaortitis (mĕs"ā-or-tī'tĭs) [" + *aorte*, aorta + *itis*, inflammation]

mesaraic, mesareic (mĕs-ă-rā'ĭk, -rī'ĭk) [Gr. *mesaraion*, the mesentery]

mesarteritis (mĕs-ăr-tĕr-ī'tĭs)

mesaticephalic (mĕs-ăt"ĭ-sĕf-ăl'ĭk) [Gr. *mesatos*, medium, + *kephale*, brain]

mesatipellic, mesatipelvic (mĕs-ăt"ĭ-pĕl'ĭk, -pĕl'vĭk) [" + *pella*, bowl]

mescaline (mĕs'kă-lēn)

mescalism (mĕs'kă-lĭzm)

mesectoderm (mĕs-ĕk'tō-derm)

mesencephalitis (mĕs"ĕn-sĕf"ă-lī'tĭs) [" + *enkephalos*, brain, + *itis*, inflammation]

mesencephalon (mĕs-ĕn-sĕf'ă-lŏn) [" + *enkephalos*, brain]

mesencephalotomy (mĕs"ĕn-sĕf"ă-lŏt'ō-mē) [" + " + *tome*, a cutting, slice]

mesenchyme (mĕs'ĕn-kīm) [" + *enchyma*, infusion]

mesenchymoma (mĕs"ĕn-kī-mō'mă)

mesenterectomy (mĕs"ĕn-tĕ-rĕk'tō-mē) [" + *enteron*, intestine, + *ektome*, excision]

mesenteric (mĕs"ĕn-tĕr'ĭk) [Gr. *mesenterikos*]

mesenteriolum (mĕs-ĕn"tĕr-ī'ō-lŭm) [L.]

mesenteriopexy (mĕs"ĕn-tĕr'ē-ō-pĕk"sē) [" + *enteron*, intestine, + *pexis*, fixation]

mesenteriorrhaphy (mĕs"ĕn-tĕr-ē-or'ă-fē) [" + " + *rhaphe*, seam]

mesenteriplication (mĕs"ĕn-tĕr"ĭ-plĭ-kā'shŭn) [" + " + L. *plicare*, to fold]

mesenteritis (mĕs"ĕn-tĕr-ī'tĭs) [" + " + *itis*, inflammation]

mesenterium (mĕs"ĕn-tē'rē-ŭm)

mesenteron (mĕs-ĕn'tĕr-ŏn)

mesentery (mĕs'ĕn-tĕr"ē) [" + *enteron*, intestine]

MESH Medical Subject Headings

mesiad (mē′zē-ăd) [″ + L. ad, toward]
mesial (mē′zē-ăl)
mesial drift
mesio- [Gr. mesos, middle]
mesiobuccal (mē″zē-ō-bŭk′kăl)
mesiobucco-occlusal (mē″zē-ō-bŭk″kō-ō-kloo′zăl)
mesiobuccopulpal (mē″zē-ō-bŭk″kō-pŭl′păl)
mesiocervical (mē″zē-ō-sĕr′vĭ-kăl)
mesioclusion (mē″zē-ō-kloo′zhŭn)
mesiodens (mē′zē-ō-dĕnz)
mesiodistal (mē″zē-ō-dĭs′tăl)
mesiogingival (mē′zē-ō-jĭn′jĭ-văl)
mesiolabial (mē″zē-ō-lā′bē-ăl)
mesiolingual (mē″zē-ō-lĭng′gwăl)
mesiolinguo-occlusal (mē″zē-ō-lĭng′gwō-ō-kloo′zăl)
mesiolinguopulpal (mē′zē-ō-lĭng″gwō-pŭl′păl)
mesion (mē′sē-ŏn) [Gr. mesos, middle]
mesiopulpal (mē″zē-ō-pŭl′păl)
mesioversion (mē″zē-ō-vĕr′zhŭn)
mesiris (mĕs-ī′rĭs)
mesmeric (mĕs-mĕr′ĭk) [Franz Anton Mesmer, Austrian physician, 1734–1815]
mesmerism (mĕs′mĕr-ĭzm)
meso- [Gr. mesos, middle]
mesoappendicitis
mesoappendix (mĕs″ō-ă-pĕn′dĭks) [Gr. mesos, middle, + L. appendix, an appendage]
mesoarium (mĕs″ō-ā′rē-ŭm)
mesoblast (mĕs′ō-blăst) [″ + blastos, germ]
mesobronchitis (mĕs″ō-brŏng-kī′tĭs)
mesocardia (mĕs″ō-kăr′dē-ă) [″ + kardia, heart]
mesocardium (mĕs-ō-kăr′dē-ŭm)
mesocarpal (mĕs″ō-kăr′păl)
mesocecum (mĕs″ō-sē′kŭm) [″ + L. caecum, blindness]
mesocele (mĕs′ō-sēl) [″ + koilia, cavity, belly]
mesocephalic (mĕs″ō-sĕ-făl′ĭk) [″ + kephale, head]

mesocephalon (mĕs″ō-sĕf′ă-lŏn)
mesocolic (mĕs″ō-kŏl′ĭk)
mesocolon (mĕs″ō-kō′lŏn) [″ + kolon, colon]
mesocolopexy (mĕs″ō-kō′lō-pĕk″sē) [″ + ″ + pexis, fixation]
mesocoloplication (mĕs″ō-kō″lō-plĭ-kā′shŭn) [″ + ″ + L. plicare, to fold]
mesocord
mesocuneiform (mĕs″ō-kū′nē-ĭ-form)
mesoderm (mĕs′ō-dĕrm) [″ + derma, skin]
   m., axial
   m., extraembryonic
   m., intermediate
   m., lateral
   m., paraxial
   m., somatic
   m., splanchnic
mesodiastolic (mĕs″ō-dī″ă-stŏl′ĭk)
mesodont (mĕs′ō-dŏnt)
mesoduodenum (mĕs″ō-dū″ō-dē′nŭm)
mesoepididymis (mĕs″ō-ĕp″ĭ-dĭd′ĭ-mĭs)
mesogastric (mĕs″ō-găs′trĭk)
mesogastrium (mĕs″ō-găs′trē-ŭm) [″ + gaster, belly]
mesoglia (mĕ-sŏg′lē-ă)
mesogluteal (mĕs″ō-gloo′tē-ăl)
mesogluteus (mĕs″ō-gloo′tē-ŭs)
mesognathion (mĕs-ŏg-nā′thē-ŏn)
mesognathous
mesohyloma (mĕs″ō-hī-lō′mă) [″ + hyle, matter, + oma, tumor]
mesoileum (mĕs″ō-ĭl′ē-ŭm)
mesojejunum (mĕs″ō-jē-jū′nŭm)
mesolymphocyte (mĕs″ō-lĭm′fō-sīt)
mesomere (mĕs′ō-mēr) [″ + meros, part]
mesometritis (mĕs-ō-mē-trī′tĭs) [″ + metra, uterus, + itis, inflammation]
mesometrium (mĕs″ō-mē′trē-ŭm)
mesomorph (mĕs′ō-morf)
meson (mĕs′ŏn, mē′sŏn) [Gr. mesos, middle]
mesonasal (mĕs″ō-nā′zăl)

mesonephric (mĕs"ō-nĕf'rĭk) [" + *nephros*, kidney]

mesonephric duct

mesonephric tubules

mesonephroma (mĕs"ō-nē-frō'mă) [" + *nephros*, kidney, + *oma*, tumor]

mesonephros (mĕs"ō-nĕf'rŏs)

mesoneuritis (mĕs-ō-nū-rī'tĭs) [" + *neuron*, nerve, + *itis*, inflammation]

meso-ontomorph (mĕs"ō-ŏn'tō-morf)

mesopexy (mĕs'ō-pĕks"ē) [" + *pexis*, fixation]

mesophilic (mĕs-ō-fĭl'ĭk) [" + *philein*, to love]

mesophlebitis (mĕs"ō-flĕ-bī'tĭs)

mesophragma (mĕs"ō-frăg'mă) [" + *phragmos*, a fencing in]

mesophryon (mĕs-ŏf'rē-ŏn) [" + *ophrys*, eyebrow]

mesopic (mĕs-ŏp'ĭk)

mesopneumon (mĕs"ō-nū'mŏn) [" + *pneumon*, lung]

mesoporphyrin

mesoprosopic (mĕs"ō-prō-sŏp'ĭk) [" + *prosopon*, face]

mesopulmonum (mĕs"ō-pŭl-mō'nŭm)

mesorchium (mĕs-or'kē-ŭm) [" + *orchis*, testicle]

mesorectum (mĕs"ō-rĕk'tŭm)

mesoridazine besylate (mĕs"ō-rĭd'ă-zēn)

mesoropter (mĕs-ō-rŏp'tĕr) [" + *horos*, boundary, + *opter*, observer]

mesorrhachischisis (mĕs"ō-ră-kĭs'kĭ-sĭs) [" + *rhachis*, spine, + *schisis*, cleavage]

mesorrhaphy (mĕs-or'ă-fē) [" + *rhaphe*, seam]

mesorrhine (mĕs'ō-rīn) [" + *rhis*, nose]

mesosalpinx (mĕs"ō-săl'pĭnks) [" + *salpinx*, tube]

mesoseme (mĕs'ō-sēm) [" + *sema*, sign]

mesosigmoid (mĕs-ō-sĭg'moyd)

mesosigmoiditis (mĕs"ō-sĭg"moy-dī'tĭs)

mesosigmoidopexy (mĕs"ō-sĭg-moy'dō-pĕk"sē)

mesoskelic (mĕs-ō-skĕl'ĭk) [" + *skelos*, leg]

mesosome (mĕs'ō-sōm) [" + *soma*, body]

mesosternum (mĕs"ō-stĕr'nŭm) [" + *sternon*, chest]

mesosystolic (mĕs"ō-sĭs-tŏl'ĭk)

mesotarsal (mĕs"ō-tăr'săl)

mesotendineum (mĕs"ō-tĕn-dĭn'ē-ŭm)

mesotendon

mesothelial (mĕs"ō-thē'lē-ăl)

mesothelioma (mĕs"ō-thē-lē-ō'mă)

mesothelium (mĕs"ō-thē'lē-ŭm) [" *epi*, at, + *thele*, nipple]

mesothenar (mĕs"ō-thē'năr) [" + *thenar*, palm]

mesothorium (mĕs"ō-thō'rē-ŭm)

mesotron

mesouranic (mĕs"ō-ū-răn'ĭk)

mesovarium (mĕs"ō-vā'rē-ŭm)

Mestinon

mestranol (mĕs'tră-nŏl)

MET *metabolic equivalent*

meta- (mĕt'ă) [Gr. *meta*, after, beyond, over]

meta-analysis

metabiosis (mĕt'ă-bī-ō'sĭs) [" + *biosis*, way of life]

metabolic (mĕt"ă-bŏl'ĭk) [Gr. *metabolikos*, changing]

metabolic balance

metabolic body size

metabolic equivalent

metabolic failure

metabolic gradient

metabolic rate

metabolimeter (mĕt"ă-bō-lĭm'ĕ-tĕr) [Gr. *meta*, after, beyond, over, + *biosis*, way of life, + *metron*, measure]

metabolism [Gr. *metabole*, change, + *-ismos*, condition]
    m., basal
    m., carbohydrate
    m., constructive
    m., destructive
    m., fat

m., general
m., protein
m., purine
m., special
metabolite (mĕ-tăb′ō-līt)
metabolize (mĕ-tăb′ō-līz) [Gr. *metabole*, change]
metacarpal [Gr. *meta*, after, beyond, over, + *karpos*, wrist]
metacarpectomy (mĕt″ă-kăr-pĕk′tō-mē) [″ + ″ + *ektome*, excision]
metacarpophalangeal (mĕt″ă-kăr″pō-fă-lăn′jē-ăl)
metacarpus (mĕt″ă-kăr′pŭs) [″ + *karpos*, wrist]
metacentric (mĕt″ă-sĕn′trĭk)
metacercaria (mĕt″ă-sĕr-kā′rē-ă)
metachromasia, metachromatism (mĕt-ă-krō-mā′zē-ă, -krōm′ă-tĭzm) [Gr. *meta*, change, + *chroma*, color]
metachromatic (mĕt″ă-krō-măt′ĭk)
metachromatic granules
metachromatic leukodystrophy
metachromophil (mĕt-ă-krōm′ō-fĭl) [″ + *chroma*, color, + *philein*, to love]
metachrosis (mĕt-ă-krō′sĭs)
metacone [Gr. *meta*, after, beyond, over, + *konos*, cone]
metaconid (mĕt-ă-kōn′ĭd)
metaconule (mĕt-ă-kōn′ūl)
metacyesis (mĕt-ă-sī-ē′sĭs) [″ + *kyesis*, pregnancy]
metagenesis [″ + *genesis*, generation, birth]
metagglutinin (mĕt″ă-gloo′tĭn-ĭn) [″ + L. *agglutinare*, glue]
Metagonimus (mĕt″ă-gŏn′ĭ-mŭs) [″ + *gonimos*, productive]
   M. yokogawai
Metahydrin
metaicteric (mĕt″ă-ĭk-tĕr′ĭk) [″ + *ikteros*, jaundice]
metainfective (mĕt″ă-ĭn-fĕk′tĭv)
metakinesis (mĕt″ă-kī-nē′sĭs)
metalbumin (mĕt-ăl-bū′mĭn)
metal fume fever
metallesthesia (mĕt″ăl-ĕs-thē′sē-ă) [Gr. *metallon*, metal, + *aisthesis*, feeling, perception]
metallic
metallic tinkling
metalloenzyme (mĕ-tăl″ō-ĕn′zīm)
metalloid (mĕt′ăl-loyd) [″ + *eidos*, form, shape]
metallophilia (mĕ-tăl″ō-fĭl′ē-ă) [″ + *philein*, to love]
metallophobia (mĕ″tăl-ō-fō′bē-ă) [″ + *phobos*, fear]
metalloporphyrin (mĕ-tăl″ō-por′fĭ-rĭn)
metalloprotein (mĕ-tăl″ō-prō′tē-ĭn)
metalloscopy (mĕt-ăl-ŏs′kō-pē) [″ + *skopein*, to examine]
metallotherapy (mĕt″ăl-ō-thĕr′ă-pē) [″ + *therapeuein*, to heal]
metallurgy (mĕt″ăl-ŭr′jē) [″ + *ergon*, work]
metamer (mĕt′ă-mĕr)
metamere (mĕt′ă-mĕr) [Gr. *meta*, after, beyond, over, + *meros*, part]
metameric (mĕt-ă-mĕr′ĭk)
metamerism (mĕ-tăm′ĕr-ĭzm)
metamorphopsia (mĕt″ă-mor-fŏp′sē-ă) [Gr. *meta*, after, beyond, over, + *morphe*, form, + *opsis*, sight, appearance, vision]
metamorphosis (mĕt″ă-mor′fō-sĭs) [″ + *morphosis*, bringing into shape]
   m., fatty
   m., platelet
   m., retrograde
   m., structural
   m., viscous
Metamucil
metamyelocyte (mĕt″ă-mī-ĕl′ō-sīt)
Metandren
metanephrine (mĕt″ă-nĕf′rĭn)
metanephrogenic (mĕt″ă-nĕf′rō-jĕn′ĭk) [″ + *nephros*, kidney, + *gennan*, to produce]
metanephros (mĕt″ă-nĕf′rŏs) [″ + *nephros*, kidney]
metaneutrophil (mĕt-ă-nū′trō-fĭl) [″ + L. *neuter*, neither, + Gr. *philein*, to love]
metaphase (mĕt′ă-fāz) [″ +

phasis, appearance]

metaphrenia (mĕt″ă-frē′nē-ă) [″ + *phren,* mind]

metaphysis (mĕ-tăf′ĭ-sĭs) [Gr. *meta,* after, beyond, over, + *phyein,* to grow]

metaphysitis (mĕt″ă-fĭs-ī′tĭs) [″ + ″ + *itis,* inflammation]

metaplasia (mĕt″ă-plā′zē-ă) [″ + *plassein,* to form]
   m., myeloid

metaplasm (mĕt′ă-plăzm)

metaplastic (mĕt-ă-plăs′tĭk) [″ + *plastikos,* formed]

metapneumonic (mĕt″ă-nū-mŏn′ĭk)

metapophysis (mĕt″ă-pŏf′ĭ-sĭs) [″ + *apophysis,* a process]

Metaprel

metaprotein

metaproterenol sulfate (mĕt″ă-prō-tĕr′ĕ-nōl)

metapsychology (mĕt″ă-sī-kŏl′ō-jē)

metaraminol bitartrate (mĕt″ă-răm′ĭ-nōl)

metarteriole (mĕt″ăr-tē′rē-ōl)

metarubricyte (mĕt″ă-roo′brĭ-sīt)

metastable [″ + L. *stabilis,* stable]

metastasis (mĕ-tăs′tă-sis) [Gr. *methistanai,* to change]

metastasize (mĕ-tăs′tă-sīz)

metastatic (mĕt″ă-stăt′ĭk)

metastatic survey

metasternum (mĕt″ă-stĕr′nŭm)

metatarsal (mĕt″ă-tăr′săl)

metatarsalgia (mĕt″ă-tăr-săl′jē-ă) [″ + *tarsos,* flat of the foot, flat surface, edge of eyelid, + *algos,* pain]

metatarsectomy (mĕt″ă-tăr-sĕk′tō-mē) [″ + ″ + *ektome,* excision]

metatarsophalangeal (mĕt″ă-tăr″sō-fă-lăn′jē-ăl) [″ + ″ + *phalanx,* line of battle]

metatarsus (mĕt″ă-tăr′sŭs) [″ + *tarsos,* flat of the foot, flat surface, edge of eyelid]

metatarsus primus varus

metatarsus varus

metathalamus (mĕt″ă-thăl′ă-mŭs)

[″ + *thalamos,* chamber]

metathesis (mĕ-tăth′ĕ-sĭs) [″ + *thesis,* placement]

metatrophia (mĕt″ă-trō′fē-ă) [″ + *trophe,* nourishment]

metatrophic

metatypical (mĕt″ă-tĭp′ĭ-kăl)

metaxalone (mĕ-tăks′ă-lōn)

Metazoa [″ + *zoon,* animal]

Metchnikoff's theory (mĕch′nĭ-kŏfs) [Elie Metchnikoff, Russian zoologist in France, 1845–1916]

metencephalon (mĕt″ĕn-sĕf′ă-lŏn) [Gr. *meta,* after, beyond, over, + *enkephalos,* brain]

meteorism (mē′tē-or-ĭzm) [Gr. *meteorizein,* to raise up]

meteoropathy (mē″tē-ĕ-rŏp′ă-thē) [″ + *pathos,* disease, suffering]

meteorotropic (mē″tē-ĕ-rō-trŏp′ĭk) [″ + *trope,* a turn]

meteorotropism (mē″tē-ĕ-rŏt′rō-pĭzm)

meter [Gr. *metron,* measure]

metergasis (mĕt″ĕr-gā′sĭs) [Gr. *meta,* change, + *ergon,* work]

metestrus (mĕ-tĕs′trŭs) [″ + L. *oistros,* mad desire]

methacholine chloride (mĕth″ă-kō′lēn)

methacycline hydrochloride

methadone hydrochloride

methallenestril (mĕth″ăl-ĕ-nĕs′trĭl)

methamphetamine hydrochloride (mĕth″ăm-fĕt′ă-mēn)

methane

methandriol (mĕth-ăn′drē-ōl)

methandrostenolone (mĕth-ăn″drō-stĕn′ō-lōn)

methanol

methantheline bromide (mĕ-thăn′thĕ-lēn)

methapyrilene fumarate (mĕth″ă-pīr′ĭ-lēn)

methaqualone hydrochloride (mĕ-thă′kwă-lōn)

metharbital (mĕ-thăr′bĭ-tăl)

methazolamide (mĕth″ă-zō′lă-mīd)

methdilazine (mĕth-dī′lă-zēn)

methemalbumin (mĕt"hĕm-ăl-bū'mĭn)
methemoglobin (mĕt-hē"mō-glō'bĭn)
[Gr. *meta*, across, + *haima*,
blood, + L. *globus*, globe]
   m. reductase
methemoglobinemia (mĕt"hē-mō-
glōb"ĭ-nē'mē-ă) [" + " + "
+ *haima*, blood]
   m., congenital
methemoglobinuria (mĕt"hē-mō-
glōb"ĭ-nū'rē-ă) [" + " + " +
ouron, urine]
methenamine (mĕth-ĕn'ă-mēn)
   m. mandelate
methene
Methergine
methicillin sodium (mĕth"ĭ-sĭl'ĭn)
methimazole (mĕth-ĭm'ă-zōl)
methiodal sodium (mĕth-ī'ō-dăl)
methionine (mĕth-ī'ō-nīn)
methisazone (mĕ-thĭs'ă-zōn)
methixene hydrochloride (mĕ-
thĭks'ēn)
methocarbamol (mĕth"ō-kăr'bă-mŏl)
method [Gr. *methodos*]
methodology (mĕth"ō-dŏl'ō-jē) [" +
logos, word, reason]
methohexital sodium (mĕth"ō-
hĕk'sĭ-tăl)
methomania (mĕth"ō-mā'nē-ă) [Gr.
methe, drunkenness, + *mania*,
madness]
methotrexate (mĕth"ō-trĕk'sāt)
methotrimeprazine (mĕth"ō-trī-
mĕp'ră-zēn)
methoxamine hydrochloride (mĕ-
thŏk'să-mēn)
methoxsalen (mĕ-thŏk'să-lĕn)
methoxyflurane (mĕ-thŏk"sē-
floo'rān)
**methoxyphenamine hydrochlo-
ride** (mĕ-thŏk"sē-fĕn'ă-mēn)
methscopolamine bromide
(mĕth"skō-pŏl'ă-mēn)
methsuximide (mĕth-sŭk'sĭ-mīd)
methyclothiazide (mĕth"ĭ-klō-thī'ă-
zīd)
methyl (mĕth'ĭl) [Gr. *methy*, wine, +
hyle, wood]

   m. alcohol
   m. ether
   m. orange
   m. purine
   m. salicylate
   m. violet
methyl alcohol poisoning
methylate (mĕth'ĭ-lāt)
methylation (mĕth"ĭ-lā'shŭn)
methylatropine nitrate (mĕth"ĭl-
ăt'rō-pēn)
methylbenzethonium chloride
(mĕth"ĭl-bĕn"zĕ-thō'nē-ŭm)
methylcellulose
methylcytosine (mĕth"ĭl-sī'tō-sĭn)
methyldopa (mĕth"ĭl-dō'pă)
methyldopate hydrochloride
(mĕth"ĭl-dō'pāt)
methylene (mĕth'ĭ-lēn)
methylene blue (mĕth'ĭ-lēn)
methylenophil (mĕth"ĭ-lĕn'ō-fĭl)
methylergonovine maleate
(mĕth"ĭl-ĕr"gō-nō'vēn)
methylmalonic acidemia
methylparaben (mĕth"ĭl-păr'ă-bĕn)
methylphenidate hydrochloride
(mĕth"ĭl-fĕn'ĭ-dāt)
methylprednisolone (mĕth"ĭl-prĕd'nĭ-
sō-lōn)
methylrosaniline chloride (mĕth"ĭl-
rō-zăn'ĭ-lĭn)
methyltestosterone (mĕth"ĭl-tĕs-
tŏs'tĕr-ōn)
methylthiouracil (mĕth"ĭl-thī"ō-ū'ră-sĭl)
methyltransferase (mĕth"ĭl-
trăns'fĕr-ās)
methyprylon (mĕth"ĭ-prī'lŏn)
methysergide maleate (mĕth"ĭ-
sĕr'jĭd)
Meticorten
Meti-Derm
metmyoglobin (mĕt-mī"ō-glō'bĭn)
metocurine iodide (mĕt"ō-kū'rēn)
metonymy (mĕ-tŏn'ĭ-mē) [Gr. *meta*,
after, beyond, over, + *onyma*,
name]
metopagus (mĕ-tŏp'ă-gŭs) [Gr. *metopon*, forehead, + *pagos*, thing
fixed]

metopic (mē-tŏp′ĭk) [Gr. *metopon*, forehead]

metopion (mē-tō′pē-ŏn)

metopism (mĕt′ō-pĭzm)

metopodynia (mĕt″ō-pō-dĭn′ē-ă) [″ + *odyne*, pain]

metoprolol tartrate

metoxenous (mĕt″ŏk-sē′nŭs) [Gr. *meta*, change, + *xenos*, host]

metoxeny (mĕt-ŏk′sĕ-nē)

metra (mē′tră) [Gr.]

metralgia (mē-trăl′jē-ă) [Gr. *metra*, uterus, + *algos*, pain]

metratome (mē′tră-tōm) [″ + *tome*, a cutting, slice]

metratomy (mē-trăt′ō-mē)

metratonia (mē″tră-tō′nē-ă)

metratrophia (mē″tră-trō′fē-ă)

metre (mē′tĕr) [Gr. *metron*, measure]

metrectasia (mē″trĕk-tā′zē-ă) [Gr. *metra*, uterus, + *ektasis*, extension]

metrectopia (mē″trĕk-tō′pē-ă) [″ + *ektopos*, displaced]

metreurynter (mē-troo-rĭn′tĕr) [″ + *eurynein*, to stretch]

metreurysis (mē-troo′rĭ-sĭs)

metria (mē′trē-ă)

metric system

metriocephalic (mĕt″rē-ō-sĕ-făl′ĭk) [Gr. *metrios*, moderate, + *kephale*, head]

metritis (mĕ-trī′tĭs) [Gr. *metra*, uterus, + *itis*, inflammation]
  m., chronic

metrizamide

metro- [Gr. *metra*, uterus]

metrocarcinoma (mē″trō-kăr-sĭ-nō′mă) [″ + *karkinos*, cancer, + *oma*, tumor]

metrocele (mē′trō-sēl) [″ + *kele*, tumor, swelling]

metrocolpocele (mē″trō-kŏl′pō-sēl) [″ + *kolpos*, vagina, + *kele*, tumor, swelling]

metrocystosis (mē″trō-sĭs-tō′sĭs) [″ + *kystis*, cyst, + *osis*, condition]

metrodynia (mē″trō-dĭn′ē-ă) [″ + *odyne*, pain]

metrofibroma (mē-trō-fī-brō′mă) [″ + L. *fibra*, fiber, + *oma*, tumor]

metromalacia (mē″trō-măl-ā′shē-ă) [″ + *malakia*, softness]

metromalacosis (mē″trō-măl-ă-kō′sĭs) [″ + ″ + *osis*, condition]

metronidazole

metronome (mĕt′rō-nōm) [Gr. *metron*, measure, + *nomos*, law]

metronoscope (mĕ-trŏn′ō-skōp)

metroparalysis (mē″trō-pă-răl′ĭ-sĭs) [Gr. *metra*, uterus, + *paralyein*, to loosen, disable]

metropathia hemorrhagica (mē″trō-păth′ē-ă hĕm″ō-răj′ĭk-ă) [″ + *pathos*, disease, suffering, + *haima*, blood, + *rhegnynai*, to burst forth]

metropathic (mē″trō-păth′ĭk)

metropathy (mē-trŏp′ă-thē)

metroperitoneal (mē″trō-pĕr″ĭ-tō-nē′ăl) [″ + *peritonaion*, stretched around or over]

metroperitonitis (mē″trō-pĕr″ĭ-tō-nī′tĭs) [″ + ″ + *itis*, inflammation]

metrophlebitis (mē″trō-flē-bī′tĭs) [″ + *phleps*, blood vessel, vein, + *itis*, inflammation]

metroplasty (mē″trō-plăs′tē) [″ + *plastikos*, formed]

metroptosis (mē-trō-tō′sĭs) [″ + *ptosis*, fall, falling]

metrorrhagia (mĕt″rō-rā′jē-ă) [″ + *rhegnynai*, to burst forth]

metrorrhea (mē″trō-rē′ă) [″ + *rhein*, to flow]

metrorrhexis (mē″trō-rĕk′sĭs) [″ + *rhexis*, rupture]

metrosalpingitis (mē″trō-săl″pĭn-jī′tĭs) [″ + *salpinx*, tube, + *itis*, inflammation]

metrosalpingography (mē″trō-săl″pĭng-gŏg′ră-fē) [″ + ″ + *graphein*, to write]

metrostaxis (mē″trō-stăk′sĭs) [″ +

staxis, a dripping]

metrostenosis (mē″trō-stĕn-ō′sĭs)
[″ + *stenosis,* act of narrowing]

metrotherapy [Gr. *metron,* measure,
+ *therapeia,* treatment]

metrotome (mē′trō-tōm) [Gr. *metra,*
uterus, + *tome,* a cutting, slice]

metrotomy (mē-trŏt′ō-mē)

metrourethrotome (mĕt″rō-ū-rē′thrō-
tōm) [Gr. *metron,* measure, + *ourethra,* urethra, + *tome,* a cutting,
slice]

-metry [Gr. *metrein,* to measure]

metyrapone (mĕ-tēr′ă-pōn)

mev *million electron volts*

Mexate

Meynert's commissure (mī′nĕrts)
[Theodor H. Meynert, Austrian neurologist, 1833–1892]

Meynet's nodosities (mā-nāz′) [Paul
C. H. Meynet, Fr. physician, 1831–
1892]

M.F.D. *minimum fatal dose*

μg. *microgram*

Mg *magnesium*

mg *milligram*

mgh *milligram hour*

MHC *major histocompatibility complex*

mho (mō)

miasm, miasma (mī′ăzm, mī-ăz′mă)
[Gr. *miasma,* stain]

miasmatic (mī″ăz-măt′ĭk)

mica (mī′kă) [L.]

mication (mī-kā′shŭn)

micella, micelle (mī-sĕl′ă, mī-sĕl′)

miconazole nitrate (mī-kŏn′ă-zōl)

micra

micracusia (mī″kră-kū′zē-ă) [Gr.
mikros, small, + *akousis,* hearing]

micrencephalon (mī″krĕn-sĕf′ă-lon)
[Gr. *mikros,* small, + *enkephalos,*
brain]

micrencephalous (mī″krĕn-sĕf′ă-lŭs)

micrencephaly (mī″krĕn-sĕf′ă-lē)

micro-, micr- [Gr. *mikros,* small]

microabscess (mī″krō-ăb′sĕs) [″ +
L. *abscessus,* a going away]

microaerophilic (mī″krō-ā′ĕr-ō-fĭl′ĭk)

[″ + *aer,* air, + *philein,* to
love]

microanalysis

microanatomy

microaneurysm (mī″krō-ăn′ū-rĭzm)
[″ + *aneurysma,* a widening]

microangiitis (mī″krō-ăn″jē-ī′tĭs)

microangiopathy (mī″krō-ăn″jē-ŏp′ă-
thē) [″ + *angeion,* vessel, +
pathos, disease, suffering]
  m., thrombotic

microangioscopy (mī″krō-ăn″jē-
ŏs′kō-pē) [″ + ″ + *skopein,* to
examine]

microbalance (mī′krō-băl″ăns)

microbe (mī′krōb) [″ + *bios,* life]

microbial (mī-krō′bē-ăl)

microbic (mī-krōb′ĭk)

microbicidal (mī-krō″bī-sī′dăl) [″ +
bios, life, + L. *cida* fr. *caedere,* to
kill]

microbicide (mī-krō′bī-sīd)

microbiology (mī″krō-bī-ŏl′ō-jē) [″ +
bios, life, + *logos,* word, reason]

microbiophobia (mī″krō-bī″ō-fō′bē-ă)
[″ + ″ + *phobos,* fear]

microbiota (mī″krō-bī-ō′tă)

microbiotic (mī″krō-bī-ŏt′ĭk)

microbism (mī′krōb-ĭzm) [″ + *bios,*
life, + *-ismos,* condition]

microblast (mī′krō-blăst) [″ +
blastos, germ]

microblepharism, microblephary
(mī″krō-blĕf′ăr-ĭzm, -ăr-ē) [″ +
blepharon, eyelid]

microbodies

microbrachia (mī″krō-brā′kē-ă) [″ +
brachion, arm]

microbrachius (mī″krō-brā′kē-ŭs)
[″ + *brachion,* arm]

microcalorie (mī″krō-kăl′ō-rē) [Gr.
mikros, small, + L. *calor,* heat]

microcardia (mī″krō-kăr′dē-ă) [″ +
kardia, heart]

microcaulia (mī″krō-kaw′lē-ă) [″ +
kaulos, penis]

microcentrum (mī″krō-sĕn′trŭm) [″ +
kentron, center]

microcephalia (mī″krō-sĕf-ā′lē-ă)
[″ + kephale, head]
microcephalic (mī″krō-sĕf-ăl′ĭk)
microcephalous (mī″krō-sĕf′ă-lŭs)
microcephalus (mī″krō-sĕf′ă-lŭs)
microcephaly (mī″krō-sĕf′ă-lē)
microcheilia (mī″krō-kī′lē-ă) [Gr.
mikros, small, + cheilos, lip]
microchemistry (mī″krō-kĕm′ĭs-trē)
[″ + chemeia, chemistry]
microchiria, microcheiria (mī″krō-
kī′rē-ă) [″ + cheir, hand]
microcinematography (mī″krō-sĭn″ĕ-
mă-tŏg′ră-fē) [″ + kinema, motion,
+ graphein, to write]
microcirculation (mī″krō-sĭr″kū-
lā′shŭn)
Micrococcaceae (mī″krō-kŏk-ā′sē-ē)
Micrococcus (mī″krō-kŏk′ŭs) [Gr.
mikros, small, + kokkos, berry]
M. albus
M. melitensis
micrococcus (mī″krō-kŏk′ŭs)
microcolon
microcoria (mī″krō-kō′rē-ă) [″ +
kore, pupil]
microcornea
microcoulomb (mī″krō-koo′lŏm)
microcrystalline (mī″krō-krĭs′tăl-
īn, -ĕn)
microcurie
microcurie-hour
microcyst (mī′krō-sĭst)
microcytase (mī″krō-sī′tās) [″ +
kytos, cell, + -ase, enzyme]
microcyte
microcythemia (mī″krō-sī-thē′mē-ă)
[″ + ″ + haima, blood]
microcytosis
microdactylia (mī″krō-dăk-tĭl′ē-ă)
[″ + daktylos, finger]
microdetermination
microdissection (mī″krō-dī-sĕk′shŭn)
[″ + L. dissectio, a cutting apart]
microdont (mī′krō-dŏnt) [″ +
odous, tooth]
microdontia (mī″krō-dŏn′shē-ă) [″ +
odous, tooth]

microdontism (mī″krō-dŏn′tĭzm) [″ +
″ + -ismos, condition]
microdose
microelectrophoresis
microembolus (mī″krō-ĕm′bō-lŭs)
[″ + embolos, plug]
microencephaly (mī″krō-ĕn-sĕf′ă-lē)
[″ + enkephalos, brain]
microenvironment
microerythrocyte (mī″krō-ĕ-rĭth′rō-sīt)
[″ + erythros, red, + kytos,
cell]
microfarad (mī-krō-făr′ăd)
microfauna (mī″krō-faw′nă)
microfibril (mī″krō-fī′brĭl)
microfiche (mī′krō-fēsh″) [Gr. mikros,
small, + Fr. fiche, index card]
microfilament (mī″krō-fĭl′ă-mĕnt)
microfilaremia (mī″krō-fĭl″ă-rē′mē-ă)
microfilaria (mī″krō-fī-lā′rē-ă)
microfilm
microflora (mī″krō-flō′ră)
microgamete (mī-krō-găm′ēt) [″ +
gametes, spouse]
microgametocyte (mī″krō-gă-mē′tō-
sīt) [″ + ″ + kytos, cell]
microgamy (mī-krŏg′ă-mē)
microgastria (mī″krō-găs′trē-ă) [″ +
gaster, stomach]
microgenia (mī″krō-jĕn′ē-ă) [″ +
geneion, chin]
microgenitalism (mī″krō-jĕn′ĭ-tăl-īzm)
[″ + L. genitalis, to beget, +
Gr. -ismos, condition]
microglia (mī-krŏg′lē-ă) [″ + glia,
glue]
microgliacyte (mī″krŏg′lē-ă-sīt) [″
+ ″ + kytos, cell]
microglioma (mī″krō-glī-ō′mă) [″ +
″ + oma, tumor]
microglossia (mī-krō-glŏs′ē-ă) [″ +
glossa, tongue]
micrognathia (mī-krō-nā′thē-ă) [″ +
gnathos, jaw]
microgonioscope (mī″krō-gō′nē-ō-
skōp) [″ + gonia, angle, +
skopein, to examine]
microgram

micrograph (mī'krō-grăf) [Gr. *mikros,* small, + *graphein,* to write]

micrography (mī-krŏg'ră-fē)

microgyria (mī-krō-jīr'ē-ă) [" + *gyros,* circle]

microgyrus (mī"krō-jī'rŭs) [" + *gyros,* circle]

microhematocrit (mī"krō-hē-măt'ō-krĭt)

microhepatia (mī"krō-hē-păt'ē-ă) [" + *hepar,* liver]

microhm (mī'krōm)

microincineration

microinjection

microinvasion (mī"krō-ĭn-vā'zhŭn)

microleakage

microlentia (mī"krō-lĕn'shē-ă)

microlesion (mī"krō-lē'zhŭn)

microleukoblast [" + *leukos,* white, + *blastos,* germ]

microliter (mī'krō-lē"tĕr)

microlith (mī'krō-lĭth) [" + *lithos,* stone]

microlithiasis (mī"krō-lĭ-thī'ă-sĭs) [" + " + *-iasis,* state or condition of]

m., pulmonary alveolar

micromanipulator

micromastia (mī-krō-măs'tē-ă)

micromazia (mī-krō-mā'zē-ă) [Gr. *mikros,* small, + *mazos,* breast]

micromelia (mī"krō-mē'lē-ă) [" + *melos,* limb]

micromelus (mī-krŏm'ē-lŭs) [" + *melos,* limb]

micromere (mī'krō-mēr) [" + *meros,* part]

micrometer (mī'krō-mē-ter; mī-krŏm'ē-tĕr)

micromethod (mī"krō-mĕth'ŏd)

micrometry (mī-krŏm'ē-trē) [" + *metron,* measure]

micromicrogram (mī"krō-mī'krō-grăm)

micromicron (mī"krō-mī'krŏn)

micromillimeter (mī-krō-mĭl'ĭ-mē-tĕr)

micromole (mī'krō-mōl)

micromolecular (mī"krō-mō-lĕk'ū-lăr)

Micromonospora (mī"krō-mō-nŏs'por-ă)

micromyces (mī-krŏm'ĭ-sēs) [Gr. *mikros,* small, + *mykes,* fungus]

micromyelia (mī"krō-mī-ē'lē-ă) [" + *myelos,* marrow]

micromyeloblast (mī-krō-mī'ĕl-ō-blăst) [" + *myelos,* marrow, + *blastos,* germ]

micromyelolymphocyte (mī"krō-mī"ĕ-lō-lĭm'fō-sīt) [" + " + L. *lympha,* lymph, + Gr. *kytos,* cell]

micron

microne (mī'krŏn)

microneedle

micronize

micronodular (mī"krō-nŏd'ū-lăr)

micronucleus (mī-krō-nū'klē-ŭs) [" + L. *nucleus,* kernel]

micronutrient (mī"krō-nū'trē-ĕnt)

micronychia (mī"krō-nĭk'ē-ă) [" + *onyx,* nail]

microorganism (mī-krō-or'găn-ĭzm) [" + *organon,* organ, + *-ismos,* condition]

m., pathologic

microparasite (mī"krō-păr'ă-sīt)

micropathology (mī"krō-păth-ŏl'ō-jē) [Gr. *mikros,* small, + *pathos,* disease, suffering, + *logos,* word, reason]

micropenis (mī"krō-pē'nĭs)

microphage, microphagus (mī'krō-fāj, mī-krŏf'ă-gŭs) [" + *phagein,* to eat]

microphagocyte (mī"krō-făg'ō-sīt) [" + " + *kytos,* cell]

microphakia (mī"krō-fā'kē-ă) [" + *phakos,* lens]

microphallus (mī-krō-făl'ŭs) [" + *phallos,* penis]

microphobia (mī-krō-fō'bē-ă) [" + *phobos,* fear]

microphone (mī'krō-fōn) [" + *phone,* voice]

microphonia (mī-krō-fō'nē-ă)

microphonoscope (mī"krō-fō'nō-skōp) [Gr. *mikros,* small, + *phone,* voice, + *skopein,* to examine]

microphotograph (mī"krō-fō'tō-grăf)

[" + *phos*, light, + *graphein*, to write]

microphthalmia (mī-krŏf-thăl′mē-ă) [" + *ophthalmos*, eye]

microphthalmus (mī-krŏf-thăl′mŭs)

microphysics (mī-krō-fĭz′ĭks)

microphyte (mī′krō-fīt) [" + *phyton*, plant]

micropia (mī-krō′pē-ă) [" + *opsis*, sight, appearance, vision]

micropipette

microplasia (mī″krō-plā′zē-ă) [" + *plassein*, to form]

microplethysmography (mī″krō-plĕth″ĭs-mŏg′ră-fē) [" + *plethysmos*, increase, + *graphein*, to write]

micropodia (mī-krō-pō′dē-ă) [" + *pous*, feet]

micropolariscope (mī″krō-pōl-ăr′ĭ-skōp)

microprobe (mī′krō-prōb)

microprojection

microprosopia (mī″krō-prō-sō′pē-ă) [" + *prosopon*, face]

micropsia (mī-krŏp′sē-ă) [" + *opsis*, sight, appearance, vision]

micropuncture (mī″krō-pŭnk′chŭr)

micropus (mī-krō′pŭs) [" + *pous*, feet]

micropyle (mī′krō-pīl) [" + *pyle*, gate]

microradiography (mī″krō-rā″dē-ŏg′ră-fē)

microrefractometer (mī″krō-rē″frăk-tŏm′ĕ-tĕr)

microrespirometer (mī″krō-rĕs″pī-rŏm′ĕ-tĕr)

microrhinia (mī″krō-rĭn′ē-ă) [" + *rhis*, nose]

microscelous (mī-krŏs′kĕ-lŭs) [" + *skelos*, leg]

microscope (mī′krō-skōp) [" + *skopein*, to examine]

    m., binocular
    m., compound
    m., dark-field
    m., electron

    m., light
    m., operating
    m., phase
    m., polarization
    m., scanning electron
    m., simple
    m., slit-lamp
    m., stereoscopic
    m., ultraviolet
    m., x-ray

microscopic, microscopical (mī-krō-skŏp′ĭk, -ĭ-kăl)

microscopy (mī-krŏs′kōp-ē)

microsecond (mī′krō-sĕk″ŭnd)

microseme (mī′krō-sēm) [Gr. *mikros*, small, + *sema*, sign]

microsmatic (mī″krŏs-măt′ĭk) [" + *osmasthai*, to smell]

microsoma (mī″krō-sō′mă) [" + *soma*, body]

microsome (mī′krō-sōm)

microsomia (mī-krō-sō′mē-ă)

microspectrophotometry (mī″krō-spĕk″trō-fō-tŏm′ĕ-trē)

microspectroscope [" + L. *spectrum*, image, + Gr. *skopein*, to examine]

microspheres

microspherocyte (mī″krō-sfē′rō-sīt) [" + *sphaira*, globe, + *kytos*, cell]

microspherocytosis (mī″krō-sfē″rō-sī-tō′sīs) [" + " + *osis*, condition]

microsphygmia (mī-krō-sfĭg′mē-ă) [" + *sphygmos*, pulse]

microsplanchnic (mī″krō-splănk′nĭk)

microsplenia (mī-krō-splē′nē-ă) [" + *splen*, spleen]

microsporid (mī-krŏs′pō-rĭd)

Microsporon (mī-krŏs′por-rŏn) [" + *sporos*, seed]

microsporosis (mī-krō-spō-rō′sīs)

Microsporum (mī″krŏs′por-ŭm)
    M. audouini
    M. canis

microstomia (mī-krō-stō′mē-ă) [" + *stoma*, mouth, opening]

microstrabismus (mī″krō-stră-bĭs′mŭs) [" + *strabismos*, a squinting] microsurgery

microsyringe

microthelia (mī″krō-thē′lē-ă) [″ + thele, nipple]

microtia (mī-krō′shē-ă) [″ + ous, ear]

microtome (mī′krō-tōm) [″ + tome, a cutting, slice]
   m., freezing
   m., sliding

microtomy (mī-krŏt′ō-mē)

microtonometer (mī″krō-tō-nŏm′ĕ-tĕr)

microtrauma (mī″krō-traw′mă)

microtropia (mī″krō-trō′pē-ă) [″ + trope, a turning]

microtubule (mī″krō-tū′būl)

microtus (mī-krō′tŭs) [″ + ous, ear]

microvascular (mī″krō-văs′kū-lăr)

microvilli (mī″krō-vĭl′ī) [L., tufts of hair]

microvolt

microwave (mī′krō-wāv)

microxycyte (mī-krŏk′sī-sīt) [Gr. mikros, small, + oxys, sharp, + kytos, cell]

microxyphil (mī-krŏk′sī-fĭl) [″ + ″ + philein, to love]

microzoon (mī″krō-zō′ŏn) [″ + zoon, animal]

micrurgy (mī′krŭr-jē) [″ + ergos, work]

miction (mĭk′shŭn)

micturate (mĭk′tū-rāt) [L. micturire]

micturition (mĭk-tū-rĭ′shŭn)

micturition syncope

MICU medical intensive care unit

MID minimum infective dose

midazolam hydrochloride

midbody (mĭd′bŏd-ē)

midbrain [AS. mid, middle, + braegen, brain]

midcarpal (mĭd-kăr′păl)

middle lobe syndrome

midge (mĭj) [ME. migge]

midget

midgut [AS. mid, middle, + gut, intestine]

midline (mĭd′lĭn)

midoccipital (mĭd″ŏk-sĭp′ĭ-tăl)

midpain (mĭd′pān)

midplane (mĭd′plān)

midriff (mĭd′rĭf) [″ + hrif, belly]

midsection (mĭd-sĕk′shŭn) [″ + L. secare, to cut]

midsternum (mĭd-stĕr′nŭm)

midstream specimen

midtarsal (mĭd-tăr′săl)

midwife [″ + wif, wife]
   m., nurse-

midwifery (mĭd-wĭf′ĕr-ē)

migraine (mī′grān) [Fr. from Gr. hemikrania, half skull]

migration (mī-grā′shŭn) [L. migrare, to move from place to place]
   m., internal, of ovum
   m. of leukocytes
   m. of testicle

migratory

Mikulicz's drain (mĭk′ū-lĭch″ĕs) [Johann von Mikulicz-Radecki, Polish surgeon, 1850–1905]

Mikulicz's mask

Mikulicz's pad

Mikulicz's syndrome

mildew [AS. mildeaw]

milia (mĭl′ē-ă)

miliaria (mĭl-ē-ā′rē-ă) [L. milium, millet]
   m. crystallina
   m. profunda
   m. rubra

miliary (mĭl′ē-ă-rē) [L. miliaris, like a millet seed]

miliary fever

miliary tubercles

miliary tuberculosis

milieu (mē-lyŭ′) [Fr.]
   m. interieur

milieu therapy

military antishock trousers

milium (mĭl′ē-ŭm) [L., millet seed]
   m., colloid

milk [AS. meolc]
   m., acidophilus
   m., butter-
   m., casein
   m., certified
   m., condensed

m., cow's
m., evaporated
m., filled
m., fortified
m., homogenized
m., instant dry nonfat
m., lactic acid evaporated
m., low fat, 1%
m., low fat, 2%
m., modified
m., mother's
m., nonfat
m. of bismuth
m., pasteurized
m., protein
m., red
m., ropy
m., skim
m., sour
m., sterilized
m., uterine
m., uviol
m., vegetable
m., vitamin D
m., whole
m., witch's
milk-alkali syndrome
milker's nodules
milk fever
milking
milk leg
Milkman's syndrome (mĭlk'mănz) [Louis A. Milkman, U.S. roentgenologist, 1895–1951]
milk of magnesia
milk teeth
milk tumor
Miller-Abbott tube [T. Grier Miller, U.S. physician, b. 1886; W. Osler Abbott, U.S. physician, 1902–1943]
milli- [L. milli, thousand]
milliammeter
milliampere (mĭl"ē-ăm'pēr)
milliampere minute
milliampere-seconds
millibar (mĭl'ĭ-băr)
millicoulomb (mĭl"ĭ-koo'lŏm)
millicurie (mĭl"ĭ-kū'rē)

millicurie hour
milliequivalent
milligram (mĭl'ĭ-grăm)
millilambert (mĭl"ĭ-lăm'bĕrt)
milliliter
millimeter
millimicrocurie (mĭl"ĭ-mī"krō-kū'rē)
millimicrogram (mĭl"ĭ-mī'krō-grăm)
millimicron (mĭl-ĭ-mī'krŏn)
millimole (mĭl'ĭ-mōl)
milling-in
millinormal (mĭl"ĭ-nor'măl)
milliosmole (mĭl"ē-ŏs'mōl)
millipede (mĭl'ĭ-pēd)
millisecond (mĭl"ĭ-sĕk'ŏnd)
millivolt (mĭl'ĭ-vōlt)
Milontin
milphae (mĭl'fē) [Gr. milphai]
milphosis (mĭl-fō'sĭs) [Gr.]
Milroy's disease (mĭl'roys) [William F. Milroy, U.S. physician, 1853–1942]
Miltown
Milwaukee brace
mimesis [Gr.]
mimetic, mimic (mī-mĕt'ĭk, mĭm'ĭk) [Gr. mimetikos]
mimmation (mī-mā'shŭn)
mimosis (mī-mō'sĭs)
min. minim; minute
Minamata disease (mĭn"ă-maw'tă)
mind [AS. gemynd]
mineral [L. minerale]
mineral acid
mineral compounds
mineralization (mĭn"ĕr-ăl-ĭ-zā'shŭn)
mineralocorticoid (mĭn"ĕr-ăl-ō-kor'tĭ-koyd)
mineral oil
mineral spring
mineral water
minification
minim (mĭn'ĭm) [L. minimum, least]
minimal (mĭn'ĭ-măl)
minimal brain damage
minimal brain dysfunction
minimal cerebral dysfunction
minimal change disease
minimal dose

minimum (mĭn'ĭ-mŭm)
minimum daily requirements
minimum lethal dose
Minin light (mĭn'ĭn) [A. V. Minin, Russian surgeon]
Minipress
Minocin
minocycline hydrochloride (mĭ-nō-sī'klēn)
minor
    m., emancipated
Minot-Murphy diet (mī'nŏt) [George R. Minot, U.S. physician, 1885–1950; William P. Murphy, U.S. physician, b. 1892]
minoxidil
Mintezol
minute volume
mio- (mī'ō) [Gr. meion, less]
miocardia (mī-ō-kăr'dē-ă) [" + kardia, heart]
Miochol
miodidymus (mī"ō-dĭd'ĭ-mŭs) [" + didymos, twin]
miolecithal (mī"ō-lĕs'ĭ-thăl) [" + lekithos, egg yolk]
mionectic (mī-ō-nĕk'tĭk) [Gr. meionektikos, disposed to taking too little]
mioplasmia
miopragia (mī-ō-prā'jē-ă) [Gr. meion, less, + prassein, to perform]
miopus (mī'ō-pŭs) [" + ops, face]
miosis (mī-ō'sĭs) [Gr. meiosis, a lessening]
Miostat
miotic
miracidium (mī"ră-sĭd'ē-ŭm) [Gr. meirakidion, lad]
miracle, medical
mire (mēr) [L. mirari, to look at]
mirror [Fr. miroir]
    m., dental
miryachit (mĭr-ē-ă-chĭt) [Russian]
mis- [AS. mis, wrong]
misanthropia (mĭs"ăn-thrō'pē-ă) [" + Gr. anthropos, man]
miscarriage [" + L. carrus, cart]
misce (mĭs'ē) [L., mix]

miscegenation (mĭs"ĕ-jē-nā'shŭn) [L. miscere, to mix, + genus, race]
miscible (mĭs'ĭ-bl)
misocainia (mĭs-ō-kī'nē-ă) [Gr. miseio, to hate, + kainos, new]
misogamy (mī-sŏg'ă-mē) [" + gamos, marriage]
misogynist (mĭs-ŏj'ĭ-nĭst) [" + gyne, woman]
misogyny (mĭs-ŏj'ĭn-ē)
misologia (mĭs-ō-lō'jē-ă) [Gr. miseio, to hate, + logos, word, reason]
misoneism (mĭs-ō-nē'ĭzm) [" + neos, new]
misopedia (mĭ-sō-pē'dē-ă) [" + Gr. pais, child]
Mist., mist. mistura
mister
mistura (mĭs-tū'ră) [L., mixture]
Mitchell's disease (mĭch'ĕlz) [Silas W. Mitchell, U.S. neurologist, 1829–1914]
mite (mīt) [AS.]
    m., follicle
    m., itch
    m., mange
    m., red
mitella (mī-tĕl'ă) [L.]
Mithracin
mithramycin (mĭth"ră-mī'sĭn)
mithridatism (mĭth'rĭ-dăt"ĭzm) [Mithridates, king of Pontus, 132–63 B.C., supposed to have acquired immunity in this fashion]
miticide (mī'tĭ-sīd) [AS. mite, mite, + L. caedere, to kill]
mitigated (mĭt'ĭ-gāt-ĕd) [L. mitigare, to soften]
mitis (mī'tĭs) [L., mild]
mitochondria (mĭt"ō-kŏn'drē-ă) [Gr. mitos, thread, + chondros, cartilage]
mitogen (mī'tō-jĕn)
mitogenesis (mī"tō-jĕn'ĕ-sĭs) [" + osis, condition, + genesis, generation, birth]
mitoma, mitome [Gr. mitos, thread]
mitomycin (mī"tō-mī'sĭn)

mitoplasm (mī'tō-plăzm) [" + plassein, to form]
mitosis (mī-tō'sĭs) [" + osis, condition]
   m., heterotypic
   m., homeotypic
mitosome (mī'tō-sōm) [Gr. mitos, thread, + soma, body]
mitotane (mī'tō-tān)
mitotic (mī-tŏt'ĭk)
mitral (mī'trăl)
mitral commissurotomy
mitral disease
mitralization (mī"trăl-ĭ-zā'shŭn)
mitral murmur
mitral orifice
mitral regurgitation
mitral stenosis
mitral valve
mitral valve prolapse
mittelschmerz (mĭt'ĕl-shmārts) [Ger.]
Mittendorf's dot [20th century U.S. physician]
mix (mĭks) [L. mixtus, to mix]
mixed [L. mixtus]
mixoscopia [Gr. mixis, intercourse, + skopein, to examine]
mixture (mĭks'tūr) [L. mistura]
MKS, mks meter-kilogram-second
ml milliliter
M.L.A. left mentoanterior
M.L.D., m.l.d. minimum lethal dose
mM millimole
mm millimeter
mmm millimicron
Mn manganese
mnemasthenia (nē"măs-thē'nē-ă) [Gr. mneme, memory, + a-, not, + sthenos, strength]
mnemic (nē'mĭk)
mnemonics (nē-mŏn'ĭks) [Gr. mnemonikos, pert. to memory]
M.O. Medical Officer
Mo molybdenum
mo. month
mobile [L. mobilis]
mobile arm support
mobile spasm

mobility [L. mobilitas]
   m., tooth
mobility training
mobilization (mō"bĭl-ĭ-zā'shŭn)
   m., stapes
mobilize (mō'bĭl-īz)
Möbius' disease (mē'bē-ŭs) [Paul J. Möbius, Ger. neurologist, 1853 – 1907]
Möbius' sign
modal (mōd'l) [L. modus, mode]
modality
Modane
Modane Soft
mode (mōd)
model
   m., animal
modeling
modem modulator-demodulator
moderated
modification (mŏd"ĭ-fĭ-kā'shŭn)
modiolus (mō-dī'ō-lŭs) [L., hub]
modulation (mŏd"ū-lā'shŭn)
modulus (mŏj'ŭ-lŭs) [L., a small measure]
modus [L., mode]
modus operandi
mogilalia (mŏj-ĭ-lā'lē-ă) [Gr. mogis, with difficulty, + lalia, chatter, prattle]
mogiphonia (mŏj-ĭ-fō'nē-ă) [" + phone, voice]
Mohrenheim's space (mor'ĕn-hīmz) [Baron J. J. Freiherr von Mohrenheim, Austrian surgeon, 1759 – 1799]
Mohs' chemosurgery technique [F. E. Mohs, U.S. surgeon, 1910 – 1979]
moiety (moy'ĕ-tē) [Fr. moitié, fr. L. medietas, middle]
moist (moyst)
mol mole
molal (mō'lăl)
molality (mō-lăl'ĭ-tē)
molar [L. molaris, grinding; moles, a mass]
molariform (mōl-ăr'ĭ-form)
molarity
molar solution
mold
molding

mole (mōl) [AS. *mael*; L. *moles*, a shapeless mass; Ger. *Mol*, abbr. for *Molekulargewicht*, molecular weight]
   m., blood
   m., Breus'
   m., carneous
   m., false
   m., fleshy
   m., hydatid
   m., pigmented
   m., stone
   m., true
   m., vascular
   m., vesicular
molecular (mō-lĕk'ū-lăr) [L. *molecula*, little mass]
molecular biology
molecular disease
molecular layer
molecular lesion
molecular weight
molecule (mŏl'ĕ-kūl) [L. *molecula*, little mass]
molimen (mō-lĭ'mĕn) [L., effort]
Mol-Iron
Moll's glands [Jacob A. Moll, Dutch oculist, 1832–1914]
mollities (mŏl-ĭsh'ē-ēz) [L.]
   m. ossium
mollusc, mollusk
Mollusca
molluscous (mŏ-lŭs'kŭs)
molluscum (mŏ-lŭs'kŭm) [L., soft]
   m. contagiosum
   m. fibrosum
molt
mol. wt. *molecular weight*
molybdenum (mō-lĭb'dĕ-nŭm)
molysmophobia (mō-lĭz"mō-fō'bē-ă) [Gr. *molysma*, stain, + *phobia*, fear]
momentum (mō-mĕn'tŭm) [L.]
monad [Gr. *monas*, a unit]
monamide (mŏn-ăm'ĭd)
monamine (mŏn-ăm'ĭn)
monarthric (mŏn-ăr'thrĭk) [Gr. *monos*, single, + *arthron*, joint]
monarthritis (mŏn"ăr-thrī'tĭs) [" +

" + *itis*, inflammation]
monarticular (mŏn-ăr-tĭk'ŭ-lăr)
monaster (mŏn-ăs'tĕr) [" + *aster*, star]
monathetosis (mŏn"ăth-ē-tō'sĭs) [" + *athetos*, not fixed, + *osis*, condition]
monatomic (mŏn"ă-tŏm'ĭk) [" + *atomos*, indivisible]
monaural (mŏn-aw'răl)
monaxonic (mŏn"ăk-sŏn'ĭk) [" + Gr. *axon*, axis]
Mondonesi's reflex (mŏn-dō-nā'zēz) [Filippo Mondonesi, It. physician]
Mondor's disease (mŏn'dorz) [Henri Mondor, Fr. physician, 1885–1962]
monecious (mŏn-ē'shŭs)
monesthetic (mŏn"ĕs-thĕt'ĭk) [Gr. *monos*, single, + *aisthesis*, feeling, perception]
monestrous (mŏn-ĕs'trŭs)
mongolian spots (mŏn-gō'lē-ăn)
mongolism
mongoloid (mŏn'gō-loyd)
monilethrix (mŏn-ĭl'ĕ-thrĭks) [L. *monile*, necklace, + Gr. *thrix*, hair]
Monilia [L. *monile*, necklace]
monilial (mō-nĭl'ē-ăl)
moniliasis (mō"nĭ-lī'ă-sĭs)
moniliform (mŏn-ĭl'ĭ-form) [" + *forma*, shape]
moniliid (mō-nĭl'ē-ĭd)
moniliosis (mō-nĭl-ē-ō'sĭs)
monitor (mŏn'ĭ-tor) [L., one who warns]
   m., blood pressure
   m., cardiac
   m., fetal
   m., Holter
   m., personal radiation
   m., temperature
mono-, mon- [Gr. *monos*, single]
monoacidic (mŏn"ō-ă-sĭd'ĭk)
monoamide
monoamine
monoamine oxidase inhibitors
monoanesthesia (mŏn"ō-ăn-ĕs-thē'sē-ă)
monobacillary (mŏn"ō-băs'ĭ-lā"rē)
monobacterial (mŏn"ō-băk-tē'rē-ăl)

monobasic (mŏn-ō-bā′sĭk) [″ + basis, a base]

monobenzone (mŏn″ō-bĕn′zōn)

monoblast (mŏn′ō-blăst) [″ + blastos, germ]

monoblastoma (mŏn″ō-blăs-tō′mă) [″ + ″ + oma, tumor]

monoblepsia (mŏn-ō-blĕp′sē-ă) [″ + blepsis, sight]

monobrachius (mŏn″ō-brā′kē-ŭs) [″ + brachion, arm]

monobromated (mŏn″ō-brō′māt-ĕd)

monocalcic (mŏn-ō-kăl′sĭk)

monocardian (mŏn-ō-kăr′dē-ăn) [″ + kardia, heart]

monocelled (mŏn′ō-sĕld)

monocephalus (mŏn″ō-sĕf′ă-lŭs) [″ + kephale, head]

monochord (mŏn′ō-kord) [″ + chorde, cord]

monochorea (mŏn″ō-kō-rē′ă) [″ + choreia, dance]

monochorionic (mŏn-ō-kor″ē-ŏn′ĭk)

monochromasy (mŏn″ō-krō-mā′sē) [″ + chroma, color]

monochromatic (mŏn″ō-krō-măt′ĭk)

monochromatism (mŏn″ō-krō′mă-tĭzm) [Gr. monos, single, + chroma, color, + -ismos, condition]

monochromatophil (mŏn″ō-krō-măt′ō-fĭl) [″ + ″ + philein, to love]

monochromator (mŏn-ō-krō′mă-tor)

Monoclate

monoclinic (mŏn″ō-klin′ĭk) [″ + klinein, to incline]

monoclonal (mŏn″ō-klōn′ăl)

monoclonal antibodies

monococcus (mŏn-ō-kŏk′ŭs) [″ + kokkos, berry]

monocontaminated (mŏn″ō-kŏn-tăm′ĭ-nāt″ĕd)

monocrotic (mŏn″ō-krŏt′ĭk) [″ + krotos, beat]

monocular (mŏn-ŏk′ū-lar) [″ + L. oculus, eye]

monoculus (mŏn-ŏk′ū-lŭs)

monocyclic (mŏn″ō-sī′klĭk)

monocyesis (mŏn″ō-sī-ē′sīs) [″ + kyesis, pregnancy]

monocyte (mŏn′ō-sīt) [″ + kytos, cell]

monocytic (mŏn-ō-sīt′ĭk)

monocytopenia (mŏn″ō-sī″tō-pē′nē-ă) [″ + kytos, cell, + penia, lack]

monocytosis (mŏn″ō-sī-tō′sīs) [″ + ″ + osis, condition]

monodactylism (mŏn-ō-dăk′tĭl-ĭzm) [″ + daktylos, finger]

monodal (mŏn-ō′dăl) [″ + hodos, road]

monodermoma (mŏn″ō-dĕr-mō′mă) [″ + derma, skin, + oma, tumor]

monodiplopia (mŏn″ō-dĭ-plō′pē-ă) [″ + diploos, double, + ops, eye]

monodromia

monoecious (mŏn-ē′shŭs) [″ + oikos, house]

monogamy (mō-nŏg′ă-mē) [″ + gamos, marriage]

monogenesis (mŏn″ō-jĕn′ĕ-sīs) [Gr. monos, single, + genesis, generation, birth]

monogerminal (mŏn″ō-jĕr′mĭ-năl)

monogony (mō-nŏg′ō-nē) [″ + gone, seed]

monograph (mŏn′ō-grăf) [″ + graphein, to write]

monogyny (mō-nŏj′ă-nē) [″ + gyne, woman]

monohybrid [″ + L. hybrida, mongrel]

monohydrated (mŏn-ō-hī′drāt-ĕd) [″ + hydor, water]

monohydric (mŏn″ō-hī′drĭk)

monoideaism,   monoideism (mŏn″ō-ī-dē′ă-ĭzm, -dē′ĭzm) [″ + idea, idea]

monoinfection (mŏn″ō-ĭn-fĕk′shŭn)

monoiodotyrosine (mŏn″ō-ī-ō″dō-tī′rō-sēn)

monolayer (mŏn″ō-lā′ĕr)

monolocular (mŏn″ō-lŏk′ū-lar) [″ + L. loculus, a small chamber]

monomania (mŏn-ō-mā'nē-ă) [" + *mania*, madness]
monomaniac
monomastigote (mŏn-ō-măs'tĭ-gōt) [" + *mastix*, whip]
monomelic (mŏn-ō-mĕl'ĭk) [" + *melos*, limb]
monomer (mŏn'ō-mĕr)
monomeric (mŏn-ō-mĕr'ĭk) [" + *meros*, part]
monometallic (mŏn"ō-mĕ-tăl'ĭk)
monomicrobic (mŏn"ō-mī-krō'bĭk)
monomolecular (mŏn"ō-mō-lĕk'ū-lăr)
monomorphic (mŏn-ō-mor'fĭk) [" + *morphe*, form]
monomyoplegia (mŏn"ō-mī"ō-plē'jē-ă) [" + *mys*, muscle, + *plege*, stroke]
monomyositis (mŏn"ō-mī-ō-sī'tĭs) [" + " + *itis*, inflammation]
mononeural (mŏn-ō-nū'răl) [" + *neuron*, nerve]
mononeuritis (mŏn"ō-nū-rī'tĭs) [" + " + *itis*, inflammation]
m. multiplex
mononeuropathy (mŏn"ō-nū-rŏp'ă-thē) [" + " + *pathos*, disease, suffering]
mononoea (mŏn"ō-nē'ă) [" + *nous*, mind]
mononuclear (mŏn-ō-nū'klē-ăr) [" + L. *nucleus*, kernel]
mononuclear phagocyte system
mononucleosis (mŏn-ō-nū"klē-ō'sĭs) [" + *nucleus*, kernel, + *osis*, condition]
m., infectious
mononucleotide (mŏn"ō-nū'klē-ō-tīd")
monoparesis (mŏn-ō-păr-ē'sĭs) [Gr. *monos*, single, + *parienai*, let fall]
monoparesthesia (mŏn"ō-păr-ĕs-thē'sē-ă) [" + *para*, alongside, past, beyond, + *aisthesis*, feeling, perception]
monopathy (mō-nŏp'ă-thē) [" + *pathos*, disease, suffering]
monophagia (mŏn-ō-fā'jē-ă) [" + *phagein*, to eat]

monophasia (mŏn-ō-fā'zē-ă) [" + *phasis*, utterance]
monophobia (mŏn-ō-fō'bē-ă) [" + *phobos*, fear]
monophthalmus (mŏn"ŏf-thăl'mŭs) [" + *ophthalmos*, eye]
monophyletic (mŏn"ō-fīl-ĕt'ĭk) [" + *phyle*, tribe]
monophyletism (mŏn"ō-fī'lĕ-tĭzm)
monophyodont (mŏn"ō-fī'ō-dŏnt) [" + *phyein*, to grow, + *odous*, tooth]
monoplasmatic (mŏn"ō-plăz-măt'ĭk) [" + LL. *plasma*, form, mold]
monoplast (mŏn"ō-plăst) [" + *plastos*, formed]
monoplegia (mŏn-ō-plē'jē-ă) [" + *plege*, stroke]
monopodia (mŏn"ō-pō'dē-ă) [" + *pous*, foot]
monopolar (mŏn-ō-pōl'ăr) [" + L. *polus*, pole]
monops (mŏn'ŏps) [" + *ops*, eye]
monopsychosis (mŏn"ō-sī-kō'sĭs) [Gr. *monos*, single, + *psyche*, mind, + *osis*, condition]
monopus (mŏn'ō-pŭs) [" + *pous*, foot]
monorchia (mŏn-or'kē-ă)
monorchid (mŏn-or'kĭd) [" + *orchis*, testicle]
monorchidism, monorchism (mŏn-or'kĭd-ĭzm, mŏn'or-kĭzm)
monorhinic (mŏn"ō-rīn'ĭk) [" + *rhis*, nose]
monosaccharide (mŏn-ō-săk'ă-rīd) [" + Sanskrit *sarkara*, sugar]
monosodium glutamate
monosome (mŏn'ō-sōm) [" + *soma*, body]
monosomy (mŏn'ō-sō"mē)
monospasm (mŏn'ō-spăzm) [" + *spasmos*, a convulsion]
monospermy (mŏn'ō-spĕr"mē) [" + *sperma*, seed]
monostotic (mŏn"ŏs-tŏt'ĭk) [" + *osteon*, bone]
monostratal (mŏn"ō-strā'tăl)

monosubstituted (mŏn"ō-sŭb'stĭ-tūt"ĕd)

monosymptomatic (mŏn"ō-sĭmp-tō-măt'ĭk) [" + symptomatikos, pert. to symptom]

monosynaptic (mŏn"ō-sī-năp'tĭk)

monosyphilide (mŏn-ō-sĭf'ĭl-īd) [" + Fr. syphilide, syphilitic lesion]

monoterminal [" + terma, a limit]

monothermia (mŏn-ō-thĕrm'ē-ă) [" + therme, heat]

monotocous (mō-nŏt'ō-kŭs) [Gr. monos, single, + tokos, birth]

Monotricha (mō-nŏt'rĭ-kă) [" + thrix, hair]

monotrichous (mŏn-ŏt'rĭ-kŭs)

monovalent (mŏn-ō-vā'lĕnt) [" + L. valere, to have power]

monoxenous (mō-nŏks'ĕn-ŭs) [" + xenos, stranger]

monoxide (mŏn-ŏk'sīd)

monozygotic (mŏn"ō-zī-gŏt'ĭk) [" + zygotos, yoked]

monozygotic twins

Monro's foramen (mŏn-rōz') [Alexander Monro, Scot. anatomist, 1737–1817]

Monro's sulcus

mons (mŏns) [L., mountain]
   m. pubis
   m. veneris

monster [L. monstrum]

monstriparity (mŏn"strĭ-păr'ĭ-tē) [" + parere, to beget, produce]

monstrosity [L. monstrositas]

Monteggia's fracture (mŏn-tĕj'ăz) [Giovanni B. Monteggia, It. surgeon, 1762–1815]

Montgomery's glands [William F. Montgomery, Ir. obstetrician, 1797–1859]

Montgomery straps

monticulus (mŏn-tĭk'ū-lŭs) [L., little mountain]
   m. cerebelli

mood [AS. mod, mind, feeling]

mood disorders

moon face

Moore's lightning streaks [Robert F. Moore, Brit. ophthalmologist, 1878–1963]

Moraxella (mor-ăx-ĕl'ă)

morbid (mor'bĭd) [L. morbidus, sick]

morbidity [L. morbidus, sick]

morbidity rate

morbific (mor-bĭf'ĭk) [" + facere, to make]

morbilli (mor-bĭl'ī) [L. morbillus, little disease]

morbilliform [" + forma, shape]

morbillous (mor-bĭl'ŭs)

morbus [L., disease]
   m. caeruleus
   m. miseriae

morcellation, morcellement (mor-sĕl-ā'shŭn, -ā-mŏn') [Fr. morceller, to subdivide]

mordant (mor'dănt) [L. mordere, to bite]

mores (mō'rāz) [L.]

Morgagni (mor-găn'yē) [Giovanni B. Morgagni, It. pathological anatomist, 1682–1771]
   M.'s caruncle
   M.'s cataract
   M.'s hydatid
   M.'s hyperostosis
   M.'s ventricle

morgagnian (mor-găn'yē-ăn)

morgagnian cyst

morgue (morg) [Fr.]

moria (mō'rē-ă) [Gr. moria, folly]

moribund (mor'ĭ-bŭnd) [L. moribundus]

morioplasty (mō'rē-ō-plăs-tē) [Gr. morion, piece, + plassein, to form]

morning care

morning sickness

morning stiffness

moron [Gr. moros, stupid]

Moro reflex [Ernst Moro, Ger. pediatrist, 1874–1951]

morphea (mor-fē'ă) [Gr. morphe, form]

morpheme (mor'fēm)

morphia

morphine (mor'fēn) [L. morphina, from Morpheus, god of sleep]
   m. sulfate

morphine poisoning
morphinism (mor″fĭn-ĭzm) [L. *morphina,* morphine, + *-ismos,* condition]
morphinomania, **morphiomania** (mor″fĭn-ō-mā′nē-ă, -fē-ō-mā′nē-ă) [″ + *mania,* madness]
morphogenesis (mor″fō-jĕn′ĕ-sĭs) [Gr. *morphe,* form, + *genesis,* generation, birth]
morphogenetic (mor″fō-jĕn-ĕt′ĭk)
morphogenetic processes
morphogenetic substance
morphography (mor-fŏg′ră-fē) [″ + *graphein,* to write]
morphology (mor-fŏl′ō-jē) [Gr. *morphe,* form, + *logos,* word, reason]
morphometry (mor-fŏm′ĕ-trē) [″ + *metron,* measure]
morphon (mor′fŏn) [Gr., forming]
morphosis (mor-fō′sĭs) [Gr., a shaping]
morpio, morpion (mor′pē-ō, -pē-ŏn) [L.]
Morquio's syndrome (mor-kē′ōz) [Louis Morquio, Uruguayan physician, 1867–1935]
morrhuate sodium injection (mor′ū-āt)
mors [L., death]
    m. putativa
    m. subita
morsal (mor′săl) [L. *morsus,* bite]
morsulus (mor′sū-lŭs) [L. dim. of *morsus,* bite]
mortal [L. *mortalis*]
mortality
mortar [L. *mortarium*]
mortician [L. *mors,* death]
mortification (mor″tĭ-fĭ-kā′shŭn) [″ + *facere,* to make]
mortinatality (mor″tĭ-nā-tăl′ĭ-tē) [″ + *natus,* birth]
mortise joint
Morton's disease, syndrome (mor′tŭnz) [Dudley J. Morton, U.S. orthopedist, 1884–1960]
Morton's foot syndrome
Morton's neuralgia [Thomas G. Morton, U.S. surgeon, 1835–1903]
Morton's neuroma
mortuary (mor′chū-ā-rē) [L. *mortuarium,* a tomb]
morula (mor′ū-lă) [L. *morus,* mulberry]
morulation (mor″ū-lā′shŭn)
moruloid (mor′ū-loyd) [″ + Gr. *eidos,* form, shape]
Morvan's disease (mor′vănz) [Augustin M. Morvan, Fr. physician, 1819–1897]
mosaic
mosaic bone
mosaicism (mō-zā′ĭ-sĭzm)
mosquito [Sp., little fly]
mosquitocide [″ + L. *caedere,* to kill]
mosquito forceps
moss
    m., sphagnum
mossy cell
mossy fibers
mother [AS. *modor*]
mother cell
mother cyst
mother liquor
mother's mark
motile (mō′tĭl) [L. *motilis,* moving]
motility (mō-tĭl′ĭ-tē)
motion (mō′shŭn) [L. *motio,* movement]
    m., active
    m., passive
motion sickness
motivation (mō″tĭ-vā′shŭn)
motive (mō′tĭv)
motofacient (mō″tō-fā′shĕnt)
motoneuron (mō″tō-nū′rŏn)
    m.'s, lower
    m.'s, peripheral
    m.'s, upper
motor [L. *motus,* moving]
motor aphasia
motor area
motor endplate
motor fibers
motorial (mō-tor′ē-ăl) [L. *motus,* moving]
motoricity (mō-tor-ĭs′ĭ-tē)

motorium (mō-tor′ē-ŭm) [L., power of motion]

motorius (mō-tor′ē-ŭs)

motor nerve

motor neuron

motor neuron disease

motorpathy (mō-tor′păth-ē) [L. *motus*, moving, + Gr. *pathos*, disease, suffering]

motor points

motor sense

motor speech area

motor unit

Motrin

mottled enamel

mottling (mŏt′lĭng) [ME. *motteley*, many colored]

moulage (moo-lăzh′) [Fr.]

mounding

mount (mownt) [ME. *mounten*, to mount]
m., x-ray

mountain fever

mountain sickness, chronic

mountant

mounting (mownt′ĭng)

mourning [AS. *murnan*]

mouse (mows)
m., joint
m., NZB

mouse unit

mouth [AS. *muth*]
m., trench

mouthrinse

mouthstick

mouthwash

movement [L. *movere*, to move]
m., active
m., ameboid
m., angular
m., associated
m., autonomic
m., bodily
m., brownian
m., ciliary
m., circus
m., disorders of
m.'s, fetal
m., gliding

m., hinge
m., jaw
m., masticatory
m., molecular
m. of restitution
m., orthodontic
m., passive
m.'s, pendular
m., peristaltic
m., respiratory
m., rotational
m.'s, saccadic
m., segmenting
m., tipping
m., vermicular
m., vibratile

moxa (mŏk′sa) [Japanese]

moxalactam disodium

Moxam

moxibustion (mŏks-ĭ-bŭs′chŭn) [″ + L. *combustus*, burned]

M.P.D. *maximum permissible dose*

M.P.H. *Master of Public Health*

M.P.N. *most probable number*

MPS *mucopolysaccharidosis*

MR *magnetic resonance*

mR *milliroentgen*

MRI *magnetic resonance imaging*

M.R.L. *medical records librarian*

mRNA *messenger RNA*

MS *multiple sclerosis*

M.S. *Master of Surgery; Master of Science*

msec *millisecond*

MSH *melanocyte-stimulating hormone*

M.S.N. *Master of Science in Nursing*

M.T. *medical technologist*

M.u. *Mache unit*

m.u. *mouse unit*

mu (mū) [Gr. *μ*, letter m]

mucedin (mū′sĕ-dĭn) [L. *mucedo*, mucus]

muciferous (mū-sĭf′ĕr-ŭs) [L. *mucus*, mucus, + *ferre*, to carry]

muciform (mū′sĭ-form) [″ + *forma*, shape]

mucigen (mū′sĭ-jĕn) [″ + Gr. *gennan*, to produce]

mucigenous (mū-sĭj′ĕn-ŭs)

mucilage (mū′sĭ-lĭj) [L. *mucilago*, moldy juice]

mucilaginous (mū-sĭl-ăj′ĭn-ŭs)

mucilago

mucilloid (mū′sĭl-loyd)
m., psyllium hydrophilic

mucin (mū′sĭn) [L. *mucus*, mucus]
m., gastric

mucinase (mū′sĭ-nās)

mucinemia (mū″sĭn-ē′mē-ă) [″ + Gr. *haima*, blood]

mucinogen (mū-sĭn′ō-jĕn) [″ + Gr. *gennan*, to produce]

mucinoid (mū′sĭn-oyd) [″ + Gr. *eidos*, form, shape]

mucinolytic (mū″sĭ-nō-lĭt′ĭk) [″ + Gr. *lysis*, dissolution]

mucinuria (mū-sĭn-ū′rē-ă) [″ + Gr. *ouron*, urine]

muciparous (mū-sĭp′ăr-ŭs) [″ + *parere*, to beget, produce]

muco- [L. *mucus*, mucus]

mucocele (mū′kō-sēl) [″ + Gr. *kele*, tumor, swelling]

mucocolpos (mū″kō-kŏl′pŏs) [″ + Gr. *kolpos*, vagina]

mucocutaneous (mū″kō-kū-tā′nē-ŭs) [″ + *cutis*, skin]

mucocutaneous lymph node syndrome

mucodermal (mū-kō-dĕr′măl) [″ + Gr. *derma*, skin]

mucoenteritis (mū″kō-ĕn-tĕr-ī′tĭs) [″ + Gr. *enteron*, intestine, + *itis*, inflammation]

mucoglobulin (mū″kō-glŏb′ū-lĭn) [″ + *globulus*, globule]

mucoid (mū′koyd) [″ + Gr. *eidos*, form, shape]

mucomembranous (mū″kō-mĕm′bră-nŭs) [″ + *membrana*, membrane]

mucoperiosteum (mū″kō-pĕr″ē-ŏs′tē-ŭm)

mucopolysaccharidase (mū″kō-pŏl″ē-săk′ă-rī-dās)

mucopolysaccharide (mū″kō-pŏl″ĭ-săk′ă-rīd)

mucopolysaccharidosis

mucopolysacchariduria (mū″kō-pŏl″ē-săk′ă-rī-dū′rē-ă)

mucoprotein (mū″kō-prō′tē-ĭn)
m., Tamm-Horsfall [Igor Tamm, U.S. microbiologist, 1922–1971; Frank L. Horsfall, Jr., U.S. physician, 1906–1971]

mucopurulent (mū-kō-pūr′ū-lĕnt) [L. *mucus*, mucus, + *purulentus*, full of pus]

mucopus (mū′kō-pŭs)

Mucor (mū′kor) [L.]

mucoriferous (mū″kor-ĭf′ĕr-ŭs) [L. *mucor*, mold, + *ferre*, to carry]

mucorin (mū′kor-ĭn)

mucormycosis (mū″kor-mī-kō′sĭs) [″ + Gr. *mykes*, fungus, + *osis*, condition]

mucorrhea [″ + *rhein*, to flow]

mucosa (mū-kō′să) [L., mucous]
m., alveolar
m., lingual
m., masticatory
m., nasal
m., oral

mucosal (mū-kō′săl)

mucosanguineous (mū″kō-săn-gwĭn′ē-ŭs) [″ + *sanguineus*, bloody]

mucosedative (mū″kō-sĕd′ă-tĭv) [″ + *sedativus*, allaying]

mucoserous (mū″kō-sēr′ŭs)

mucosin (mū′kō-sĭn)

mucositis (mū″kō-sī′tĭs) [″ + Gr. *itis*, inflammation]

mucosocutaneous (mū-kō″sō-kū-tā′nē-ŭs)

mucostatic (mū″kō-stăt′ĭk) [″ + *statikos*, standing]

mucous (mū′kŭs)

mucous colitis

mucous membrane

mucous polypus

mucoviscidosis (mū″kō-vĭs″ĭ-dō′sĭs)

mucro (mū′krō) [L., a sharp point]

mucus (mū′kŭs) [L.]

mulatto (mū-lăt′tō) [Sp. *mulato*, of mixed breed]

muliebria (mū"lē-ĕb'rē-ă) [L.]
muliebrity (mū"lē-ĕb'rĭ-tē) [L. *mulie-britas*]
mull (mŭl)
Müller, Heinrich (mĭl'ĕr) [Ger. anatomist, 1820 – 1864]
    M.'s fibers
    M.'s muscle
    M.'s trigone
Müller, Johannes P. (mĭl'ĕr) [Ger. physician, 1801 – 1858]
    M.'s ducts
    M.'s ring
    M.'s tubercle
mult-, multi- [L. *multus*]
multangular
multangular bone, greater
multangular bone, lesser
multiallelic (mŭl"tē-ă-lĕl'ĭk)
multiarticular (mŭl"tē-ăr-tĭk'ū-lăr) [L. *multus*, many, + *articulus*, joint]
multicapsular (mŭl"tĭ-kăp'sū-lăr) [" + *capsula*, a little box]
multicellular (mŭl"tĭ-sĕl'ū-lăr) [" + *cellula*, small chamber]
Multiceps
multicuspid, multicuspidate (mŭl"tĭ-kŭs'pĭd, -pī-dăt) [" + *cuspis*, point]
multifactorial
multifamilial (mŭl"tĭ-fă-mĭl'ē-ăl)
multifid (mŭl"tĭ-fĭd) [" + *fidus*, from *findere*, to split]
multifocal (mŭl"tĭ-fō'kăl)
multiform (mŭl'tĭ-form) [" + *forma*, shape]
multiglandular (mŭl"tĭ-glănd'ū-lăr) [" + *glandula*, a little acorn]
multigravida (mŭl"tĭ-grăv'ĭ-dă) [" + *gravida*, pregnant]
multi-infection (mŭl"tĭ-ĭn-fĕk'shŭn) [L. *multus*, many, + *infectio*, an infection]
multilobular (mŭl"tĭ-lŏb'ū-lăr) [" + *lobulus*, a small lobe]
multilocular (mŭl"tĭ-lŏk'ū-lăr) [" + *loculus*, a cell]
multimammae (mŭl"tĭ-măm'mē) [" + *mamma*, breast]

multinodal (mŭl-tĭ-nō'dăl)
multinodular (mŭl-tĭ-nŏd'ū-lăr) [" + *nodulus*, little knot]
multinuclear, multinucleate (mŭl-tĭ-nū'klē-ăr, -āt)
multipara (mŭl-tĭp'ă-ră) [" + *parere*, to beget, produce]
    m., grand
multiparity (mŭl-tĭ-păr'ĭ-tē)
multiparous (mŭl-tĭp'ăr-ŭs)
multipartial (mŭl"tĭ-păr'shăl)
multiphasic screening
multiple (mŭl'tĭ-pl) [L. *multiplex*, many folded]
multiple drug resistance
multiple endocrine neoplasia
multiple myeloma
multiple personality
multiple sclerosis
multiple systems organ failure
multiplexor
multipolar (mŭl-tĭ-pōl'ăr) [L. *multus*, many, + *polus*, a pole]
multirooted
multisynaptic (mŭl"tē-sĭ-năp'tĭk)
multiterminal [" + Gr. *terma*, a limit]
multivalent (mŭl-tĭ-vā'lĕnt) [" + *valere*, to have power]
mummification (mŭm"mĭ-fĭ-kā'shŭn) [Arabian *mumiyaa*, mummy, + L. *facere*, to make]
mumps (mŭmps)
mumps skin test antigen
Mumpsvax
mumps virus vaccine live
mumps virus vaccine live attenuated
Munchausen syndrome (mĕn-chow'zĕn) [Baron Karl F. H. von Munchausen, fictional 18th century baron created by Rudolph Raspe]
mural (mū'răl) [L. *murus*, a wall]
muramidase
Murchison-Pel-Ebstein fever (mŭr'chĭ-sŏn-pĕl-ĕb'stĭn) [Charles Murchison, Brit. physician, 1830 – 1879; Pieter K. Pel, Dutch physician, 1852 –

1919; Wilhelm Ebstein, Ger. physician, 1836–1912]
murdering while asleep
muriate (mūr′ē-āt) [L. *muria*, brine]
muriatic acid (mū″rē-ăt′ĭk)
murine (mū′rĭn) [L. *mus*, mouse]
murmur [L.]
  m., aneurysmal
  m., aortic obstructive
  m., aortic regurgitant
  m., apex
  m., arterial
  m., Austin Flint
  m., bronchial
  m., cardiac
  m., cardiopulmonary
  m., continuous
  m., crescendo
  m., Cruveilhier-Baumgarten
  m., diastolic
  m., Duroziez'
  m., ejection
  m., endocardial
  m., exocardial
  m., Flint's
  m., friction
  m., functional
  m., Gibson
  m., Graham Steell's
  m., heart
  m., hemic
  m., machinery
  m., mitral
  m., musical
  m., organic
  m., pansystolic
  m., pericardial
  m., physiologic
  m., prediastolic
  m., presystolic
  m., pulmonary
  m., regurgitant
  m., seagull
  m., Still's
  m., systolic
  m., to-and-fro
  m., tricuspid
  m., vascular

  m., vesicular
Murphy's button [John B. Murphy, U.S. surgeon, 1857–1916]
Murphy's sign
Mus (mŭs) [L., mouse]
  M. musculus
Musca (mŭs′kă) [L., fly]
  M. domestica
muscae volitantes (mŭs′sē vŏl-ĭ-tăn′tēz) [L., flitting flies]
muscarine (mŭs′kă-rĭn) [L. *muscarius*, pert. to flies]
muscegenetic (mŭs″ē-jĕ-nĕt′ĭk) [L. *musca*, fly, + Gr. *genesis*, generation, birth]
muscicide (mŭs′ĭ-sīd) [″ + *caedere*, to kill]
muscle (mŭs′ĕl) [L. *musculus*]
  m., abductor
  m., adductor
  m., antagonistic
  m.'s, antigravity
  m., appendicular
  m., arrector pili
  m., articular
  m., axial
  m., bipennate
  m., constrictor, of pharynx
  m., digastric
  m., extensor
  m.'s, extraocular eye
  m., extrinsic
  m., fixation
  m., flexor
  m., fusiform
  m., intrinsic
  m., involuntary
  m.'s, mastication
  m.'s, mimetic
  m., multipennate
  m., nonstriated
  m., papillary
  m., pectinate
  m., postaxial
  m., preaxial
  m., skeletal
  m., smooth
  m., somatic

m., sphincter
m., sphincter, of urinary bladder
m., striated
m.'s, synergistic
m., unipennate
m., unstriated
m., voluntary
muscle compartment syndrome
muscle cramps
**muscle fiber types, fast twitch and
slow twitch**
muscle soreness
muscular [L. *muscularis*]
muscular contractions, graduated
muscular dystrophy
muscularis (mŭs-kū-lā'rĭs) [L.]
m. mucosae
muscularity
muscularize (mŭs'kū-lăr-īz)
musculature [L. *musculus*, muscle]
musculin
musculo- [L. *musculus*, muscle]
musculoaponeurotic (mŭs-kū-lō-
ăp"ō-nū-rŏt'ĭk)
musculocutaneous (mŭs"kū-lō-kū-
tān'ē-ŭs) [" + *cutis*, skin]
musculofascial (mŭs"kū-lō-făsh'ē-ăl)
musculomembranous (mŭs"kū-lō-
mĕm'brăn-ŭs)
musculophrenic (mŭs"kū-lō-frĕn'ĭk)
musculoskeletal (mŭs"kū-lō-skĕl'ē-tăl)
musculospiral (mŭs"kū-lō-spī'răl) [" +
spira, coil]
musculotendinous
musculotropic (mŭs"kū-lō-trŏp'ĭk) [" +
Gr. *tropikos*, turning]
musculus [L., muscle]
mushbite (mŭsh'bīt)
mushroom [Fr. *mousseron*]
mushroom and toadstool poisoning
musicogenic (mū"zĭ-kō-jĕn'ĭk) [L. *mu-
sica*, music, + *gennan*, to produce]
musicogenic epilepsy
musicomania [" + Gr. *mania*,
madness]
musicotherapy [" + *therapeia*,
treatment]
musk (mŭsk) [Sanskrit *muska*, testicle]

mussel
mussel poisoning
Musset's sign (mū-sāz') [Louis C. A. de
Musset, Fr. poet, 1810–1857]
mussitation (mŭs-sĭ-tā'shŭn) [L. *mussi-
tare*, to matter]
mustard [Fr. *moustarde*]
m., nitrogen
mustard gas
Mustargen
mutacism (mū'tă-sĭzm)
mutagen (mū'tă-jĕn) [L. *mutare*, to
change, + Gr. *gennan*, to pro-
duce]
mutagenesis (mū"tă-jĕn'ĕ-sĭs)
mutagenicity (mū"tă-jĕ-nĭs'ĭ-tē)
mutant (mū'tănt) [L. *mutare*, to change]
mutase (mū'tās) [" + *ase*, enzyme]
mutation (mū-tā'shŭn)
m., induced
m., natural
m., somatic
mute (mūt) [L. *mutus*, dumb]
m., deaf
mutilate [L. *mutilatus*, to maim]
mutilation (mū"tĭ-lā'shŭn)
mutism (mū'tĭzm) [L. *mutus*, dumb]
m., akinetic
m., hysterical
mutualism (mū'tū-ăl-ĭzm) [L. *mutuus*, ex-
changed]
mutualist (mū'tū-ăl-ĭst)
M.V. *Medicas Veterinarius*
mv *millivolt*
M.W.I.A. *Medical Women's International Association*
my-, myo- [Gr. *mys*, muscle]
myalgia (mī-ăl'jē-ă) [" + *algos*,
pain]
Myambutol
myasis (mī-ā'sĭs) [Gr. *myia*, a fly]
myasthenia (mī-ăs-thē'nē-ă) [Gr. *mys*,
muscle, + *astheneia*, weakness]
m., angiosclerotic
m. cordis
m. gastrica
m. gravis
myasthenic

myatonia (mī-ă-tō'nē-ă)
m. congenita
myatrophy (mī-ăt'rō-fē)
myc-, myco- [Gr. *mykes*, fungus]
mycelioid (mī-sē'lē-oyd) [" +
helos, nail, + *eidos*, form, shape]
mycelium (mī-sē'lē-ŭm) [Gr. *mykes*,
fungus, + *helos*, nail]
mycetes (mī-sē'tēz)
mycethemia (mī-sĕ-thē'mē-ă) [" +
haima, blood]
mycetism, mycetismus (mī'sĕ-tĭzm,
mī-sĕ-tĭz'mŭs) [" + *-ismos*, condition]
mycetogenetic (mī-sē"tō-jĕn-ĕt'ĭk)
[" + *gennan*, to produce]
mycetoma (mī-sĕ-tō'mă) [" +
oma, tumor]
Mycifradin
mycobacteriosis (mī"kō-băk-tē"rē-ō'sĭs)
Mycobacterium [" + *bakterion*,
little rod]
　M., atypical
　M. balnei
　M. bovis
　M. kansasii
　M. leprae
　M. marinum
　M. tuberculosis
mycocidin (mī"kō-sī'dĭn)
mycoderma [Gr. *mykos*, mucus, +
derma, skin]
mycodermatitis (mī"kō-dĕr"mă-tī'tĭs)
mycodermomycosis (mī"kō-dĕr"mō-mī-kō'sĭs)
mycohemia (mī"kō-hē'mē-ă) [Gr.
mykes, fungus, + *haima*, blood]
mycoid (mī'koyd) [" + *eidos*, form,
shape]
mycology (mī-kŏl'ō-jē) [" + *logos*,
word, reason]
mycomyringitis (mī"kō-mĭr-ĭn-jī'tĭs)
[" + L. *myringa*, drum membrane,
+ *itis*, inflammation]
mycophthalmia (mī-kŏf-thăl'mē-ă)
mycoplasmas
mycoprecipitin (mī"kō-prē-sĭp'ĭ-tĭn)

mycosis (mī-kō'sĭs) [" + *osis*, condition]
　m. fungoides
　m., superficial
　m., systemic
mycostasis (mī-kŏs'tă-sĭs) [Gr. *mykes*,
fungus, + *stasis*, standing still]
mycostat (mī'kō-stăt) [" + *statikos*,
standing]
Mycostatin
mycotic (mī-kŏt'ĭk)
mycotoxicosis (mī"kō-tŏk"sī-kō'sĭs)
[" + *toxikon*, poison, + *osis*,
condition]
mycotoxinization (mī"kō-tŏk"sĭn-ī-zā'shŭn)
mycotoxins
mycterophonia (mĭk"tĕr-ō-fō'nē-ă)
[Gr. *mykter*, nostril, + *phone*,
voice]
mydaleine (mīd-ă'lē-ēn) [Gr. *mydaleos*, moldy]
Mydfrin
Mydriacyl
mydriasis (mĭd-rī'ă-sĭs) [Gr.]
　m., alternating
　m., paralytic
　m., spastic
　m., spinal
mydriatic (mĭd-rē-ăt'ĭk)
myectomy (mī-ĕk'tō-mē) [Gr. *mys*, muscle, + *ektome*, excision]
myectopia (mī-ĕk-tō'pē-ă) [" +
ek, out, + *topos*, place]
myelalgia (mī-ĕl-ăl'jē-ă) [Gr. *myelos*,
marrow, + *algos*, pain]
myelanalosis (mī"ĕl-ăn"ăl-ō'sĭs) [" +
analosis, wasting]
myelapoplexy (mī"ĕl-ăp'ō-plĕks-ē)
[" + *apoplexia*, to cripple by a
stroke]
myelasthenia (mī"ĕl-ăs-thē'nē-ă) [Gr.
myelos, marrow, + *astheneia*,
weakness]
myelatelia (mī"ĕl-ă-tē'lē-ă) [" +
ateleia, imperfection]
myelatrophy (mī-ĕl-ăt'rō-fē) [" +
atrophia, atrophy]

myelauxe (mī-ĕl-awks'ē) [" + auxe, increase]

myelemia (mī-ĕl-ē'mē-ă) [" + haima, blood]

myelencephalon (mī"ĕl-ĕn-sĕf'ă-lŏn) [Gr. myelos, marrow, + enkephalos, brain]

myelic

myelin

myelination (mī"ĕl-ĭn-ā'shŭn) [Gr. myelos, marrow]

myelinic (mī-ĕl-ĭn'ĭk)

myelinization (mī"ĕl-ĭn-ĭ-zā'shŭn)

myelinoclasis (mī"ĕ-lĭn-ŏk'lă-sĭs) [" + klasis, breaking]

myelinogenesis (mī"ĕ-lĭn"ō-jĕn'ĕ-sĭs) [" + genesis, generation, birth]

myelinogenetic (mī"ĕl-ĭn-ō-jĕn-ĕt'ĭk) [" + gennan, to produce]

myelinolysis (mī"ĕ-lĭn-ŏl'ĭ-sĭs) [" + lysis, dissolution]

myelinosis (mī"ĕl-ĭn-ō'sĭs) [" + osis, condition]

myelitic (mī-ĕl-ĭt'ĭk)

myelitis (mī-ĕ-lī'tĭs) [" + itis, inflammation]

   m., acute

   m., ascending, acute

   m., bulbar

   m., central

   m., compression

   m., descending

   m., disseminated

   m., focal

   m., hemorrhagic

   m., sclerosing

   m., transverse

   m., transverse, acute

   m., traumatic

myelo- [Gr. myelos, marrow]

myeloblast (mī'ĕl-ō-blăst) [" + blastos, germ]

myeloblastemia (mī"ĕl-ō-blăst-ē'mē-ă) [" + " + haima, blood]

myeloblastoma (mī"ĕl-ō-blăst-ō'mă) [" + " + oma, tumor]

myeloblastosis (mī"ĕ-lō-blăs-tō'sĭs) [" + " + osis, condition]

myelocele (mī'ĕ-lō-sēl) [" + kele, tumor, swelling]

myelocyst (mī'ĕl-ō-sĭst) [" + kystis, bladder]

myelocystocele (mī"ĕl-ō-sĭst'ō-sēl) [" + " + kele, tumor, swelling]

myelocystomeningocele (mī"ĕl-ō-sĭst"ō-mĕn-ĭn'gō-sēl) [" + kystis, bladder, + meninx, membrane, + kele, tumor, swelling]

myelocyte (mī'ĕl-ō-sīt) [" + kytos, cell]

myelocythemia (mī"ĕl-ō-sī-thē'mē-ă) [" + " + haima, blood]

myelocytic (mī"ĕl-ō-sīt'ĭk)

myelocytosis (mī"ĕl-ō-sī-tō'sĭs) [" + " + osis, condition]

myelodiastasis (mī"ĕl-ō-dī-ăs'tă-sĭs) [Gr. myelos, marrow, + diastasis, separation]

myelodysplasia (mī"ĕl-ō-dĭs-plā'zē-ă) [" + dys, bad, difficult, painful, disordered, + plassein, to form]

myeloencephalic (mī"ĕl-ō-ĕn-sĕf-ăl'ĭk) [" + enkephalos, brain]

myeloencephalitis (mī"ĕl-ō-ĕn-sĕf"ă-lī'tĭs) [" + " + itis, inflammation]

myelofibrosis (mī"ĕ-lō-fī-brō'sĭs)

myelogenesis (mī"ĕl-ō-jĕn'ĕ-sĭs) [" + genesis, generation, birth]

myelogenic, myelogenous (mī-ĕ-lō-jĕn'ĭk, -lŏj'ĕn-ŭs) [" + gennan, to produce]

myelogeny (mī"ĕ-lŏj'ĕ-nē)

myelogram (mī'ĕ-lō-grăm) [" + gramma, letter, piece of writing]

myelography (mī-ĕ-lŏg'ră-fē) [" + graphein, to write]

   m., air

myeloid (mī'ĕ-loyd) [" + eidos, form, shape]

myeloidosis (mī"ĕ-loy-dō'sĭs) [" + " + osis, condition]

myelolymphangioma (mī"ĕ-lō-lĭm-făn"jē-ō'mă)

myelolymphocyte (mī"ĕ-lō-lĭmf'ō-sīt) [" + L. lympha, lymph, + Gr. kytos, cell]

myelolysis (mī"ĕ-lŏl'ĭs-sĭs) [" + lysis, dissolution]

myeloma (mī-ĕ-lō'mă) [" + oma, tumor]

  m., multiple

myelomalacia (mī"ĕ-lō-mă-lā'sē-ă) [Gr. myelos, marrow, + malakia, softening]

myelomatosis (mī"ĕl-ō-mă-tō'sĭs)[" + oma, tumor, + osis, condition]

myelomenia (mī-ĕ-lō-mē'nē-ă) [" + men, month]

myelomeningitis (mī"ĕ-lō-mĕn-ĭn-jī'tĭs) [" + meninx, membrane, + itis, inflammation]

myelomeningocele (mī"ĕ-lō-mĕn-ĭn'gō-sēl) [" + " + kele, tumor, swelling]

myelomere (mī'ĕ-lō-mēr) [" + meros, part]

myelomyces (mī"ĕ-lō-mī'sēs) [" + mykes, fungus]

myeloneuritis (mī"ĕ-lō-nū-rī'tĭs) [" + neuron, nerve, + itis, inflammation]

myelopathy (mī-ĕ-lŏp'ă-thē) [" + pathos, disease, suffering]

  m., ascending

  m., descending

  m., focal

  m., sclerosing

  m., transverse

  m., traumatic

myelopetal (mī-ĕ-lŏp'ĕt-ăl) [" + L. petere, to seek for]

myelophage (mī'ĕ-lō-fāj) [" + phagein, to eat]

myelophthisis (mī-ĕ-lŏf'thĭ-sĭs) [" + phthisis, a wasting]

myeloplast (mī'ĕ-lō-plăst) [" + plastos, formed]

myeloplax [Gr. myelos, marrow, + plax, plate]

myeloplaxoma (mī"ĕ-lō-plăk-sō'mă) [" + " + oma, tumor]

myeloplegia (mī"ĕl-ō-plē'jē-ă) [" + plege, stroke]

myelopoiesis (mī"ĕl-ō-poy-ē'sĭs) [" + poiein, to form]

  m., ectopic

  m., extramedullary

myelopore

myeloproliferative (mī"ĕ-lō-prō-lĭf"ĕr-ā'tĭv)

myeloradiculitis (mī"ĕ-lō-ră-dĭk"ū-lī'tĭs) [" + L. radiculus, rootlet, + Gr. itis, inflammation]

myeloradiculodysplasia (mī"ĕ-lō-ră-dĭk"ū-lō-dĭs-plā'sē-ă) [" + " + Gr. dys, bad, difficult, painful, disordered, + plassein, to form]

myeloradiculopathy (mī"ĕ-lō-ră-dĭk"ū-lŏp'ă-thē) [" + " + Gr. pathos, disease, suffering]

myelorrhagia (mī-ĕ-lō-rā'jē-ă) [" + rhegnynai, to burst forth]

myelorrhaphy (mī-ĕl-or'ă-fē) [" + rhaphe, seam]

myelosarcoma (mī"ĕl-ō-săr-kō'mă) [" + sarx, flesh, + oma, tumor]

myelosarcomatosis (mī"ĕ-lō-săr-kō"mă-tō'sĭs) [" + " + " + osis, condition]

myeloschisis (mī"ĕ-lŏs'kĭ-sĭs) [" + schisis, cleavage]

myelosclerosis (mī"ĕ-lō-sklĕr-ō'sĭs) [" + sklerosis, a hardening]

myelosis (mī-ĕ-lō'sĭs) [" + osis, condition]

  m., erythremic

myelospongium (mī"ĕ-lō-spŏn'jē-ŭm) [Gr. myelos, marrow, + spongos, sponge]

myelosuppressive (mī"ĕ-lō-sū-prĕs'ĭv)

myelosyphilis (mī"ĕ-lō-sĭf'ĭ-lĭs)

myelosyringosis (mī"ĕ-lō-sĭr"ĭng-gō'sĭs) [" + syrinx, pipe, + osis, condition]

myelotome (mī-ĕl'ō-tōm) [" + tome, a cutting, slice]

myelotomy (mī-ĕl-ŏt'ō-mē)

myelotoxic (mī-ĕl-ō-tŏk'sĭk) [" + toxikon, poison]

myelotoxin (mī"ĕl-ō-tŏk'sĭn)

myenteric (mī"ĕn-tĕr'ĭk) [Gr. mys, muscle, + enteron, intestine]

myenteric reflex
myenteron (mī-ĕn'tĕr-ŏn)
Myerson's sign
myesthesia (mī"ĕs-thē'zē-ă) [" +
aisthesis, feeling, perception]
myiasis (mī'ă-sĭs) [Gr. myia, fly, +
-sis, condition]
myiocephalon (mī"yō-sĕf'ă-lŏn) [" +
kephale, head]
myiodesopsia (mī"ē-ō-dĕs-ŏp'sē-ă)
[Gr. myiodes, flylike, + opsis,
sight, appearance, vision]
myiosis (mī-yō'sĭs) [" + osis, condi-
tion]
myitis (mī-ī'tĭs) [Gr. mys, muscle, +
itis, inflammation]
Mylaxen
Myleran
Mylicon
mylodus
mylohyoid (mī"lō-hī'oyd) [Gr. myle,
mill, + hyoid, U-shaped]
myo- [Gr. mys, muscle]
myoalbumin (mī"ō-ăl-bū'mĭn) [" +
L. albus, white]
myoalbumose (mī"ō-ăl'bū-mōs)
myoarchitectonic (mī"ō-ăr"kĭ-tĕk-
tŏn'ĭk) [Gr. mys, muscle, + archi-
tekton, master workman]
myoatrophy (mī-ō-ăt'rō-fē)
myoblast (mī'ō-blăst) [" + blastos,
germ]
myoblastoma (mī"ō-blăs-tō'mă) ["
+ " + oma, tumor]
myobradia (mī"ō-brā'dē-ă) [" +
bradys, slow]
myocardial, myocardiac (mī-ō-
kăr'dē-ăl, -ăk) [" + kardia, heart]
myocardial infarction
myocardial insufficiency
myocardiograph (mī"ō-kăr'dē-ō-
grăf) [" + " + graphein, to
write]
myocardiopathy (mī"ō-kăr"dē-ŏp'ă-
thē) [" + " + pathos, disease,
suffering]
myocardiosis (mī"ō-kăr-dē-ō'sĭs) ["
+ " + osis, condition]

myocarditis (mī"ō-kăr-dī'tĭs) [" +
kardia, heart, + itis, inflammation]
  m., acute primary
  m., acute secondary
  m., acute septic
  m., chronic
  m., fragmentation
  m., indurative
myocardium (mī-ō-kăr'dē-ŭm) [" +
kardia, heart]
myocardosis (mī"ō-kăr-dō'sĭs) [" +
" + osis, condition]
myocele (mī'ō-sēl) [" + kele,
tumor, swelling]
myocelialgia (mī"ō-sē-lē-ăl'jē-ă) [" +
koilia, cavity, belly, + algos, pain]
myocelitis (mī"ō-sē-lī'tĭs) [" + "
+ itis, inflammation]
myocellulitis (mī"ō-sĕl-ū-lī'tĭs) [" +
L. cellula, little chamber, + Gr. itis,
inflammation]
myoceptor (mī'ō-sĕp"tor) [" + L.
capere, to take]
myocerosis (mī"ō-sē-rō'sĭs) [" +
keros, wax]
myochorditis (mī"ō-kor-dī'tĭs) [" +
chorde, cord, + itis, inflammation]
myochrome (mī'ō-krōm) [" +
chroma, color]
myochronoscope (mī"ō-krō'nō-skōp)
[" + chronos, time, + skopein,
to examine]
myocinesimeter (mī"ō-sĭn"ĕ-sĭm'ĕ-tĕr)
myoclonia (mī-ō-klō'nē-ă) [" +
klonos, tumult]
myoclonus (mī-ŏk'lō-nŭs)
  m. multiplex
  m., palatal
myocoele (mī'ō-sēl) [" + koila,
hollow]
myocolpitis (mī"ō-kŏl-pī'tĭs) [" +
kolpos, vagina, + itis, inflamma-
tion]
myocomma (mī-ō-kŏm'mă) [" +
komma, cut]
myocrismus (mī-ō-krĭs'mŭs) [" +
krizein, to creak]
myocyte (mī'ō-sīt) [" + kytos, cell]

myocytoma (mī″ō-sī-tō′mă) [″ + ″ + oma, tumor]

myodemia (mī-ō-dē′mē-ă) [″ + demos, fat]

myodesopsia (mī″ō-dĕs-ŏp′sē-ă) [Gr. myiodes, flylike, + opsis, sight, appearance, vision]

myodiastasis (mī″ō-dī-ăs′tă-sĭs) [Gr. mys, muscle, + diastasis, separation]

myodiopter (mī″ō-dī-ŏp′tĕr)

myodynamia (mī″ō-dī-năm′ē-ă) [″ + dynamis, force]

myodynamometer (mī″ō-dī″nă-mŏm′ĕt-ĕr) [″ + ″ + metron, measure]

myodynia (mī″ō-dĭn′ē-ă) [″ + odyne, pain]

myodystonia (mī″ō-dĭs-tō′nē-ă) [″ + dys, bad, difficult, painful, disordered, + tonos, act of stretching, tension, tone]

myodystrophy (mī″ō-dĭs′trō-fē) [″ + ″ + trophe, nutrition]

myoedema (mī″ō-ĕ-dē′mă) [″ + oidema, swelling]

myoelastic

myoelectric

myoelectric prosthesis

myoendocarditis (mī″ō-ĕn″dō-kăr-dī′tĭs) [″ + endon, within, + kardia, heart, + itis, inflammation]

myoepithelial (mī″ō-ĕp″ī-thē′lē-ăl)

myoepithelial cells

myoepithelioma (mī″ō-ĕp″ī-thē″lē-ō′mă) [″ + epi, upon, + thele, nipple, + oma, tumor]

myoepithelium (mī″ō-ĕp″ī-thē′lē-ŭm) [″ + ″ + thele, nipple]

myofasciitis (mī″ō-făs″ē-i′tĭs) [″ + L. fascia, band, + Gr. itis, inflammation]

myofibril, myofibrilla (mī-ō-fī′brĭl, -fī-brĭl′lă) [″ + L. fibrilla, a small fiber]

myofibroma (mī″ō-fī-brō′mă) [″ + L. fibra, fiber, + Gr. oma, tumor]

myofibrosis (mī″ō-fī-brō′sĭs) [″ + ″ + Gr. osis, condition]

myofibrositis (mī″ō-fī″brō-sī′tĭs) [Gr. mys, muscle, + L. fibra, fiber, + Gr. itis, inflammation]

myofilament (mī″ō-fĭl′ă-mĕnt)

myofunctional (mī″ō-fŭnk′shŭn-ăl)

myogelosis (mī″ō-jē-lō′sĭs) [″ + L. gelare, to congeal]

myogen (mī′ō-jĕn) [″ + gennan, to produce]

myogenesis (mī-ō-jĕn′ĕ-sĭs) [″ + genesis, generation, birth]

myogenetic, myogenic (mī-ō-jĕn′ĕt′ĭk, mī-ō-jĕn′ĭk) [″ + gennan, to produce]

myoglia (mī-ŏg′lē-ă) [″ + glia, glue]

myoglobin

myoglobinuria (mī″ō-glō″bĭn-ū′rē-ă)

myoglobulin (mī″ō-glŏb′ū-lĭn) [″ + L. globulus, globule]

myognathus (mī-ŏg′nă-thŭs) [″ + gnathos, jaw]

myogram [″ + gramma, letter, piece of writing]

myograph (mī′ō-grăf) [″ + graphein, to write]

myographic (mī-ō-grăf′ĭk)

myographic tracing

myography (mī-ŏg′ră-fē)

myohematin (mī″ō-hĕm′ă-tĭn)

myohemoglobin (mī″ō-hē″mō-glō′bĭn)

myohysterectomy (mī″ō-hĭs-tĕr-ĕk′tō-mē) [Gr. mys, muscle, + hystera, womb, + ektome, excision]

myoid (mī′oyd) [″ + eidos, form, shape]

myoidema (mī-oy-dē′mă) [″ + oidema, swelling]

myoischemia (mī″ō-ĭs-kē′mē-ă) [″ + ischein, to hold back, + haima, blood]

myokerosis (mī″ō-kē-rō′sĭs) [″ + keros, wax, + osis, condition]

myokinase (mī″ō-kĭn′ās)

myokinesimeter (mī″ō-kĭn″ē-sĭm′ĕ-tĕr) [″ + kinesis, motion, + metron, measure]

myokinesis (mī"ō-kĭn-ē'sĭs) [" +
kinesis, motion]
myokymia (mī-ō-kīm'ē-ă) [" +
kyma, wave]
myolemma (mī"ō-lĕm'ă) [" +
lemma, sheath]
myolipoma (mī"ō-lĭ-pō'mă) [" +
lipos, fat, + *oma,* tumor]
myology (mī-ŏl'ō-jē) [" + *logos,*
word, reason]
myolysis (mī-ŏl'ĭ-sĭs) [" + *lysis,* dis-
solution]
myoma (mī-ō'mă) [" + *oma,* tumor]
 m., nonstriated
 m. striocellulare
 m. telangiectodes
 m. uteri
myomalacia (mī"ō-mă-lā'sē-ă) [Gr.
mys, muscle, + *malakia,* softening]
 m. cordis
myomatosis (mī"ō-mă-tō'sĭs) [" +
oma, tumor, + *osis,* condition]
myomatous (mī-ō'mă-tŭs)
myomectomy (mī"ō-mĕk'tō-mē) [" +
oma, tumor, + *ektome,* excision]
myomelanosis (mī"ō-mĕl-ă-nō'sĭs)
[" + *melanosis,* blackening]
myomere (mī'ō-mēr) [" + *meros,*
part]
myometer (mī-ŏm'ĕt-ĕr) [" + *metron,* measure]
myometritis (mī"ō-mē-trī'tĭs) [" +
metra, uterus, + *itis,* inflammation]
myometrium (mī"ō-mē'trē-ŭm)
myomohysterectomy (mī-ō"mō-hĭst-
tĕr-ĕk'tō-mē) [" + *oma,* tumor,
+ *hystera,* womb, + *ektome,*
excision]
myomotomy (mī"ō-mŏt'ō-mē) [" +
" + *tome,* a cutting, slice]
myon [Gr. *mys,* muscle]
myonarcosis (mī"ō-năr-kō'sĭs) [" +
narkosis, action of benumbing]
myonecrosis (mī"ō-nĕ-krō'sĭs) [" +
nekrosis, state of death]
myonephropexy (mī"ō-nĕf'rō-
pĕk"sē) [" + *nephros,* kidney, +
pexis, fixation]

myoneural
myoneuralgia (mī"ō-nū-răl'jē-ă) [" +
neuron, nerve, + *algos,* pain]
myoneural junction
myoneurasthenia (mī"ō-nūr"ăs-
thē'nē-ă) [" + " + *astheneia,*
weakness]
myoneuroma (mī"ō-nū-rō'mă) [" +
" + *oma,* tumor]
myonosus (mī-ŏn'ō-sŭs) [" +
nosos, disease]
myonymy (mī-ŏn'ĭ-mē) [" +
onoma, name]
myopachynsis (mī"ō-păk-ĭn'sĭs) [" +
pachynsis, thickening]
myopalmus (mī-ō-păl'mŭs) [" +
palmos, a twitching]
myoparalysis (mī"ō-pă-răl'ĭ-sĭs)
myoparesis (mī"ō-păr'ĕ-sĭs)
myopathic (mī-ō-păth'ĭk) [" +
pathos, disease, suffering]
myopathic facies
myopathy (mī-ŏp'ă-thē)
 m., centronuclear
 m., cortisone
 m., distal
 m., facial
 m., metabolic
 m., myotubular
 m., nemaline
 m., ocular
 m., thyrotoxic
myope (mī'ōp) [Gr. *myein,* to shut, +
ops, eye]
myopericarditis (mī"ō-pĕr-ĭ-kar-dī'tĭs)
[Gr. *mys,* muscle, + *peri,* around,
+ *kardia,* heart, + *itis,* inflam-
mation]
myophage (mī'ō-fāj) [" + *phagein,* to eat]
myophone (mī'ō-fōn) [" + *phone,*
voice]
myopia [Gr. *myein,* to shut, + *ops,*
eye]
 m., axial
 m., chromic
 m., curvature
 m., index

m., malignant
m., pernicious
m., prodromal
m., progressive
m., stationary
m., transient
myopic (mī-ŏp′ĭk)
myopic crescent
myoplasm (mī′ō-plăzm) [Gr. *mys*, muscle, + LL. *plasma*, form, mold]
myoplastic (mī′ō-plăs′tĭk) [″ + *plassein*, to form]
myoplasty (mī-ō-plăs″tē)
myopolar (mī″ō-pō′lăr)
myoporthosis (mī″ŏp-or-thō′sĭs)
myoprotein (mī″ō-prō′tēn)
myopsis (mī-ŏp′sĭs)
myopsychopathy (mī″ō-sī-kŏp′ă-thē) [″ + *psyche*, mind, + *pathos*, disease, suffering]
myoreceptor (mī″ō-rē-sĕp′tor)
myorrhaphy (mī-or′ă-fē) [Gr. *mys*, muscle, + *rhaphe*, seam]
myorrhexis (mī-or-ĕk′sĭs) [″ + *rhexis*, a rupture]
myosalgia (mī-ō-săl′jē-ă) [″ + *algos*, pain]
myosalpingitis (mī″ō-săl-pĭn-jī′tĭs) [″ + *salpinx*, tube, + *itis*, inflammation]
myosarcoma (mī″ō-sar-kō′mă) [″ + *sarx*, flesh, + *oma*, tumor]
myosclerosis (mī″ō-sklĕr-ō′sĭs) [″ + *skleros*, hardening]
myoseism (mī′ō-sīzm) [″ + *seismos*, shake, + *-ismos*, condition]
myosin [Gr. *mys*, muscle]
myosinase (mī″ō-sĭn-ās′)
myosinogen (mī″ō-sĭn′ō-jĕn) [Gr. *mys*, muscle, + *gennan*, to produce]
myosinose (mī-ŏs′ĭn-ōs)
myosinuria (mī″ō-sĭn-ū′rē-ă)
myositis (mī-ō-sī′tĭs) [″ + *itis*, inflammation]
m., epidemic
m. fibrosa
m., interstitial
m., multiple

m. ossificans
m., parenchymatous
m. purulenta
m., traumatic
m. trichinosa
myospasm (mī′ō-spăzm) [″ + *spasmos*, a convulsion]
myosteoma (mī-ŏs″tē-ō′mă) [″ + *osteon*, bone, + *oma*, tumor]
myosthenometer (mī″ō-sthĕn-ŏm′ĕ-tĕr) [″ + *sthenos*, strength, + *metron*, measure]
myostroma (mī″ō-strō′mă) [″ + *stroma*, mattress]
myosuria (mī-ō-sū′rē-ă) [″ + *ouron*, urine]
myosuture (mī″ō-sū′chūr) [″ + L. *sutura*, seam]
myosynizesis (mī″ō-sĭn″ĭ-zē′sĭs) [Gr. *mys*, muscle, + *synizesis*, sitting together]
myotactic (mī″ō-tăk′tĭk) [″ + L. *tactus*, touch]
myotasis (mī-ŏt′ă-sĭs) [″ + *tasis*, stretching]
myotatic
myotatic reflex
myotenontoplasty (mī″ō-tĕn-ŏn′tō-plăst″ē) [″ + *tenon*, tendon, + *plassein*, to form]
myotenositis (mī″ō-tĕn-ō-sī′tĭs) [″ + ″ + *itis*, inflammation]
myotenotomy (mī″ō-tĕn-ŏt′ō-mē) [″ + ″ + *tome*, a cutting, slice]
myothermic (mī″ō-thĕrm′ĭk) [″ + *therme*, heat]
myotic (mī-ŏt′ĭk)
myotility (mī-ō-tĭl′ĭ-tē) [Gr. *mys*, muscle]
myotome (mī′ō-tōm) [″ + *tome*, a cutting, slice]
myotomy (mī-ŏt′ō-mē)
myotonia (mī″ō-tō′nē-ă) [″ + *tonos*, act of stretching, tension, tone]
m. atrophica
m. congenita
m. dystrophica
myotonic
myotonoid (mī-ŏt′ō-noyd)

myotonometer   (mī″ō-tō-nŏm′ĕt-ĕr)
[″ + *tonos*, act of stretching, tension, tone, + *metron*, measure]
myotonus   (mī-ŏt′ō-nŭs)
myotony   (mī-ŏt′ō-nē)
myotrophy   (mī-ŏt′rō-fē)   [″ + *trophe*, nourishment]
myotropic   (mī″ō-trŏp′ĭk)   [″ + *trope*, a turn]
myotube   (mī′ō-tūb)
myovascular   (mī″ō-văs′kū-lăr)
myriachit   (mĭr-ē′ă-chīt) [Russian]
Myriapoda   (mĭr-ē-ăp′ō-dă)   [Gr. *myrios*, numberless, + *pous*, foot]
myriapodiasis   (mĭr″ē-ăp-ō-dī′ă-sĭs)
myricin   (mĭr′ĭ-sĭn)
myringa   (mĭr-ĭn′gă) [L.]
myringectomy   (mĭr-ĭn-jĕk′tō-mē) [″ + Gr. *ektome*, excision]
myringitis   (mĭr-ĭn-jī′tĭs) [L. *myringa*, drum membrane, + Gr. *itis*, inflammation]
    m. bullosa
myringodectomy   (mĭr-ĭn″gō-dĕk′tō-mē) [″ + Gr. *ektome*, excision]
myringomycosis   (mĭr-ĭn″gō-mī-kō′sĭs) [″ + Gr. *mykes*, fungus, + *osis*, condition]
myringoplasty   (mĭr-ĭn′gō-plăst″ē) [″ + Gr. *plassein*, to form]
myringoscope   (mĭr-ĭn′gō-skōp) [″ + Gr. *skopein*, to examine]
myringotome   (mĭ-rĭn′gō-tōm) [″ + Gr. *tome*, a cutting, slice]
myringotomy   (mĭr-ĭn-gŏt′ō-mē)
myrmecia   (mŭr-mē′shē-ă) [Gr. *myrmex*, ant]
myrrh   (mŭr) [Gr. *myrra*]
mysophilia   (mī″sō-fīl′ē-ă)
mysophobia   (mī″sō-fō′bē-ă)   [Gr. *mysos*, filth, + *phobos*, fear]
mytacism   (mī′tă-sĭzm) [Gr. *mytakismos* from Gr. letter μ]
mythomania   (mĭth″ō-mā′nē-ă) [Gr. *mythos*, myth, + *mania*, madness]
mythophobia   (mĭth″ō-fō′bē-ă) [″ + *phobos*, fear]
mytilotoxin   (mĭt″ĭ-lō-tŏk′sĭn)

myxadenitis   (mĭks″ăd-ĕn-ī′tĭs)   [Gr. *myxa*, mucus, + *aden*, gland, + *itis*, inflammation]
    m. labialis
myxadenoma   (mĭks″ăd-ē-nō′mă)
[″ + ″ + *oma*, tumor]
myxangitis   (mĭks″ăn-jī′tĭs) [″ + *angeion*, vessel, + *itis*, inflammation]
myxasthenia   (mĭks″ăs-thē′nē-ă) [″ + *astheneia*, weakness]
myxedema   (mĭks-ĕ-dē′mă) [Gr. *myxa*, mucus, + *oidema*, swelling]
    m., childhood
    m., operative
    m., pituitary
myxedematoid   (mĭks-ĕ-dēm′ă-toyd)
[Gr. *myxa*, mucus, + *oidema*, swelling, + *eidos*, form, shape]
myxedematous   (mĭks-ĕ-dēm′ă-tŭs)
myxemia   (mĭks-ē′mē-ă)   [″ + *haima*, blood]
myxiosis   (mĭks-ē-ō′sĭs) [″ + *osis*, condition]
myxo-, myx-   [Gr. *myxa*]
myxoadenoma   (mĭks″ō-ăd-ē-nō′mă)
[″ + *aden*, gland, + *oma*, tumor]
Myxobacterales   (mĭks″ō-băk-tĕ-rā′lēz)
myxochondrofibrosarcoma
(mĭks″ō-kŏn″drō-fī″brō-săr-kō′mă)
myxochondroma   (mĭks″ō-kŏn-drō′mă)
myxocystoma   (mĭks″ō-sĭs-tō′mă) [Gr. *myxa*, mucus, + *kystis*, cyst, + *oma*, tumor]
myxocyte   (mĭk′sō-sīt) [″ + *kytos*, cell]
myxoedema   (mĭks″ē-dē′mă) [″ + *oidema*, swelling]
myxoenchondroma   (mĭks″ō-ĕn-kŏn-drō′mă) [″ + *en*, in, + *chondros*, cartilage, + *oma*, tumor]
myxofibroma   (mĭks″ō-fī-brō′mă) [″ + L. *fibra*, fiber, + Gr. *oma*, tumor]
myxofibrosarcoma   (mĭk″sō-fī″brō-săr-kō′mă) [″ + ″ + Gr. *sarx*, flesh, + *oma*, tumor]

myxoglioma (mĭk″sō-glĭ-ō′mă) [Gr. myxa, mucus, + glia, glue, + oma, tumor]

myxoid (mĭk′soyd) [″ + eidos, form, shape]

myxoinoma (mĭk″sō-ĭn-ō′mă)

myxolipoma (mĭk″sō-lĭ-pō′mă) [″ + lipos, fat, + oma, tumor]

myxoma (mĭk-sō′mă) [″ + oma, tumor]

    m., cartilaginous

    m., cystic

    m., enchondromatous

    m., erectile

    m., fibrous

    m., intracanalicular, of mamma

    m., odontogenic

    m., telangiectatic, vascular

myxomatosis (mĭk″sō-mă-tō′sĭs) [″ + ″ + osis, condition]

Myxomycetes (mĭk″sō-mī-sē′tēz) [Gr. myxa, mucus, + mykes, fungus]

myxomyoma (mĭks-ō-mī-ō′mă) [″ + mys, muscle, + oma, tumor]

myxoneuroma (mĭks″ō-nū-rō′mă) [″ + neuron, nerve, + oma, tumor]

myxopapilloma (mĭk″sō-păp″ĭl-ō′mă) [″ + L. papilla, nipple, + Gr. oma, tumor]

myxopoiesis (mĭk″sō-poy-ē′sĭs) [″ + poiesis, creation]

myxorrhea (mĭk-sō-rē′ă) [″ + rhein, to flow]

    m. gastrica

    m. intestinalis

myxosarcoma (mĭk″sō-săr-kō′mă) [″ + sarx, flesh, + oma, tumor]

myxosarcomatous (mĭk″sō-săr-kō′mă-tŭs)

myxospore (mĭks′ō-spor) [″ + sporos, seed]

Myxosporidia (mĭks-ō-spor-ĭd′ē-ă)

myxoviruses

myzesis (mī-zē′sĭs) [Gr. myzan, to suck]

Myzomyia (mī″zō-mī′ă) [″ + myia, fly]

Myzorhynchus (mī″zō-rĭng′kŭs) [″ + rhynchos, snout]

N

N *nitrogen; normal*
n *index of refraction; nasal; number*
n_1, n_2, n_3 . . . n_n
^{15}N *radioactive isotope of nitrogen*
NA *nicotinic acid; Nomina Anatomica; numerical aperture; nurse's aide*
N.A.A.C.O.G. *Nurses Association of the American College of Obstetricians and Gynecologists*
Na [L.] *natrium, sodium*
nabothian cysts (nă-bō'thē-ăn)
NaBr *sodium bromide*
NaCl *sodium chloride*
NaClO *sodium hypochlorite*
Na_2CO_3 *sodium carbonate*
nacreous (nā'krē-ŭs) [L. *nacer*, mother of pearl]
NAD *nicotinamide adenine dinucleotide*
NAD^+ *oxidized NAD*
N.A.D. *no appreciable disease*
NADH *reduced NAD^+*
NADH-diaphorase
NADP *nicotinamide adenine dinucleotide phosphate*
$NADP^+$ *oxidized NADP*
Naegele's obliquity (nā'gě-lēz) [Franz Carl Naegele, Ger. obstetrician, 1777–1851]
Naegele's pelvis
Naegele's rule
NaF *sodium fluoride*
Nafcil
nafcillin sodium (năf-sĭl'ĭn)
$NaHCO_3$ *sodium bicarbonate*
$NaHSO_3$ *sodium bisulfite*
nail [AS. *naegel*]
    n., eggshell
    n., hang
    n., ingrown
    n., intermedullary
    n., reedy

    n., Smith-Petersen
    n., spoon
nailbed
nail biting
nail fold
nail groove
nail matrix
nail-patella syndrome
nail root
nail wall
Naja-naja
naked (nā'kĕd) [As. *naced*, nude]
Nalfon
nalidixic acid
Nalline
nalorphine hydrochloride (năl-or'fēn)
naloxone hydrochloride (năl-ŏks'ōn)
NANDA *North American Nursing Diagnosis Association*
nandrolone decanoate (năn'drō-lōn)
nandrolone phenpropionate
nanism (nā'nĭzm) [L. *nanus*, dwarf, + Gr. *-ismos*, condition]
    n., symptomatic
nano- (nā'nō) [L. *nanus*, dwarf]
nanocephalism (nā-nō-sěf'ăl-ĭzm) [" + Gr. *kephale*, head, + *-ismos*, condition]
nanocephalous (nā-nō-sěf'ă-lŭs)
nanocormia (nā"nō-kor'mē-ă) [L. *nanus*, dwarf, + Gr. *kormos*, trunk]
nanocurie (nā"nō-kū'rē)
nanogram
nanoid (nā'noyd) [" + Gr. *eidos*, form, shape]
nanomelus (nā-nŏm'ě-lŭs) [" + Gr. *melos*, limb]
nanometer (nā"nō-mē'těr)
nanophthalmos (năn"ŏf-thăl'mŭs)

[" + *ophthalmos*, eye]
nanosecond (nă"nō-sĕk'ŏnd)
nanosoma, nanosomia (nă"nō-sō'mă, nănō-sō'mē-ă) [L. *nanus*, dwarf, + Gr. *soma*, body]
nanosomus (nā-nō-sō'mŭs)
nanous (nā'nŭs) [L. *nanus*, dwarf]
nanukayami (nă"nŭ-kă-yă'mē)
nanus (nā'nŭs) [L.]
NaOH *sodium hydroxide*
nap (năp) [AS. *hnappian*, nap]
napalm (nā'pălm) [from *naphthene* + *palmitate*]
napalm burn
nape (nāp, năp) [origin uncertain]
napex (nā'pĕks) [origin uncertain]
naphazoline hydrochloride (năf-ăz'ō-lēn)
naphtha (năf'thă)
naphthalene (năf'thă-lēn)
naphthol (năf'thōl)
napiform (nā'pĭ-form) [L. *napus*, turnip, + *forma*, shape]
N.A.P.N.A.P. *National Association of Pediatric Nurse Associates and Practitioners*
N.A.P.N.E.S. *National Association for Practical Nurse Education and Services*
naprapathy (nă-prăp'ăth-ē) [Bohemian *napravit*, correction, + Gr. *pathos*, disease, suffering]
Naprosyn
N.A.P.T. *National Association of Physical Therapists*
Naqua
Narcan
narcissism (năr-sĭs'ĭzm) [Narcissus, a Gr. mythical character who fell in love with his own reflection]
narcissistic (năr-sĭs-sĭst'ĭk)
narcissistic object choice
narco- [Gr. *narkoun*, to benumb]
narcoanalysis (năr"kō-ă-năl'ĭ-sĭs) [" + *analyein*, to dissolve]
narcoanesthesia (năr"kō-ăn-ĕs-thē'zē-ă)
narcohypnia (năr"kō-hĭp'nē-ă) [Gr. *narkoun*, to benumb, + *hypnos*, sleep]
narcohypnosis (năr"kō-hĭp-nō'sĭs)
narcolepsy (năr'kō-lĕp"sē) [Gr. *narkoun*, to benumb, + *lepsis*, seizure]
narcoleptic (năr-kō-lĕp'tĭk) [" + *lepsis*, seizure]
narcomatous (năr-kō'mă-tŭs) [Gr. *narkoun*, to benumb]
narcosis [NL. fr. Gr. *narkosis*, action of benumbing]
    n., basal
    n., medullary
narcosynthesis (năr"kō-sĭn'thĕ-sĭs) [" + *synthesis*, synthesis]
narcotic [Gr. *narkotikos*, benumbing]
narcotic addict
narcotic poisoning
narcotism (năr'kō-tĭzm) [" + *-ismos*, condition]
narcotize [Gr. *narkotikos*, benumbing]
Nardil
naris (nā'rĭs) [L.]
    n., anterior
    n., posterior
narrowing
NASA *National Aeronautics and Space Administration*
nasal (nā'zl) [L. *nasus*, nose]
nasal bleeding
nasal bones
nasal cartilages
nasal cavity
nasal concha
nasal douche
nasal feeding
nasal fossa
nasal gavage
nasal height
nasal index
nasal line
nasal meatus
nasal obstruction
nasal reflex
nasal septum
nasal sinuses, accessory
nasal width
nascent (năs'ĕnt; nā'sĕnt) [L. *nascens*, born]

nasioiniac (nã″zē-ō-īn′ē-ăk) [L. *nasus*, nose, + Gr. *inion*, back of the head]

nasion (nã′zē-ōn) [L. *nasus*, nose]

nasitis (nă-zī′tĭs) [″ + Gr. *itis*, inflammation]

Nasmyth's membrane (năz′mĭths) [Alexander Nasmyth, Scottish dental surgeon, died 1847]

naso- [L. *nasus*, nose]

nasoantral (nã″zō-ăn′trăl) [″ + Gr. *antrum*, cavity]

nasoantritis (nã″zō-ăn-trī′tĭs) [″ + ″ + *itis*, inflammation]

nasociliary (nã″zō-sĭl′ē-ār-ē)

nasofrontal [″ + *frontalis*, forehead]

nasogastric tube (nã″zō-găs′trĭk) [″ + Gr. *gaster*, belly]

nasolabial [″ + *labium*, lip]

nasolacrimal (nã″zō-lăk′rĭm-ăl) [″ + *lacrima*, tear]

nasology (nă-zŏl′ō-jē) [″ + Gr. *logos*, word, reason]

nasomental (nã″zō-měn′tăl) [″ + *mentum*, chin]

nasomental reflex

naso-oral (nã″zō-ō′răl) [″ + *oralis*, pert. to the mouth]

nasopalatine (nã″zō-păl′ă-tīn) [L. *nasus*, nose, + *palatum*, palate]

nasopharyngeal (nã″zō-făr-ĭn′jē-ăl) [″ + Gr. *pharynx*, throat]

nasopharyngitis (nã″zō-făr-ĭn-jī′tĭs) [″ + ″ + *itis*, inflammation]

nasopharyngography

nasopharynx (nã″zō-făr′ĭnks) [L. *nasus*, nose, + Gr. *pharynx*, throat]

nasorostral (nã″zō-rŏs′trăl) [″ + *rostralis*, resembling a beak]

nasoscope (nã′zō-skōp) [″ + Gr. *skopein*, to examine]

nasoseptitis (nã″zō-sĕp-tī′tĭs) [″ + *saeptum*, partition, + Gr. *itis*, inflammation]

nasosinusitis (nã″zō-sī″nū-sī′tĭs) [″ + *sinus*, cavity]

nasospinale (nã″zō-spīn′ăl-ē)

nasus (nã′sŭs) [L.]

Natacyn

natal (nã′tăl) [L. *natus*, birth; *nates*, buttocks]

natality [L. *natalis*, birth]

natamycin (năt″ă-mī′sĭn)

natant (nã′tănt) [L. *natare*, to swim]

nates (nã′tēz) [L.]

natimortality (nã″tĭ-mor-tăl′ĭ-tē) [L. *natus*, birth, + *mortalitas*, death]

National Formulary

National League for Nursing

National Organization for Rare Disorders

native (nã′tĭv) [L. *nativus*]

Native American

natremia (nă-trē′mē-ă) [L. *natrium*, sodium, + Gr. *haima*, blood]

natrium (nã′trē-ŭm) [L.]

natriuresis (nã″trē-ū-rē′sĭs) [″ + Gr. *ouresis*, make water]

natriuretic (nã″trē-ūr-ĕt′ĭk)

natron

natural [L. *natura*, nature]

natural childbirth

natural killer cells

natural selection

nature and nurture

Naturetin

naturopath (nã′tūr-ō-păth) [″ + Gr. *pathos*, disease, suffering]

naturopathy (nã″tūr-ŏp′ă-thē)

nausea (naw′sē-ă) [Gr. *nausia*, seasickness]
    n. gravidarum
    n. navalis

nauseant (naw′shē-ănt, naw′sē-ănt)

nauseate (naw′shē-āt, naw′sē-āt)

nauseous (naw′shŭs, naw′shē-ŭs)

Navane Hydrochloride

navel (nã′vĕl) [AS. *nafela*]

navicula (nă-vĭk′ū-lă) [L. *navicula*, boat]

navicular (nă-vĭk′ū-lăr)

navicular fossa

Nb *niobium*

nc *nanocurie*

N.C.A.P. *National Coalition for Action*

in Politics
N.C.I. *National Cancer Institute*
Nd *neodymium*
N.D.A. *National Dental Association*
Ne *neon*
near-death experience
near point
nearsight
nearsighted
nearsightedness
nearthrosis (nē″ăr-thrō′sĭs) [Gr. *neos,* new, + *arthron,* joint, + *osis,* condition]
Nebcin
nebula (nĕb′ū-lă) [L., mist, cloud]
nebulization
nebulizer (nĕb′ū-lī″zĕr) [L. *nebula,* mist]
Necator (nē-kā′tor) [L., murderer]
  N. americanus
necatoriasis (nē-kā″tō-rī′ă-sĭs)
neck [AS. *hnecca,* nape]
  n., anatomical, of humerus
  n., Madelung's
  n. of femur
  n. of mandible
  n. of tooth
  n. of uterus
  n., surgical, of humerus
  n., webbed
  n., wry-
neck conformer
necklace, Casal's
neck-righting reflex
necrectomy (nē-krĕk′tō-mē) [Gr. *nekros,* dead body, + *ektome,* excision]
necro- [Gr. *nekros,* dead body]
necrobiosis (nĕk-rō-bī-ō′sĭs) [″ + *biosis,* life]
  n. lipoidica diabeticorum
necrobiotic (nĕ″krō-bī-ŏt′ĭk)
necrocytosis (nĕ″krō-sī-tō′sĭs) [″ + *kytos,* cell, + *osis,* condition]
necrocytotoxin (nĕk″rō-sī″tō-tŏks′ĭn)
necrogenic, necrogenous (nĕ-krō-jĕn′ĭk, -krŏj′ĕn-ŭs) [″ + *gennan,* to produce]
necrologist (nĕk-rŏl′ō-jĭst) [″ +

logos, word, reason]
necrology (nĕk-rŏl′ō-jē)
necrolysis (nĕ-krŏl′ĭ-sĭs) [″ + *lysis,* dissolution]
necromania (nĕk-rō-mā′nē-ă) [″ + *mania,* madness]
necrometer (nĕk-rŏm′ĕt-ĕr) [″ + *metron,* measure]
necromimesis (nĕk″rō-mĭ-mē′sĭs) [″ + *mimesis,* imitation]
necronectomy (nĕk-rō-nĕk′tō-mē) [″ + *ektome,* excision]
necroparasite (nĕk″rō-păr′ă-sīt) [″ + *para,* alongside, past, beyond, + *sitos,* food]
necrophagous (nĕ-krŏf′ă-gŭs) [″ + *phagein,* to eat]
necrophile (nĕk′rō-fĭl) [″ + *philein,* to love]
necrophilia (nĕk″rō-fĭl′ē-ă) [″ + *philein,* to love]
necrophilic (nĕk″rō-fĭl′ĭk) [″ + *philein,* to love]
necrophilism (nĕk-rŏf′ĭl-ĭzm)
necrophilous (nĕk-rŏf′ĭl-ŭs)
necrophobia (nĕk-rō-fō′bē-ă) [″ + *phobos,* fear]
necropneumonia (nĕk″rō-nū-mō′nē-ă) [″ + *pneumon,* lung]
necropsy (nĕk′rŏp-sē) [″ + *opsis,* sight, appearance, vision]
necrosadism (nĕk″rō-sā′dĭzm) [″ + *sadism*]
necroscopy (nĕ-krŏs′kō-pē) [″ + *skopein,* to examine]
necrose (nĕk-rōs′) [Gr. *nekroun,* to make dead]
necrosin
necrosis (nĕ-krō′sĭs) [Gr. *nekrosis,* state of death]
  n., anemic
  n., aseptic
  n., Balser's fatty
  n., caseous
  n., central
  n., cheesy
  n., coagulation
  n., colliquative

n., dry
n., embolic
n., fat
n., fibrinous
n., focal
n., gummatous
n., ischemic
n., liquefactive
n., medial
n., moist
n., postpartum pituitary
n., putrefactive
n., subcutaneous fat, of newborn
n., superficial
n., thrombotic
n., total
n. ustilaginea
n., Zenker's
necrospermia (něk-rō-spěr'mē-ǎ) [" + *sperma*, seed]
necrotic [Gr. *nekrotikos*, dead]
necrotizing (něk'rō-tīz"ǐng)
necrotomy (nē-krǒt'ō-mē) [" + *tome*, a cutting, slice]
necrotoxin (něk"rō-tǒk'sǐn) [" + *toxikon*, poison]
need
needle [AS. *naedl*]
n., aneurysm
n., aspirating
n., atraumatic
n., cataract
n., discission
n., Hagedorn
n., hypodermic
n., knife
n., ligature
n., obturator
n., Reverdin's
n., stop
NEF *Nurses Educational Funds*
NEFA *nonesterified fatty acids*
negation (nē-gā'shǔn) [L. *negare*, to deny]
negative (něg'ǎ-tǐv) [L. *negare*, to deny]
negative culture
negative electrode

negative glow
negative sign
negativism
negatron (něg'ǎ-trǒn)
NegGram
Negri bodies (nā'grē) [Adelchi Negri, It. physician, 1876–1912]
Neisseria (nī-sē'rē-ǎ) [Albert Neisser, Ger. physician, 1855–1916]
N. catarrhalis
N. gonorrhoeae
N. meningitidis
N. sicca
Neisseriaceae (nīs-sē"rē-ā'sē-ē)
Nélaton's line (nā-lǎ-tǒnz') [Auguste Nélaton, Fr. surgeon, 1807–1873]
nemathelminth (něm"ǎ-thěl'mǐnth) [Gr. *nema*, thread, + *helmins*, worm]
Nemathelminthes (něm"ǎ-thěl-mǐn'thēz)
nematocide (něm'ǎ-tō-sīd") [Gr. *nema*, thread, + L. *caedere*, to kill]
nematocyst (něm'ǎ-tō-sǐst) [" + *kystis*, bladder]
Nematoda (něm"ǎ-tō'dǎ) [" + *eidos*, form, shape]
nematode (něm'ǎ-tōd) [Gr. *nema*, thread, + *eidos*, form, shape]
nematodiasis (něm"ǎ-tō-dī'ǎ-sǐs) [" + " + -*iasis*, state or condition of]
nematoid (něm'ǎ-toyd)
nematology (něm"ǎ-tǒl'ō-jē)
nematospermia (něm"ǎ-tō-spěr'mē-ǎ) [" + *sperma*, seed]
Nembutal (něm'bū-tǎl)
neo- [Gr. *neos*]
neoantigen (nē"ō-ǎn'tǐ-jěn) [" + *anti*, against, + *gennan*, to produce]
neoarthrosis (nē"ō-ǎr-thrō'sǐs) [" + *arthron*, joint, + *osis*, condition]
Neo-Betalin 12
neobiogenesis (nē"ō-bī"ō-jěn'ě-sǐs) [" + *bios*, life, + *genesis*, generation, birth]
Neobiotic

neoblastic [" + *blastos*, germ]

neocerebellum (nē″ō-sĕr-ĕ-bĕl′ŭm) [Gr. *neos*, new, + L. *cerebellum*, little brain]

neocinetic (nē″ō-sī-nĕt′ĭk) [" + *kinetikos*, pert. to movement]

neocortex (nē″ō-kor′tĕks)

neodymium (nē″ō-dĭm′ē-ŭm)

neofetus (nē-ō-fē′tŭs) [" + L. *foetus*, offspring]

neoformation (nē″ō-for-mā′shŭn) [" + L. *formatio*, a shaping]

neogala (nē-ōg′ă-lă) [" + *gala*, milk]

neogenesis (nē-ō-jĕn′ē-sĭs) [" + *genesis*, generation, birth]

neogenetic (nē″ō-jĕn-ĕt′ĭk)

neohymen (nē-ō-hī′mĕn) [Gr. *neos*, new, + *hymen*, membrane]

neolalism (nē″ō-lăl′ĭzm) [" + *laleo*, to chatter]

neologism (nē-ōl′ō-jĭzm) [" + *logos*, word, reason, + *-ismos*, condition]

neomembrane (nē-ō-mĕm′brān) [" + L. *membrana*, membrane]

neomorph (nē′ō-morf) [" + *morphe*, form]

neomycin sulfate (nē″ō-mī′sĭn) [" + *mykes*, fungus]

neon (nē′ŏn) [Gr. *neos*, new]

neonatal (nē″ō-nā′tăl) [" + L. *natus*, born]

neonate (nē′ō-nāt)

neonatologist (nē″ō-nā-tŏl′ō-jĭst) [" + " + Gr. *logos*, word, reason]

neonatology (nē″ō-nā-tŏl′ō-jē)

neon gas

neopallium (nē″ō-păl′ē-ŭm) [Gr. *neos*, new, + L. *pallium*, cloak]

neopathy (nē-ŏp′ă-thē) [" + *pathos*, disease, suffering]

neophilism (nē-ŏf′ĭl-ĭzm) [" + *philein*, to love, + *-ismos*, condition]

neophobia (nē″ō-fō′bē-ă) [" + *phobos*, fear]

neophrenia (nē″ō-frē′nē-ă) [" + *phren*, mind]

neoplasia (nē″ō-plā′zē-ă) [" + *plassein*, to form]

neoplasm (nē′ō-plăzm) [" + LL. *plasma*, form, mold]
  n., benign
  n., histoid
  n., malignant
  n., mixed
  n., multicentric
  n., organoid
  n., unicentric

neoplastic (nē″ō-plăs′tĭk) [Gr. *neos*, new, + *plastikos*, formed]

neoplasty (nē′ō-plăs-tē) [" + *plassein*, to form]

neostigmine (nē-ō-stĭg′mĭn)
  n. bromide
  n. methylsulfate

neostomy (nē-ŏs′tō-mē) [" + *stoma*, mouth, opening]

neostriatum (nē″ō-strī-ā′tŭm) [" + L. *striatum*, grooved]

Neo-Synephrine Hydrochloride (nē″ō-sĭn-ĕf′rĭn)

neoteny (nē-ŏt′ĕ-nē) [" + *teinein*, to extend]

neothalamus (nē″ō-thăl′ă-mŭs) [" + L. *thalamus*, thalamus]

nephelometer (nĕf″ĕl-ŏm′ĕ-ter) [Gr. *nephele*, mist, + *metron*, measure]

nephelometry (nĕf″ĕl-ŏm′ĕ-trē)

nephelopia (nĕf″ē-lō′pē-ă) [Gr. *nephele*, mist, + *ops*, eye]

nephr- [Gr. *nephros*, kidney]

nephradenoma (nĕf″răd-ē-nō′mă) [Gr. *nephros*, kidney, + *aden*, gland, + *oma*, tumor]

nephralgia (nĕ-frăl′jē-ă) [" + *algos*, pain]

nephralgic (nĕ-frăl′jĭk)

nephrapostasis (nĕf″ră-pŏs′tă-sĭs) [" + *apostasis*, suppuration]

nephratony (nē-frăt′ō-nē) [" + *a*, not, + *tonos*, act of stretching, tension, tone]

nephrauxe (nĕf-rawks′ē) [" + *auxe*, increase]

nephrectasia, nephrectasis, nephrectasy (nĕf-rĕk-tā'zē-ă, -rĕk'tă-sĭs, -tă-sē) [Gr. *nephros*, kidney, + *ektasis*, distention]

nephrectomize (nĕ-frĕk'tō-mīz) [" + *ektome*, excision]

nephrectomy (nĕ-frĕk'tō-mē) [" + *ektome*, excision]
  n., abdominal
  n., paraperitoneal

nephrelcosis (nĕf-rĕl-kō'sĭs) [Gr. *nephros*, kidney, + *helkosis*, ulceration]

nephrelcus (nĕf-rĕl'kŭs)

nephremia (nĕf-rē'mē-ă) [" + *haima*, blood]

nephremphraxis (nĕf"rĕm-frăks'ĭs) [" + *emphraxis*, obstruction]

nephric (nĕf'rĭk) [Gr. *nephros*, kidney]

nephridium (nĕ-frĭd'ē-ŭm) [Gr. *nephridios*, pert. to the kidney]

nephritic (nē-frĭt'ĭk)

nephritis (nĕf-rī'tĭs) [" + *itis*, inflammation]
  n., acute
  n., chronic
  n., glomerular
  n., interstitial
  n., salt-losing
  n., scarlatinal
  n., suppurative
  n., transfusion

nephritogenic (nĕ-frīt"ō-jĕn'ĭk) [" + *gennan*, to produce]

nephro- [Gr. *nephros*, kidney]

nephroabdominal (nĕf"rō-ăb-dŏm'ĭ-năl) [" + L. *abdominalis*, abdomen]

nephroblastoma (nĕf"rō-blăs-tō'mă) [" + *blastos*, germ, + *oma*, tumor]

nephrocalcinosis (nĕf-rō"kăl"sĭn-ō'sĭs) [" + L. *calx*, lime, + Gr. *osis*, condition]

nephrocapsectomy (nĕf"rō-kăp-sĕk'tō-mē) [" + L. *capsula*, capsule, + Gr. *ektome*, excision]

nephrocardiac (nĕf"rō-kăr'dē-ăk) [" + *kardia*, heart]

nephrocele (nĕf'rō-sēl) [" + *kele*, tumor, swelling]

nephrocolic (nĕf"rō-kŏl'ĭk) [Gr. *nephros*, kidney, + *kolikos*, colic]

nephrocolopexy (nĕf"rō-kŏl'ō-pĕks"ē) [" + Gr. *kolon*, colon, + *pexis*, fixation]

nephrocoloptosis (nĕf"rō-kō"lŏp-tō'sĭs) [" + " + *ptosis*, fall, falling]

nephrocystanastomosis (nĕf"rō-sĭst-ă-năs"tō-mō'sĭs) [" + *kystis*, bladder, + *anastomosis*, outlet]

nephrocystitis (nĕf"rō-sĭs-tī'tĭs) [" + " + *itis*, inflammation]

nephrocystosis (nĕf"rō-sĭs-tō'sĭs) [" + " + *osis*, condition]

nephroerysipelas (nĕf"rō-ĕr"ĭ-sĭp'ĕ-lăs) [" + *erythros*, red, + *pella*, skin]

nephrogenetic (nĕf"rō-jĕn-ĕt'ĭk) [" + *gennan*, to produce]

nephrogenic

nephrogenous (nĕ-frŏj'ĕ-nŭs)

nephrogram

nephrography (nĕ-frŏg'ră-fē) [" + *graphein*, to write]

nephrohydrosis (nĕf"rō-hī-drō'sĭs) [" + *hydor*, water, + *osis*, condition]

nephrohypertrophy (nĕf"rō-hī-pĕr'trō-fē) [" + *hyper*, over, above, excessive, + *trophe*, nourishment]

nephroid (nĕf'royd) [" + *eidos*, form, shape]

nephrolith (nĕf'rō-lĭth) [" + *lithos*, stone]

nephrolithiasis (nĕf"rō-lĭth-ī'ă-sĭs)

nephrolithotomy (nĕf"rō-lĭth-ŏt'ō-mē) [" + *lithos*, stone, + *tome*, a cutting, slice]

nephrology (nē-frŏl'ō-jē) [" + *logos*, word, reason]

nephrolysine (nē-frŏl'ĭ-sīn) [" + *lysis*, dissolution]

nephrolysis (nē-frŏl'ĭ-sĭs) [" + *lysis*, dissolution]

nephroma (nĕ-frō'mă) [" + oma, tumor]

nephromalacia (nĕf"rō-mă-lā'sē-ă) [" + malakia, softening]

nephromegaly (nĕf"rō-mĕg'ă-lē) [" + megas, great]

nephromere (nĕf'rō-mēr) [" + meros, part]

nephron (nĕf'rŏn) [Gr. nephros, kidney]

nephroncus (nĕf-rŏn'kŭs) [" + onkos, bulk, mass]

nephroparalysis (nĕf"rō-păr-ăl'ĭ-sĭs) [" + paralyein, to loosen, disable]

nephropathy (nē-frŏp'ă-thē) [" + pathos, disease, suffering]
   n., analgesic
   n., hypercalcemic
   n., hypokalemic
   n., membranous

nephropexy (nĕf'rō-pĕks-ē) [" + pexis, fixation]

nephrophthisis (nĕ-frŏ'thĭ-sĭs) [" + phthisis, a wasting]

nephroptosis (nĕf"rŏp-tō'sĭs) [" + ptosis, fall, falling]

nephropyelitis (nĕf"rō-pī-ĕl-ī'tĭs) [" + pyelos, pelvis, + itis, inflammation]

nephropyelography (nĕf"rō-pī"ĕ-lŏg'ră-fē) [" + pyelos, pelvis, graphein, to write]

nephropyeloplasty (nĕf"rō-pī'ĕ-lō-plăs"tē) [" + " + plassein, to form]

nephropyosis (nĕf"rō-pī-ō'sĭs) [" + pyosis, suppuration]

nephrorrhagia (nĕf-ror-ā'jē-ă) [" + rhegnynai, to burst forth]

nephrorrhaphy (nĕf-ror'ă-fē) [" + rhaphe, seam]

nephros (nĕf'rŏs) [Gr.]

nephrosclerosis (nĕf"rō-sklĕ-rō'sĭs) [" + sklerosis, a hardening]
   n., arterial
   n., arteriolar
   n., malignant

nephrosis (nĕf-rō'sĭs) [Gr. nephros, kidney, + osis, condition]

   n., lipoid

nephrosonephritis (nĕ-frō"sō-nĕ-frī'tĭs) [" + osis, condition, + nephros, kidney, + itis, inflammation]

nephrospasis (nĕf"rō-spăs'ĭs) [" + Gr. span, to draw]

nephrostoma (nĕ-frŏs'tō-mă) [" + stoma, mouth, opening]

nephrostomy (nĕ-frŏs'tō-mē)

nephrotic (nĕ-frŏt'ĭk) [Gr. nephros, kidney]

nephrotic syndrome
   n.s., idiopathic

nephrotome (nĕf'rō-tōm) [" + tome, a cutting, slice]

nephrotomogram (nĕf"rō-tō'mō-grăm)

nephrotomography (nĕf"rō-tō-mŏg'ră-fē) [" + tomos, slice, section, + graphein, to write]

nephrotomy (nĕ-frŏt'ō-mē) [" + tome, a cutting, slice]

nephrotoxin (nĕf"rō-tŏk'sĭn) [" + toxikon, poison]

nephrotresis (nĕf-rō-trē'sĭs) [" + tresis, piercing]

nephrotropic (nĕf"rō-trŏp'ĭk) [" + tropos, turning]

nephrotuberculosis (nĕf"rō-tū-bĕr"kū-lō'sĭs) [" + tuberculum, a little swelling, + osis, condition]

nephrotyphoid (nĕf"rō-tī'foyd) [" + typhos, stupor, + eidos, form, shape]

nephroureterectomy (nĕf"rō-ū-rē"tĕr-ĕk'tō-mē) [" + oureter, ureter, + ektome, excision]

nephrourography

nephrydrosis (nĕf"rĭ-drō'sĭs) [" + hydor, water, + osis, condition]

Neptazane

neptunium [planet Neptune]

nerve [L. nervus, sinew; Gr. neuron, sinew]
   n.'s, accelerator
   n., acoustic
   n., adrenergic

n., afferent
n., autonomic
n., cerebrospinal
n., cholinergic
n., cranial
n., depressor
n., efferent
n., excitatory
n., excitoreflex
n., facial
n., gangliated
n., glossopharyngeal
n., inhibitory
n., mixed
n., motor
n.'s, olfactory
n., optic
n., parasympathetic
n., peripheral
n., pilomotor
n., pressor
n., secretory
n., sensory
n., somatic
n., spinal
n., splanchnic
n., sudomotor
n., sympathetic
n., trigeminal
n., trophic
n., vagus
n., vasoconstrictor
n., vasodilator
n., vasomotor
n., vasosensory
nerve block
nerve cell
nerve ending
nerve entrapment syndrome
nerve fiber
n.f., adrenergic
n.f., arcuate
n.f., association
n.f., cholinergic
n.f.'s, climbing, of cerebellum
n.f., collateral
n.f., commissural
n.f., myelinated
n.f., nonmedullated

n.f., postganglionic
n.f., preganglionic
n.f., projection
nerve fibril
nerve growth factor
nerve impulse
nerve plexus
nerve trunk
nervi
n. terminales
nervimotility (nĕr″vĭ-mō-tĭl′ĭ-tē) [L.
nervus, nerve, + motilis, moving]
nervimotor (nĕr″vĭ-mō′tor) [″ +
motus, moving]
nervo- [L. nervus, nerve]
nervomuscular [″ + musculus, a
muscle]
nervone
nervous [L. nervosus]
nervous breakdown
nervous debility
nervous impulse
nervousness
nervous prostration
nervous system
nervous tissue
nervus [L.]
n. erigens
n. intermedius
n. nervorum
n. vasorum
Nesacaine
nesidiectomy (nē-sĭd″ē-ĕk′tō-mē) [Gr.
nesidion, islet, + ektome, excision]
nesidioblastoma (nē-sĭd″ē-ō-blăs-
tō′mă) [″ + blastos, germ, +
oma, tumor]
nesslerize (nĕs′lĕr-īz)
Nessler's reagent (nĕs′lĕrz) [A.
Nessler, Ger. chemist, 1827–1905]
nest
n., cancer
n., cell
nesteostomy (nĕs″tē-ŏs′tō-mē) [Gr.
nestis, jejunum, + stoma, mouth,
opening]
nestiatria (nĕs″tē-ā′trē-ă) [Gr. nestis,
fasting, + iatreia, medical treat-
ment]

n. et m. *nocte et mane,* night and morning

net reproductive rate

ne tr. s. num. *ne tradas sine nummo,* do not deliver unless paid

nettle

nettle rash [AS. *netel*]

network [AS. *net,* net, + *wyrcan,* to work]

Neumann's disease (noy'mănz) [Isidor Neumann, Austrian dermatologist, 1832–1906]

neurad (nū'răd) [" + L. *-ad,* toward]

neuragmia (nū-răg'mē-ă) [Gr. *neuron,* nerve, sinew, + *agmos,* break]

neural (nū'răl) [L. *neuralis*]

neural crest

neural fold

neuralgia (nū-răl'jē-ă) [Gr. *neuron,* nerve, sinew, + *algos,* pain]

  n., cardiac

  n., degenerative

  n., facial

  n., facialis vera

  n., Fothergill's

  n., geniculate

  n., glossopharyngeal

  n., hallucinatory

  n., Hunt's

  n., idiopathic

  n., intercostal

  n., mammary

  n., Morton's

  n., nasociliary

  n., occipital

  n., otic

  n., reminiscent

  n., sphenopalatine

  n., stump

  n., symptomatic

  n., trifacial

  n., trigeminal

neuralgic (nū-răl'jĭk) [Gr. *neuron,* nerve, sinew, + *algos,* pain]

neuralgiform (nū-răl'jĭ-form) [" + " + L. *forma,* form]

neural plate

neural spine

neural tube

neural tube defects

neuramebimeter (nū″răm-ē-bĭm'ĕt-ĕr) [" + *amoibe,* response, + *metron,* measure]

neuraminidase (nūr-ăm'ĭn-ĭ-dās″)

neuranagenesis (nū″răn-ă-jĕn'ĕ-sĭs) [" + *anagennan,* to regenerate]

neurapophysis (nū″ră-pŏf'ĭ-sĭs [" + *apo,* from, + *physis,* growth]

neurapraxia (nū″ră-prăks'ē-ă) [" + *apraxia,* nonactive]

neurarchy (nū'răr-kē) [" + *arche,* rule]

neurarthropathy (nū″răr-thrŏp'ă-thē) [" + *arthron,* joint, + *pathos,* disease, suffering]

neurasthenia (nū″răs-thē'nē-ă) [" + *astheneia,* weakness]

neurasthenic (nū-răs-thē'nĭk)

neuratrophia, neuratrophy (nū-ră-trō'fē-ă, -răt'rō-fē) [" + *atrophia,* a wasting]

neuraxis (nū-răk'sĭs) [" + L. *axon,* axis]

neuraxitis (nū-răks-ī'tĭs) [" + " + *itis,* inflammation]

  n., epidemic

neuraxon(e) (nū-răks'ŏn)

neurectasia, neurectasis, neurectasy (nū″rĕk-tā'sē-ă, -rĕk'tă-sĭs, -rĕk'tă-sē) [" + *ektasis,* a stretching]

neurectomy (nū-rĕk'tō-mē) [" + *ektome,* excision]

neurectopia, neurectopy (nū-rĕk-tō'pē-ă, nūr-ĕk'tō-pē) [" + *ek,* out, + *topos,* place]

neurenteric (nū-rĕn-tĕr'ĭk [" + *enteron,* intestine]

neurenteric canal

neurepithelium (nūr″ĕp-ĭ-thē'lē-ŭm) [" + *epi,* upon, + *thele,* nipple]

neurergic (nū-rĕr'jĭk) [" + *ergon,* work]

neurexeresis (nūr″ĕks-ĕr'ĕ-sĭs) [" + *exairein,* to draw out]

neuriatry (nū-rī'ă-trē) [" + *iatreia,*

medication]

neurilemma (nū'rĭ-lĕm"mă) [" + *lemma*, husk]

neurilemmitis (nū"rĭ-lĕm-mī'tĭs) [" + " + *itis*, inflammation]

neurilemmosarcoma (nū"rĭ-lĕm"ō-săr-kō'mă)

neurilemoma,   neurilemmoma (nū"rĭ-lĕm-ō'mă) [" + *eilema*, tight sheath, + *oma*, tumor]

neurimotility (nū"rĭ-mō-tĭl'ĭ-tē) [" + *motilus*, moving]

neurimotor [" + L. *motor*, a mover]

neurinoma (nū-rĭ-nō'mă) [" + *oma*, tumor]

neurinomatosis (nū"rĭ-nō-mă-tō'sĭs) [" + " + *osis*, condition]

neurite (nū'rīt) [Gr. *neuron*, sinew]

neuritis (nū-rī'tĭs) [" + *itis*, inflammation]
   n., adventitial
   n., ascending
   n., axial
   n., degenerative
   n., descending
   n., dietetic
   n., diphtheritic
   n., disseminated
   n., endemic
   n., interstitial
   n., intraocular
   n. migrans
   n., multiple
   n. nodosa
   n., optic
   n., parenchymatous
   n., peripheral
   n., retrobulbar
   n., rheumatic
   n., sciatic
   n., segmental
   n., senile
   n., sympathetic
   n., tabetic
   n., toxic
   n., traumatic

neuro- [Gr. *neuron*, nerve, sinew]

neuroallergy (nū"rō-ăl'ĕr-jē) [" + *allos*, other, + *ergon*, work]

neuroanastomosis (nū"rō-ă-năs"tō-mō'sĭs) [" + *anastomosis*, opening]

neuroanatomy (nū"rō-ăn-ăt'ō-mē)

neuroarthritism (nū"rō-ăr'thrĭ-tĭzm) [" + *arthron*, joint, + *-ismos*, condition]

neuroarthropathy (nū"rō-ăr-thrŏp'ăth-ē) [" + " + *pathos*, disease, suffering]

neuroastrocytoma (nū"rō-ăs"trō-sī-tō'mă) [" + *kytos*, cell, + *oma*, tumor]

neurobiology (nū"rō-bī-ŏl'ō-jē) [" + *bios*, life, + *logos*, word, reason]

neurobiotaxis (nū"rō-bī-ō-tăk'sĭs) [" + *bios*, life, + *taxis*, order]

neuroblast (nū'rō-blăst) [" + *blastos*, germ]

neuroblastoma (nū"rō-blăs-tō'mă) [" + " + *oma*, tumor]

neurocanal (nū"rō-kă-năl') [" + L. *canalis*, passage]

neurocardiac (nū"rō-kăr'dē-ăk) [" + *kardia*, heart]

neurocele (nū'rō-sēl) [" + *koilia*, cavity, belly]

neurocentral (nū"rō-sĕn'trăl) [" + *kentron*, center]

neurocentrum (nū"rō-sĕn'trŭm)

neurochemistry (nū"rō-kĕm'ĭs-trē)

neurochitin (nū"rō-kī'tĭn)

neurochorioretinitis (nū"rō-kō"rē-ō-rĕ"tĭn-ī'tĭs) [Gr. *neuron*, nerve, sinew, + *chorion*, skin, + L. *retina*, retina, + Gr. *itis*, inflammation]

neurochoroiditis (nū"rō-kō-roy-dī'tĭs) [" + " + *eidos*, form, shape, + *itis*, inflammation]

neurocirculatory (nū"rō-sŭr'kū-lă-tō"rē) [" + L. *circulatio*, circulation]

neurocirculatory asthenia

neurocladism (nū-rŏk'lă-dĭzm) [" + Gr. *klados*, a young branch]

neuroclonic (nū"rō-klŏn'ĭk) [" + *klonos*, spasm]

neurocoele (nū'rō-sēl) [" + *koilia*,

cavity, belly]

neurocranium (nū″rō-krā′nē-ŭm) [″ + kranion, skull]

neurocrine (nū′rō-krĭn) [″ + krinein, to secrete]

neurocutaneous (nū″rō-kū-tā′nē-ŭs) [″ + L. cutis, skin]

neurocyte (nū′rō-sīt) [″ + kytos, cell]

neurocytolysis (nū″rō-sī-tŏl′ĭ-sĭs) [″ + kytos, cell, + lysis, dissolution]

neurocytoma (nū″rō-sī-tō′mă) [″ + ″ + oma, tumor]

neurodealgia (nū-rō″dē-ăl′jē-ă) [Gr. neurodes, retina, + algos, pain]

neurodegenerative

neurodendrite, neurodendron (nū″rō-dĕn′drīt, -drŏn) [Gr. neuron, sinew, + dendron, tree]

neurodermatitis (nū″rō-dĕr-mă-tī′tĭs) [″ + derma, skin, + itis, inflammation]
n., disseminated

neurodermatosis (nū″rō-dĕr-mă-tō′sĭs) [″ + ″ + osis, condition]

neurodermatrophia (nū″rō-dĕrm″ă-trōf′ē-ă)

neurodiagnosis (nū″rō-dī-ăg-nō′sĭs)

neurodynamic (nū″rō-dī-năm′ĭk)

neurodynia (nū″rō-dĭn′ē-ă) [Gr. neuron, nerve, + odyne, pain]

neuroectoderm (nū″rō-ĕk′tō-dĕrm) [″ + ektos, out of, + derma, skin]

neuroencephalomyelopathy (nū″rō-ĕn-sĕf″ă-lō-mī″ĕ-lŏp′ă-thē) [″ + enkephalos, brain, + myelos, marrow, + pathos, disease, suffering]

neuroendocrine (nū″rō-ĕn′dō-krĭn)

neuroendocrinology (nū″rō-ĕn″dō-krī-nŏl′ō-jē) [″ + endon, within, + krinein, to secrete, + logos, word, reason]

neuroenteric (nū″rō-ĕn-tĕr′ĭk)

neuroepidermal (nū″rō-ĕp-ĭ-dĕr′măl) [″ + epi, upon, + derma, skin]

neuroepithelioma (nū″rō-ĕp″ĭ-thē-lē-ō′mă) [″ + ″ + thele, nipple, + oma, tumor]

neuroepithelium (nū″rō-ĕp″ĭ-thē′lē-ŭm)

neurofibril, neurofibrilla (nū-rō-fĭ′brĭl, -fĭ-brĭl′ă) [″ + L. fibrilla, a small fiber]

neurofibroma (nū″rō-fĭ-brō′mă) [Gr. neuron, nerve, + L. fibra, fiber, + Gr. oma, tumor]

neurofibromatosis (nū″rō-fĭ-brō″mă-tō′sĭs) [″ + ″ + ″ + osis, condition]

neurofibrosarcoma (nū″rō-fĭ″brō-săr-kō′mă) [″ + ″ + Gr. sarx, flesh, + oma, tumor]

neurofibrositis (nū″rō-fĭ″brō-sī′tĭs) [″ + ″ + Gr. itis, inflammation]

neurogangliitis (nū″rō-găn-glē-ī′tĭs) [″ + ganglion, knot, + itis, inflammation]

neuroganglion (nū″rō-găn′glē-ŏn)

neurogastric (nū″rō-găs′trĭk) [″ + gaster, belly]

neurogenesis (nū″rō-jĕn′ĕ-sĭs) [″ + genesis, generation, birth]

neurogenetic (nūr″ō-jĕn-ĕt′ĭk)

neurogenic, neurogenous (nū-rō-jĕn′ĭk, -rŏj′ĕn-ŭs)

neuroglia (nū-rŏg′lē-ă) [″ + glia, glue]

neurogliacyte (nū-rŏg′lē-ă-sīt) [″ + ″ + kytos, cell]

neuroglial (nū-rŏg′lē-ăl)

neuroglioma (nū″rō-glī-ō′mă) [Gr. neuron, nerve, + glia, glue, + oma, tumor]
n., ganglionare

neurogliomatosis (nū″rō-glī″ō-mă-tō′sĭs) [″ + ″ + ″ + osis, condition]

neurogliosis (nū-rŏg″lē-ō′sĭs) [″ + ″ + osis, condition]

neurogram (nū′rō-grăm)

neurography (nū-rŏg′ră-fē) [″ + graphein, to write]

neurohematology (nū″rō-hĕm″ă-tŏl′ō-jē) [″ + *haima*, blood, + *logos*, word, reason]

neurohistology (nū″rō-hĭs-tŏl′ō-jē) [″ + *histos*, tissue, + *logos*, word, reason]

neurohormone (nū-rō-hor″mōn) [″ + *hormon*, urging on]

neurohumor (nū-rō-hū′mor)

neurohypophysis (nū″rō-hī-pŏf′ĭs-ĭs) [″ + *hypo*, under, beneath, below, + *physis*, growth]

neuroid (nū′royd) [″ + *eidos*, form, shape]

neuroinduction (nū″rō-ĭn-dŭk′shŭn) [″ + L. *inductus*, leading]

neurokeratin (nū″rō-kĕr′ă-tĭn) [″ + *keras*, horn]

neurokyme (nū′rō-kīm) [″ + *kyma*, wave]

neurolemma

neurolemmitis (nū″rō-lĕ-mī′tĭs) [″ + *lemma*, husk]

neurolemmoma (nū″rō-lĕ-mō′mă) [″ + ″ + *oma*, tumor]

neuroleptanesthesia (nū″rō-lĕp″tăn-ĕs-thē′zēă) [″ + *leptos*, slender, + *-an*, not, + *aisthesis*, feeling, perception]

neuroleptic (nū″rō-lĕp′tĭk) [″ + *lepsis*, a taking hold]

neuroleptic anesthesia

neuroleptic drugs

neuroleptic malignant syndrome

neurologic, neurological (nū-rō-lŏj′ĭk, -ĭ-kăl) [″ + *logos*, word, reason]

neurologist (nū-rŏl′ō-jĭst)

neurology (nū-rŏl′ō-jē) [″ + *logos*, word, reason]
n., clinical

neurolymphomatosis (nū″rō-lĭm″fō-mă-tō′sĭs) [″ + L. *lympha*, lymph, + Gr. *oma*, tumor, + *osis*, condition]

neurolysin (nū-rŏl′ĭs-ĭn) [″ + *lysis*, dissolution]

neurolysis (nū-rŏl′ĭs-ĭs)

neurolytic (nū-rō-lĭt′ĭk)

neuroma (nū-rō′mă) [″ + *oma*, tumor]
n., acoustic
n., amputation
n., amyelinic
n., appendiceal
n. cutis
n., cystic
n., false
n., ganglionated
n., multiple
n., myelinic
n., plexiform
n. telangiectodes
n., traumatic

neuromalacia (nū″rō-măl-ā′sē-ă) [″ + *malakia*, softening]

neuromatosis (nū-rō″mă-tō′sĭs) [″ + *oma*, tumor, + *osis*, condition]

neuromatous (nū-rō″mă-tŭs)

neuromechanism (nū″rō-mĕk′ăn-ĭzm)

neuromere (nū′rō-mēr) [″ + *meros*, part]

neuromimesis (nū″rō-mī-mē′sĭs) [″ + *mimesis*, imitation]

neuromuscular (nū″rō-mŭs′kū-lăr) [″ + L. *musculus*, a muscle]

neuromyasthenia (nū″rō-mī″ăs-thē′nē-ă) [″ + *mys*, muscle, + *astheneia*, weakness]

neuromyelitis (nū″rō-mī-ĕl-ī′tĭs) [″ + *myelos*, marrow, + *itis*, inflammation]
n. optica

neuromyopathic (nū″rō-mī″ō-păth′ĭk) [″ + *mys*, muscle, + *pathos*, disease, suffering]

neuromyositis (nū″rō-mī″ō-sī′tĭs) [″ + ″ + *itis*, inflammation]

neuron (nū′rŏn) [Gr. *neuron*, nerve, sinew]
n., afferent
n., associative
n., bipolar
n., central
n., commissural
n., efferent
n., motor

n., motor, lower
n., motor, upper
n., multipolar
n., peripheral
n., postganglionic
n., preganglionic
n., sensory
n., unipolar

neuronal (nū′rō-năl)

neurone (nū′rōn)

neuronephric (nū″rō-nĕf′rĭk) [″ + nephros, kidney]

neuronevus (nū″rō-nē′vŭs)

neuronitis (nū-rō-nī′tĭs) [Gr. neuron, nerve, + itis, inflammation]

neuronophage (nū-rŏn′ō-fāj) [″ + phagein, to eat]

neuronophagia, neuronophagy (nū-rŏn″ō-fā′jē-ă, -ŏf′ă-jē)

neuro-ophthalmology (nū″rō-ŏf″thăl-mŏl′ō-jē) [″ + ophthalmos, eye, + logos, word, reason]

neuro-optic (nū″rō-ŏp′tĭk) [″ + optikos, pert. to vision]

neuropacemaker

neuropapillitis (nū″rō-păp″ĭ-lī′tĭs) [″ + L. papilla, nipple, + Gr. itis, inflammation]

neuroparalysis (nū″rō-pă-răl′ĭ-sĭs) [″ + paralyein, to loosen, disable]

neuropathic (nū-rō-păth′ĭk) [″ + pathos, disease, suffering]

neuropathogenesis (nū″rō-păth″ō-jĕn′ĕ-sĭs) [″ + ″ + genesis, generation, birth]

neuropathogenicity (nū″rō-păth″ō-jĕ-nĭs′ĭ-tē) [″ + pathos, disease, suffering, + gennan, to produce]

neuropathology (nū″rō-pă-thŏl′ō-jē) [″ + ″ + logos, word, reason]

neuropathy (nū-rŏp′ă-thē)
n., ascending
n., descending
n., entrapment
n., hypertrophic mono-
n., optic

neuropharmacology (nū″rō-făr″mă-kŏl′ō-jē) [″ + pharmakon, drug, + logos, word, reason]

neurophilic (nū″rō-fĭl′ĭk) [″ + philos, love]

neurophonia (nū″rō-fō′nē-ă) [Gr. neuron, nerve, + phone, voice]

neurophthalmology (nū″rŏf-thăl-mŏl′ō-jē) [″ + ophthalmos, eye, + logos, word, reason]

neurophthisis (nū-rŏf′thī-sĭs) [″ + phthisis, wasting]

neurophysin (nū″rō-fī′zĭn)

neurophysiological treatment approach

neurophysiology (nū″rō-fĭz-ē-ōl′ō-jē) [″ + physis, growth, + logos, word, reason]

neuropil (nū′rō-pĭl) [″ + pilos, felt]

neuroplasm (nū′rō-plăzm) [″ + LL. plasma, form, mold]

neuroplasmic (nū″rō-plăz′mĭk)

neuroplasty (nū′rō-plăs″tē) [″ + plassein, to form]

neuropodia (nū″rō-pō′dē-ă) [″ + podion, little feet]

neuropore (nū′rō-pōr″) [″ + poros, passage]

neuropotential (nū″rō-pō-tĕn′shăl) [″ + L. potentia, power]

neuropraxia [″ + Gr. praxis, action]

neuropsychiatrist (nū″rō-sī-kī′ă-trĭst) [″ + psyche, mind, + iatreia, healing]

neuropsychiatry (nū″rō-sī-kī′ă-trē)

neuropsychopathy (nū″rō-sī-kŏp′ăth-ē) [″ + ″ + pathos, disease, suffering]

neuropsychopharmacology (nū″rō-sī″kō-făr″mă-kŏl′ō-jē) [″ + ″ + pharmakon, drug, + logos, word, reason]

neuroradiography (nū″rō-rā″dē-ŏg′ră-fē) [″ + L. radius, ray, + Gr. graphein, to write]

neuroradiology (nū″rō-rā″dē-ŏl′ō-jē) [″ + ″ + Gr. logos, word, reason]

neurorelapse (nū″rō-rē-lăps′) [Gr.

neuron, nerve, sinew, + L. *re-lapsus,* fallen back]

neuroretinitis (nū″rō-rĕt″ĭn-ī′tĭs) [″ + L. *retina,* retina, + Gr. *itis,* inflammation]

neuroretinopathy (nū″rō-rĕt″ĭ-nŏp′ă-thē) [″ + ″ + Gr. *pathos,* disease, suffering]

neuroroentgenography (nū″rō-rĕnt″gĕn-ŏg′ră-fē) [″ + *roentgen* + Gr. *graphein,* to write]

neurorrhaphy (nū-ror′ă-fē) [″ + *rhaphe,* seam]

neurosarcokleisis (nū″rō-săr″kō-klī′sĭs) [″ + *sarx,* flesh, + *kleisis,* closure]

neurosarcoma (nū″rō-săr-kō′mă) [″ + ″ + *oma,* tumor]

neuroscience (nū″rō-sī′ĕns)

neurosclerosis (nū″rō-sklĕ-rō′sĭs) [″ + *sklerosis,* a hardening]

neurosecretion (nū″rō-sē-krē′shŭn) [″ + L. *secretio,* separation]

neurosensory (nū″rō-sĕn′sō-rē) [″ + L. *sensorius,* pert. to a sensation]

neurosis (nū-rō′sĭs) [″ + *osis,* condition]
   n., accident
   n., anxiety
   n., association
   n., cardiac
   n., compensation
   n., compulsion
   n., craft
   n., expectation
   n., fatigue
   n., obsessional
   n., occupational
   n., pension
   n., sexual
   n., traumatic
   n., war

neuroskeletal (nū″rō-skĕl′ĕ-tăl) [Gr. *neuron,* nerve, + *skeleton,* a dried-up body]

neuroskeleton (nū″rō-skĕl′ĕ-tŏn) [″ + *skeleton,* a dried-up body]

neurosome (nū′rō-sōm) [″ + *soma,* body]

neurospasm (nū′rō-spăzm) [″ + *spasmos,* a convulsion]

neurosplanchnic (nū″rō-splăngk′nĭk) [″ + *splanchnikos,* pert. to the viscera]

neurospongioma (nū″rō-spŏn″jē-ō′mă) [″ + *spongos,* sponge, + *oma,* tumor]

Neurospora (nū-rŏs′pō-ră)

neurosurgeon (nū″rō-sŭr′jŭn)

neurosurgery [Gr. *neuron,* nerve, sinew, + L. *chirurgia,* hand, + *ergon,* work]

neurosuture (nū″rō-soo′chūr) [″ + L. *sutura,* seam]

neurosyphilis (nū″rō-sĭf′ĭ-lĭs)
   n., asymptomatic
   n., meningovascular
   n., paretic
   n., tabetic

neurotendinous (nū″rō-tĕn′dĭ-nŭs) [″ + L. *tendinosus,* tendinous]

neurotension (nū″rō-tĕn′shŭn) [″ + L. *tensio,* a stretching]

neurothecitis (nū″rō-thē-sī′tĭs) [″ + *theke,* sheath, + *itis,* inflammation]

neurothele (nū″rō-thē′lē) [″ + *thele,* nipple]

neurotherapeutics (nū″rō-thĕr-ă-pū′tĭks) [″ + *therapeutike,* treatment]

neurotherapy (nū″rō-thĕr′ă-pē) [″ + *therapeia,* treatment]

neurotic (nū-rŏt′ĭk) [Gr. *neuron,* nerve, sinew]

neurotic disorder

neuroticism (nū-rŏt′ĭ-sĭzm) [″ + *-ismos,* condition]

neurotization (nū″rŏt-ī-zā′shŭn) [Gr. *neuron,* nerve, sinew]

neurotmesis (nū″rŏt-mē′sĭs) [″ + *tmesis,* cutting]

neurotology (nū″rō-tŏl′ō-jē) [″ + *ous,* ear, + *logos,* word, reason]

neurotome (nū′rō-tōm)

neurotomy (nū-rŏt′ō-mē) [″ + *tome,* a cutting, slice]

neurotonic (nū″rō-tŏn′ĭk) [″ + *tonos,* act of stretching, tension, tone]

neurotony (nū-rŏt′ō-nē)
neurotoxic (nū″rō-tŏks′ĭk) [″ + toxikon, poison]
neurotoxicity (nū″rō-tŏk-sĭs′ĭ-tē) [″ + toxikon, poison]
neurotoxin (nū″rō-tŏks′ĭn)
neurotransmitter (nū″rō-trăns′mĭt-ĕr)
neurotrauma (nū-rō-traw′mă) [″ + trauma, wound]
neurotripsy (nū″rō-trĭp′sē) [″ + tripsis, a rubbing, friction]
neurotrophasthenia (nū″rō-trŏf-ăs-thē′nē-ă) [″ + trophe, nourishment, + astheneia, weakness]
neurotrophic
neurotrophy (nū-rŏt′rō-fē)
neurotropism (nū-rŏt′rō-pĭzm) [Gr. neuron, nerve, + trope, a turning, + -ismos, condition]
neurotropy (nū-rŏt′rō-pē)
neurotrosis (nū″rō-trō′sĭs) [″ + trosis, a wound]
neurotubule (nū″rō-too′būl) [″ + L. tubulus, a tubule]
neurovaccine (nū″rō-văk′sēn)
neurovaricosis (nū″rō-văr″ĭ-kō′sĭs) [″ + L. varicosus, pert. to a swollen vein, + osis, condition]
neurovascular (nū″rō-văs′kū-lar) [″ + L. vasculus, a small vessel]
neurovegetative (nū″rō-vĕj′ĕ-tā″tĭv)
neurovirus (nū″rō-vī′rŭs)
neurovisceral (nū″rō-vĭs′ĕr-ăl) [″ + L. viscera, body organs]
neurula (nū′roo-lă)
neurulation (nū″roo-lā′shŭn)
neutral (nū′trăl) [L. neutralis, neither]
neutral fat
neutralization (nū″trăl-ĭ-zā′shŭn)
neutralize (nū′trăl-īz)
neutral point
neutral red
neutral warmth
neutrino (nū-trē′nō)
neutroclusion (nū″trō-kloo′zhŭn) [L. neuter, neither, + occludo, to close]
neutrocyte (nū′trō-sīt) [″ + Gr. kytos, cell]

neutrocytopenia (nū″trō-sī″tō-pē′nē-ă) [″ + ″ + penia, lack]
neutrocytosis (nū″trō-sī-tō′sĭs) [″ + ″ + osis, condition]
neutron (nū′trŏn) [L. neuter, neither]
neutron capture analysis
neutropenia (nū-trō-pē′nē-ă) [″ + Gr. penia, lack]
  n., malignant
neutrophil(e) (nū′trō-fĭl, -fĭl) [″ + Gr. philein, to love]
neutrophilia (nū″trō-fĭl′ē-ă)
neutrophilic, neutrophilous (nū-trō-fĭl′ĭk, -trŏf′ĭ-lŭs) [″ + Gr. philein, to love]
neutrotaxis (nū″trō-tăk′sĭs) [neutrophil + Gr. taxis, arrangement]
nevocarcinoma (nē″vō-kăr″sĭ-nō′mă) [L. naevus, birthmark, + Gr. karkinos, crab, + oma, tumor]
nevoid (nē′voyd) [″ + Gr. eidos, form, shape]
nevolipoma (nē″vō-lĭ-pō′mă) [″ + Gr. lipos, fat, + oma, tumor]
nevose (nē′vōs) [L. naevus, birthmark]
nevoxanthoendothelioma (nē″vō-zăn″thō-ĕn″dō-thē″lē-ō′mă) [″ + xanthos, yellow, + endon, within, + thele, nipple, + oma, tumor]
nevus (nē′vŭs) [L. naevus, birthmark]
  n. angiectodes
  n. angiomatodes
  n. araneus
  n., blue
  n., blue rubber bleb
  n., capillary
  n. comedonicus
  n., connective tissue
  n., cutaneous
  n., epidermal
  n. flammeus
  n., hairy
  n., halo
  n., intradermal
  n., Ito's
  n., junction
  n. lipomatodes
  n. maternus
  n., melanocytic

n., nevocytic
n., Ota's
n. pigmentosus
n. pilosus
n., sebaceous
n., spider
n. spilus
n. spongiosus albus mucosae
n., strawberry
n., telangiectatic
n. unius lateris
n. vascularis
n. venosus
n. verrucosus
n., white sponge
newborn
Newcastle disease (nū'kăs-ĕl) [New-castle, England]
new growth
newton
newton meter
nexus (nĕk'sŭs) [L., bond]
NF *National Formulary*
N.F.L.P.N. *National Federation of Licensed Practical Nurses*
ng *nanogram*
NG tube *nasogastric* tube
NH₃ *ammonia*
NH₄⁺ *univalent ammonium radical*
NH₄Br *ammonium bromide*
NH₄Cl *ammonium chloride*
N.H.I. *National Heart Institute*
N.H.L.I. *National Heart and Lung Institute*
NH₄NO₃ *ammonium nitrate*
NH₄OH *ammonium hydroxide*
Ni *nickel*
niacin (nī'ă-sĭn)
niacinamide (nī"ă-sĭn-ăm'ĭd)
N.I.A.I.D. *National Institute of Allergy and Infectious Diseases*
N.I.A.M.D. *National Institute of Arthritis and Metabolic Diseases*
nib (nĭb)
niche (nĭch) [Fr.]
n., enamel
N.I.C.H.H.D. *National Institute of Child Health and Human Development*

nickel
n. carbonyl
nicking
niclosamide (nĭ-klō'să-mīd)
Nicobid
Nicolar
Nicolas-Favre disease (nē"kō-lă-făv'r) [Josef Nicolas, b. 1868, and M. Favre, 1876–1954, Fr. physicians]
nicotinamide (nĭk"ō-tĭn'ă-mīd)
n. adenine dinucleotide
n. adenine dinucleotide-dehydrogenase
n. adenine dinucleotide-diaphorase
n. adenine dinucleotide phosphate
n. adenine diphosphate
nicotine (nĭk'ō-tēn, -tĭn) [L. *nicotiana*, tobacco]
nicotine poisoning, acute
nicotinic acid (nĭk"ō-tĭn'ĭk)
nicotinism (nĭk'ō-tĭn-ĭzm)
nictation [L. *nictitare*, to wink]
nictitate (nĭk'tĭ-tāt)
nictitating (nĭk'tĭ-tāt-ĭng)
nictitating membrane
nictitating spasm
nictitation [L. *nictitare*, to wink]
nidal (nī'dăl) [L. *nidus*, nest]
nidation (nī-dā'shŭn)
N.I.D.R. *National Institute of Dental Research*
nidus (nī'dŭs) [L., nest]
n. avis cerebelli
n. hirundinis
Niemann-Pick disease (nē'măn-pĭk) [Albert Niemann, Ger. pediatrician, 1880–1921; Ludwig Pick, Ger. physician, 1868–1935]
night blindness
Nightingale, Florence (nīt'ĭn-gāl) [Brit. philanthropist, 1820–1910]
Nightingale Pledge
nightmare (nīt'măr) [AS. *nyht*, night, + *mara*, a demon]
nightshade (nīt'shād) [AS. *nihtscada*]
n., deadly
night sweat [AS. *nyht*, night, + *swat*, sweat]

night terrors [" + L. *terrere*, to frighten]
night vision
nightwalking
N.I.G.M.S. *National Institute of General Medical Sciences*
nigra (nī'grä) [L., black]
nigri-, nigro- [L. *nigra*, black]
nigricans (nī'grī-kăns)
nigrities (nī-grĭsh'ĭ-ēz)
   n. linguae
nigrosin (nī'grō-sĭn)
nigrostriatal (nī‴grō-strī-ā'tăl)
NIH *National Institutes of Health*
nihilism (nī'ĭ-lĭzm) [L. *nihil*, nothing, + Gr. *-ismos*, condition]
nikethamide (nī-kĕth'ă-mīd)
Nikolsky's sign (nī-kŏl'skēz) [Pyotr Nikolsky, Russ. dermatologist, 1855 – 1940]
Nilstat
N.I.M.H. *National Institute of Mental Health*
N.I.N.D.B. *National Institute of Neurological Diseases and Blindness*
ninth cranial nerve
niobium (nī-ō'bē-um) [Legendary Gr. woman, Niobe, who was turned into stone]
niphablepsia (nĭf‴ă-blĕp'sē-ă) [Gr. *nipha*, snow, + *ablepsia*, blindness]
niphotyphlosis (nĭf‴ō-tĭf-lō'sĭs) [" + *typhlosis*, blindness]
nipple (nĭp'l) [AS. *neble*, a little protuberance]
   n., crater
   n., retracted
nipple shield
Nipride
Nisentil
Nissl bodies (nĭs'l) [Franz Nissl, Ger. neurologist, 1860 – 1919]
nisus (nī'sŭs) [L.]
nit (nĭt) [AS. *hnitu*]
niter (nī'ter) [Gr. *nitron*, salt]
niton (nī'tŏn)
nitr- [Gr. *nitron*, salt]

nitrate (nī'trāt) [L. *nitratum*]
nitrated
nitration
nitre (nī'tĕr) [Fr.]
nitremia (nī-trē'mē-ă)
nitric acid
   n.a., fuming
nitric acid poisoning
nitridation (nī-trī-dā'shŭn)
nitride (nī'trīd)
nitrification (nī‴trī-fĭ-kā'shŭn)
nitrifying (nī'trī-fī‴ĭng)
nitrifying bacteria
nitrile (nī'trĭl)
nitrite (nī'trīt) [Gr. *nitron*, salt]
nitritoid (nī'trī-toyd) [" + *eidos*, form, shape]
   n. crisis
nitrituria (nī-trī-tū'rē-ă) [" + *ouron*, urine]
nitro- [Gr. *nitron*, salt]
nitrobenzene (nī‴trō-bĕn'zēn)
nitroblue tetrazolium test
nitrocellulose (nī‴trō-sĕl'ū-lōs)
nitrofurantoin (nī‴trō-fū-răn'tō-ĭn)
nitrofurazone (nī‴trō-fū'ră-zōn)
nitrogen (nī'trō-jĕn) [Fr. *nitrogene*]
   n. monoxide
   n. mustards
   n., nonprotein
nitrogenase (nī'trō-jĕn-ās) [*nitrogen* + *-ase*, enzyme]
nitrogen balance
nitrogen cycle
nitrogen equilibrium
nitrogen fixation
nitrogen lag
nitrogen narcosis
nitrogenous (nī-trŏj'ĕn-ŭs)
nitroglycerin (nī‴trō-glĭs'ĕr-ĭn) [Gr. *nitron*, salt, + *glycerin*]
nitroglycerin tablets
nitromersol (nī‴trō-mĕr'sŏl)
nitrometer (nī-trŏm'ĕ-tĕr) [*nitrogen* + Gr. *metron*, measure]
nitromuriatic acid (nī‴trō-mū-rē-ăt'ĭk) [" + L. *muriaticus*, briny]
Nitrong

Nitropress
Nitrosomonas
nitrous (nī′trŭs) [Gr. *nitron*, salt]
nitrous acid
nitrous oxide
NK cells *natural killer cells*
N.L.N. *National League for Nursing*
NMRI *Naval Medical Research Institute; nuclear magnetic resonance imaging*
NMR spectroscopy *nuclear magnetic resonance spectroscopy*
N.M.S.S. *National Multiple Sclerosis Society*
N.N.D. *New and Nonofficial Drugs*
No *nobelium*
N₂O N_2O *nitrous oxide*
N₂O₃ N_2O_3 *nitrogen trioxide*
N₂O₅ N_2O_5 *nitrogen pentoxide*
no. [L.] *numero*, to the number of
nobelium (nō-bē′lē-ŭm) [Named for Nobel Institute, where it was first isolated]
Nobel prize [Alfred B. Nobel, Swedish chemist and philanthropist, 1833–1896]
Nocardia [Edmund I. E. Nocard, Fr. veterinary pathologist, 1850–1903]
　　N. asteroides
　　N. brasiliensis
nocardial (nō-kăr′dē-ăl)
nocardiosis
noci- (nō′sē) [L. *nocere*, to injure]
nociassociation (nō″sē-ă-sō″sē-ā′shŭn) [″ + *ad*, to, + *socius*, companion]
nociceptive (nō″sĭ-sĕp′tĭv) [″ + *ceptus*, receiving]
nociceptive impulses
nociceptive reflex
nociceptor (nō″sē-sĕp′tor) [″ + L. *receptor*, receiver]
noci-influence (nō″sē-ĭn′floo-ĕns) [″ + *influence*]
nociperception (nō″sĭ-pĕr-sĕp′shŭn) [″ + *perceptio*, apprehension]
"no code" orders
noct. [L.] *nocte*, night
noctalbuminuria (nŏk″tăl-bū-mĭn-ū′rē-

ă) [L. *nocte*, at night, + *albumen*, white of egg, + Gr. *ouron*, urine]
noctambulation (nŏk″tăm-bū-lā′shŭn) [″ + *ambulare*, to move about]
noctambulism (nŏk-tăm′bū-lĭzm) [″ + ″ + Gr. *-ismos*, condition]
Noctec
noctiphobia (nŏk″tĭ-fō′bē-ă) [″ + Gr. *phobos*, fear]
nocturia (nŏk-tū′rē-ă) [″ + Gr. *ouron*, urine]
nocturnal [L. *nocturnus*, at night]
nocturnal emission
nocturnal enuresis
nocturnal penile tumescence
nocuous (nŏk′ū-ŭs) [L. *nocuus*]
nodal (nō′dăl) [L. *nodus*, knot]
nodal points
nodal rhythm
nodding (nŏd′ĭng)
nodding spasm
node (nōd) [L. *nodus*, knot]
　　n., Aschoff's
　　n., atrioventricular
　　n., A-V
　　n., Bouchard's
　　n., Flack's
　　n.'s, Haygarth's
　　n.'s, Heberden's
　　n., hemal
　　n., Hensen's
　　n., lymph
　　n.'s, Meynet's
　　n.'s of Ranvier
　　n.'s, Osler's
　　n.'s, Parrot's
　　n., piedric
　　n., Schmorl's
　　n., sentinel
　　n., signal
　　n., singer's
　　n., sinoatrial
　　n., sinoauricular
　　n., sinus
　　n., syphilitic
　　n., teacher's
　　n., Troisier's
　　n., Virchow

nodi (nō'dī)
no diagnosis
nodose (nō'dōs) [L. *nodosus,* knotted]
nodosity (nō-dòs'ĭ-tē) [L. *nodositas,* a knot]
nodular (nŏd'ū-lăr)
nodulation (nŏd"ū-lā'shŭn)
nodule (nŏd'ūl) [L. *nodulus,* little knot]
   n.'s, aggregate
   n.'s, Albini's
   n., apple jelly
   n.'s, Arantius'
   n., Aschoff's
   n.'s, cortical
   n.'s, Gamna
   n., lymph
   n., lymphatic
   n., milker's
   n.'s, Morgagni
   n.'s of semilunar valve
   n., rheumatic
   n., Schmorl's
   n.'s, siderotic
   n., Sister Mary Joseph
   n., solitary
   n.'s, subcutaneous
   n.'s, surfer's
   n.'s, typhoid
   n.'s, typhus
nodulus (nŏd'ū-lŭs) [L.]
nodus (nō'dŭs) [L.]
noematachograph (nō-ē"mă-tăk'ō-grăf) [Gr. *noema,* thought, + *tachys,* swift, + *graphein,* to write]
noematachometer (nō-ē"mă-tăk-ŏm'ĕ-tĕr) [" + " + *metron,* measure]
noematic (nō"ē-măt'ĭk) [Gr. *noema,* thought]
noesis (nō-ē'sĭs) [Gr. *noesis,* thought]
Noguchia (nō-goo'chē-ă) [Hideyo Noguchi, Japanese bacteriologist in U.S., 1876–1928]
noise [O. Fr. *noise,* strife, brawl]
noli me tangere (nō"lē-mē-tăn'jĕ-rē) [L., touch me not]
Noludar
Nolvadex

noma (nō'mă) [Gr. *nome,* a spreading]
   n. pudendi
nomadism [Gr. *nomas,* roaming about]
nomenclature (nō'mĕn-klā"chūr) [L. *nomen,* name, + *calare,* to call]
   n., binomial
Nomina Anatomica (nō'mĭ-nă ăn-ă-tŏm'ĭ-kă) [" + Gr. *anatome,* dissection]
nomogram (nŏm'ō-grăm) [Gr. *nomos,* law, + *gramma,* letter, piece of writing]
nomography (nō-mŏg'ră-fē) [" + *graphein,* to write]
nomotopic (nō-mō-tŏp'ĭk) [" + *topos,* place]
nona-, non [L. *nonus,* ninth]
nonan (nō'năn)
noncompliance
non compos mentis (nŏn kŏm'pòs mĕn'tĭs) [L.]
nonconductor [L. *non,* not, + *con,* with, + *ductor,* a leader]
nondisjunction
nonelectrolyte [" + *electron,* amber, + *lytos,* dissolved]
nonigravida (nō"nĭ-gră'vĭ-dă) [L. *nonus,* ninth, + *gravida,* pregnant]
noninvasive
noninvasive neoplasm
nonipara (nō-nĭp'ăr-ă) [" + *parere,* to beget, produce]
nonlaxative diet
nonmedullated (nŏn-mĕd'ū-lāt"ĕd) [L. *non,* not, + *medulla,* marrow]
nonmyelinated (nŏn-mī'ĕ-lĭ-nāt"ĕd) [" + *myelos,* marrow]
non-nucleated (nŏn-nū'klē-āt"ĕd) [" + *nucleatus,* having a kernel]
nonocclusion (nŏn"ō-kloo'zhŭn) [" + *occlusio,* occlusion]
nonopaque (nŏn"ō-pāk')
nonose (nŏn'ōs) [L. *nonus,* ninth]
nonoxynol (nō-nŏks'ĭ-nŏl)
   n. 9
nonparous (nŏn-păr'ŭs) [L. *non,* not, + *parere,* to beget, produce]
nonpolar [" + *polus,* a pole]

nonpolar compound
nonproprietary name
nonprotein [L. *non*, not, + Gr. *protos*, first]
nonprotein nitrogen
non rep. [L.] *non repetatur*, do not repeat
nonrestraint (nŏn″rē-strănt′) [L. *non*, not, + *re*, back, + *stringere*, to bind back]
nonrotation (nŏn″rō-tā′shŭn) [″ + *rotare*, to turn]
  n. of intestine
nonsecretor (nŏn″sē-krē′tor) [″ + *secretio*, separation]
nonseptate (nŏn-sĕp′tāt) [″ + *septum*, a partition]
nonsexual (nŏn-sĕk′shū-ăl)
nonspecific
nonspecific urethritis
nontoxic (nŏn-tŏk′sĭk) [Gr. *non*, not, + Gr. *toxikon*, poison]
nontoxic substances
nonunion (nŏn-ūn′yŭn) [″ + *unio*, oneness]
nonus [L.]
nonvalent (nŏn-vā′lĕnt) [L. *non*, not, + *valens*, powerful]
nonviable (nŏn-vī′ă-bl) [″ + *via*, life]
nonyl
nookleptia (nō-ō-klĕp′tē-ă) [Gr. *nous*, mind, + *kleptein*, to steal]
Noonan's syndrome [Jacqueline A. Noonan, U.S. cardiologist, b. 1921]
noopsyche (nō′ō-sī″kē) [Gr. *nous*, mind, + *psyche*, soul]
noradrenalin bitartrate (nor″ă-drĕn′ă-lĭn)
NORD *National Organization for Rare Disorders*
nordefrin hydrochloride (nor-dĕf′rĭn)
norepinephrine (nor-ĕp″ĭ-nĕf′rĭn)
  n. bitartrate
norethandrolone (nor″ĕth-ăn′drō-lōn)
norethindrone (nor-ĕth′ĭn-drōn)

norethynodrel (nor″ĕ-thī′nō-drĕl)
Norflex
norflurane (nor-floor′ān)
norgestrel (nor-jĕs′trĕl)
Norisodrine Aerotrol
Norlutate
Norlutin
norm [L. *norma*, rule]
norma [L., rule]
  n., anterior
  n. basilaris
  n. facialis
  n. frontalis
  n., inferior
  n. lateralis
  n. occipitalis
  n. sagittalis
  n., superior
  n. ventralis
  n. verticalis
normal (nor′măl) [L. *normalis*, according to pattern]
normalization (nor″măl-ĭ-zā′shŭn) [L. *normalis*, according to pattern]
normal salt
normal solution
normergic (nor-mĕr′jĭk)
normetanephrine (nor-mĕt″ă-nĕf′rĭn)
normo- [L. *norma*, rule]
normoblast (nor′mō-blăst) [″ + Gr. *blastos*, germ]
normoblastosis (nor″mō-blăs-tō′sĭs) [″ + ″ + *osis*, condition]
normocalcemia (nor″mō-kăl-sē′mē-ă)
normocapnia (nor″mō-kăp′nē-ă)
normocapnic (nor″mō-kăp′nĭk)
normocholesterolemia (nor″mō-kō-lĕs″tĕr-ō-lē′mē-ă)
normochromasia (nor″mō-krō-mā′zē-ă) [″ + Gr. *chroma*, color]
normochromia (nor″mō-krō′mē-ă)
normocyte (nor′mō-sīt) [″ + Gr. *kytos*, cell]
normocytosis (nor″mō-sī-tō′sĭs) [″ + ″ + *osis*, condition]
normoerythrocyte (nor″mō-ĕ-rĭth′rō-sīt) [″ + Gr. *erythros*, red, + *kytos*, cell]

normoglycemia (nor″mō-glī-sē′mē-ă) [″ + Gr. *glykys*, sweet, + *haima*, blood]
normoglycemic (nor″mō-glī-sē′mĭk)
normokalemia (nor″mō-kă-lē′mē-ă)
normo-orthocytosis (nor″mō-or″thō-sī-tō′sĭs) [L. *norma*, rule, + Gr. *orthos*, straight, + *kytos*, cell, + *osis*, condition]
normoskeocytosis (nor″mō-skē″ō-sī-tō′sĭs) [″ + *skaios*, left, + *kytos*, cell, + *osis*, condition]
normospermic (nor″mō-spĕr′mĭk) [″ + *sperma*, seed]
normosthenuria (nor″mō-sthĕn-ū′rē-ă) [″ + Gr. *sthenos*, strength, + *ouron*, urine]
normotensive (nor″mō-tĕn′sĭv)
normothermia (nor″mō-thĕr′mē-ă) [″ + Gr. *therme*, heat]
normotonic (nor″mō-tŏn′ĭk) [″ + Gr. *tonos*, act of stretching, tension, tone]
normotopia (nor″mō-tō′pē-ă) [″ + Gr. *topos*, place]
normotopic (nor″mō-tŏp′ĭk)
normovolemia (nor″mō-vō-lē′mē-ă) [″ + *volumen*, volume, + Gr. *haima*, blood]
Norpace
Norpramin
Norrie's disease [G. Norrie, Danish ophthalmologist, 1855–1941]
nortriptyline hydrochloride (nor-trĭp′tĭ-lēn)
Norwalk agent [virus first identified in Norwalk, Ohio, U.S.A.]
Norwegian itch
noscapine (nŏs′kă-pēn)
nose [AS. *nosw*]
  n., bridge of
  n., foreign body in
  n., hammer
  n., saddle
nosebleed
Nosema (nō-sē′mă)
nosepiece (nōz′pēs)
nosetiology (nŏs″ē-tē-ŏl′ō-jē) [Gr.

nosos, disease, + *aitia*, cause, + *logos*, word, reason]
nosh
noso- [Gr. *nosos*, disease]
nosochthonography (nŏs″ŏk-thō-nŏg′ră-fē) [″ + *chthon*, earth, + *graphein*, to write]
nosocomial (nŏs″ō-kō′mē-ăl) [″ + *komeion*, to care for]
nosocomial infection
nosogenesis, nosogeny (nŏs″ō-jĕn′ĕ-sĭs, nō-sŏj′ĕn-ē) [Gr. *nosos*, disease, + *genesis*, generation, birth; *gennan*, to produce]
nosogeography (nŏs″ō-jē-ŏg′ră-fē) [″ + *ge*, earth, + *graphein*, to write]
nosography (nō-sŏg′ră-fē) [″ + *graphein*, to write]
nosohemia (nŏs-ō-hē′mē-ă) [″ + *haima*, blood]
nosology (nō-sŏl′ō-jē) [″ + *logos*, word, reason]
nosomania (nŏs″ō-mā′nē-ă) [″ + *mania*, madness]
nosomycosis (nŏs″ō-mī-kō′sĭs) [″ + *mykes*, fungus, + *osis*, condition]
nosonomy (nō-sŏn′ō-mē) [″ + *nomos*, law]
nosophilia (nŏs″ō-fĭl′ē-ă) [″ + *philein*, to love]
nosophobia (nŏ″sō-fō′bē-ă) [″ + *phobos*, fear]
nosophyte (nŏs′ō-fīt) [″ + *phyton*, plant]
nosopoietic (nŏs″ō-poy-ĕt′ĭk) [″ + *poiein*, to form]
Nosopsyllus (nŏs″ō-sĭl′ŭs) [″ + *psylla*, flea]
  N. fasciatus
nosotaxy (nŏs′ō-tăk″sē) [″ + *taxis*, arrangement]
nosotherapy (nŏs″ō-thĕr′ă-pē) [″ + *therapeia*, treatment]
nosotoxic (nŏs″ō-tŏk′sĭk [″ + *toxikon*, poison]
nosotoxicosis (nŏs″ō-tŏk″sī-kō′sĭs) [″ + ″ + *osis*, condition]

nosotrophy (nō-sŏt'rō-fē) [" + trophe, nourishment]

nosotropic (nō"sō-trŏp'ĭk) [" + tropos, turning]

nostalgia (nŏs-tăl'jē-ă) [Gr. nostos, a return home, + algos, pain]

nostomania (nŏs"tō-mā'nē-ă) [" + mania, madness]

nostril [AS. nosu, nose, + thyrel, a hole]

nostril reflex

nostrum (nŏs'trŭm) [L., our]

notal (nō'tăl) [Gr. noton, back]

notalgia (nō-tăl'jē-ă) [" + algos, pain]

notancephalia (nō"tăn-sĕ-fā'lē-ă) [" + -an, not, + kephale, head]

notanencephalia (nō"tăn-ĕn-sĕ-fā'lē-ă) [" + " + enkephalos, brain]

notch (nŏch)
  n., acetabular
  n., aortic
  n., cardiac
  n., cerebellar, anterior and posterior
  n., clavicular
  n., costal
  n., cotyloid
  n., ethmoidal
  n., frontal
  n., interclavicular
  n., jugular (of occipital bone)
  n., jugular (of sternum)
  n., labial
  n., mandibular
  n., manubrial
  n., nasal
  n. of Rivinus
  n., pancreatic
  n., parotid
  n., radial
  n., scapular
  n., sciatic, greater
  n., sciatic, lesser
  n., semilunar
  n., sphenopalatine
  n., tentorial
  n., thyroid

  n., tympanic
  n., ulnar
  n., umbilical
  n., vertebral

note [L. nota, a mark]

note blindness

notencephalocele (nō"tĕn-sĕf'ăl-ō-sēl) [Gr. noton, back, + enkephalos, brain, + kele, tumor, swelling]

notencephalus (nō"tĕn-sĕf'ă-lŭs) [" + enkephalos, brain]

nothing by mouth

notifiable diseases

noto- [Gr. noton, back]

notochord (nō'tō-kord) [" + chorde, cord]

notogenesis (nō"tō-jĕn'ĕ-sĭs) [" + genesis, generation, birth]

notomelus (nō-tŏm'ĕ-lŭs) [" + melos, limb]

noumenal (nū'mē-năl) [Gr. nooumenon, a thing perceived]

noumenon (nū'mē-nŏn) [Gr. nooumenon]

nourishment [L. nutrire, to nurse]

Novafed

Novocain

noxa (nŏk'să) [L., injury]

noxious (nŏk'shŭs) [L. noxius, injurious]

NP neuropsychiatrist; neuropsychiatry; nucleoprotein; nursing practice; nurse practitioner; nursing procedure;

Np neptunium

NPC nodal premature complex

NPH insulin neutral protamine Hagedorn insulin

NPN nonprotein nitrogen

n.p.t. normal pressure and temperature

NR nodal rhythm

NREM sleep nonrapid eye movement sleep

N.R.M.S. National Registry of Medical Secretaries

ns nanosecond; nonsignificant

NSA Neurosurgical Society of America

NSCC National Society for Crippled Children

NSD *nominal standard dose*

nsec *nanosecond*

N.S.N.A. *National Student Nurses' Association*

NSPB *National Society for the Prevention of Blindness*

NSR *normal sinus rhythm*

NT *nodal tachycardia*

Nt *niton*

nth (ĕnth)

Nubain

nubecula (nū-bĕk'ū-lă) [L., little cloud]

nubile (nū'bǐl) [L. *nubere*, to marry]

nubility (nū-bǐl'ǐ-tē)

nucha (nū'kă) [L.]

nuchal (nū'kăl) [L. *nucha*, back of neck]

Nuck's canal (nŭks) [Anton Nuck, Dutch anatomist, 1650–1692]

nuclear (nū'klē-ăr) [L. *nucleus*, a kernel]

nuclear antigen

nuclear arc

nuclear envelope

nuclear family

nuclear magnetic resonance imaging

nuclear medicine

nuclear winter

nuclease (nū'klē-ās) [L. *nucleus*, kernel, + -*ase*, enzyme]

nucleate (nū'klē-āt) [L. *nucleatus*, having a kernel]

nucleic acid

nucleiform (nū'klē-ǐ-form) [L. *nucleus*, kernel, + *forma*, shape]

nuclein (nū'klē-ǐn) [L. *nucleus*, a kernel]

nucleinase

nuclein bases

nucleo- [L. *nucleus*]

nucleocapsid (nū"klē-ō-kăp'sǐd)

nucleochylema (nū"klē-ō-kī-lē'mă) [" + Gr. *chylos*, juice]

nucleochyme (nū'klē-ō-kīm) [" + Gr. *chymos*, juice]

nucleofugal (nū-klē-ŏf'ū-găl) [" + *fugere*, to flee]

nucleohistone (nū"klē-ŏ-hǐs'tŏn, -tōn) [" + *histos*, tissue]

nucleoid (nū'klē-oyd) [" + Gr. *eidos*, form, shape]

nucleolar (nū-klē'ō-lăr) [L. *nucleolus*, a little kernel]

nucleoli (nū-klē'ō-lī)

nucleoliform (nū-klē-ō'lǐ-form) [" + *forma*, shape]

nucleoloid (nū'klē-ō-loyd)

nucleolonema (nū"klē-ō"lō-nē'mă) [" + Gr. *nema*, thread]

nucleolus (nū-klē'ō-lŭs) [L., little kernel]

nucleomicrosome (nū"klē-ō-mī'krō-sōm) [L. *nucleus*, kernel, + Gr. *mikros*, tiny, + *soma*, body]

nucleons (nū'klē-ŏnz)

nucleopetal (nū-klē-ŏp'ĕ-tăl) [L. *nucleus*, kernel, + *petere*, to seek]

nucleophilic (nū"klē-ō-fǐl'ǐk) [" + *philein*, to love]

nucleoplasm (nū'klē-ō-plăzm") [" + LL. *plasma*, form, mold]

nucleoplasmic

nucleoplasmic index

nucleoprotein (nū"klē-ō-prō'tē-ǐn) [" + Gr. *protos*, first]

nucleoreticulum (nū"klē-ō-rē-tǐk'ū-lŭm) [" + *reticulum*, network]

nucleosidase (nū"klē-ō-sī'dās)

nucleoside

nucleospindle (nū"klē-ō-spǐn'dl)

nucleotidase (nū"klē-ŏt'ǐ-dās)

5'-nucleotidase

nucleotide (nū'klē-ō-tīd) [L. *nucleus*, kernel]

nucleotidyl (nū"klē-ō-tīd'ǐl)

nucleotidyltransferase (nū"klē-ō-tīd'ǐl-trăns'fĕr-ās)

nucleotoxin [" + Gr. *toxikon*, poison]

nucleus (nū'klē-ŭs) [L., kernel]

  n., abducens

  n., ambiguous

  n., amygdaloid

  n., angular

  n., anterior, of thalamus

  n., arcuate

  n., atomic

  n., auditory

  n., Bechterew's, Bekhterev's

n., caudate
n., central, of thalamus
n., centromedian
n., cerebellar
n., cochlear, dorsal
n., cochlear, ventral
n., cornucommissural, posterior
n., cuneate
n., Deiters'
n., dentate
n., diploid
n., dorsal, of spinal cord
n., dorsal motor, of vagus
n., dorsal sensory, of vagus
n., ectoblastic
n., Edinger-Westphal
n., emboliform
n., facial motor
n., fastigial
n., fertilization
n., free
n. funiculi gracilis
n., germinal
n., globose
n., gonad
n. gracilis
n., habenular
n., haploid
n., hypoglossal
n., hypothalamic
n., interpeduncular
n., interstitial, of Cajal
n., intraventricular
n., lenticular
n. lentis
n., masticatory
n., mesencephalic tract
n., mother
n., motor
n., motor, of trigeminal nerve
n., oculomotor
n. of Burdach
n. of origin
n. of termination
n., olivary, inferior
n., olivary, superior
n., paraventricular
n., pontine

n., principal trigeminal sensory
n. pulposus
n., pyramidal
n., red
n., reproductive
n., reticular
n. ruber
n., salivatory, inferior
n., salivatory, superior
n., segmentation
n., sensory
n., sensory, of trigeminal nerve
n., sperm
n., subthalamic
n., supraoptic
n., thalamic
n., thoracic
n., trigeminal spinal
n., vesicular
n., vestibular
n., vitelline
n., white
n., yolk
nuclide (nū'klīd)
nude [L. *nudus*, naked]
nude mice
nudism
nudo- [L. *nudus*]
nudomania (nū"dō-mā'nē-ă) [" + Gr. *mania*, madness]
nudophobia (nū"dō-fō'bē-ă) [" + Gr. *phobos*, fear]
Nuel's space (nū'ĕlz) [Jean P. Nuel, Bel. oculist, 1847–1920]
Nuhn's glands (noonz) [Anton Nuhn, Ger. anatomist, 1814–1889]
null hypothesis
nulligravida
nullipara (nŭl-ĭp'ă-ră) [L. *nullus*, none, + *parere*, to beget, produce]
nulliparity (nŭl"ĭ-păr'ĭ-tē)
nulliparous (nŭl-lĭp'ăr-ŭs)
nullisomatic (nŭl"ĭ-sō-măt'ĭk) [" + Gr. *soma*, body]
numb (nŭm)
number [L. *numerus*, number]
n., atomic
n., Avogadro's

n., hardness
n., mass
numbness
numeral (nū'mĕr-ăl) [L. *numerus*, number]
nummiform (nŭm'mĭ-form) [L. *nummus*, a coin, + *forma*, shape]
nummular (nŭm'ū-lăr) [L. *nummus*, coin]
nummulation (nŭm-ū-lā'shŭn)
Numorphan
nunnation (nŭn-ā'shŭn) [Heb. *nun*, letter N]
nurse [L. *nutrix*, nurse]
n., charge
n., clinical (nurse) specialist
n., community health
n., dental
n., epidemiologist
n., flight
n., general duty
n., graduate
n., head
n., health
n., infection control
n., licensed practical
n., practical
n., prescribing
n., private duty
n.'s, probationer
n., public health
n., registered
n., school
n., scrub
n., special
n., specialist
n., student
n., trained
n., visiting
n., wet
nurse anesthetist
nurse clinician
nurse-midwife
nurse practitioner
nursery
n., day
nurse's aide
nursing
nursing assessment

nursing audit
nursing diagnosis
nursing histories
nursing intervention
nursing process
nutation (nū-tā'shŭn) [L. *nutatio*]
nutgall (nŭt'gawl)
Nutracort
nutrient (nū'trē-ĕnt) [L. *nutriens*]
nutrilite (nū'trĭ-līt)
nutriment (nū'trĭ-mĕnt) [L. *nutrimentum*, nourishment]
nutrition (nū-trĭ'shŭn) [L. *nutritio*, nourish]
nutritional (nū-trĭsh'ŭn-ăl)
nutritional adequacy
nutritious (nū-trĭsh'ŭs) [L. *nutritius*]
nutritive (nū'trĭ-tĭv)
nutritive enema
nutriture (nū'trĭ-tūr)
nux vomica (nŭks vŏm'ĭ-kă)
nyctalbuminuria (nĭk"tăl-bū"mĭn-ū'rē-ă) [Gr. *nyx*, night, + L. *albus*, white, + Gr. *ouron*, urine]
nyctalgia (nĭk-tăl'jē-ă) [" + *algos*, pain]
nyctalopia (nĭk-tă-lō'pē-ă) [" + *alaos*, blind, + *ops*, eye]
nyctamblyopia (nĭk"tăm-blē-ō'pē-ă) [Gr. *nyx*, night, + *amblyopia*, poor sight]
nyctaphonia (nĭk-tă-fō'nē-ă) [" + *a*, not, + *phone*, voice]
nycterine (nĭk'tĕr-īn) [Gr. *nykterinos*, by night]
nycthemerus (nĭk-thĕm'ĕ-rŭs) [Gr. *nychthemeros*]
nycto- (nĭk'tō) [Gr. *nyx*, night]
nyctohemeral (nĭk"tō-hĕm'ĕr-ăl)
nyctophilia (nĭk"tō-fĭl'ē-ă) [Gr. *nyx*, night, + *philein*, to love]
nyctophobia (nĭk"tō-fō'bē-ă) [" + *phobos*, fear]
nyctophonia (nĭk"tō-fō'nē-ă) [" + *phone*, voice]
nyctotyphlosis (nĭk"tō-tĭf-lō'sĭs) [" + *typhlosis*, blindness]
nycturia (nĭk-tū'rē-ă) [" + *ouron*, urine]

Nydrazid
nylidrin hydrochloride (nĭl'ĭ-drĭn)
nymph (nĭmf) [Gr. *nymphe*, a maiden]
nympha [Gr. *nymphe*, a maiden]
nymphectomy (nĭm-fĕk'tō-mē) [" +
ektome, excision]
nymphitis (nĭm-fī'tĭs) [" + *itis*, in-
flammation]
nympho- (nĭm'fō) [Gr. *nymphe*, a
maiden]
nymphocaruncular sulcus (nĭm"fō-
kăr-ŭn'kū-lăr sŭl'kŭs) [" + L. *caruncula*, little mass of flesh, + *sulcus*, a
groove]
nymphohymenal sulcus (nĭm"fō-
hī'mĕn-ăl sŭl'kŭs) [" + *hymen*,
membrane, + *sulcus*, a groove]
nympholepsy (nĭm'fō-lĕp"sē) [" +
lepsis, a seizure]
nymphomania (nĭm"fō-mā'nē-ă)
[" + *mania*, madness]
nymphomaniac (nĭm"fō-mā'nē-ăk)
[" + *mania*, madness]
nymphoncus (nĭm-fŏn'kŭs) [" +
onkos, bulk, mass]
nymphotomy (nĭm-fŏt'ō-mē) [" +
tome, a cutting, slice]
nystagmic (nĭs-tăg'mĭk) [Gr. *nystagmos*, to nod]
nystagmiform (nĭs-tăg'mĭ-form) [" +
L. *forma*, shape]

nystagmograph (nĭs-tăg'mō-grăf)
[" + *graphein*, to write]
nystagmoid (nĭs-tăg'moyd) [" +
eidos, form, shape]
nystagmus (nĭs-tăg'mŭs) [Gr. *nystagmos*, to nod]
n., aural
n., Cheyne's
n., convergence
n., dissociated
n., end-position
n., fixation
n., jerk
n., labyrinthine
n., latent
n., lateral
n., miner's
n., opticokinetic
n., pendular
n., retraction
n., rhythmic
n., rotatory
n., vertical
n., vestibular
n., voluntary
nystatin (nĭs'tă-tĭn)
nystaxis (nĭs-tăk'sĭs) [Gr.]
Nysten's law (nē-stănz') [Pierre Hubert
Nysten, Fr. pediatrician, 1774 – 1817]
nyxis (nĭk'sĭs) [Gr.]
NZB mouse *New Zealand black* mouse

O

O octarius, pint; [L.] oculus, eye; oxygen; a particular blood type
o- ortho-
O₂ oxygen
O₃ ozone
O.A. occiput anterior
oakum (ō'kŭm) [AS. acumba, tow]
oarialgia (ō"ār-ē-ăl'jē-ă) [Gr. oarion, little egg, + algos, pain]
oario-, oari- [Gr. oarion, little egg]
oasis (ō-ā'sĭs) [Gr., a fertile area in an arid region]
oasthouse urine disease
oat [AS. ate, oat]
oath [AS. ooth]
oatmeal [AS. ate, oat, + mele, meal]
OB obstetrics
obcecation (ŏb"sē-kā'shŭn)
obdormition (ŏb-dor-mĭsh'ŭn) [L. ob, towards, + dormire, to sleep]
obduction (ŏb-dŭk'shŭn) [" + ducere, to lead]
obelion (ō-bē'lē-ŏn) [Gr. obelos, a spit]
obese (ō-bēs') [L. obesus]
obesity (ō-bē'sĭ-tē) [L. obesitas, corpulence]
   o., endogenous
   o., exogenous
   o., hypothalamic
   o., morbid
obex (ō'bĕks) [L., a band]
obfuscation (ŏb-fŭs-kā'shŭn) [L. obfuscare, to darken]
object [L. objectus]
object blindness
objective (ŏb-jĕk'tĭv)
   o., achromatic
   o., apochromatic
   o., immersion
objective sign

objective symptoms
object relations
obligate (ŏb'lĭ-gāt) [L. obligatus]
oblique (ō-blēk', ō-blīk') [L. obligatus]
obliquimeter (ŏb"lĭ-kwĭm'ĕt-ĕr) [" + Gr. metron, measure]
obliquity (ŏb-lĭk'wĭ-tē) [L. obliquus, slanting]
   o., Litzmann's
   o., Naegele's
   o. of pelvis
   o., Roederer's
obliquus (ŏb-lĭk'wŭs) [L.]
obliquus reflex
obliteration (ŏb-lĭt"ĕr-ā'shŭn) [L. obliterare, to remove]
Oblomov syndrome [After Ilya Ilych Oblomov, a character in Ivan Goncharov's 19th century novel who would not get out of bed]
oblongata (ŏb"lŏng-gā'tă) [L. oblongus, long]
obmutescence (ŏb"mū-tĕs'ĕns) [L. obmutescere, to become dumb]
obscure (ŏb-skūr') [L. obscurus, hide]
observerscope (ŏb-zĕr'vĕr-skōp)
obsession [L. obsessus, besiege]
   o., impulsive
   o., inhibitory
obsessional neurosis
obsessive-compulsive
obsolescence [L. obsolescere, to grow old]
obstetric (ŏb-stĕt'rĭk) [L. obstetrix, midwife]
obstetrician (ŏb-stĕ-trĭsh'ăn)
obstetrics (ŏb-stĕt'rĭks) [L. obstetrix, midwife]
obstipation (ŏb"stĭ-pā'shŭn) [L. obstipatio]
obstruction (ŏb-strŭk'shŭn)

509

o., aortic
o., intestinal
obstructive lung disease, chronic
obstruent (ŏb'stroo-ĕnt) [L. *obstruens*]
obtund (ŏb-tŭnd') [L. *obtundere*, to beat against]
obtundent (ŏb-tŭn'dĕnt) [L. *obtundens*]
obturation (ŏb-tūr-ā'shŭn) [L. *obturare*, to stop up]
obturator (ŏb'tū-rā"tor)
obturator foramen
obturator membrane
obturator muscles
obturator sign
obtuse (ŏb-tūs') [L. *obtusus*]
obtusion (ŏb-tū'zhŭn)
O.C. *oral contraceptive*
Occam's razor (ŏck'hăms) [William of Occam, or Ockham, Brit. Franciscan and philosopher, c. 1285–1350]
occipital (ŏk-sĭp'ĭ-tăl) [L. *occipitalis*]
occipital bone
occipitalis (ŏk-sĭp"ĭ-tā'lĭs) [L.]
occipitalization (ŏk-sĭp"ĭ-tăl-ĭ-zā'shŭn)
occipital lobe
occipito- [L. *occiput*]
occipitoatloid (ŏk-sĭp"ĭ-tō-ăt'loyd)
occipitoaxoid (ŏk-sĭp"ĭ-tō-ăk'soyd)
occipitobregmatic (ŏk-sĭp"ĭ-tō-brĕg-măt'ĭk)
occipitocervical (ŏk-sĭp"ĭ-tō-sĕr'vĭ-kăl)
occipitofacial (ŏk-sĭp"ĭ-tō-fā'shăl)
occipitofrontal (ŏk-sĭp"ĭ-tō-frŏn'tăl)
occipitomastoid (ŏk-sĭp"ĭ-tō-măs'toyd)
occipitomental (ŏk-sĭp"ĭ-tō-mĕn'tăl)
occipitoparietal (ŏk-sĭp"ĭ-tō-pă-rī'ĕ-tăl)
occipitotemporal (ŏk-sĭp"ĭ-tō-tĕm'pō-răl)
occipitothalamic (ŏk-sĭp"ĭ-tō-thă-lăm'ĭk)
occiput (ŏk'sĭ-pŭt) [L.]
occlude (ō-klūd') [L. *occludere*, to shut up]
occlusal (ō-kloo'zăl)
occlusal plane
occlusal surface

occlusal wear
occlusion (ŏ-kloo'zhŭn) [L. *occlusio*]
o., abnormal
o., adjusted
o., balanced
o., centric
o., coronary
o., eccentric
o., habitual
o., traumatic
o., working
occlusive (ŏ-kloo'sĭv)
occlusive dressing
occlusometer (ŏk"loo-sŏm'ĕ-tĕr)
occult (ŭ-kŭlt') [L. *occultus*]
occult blood
occult blood test
occupational therapist
occupational therapist assistant
occupational therapy
occupational therapy aide
occupational neurosis
ochlesis (ŏk-lē'sĭs) [Gr., crowding]
ochlophobia (ŏk"lō-fō'bē-ă) [Gr. *ochlos*, crowd, + *phobos*, fear]
ochrometer (ō-krŏm'ĕt-ĕr) [Gr. *ochros*, pale yellow + *metron*, measure]
ochronosis (ō-krō-nō'sĭs) [" + *nosos*, disease]
OCT *oxytocin challenge test*
octa-, octo- [Gr. *okto*, L. *octo*]
octahedron (ŏk-tă-hē'drŏn)
octamethyl pyrophosphoramide (ŏk"tă-mĕth'ĭl pĭr"ō-fŏs-for'ă-mīd)
octan (ŏk'tăn) [L. *octo*, eight]
octane (ŏk'tăn)
octapeptide (ŏk"tă-pĕp'tĭd)
octaploid (ŏk'tă-ployd)
octaploidy (ŏk'tă-ploy"dē)
octarius (ŏk-tā'rē-ŭs) [L.]
octavalent (ŏk"tă-vā'lĕnt) [L. *octo*, eight, + *valeo*, to have power]
octigravida (ŏk"tĭ-grăv'ĭ-dă) [" + *gravida*, pregnant]
octipara (ŏk-tĭp'ă-ră) [" + L. *parere*, to beget, produce]
octogenarian (ŏk"tō-jĕn-ĕr'ē-ĕn) [L. *octogenarius*, containing eighty]

ocular (ŏk'ū-lăr) [L. *oculus*, eye]
oculi (ŏk'ū-lī)
oculinium
oculist (ŏk'ū-lĭst)
oculo- (ŏk'ū-lō) [L. *oculus*, eye]
oculocardiac reflex
oculocephalogyric reflex (ŏk"ū-lō-sĕf"ă-lō-jī'rĭk)
oculocerebrorenal syndrome
oculocutaneous (ŏk"ū-lō-kū-tā'nē-ŭs)
oculofacial (ŏk"ū-lō-fā'shē-ăl)
oculogyration (ŏk"ū-lō-jī-rā'shŭn) [" + Gr. *gyros*, circle]
oculogyria (ŏk"ū-lō-jī'rē-ă)
oculogyric (ŏk"ū-lō-jī'rĭk)
oculogyric crisis
oculomotor (ŏk"ū-lō-mō'tor) [" + *motor*, mover]
oculomotorius (ŏk"ū-lō-mō-tō'rē-ŭs) [L.]
oculomotor nerve
oculomycosis (ŏk"ū-lō-mī-kō'sĭs) [" + Gr. *mykes*, fungus, + *osis*, condition]
oculonasal (ŏk"ū-lō-nā'săl) [" + *nasus*, nose]
oculopupillary (ŏk"ū-lō-pū'pĭ-lăr-ē)
oculoreaction (ŏk"ū-lō-rē-ăk'shŭn) [L. *oculus*, eye, + *re*, back, + *actus*, acting]
oculozygomatic (ŏk"ū-lō-zī"gō-măt'ĭk) [" + Gr. *zygon*, yoke]
oculozygomatic line
oculus (ŏk'ū-lūs) [L.]
  o. dexter
  o. sinister
  o. uterque
O.D. *oculus dexter*; Doctor of Optometry; overdose
OD'd
odaxesmus (ō"dăk-sĕz'mŭs) [Gr. *odaxesmos*, an irritation]
odaxetic (ō"dăk-sĕt'ĭk)
Oddi's sphincter (ŏd'ēz) [Ruggero Oddi, It. physician, 1864–1913]
odditis (ŏd-dī'tĭs) [*Oddi* + Gr. *itis*, inflammation]
odogenesis (ō"dō-jĕn'ĕ-sĭs) [Gr.

hodos, pathway, + *genesis*, generation, birth]
odont-, odonto- [Gr. *odous*, tooth]
odontagra (ō-dŏn-tă'gră) [Gr. *odous*, tooth, + *agra*, seizure]
odontalgia (ō-dŏn-tăl'jē-ă) [" + *algos*, pain]
  o., phantom
odontatrophy (ō"dŏn-tăt'rō-fē) [" + *atrophia*, atrophy]
odontectomy (ō-dŏn-tĕk'tō-mē) [" + *ektome*, excision]
odonterism (ō-dŏn'tĕr-ĭzm) [" + *erismos*, quarrel]
odontia (ō-dŏn'shē-ă) [Gr. *odous*, tooth]
odontic (ō-dŏn'tĭk) [Gr. *odous*, tooth]
odontitis (ō"dŏn-tī'tĭs) [" + *itis*, inflammation]
odontoblast (ō-dŏn'tō-blăst) [" + *blastos*, germ]
odontoblastoma [" + " + *oma*, tumor]
odontobothrion (ō-dŏn"tō-bŏth'rē-ŏn) [" + *bothrion*, pit]
odontobothritis [" + " + *itis*, inflammation]
odontocele (ō-dŏn'tō-sēl) [" + *kele*, tumor, swelling]
odontochirurgical (ō-dŏn"tō-kī-rŭr'jĭ-kăl) [" + *chirurgia*, surgery]
odontoclasis (ō"dŏn-tŏk'lă-sĭs) [" + *klasis*, fracture]
odontoclast
odontodynia (ō-dŏn"tō-dĭn'ē-ă) [" + *odyne*, pain]
odontogenesis, odontogeny (ō-dŏn"tō-jĕn'ĕ-sĭs, -tŏj'ĕn-ē) [" + *genesis*, generation, birth]
  o. imperfecta
odontograph (ō-dŏn'tō-grăf) [" + *graphein*, to write]
odontography (ō-dŏn-tŏg'ră-fē)
odontoid (ō-dŏn'toyd) [" + *eidos*, form, shape]
odontoid process
odontolith (ō-dŏn'tō-lĭth) [" + *lithos*, stone]

odontologist (ō″dŏn-tŏl′ō-jĭst)
odontology (ō″dŏn-tŏl′ō-jē) [″ +
logos, word, reason]
odontolysis (ō-dŏn-tŏl′ĭ-sĭs) [″ +
lysis, dissolution]
odontoma (ō″dŏn-tō′mă) [″ +
oma, tumor]
    o., ameloblastic
    o., composite
    o., coronary
    o., follicular
    o., radicular
odontonecrosis (ō-dŏn″tō-nē-krō′sĭs)
[″ + nekrosis, state of death]
odontonomy (ō″dŏn-tŏn′ō-mē) [″ +
onoma, name]
odontopathy (ō-dŏn-tŏp′ă-thē) [″ +
pathos, disease, suffering]
odontophobia (ō-dŏn″tō-fō′bē-ă)
[″ + phobos, fear]
odontoprisis (ō-dŏn″tō-prī′sĭs) [″ +
prisis, sawing]
odontorrhagia (ō-dŏn″tō-rā′jē-ă)
[″ + rhegnynai, to burst forth]
odontoschism (ō-dŏn′tō-skĭzm) [″ +
schisma, cleft]
odontoscopy (ō″dŏn-tŏs′kō-pē)
[″ + skopein, to examine]
odontosis (ō-dŏn-tō′sĭs) [″ + osis,
condition]
odontotherapy (ō-dŏn″tō-thĕr′ă-pē)
[″ + therapeia, treatment]
odontotripsis (ō-dŏn″tō-trĭp′sĭs) [″ +
tripsis, a rubbing, friction]
odor (ō′dĕr) [L.]
odorant (ō′dor-ănt)
odoriferous (ō″dor-ĭf′ĕ-rŭs) [L. odor,
smell, + ferre, to bear]
odorimetry
odoriphore (ō-dor′ĭ-for) [″ + Gr.
phoros, bearing]
odorography (ō″dor-ŏg′ră-fē) [″ +
Gr. graphein, to write]
odorous [L. odor, smell]
odynacusis (ō″dĭn-ă-kū′sĭs) [Gr. odyne,
pain, + akousis, hearing]
-odynia (ō-dĭn′ē-ă) [Gr. odyne, pain]
odynometer (ō″dĭn-om′ĕt-ĕr) [″ +

metron, measure]
odynophagia (ŏd″ĭn-ō-fā′jē-ă) [″ +
phagein, to eat]
odynophobia (ŏd″ĭn-ō-fō′bē-ă) [″ +
phobos, fear]
Oedipus complex (ĕd′ĭ-pŭs) [Oe-
dipus, a character in Gr. tragedy who
unwittingly fell in love with his mother,
Jocasta, killed his father in jealousy, and
married his mother]
oenology (ē-nŏl′ō-jē) [Gr. oinos, wine,
+ logos, word, reason]
oersted (ĕr′stĕd) [Hans Christian
Oersted, Danish physicist, 1777–
1851]
oesophagostomiasis (ē-sŏf″ă-gō-
stō-mī′ă-sĭs) [Gr. oisophagos, gullet,
+ stoma, mouth, opening, +
-iasis, state or condition of]
Oesophagostomum (ē-sŏf″ă-gŏs′tō-
mŭm) [Gr. oisophagos, gullet, +
stoma, mouth, opening]
    O. apiostomum
oestrus
Oestrus ovis
O.F.D. object film distance
official
officinal (ŏf-ĭs′ĭn-ăl) [L. officina, shop]
Ogen
Ogilvie's syndrome [Sir William H.
Ogilvie, 20th century Brit. physician]
Oguchi's disease (ō-goot′chēz)
[Chuta Oguchi, Japanese ophthalmologist, 1875–1945]
OH⁻ the hydroxyl ion
ohm (ōm)
ohmammeter (ōm′ăm-mē″tĕr)
Ohm's law [George S. Ohm, Ger.
physicist, 1787–1854]
ohmmeter (ōm′mē-tĕr)
-oid [Gr. eidos, form, shape]
oikofugic (oy″kō-fū′jĭk) [Gr. oikos,
house, + L. fugere, to flee]
oikomania (oy″kō-mā′nē-ă) [″ +
mania, madness]
oikophobia (oy″kō-fō′bē-ă)
oil (oyl) [L. oleum]
    o.'s, essential

o.'s, fixed

ointment (oynt'měnt) [Fr. *oignement*]
o., hydrophilic
o., white
o., yellow

O.L. [L.] *oculus laevus*, left eye

ol. [L.] *oleum*, oil

O.L.A. [L. *occipito laevo anterior*]

olea (ō'lē-ă) [L.]

oleaginous (ō-lē-ăj'ĭ-nŭs) [L. *oleaginus*]

oleander (ō"lē-ăn'děr)

oleate (ō'lē-āt) [L. *oleatum*]

oleatum (ō-lē-ā'tŭm) [L.]

olecranal (ō-lěk'răn-ăl) [Gr. *olekranon*, elbow]

olecranarthritis (ō-lěk"răn-ăr-thrī'tĭs) [" + *arthron*, joint, + *itis*, inflammation]

olecranarthrocace (ō-lěk"răn-ăr-thrŏk'ă-sē) [" + " + *kake*, badness]

olecranarthropathy (ō-lěk"răn-ăr-thrŏp'ă-thē) [" + " + *pathos*, disease, suffering]

olecranoid (ō-lěk'ră-noyd) [" + *eidos*, form, shape]

olecranon (ō-lěk'răn-ŏn) [Gr., elbow]
o., fracture of

oleic (ō-lē'ĭk) [L. *oleum*, oil]

oleic acid

olein (ō'lē-ĭn) [L. *oleum*, oil]

oleo- [L. *oleum*, oil]

oleoarthrosis (ō"lē-ō-ăr-thrō'sĭs) [" + Gr. *arthron*, joint, + *osis*, condition]

oleogranuloma (ō"lē-ō-grăn"ū-lō'mă) [" + L. *granulum*, little grain, + Gr. *oma*, tumor]

oleoinfusion (ō"lē-ō-ĭn-fū'zhun) [" + *in*, into, + *fusus*, poured]

oleoma (ō"lē-ō'mă) [" + Gr. *oma*, tumor]

oleomargarine (ō"lē-ō-măr'jă-rĭn) [" + *margarine*]

oleometer (ō"lē-ŏm'ĕ-tĕr)

oleoresin (ō"lē-ō-rĕz'ĭn) [" + *resina*, resin]

oleosaccharum (ō-lē-ō-săk'ă-rŭm)

[" + *saccharum*, sugar]

oleostearate (ō"lē-ō-stē'ăr-āt)

oleosus (ō"lē-ō'sŭs) [L.]

oleotherapy (ō"lē-ō-thĕr'ă-pē) [L. *oleum*, oil, + Gr. *therapeia*, treatment]

oleothorax (ō-lē-ō-thō'răks) [" + Gr. *thorax*, chest]

oleovitamin (ō"lē-ō-vī'tă-mĭn)
o. A and D

oleum (ō'lē-ŭm) [L.]
o. morrhuae
o. olivea
o. percomorphum
o. ricini

olfactie (ŏl-făk'tē)

olfaction (ŏl-făk'shŭn) [L. *olfacere*, to smell]

olfactive (ŏl-făk'tĭv) [L. *olfacere*, to smell]

olfactology (ŏl-făk-tŏl'ō-jē) [" + Gr. *logos*, word, reason]

olfactometer (ŏl"făk-tŏm'ĕt-ĕr) [" + Gr. *metron*, measure]

olfactory (ŏl-făk'tō-rē)

olfactory area

olfactory bulb

olfactory cortex

olfactory esthesioneuroma

olfactory lobe

olfactory membrane

olfactory nasal sulcus

olfactory nerves

olfactory organ

olfactory striae

olfactory tract

olfactory trigone

olfactory tubercle

oligemia (ŏl-ĭg-ē'mē-ă) [Gr. *oligos*, little, + *haima*, blood]

oligergasia (ŏl-ĭ-gĕr-gā'sē-ă)

oligo-, olig- [Gr. *oligos*, little]

oligoamnios (ŏl"ĭ-gō-ăm'nē-ŏs) [" + *amnion*, lamb]

oligocholia (ŏl"ĭ-gō-kō'lē-ă) [" + *chole*, bile]

oligochromemia (ŏl"ĭg-ō-krō-mē'mē-ă) [" + *chroma*, color, +

haima, blood]

oligochylia   (ŏl″ĭ-gō-kī′lē-ă) [" + chylos, juice]

oligochymia   (ŏl″ĭg-ō-kī′mē-ă) [" + chymos, juice]

oligocystic   (ŏl-ĭ-gō-sĭs′tĭk) [" + kystis, a bladder]

oligodactylia   (ŏl-ĭ-gō-dăk-tĭl′ē-ă) [" + daktylos, finger]

oligodendroblast   (ŏl″ĭ-gō-dĕn′drō-blăst) [" + Gr. dendron, tree, + blastos, germ]

oligodendroblastoma   (ŏl″ĭ-gō-dĕn″drō-blăs-tō′mă) [" + " + " + oma, tumor]

oligodendrocyte   [" + " + kytos, cell]

oligodendroglia   (ŏl″ĭ-gō-dĕn-drŏg′lē-ă) [" + " + glia, glue]

oligodendroglioma   (ŏl″ĭ-gō-dĕn″drō-glī-ō′mă) [" + " + " + oma, tumor]

oligodipsia   (ŏl″ĭ-gō-dĭp′sē-ă) [" + dipsa, thirst]

oligodontia   (ŏl″ĭ-gō-dŏn′shē-ă) [" + odont, tooth]

oligodynamic   (ŏl″ĭ-gō-dī-năm′ĭk) [" + dynamis, power]

oligogalactia   (ŏl″ĭ-gō-găl-ăk′tē-ă) [" + galaktos, milk]

oligohemia   (ŏl″ĭ-gō-hē′mē-ă) [" + haima, blood]

oligohydramnios   (ŏl″ĭg-ō-hī-drăm′nē-ŏs) [" + hydor, water, + amnion, amnion]

oligolecithal   (ŏl″ĭg-gō-lĕs′ĭ-thăl) [" + lethikos, yolk]

oligoleukocythemia   (ŏl″ĭ-gō-lū″kō-sī-thē′mē-ă) [Gr. oligos, little, + leukos, white, + kytos, cell, + haima, blood]

oligomastigate   (ŏl″ĭ-gō-măs′tĭ-gāt) [" + mastix, whip]

oligomenorrhea   (ŏl″ĭ-gō-mĕn″ō-rē′ă) [" + men, month, + rhein, to flow]

oligomorphic   (ŏl″ĭ-gō-mor′fĭk) [" + morphe, form]

oligonucleotide   (ŏl″ĭ-gō-nū′klē-ō-tīd) [" + nucleotide]

oligophosphaturia   (ŏl″ĭ-gō-fŏs-fă-tū′rē-ă) [" + phosphas, phosphate, + ouron, urine]

oligophrenia   (ŏl″ĭg-ō-frē′nē-ă) [" + phren, mind]

   o., phenylpyruvic

oligoplastic   (ŏl″ĭ-gō-plăs′tĭk) [" + Gr. plassein, to form]

oligopnea   (ŏl-ĭ-gŏp′nē-ă) [" + pnoia, breath]

oligoposy   (ŏl-ĭ-gŏp′ō-sē) [" + posis, drink]

oligoptyalism   (ŏl-ĭ-gō-tī′ă-lĭzm) [" + ptyalon, saliva]

oligoria   (ŏl-ĭ-gor′ē-ă) [Gr., negligence]

oligosaccharide   (ŏl″ĭ-gō-săk′ă-rīd)

oligosialia   (ŏl″ĭ-gō-sī-ā′lē-ă) [Gr. oligos, little, + sialon, saliva]

oligospermia   (ŏl″ĭ-gō-spĕr′mē-ă) [" + sperma, seed]

oligosynaptic   (ŏl″ĭ-gō-sĭn-ăp′tĭk) [" + Gr. synapsis, point of contact]

oligotrichia   (ŏl″ĭ-gō-trĭk′ē-ă) [" + thrix, hair]

oligotrophy   (ŏl-ĭ-gŏt′rō-fē) [" + trophe, nourishment]

oligozoospermatism, oligozoospermia   (ŏl″ĭ-gō-zō″ō-spĕr′mă-tĭzm, -spĕr′mē-ă) [" + " + -ismos, condition]

oliguresis   (ŏl-ĭg-ū-rē′sĭs) [" + ouresis, urination]

oliguria   (ŏl-ĭg-ū′rē-ă) [" + ouron, urine]

oliva   (ō-lī′vă) [L., olive]

olivary   [L. oliva, olive]

olivary body

olive   (ŏl′ĭv) [L. oliva, olive]

   o., accessory

   o., inferior

   o., superior

olive oil

olivifugal   (ŏl″ĭ-vĭf′ū-găl) [" + fugerea, to flee]

olivipetal   (ŏl″ĭ-vĭp′ĕ-tăl) [" + peter, to seek]

olivopontocerebellar (ŏl″ĭ-vō-pŏn″tō-sĕr″ĕ-bĕl′ăr)
Ollier, Léopold L. X. E. (ŏl″ē-ā′) [Fr. surgeon, 1830–1900]
O.'s disease
O. layer
O.-Thiersch graft [Karl Thiersch, Ger. surgeon, 1822–1895]
-ology [Gr. *logos*, word, reason]
olophonia (ŏl-ō-fōn′ē-ă) [Gr. *oloos*, destroyed, + *phone*, voice]
O.L.P. [L. *occipitolaeva posterior*]
o.m. [L.] *omni mane*, every morning
omagra (ō-mă′gră) [Gr. *omos*, shoulder, + *agra*, seizure]
omalgia (ō-măl′jē-ă) [″ + *algos*, pain]
omasitis (ō-mă-sī′tĭs)
omasum (ō-mă′sŭm) [L.]
ombrophobia (ŏm-brō-fō′bē-ă) [Gr. *ombros*, rain, + *phobos*, fear]
omega-3 fatty acids (ω3)
omenta (ō-mĕn′tă)
omental (ō-mĕn′tăl) [L. *omentum*, covering]
omental bursa
omentectomy (ō-mĕn-tĕk′tō-mē) [″ + Gr. *ektome*, excision]
omentitis (ō-mĕn-tī′tĭs) [″ + Gr. *itis*, inflammation]
omentofixation (ō-mĕn″tō-fĭk-sā′shŭn)
omentopexy (ō-mĕn′tō-pĕks″ē) [″ + Gr. *pexis*, fixation]
omentoplasty (ō-mĕn′tō-plăs″tē) [L. *omentum*, covering, + Gr. *plassein*, to form]
omentorrhaphy (ō-mĕn-tor′ră-fē) [″ + Gr. *rhaphe*, seam]
omentosplenopexy (ō-mĕn″tō-splē′nō-pĕks-ē) [″ + Gr. *splen*, spleen, + *pexis*, fixation]
omentotomy (ō-mĕn-tŏt′ō-mē) [″ + Gr. *tome*, a cutting, slice]
omentovolvulus (ō-mĕn″tō-vŏl′vū-lŭs) [″ + *volvere*, to roll]
omentum (ō-mĕn′tŭm) [L., a covering]
o., gastrocolic

o., gastrohepatic
o., greater
o., lesser
omentumectomy (ō-mĕn″tŭm-ĕk′tō-mē) [″ + Gr. *ektome*, excision]
omitis (ō-mī′tĭs) [Gr. *omos*, shoulder, + *itis*, inflammation]
OML *orbitomeatal line*
Ommaya reservoir [A.K. Ommaya, contemporary U.S. neurosurgeon]
omn. bih. [L.] *omni bihora*, every two hours
omn. hor. [L.] *omni hora*, every hour
omni- (ŏm′nĭ) [L. *omnis*]
Omnipen
Omnipen-N
omnipotence of thought
omnivorous (ŏm-nĭv′ō-rŭs) [L. *omnis*, all, + *vorare*, to eat]
omn. noct. [L.] *omni nocte*, every night
omn. quad. hor. [L.] *omni quadrante hora*, every quarter of an hour
omo- [Gr. *omos*, shoulder]
omoclavicular (ō″mō-klă-vĭk′ū-lăr)
omodynia (ō-mō-dĭn′ē-ă) [Gr. *omos*, shoulder, + *odyne*, pain]
omohyoid (ō-mō-hī′oyd)
omophagia (ō-mō-fā′jē-ă) [Gr. *omos*, raw, + *phagein*, to eat]
omphal-, omphalo- [Gr. *omphalos*, navel]
omphalectomy (ŏm-făl-ĕk′tō-mē) [″ + *ektome*, excision]
omphalelcosis (ŏm″făl-ĕl-kō′sĭs) [″ + *helkosis*, ulceration]
omphalic (ŏm-făl′ĭk) [Gr. *omphalikos*, navel]
omphalitis (ŏm-făl-ī′tĭs) [″ + *itis*, inflammation]
omphaloangiopagus (ŏm″făl-ō-ăn″jē-ŏp′ă-gŭs) [″ + *angeion*, vessel, + *pagos*, thing fixed]
omphalocele (ŏm-făl′ō-sēl) [″ + *kele*, tumor, swelling]
omphalochorion (ŏm″fă-lō-kō′rē-ŏn)
omphalomesenteric (ŏm″făl-ō-mĕs-ĕn-tĕr′ĭk) [″ + *mesenterion*, mesentery]

omphaloncus (ŏm"făl-ŏn'kŭs) [" + onkos, bulk, mass]

omphalopagus (ŏm"fă-lŏp'ă-gŭs) [" + pagos, thing fixed]

omphalophlebitis (ŏm"făl-ō-flĕ-bī'tĭs) [" + phleps, blood vessel, vein, + itis, inflammation]

omphalorrhagia (ŏm"făl-ō-rā'jē-ă) [" + rhegnynai, to burst forth]

omphalorrhea (ŏm"făl-ō-rē'ă) [" + rhein, to flow]

omphalorrhexis (ŏm"făl-ō-rĕk'sĭs) [" + rhexis, rupture]

omphalos (ŏm'făl-ŏs) [Gr.]

omphalosite (ŏm"fă-lō-sīt") [" + sitos, food]

omphalospinous (ŏm"făl-ō-spī'nŭs) [" + L. spina, thorn]

omphalotomy (ŏm-făl-ŏt'ō-mē) [" + tome, a cutting, slice]

omphalotripsy (ŏm"făl-ō-trĭp'sē) [" + tripsis, a rubbing, friction]

omphalus (ŏm'fă-lŭs) [Gr. omphalos]

ON orthopedic nurse

o.n. [L.] omni nocte, every night

onanism (ō'năn-ĭzm) [So named because it was practiced by the Biblical character Onan, son of Judah]

onanist (ō'nă-nĭst)

Onanoff's reflex (ŏn-ă-nŏfs') [Jacques Onanoff, Fr. physician, b. 1859]

Onchocerca (ŏng"kō-sĕr'kă) [Gr. onkos, barbed hook, + kerkos, tail]

O. volvulus

onchocerciasis (ŏng"kō-sĕr-kī'ă-sĭs) [" + " + -iasis, state or condition of]

onco- [Gr. onkos, bulk, mass]

Oncocerca

oncocercosis

oncocyte (ŏn'kō-sīt) [" + kytos, cell]

oncocytoma (ŏng"kō-sī-tō'mă) [" + " + oma, tumor]

oncofetal (ŏng"kō-fē'tăl)

oncogene (ŏng'kō-jēn) [" + gen-

nan, to produce]

oncogenesis (ŏng"kō-jĕn'ĕ-sĭs) [" + genesis, generation, birth]

oncogenic (ŏng"kō-jĕn'ĭk)

oncogenic virus

oncograph (ŏng'kō-grăf) [Gr. onkos, bulk, mass, + graphein, to write]

oncoides (ŏng-koy'dēz) [" + eidos, form, shape]

oncology (ŏng-kŏl'ō-jē) [" + logos, word, reason]

oncolysis (ŏng-kŏl'ĭ-sĭs) [" + lysis, dissolution]

oncolytic (ŏng"kō-lĭt'ĭk)

oncometer (ŏng-kŏm'ĕt-ĕr) [" + metron, measure]

oncometric (ŏng"kō-mĕt'rĭk)

oncometry

oncosis (ŏng-kō'sĭs) [" + osis, condition]

oncosphere (ŏng'kō-sfēr) [" + sphaira, sphere]

oncotherapy (ŏng"kō-thĕr'ă-pē) [" + therapeia, treatment]

oncothlipsis (ŏng"kō-thlĭp'sĭs) [" + thlipsis, pressure]

oncotic (ŏng-kŏt'ĭk) [Gr. onkos, bulk, mass]

oncotic pressure, colloidal

oncotomy (ŏng-kŏt'ō-mē) [" + tome, a cutting, slice]

oncotropic (ŏng"kō-trŏp'ĭk) [" + tropos, a turning]

Oncovin

oncovirus (ŏn'kō-vī"rŭs) [" + virus]

Ondine's curse [Fr. Undine, mythical water nymph whose human lover was cursed to continuous sleep]

oneir(o)- (ō-nī'rō) [Gr. oneiros, dream]

oneiric (ō-nī'rĭk) [Gr. oneiros, dream]

oneirism (ō-nī'rĭzm) [" + -ismos, condition]

oneirodynia (ō-nī"rō-dĭn'ē-ă) [" + odyne, pain]

oneirogmus (ō"nī-rŏg'mŭs) [Gr. oneirogmos, an effusion during sleep]

oneirology (ō"nī-rŏl'ō-jē) [Gr. oneiros, dream, + logos, word, reason]

oneiroscopy (ō"nī-rŏs'kō-pē) [" + skopein, to examine]

oniomania (ō"nē-ō-mā'nē-ă) [Gr. onios, for sale, + mania, madness]

onion (ŭn'yŭn) [AS. oignon]

onkinocele (ŏng-kĭn'ō-sēl) [Gr. onkos, bulk, mass, + inos, fiber, + kele, tumor, swelling]

onlay

onomatology (ŏn"ō-mă-tŏl'ō-jē) [Gr. onoma, name, + logos, word, reason]

onomatomania (ŏn"ō-mă"tō-mā'nē-ă) [" + mania, madness]

onomatophobia (ŏn"ō-mă"tō-fō'bē-ă) [" + phobos, fear]

onomatopoiesis (ŏn"ō-mă"tō-poy-ē'sĭs) [Gr. onoma, name, + poiein, to make]

ontogenesis (ŏn"tō-jĕn'ĕ-sĭs)

ontogenetic (ŏn"tō-jĕ-nĕt'ĭk)

ontogeny (ŏn-tŏj'ĕn-ē) [Gr. on, being, + gennan, to produce]

onych(o)- [Gr. onyx, nail]

onychalgia (ŏn"ĭ-kăl'jē-ă) [" + algos, pain]
    o. nervosa

onychatrophia (ō"nĭk-ă-trō'fē-ă) [" + trophe, nourishment]

onychauxis (ŏn"ĭ-kawk'sĭs) [" + auxein, to increase]

onychectomy (ŏn"ĭ-kĕk'tō-mē) [" + ektome, excision]

onychia (ō-nĭk'ē-ă) [Gr. onyx, nail]
    o. craquele
    o. lateralis
    o. maligna
    o. parasitica
    o., piannic
    o. punctata

onychitis (ŏn"ĭ-kī'tĭs) [" + itis, inflammation]

onychocryptosis (ŏn"ĭ-kō-krĭp-tō'sĭs) [" + kryptein, to conceal]

onychodystrophy (ŏn"ĭ-kō-dĭs'trō-fē) [" + dys, bad, difficult, painful, disordered, + trophe, nutrition]

onychogenic (ŏn"ĭ-kō-jĕn'ĭk) [" + gennan, to produce]

onychograph (ŏn-ĭk'ō-grăf) [" + graphein, to write]

onychogryposis (ŏn"ĭ-kō-grī-pō'sĭs) [" + gryposis, a curving]

onychoheterotopia (ŏn"ĭ-kō-hĕt"ĕr-ō-tō'pē-ă) [" + heteros, other, + topos, place]

onychoid (ŏn'ĭ-koyd) [" + eidos, form, shape]

onycholysis (ŏn"ĭ-kŏl'ĭ-sĭs) [" + lysis, dissolution]

onychoma (ŏn-ĭ-kō'mă) [" + oma, tumor]

onychomadesis (ŏn'ĭ-kō-mă-dē'sĭs) [Gr. onyx, nail, + madesis, loss of hair]

onychomalacia (ŏn"ĭ-kō-mă-lā'sē-ă) [" + malakia, softening]

onychomycosis (ŏn"ĭ-kō-mī-kō'sĭs) [" + mykes, fungus, + osis, condition]

onycho-osteodysplasia (ŏn"ĭ-kō-ŏs"tē-ō-dĭs-plā'zē-ă)

onychopathology (ŏn"ĭ-kō-pă-thŏl'ō-jē) [" + pathos, disease, suffering, + logos, word, reason]

onychopathy (ŏn-ĭ-kŏp'ăth-ē) [" + pathos, disease, suffering]

onychophagy (ŏn-ĭ-kŏf'ă-jē) [" + phagein, to eat]

onychophosis (ŏn"ĭk-ō-fō'sĭs)

onychophyma (ŏn"ĭ-kō-fī'mă) [" + phyma, a growth]

onychoptosis (ŏn"ĭk-ŏp-tō'sĭs) [" + ptosis, fall, falling]

onychorrhexis (ŏn"ĭ-kō-rĕk'sĭs) [" + rhexis, a rupture]

onychoschizia (ŏn"ĭ-kō-skĭz'ē-ă) [" + schizein, to split]

onychosis (ŏn-ĭ-kō'sĭs) [" + osis, condition]

onychotillomania (ŏn"ĭ-kō-tĭl"ō-mā'nē-ă) [" + tillein, to pluck, + mania, insanity]

onychotomy (ŏn"ĭ-kŏt'ō-mē) [" + tome, a cutting, slice]

onychotrophy (ŏn-ĭ-kŏt'rō-fē) [" +

trophe, nourishment]

onyx (ŏn′ĭks) [Gr., nail]

onyxis (ō-nĭk′sĭs)

onyxitis (ŏn-ĭk-sī′tĭs) [″ + *itis*, inflammation]

oo- (ō-ō) [Gr. *oon*, egg]

ooblast (ō′ō-blăst) [″ + *blastos*, germ]

oocyesis (ō″ō-sī-ē′sĭs) [″ + *kyesis*, pregnancy]

oocyst (ō′ō-sĭst) [Gr. *oon*, egg, + *kystis*, bladder]

oocytase (ō″ō-sī′tās) [″ + *kytos*, cell, + *-ase*, enzyme]

oocyte (ō′ō-sīt) [″ + *kytos*, cell]
   o., primary
   o., secondary

oocytin (ō″ō-sī′tĭn)

oogenesis (ō″ō-jĕn′ĕ-sĭs) [″ + *genesis*, generation, birth]

oogenetic (ō″ō-jĕ-nĕt′ĭk)

oogonium (ō″ō-gō′nē-ŭm) [″ + *gone*, seed]

ookinesis (ō″ō-kĭn-ē′sĭs) [″ + *kinesis*, motion]

ookinete (ō″ō-kī-nēt′) [″ + *kinetos*, motile]

oolemma (ō″ō-lĕm′ă) [″ + *lemma*, sheath]

oophagy (ō-ŏf′ă-jē) [″ + *phagein*, to eat]

oophor- [NL. *oophoron*, ovary]

oophoralgia (ō″ŏf-ō-răl′jē-ă) [″ + Gr. *algos*, pain]

oophorauxe (ō″ŏf-ō-rawks′ē) [″ + Gr. *auxein*, to increase]

oophorectomy (ō″ŏf-ō-rĕk′tō-mē) [″ + Gr. *ektome*, excision]

oophoritis (ō″ŏf-ō-rī′tĭs) [″ + Gr. *itis*, inflammation]
   o., follicular

oophorocystectomy (ō-ŏf″ō-rō-sĭs-tĕk′tō-mē) [″ + Gr. *kystis*, cyst, + *ektome*, excision]

oophorocystosis (ō-ŏf″ō-rō-sĭs-tō′sĭs) [NL. *oophoron*, ovary, + Gr. *kystis*, cyst, + *osis*, condition]

oophorohysterectomy (ō-ŏf″ō-rō-hĭs″tĕr-ĕk′tō-mē) [″ + Gr. *hystera*,

womb, + *ektome*, excision]

oophoroma (ō-ŏf″ō-rō′mă) [″ + Gr. *oma*, tumor]

oophoron (ō-ŏf′ō-rŏn) [NL., ovary]

oophoropathy (ō-ŏf″or-ŏp′ă-thē) [″ + Gr. *pathos*, disease, suffering]

oophoropeliopexy (ō-ŏf″ō-rō-pē′lē-ō-pĕk″sē) [″ + Gr. *pellis*, pelvis, + *pexis*, fixation]

oophoropexy (ō-ŏf″ō-rō-pĕk′sē) [″ + Gr. *pexis*, fixation]

oophoroplasty (ō-ŏf′ō-rō-plăs″tē) [″ + Gr. *plassein*, to form]

oophorosalpingectomy (ō-ŏf″ō-rō-săl-pĭn-jĕk′tō-mē) [″ + Gr. *salpinx*, tube, + *ektome*, excision]

oophorosalpingitis (ō-ŏf″or-ō-săl″pĭn-jī′tĭs) [″ + ″ + Gr. *itis*, inflammation]

oophorostomy (ō-ŏf″ō-rŏs′tō-mē) [″ + Gr. *stoma*, mouth, opening]

oophorotomy (ō-ŏf″ō-rŏt′ō-mē) [″ + Gr. *tome*, a cutting, slice]

oophorrhagia (ō″ŏf-ō-rā′jē-ă) [″ + Gr. *rhegnynai*, to burst forth]

oophorrhaphy (ō-ŏf-or′ă-fē) [″ + Gr. *rhaphe*, seam]

ooplasm (ō″ō-plăzm) [Gr. *oon*, egg, + LL. *plasma*, form, mold]

oosperm (ō′ō-spĕrm) [″ + *sperma*, seed]

oosporangium (ō″ō-spō-răn′jē-ŭm)

oospore (ō′ō-spor) [″ + *sporos*, seed]

ootheca (ō-ō-thē′kă) [Gr. *ootheke*, ovary]

oothecohysterectomy (ō-ō-thē″kō-hĭs″tĕr-ĕk′tō-mē) [Gr. *ootheke*, ovary, + *hystera*, womb, + *ektome*, excision]

ootid (ō′ō-tĭd)

OP operative procedure; outpatient

O.P. occiput position

opacification (ō-păs″ĭ-fĭ-kā′shŭn) [L. *opacitas*, shadiness, + *facere*, to make]

opacity (ō-păs′ĭ-tē) [L. *opacitas*, shadiness]

opalescent (ō"păl-ĕs'ĕnt)
opaque (ō-pāk') [L. *opacus*, dark]
OPC *outpatient clinic*
OPD *outpatient department*
open [AS.]
open heart surgery
opening
  o., aortic
  o., cardiac
  o., pyloric
open reduction
operable (ŏp'ĕr-ă-bl) [L. *operor*, to work]
operant conditioning
operate (ŏp'ĕr-āt) [L. *operatus*, worked]
operation (ŏp-ĕr-ā'shŭn) [L. *operatio*, a working]
  o., ablative
  o., cosmetic
  o., exploratory
  o., flap
  o., major
  o., minor
  o., plastic
  o., radical
  o., reconstructive
  o., subtotal
operative (ŏp'ĕr-ă-tĭv) [L. *operativus*, working]
operative dentistry
operator (ŏp'ĕr-ā-tor)
opercular (ō-pĕr'kū-lăr) [L. *operculum*, a cover]
operculitis (ō-pĕr"kū-lī'tĭs) [" + Gr. *itis*, inflammation]
operculum (ō-pĕr'kū-lŭm) [L., a cover]
  o., dental
  o., trophoblastic
operon (ŏp'ĕr-ŏn)
ophiasis (ō-fī'ă-sĭs) [Gr. *ophis*, snake]
ophidiasis (ō-fī-dī'ă-sĭs)
ophidiophobia (ō-fĭd"ē-ō-fō'bē-ă) [Gr. *ophidion*, snake, + *phobos*, fear]
ophidism (ō'fĭd-ĭzm) [" + *-ismos*, condition]
ophiotoxemia (ō"fē-ō-tŏk-sē'mē-ă) [" + *toxikon*, poison, +

haima, blood]
ophritis, ophryitis (ŏf-rī'tĭs, -rē-ī'tĭs) [Gr. *ophrys*, eyebrow, + *itis*, inflammation]
ophryon (ŏf'rē-ŏn)
ophryosis (ŏf"rē-ō'sĭs) [" + *osis*, condition]
Ophthaine
Ophthalgan
ophthalmagra (ŏf"thăl-măg'ră) [Gr. *ophthalmos*, eye, + *agra*, seizure]
ophthalmalgia (ŏf"thăl-măl'jē-ă) [" + *algos*, pain]
ophthalmatrophy (ŏf-thăl-măt'rō-fē) [" + *atrophia*, a wasting]
ophthalmectomy (ŏf-thăl-mĕk'tō-mē) [" + *ektome*, excision]
ophthalmencephalon (ŏf"thăl-mĕn-sĕf'ă-lŏn) [" + *enkephalos*, brain]
ophthalmia (ŏf-thăl'mē-ă) [Gr. *ophthalmos*, eye]
  o., catarrhal
  o., Egyptian
  o., electric
  o., gonorrheal
  o., granular
  o., metastatic
  o. neonatorum
  o., neuroparalytic
  o., phlyctenular
  o., purulent
  o., scrofulous
  o., spring
  o., sympathetic
  o., varicose
ophthalmiatrics (ŏf"thăl-mē-ăt'rĭks) [" + *iatreia*, treatment]
ophthalmic (ŏf-thăl'mĭk)
ophthalmic nerve
ophthalmic reaction
ophthalmitis (ŏf"thăl-mī'tĭs) [" + *itis*, inflammation]
ophthalmo- [Gr. *ophthalmos*, eye]
ophthalmoblennorrhea (ŏf-thăl"mō-blĕn"ō-rē'ă) [" + *blenna*, mucus, + *rhein*, to flow]
ophthalmocele (ŏf-thăl'mō-sēl) [" + *kele*, tumor, swelling]
ophthalmocopia (ŏf-thăl"mō-kō'pē-ă)

[" + *kopos,* fatigue]

ophthalmodesmitis (ŏf-thăl″mō-dĕs-mī′tĭs) [" + *desmos,* ligament, + *itis,* inflammation]

ophthalmodiagnosis (ŏf-thăl″mō-dī″ăg-nō′sĭs) [" + *dia,* through, + *gnosis,* knowledge]

ophthalmodiaphanoscope (ŏf-thăl″mō-dī-ă-făn′ō-skōp) [" + " + *phainein,* to appear, + *skopein,* to examine]

ophthalmodonesis (ŏf-thăl″mō-dō-nē′sĭs) [" + *donesis,* trembling]

ophthalmodynamometer (ŏf-thăl″mō-dī″nă-mŏm′ĕ-tĕr) [" + *dynamis,* power, + *metron,* measure]

ophthalmodynamometry (ŏf-thăl″mō-dī″nă-mŏm′ĕ-trē)

ophthalmodynia (ŏf-thăl″mō-dĭn′ē-ă) [" + *odyne,* pain]

ophthalmoeikonometer (ŏf-thăl″mō-ī″kō-nŏm′ĕ-tĕr) [" + *eikon,* image, + *metron,* measure]

ophthalmofundoscope (ŏf-thăl″mō-fŭn′dō-skōp) [" + L. *fundus,* base, + Gr. *skopein,* to examine]

ophthalmography (ŏf″thăl-mŏg′răf-ē) [" + *graphein,* to write]

ophthalmogyric (ŏf-thăl″mō-jī′rĭk) [" + *gyros,* circle]

ophthalmolith (ŏf-thăl′mō-lĭth) [" + *lithos,* stone]

ophthalmologist (ŏf-thăl-mŏl′ō-jĭst) [" + *logos,* word, reason]

ophthalmology (ŏf-thăl-mŏl′ō-jē) [" + *logos,* word, reason]

ophthalmomalacia (ŏf-thăl″mō-măl-ā′sē-ă) [" + *malakia,* softening]

ophthalmometer (ŏf-thăl-mŏm′ĕt-ĕr) [" + *metron,* measure]

ophthalmometry (ŏf-thăl-mŏm′ĕt-rē)

ophthalmomycosis (ŏf-thăl″mō-mī-kō′sĭs) [" + *mykes,* fungus, + *osis,* condition]

ophthalmomyiasis (ŏf-thăl″mō-mī-ī′yă-sĭs) [Gr. *ophthalmos,* eye, + *myia,* a fly, + *-iasis,* state or condition of]

ophthalmomyitis (ŏf-thăl″mō-mī-ī′tĭs) [" + *mys,* muscle, + *itis,* inflammation]

ophthalmomyositis (ŏf-thăl″mō-mī″ō-sī′tĭs)

ophthalmomyotomy (ŏf-thăl″mō-mī-ŏt′ō-mē) [" + *mys,* muscle, + *tome,* a cutting, slice]

ophthalmoneuritis (ŏf-thăl″mō-nū-rī′tĭs) [" + *neuron,* sinew, + *itis,* inflammation]

ophthalmophlebotomy (ŏf-thăl″mō-flē-bŏt′ō-mē) [" + *phleps,* blood vessel, vein, + *tome,* a cutting, slice]

ophthalmophthisis (ŏf″thăl-mŏf′thī-sĭs) [" + *phthisis,* wasting]

ophthalmoplasty (ŏf-thăl′mō-plăs″tē) [" + *plassein,* to form]

ophthalmoplegia (ŏf-thăl″mō-plē′jē-ă) [" + *plege,* stroke]

  o. externa

  o. interna

  o., nuclear

  o., Parinaud's

  o. partialis

  o. progressiva

  o. totalis

ophthalmoptosis (ŏf-thăl″mŏp-tō′sĭs) [" + *ptosis,* fall, falling]

ophthalmoreaction (ŏf-thăl″mō-rē-ăk′shŭn) [" + L. *re,* back, + *actus,* acted]

ophthalmorrhagia (ŏf-thăl″mō-rā′jē-ă) [" + *rhegnynai,* to burst forth]

ophthalmorrhea (ŏf-thăl″mō-rē′ă) [" + *rhein,* to flow]

ophthalmorrhexis (ŏf-thăl″mō-rĕk′sĭs) [" + *rhexis,* rupture]

ophthalmoscope (ŏf-thăl′mō-skōp) [" + *skopein,* to examine]

ophthalmoscopy (ŏf-thăl-mŏs′kō-pē)

  o., medical

  o., metric

ophthalmospasm (ŏf-thăl′mō-spăsm)

ophthalmostasis (ŏf″thăl-mŏs′tă-sĭs) [Gr. *ophthalmos,* eye, + *stasis,*

standing still]
ophthalmostat (ŏf-thăl'mō-stăt)[" + statikos, standing]
ophthalmostatometer (ŏf-thăl"mō-stăt-ŏm'ĕt-ĕr) [" + " + metron, measure]
ophthalmosynchysis (ŏf-thăl"mō-sĭn'kĭ-sĭs) [" + synchisis, a mixing]
ophthalmothermometer (ŏf-thăl"mō-thĕr-mŏm'ĕt-ĕr) [" + therme, heat, + metron, measure]
ophthalmotomy (ŏf"thăl-mŏt'ō-mē) [" + tome, a cutting, slice]
ophthalmotonometer (ŏf-thăl"mō-tō-nŏm'ĕt-ĕr) [" + tonos, act of stretching, tension, tone, + metron, measure]
ophthalmotoxin (ŏf-thăl"mō-tŏk'sĭn) [" + toxikon, poison]
ophthalmotrope (ŏf-thăl'mō-trōp) [" + trope, a turning]
ophthalmotropometer (ŏf-thăl"mō-trō-pŏm'ĕt-ĕr) [" + " + metron, measure]
ophthalmovascular (ŏf-thăl"mō-văs'kū-lăr) [" + L. vasculum, a small vessel]
ophthalmoxerosis (ŏf-thăl"mō-zē-rō'sĭs) [" + xeros, dry, + osis, condition]
ophthalmoxyster (ŏf-thăl"mŏks-ĭs'tĕr) [" + xyster, scraper]
Ophthetic
opiate (ō'pē-ăt)
opiate abstinence syndrome
opiate poisoning
opiate receptor
opioid (ō'pē-oyd) [L. opium, opium, + Gr. eidos, form, shape]
opioid peptides, endogenous
opiomania (ō"pē-ō-mā'nē-ă) [" + Gr. mania, madness]
opiophagism (ō"pē-ŏf'ă-jĭzm) [" + Gr. phagein, to eat]
opisthenar (ō-pĭs'thē-năr) [Gr. opisthen, behind, in the rear, + thenar, palm]
opisthiobasial (ō-pĭs"thē-ō-bā'sē-ăl)

opisthion (ō-pĭs'thē-ŏn) [NL. fr. Gr. opisthen, back, in the rear]
opisthionasial (ō-pĭs"thē-ō-nā'zē-ăl)
opistho-, opisth- [Gr. opisthen, behind, in the rear]
opisthognathism (ō"pĭs-thō'nă-thĭzm) [" + gnathos, jaw, + -ismos, condition]
opisthoporeia (ō-pĭs"thō-pō-rē'ă) [" + poreia, walk]
opisthorchiasis (ō"pĭs-thor-kī'ă-sĭs)
Opisthorchis (ō"pĭs-thor'kĭs) [" + orchis, testicle]
  O. felineus
  O. sinensis
opisthotic (ō"pĭs-thŏt'ĭk) [Gr. opisthen, behind, in the rear, + ous, ear]
opisthotonoid (ō"pĭs-thŏt'ō-noyd) [" + tonos, act of stretching, tension, tone, + eidos, form, shape]
opisthotonos (ō"pĭs-thŏt'ō-nŏs) [" + tonos, act of stretching, tension, tone]
opium (ō'pē-ŭm) [L.]
opium poisoning
opiumism (ō'pē-ŭm-ĭzm)
opo- [Gr. opos, juice]
opocephalus (ō"pō-sĕf'ă-lŭs) [Gr. ops, face, + kephale, head]
opodidymus (ō"pō-dĭd'ĭ-mŭs) [" + didymos, twin]
Oppenheim's disease (ŏp'ĕn-hīmz) [Hermann Oppenheim, Ger. neurologist, 1858–1919]
Oppenheim's gait
oppilation (ŏp"ĭ-lā'shŭn) [L. oppilatio, an obstruction]
opponens (ō-pō'nĕns) [L.]
opponens splint
opportunistic infections
opposition
opsialgia (ŏp"sē-ăl'jē-ă) [Gr. ops, face, + algos, pain]
opsin (ŏp'sĭn)
opsinogen (ŏp-sĭn'ō-jĕn)
opsinogenous (ŏp"sĭn-ŏj'ĕn-ŭs)
opsiometer (ŏp"sē-ŏm'ĕ-tĕr)
opsiuria (ŏp-sē-ū'rē-ă) [Gr. opse, late, + ouron, urine]

opsoclonus
opsogen (ŏp'sō-jĕn)
opsomania (ŏp"sō-mā'nē-ă) [Gr.
opson, food, + *mania*, madness]
opsonic (ŏp-sŏn'ĭk) [Gr. *opsonein*, to
purchase victuals]
opsonification (ŏp-sŏn"ĭ-fĭ-kā'shŭn)
opsonin (ŏp-sō'nĭn) [Gr. *opsonein*, to
purchase victuals]
   o., immune
opsonization (ŏp"sō-nĭ-zā'shŭn)
opsonize (ŏp'sō-nīz) [Gr. *opsonein*, to
purchase victuals]
opsonocytophagic (ŏp"sŏn-ō-sī"tō-
fā'jĭk) [" + *kytos*, cell, + *phagein*, to eat]
opsonometry (ŏp-sō-nŏm'ĕt-rē)
[" + *metron*, measure]
opsonophilia (ŏp"sō-nō-fĭl'ē-ă) [" +
philein, to love]
opsonophilic
opsonotherapy (ŏp"sō-nō-thĕr'ă-pē)
Optacon Optical to Tactile Converter
optesthesia (ŏp"tĕs-thē'zē-ă) [Gr. *optikos*, optical, + *aisthesis*, feeling,
perception]
optic (ŏp'tĭk) [Gr. *optikos*]
optical (ŏp'tĭ-kăl) [Gr. *optikos*; L. *op-
ticus*]
optical activity
optic chiasm
optic disk
optic foramen
optician (ŏp-tĭsh'ăn)
opticianry (ŏp-tĭsh'ăn-rē)
opticist (ŏp'tĭ-sĭst)
optic nerve
optic neuropathy
optico- [Gr. *optikos*]
opticociliary (ŏp"tĭ-kō-sĭl'ē-ăr-ē)
opticokinetic (ŏp"tĭ-kō-kĭ-nĕt'ĭk) [" +
kinesis, motion]
opticonasion (ŏp"tĭ-kō-nā'sē-ŏn)
opticopupillary (ŏp"tĭ-kō-pū'pĭl-ĕr"ē)
optic papilla
optics (ŏp'tĭks) [Gr. *optikos*, pert. to vi-
sion]
optic tract

Optimine
optimum (ŏp'tĭ-mŭm) [L. *optimus*, best]
optimum temperature
opto- [Gr. *optos*, seen]
optogram (ŏp'tō-grăm) [Gr. *optos*,
seen, + *gramma*, letter, piece of
writing]
optokinetic (ŏp"tō-kī-nĕt'ĭk) [" +
kinesis, motion]
optomeninx (ŏp"tō-mē'nĭngks) [" +
meninx, membrane]
optometer (ŏp-tŏm'ĕt-ĕr) [" +
metron, measure]
optometrist (ŏp-tŏm'ĕt-rĭst)
optometry (ŏp-tŏm'ĕt-rē)
optomyometer (ŏp"tō-mī-ŏm'ĕt-ĕr)
[" + *mys*, muscle, + *metron*, a
measure]
optophone (ŏp'tō-fōn) [" +
phone, voice]
optostriate (ŏp-tō-strī'āt) [" + L.
striatus, grooved]
optotype (ŏp'tō-tīp)
OR operating room
ora (ō'ră) [L.]
   o. serrata retinae
orad (ō'răd) [L. *oris*, mouth, + *ad*,
toward]
Oragrafin Sodium
oral (or'ăl) [L. *oralis*]
oral contraceptive
oral diagnosis
orale (ō-rā'lē)
orality (ō-răl'ĭ-tē)
oralogy (ō-răl'ō-jē) [" + Gr. *logos*,
word, reason]
oral rehydration solutions
oral rehydration therapy
orange, methyl
Orasone
Ora-Testryl
orb [L. *orbis*, circle, disk]
orbicular (or-bĭk'ū-lăr) [L. *orbiculus*, a
small circle]
orbicular bone
orbiculare (or-bĭk"ū-lā'rē)
orbicular muscle
orbicular process

orbiculus (or-bĭk'ū-lŭs) [L., little circle]
　o. ciliaris
　o. oculi
　o. oris
orbit (or'bĭt) [L. *orbita*, track]
orbita (or'bĭ-tă) [L.]
orbital (or'bĭ-tăl) [L. *orbitalis*]
orbitale
orbitomeatal line
orbitonasal (or"bĭ-tō-nā'zăl)
orbitonometer (or"bĭ-tō-nŏm'ĕ-tĕr)
orbitonometry (or"bĭ-tō-nŏm'ĕ-trē)
orbitopagus (or"bĭ-tŏp'ă-gŭs) [L. *orbita*, track, + Gr. *pagos*, thing fixed]
orbitotomy (or-bĭ-tŏt'ō-mē) [" + Gr. *tome*, a cutting, slice]
orcein (or-sī'ĭn)
orchectomy (or-kĕk'tō-mē) [Gr. *orchis*, testicle, + *ektome*, excision]
orcheoplasty (or'kē-ō-plăs"tē) [" + *plassein*, to form]
orchialgia (or-kē-ăl'jē-ă) [" + *algos*, pain]
orchichorea (or"kĭ-kō-rē'ă) [" + *choreia*, dance]
orchidalgia (or-kĭ-dăl'jē-ă) [" + *algos*, pain]
orchidectomy (or"kĭ-dĕk'tō-mē) [" + *ektome*, excision]
orchidic (or-kĭd'ĭk)
orchiditis (or"kĭ-dī'tĭs) [" + *itis*, inflammation]
orchido- [Gr. *orchidion*]
orchidoncus (or-kĭ-dŏng'kŭs) [" + *onkos*, bulk, mass]
orchidopexy (or'kĭd-ō-pĕk"sē) [" + *pexis*, fixation]
orchidoplasty (or'kĭd-ō-plăs"tē) [" + *plassein*, to form]
orchidoptosis (or"kĭd-ŏp-tō'sĭs) [" + *ptosis*, fall, falling]
orchidorrhaphy (or"kĭ-dor'ă-fē) [" + *rhaphe*, seam]
orchidotomy (or-kĭd-ŏt'ō-mē) [" + *tome*, a cutting, slice]
orchiectomy (or"kē-ĕk'tō-mē) [" + *ektome*, excision]

orchiepididymitis (or"kē-ĕp"ĭ-dĭd"ĭ-mī'tĭs) [" + *epi*, upon, + *didymos*, testis, + *itis*, inflammation]
orchilytic (or"kĭ-lĭt'ĭk) [" + *lysis*, dissolution]
orchiocele (or'kē-ō-sēl) [" + *kele*, tumor, swelling]
orchiodynia (or"kē-ō-dĭn'ē-ă) [" + *odyne*, pain]
orchioncus (or"kē-ŏng'kŭs) [" + *onkos*, bulk, mass]
orchioneuralgia (or"kē-ō-nū-răl'jē-ă) [" + *neuron*, sinew, + *algos*, pain]
orchiopathy (or"kē-ŏp'ăth-ē) [" + *pathos*, disease, suffering]
orchiopexy (or"kē-ō-pĕk'sē) [" + *pexis*, fixation]
orchioplasty (or'kē-ō-plăs"tē) [" + *plassein*, to form]
orchiorrhaphy (or"kē-or'ră-fē) [" + *rhaphe*, seam]
orchioscheocele (or"kē-ōs'kē-ō-sēl) [" + *oscheon*, scrotum, + *kele*, tumor, swelling]
orchioscirrhus (or"kē-ō-skĭr'rŭs) [" + *skirros*, hard]
orchiotomy (or"kē-ŏt'ō-mē) [" + *tome*, a cutting, slice]
orchis (or'kĭs) [Gr.]
orchitic (or-kĭt'ĭk)
orchitis (or-kī'tĭs) [" + *itis*, inflammation]
　o., gonorrheal
　o., metastatic
　o., syphilitic
　o., tuberculous
orchitolytic (or"kĭt-ō-lĭt'ĭk) [" + *lysis*, dissolution]
orchotomy (or-kŏt'ō-mē) [" + *tome*, a cutting, slice]
orcin, orcinol (or'sĭn, -ŏl)
order [L. *ordo*, a row, series]
orderly (or'dĕr-lē)
ordinate (or'dĭ-năt)
ordure (or'dūr)
Oretic
Oreton-Methyl

orexia (ō-rĕk'sē-ă) [Gr. *orexis*]
orexigenic (ō-rĕk"sĭ-jĕn'ĭk) [Gr. *orexis*, appetite, + *gennan*, to produce]
oreximania (ō-rĕk"sĭ-mā'nē-ă) [" + *mania*, madness]
orf
organ (or'găn) [Gr. *organon*; L. *organum*]
    o., accessory
    o., acoustic
    o., enamel
    o., end
    o., excretory
    o., Golgi's
    o., gustatory
    o. of Corti
    o. of Giraldès
    o. of Jacobson
    o. of Ruffini
    o.'s of Zuckerkandl
    o., reproductive
    o., sense
    o., sex
    o.'s, special sense
    o., spiral
    o., target
    o., vestigial
    o., vomeronasal
    o., Weber's
organelle (or"găn-ĕl')
organic (or-găn'ĭk) [Gr. *organikos*]
organic acid
organic brain syndromes
organic chemistry
organic disease
organic dust toxic syndrome
organicism (or-găn'ĭ-sĭzm)
organicist (or-găn'ĭ-sĭst)
organic psychoses
organism (or'găn-ĭzm) [Gr. *organon*, organ, + *-ismos*, condition]
organization (or"găn-ĭ-zā'shŭn)
organization center
organize (or'găn-īz)
organo- (or'gă-nō)
organoferric (or"gă-nō-fĕr'ĭk)
organogel (or-găn'ō-jĕl)
organogenesis (or"găn-ō-jĕn'ĕ-sĭs) [" + *genesis*, generation, birth]

organogeny (or"gă-nŏj'ĕ-nē)
organography (or-găn-ŏg'ră-fē) [" + *graphein*, to write]
organoid [" + *eidos*, form, shape]
organoleptic (or"găn-ō-lĕp'tĭk) [" + *lepsis*, a seizure]
organology (or-gă-nŏl'ō-jē) [" + *logos*, word, reason]
organoma (or-gă-nō'mă) [" + *oma*, tumor]
organomegaly (or"gă-nō-mĕg'ă-lē) [" + *megas*, large]
organomercurial (or"gă-nō-mĕr-kū'rē-ăl)
organometallic (or-gă-nō-mĕ-tăl'ĭk)
organon (or'gă-nŏn) [Gr.]
organonomy (or"gă-nŏn'ō-mē) [" + *nomos*, law]
organopathy (or"gă-nŏp'ă-thē) [" + *pathos*, disease, suffering]
organopexy (or'găn-ō-pĕk"sē) [" + *pexis*, fixation]
organophilic (or"gă-nō-fĭl'ĭk) [" + *philos*, love]
organoscopy (or-gă-nŏs'kō-pē) [" + *skopein*, to examine]
organotherapy (or"găn-ō-thĕr'ă-pē) [" + *therapeia*, treatment]
organotrope, organotropic (or-găn'ō-trōp, -găn-ō-trōp'ĭk) [" + *tropos*, turning]
organotrophic (or"gă-nō-trŏf'ĭk) [" + *trophe*, nutrition]
organotropism (or"gă-nŏt'rō-pĭzm) [" + *trope*, a turn, + *-ismos*, condition]
organ perfusion system
organ-specific (or'găn-spĕ-sĭf'ĭk)
organum [L.]
    o. auditus
    o. gustus
    o. olfactus
    o. spirale
    o. vestibulocochleare
    o. visus
    o. vomeronasale
orgasm (or'găzm) [Gr. *orgasmos*, swelling]
Oriental sore

orientation (or"ē-ĕn-tā'shŭn) [L. *oriens*, to arise]

orifice (or'ĭ-fĭs) [L. *orificium*]
o., anal
o., atrioventricular
o., cardiac
o., mitral
o., oral
o., pyloric
o., ureteric
o., urethral, external
o., urethral, internal

orificial (or"ĭ-fĭ'shăl) [L. *orificium*, outlet]

orificium (or"ĭ-fĭsh'ē-ŭm) [L.]

origin (or'ĭ-jĭn) [L. *origo*, beginning]
o., deep
o., superficial

Orimune

Orinase

Ormond's disease

ornithine (or'nĭ-thĭn)

Ornithodoros (or"nĭ-thŏd'ō-rōs)

ornithosis (or"nĭ-thō'sĭs) [Gr. *ornithos*, bird, + *osis*, condition]

orodiagnosis (or"ō-dĭ-ăg-nō'sĭs) [Gr. *oros*, serum, + *dia*, through, + *gnosis*, knowledge]

orofacial (or"ō-fā'shē-ăl) [L. *oris*, mouth, + *facies*, face]

orofaciodigital syndrome

orolingual (or"ō-lĭng'gwăl) [L. *oris*, mouth, + *lingua*, tongue]

oromeningitis (or"ō-mĕn"ĭn-jī'tĭs) [" + Gr. *meninx*, membrane, + *itis*, inflammation]

oronasal (or"ō-nā'zăl) [" + *nasus*, nose]

oropharynx (or"ō-făr'ĭnks) [" + Gr. *pharynx*, throat]

orosomucoid (or"ŏ-sō-mū'koyd)

orotherapy (or"ō-thĕr'ă-pē) [" + Gr. *therapeia*, treatment]

orotic acid

orotic aciduria

Oroya fever [Oroya, a region of Peru]

orphan drugs

orphenadrine citrate (or-fĕn'ă-drēn)

orrhology (or-ŏl'ō-jē) [Gr. *orrhos*, blood serum, + *logos*, word, reason]

orrhomeningitis (or"ō-mĕn"ĭn-jī'tĭs) [" + *meninx*, membrane, + *itis*, inflammation]

orrhoreaction (or"ō-rē-ăk'shŭn) [" + *re*, back, + *actus*, acted]

orrhorrhea (or"ō-rē'ă) [" + *rhein*, to flow]

orrhotherapy (or"rō-thĕr'ă-pē) [" + *therapeia*, treatment]

orris root (or'ĭs)

ORT *oral rehydration therapy*

orthergasia (or"thĕr-gă'zē-ă) [Gr. *orthos*, straight, + *ergon*, work]

orthesis (or-thē'sĭs)

orthetics (or-thĕt'ĭks)

orthetist (or'thĕ-tĭst)

ortho- [Gr. *orthos*, straight]

orthoacid (or"thō-ăs'ĭd)

orthobiosis (or"thō-bī-ō'sĭs) [" + *bios*, life]

orthocephalic (or"thō-sē-făl'ĭk) [" + *kephale*, head]

orthochorea (or"thō-kō-rē'ă) [" + *choreia*, dance]

orthochromatic (or"thō-krō-măt'ĭk) [" + *chroma*, color]

orthochromophil (or"thō-krō'mō-fĭl) [" + " + *philein*, to love]

orthocytosis (or"thō-sī-tō'sĭs) [" + *kytos*, cell, + *osis*, condition]

orthodentin (or"thō-dĕn'tĭn)

orthodiagraph (or"thō-dī'ă-grăf) [" + *dia*, through, + *graphein*, to write]

orthodigita (or"thō-dĭj'ĭ-tă) [" + L. *digitus*, finger, toe]

orthodontia (or"thō-dŏn'shē-ă) [" + *odous*, tooth]

orthodontics (or"thō-dŏn'tĭks)

orthodontist

orthodromic (or"thō-drŏm'ĭk) [Gr. *orthodromein*, to run straight forward]

orthogenesis (or"thō-jĕn'ĕ-sĭs) [Gr. *orthos*, straight, + *genesis*, generation, birth]

orthogenic

orthogenics (or"thō-jĕn'ĭks)

orthograde (or'thō-grād) [" + L.

gradi, to walk]
orthokinetic cuff
orthokinetics
orthomelic (or″thō-mē′lĭk) [″ + *melos*, limb]
orthometer (or-thŏm′ĕ-tĕr) [″ + *metron*, measure]
orthomolecular (or″thō-mō-lĕk′ū-lăr)
orthomolecular psychiatry
orthomyxoviruses (or″thō-mĭk″sō-vī′rŭs-ĕs)
Ortho-Novum
orthopedia (or″thō-pē′dē-ă) [Gr. *orthos*, straight, + *pais*, child]
orthopedic (or″thō-pē′dĭk)
orthopedics (or″thō-pē′dĭks) [″ + *pais*, child]
orthopedic surgery
orthopedist (or″thō-pē′dĭst)
orthopercussion (or″thō-pĕr-kŭsh′ŭn) [″ + L. *percussio*, a striking]
orthophoria (or″thō-fō′rē-ă) [″ + *pherein*, to bear]
orthophrenia (or″thō-frē′nē-ă) [″ + *phren*, mind]
orthopnea (or″thŏp′nē-ă) [″ + *pnoia*, breath]
orthopneic position (or″thŏp-nē′ĭk)
Orthopoxvirus
orthopraxis (or″thō-prăk′sĭs) [″ + *prassein*, to make]
orthopsychiatry (or″thō-sī-kī′ă-trē) [″ + *psyche*, soul, + *iatreia*, treatment]
orthoptic (or-thŏp′tĭk) [″ + *optikos*, pert. to vision]
orthoptics
orthoptic training
orthoroentgenography (or″thō-rĕnt-gĕn-ŏg′ră-fē)
orthoscopic (or″thō-skŏp′ĭk)
orthoscopy (or-thŏs′kō-pē)
orthosis [Gr., straightening]
orthostatic (or″thō-stăt′ĭk) [Gr. *orthos*, straight, + *statikos*, causing to stand]
orthostatic hypotension
orthostatism (or″thō-stăt″ĭzm) [″ + ″ + *-ismos*, condition]

orthotast (or′thō-tăst) [″ + *tassein*, to arrange]
orthotic [Gr. *orthosis*, straightening]
orthotics (or-thŏt′ĭks)
orthotist (or′thō-tĭst) [Gr. *orthosis*, straightening]
orthotonos, orthotonus (or-thŏt′ō-nŏs, -nŭs) [″ + *tonos*, act of stretching, tension, tone]
orthotopic (or″thō-tŏp′ĭk)
orthovoltage (or″thō-vŏl′tĭj)
orthropsia (or-thrŏp′sē-ă) [Gr. *orthros*, time near dawn, + *opsis*, sight, appearance, vision]
orthuria (orth-ū′rē-ă) [Gr. *orthos*, straight, + *ouron*, urine]
O.S., o.s. [L.] *oculus sinister*, left eye
Os *osmium*
os (ōs) [L.]
   o. uteri
   o. uteri externum
   o. uteri internum
   o. ventriculi
os (ŏs) [L.]
   o. calcis
   o. coxae
   o. hamatum
   o. hyoideum
   o. ilii
   o. innominatum
   o. magnum
   o. orbiculare
   o. peroneum
   o. planum
   o. pubis
   o. scaphoideum
   o. temporale
   o. trigonum
   o. unguis
   o. vesalianum
osazone (ō′să-zōn)
oscedo (ŏs-sē′dō) [L.]
oscheal (ŏs′kē-ăl) [Gr. *oscheon*, scrotum]
oscheitis (ŏs-kē-ī′tĭs) [″ + *itis*, inflammation]
oschelephantiasis (ŏsk″ĕl-ĕ-făn-tī′ă-sĭs)
oscheo- [Gr. *oscheon*]

oscheocele (ŏs'kē-ō-sēl) [" + *kele*, tumor, swelling]

oscheohydrocele (ŏs"kē-ō-hī'drō-sēl) [" + *hydor*, water, + *kele*, tumor, swelling]

oscheolith (ŏs'kē-ō-lĭth) [" + *lithos*, stone]

oscheoma (ŏs-kē-ō'mă) [" + *oma*, tumor]

oscheoncus (ŏs"kē-ōng'kŭs) [" + *onkos*, bulk, mass]

oscheoplasty (ŏs'kē-ō-plăs"tē) [" + *plassein*, to form]

oschitis (ŏs-kī'tĭs)

oscillation (ŏs"sĭl-ā'shŭn) [L. *oscillare*, to swing]

oscillator (ŏs'ĭ-lā"tor)

oscillogram (ŏs'ĭl-ō-grăm) [" + Gr. *gramma*, letter, piece of writing]

oscillograph (ŏs'ĭl-ō-grăf) [" + Gr. *graphein*, to write]

oscillometer (ŏs-ĭl-ŏm'ĕt-ĕr) [" + Gr. *metron*, measure]

oscillometry (ŏs-ĭl-ŏm'ĕ-trē)

oscillopsia

oscilloscope (ō-sĭl'ō-skōp) [L. *oscillare*, to swing, + Gr. *skopein*, to examine]

Oscinidae

oscitation (ŏs-ĭ-tā'shŭn) [L. *oscitatio*]

osculation [L. *osculum*, little mouth, kiss]

osculum (ŏs'kū-lŭm) [L.]

Osgood-Schlatter disease (ŏz-good-shlăt'ĕr) [Robert B. Osgood, U.S. orthopedist, 1873–1956; Carl Schlatter, Swiss surgeon, 1864–1934]

OSHA *Occupational Safety and Health Administration*

-osis [Gr.]

Osler, Sir William (ŏs'lĕr) [Canadian-born physician, 1849–1919]
    O.'s disease
    O.'s maneuver
    O.'s nodes
    O.- Vaquez disease
    O.- Weber-Rendu disease [Frederick P. Weber, Brit. physician, 1863–1962; Henri J. L. M. Rendu, Fr. physician, 1844–1902]

osmate

osmatic (ŏz-măt'ĭk) [Gr. *osmasthai*, to smell]

osmesis (ŏz-mē'sĭs) [Gr. *osmesis*, smelling]

osmesthesia (ŏz"mĕs-thē'zē-ă) [Gr. *osme*, odor, + *aisthesis*, feeling, perception]

osmic acid (ŏz'mĭk)

osmicate (ŏz'mĭ-kāt)

osmics (ŏz'mĭks) [Gr. *osme*, odor]

osmidrosis (ŏz-mĭ-drō'sĭs) [" + *hidros*, sweat]

osmiophilic (ŏz"mē-ō-fĭl'ĭk)

osmiophobic (ŏz"mē-ō-fō'bĭk)

Osmitrol

osmium (ŏz'mē-ŭm) [Gr. *osme*, smell]
    o. tetroxide

osmo- [Gr. *osme*, odor; *osmos*, impulse]

osmodysphoria (ŏz-mō-dĭs-fō'rē-ă) [Gr. *osme*, odor, + *dys*, bad, difficult, painful, disordered, + *pherein*, to bear]

osmolagnia (ŏz"mō-lăg'nē-ă) [" + *lagneia*, lust]

osmolality (ŏs"mō-lăl'ĭ-tē)
    o., serum
    o., urine

osmolar (ŏz-mō'lăr)

osmolarity (os"mō-lăr'ĭ-tē)

osmology (ŏz-mŏl'ō-jē) [Gr. *osme*, odor, + *logos*, word, reason; Gr. *osmos*, impulse, + *logos*, word, reason]

osmometer (ŏz-mŏm'ĕt-ĕr) [" + *metron*, measure; Gr. *osmos*, impulse, + *metron*, measure]

osmonosology (ŏz"mō-nō-sŏl'ō-jē) [" + *nosos*, disease, + *logos*, word, reason]

osmophilic (ŏz"mō-fĭl'ĭk) [Gr. *osmos*, impulse, + *philos*, love]

osmophore (ŏz"mō-for) [" + *phoros*, bearing]

osmoreceptor (ŏz"mō-rē-sĕp'tor)

osmoregulation (ŏz"mō-rĕg"ū-lā'shŭn)

osmose (ŏz'mōs) [Gr. *osmos*, impulse]

osmosis (ŏz-mō'sĭs) [Gr. *osmos*, im-

pulse, + *osis*, condition]
osmotherapy (ŏz"mō-thĕr'ă-pē)
[" + *therapeia*, treatment]
osmotic (ŏz-mŏt'ĭk) [Gr. *osmos*, impulse]
osmotic pressure
osphresiolagnia (ŏs-frē"zē-ō-lăg'nē-ă) [Gr. *osphresis*, smell, + *lagneia*, lust]
osphresiology (ŏs"frē-zē-ŏl'ō-jē) [" + *logos*, word, reason]
osphresiometer (ŏs"frē-zē-ŏm'ĕt-ĕr) [" + *metron*, measure]
osphresis (ŏs-frē'sĭs) [Gr.]
osphretic (ŏs-frĕt'ĭk)
osphus (ŏs'fŭs) [Gr. *osphys*]
osphyalgia (ŏs-fē-ăl'jē-ă) [" + *algos*, pain]
osphyitis (ŏs-fē-ī'tĭs) [" + *itis*, inflammation]
osphyomyelitis (ŏs"fē-ō-mī"ĕl-ī'tĭs) [" + *myelos*, marrow, + *itis*, inflammation]
ossa (ŏs'ă) [L., bones]
ossein (ŏs'ē-ĭn) [L. *ossa*, bones]
osseocartilaginous (ŏs"ē-ō-kăr"tĭ-lăj'ĭ-nŭs)
osseofibrous (ŏs"ē-ō-fī'brŭs) [" + *fibra*, fiber]
osseointegration
osseomucin (ŏs"ē-ō-mū'sĭn)
osseous (ŏs'ē-ŭs) [L. *osseus*, bony]
ossicle (ŏs'ĭ-kl) [L. *ossiculum*, little bone]
o.'s, auditory
ossicula (ŏ-sĭk'ū-lă) [L.]
ossiculectomy (ŏs"ĭk-ū-lĕk'tō-mē) [L. *ossiculum*, little bone, + Gr. *ektome*, excision]
ossiculotomy (ŏ"sĭk-ū-lŏt'ō-mē) [" + Gr. *tome*, a cutting, slice]
ossiculum (ŏ-sĭk'ū-lŭm) [L.]
ossiferous (ŏs-ĭf'ĕr-ŭs) [L. *os*, bone, + *ferre*, to bear]
ossific (ŏs-ĭf'ĭk) [" + *facere*, to make]
ossification (ŏs"ĭ-fĭ-kā'shŭn) [" + *facere*, to make]
o., endochondral
o., intramembranous
o., pathologic

o., periosteal
ossifluence (ŏ-sĭf'lū-ĕns)
ossiform (ŏs'ĭ-form)
ossify (ŏs'ĭ-fī) [" + *facere*, to make]
ostalgia (ŏs-tăl'jē-ă) [Gr. *osteon*, bone, + *algos*, pain]
osteal (ŏs'tē-ăl)
ostealgia (ŏs'tē-ăl'jē-ă) [" + *algos*, pain]
osteanagenesis (ŏs"tē-ăn-ă-jĕn'ē-sĭs) [" + *ana*, on, + Gr. *genesis*, generation, birth]
ostearthrotomy (ŏs"tē-ăr-thrŏt'ō-mē) [" + *arthron*, joint, + *tome*, a cutting, slice]
ostectomy, osteectomy (ŏs-tĕk'tō-mē, -tē-ĕk'tō-mē) [" + *ektome*, excision]
osteectopia (ŏs"tē-ĕk-tō'pē-ă) [" + *ektopos*, out of place]
osteitis (ŏs-tē-ī'tĭs) [" + *itis*, inflammation]
o., condensing
o. deformans
o. fibrosa cystica generalistata
o. fragilitans
o., gummatous
o., rarefying
o., sclerosing
ostembryon (ŏs-tĕm'brē-ŏn) [Gr. *osteon*, bone, + *embryon*, to swell inside]
ostemia (ŏs-tē'mē-ă) [" + *haima*, blood]
ostempyesis (ŏs"tĕm-pī-ē'sĭs) [" + *empyesis*, suppuration]
osteo- [Gr. *osteon*, bone]
osteoanagenesis (ŏs"tē-ō-ăn"ă-jĕn'ē-sĭs) [" + Gr. *ana*, again, + Gr. *genesis*, generation, birth]
osteoanesthesia (ŏs"tē-ō-ăn"ĕs-thē'zē-ă) [" + *an-*, not, + *aisthesis*, feeling, perception]
osteoaneurysm (ŏs"tē-ō-ăn'ū-rĭzm) [" + *aneurysma*, a widening]
osteoarthritis (ŏs"tē-ō-ăr-thrī'tĭs) [" + *arthron*, joint, + *itis*, inflammation]
osteoarthropathy (ŏs"tē-ō-ăr-

thrŏp′ă-thē) [″ + ″ + *pathos*, disease, suffering]

o., hypertrophic pulmonary

osteoarthrosis (ŏs″tē-ō-ăr-thrō′sĭs) [″ + ″ + *osis*, condition]

osteoarthrotomy (ŏs″tē-ō-ăr-thrŏt′ō-mē) [″ + ″ + *tome*, a cutting, slice]

osteoblast (ŏs′tē-ō-blăst) [Gr. *osteon*, bone, + *blastos*, germ]

osteoblastoma (ŏs″tē-ō-blăs-tō′mă) [″ + ″ + *oma*, tumor]

osteocampsia (ŏs″tē-ō-kămp′sē-ă) [″ + *kamptein*, to bend]

osteocarcinoma (ŏs″tē-ō-kăr-sĭn-ō′mă) [″ + *karkinos*, cancer, + *oma*, tumor]

osteocartilaginous (ŏs″tē-ō-kăr″tĭ-lăj′ĭ-nŭs)

osteocele (ŏs′tē-ō-sēl) [″ + *kele*, tumor, swelling]

osteocephaloma (ŏs″tē-ō-sĕf″ă-lō′mă) [″ + *kephale*, head, + *oma*, tumor]

osteochondral (ŏs″tē-ō-kŏn′drăl)

osteochondritis (ŏs″tē-ō-kŏn-drī′tĭs) [″ + *chondros*, cartilage, + *itis*, inflammation]

o. deformans juvenilis

o. dissecans

osteochondrodystrophy (ŏs″tē-ō-kŏn″drō-dĭs′trō-fē) [″ + ″ + *dys*, bad, difficult, painful, disordered, + *trephein*, to nourish]

o., familial

osteochondrolysis (ŏs″tē-ō-kŏn-drŏl′ĭ-sĭs) [″ + ″ + *lysis*, dissolution]

osteochondroma (ŏs″tē-ō-kŏn-drō′mă) [″ + ″ + *oma*, tumor]

osteochondromatosis (ŏs″tē-ō-kŏn″drō-mă-tō′sĭs) [″ + ″ + ″ + *osis*, condition]

osteochondrosarcoma (ŏs″tē-ō-kŏn″drō-săr-kō′mă) [″ + ″ + *sarx*, flesh, + *oma*, tumor]

osteochondrosis (ŏs″tē-ō-kŏn-drō′sĭs) [″ + ″ + *osis*, condition]

o. deformans tibiae

osteochondrous (ŏs″tē-ō-kŏn′drŭs)

osteoclasia, osteoclasis (ŏs″tē-ō-klā′zē-ă, -ŏk′lă-sĭs) [″ + *klasis*, a breaking]

osteoclast (ŏs′tē-ō-klăst) [″ + *klan*, to break]

osteoclast activating factor

osteoclastic (ŏs″tē-ō-klăs′tĭk)

osteoclastoma (ŏs″tē-ō-klăs-tō′mă) [″ + ″ + *oma*, tumor]

osteoclasty (ŏs′tē-ō-klăs″tē)

osteocope (ŏs′tē-ō-kōp) [″ + *kopos*, pain]

osteocopic (ŏs″tē-ō-kŏp′ĭk)

osteocranium (ŏs″tē-ō-krā′nē-ŭm) [″ + *kranion*, skull]

osteocystoma (ŏs″tē-ō-sĭs-tō′mă) [″ + *kystis*, sac, bladder, + *oma*, tumor]

osteocyte (ŏs′tē-ō-sīt″) [″ + *kytos*, cell]

osteodensitometer

osteodentin

osteodermia (ŏs″tē-ō-dĕr′mē-ă) [″ + *derma*, skin]

osteodesmosis (ŏs″tē-ō-dĕs-mō′sĭs) [″ + *desmos*, tendon, + *osis*, condition]

osteodiastasis (ŏs″tē-ō-dĭ-ăs′tă-sĭs) [″ + *diastasis*, separation]

osteodynia (ŏs″tē-ō-dĭn′ē-ă) [″ + *odyne*, pain]

osteodystrophia (ŏs″tē-ō-dĭs-trō′fē-ă) [″ + *dys*, bad, difficult, painful, disordered, + *trophe*, nourishment]

osteodystrophy (ŏs″tē-ō-dĭs′trō-fē)

o., renal

osteoectomy (ŏs″tē-ō-ĕk′tō-mē) [″ + *ektome*, excision]

osteoepiphysis (ŏs″tē-ō-ē-pĭf′ĭs-ĭs) [″ + *epi*, upon, + *physis*, growth]

osteofibroma (ŏs″tē-ō-fĭ-brō′mă) [″ + L. *fibra*, fiber, + Gr. *oma*, tumor]

osteogen (ŏs′tē-ō-jĕn) [″ + *gennan*, to produce]

osteogenesis, osteogeny (ŏs″tē-ō-

jĕn'ĕ-sĭs, -ŏj'ĕ-nē)
o. imperfecta

osteogenic

osteography (ŏs"tē-ŏg'răf-ē) [Gr. *osteon*, bone, + *graphein*, to write]

osteohalisteresis (ŏs"tē-ō-hăl-ĭs"tĕr-ē'sĭs) [" + *hals*, salt, + *sterein*, to deprive]

osteoid (ŏs'tē-oyd) [" + *eidos*, form, shape]

osteolipochondroma (ŏs"tē-ō-lĭ-pō"kŏn-drō'mă) [" + *lipos*, fat, + *chondros*, cartilage, + *oma*, tumor]

osteologist (ŏs"tē-ŏl'ō-jĭst) [" + *logos*, word, reason]

osteology (ŏs-tē-ŏl'ō-jē) [" + *logos*, word, reason]

osteolysis (ŏs"tē-ŏl'ĭ-sĭs) [" + *lysis*, dissolution]

osteolytic (ŏs"tē-ō-lĭt'ĭk)

osteoma (ŏs-tē-ō'mă) [" + *oma*, tumor]

   o., cancellous
   o., cavalryman's
   o. cutis
   o., dental
   o. durum, eburneum
   o. medullare
   o., osteoid
   o. spongiosum

osteomalacia (ŏs"tē-ō-măl-ā'shē-ă) [Gr. *osteon*, bone, + *malakia*, softening]

osteomalacic (ŏs"tē-ō-măl-ā'sĭk) [" + *malakia*, softening]

osteomatoid (ŏs-tē-ō'mă-toyd) [" + *oma*, tumor, + *eidos*, form, shape]

osteomatosis (ŏs"tē-ō"mă-tō'sĭs) [" + " + *osis*, condition]

osteomere (ŏs'tē-ō-mēr) [" + *meros*, part]

osteometry (ŏs-tē-ŏm'ĕt-rē) [" + *metron*, measure]

osteomyelitis (ŏs"tē-ō-mī"ĕl-ī'tĭs) [" + *myelos*, marrow, + *itis*, inflammation]

osteomyelodysplasia (ŏs"tē-ō-mī"ĕ-

lō-dĭs-plā'sē-ă) [" + " + *dys*, bad, difficult, painful, disordered, + *plassein*, to form]

osteon (ŏs'tē-ŏn) [Gr., bone]

osteoncus (ŏs-tē-ŏng'kŭs) [" + *onkos*, bulk, mass]

osteonecrosis (ŏs"tē-ō-nē-krō'sĭs) [" + *nekrosis*, state of death]

osteonectin

osteoneuralgia (ŏs"tē-ō-nū-răl'jē-ă) [" + *neuron*, nerve, + *algos*, pain]

osteopath (ŏs'tē-ō-păth) [" + *pathos*, disease, suffering]

osteopathic (ŏs"tē-ō-păth'ĭk)

osteopathology (ŏs"tē-ō-păth-ŏl'ō-jē) [" + *pathos*, disease, suffering, + *logos*, word, reason]

osteopathy (ŏs-tē-ŏp'ă-thē) [" + *pathos*, disease, suffering]

osteopecilia (ŏs"tē-ō-pē-sĭl'ē-ă) [" + *poikilia*, spottedness]

osteopedion (ŏs"tē-ō-pē'dē-ŏn) [" + *paidion*, child]

osteopenia (ŏs"tē-ō-pē'nē-ă) [" + *penia*, lack]

osteoperiosteal (ŏs"tē-ō-pĕr"ē-ŏs'tē-ăl) [" + *peri*, around, + *osteon*, bone]

osteoperiostitis (ŏs"tē-ō-pĕr"ē-ŏs-tī'tĭs) [" + " + *itis*, inflammation]

osteopetrosis (ŏs"tē-ō-pē-trō'sĭs) [" + *petra*, stone, + *osis*, condition]

osteophage (ŏs'tē-ō-fāj) [" + *phagein*, to eat]

osteophagia (ŏs"tē-ō-fā'jē-ă)

osteophlebitis (ŏs"tē-ō-flē-bī'tĭs) [" + *phleps*, blood vessel, vein, + *itis*, inflammation]

osteophone (ŏs'tē-ō-fōn") [Gr. *osteon*, bone, + *phone*, voice]

osteophony (ŏs"tē-ŏf'ō-nē)

osteophore (ŏs'tē-ō-for) [" + *pherein*, to carry]

osteophyma (ŏs"tē-ō-fī'mă) [" + *phyma*, growth]

osteophyte (ŏs'tē-ō-fīt) [" + *phy-*

ton, plant]

osteoplaque (ŏs′tē-ō-plăk)

osteoplast (ŏs′tē-ō-plăst) [″ + plastos, formed]

osteoplastic (ŏs″tē-ō-plăs′tĭk) [″ + plastikos, formed]

osteoplasty (ŏs′tē-ō-plăs″tē) [″ + plassein, to form]

osteopoikilosis (ŏs″tē-ō-poy″kī-lō′sĭs) [″ + poikilos, spotted]

osteoporosis (ŏs″tē-ō-por-ō′sĭs) [″ + poros, passage, + osis, condition]
   o. circumscripta cranii
   o. of disuse
   o., posttraumatic

osteoporotic (ŏs″tē-ō-por-ŏt′ĭk)

osteoradionecrosis (ŏs″tē-ō-rā″dē-ō-nĕ-krō′sĭs) [Gr. osteon, bone, + L. radiatio, radiation, + Gr. nekrosis, state of death]

osteorrhagia (ŏs″tē-ō-rā′jē-ă) [″ + rhegnynai, to burst forth]

osteorrhaphy (ŏs-tē-or′ă-fē) [″ + rhaphe, seam]

osteosarcoma (ŏs″tē-ō-săr-kō′mă) [″ + sarx, flesh, + oma, tumor]

osteosarcomatous (ŏs″tē-ō-săr-kō′măt-ŭs)

osteosclerosis (ŏs″tē-ō-sklē-rō′sĭs) [″ + skleros, hard, + osis, condition]
   o. congenita

osteoscope (ŏs′tē-ō-skōp) [″ + skopein, to examine]

osteoseptum (ŏs″tē-ō-sĕp′tŭm) [″ + L. septum, a partition]

osteosis (ŏs″tē-ō′sĭs) [″ + osis, condition]
   o. cutis

osteospongioma (ŏs″tē-ō-spŏn″jē-ō′mă) [″ + spongos, sponge, + oma, tumor]

osteosteatoma (ŏs″tē-ō-stē″ă-tō′mă) [″ + stear, fat, + oma, tumor]

osteostixis (ŏs″tē-ō-stĭk′sĭs) [″ + stixis, a puncture]

osteosuture (ŏs″tē-ō-sū′chŭr) [″ + L. sutura, seam]

osteosynovitis (ŏs″tē-ō-sĭn″ō-vī′tĭs) [″ + syn, with, + oon, egg, + itis, inflammation]

osteosynthesis (ŏs″tē-ō-sĭn′thē-sĭs) [″ + synthesis, a joining]

osteotabes (ŏs″tē-ō-tā′bēz) [″ + L. tabes, wasting disease]

osteotelangiectasia (ŏs″tē-ō-tĕl-ăn″jē-ĕk-tā′zē-ă) [″ + telos, end, + angeion, vessel, + ektasis, a stretching]

osteothrombosis (ŏs″tē-ō-thrŏm-bō′sĭs) [″ + thrombosis, a clotting]

osteotome (ŏs′tē-ō-tōm) [″ + tome, a cutting, slice]

osteotomoclasis (ŏs″tē-ō-tō-mŏk′lă-sĭs) [Gr. osteon, bone, + tomos, slice, section, + klasis, breaking]

osteotomy (ŏs-tē-ŏt′ō-mē) [″ + tome, a cutting, slice]
   o., cuneiform
   o., linear
   o., Macewen's
   o., subtrochanteric
   o., transtrochanteric

osteotribe (ŏs′tē-ō-trīb″) [″ + tribein, to rub]

osteotrite (ŏs′tē-ō-trīt) [″ + tribein, to grind or rub]

osteotrophy (ŏs-tē-ŏt′rō-fē) [″ + trophe, nutrition]

osteotylus (ŏs″tē-ŏt′ĭ-lŭs) [″ + tylos, callus]

osteotympanic (ŏs″tē-ō-tĭm-păn′ĭk)

ostial (ŏs′tē-ăl) [L. ostium, a little opening]

ostitis (ŏs-tī′tĭs) [″ + itis, inflammation]

ostium (ŏs′tē-ŭm) [L.]
   o. abdominale tubae uterinae
   o. arteriosum
   o. internum
   o. pharyngeum
   o. primum
   o. primum defect
   o. secundum

o. secundum defect
o. tympanicum
o. urethrae externum
o. uteri
o. uterinum tubae
o. vaginae

ostomate (ŏs'tō-māt) [L. *ostium*, little opening]

ostomy (ŏs'tō-mē)

ostosis (ŏs-tō'sĭs)

ostraceous (ŏs-trā'shŭs)

ostraco-, ostrac- [Gr. *ostrakon*, shell]

ostreotoxismus (ŏs"trē-ō-tŏks-ĭz'mŭs) [Gr. *ostreon*, oyster, + *toxikon*, poison]

O.T. *occupational therapy*

otacoustic (ō"tă-koo'stĭk) [Gr. *otakousteo*, to listen]

otalgia (ō-tăl'jē-ă) [Gr.]

otantritis (ō"tăn-trī'tĭs) [Gr. *otos*, ear, + L. *antrum*, sinus, + Gr. *itis*, inflammation]

O.T.C. *over the counter*

OTD *organ tolerance dose*

otectomy (ō-tĕk'tō-mē) [Gr. *otos*, ear, + *ektome*, excision]

othelcosis (ō-thĕl-kō'sĭs) [" + *helkosis*, ulceration]

othematoma (ŏt"hē-mă-tō'mă) [" + *haima*, blood, + *oma*, tumor]

othemorrhea (ŏt-hĕm"ō-rē'ă) [" + " + *rhein*, to flow]

othygroma (ŏt-hī-grō'mă) [" + *hygros*, moist, + *oma*, tumor]

otic (ō'tĭk) [Gr. *otikos*]

oticodinia (ō"tĭ-kō-dĭn'ē-ă) [Gr. *otikos*, aural, + *dine*, whirl]

otitic (ō-tĭt'ĭk)

otitis (ō-tī'tĭs) [Gr. *otos*, ear, + *itis*, inflammation]

o., aero-
o., aviation
o. externa
o., furuncular
o. interna, labyrinthica
o. labyrinthica
o. mastoidea
o. media
o. media with effusion
o. mycotica
o. parasitica
o. sclerotica

oto-, ot- [Gr. *otos*, ear]

otoantritis (ō"tō-ăn-trī'tĭs) [" + *antron*, cavity, + *itis*, inflammation]

otoblennorrhea (ō"tō-blĕn"ō-rē'ă) [" + *blenna*, mucus, + *rhein*, to flow]

otocatarrh (ō"tō-kă-tăr) [" + *katarrhein*, to flow down]

otocephalus (ō"tō-sĕf'ă-lŭs)

otocephaly (ō"tō-sĕf'ă-lē) [" + *kephale*, head]

otocleisis (ō-tō-klī'sĭs) [" + *kleisis*, closure]

otoconium (ō"tō-kō'nē-ŭm) [" + *konis*, dust]

otocyst (ō'tō-sĭst) [" + *kystis*, sac, bladder]

otodynia (ō"tō-dĭn'ē-ă) [" + *odyne*, pain]

otoganglion (ō"tō-găng'glē-ŏn) [" + *ganglion*, ganglion]

otogenic, otogenous (ō"tō-jĕn'ĭk, ō-tŏj'ĕn-ŭs) [" + *gennan*, to produce]

otography (ō-tŏg'ră-fē) [" + *graphein*, to write]

otolaryngologist (ō"tō-lar"ĭn-gŏl'ō-jĭst) [" + *larynx*, larynx, + *logos*, word, reason]

otolaryngology (ō"tō-lar"ĭn-gŏl'ō-jē)

otolith (ō'tō-lĭth) [" + *lithos*, stone]

otological (ō"tō-lŏj'ĭ-kăl) [" + *logos*, word, reason]

otologist (ō-tŏl'ō-jĭst)

otology (ō-tŏl'ō-jē) [Gr. *otos*, ear, + *logos*, word, reason]

otomassage [" + *massein*, to knead]

otomucormycosis (ō"tō-mū"kor-mī-kō'sĭs) [" + L. *mucor*, mold, + Gr. *mykes*, fungus, + *osis*, condition]

otomyasthenia (ō"tō-mī"ăs-thē'nē-ă) [" + *mys*, muscle, + *asthe-*

neia, weakness]

otomyces (ō″tō-mī′sēz) [″ +
mykes, fungus]

otomycosis (ō″tō-mī-kō′sĭs) [″ + ″
+ osis, condition]

otoncus (ō-tŏng′kŭs) [″ + onkos,
bulk, mass]

otonecrectomy, otonecronectomy
(ō″tō-nē-krĕk′tō-mē,   ō″tō-nē″krŏ-
nĕk′tō-mē) [″ + nekros, dead
body, + ektome, excision]

otoneuralgia (ō″tō-nū-răl′jē-ă) [″ +
neuron, sinew, + algos, pain]

otoneurasthenia   (ō″tō-nū″răs-
thē′nē-ă) [″ + ″ + astheneia,
weakness]

otoneurology (ō″tō-nū-rŏl′ō-jē) [″ +
″ + logos, word, reason]

otopathy   (ō-tŏp′ă-thē)   [″ +
pathos, disease, suffering]

otopharyngeal   (ō″tō-făr-ĭn′jē-ăl)
[″ + pharynx, throat]

otopharyngeal tube

otoplasty (ō′tō-plăs″tē) [″ + plassein, to form]

otopolypus   (ō″tō-pŏl′ĭ-pŭs)[″ +
poly, many, + pous, foot]

otopyorrhea (ō″tō-pī″ō-rē′ă) [″ +
pyon, pus, + rhein, to flow]

otopyosis (ō″tō-pī-ō′sĭs) [″ + ″
+ osis, condition]

otorhinolaryngology   (ō″tō-rī″nō-
lăr″ĭn-gŏl′ō-jē) [″ + rhis, nose,
+ larynx, larynx, + logos, word,
reason]

otorhinology (ō″tō-rī-nŏl′ō-jē) [″ +
″ + logos, word, reason]

otorrhagia (ō-tō-rā′jē-ă) [Gr. otos, ear,
+ rhegnynai, to burst forth]

otorrhea (ō″tō-rē′ă) [″ + rhein,
flow]

otosalpinx (ō″tō-săl′pĭnks) [″ +
salpinx, tube]

otoscleronectomy   (ō″tō-sklē″rō-
nĕk′tō-mē) [″ + skleros, hard, +
ektome, excision]

otosclerosis (ō″tō-sklē-rō′sĭs) [″ +
sklerosis, a hardening]

otoscope (ō′tō-skōp) [″ + skopein,
to examine]

otoscopy (ō-tŏs′kō-pē)

otosis (ō-tō′sĭs) [″ + osis, condition]

otosteal (ō-tŏs′tē-ăl) [″ + osteon,
bone]

ototomy (ō-tŏt′ō-mē) [″ + tome, a
cutting, slice]

ototoxic (ō″tō-tŏk′sĭk) [″ + toxikon, poison]

ototoxicity (ō″tō-tŏks-ĭs′ĭ-tē)

O.T.R. occupational therapist, registered

Otrivin Hydrochloride

Otto pelvis (ŏt′ō) [Adolph W. Otto,
Ger. surgeon, 1786–1845]

O.U., o.u. [L.] oculus uterque, for each
eye

ouabain (wă-bā′ĭn)

oulitis (oo-lī′tĭs) [Gr. oulon, gum, +
itis, inflammation]

oulorrhagia (oo-lō-rā′jē-ă) [″ +
rhegnynai, to burst forth]

ounce (owns) [L. uncia, a twelfth]
o., fluid

outcome

outflow
o., craniosacral
o., thoracolumbar

outlet
o., pelvic

outpatient

outpocketing

output (owt′poot)
o., cardiac
o., energy
o., stroke
o., urinary

outrigger

ova (ō′vă) [L. ovum, egg]

oval (ō′văl) [L. ovalis, egg shaped]

ovalbumin (ō″văl-bū′mĭn) [″ + albumen, white of egg]

ovalocyte (ō′văl-ō-sīt″) [″ + Gr.
kytos, cell]

ovalocytosis (ō-văl″ō-sī-tō′sĭs) [″ +
″ + osis, condition]

oval window

ovaralgia, ovarialgia (ŏ″văr-ăl′jē-ă, -ē-ăl′jē-ă) [NL. *ovarium*, ovary, + Gr. *algos*, pain]

ovarian (ō-vā′rē-ăn) [NL. *ovarium*, ovary]

ovarian cyst

ovariectomy (ō″vā-rē-ĕk′tō-mē) [″ + Gr. *ektome*, excision]

ovario- [NL. *ovarium*, ovary]

ovariocele (ō-vā′rē-ō-sēl) [″ + Gr. *kele*, tumor, swelling]

ovariocentesis (ō-vā″rē-ō-sĕn-tē′sĭs) [″ + Gr. *kentesis*, puncture]

ovariocyesis (ō-vā″rē-ō-sī-ē′sĭs) [″ + Gr. *kyesis*, pregnancy]

ovariodysneuria (ō-vā″rē-ō-dĭs-nū′rē-ă) [″ + Gr. *dys*, bad, difficult, painful, disordered, + *neuron*, sinew]

ovariogenic (ō-vā″rē-ō-jĕn′ĭk) [″ + gennan, to produce]

ovariohysterectomy (ō-vā″rē-ō-hĭs″tĕr-ĕk′tō-mē) [″ + Gr. *hystera*, womb, + *ektome*, excision]

ovariopathy (ō-vā″rē-ŏp′ă-thē) [″ + pathos, disease, suffering]

ovariopexy (ō-vā″rē-ō-pĕk′sē) [″ + pexis, fixation]

ovariorrhexis (ō-vā″rē-ō-rĕk′sĭs) [″ + Gr. *rhexis*, a rupture]

ovariosalpingectomy (ō-vā″rē-ō-săl″pĭn-jĕk′tō-mē) [″ + Gr. *salpinx*, tube, + *ektome*, excision]

ovariosteresis (ō-vā″rē-ō-stĕr-ē′sĭs) [″ + Gr. *steresis*, loss]

ovariostomy (ō-vā″rē-ŏs′tō-mē) [″ + Gr. *stoma*, mouth, opening]

ovariotexy

ovariotomy (ō-vā″rē-ŏt′ō-mē) [NL. *ovarium*, ovary, + Gr. *tome*, a cutting, slice]

ovariotubal (ō-vā″rē-ō-tū′băl) [″ + *tuba*, a narrow duct]

ovariprival (ō-vā″rĭ-prī′văl) [″ + privare, to remove]

ovaritis (ō″vă-rī′tĭs) [″ + Gr. *itis*, inflammation]

ovarium (ō-vā′rē-ŭm) [LL.]

ovary (ō′vă-rē) [NL. *ovarium*, ovary]

overbite

Ovcon

overclosure

overcompensation

overcorrection

overdenture

overdetermination

overdose

overeruption

overexertion

overextension

overflow

overgrowth

overhang

overhydration

overjet

overlap

overlay
   o., psychogenic

overproduction

overresponse

overriding

overtoe

overtone

overvalued idea

overventilation

ovi- [L. *ovum*, egg]

ovi albumin (ō″vē-ăl-bū′mĭn) [L.]

ovicide (ō′vĭ-sīd) [L. *ovum*, egg, + caedere, to kill]

oviduct (ō′vĭ-dŭkt) [″ + ductus, a path]

oviferous (ō-vĭf′ĕr-ŭs) [″ + ferre, to bear]

oviform (ō′vĭ-form) [″ + forma, shape]

ovigenesis [″ + Gr. *genesis*, generation, birth]

ovigerm (ō′vĭ-jĕrm) [″ + germen, a bud]

ovination (ō″vĭ-nā′shŭn) [L. *ovinus*, of a sheep]

ovine (ō′vīn) [L. *ovinus*, of a sheep]

ovinia (ō-vĭn′ē-ă) [L. *ovinus*, of a sheep]

oviparity (ō″vĭ-păr′ĭ-tē)

oviparous (ō-vĭp′ăr-ŭs) [L. *ovum*, egg, + parere, to beget, produce]

oviposition [" + *ponere*, to place]
ovipositor (ō″vĭ-pŏs′ĭ-tor)
ovisac (ō′vĭ-săk)
ovo- [L. *ovum*, egg]
ovocenter
ovocyte (ō′vō-sīt) [" + *kytos*, cell]
ovoflavin (ō″vō-flā′vĭn) [" + *flavus*, yellow]
ovogenesis (ō″vō-jĕn′ĕ-sĭs) [" + Gr. *genesis*, generation, birth]
ovoglobulin (ō″vō-glŏb′ū-lĭn) [" + *globulus*, globule]
ovogonium (ō″vō-gō′nē-ŭm)
ovoid (ō′voyd) [L. *ovum*, egg, + Gr. *eidos*, form, shape]
ovomucin (ō″vō-mū′sĭn)
ovomucoid (ō″vō-mū′koyd) [" + *mucus*, mucus, + Gr. *eidos*, form, shape]
ovoplasm (ō′vō-plăzm) [" + LL. *plasma*, form, mold]
ovotestis (ō″vō-tĕs′tĭs)
ovovitellin (ō″vō-vī-tĕl′ĭn) [" + *vitellus*, yolk]
ovoviviparous (ō″vō-vī-vĭp′ă-rŭs) [" + *vivus*, alive, + *parere*, to beget, produce]
Ovral
Ovrette
ovula (ŏv′ū-lă) [L.]
ovular (ō′vū-lăr) [L. *ovulum*, little egg]
ovulation (ŏv″ū-lā′shŭn) [L. *ovulum*, little egg]
ovulatory (ŏv′ū-lă-tō″rē)
ovule (ō′vūl) [L. *ovulum*]
Ovulen
ovulogenous (ō-vū-lŏj′ĕn-ŭs)
ovulum (ŏv′ū-lŭm) [L. *ovulum*, little egg]
ovum (ō′vŭm) [L., egg]
   o., alecithal
   o., centrolecithal
   o., holoblastic
   o., human
   o., isolecithal
   o., meroblastic
   o., permanent
   o., primordial
   o., telolecithal

Owren's disease
oxacillin (ŏks″ă-sĭl′ĭn)
   o. sodium
oxalacetic acid (ŏks″ăl-ă-sē′tĭk)
oxalate (ŏk′să-lāt) [Gr. *oxalis*, sorrel]
   o., potassium
oxalemia (ŏk″să-lē′mē-ă) [" + *haima*, blood]
oxalic acid (ŏks-ăl′ĭk)
oxalic acid poisoning
oxalism (ŏks′ăl-ĭzm) [Gr. *oxalis*, sorrel, + -*ismos*, condition]
oxalosis
oxaluria (ŏk-să-lū′rē-ă) [" + *ouron*, urine]
oxalylurea (ŏk″săl-ĭl-ū-rē′ă)
oxandrolone (ŏk-săn′drō-lōn)
oxazepam (ŏk-săz′ĕ-păm)
oxidant (ŏk′sī-dănt)
oxidase (ŏk′sī-dās) [Gr. *oxys*, sharp]
   o., cytochrome
oxidation (ŏk′sī-dā′shŭn) [Gr. *oxys*, sharp]
oxidation-reduction reaction
oxide (ŏk′sīd)
oxidize (ŏk′sī-dīz)
oxidoreductase (ŏk″sī-dō-rē-dŭk′tās)
oxim, oxime (ŏk′sīm)
oximeter (ŏk-sīm′ĕ-ter) [Gr. *oxys*, sharp, + *metron*, measure]
   o., ear
oxonemia (ŏk″sō-nē′mē-ă) [L. *oxone*, acetone, + Gr. *haima*, blood]
oxophenarsine hydrochloride
oxprenolol hydrochloride (ŏks-prĕn′ō-lōl)
oxtriphylline (ŏks-trĭf′ĭ-lēn)
oxy- [Gr. *oxys*]
oxyacoia (ŏk″sē-ă-koy′ă)
oxyacusis (ŏk″sē-ă-kū′sĭs) [Gr. *oxys*, sharp, + *akousis*, hearing]
oxybenzene (ŏk″sē-bĕn′zēn)
oxybenzone (ŏk″sē-bĕn′zōn)
oxyblepsia (ŏk″sē-blĕp′sē-ă) [Gr. *oxys*, sharp, + *blepsis*, vision]
oxybutyria (ŏk″sē-bū-tĭr′ē-ă)
oxycalcium (ŏk″sē-kăl′sē-ŭm)
Oxycel

oxycephalous (ŏk-sē-sĕf'ă-lŭs) [Gr. *oxys*, sharp, + *kephale*, head]

oxycephaly (ŏk"sē-sĕf-ă'lē-ă, -sĕf'ă-lē)

oxychloride (ŏk"sē-klō'rīd) [Gr. *oxys*, sharp, + *chloros*, green]

oxychromatic (ŏk"sē-krō-măt'ĭk) [" + *chroma*, color]

oxychromatin (ŏk"sē-krō'mă-tĭn)

oxycinesia (ŏk"sē-sĭ-nē'zē-ă) [" + *kinesis*, motion]

oxyecoia (ŏk"sē-ē-koy'ă) [" + *akoe*, hearing]

oxyesthesia (ŏk"sē-ĕs-thē'zē-ă) [" + *aisthesis*, feeling, perception]

oxygen (ŏk'sĭ-jĕn) [Gr. *oxys*, sharp, + *gennan*, to produce]

oxygen, transtracheal

oxygenase (ŏk'sĭ-jĕn-ās") [Gr. *oxys*, sharp, + *gennan*, to produce, + *-ase*, enzyme]

oxygenate (ŏk'sĭ-jĕn-āt)

oxygenation (ŏk'sĭ-jĕn-ā'shŭn)

  o., hyperbaric

oxygenator (ŏk'sĭ-jĕ-nā'tor)

  o., bubble

  o., rotating disk

  o., screen

oxygen capacity

oxygen content

oxygen debt or deficit

oxygen dissociation curve

oxygenic (ŏk"sĭ-jĕn'ĭk) [" + *gennan*, to produce]

oxygenize

oxygen radicals

oxygen saturation

oxygen tent

oxygen therapy

oxygen toxicity

oxygeusia (ŏk"sē-gū'sē-ă) [Gr. *oxys*, sharp, + *geusis*, taste]

oxyhematin (ŏk"sē-hĕm'ă-tĭn)

oxyhematoporphyrin (ŏk"sē-hĕm"ă-tō-por'fĭ-rĭn)

oxyhemoglobin (ŏk"sē-hē"mō-glō'bĭn) [" + *haima*, blood, + L. *globus*, a sphere]

oxyhemoglobinometer (ŏk"sē-hē"mō-glō"bĭn-ŏm'ĕt-ĕr) [" + " + " + Gr. *metron*, measure]

oxyhydrocephalus (ŏk"sē-hī-drō-sĕf'ăl-ŭs) [" + *hydor*, water, + *kephale*, brain]

oxyiodide (ŏk"sē-ī'ō-dīd) [" + *ioeides*, violet colored]

oxylalia (ŏk"sē-lā'lē-ă) [" + *lalian*, chatter, prattle]

Oxylone

oxymetazoline hydrochloride (ŏk"sē-mĕt-ăz'ō-lēn)

oxymetholone (ŏk"sē-mĕth'ō-lōn)

oxymorphone hydrochloride (ŏk"sē-mor'fōn)

oxymyoglobin (ŏk"sē-mī"ō-glō'bĭn)

oxyntic (ŏk-sĭn'tĭk) [Gr. *oxynein*, to make acid]

oxyopia (ŏk"sē-ō'pē-ă) [Gr. *oxys*, sharp, + *ops*, sight]

oxyopter (ŏk"sē-ŏp'tĕr)

oxyosmia (ŏk"sē-ŏz'mē-ă) [" + *osme*, odor]

oxyosphresia (ŏk"sē-ŏs-frē'zē-ă) [" + *osphresis*, smell]

oxypathia, oxypathy (ŏk"sē-păth'ē-ă, -sĭp'ăth-ē) [" + *pathos*, disease, suffering]

oxyperitoneum (ŏk"sĭ-pĕr-ĭ-tō-nē'ŭm) [" + *peritonaion*, stretched around or over]

oxyphenbutazone (ŏk"sē-fĕn-bū'tă-zōn)

oxyphencyclimine hydrochloride (ŏk"sē-fĕn-sī'klĭ-mēn)

oxyphil(e) (ŏk'sē-fĭl, -fīl) [" + *philein*, to love]

oxyphilous (ŏk-sĭf'ĭl-ŭs)

oxyphonia (ŏk"sē-fō'nē-ă)

oxypurine (ŏk"sē-pū'rēn) [" + L. *purus*, pure, + *urina*, urine]

oxyrhine (ŏk'sē-rīn) [" + *rhis*, nose]

oxytalan (ŏks-ĭt'ă-lăn)

oxytetracycline (ŏks"ē-tĕt"ră-sī'klēn)

oxytocia (ŏk"sē-tō'sē-ă) [" + *tokos*, childbirth]

oxytocic (ŏk″sē-tō′sĭk)
oxytocic principle
oxytocin [injection] (ŏk″sē-tō′sĭn)
oxytocin challenge test
oxyuriasis (ŏk″sē-ū-rī′ăs-ĭs) [Gr. *oxys,* sharp, + *oura,* tall, + *-iasis,* state or condition of]
oxyuricide (ŏk″sē-ū′rĭ-sīd) [″ + ″ + L. *caedere,* to kill]
oxyurid (ŏk″sē-ūr′ĭd)
Oxyuris [″ + *oura,* tail]
   O. vermicularis
Oxyuroidea (ŏk″sē-ū″roy-dē′ă)
oyster [AS. *oistre*]
oz. *ounce*

oz. ap. *ounce apothecary's*
oz. av. *ounce avoirdupois*
ozena (ō-zē′nă) [Gr. *oze,* stench]
ozochrotia (ō″zō-krō′shē-ă) [″ + *chros,* skin]
ozonator (ō′zō-nā″tor)
ozone (ō′zōn) [Gr. *ozein,* to smell]
ozonization (ō″zō-nī-zā′shŭn)
ozonize (ō′zō-nīz) [Gr. *ozein,* to smell]
ozonometer (ō″zō-nŏm′ĕt-ĕr) [Gr. *oze,* stench, + *metron,* measure]
ozonoscope (ō-zō′nō-skōp) [″ + *skopein,* to examine]
ozostomia (ō″zō-stō′mē-ă) [″ + *stoma,* mouth, opening]

P

P *phosphorus; position; posterior; postpartum; pressure; pulse; pupil*

p *page; probability; pupil*

p̄- *para-*

p̄ *after- or post-*

P₁ *first parental generation; first pulmonic heart sound*

P₂ *pulmonic second sound*

³²P *radioactive isotope of phosphorus*

PA *pulmonary artery*

P.A. *physician's assistant*

Pa *protactinium*

P-A, p-a *posteroanterior*

P & A *percussion and auscultation*

PABA

Pabanol

Pablum (păb'lŭm)

pabular (păb'ū-lăr) [L. *pabulum*, food]

pabulum (păb'ū-lŭm) [L.]

PAC *premature atrial contraction*

PA catheter

pacchionian bodies (păk″ē-ō'nē-ăn) [Antonio Pacchioni, It. anatomist, 1665–1726]

pacchionian depressions

pacemaker (pās'māk-ĕr) [L. *passus*, a step, + AS. *macian*, to make]
  p., cardiac, artificial
  p., demand
  p., ectopic
  p., external
  p., fixed rate
  p., mediastinal
  p., permanent
  p., programmable
  p., temporary
  p., transthoracic
  p., transvenous
  p., wandering

pacer

pachismus (păk-ĭz'mŭs) [Gr. *pachys*,

thick, + *-ismos*, condition]

pachy-, pach- [Gr. *pachys*, thick]

pachyacria, pachyakria (păk″ē-ā'krē-ă) [Gr. *pachys*, thick, + *akron*, end]

pachyblepharon (păk″ē-blĕf'ă-rŏn) [″ + *blepharon*, eyelid]

pachyblepharosis (păk″ē-blĕf″ă-rō'sĭs)

pachycephalic (păk″ē-sĕ-făl'ĭk) [″ + *kephale*, brain]

pachycephalous (păk″ē-sĕf'ă-lŭs)

pachycephaly (păk″ē-sĕf'ă-lē)

pachycheilia (păk″ē-kī'lē-ă) [″ + *cheilos*, lip]

pachycholia (păk″ē-kō'lē-ă) [″ + *chole*, bile]

pachychromatic (păk″ē-krō-măt'ĭk) [″ + *chroma*, color]

pachycolpismus (păk″ē-kŏl-pīz'mŭs) [″ + *kolpos*, vagina, + *-ismos*, condition]

pachydactylia, pachydactyly (păk″ē-dăk-tĭl'ē-ă, -dăk'tĭ-lē) [″ + *daktylos*, finger]

pachyderma (păk-ē-dĕr'mă) [″ + *derma*, skin]
  p. circumscripta
  p. laryngis
  p. lymphangiectatica
  p., occipital
  p. vesicae

pachydermatocele (păk″ē-dĕr-măt'ō-sēl) [″ + ″ + *kele*, tumor, swelling]

pachydermatosis (păk″ē-dĕr″mă-tō'sĭs) [″ + ″ + *osis*, condition]

pachydermatous (păk-ē-dĕr'mă-tŭs) [″ + *derma*, skin]

pachydermoperiostosis (păk″ē-dĕr″mō-pĕr″ē-ŏs-tō'sĭs)

pachyemia (păk-ē-ē'mē-ă) [Gr. *pachys*, thick, + *haima*, blood]

pachyglossia (păk"ē-glŏs'sē-ă) [" + *glossa*, tongue]

pachygnathous (pă-kĭg'năth-ŭs) [" + *gnathos*, jaw]

pachygyria (păk-ē-jī'rē-ă) [" + *gyros*, a circle]

pachyhematous (păk-ē-hĕm'ă-tŭs) [" + *haima*, blood]

pachyleptomeningitis (păk-ē-lĕp"tō-mĕn"ĭn-jī'tĭs) [" + *leptos*, thin, + *meninx*, membrane, + *itis*, inflammation]

pachylosis (păk-ē-lō'sĭs) [" + *osis*, condition]

pachymenia (păk-ē-mē'nē-ă) [" + *hymen*, membrane]

pachymeningitis (păk-ē-mĕn"ĭn-jī'tĭs) [" + *meninx*, membrane, + *itis*, inflammation]
    p., external
    p., hemorrhagic
    p., internal
    p., spinal

pachymeningopathy (păk"ē-mĕn"ĭn-gŏp'ă-thē) [" + " + *pathos*, disease, suffering]

pachymeninx (păk-ē-mē'nĭnks) [" + *meninx*, membrane]

pachynema (păk-ē-nē'mă) [" + *nema*, thread]

pachynsis (pă-kĭn'sĭs) [Gr.]

pachyonychia (păk"ē-ō-nĭk'ē-ă) [Gr. *pachys*, thick, + *onyx*, nail]
    p. congenita

pachyostosis (păk"ē-ŏs-tō'sĭs) [" + *osteon*, bone, + *osis*, condition]

pachyotia (păk-ē-ō'shē-ă) [" + *ous*, ear]

pachypelviperitonitis (păk"ē-pĕl"vĭ-pĕr"ĭ-tō-nī'tĭs) [" + L. *pelvis*, basin, + Gr. *peritonaion*, stretched around or over, + *itis*, inflammation]

pachyperiostitis (păk"ē-pĕr"ē-ŏs-tī'tĭs) [" + *periosteon*, periosteum, + *itis*, inflammation]

pachyperitonitis (păk"ē-pĕr"ĭ-tō-nī'tĭs) [" + " + *itis*, inflammation]

pachypleuritis (păk-ē-plū-rī'tĭs) [" + *pleura*, side, + *itis*, inflammation]

pachypodous (pă-kĭp'ō-dŭs) [" + *pous*, foot]

pachyrhinic (păk"ē-rī'nĭk) [" + *rhis*, nose]

pachysalpingitis (păk"ē-săl"pĭn-jī'tĭs) [" + *salpinx*, tube, + *itis*, inflammation]

pachysalpingoovaritis (păk"ē-săl-pĭng"gō-ō"văr-ī'tĭs) [" + " + NL. *ovarium*, ovary, + Gr. *itis*, inflammation]

pachysomia (păk-ē-sō'mē-ă) [Gr. *pachys*, thick, + *soma*, body]

pachytene (păk'ē-tēn) [" + *tainia*, band]

pachytrichous

pachyvaginalitis (păk"ē-văj"ĭn-ă-lī'tĭs) [" + L. *vagina*, sheath, + Gr. *itis*, inflammation]

pachyvaginitis (păk"ē-văj"ĭn-ī'tĭs)

pacifier

pacing (pās'ĭng) [L. *passus*, a step]

pacing code

pacing wire

pacinian corpuscles (pă-sĭn'ē-ăn) [Filippo Pacini, It. anatomist, 1812–1883]

pack (păk) [AS. *pak*]
    p., cold
    p., dry
    p., full
    p., half
    p., hot
    p., ice
    p., one-sheet
    p., partial
    p., periodontal
    p., three-quarter
    p., umbrella
    p., wet-dry
    p., wet-sheet

package insert

packed cells

packer (păk'ĕr)

packing (păk'ĭng)
PaCO₂
pad (păd)
   p., abdominal
   p., dinner
   p., fat
   p., kidney
   p.'s, knuckle
   p., Malgaigne's
   p., Mikulicz's
   p., perineal
   p., sucking
   p., surgical
Paget, Sir James (păj'ĕt) [Brit. surgeon, 1814–1899]
   P.'s disease
   P.'s disease, extramammary
   P.'s disease, mammary
pagetoid (paj'ĕ-toyd) [Paget + Gr. eidos, form, shape]
page turner
Pagitane Hydrochloride
pagophagia [Gr. pagos, frost, + phagein, to eat]
-pagus [Gr. pagos, thing fixed]
PAH PAHA, para-aminohippuric acid
pain (pān) [L. poena, a fine, a penalty]
   p., abdominal
   p., aching
   p., acute
   p.'s, after-
   p., agonizing
   p., angina pectoris
   p., appendicitis
   p.'s, bearing-down
   p., boring
   p., Brodie's
   p., burning
   p., cardiac
   p., causalgic
   p., central
   p., cephalgic
   p., chest
   p., chronic
   p., chronic intractable
   p., cramplike
   p., dental
   p.'s, dilating

p., dull
p., ear
p., eccentric
p., epigastric
p.'s, expulsive
p., false
p., fulgurant
p., gallbladder
p., gas
p., gastralgic
p., girdle
p.'s, growing
p., head
p., heterotopic
p., homotopic
p., hunger
p., hypogastric
p., imperative
p., inflammatory
p., intermenstrual
p., intractable
p.'s, labor
p., lancinating
p., lightning
p., lingual
p., lung
p., menstrual
p., mental
p., middle
p., migraine
p., mind
p., mobile
p., movement
p., neuralgic
p., night
p., noise
p., objective
p., organic
p., osteocopic
p., parenchymatous
p., paresthesic
p., phantom limb
p., postprandial
p., precordial
p., premonitory
p., pseudomyelic
p., psychic
p., psychogenic

p., psychosomatic
p., pulmonary
p., rectal, constant
p., referred
p., remittent
p., rest
p., root
p., shifting
p.'s, spot
p.'s, starting
p., subdiaphragmatic
p., subjective
p., sympathetic
p., tenesmic
p., terebrant
p., thermalgesic
p., thoracic
p., throbbing
p., tongue
p., tracheal
p., wandering
paint (pānt)
   p., Castellani's
painters' colic
pair
   p., base
PAL *posterior axillary line*
palatable (păl'ăt-ă-bl) [L. *palatum,* palate]
palatal (păl'ă-tăl)
palatal reflex
palate (păl'ăt) [L. *palatum,* palate]
   p., artificial
   p., bony
   p., cleft
   p., falling
   p., gothic
   p., hard
   p., pendulous
   p., primary
   p., secondary
   p., soft
palate bones
palatiform (pă-lăt'ĭ-form) [L. *palatum,* palate, + *forma,* form]
palatine (păl'ă-tīn) [L. *palatinus*]
palatine arches
palatine artery, greater

palatine bone
palatitis (păl-ăt-ī'tĭs) [L. *palatum,* palate, + Gr. *itis,* inflammation]
palatoglossal (păl″ă-tō-glŏs'ăl)
palatoglossus (păl″ă-tō-glŏs'ŭs) [″ + Gr. *glossa,* tongue]
palatognathous (păl″ă-tŏg'nă-thŭs) [″ + Gr. *gnathos,* jaw]
palatograph (păl'ă-tō-grăf)
palatography (păl″ă-tŏg'ră-fē) [″ + Gr. *graphein,* to write]
palatomaxillary (păl″ă-tō-măk'sĭ-lĕr″ē)
palatomyograph (păl″ă-tō-mī'ō-grăf) [″ + Gr. *mys,* muscle, + *graphein,* to write]
palatonasal (păl″ă-tō-nā'zăl)
palatopharyngeal (păl″ă-tō-fă-rĭn'jē-ăl)
palatopharyngeus (păl″ăt-ō-făr″ĭn-jē'ŭs) [″ + Gr. *pharynx,* throat]
palatopharyngoplasty
palatoplasty (păl'ăt-ō-plăs″tē) [″ + Gr. *plassein,* to form]
palatoplegia (păl″ă-tō-plē'jē-ă) [″ + Gr. *plege,* stroke]
palatorrhaphy (păl-ă-tor'ă-fē) [″ + Gr. *rhaphe,* seam]
palatosalpingeus (păl″ă-tō-săl-pĭn'jē-ŭs) [″ + Gr. *salpinx,* tube]
palatoschisis (păl-ă-tŏs'kĭ-sĭs) [″ + *schisis,* cleavage]
palatum (păl-ă'tŭm) [L.]
paleencephalon, paleoencephalon (pā″lē-ĕn-sĕf'ă-lŏn, -ō-ĕn-sĕf'ă-lŏn) [Gr. *palaios,* old, + *enkephalos,* brain]
paleo- [Gr. *palaios,* old, ancient]
paleocerebellum (păl″ē-ō-sĕr″ĕ-bĕl'ŭm) [Gr. *palaios,* old, + L. *cerebellum,* little brain]
paleogenesis (pā″lē-ō-jĕn'ĕ-sĭs) [″ + *genesis,* generation, birth]
paleogenetic (pā″lē-ō-jĕn-ĕt'ĭk) [″ + *gennan,* to produce]
paleokinetic (pā″lē-ō-kĭ-nĕt'ĭk) [″ + Gr. *kinetikos,* concerning movement]
paleontology (pā″lē-ŏn-tŏl'ō-jē)

[" + *onta*, existing things, + *logos*, word, reason]

paleopathology (pā″lē-ō-pă-thŏl′ō-jē) [" + *pathos*, disease, suffering, + *logos*, word, reason]

paleostriatal (pā″lē-ō-strī-ā′tăl) [" + L. *striatus*, ridged]

paleostriatum (pā″lē-ō-strī-ā′tŭm)

paleothalamus (pā″lē-ō-thăl′ă-mŭs) [" + *thalamos*, chamber]

pali-, palin- [Gr. *palin*, backward, again]

palikinesia (păl″ĭ-kĭn-ē′zē-ă) [" + *kinesis*, motion]

palilalia (păl-ĭ-lā′lē-ă) [" + *lalia*, chatter, prattle]

palinal (păl′ĭn-ăl) [Gr. *palin*, backward]

palindromia (păl-ĭn-drŏ′mē-ă) [" + *dromos*, a running]

palindromic (păl-ĭn-drŏm′ĭk)

palindromic rheumatism

palinesthesia (păl″ĭn-ĕs-thē′zē-ă) [Gr. *palin*, again, + *aisthesis*, feeling, perception]

palingenesis (păl″ĭn-jĕn′ĕ-sĭs) [" + *genesis*, generation, birth]

palingraphia (păl″ĭn-grăf′ē-ă) [" + *graphein*, to write]

palinopsia [" + *opsis*, sight, appearance, vision]

paliphrasia (păl-ĭ-frā′zē-ă) [" + *phrasis*, diction]

palladium (pă-lā′dē-ŭm) [L.]

pallanesthesia (păl″ăn-ĕs-thē′zē-ă) [Gr. *pallein*, to shake, + *anaisthesia*, anesthesia]

pallescence (păl-lĕs′ĕns) [L. *pallescere*, to grow pale]

pallesthesia (păl-ĕs-thē′zē-ă) [Gr. *pallein*, to shake, + *aisthesis*, feeling, perception]

palliate (păl′ē-āt) [L. *palliatus*, cloaked]

palliative (păl′ē-ā″tĭv)

pallid (păl′ĭd) [L. *pallidus*, pale]

pallidal (păl′ĭ-dăl)

pallidectomy (păl″ĭ-dĕk′tō-mē) [L. *pallidum*, pallidum, + Gr. *ektome*, excision]

pallidoansotomy (păl″ĭ-dō-ăn-sŏt′ō-mē) [" + *ansa*, a handle, + Gr. *tome*, a cutting, slice]

pallidotomy (păl″ĭ-dŏt′ō-mē) [" + Gr. *tome*, a cutting, slice]

pallidum (păl′ĭ-dŭm) [L.]

pallium (păl′ē-ŭm) [L., cloak]

pallor (păl′or) [L.]

palm [L. *palma*, hand]

palma (păl′mă) [L.]

palmar (păl′măr)

palmar cuff

palmar grasp reflex

palmaris (păl-mā′rĭs)

palmar reflex

palmature (păl′mă-tūr) [L. *palma*, hand]

palm-chin reflex

palmic (păl′mĭk) [Gr. *palmikos*]

palmitic acid (păl-mĭt′ĭk)

palmitin (păl′mĭ-tĭn)

palmomental reflex

palmoplantar (păl″mō-plăn′tăr)

palmus (păl′mŭs) [Gr. *palmos*, pulsation, quivering]

palpable (păl′pă-bl) [L. *palpabilis*, stroke, touch]

palpate (păl′pāt) [L. *palpare*, to touch]

palpation (păl-pā′shŭn) [L. *palpatio*]
  p., light-touch

palpatopercussion (păl″pă-tō-pĕr-kŭsh′ŭn)

palpebra (păl′pĕ-bră) [L.]
  p. inferior
  p. superior

palpebral (păl′pĕ-brăl)

palpebral cartilages

palpebral commissure

palpebral fissure

palpebral ligament

palpebral muscles

palpebrate (păl′pĕ-brāt) [L. *palpebrare; palpebra*, eyelid]

palpebritis (păl″pĕ-brī′tĭs) [L. *palpebra*, eyelid, + Gr. *itis*, inflammation]

palpitant (păl′pĭ-tănt) [L. *palpitare*, to quiver]

palpitate (păl′pĭ-tāt) [L. *palpitatus*, throbbing]

palpitation (păl-pĭ-tā′shŭn)
  p., arterial

palsy (pawl′zē) [ME. *palesie*, from L. *paralysis*]
  p., Bell's
  p., birth
  p., bulbar
  p., cerebral
  p., crutch
  p., diver's
  p., Erb's
  p., facial
  p., lead
  p., night
  p., progressive supranuclear
  p., Saturday night
  p., scrivener's
  p., shaking
  p., wasting

paludal (păl′ū-dăl) [L. *palus*, a marsh]

paludism (păl′ū-dĭzm) [″ + Gr. *-ismos*, condition]

palynology [Gr. *palumein*, to sprinkle, + *logos*, word, reason]

Pamelor

Pamine

pampiniform (păm-pĭn′ĭ-form) [L. *pampinus*, tendril, + *forma*, shape]

pampiniform plexus

pampinocele (păm-pĭn′ō-sēl) [″ + Gr. *kele*, tumor, swelling]

panacea (păn-ă-sē′ă) [Gr. *panakeia*, universal remedy]

panagglutinable (păn″ă-gloo′tĭ-nă-b′l) [Gr. *pan*, all, + L. *agglutinare*, to glue to]

panagglutinin (păn″ă-glū′tĭn-ĭn) [Gr. *pan*, all, + L. *agglutinare*, to glue to]

panangiitis (păn″ăn-jē-ī′tĭs) [″ + *angeion*, vessel, + *itis*, inflammation]

panaris (păn′ă-rĭs) [L. *panaricium*, disease of the fingernail]

panarteritis (păn″ăr-tĕ-rī′tĭs) [Gr. *par*, all, + *arteria*, artery, + *itis*, inflammation]

panarthritis (păn″ăr-thrī′tĭs) [″ + *arthron*, joint, + *itis*, inflammation]

panasthenia (păn″ăs-thē′nē-ă) [″ + *astheneia*, weakness]

panatrophy (păn-ăt′rō-fē) [″ + *a-*, not, + *trophe*, nourishment]

panblastic (păn-blăs′tĭk) [″ + *blastos*, germ]

pancarditis (păn-kăr-dī′tĭs) [″ + *kardia*, heart, + *itis*, inflammation]

panchreston (păn-krē′stŏn) [″ + *chrestos*, useful]

panchromia (păn-krō′mē-ă) [″ + *chroma*, color]

Pancoast syndrome [H. K. Pancoast, U.S. physician, 1875–1939]

pancolectomy (păn″kō-lĕk′tō-mē) [Gr. *pan*, all, + *kolon*, colon, + *ektome*, excision]

pancreas (păn′krē-ăs) [″ + *kreas*, flesh]
  p., accessory
  p., annular
  p. divisum
  p., dorsal
  p., lesser
  p., transplantation of
  p., ventral
  p., Willis'

pancreatalgia (păn″krē-ă-tăl′jē-ă) [″ + *kreas*, flesh, + *algos*, pain]

pancreatectomy (păn″krē-ăt-ĕk′tō-mē) [″ + ″ + *ektome*, excision]

pancreatemphraxis (păn″krē-ăt-ĕm-frăk′sĭs) [″ + ″ + *emphraxis*, stoppage]

pancreathelcosis (păn″krē-ăth″ĕl-kō′sĭs) [″ + ″ + *helkosis*, ulceration]

pancreatic (păn″krē-ăt′ĭk) [Gr. *pan*, all, + *kreas*, flesh]

pancreatic duct

pancreatic juice

pancreaticocholecystostomy (păn″ krē-ăt″ĭ-kō-kō″lē-sĭs-tŏs′tō-mē) [Gr. *pan*, all, + *kreas*, flesh, +

chole, bile,   +   *kystis*, bladder, + *stoma*, mouth, opening]

pancreaticoduodenal (păn″krē-ăt″ĭ-kō-dū-ō-dē′năl) [″   +   ″   +   L. *duodeni*, twelve]

pancreaticoduodenostomy (păn″krē-ăt″ĭ-kō-dū″ō-dē-nŏs′tō-mē) [″   +   ″   +   ″   +   Gr. *stoma*, mouth, opening]

pancreaticoenterostomy (păn″krē-ăt″ĭ-kō-ĕn″tĕr-ŏs′tō-mē) [″   +   ″   +   *enteron*, intestine,   +   *stoma*, mouth, opening]

pancreaticogastrostomy (păn″krē-ăt″ĭ-kō-găs-trŏs′tō-mē) [″   +   ″   +   *gaster*, belly,   +   *stoma*, mouth, opening]

pancreaticojejunostomy (păn″krē-ăt″ĭ-kō-jē″jū-nŏs′tō-mē) [″   +   ″   +   L. *jejunum*, empty,   +   Gr. *stoma*, mouth, opening]

pancreatin (păn′krē-ă-tĭn) [Gr. *pan*, all,   +   *kreas*, flesh]

pancreatitis (păn″krē-ă-tī′tĭs) [″   +   ″   +   *itis*, inflammation]

    p., acute
    p., acute hemorrhagic
    p., calcareous
    p., centrilobar
    p., chronic
    p., interstitial
    p., perilobar
    p., purulent
    p., suppurative

pancreatoduodenectomy (păn″krē-ă-tō-dū″ō-dē-nĕk′tō-mē) [Gr. *pan*, all,   +   *kreas*, flesh,   +   L. *duodeni*, twelve,   +   Gr. *ektome*, excision]

pancreatoduodenostomy (păn″krē-ă-tō-dū″ō-dē-nŏs′tō-mē) [″   +   ″   +   ″   +   *stoma*, mouth, opening]

pancreatogenic, pancreatogenous (păn″krē-ă-tō-jĕn′ĭk, -tŏj′ĕ-nŭs) [″   +   ″   +   *gennan*, to produce]

pancreatography (păn″krē-ă-tŏg′ră-fē) [″   +   ″   +   *graphein*, to write]

pancreatolith (păn″krē-ăt′ō-lĭth) [″   +   ″   +   *lithos*, stone]

pancreatolithectomy (păn″krē-ăt-ō-lĭth-ĕk′tō-mē) [″   +   ″   +   ″   +   *ektome*, excision]

pancreatolithiasis (păn″krē-ă-tō-lĭ-thī′ă-sĭs) [″   +   ″   +   ″   +   *-iasis*, state or condition of]

pancreatolithotomy (păn″krē-ăt-ō-lĭth-ŏt′ō-mē) [″   +   ″   +   ″   +   *tome*, a cutting, slice]

pancreatolysis (păn″krē-ă-tŏl′ĭ-sĭs) [″   +   ″   +   *lysis*, dissolution]

pancreatolytic (păn″krē-ăt-ō-lĭt′ĭk)

pancreatomy (păn-krē-ăt′ō-mē) [″   +   ″   +   *tome*, a cutting, slice]

pancreatoncus (păn-krē-ăt-ŏng′kŭs) [″   +   ″   +   *onkos*, bulk, mass]

pancreatopathy (păn″krē-ă-tŏp′ă-thē) [″   +   ″   +   *pathos*, disease, suffering]

pancreatotomy (păn″krē-ă-tŏt′ō-mē) [″   +   ″   +   *tome*, a cutting, slice]

pancreatotropic (păn-krē″ă-tō-trŏp′ĭk) [″   +   ″   +   *tropikos*, turning]

pancreectomy (păn″krē-ĕk′tō-mē) [″   +   ″   +   *ektome*, excision]

pancrelipase (păn″krē-lī′pās)

pancreolithotomy (păn″krē-ō-lĭth-ŏt′ō-mē) [″   +   *kreas*, flesh,   +   *lithos*, stone,   +   *tome*, a cutting, slice]

pancreolysis (păn″krē-ŏl′ĭ-sĭs) [″   +   ″   +   *lysis*, dissolution]

pancreolytic (păn″krē-ō-lĭt′ĭk) [″   +   ″   +   *lysis*, dissolution]

pancreopathy (păn″krē-ŏp′ă-thē) [″   +   ″   +   *pathos*, disease, suffering]

pancreoprivic (păn″krē-ō-prīv′ĭk)

pancreozymin-cholecystokinin

pancuronium bromide (păn″kū-rō′nē-ŭm)

pancytopenia (păn″sī-tō-pē′nē-ă) [″   +   *kytos*, cell,   +   *penia*, lack]

pandemia (păn-dē′mē-ă) [″   +   *demos*, the people]

pandemic (păn-dĕm′ĭk)

pandiculation (păn″dĭk-ū-lā′shŭn) [L. *pandiculari*, to stretch one's self]

panel

panencephalitis (păn″ĕn-sĕf″ă-lī′tĭs) [Gr. *pan*, all, + *enkephalos*, brain, + *itis*, inflammation]

panendoscope (păn-ĕn′dō-skōp) [″ + *endon*, within, + *skopein*, to view]

panesthesia (păn″ĕs-thē′zē-ă) [″ + *aisthesis*, feeling, perception]

Paneth, cells of (pă′nāt) [Josef Paneth, Ger. physician, 1857–1890]

pang

pangamic acid

pangenesis (păn″jĕn′ĕ-sĭs) [″ + *genesis*, generation, birth]

panglossia (păn-glŏs′sē-ă) [Gr.]

panhidrosis (păn″hĭd-rō′sĭs) [Gr. *pan*, all, + *hidros*, sweat]

panhyperemia (păn″hī-pĕr-ē′mē-ă) [″ + *hyper*, over, above, excessive, + *haima*, blood]

panhypopituitarism (păn-hī″pō-pī-tū′ĭ-tăr-ĭzm) [″ + *hypo*, under, beneath, below, + L. *pituita*, mucus, + Gr. *-ismos*, condition]

panhysterectomy (păn″hĭs-tĕr-ĕk′tō-mē) [″ + *hystera*, womb, + *ektome*, excision]

panhysterocolpectomy (păn-hĭs″tĕr-ō-kŏl-pĕk′tō-mē) [″ + ″ + *kolpos*, vagina, + *ektome*, excision]

panhystero-oophorectomy (păn-hĭs″tĕr-ō-ō″ŏf-ō-rĕk′tō-mē) [″ + ″ + NL. *oophoron*, ovary, + Gr. *ektome*, excision]

panhysterosalpingectomy (păn-hĭs″tĕr-ō-săl″pĭn-jĕk′tō-mē) [″ + ″ + *salpinx*, tube, + *ektome*, excision]

panhysterosalpingo-oophorectomy (păn-hĭs″tĕr-ō-săl″pĭng-gō-ō″ŏf-ō-rĕk′tō-mē) [″ + ″ + ″ + NL. *oophoron*, ovary, + Gr. *ektome*, excision]

panic (păn′ĭk)
   p., homosexual

panic attack

panic disorder

panimmunity (păn″ĭ-mū′nĭ-tē) [″ + L. *immunitas*, immunity]

panis (păn′ĭs) [L.]

Panmycin

panmyeloid (păn-mī′ĕ-loyd) [″ + *myelos*, marrow, + *eidos*, form, shape]

panmyelophthisis (păn″mī-ĕl-ŏf′thĭ-sĭs) [″ + *myelos*, marrow, + *phthisis*, a wasting]

panmyelosis (păn″mī-ĕl-ō′sĭs) [″ + ″ + *osis*, condition]

panneuritis (păn″ū-rī′tĭs) [″ + *neuron*, sinew, + *itis*, inflammation]
   p. epidemica

panniculitis (păn-ĭk″ū-lī′tĭs) [L. *panniculus*, a small piece of cloth, + *itis*, inflammation]
   p., nodular nonsuppurative
   p., relapsing febrile nodular nonsuppurative

panniculus (păn-ĭk′ū-lŭs) [L., a small piece of cloth]
   p. adiposus
   p. carnosus

pannus (păn′ŭs) [L., cloth]
   p. carateus
   p. carnosus
   p. crassus
   p. degenerativus
   p., phlyctenular
   p. siccus
   p. tenuis

panodic (pă-nŏd′ĭk)

panography (păn-nŏg′ră-fē)

panophobia (păn-ō-fō′bē-ă) [Gr. *pan*, all, + *phobos*, fear]

panophthalmia, panophthalmitis (păn-ŏf-thăl′mē-ă, -thăl-mī′tĭs) [″ + *ophthalmos*, eye, + *itis*, inflammation]

panoptic (păn-ŏp′tĭk) [″ + *optikos*, vision]

panoptic stain

panoptosis (păn-ŏp-tō′sĭs) [″ + *ptosis*, fall, falling]

pan-oral radiography

panosteitis (păn″ŏs-tē-ī′tĭs) [Gr. *pan*, all, + *osteon*, bone, + *itis*, inflammation]

panotitis (păn-ō-tī′tĭs) [″ + *ous*, ear, + *itis*, inflammation]

Panoxyl

panphobia (păn-fō′bē-ă) [″ + *phobos*, fear]

panplegia (păn-plē′jē-ă) [″ + *plege*, stroke]

pansclerosis (păn″sklē-rō′sĭs) [″ + *sklerosis*, a hardening]

pansinusitis (păn″sī-nŭs-ī′tĭs) [″ + *sinus*, cavity, + *itis*, inflammation]

pansphygmograph (păn-sfĭg′mō-grăf) [″ + *sphygmos*, pulse, + *graphein*, to write]

Panstrongylus (păn-strŏn′jĭ-lŭs)
P. megistus

pansystolic

pant [ME. *panten*]

pant-, panto- [Gr. *pantos*, all]

pantachromatic (păn″tă-krō-măt′ĭk) [″ + *achromatos*, colorless]

pantalgia (păn-tăl′jē-ă) [″ + *algos*, pain]

pantamorphia (păn″tă-mor′fē-ă) [″ + *a-*, not, + *morphe*, form]

pantanencephaly (păn″tăn-ĕn-sĕf′ă-lē) [″ + *an-*, not, + *enkephalos*, brain]

pantankyloblepharon (păn-tăng″kĭ-lō-blĕf′ă-rŏn) [″ + *ankyle*, noose, + *blepharon*, lid]

pantatrophia, pantatrophy (păn-tă-trō′fē-ă, -tăt′rō-fē) [″ + *atrophia*, atrophy]

Panteric

pantetheine (păn-tĕ-thē′ĭn)

panthodic (păn-thŏd′ĭk) [″ + *hodos*, way]

panting (pănt′ĭng) [ME. *panten*]

pantograph (păn′tō-grăf) [Gr. *pantos*, all, + *graphein*, to write]

pantomography (păn″tō-mŏg′ră-fē)

pantomorphia (păn″tō-mor′fē-ă) [″ + *morphe*, form]

Pantopaque

pantophobia (păn-tō-fō′bē-ă) [″ + *phobos*, fear]

pantoscopic (păn″tō-skŏp′ĭk) [″ + *skopein*, to examine]

pantoscopic glasses

pantothenate (păn-tō′thĕn-āt)

pantothenic acid (păn-tō-thĕn′ĭk)

pantothermia (păn″tō-thĕr′mē-ă) [″ + *therme*, heat]

pantropic (păn-trō′pĭk, -trŏp′ĭk) [″ + *tropos*, turning]

panturbinate (păn-tŭr′bĭ-nāt) [″ + L. *turbinatus*, shaped like a top]

Panwarfin

panzootic (păn″zō-ŏt′ĭk) [″ + *zoon*, animal]

PaO₂

pap (păp) [L. *pappa*, infant's sound for food]

papain (pă-pā′ĭn)

Papanicolaou test [George Papanicolaou, U.S. scientist, 1883–1962]

papaverine hydrochloride (pă-păv′ĕr-ēn) [L., poppy]

papaya (pă-pă′yă) [Sp. Amerind.]

paper [L. *papyrus*, paper]
　p., articulating
　p., bibulous
　p., blistering
　p., filter
　p., indicator
　p., litmus
　p., occluding
　p., test

papilla (pă-pĭl′ă) [L.]
　p., acoustic
　p., Bergmeister's
　p., circumvallate
　p., clavate
　p., conical
　p., dental
　p., dermal
　p., duodenal
　p., filiform
　p., foliate
　p., fungiform
　p., gingival
　p., gustatory

p., incisive
p., interdental
p., interproximal
p., lacrimal
p., lenticular
p., lingual
p., mammae
p. of corium
p. of hair
p. of Vater
p., optic
p., palatine
p., parotid
p. pili
p., renal
p., tactile
p., taste
p., urethral
p., vallate
papillary (păp′ĭ-lăr-ē) [L. *papilla*, nipple]
papillary ducts of Bellini
papillary layer
papillary muscles
papillary tumor
papillate (păp′ĭ-lāt) [L. *papilla*, nipple]
papillectomy (păp″ĭ-lĕk′tō-mē) [″ + Gr. *ektome*, excision]
papilledema (păp″ĭl-ĕ-dē′mă) [″ + Gr. *oidema*, swelling]
papilliferous (păp″ĭ-lĭf′ĕr-ŭs) [″ + *ferre*, to carry]
papilliform (pă-pĭl′ĭ-form) [″ + *forma*, shape]
papillitis (păp-ĭ-lī′tĭs) [″ + Gr. *itis*, inflammation]
papilloadenocystoma (păp″ĭl-ō-ăd″ē-nō-sĭs-tō′mă) [″ + Gr. *aden*, gland, + *kystis*, a cyst, + *oma*, tumor]
papillocarcinoma (păp″ĭl-ō-kăr-sĭ-nō′mă) [″ + Gr. *karkinos*, crab, + *oma*, tumor]
papilloma (păp-ĭ-lō′mă) [″ + Gr. *oma*, tumor]
p. durum
p., fibroepithelial
p., hard

p., Hopmann's
p., intracystic
p. molle
p., soft
p., villous
papillomatosis (păp″ĭ-lō-mă-tō′sĭs) [″ + Gr. *oma*, tumor, + *osis*, condition]
papillomaviruses
papilloretinitis (păp″ĭ-lō-rĕt-ĭn-ī′tĭs) [″ + *rete*, net, + Gr. *itis*, inflammation]
papovaviruses (păp″ō-vă-vī′rŭs-ĕs) [*papilloma*, + *polyoma*, + *vacuolating agent* + *virus*]
pappataci fever
pappose (păp′pōs) [L. *pappus*, down]
pappus [L.]
paprika (păp′rĭ-kă, păp-rē′kă) [Gr. *peperi*, pepper]
Pap smear; Pap test
papula (păp′ū-lă) [L.]
papular (păp′ū-lĕr)
papular fever
papulation (păp-ū-lā′shŭn)
papule (păp′ūl) [L. *papula*, pimple]
p., dry
p., moist
p., mucous
p.'s, split
papuliferous (păp″ū-lĭf′ĕr-ŭs) [L. *papula*, pimple, + *ferre*, to bear]
papulo- [L. *papula*, pimple]
papuloerythematous (păp″ū-lō-ĕr″ĕ-thĕm′ă-tŭs) [″ + Gr. *erythema*, redness]
papulopustular (păp″ū-lō-pŭs′tū-lăr) [″ + *pustula*, blister]
papulosis (păp-ū-lō′sĭs) [″ + Gr. *osis*, condition]
papulosquamous (păp″ū-lō-skwā′mŭs) [″ + *squamosus*, scalelike]
papulovesicular (păp″ū-lō-vē-sĭk′ū-lăr) [″ + *vesicula*, a tiny bladder]
papyraceous (păp-ĭ-rā′shŭs) [L.]
par [L., equal]
para [L. *parere*, to beget, produce]
para-, par- [Gr. *para*, alongside, past,

beyond; L. *par*, equal, pair]
para-actinomycosis
para-aminobenzoic acid (păr″ă-ăm″ĭ-nō-bĕn-zō′ĭk)
para-aminohippuric acid
para-aminosalicylic acid (păr″ă-ăm″ĭ-nō-săl″ĭ-sĭl′ĭk)
para-anesthesia (păr″ă-ăn-ĕs-thē′zē-ă) [″ + *an-*, negative, + *aisthesis*, feeling, perception]
para-aortic bodies
para-appendicitis (păr″ă-ă-pĕn″dĭ-sī′tĭs) [″ + L. *appendix*, appendix, + Gr. *itis*, inflammation]
parabionts (păr-ăb′ē-ŏnts) [″ + *bioun*, to live]
parabiosis (păr″ă-bī-ō′sĭs) [″ + *biosis*, living]
parabiotic (păr″ă-bī-ŏt′ĭk)
parablepsia, parablepsis (păr″ă-blĕp′sē-ă, -sĭs) [Gr. *para*, alongside, past, beyond, + *blepsis*, vision]
parabulia (păr″ă-bū′lē-ă) [″ + *boule*, will]
paracanthoma (păr″ă-kăn-thō′mă) [Gr. *para*, alongside, past, beyond, + *akantha*, thorn, + *oma*, tumor]
paracasein (păr-ă-kā′sē-ĭn)
Paracelsus (păr-ă-sĕl′sŭs) [Philippus Aureolus Theophrastus Bombastus von Hohenheim, 1493–1541]
paracenesthesia (păr″ă-sē″nĕs-thē′zē-ă) [Gr. *para*, alongside, past, beyond, + *koinos*, common, + *aisthesis*, feeling, perception]
paracentesis (păr″ă-sĕn-tē′sĭs) [Gr. *para*, alongside, past, beyond, + *kentesis*, a puncture]
  p., abdominal
  p. capitis
  p. cordis
  p. pericardii
  p. pulmonis
  p. thoracis
  p. tunicae vaginalis
  p. tympani
  p. vesicae

paracentetic (păr″ă-sĕn-tĕt′ĭk)
paracentral (păr″ă-sĕn′trăl) [″ + L. *centralis*, center]
paracentral lobule
paracephalus (păr″ă-sĕf′ă-lŭs) [″ + *kephale*, head]
parachlorophenol (păr″ă-klō″rō-fē′nŏl)
  p., camphorated
paracholera (păr″ă-kŏl′ĕr-ă) [″ + L. *cholera*, cholera]
paracholia (păr″ă-kō′lē-ă [″ + *chole*, bile]
parachordal (păr-ă-kor′dăl) [Gr. *para*, alongside, past, beyond, + *chorde*, cord]
parachordal cartilage
parachromatism (păr″ă-krō′mă-tĭzm) [″ + *chroma*, color, + *-ismos*, condition]
parachromatopsia (păr″ă-krō-mă-tŏp′sē-ă) [″ + ″ + *opsis*, sight, appearance, vision]
parachute reflex (reaction)
paracinesia, paracinesis (păr″ă-sī-nē′zē-ă, -sĭs) [″ + *kinesis*, motion]
paracme (păr-ăk′mē) [″ + *akme*, point]
Paracoccidioides (păr″ă-kŏk-sĭd″ē-oy′dēz)
  P. brasiliensis
paracoccidioidomycosis (păr″ă-kŏk-sĭd″ē-ŏy″dō-mĭ-kō′sĭs)
paracolitis (păr″ă-kō-lī′tĭs)
paracolpitis (păr″ă-kŏl-pī′tĭs) [″ + *kolpos*, vagina, + *itis*, inflammation]
paracolpium (păr″ă-kŏl′pē-ŭm)
paracone (păr′ă-kōn) [″ + *konos*, cone]
paraconid (păr″ă-kō′nĭd)
paracousis (păr″ă-koo′sĭs)
paracrine control
paracrisis (păr-ăk′rī-sĭs, păr″ă-krī′sĭs) [″ + *krinein*, to secrete]
paracusia, paracusis (păr″ă-kū′sē-ă, -kū′sĭs) [″ + *akousis*, hearing]
  p. acris

p. duplicata
p. loci
p. willisiana

paracystic (păr″ă-sĭs′tĭk) [Gr. *para*, alongside, past, beyond, + *kystis*, bladder]

paracystitis (păr″ă-sĭs-tī′tĭs) [″ + ″ + *itis*, inflammation]

paracystium (păr-ă-sĭs′tē-ŭm)

paracytic (păr″ă-sĭt′ĭk) [″ + *kytos*, cell]

paradenitis (păr″ăd-ĕn-ī′tĭs) [″ + *aden*, gland, + *itis*, inflammation]

paradental (păr″ă-dĕn′tăl) [″ + L. *dens*, tooth]

paradentium (păr″ă-dĕn′shē-ŭm)

paradidymal (păr″ă-dĭd′ĭ-măl) [″ + *didymos*, testicle]

paradidymis (păr-ă-dĭd′ĭ-mĭs) [″ + *didymos*, testicle]

Paradione

paradipsia (păr″ă-dĭp′sē-ă) [″ + *dipsa*, thirst]

paradox, Weber's

paradoxic, paradoxical (păr″ă-dŏk′sĭk, -sĭ-kăl) [Gr. *paradoxos*, conflicting with expectation]

paradoxical respiration

paraequilibrium (păr″ă-ē″kwĭ-lĭb′rē-ŭm)

paraffin (păr′ă-fĭn) [L. *parum*, too little, + *affinis*, neighboring]
p., hard
p., liquid
p., soft
p., white soft
p., yellow soft

paraffinoma (păr″ă-fĭn-ō′mă) [″ + Gr. *oma*, tumor]

paraffinum (păr-ă-fē′nŭm) [L.]

Paraflex

paraformaldehyde (păr″ă-for-măl′dĕ-hīd)

paragammacism (păr″ă-găm′mă-sĭzm) [″ + *gamma*, Gr. letter G, + *-ismos*, condition]

paraganglia (păr″ă-găng′lē-ă) [″ + *ganglion*, knot]

paraganglioma (păr″ă-găng-lē-ō′mă) [″ + ″ + *oma*, tumor]

paraganglion (păr″ă-găng′lē-ŏn) [″ + *ganglion*, knot]

parageusia, parageusis (păr-ă-gū′sē-ă, -sĭs) [″ + *geusis*, taste]

paraglossa (păr-ă-glŏs′să) [″ + *glossa*, tongue]

paraglossia (păr-ă-glŏs′sē-ă)

paragnathus (păr-ăg′nă-thŭs) [″ + *gnathos*, jaw]

paragonimiasis (păr″ă-gŏn″ĭ-mī′ă-sĭs) [*Paragonimus* + *-iasis*, state or condition of]

Paragonimus (păr″ă-gŏn′ĭ-mŭs)
P. westermani

paragrammatism

paragranuloma (păr″ă-grăn″ū-lō′mă) [Gr. *para*, alongside, past, beyond, + L. *granulum*, little grain, + Gr. *oma*, tumor]

paragraphia (păr-ă-grăf′ē-ă) [″ + *graphein*, to write]

parahemophilia (păr-ă-hē″mō-fĭl′ē-ă) [″ + *haima*, blood, + *philein*, to love]

parahepatic (păr-ă-hĕ-păt′ĭk) [″ + *hepar*, liver]

parahepatitis (păr″ă-hĕp″ă-tī′tĭs) [″ + ″ + *itis*, inflammation]

parahormone [″ + *hormaein*, to set in motion]

parahypnosis [″ + *hypnos*, sleep]

parahypophysis (păr″ă-hī-pŏf′ĭ-sĭs) [″ + *hypophysis*, an undergrowth]

parainfection [″ + L. *in*, into, + *facere*, to make]

parainfluenza viruses

parakeratosis (păr″ă-kĕr″ă-tō′sĭs) [″ + *keras*, horn, + *osis*, condition]
p. ostracea
p. psoriasiformis
p. scutularis

parakinesia

Paral

paralalia (păr″ă-lā′lē-ă) [″ + *lalia*,

chatter, prattle]
    p. literalis
paralambdacism (păr″ă-lăm′dă-sĭzm)
    [″ + *lambda*, Gr. letter L, +
    -ismos, condition]
paralbumin (păr″ăl-bū′mĭn) [″ + L.
    albumen, white of egg]
paraldehyde (păr-ăl′dĕ-hīd)
paraldehyde poisoning
paraldehydism (păr-ăl′dĕ-hīd″ĭzm)
paralepsy (păr′ă-lĕp″sē) [″ +
    lepsis, seizure]
paralexia (păr″ă-lĕk′sē-ă) [″ +
    lexis, speech]
paralgesia (păr″ăl-jē′zē-ă) [″ +
    algesis, sense of pain]
paralgia (păr-ăl′jē-ă) [″ + *algos*,
    pain]
parallactic
parallagma (păr″ăl-ăg′mă) [Gr., alter-
    nation]
parallax (păr′ă-lăks) [Gr. *parallaxis*,
    change of position]
    p., binocular
    p., heteronymous
    p., homonymous
parallelism (păr′ă-lĕl″ĭzm)
parallelometer (păr″ă-lĕl-ŏm′ĕ-tĕr)
parallergic (păr″ă-lĕr′jĭk)
parallergy (păr-ăl′ĕr-jē)
paralogia (păr″ă-lō′jē-ă) [Gr. *para*,
    alongside, past, beyond, + *logos*,
    word, reason]
    p., benign
paralogy (pă-răl′ō-jē)
paralysis (pă-răl′ĭ-sĭs) [Gr. *paralyein*,
    to loosen, disable]
    p., acoustic
    p., acute ascending spinal
    p., acute atrophic
    p., acute infectious
    p. agitans
    p., alcoholic
    p., anesthesia
    p., anterior spinal
    p., arsenical
    p., ascending
    p., association

p., asthenic bulbar
p., atrophic spinal
p., Bell's
p., birth
p., brachial
p., brachiofacial
p., bulbar
p., central
p., cerebral spastic, infantile
p., complete
p., compression
p., conjugate
p., crossed
p., crutch
p., decubitus
p., diphtheritic
p., diver's
p., Duchenne's
p., Duchenne-Erb
p., exhaustion
p., facial
p., familial periodic
p., flaccid
p., general
p., ginger
p., glossolabial
p., Gubler's
p., histrionic
p., hyperkalemic periodic
p., hypokalemic periodic
p., hysteric
p., immunological
p., incomplete
p., infantile
p., infantile cerebral ataxic
p., infantile spinal
p., infectious bulbar
p., ischemic
p., jake
p., Jamaica ginger
p., Klumpke's
p., Kussmaul's
p., labial
p., Landry's
p., lead
p., local
p., mimetic
p., mixed

p., muscular
p., musculospiral
p., normokalemic periodic
p., nuclear
p., obstetrical
p., ocular
p. of accommodation
p. periodica paramyotonia
p., phonetic
p., postdiphtheritic
p., posticus
p., Pott's
p., primary periodic
p., progressive bulbar
p., pseudobulbar
p., pseudohypertrophic muscular
p., radial
p., Saturday night
p., sensory
p., sleep
p., spastic
p., spinal
p., supranuclear
p., tick-bite
p., Todd's
p., tourniquet
p., vasomotor
p., Volkmann's
p., wasting
paralytic (păr″ă-lĭt′ĭk) [Gr. paralytikos]
paralytic dementia
paralytic ileus
paralyzant (păr′ă-lĭz″ănt) [Fr. paralyser, paralyze]
paralyze (păr′ă-līz) [Fr. paralyse]
paralyzer (păr′ă-līz″ĕr)
paramagnetic (păr″ă-măg-nĕt′ĭk)
paramania (păr″ă-mā′nē-ă) [Gr. para, alongside, past, beyond, + mania, madness]
paramastigote (păr″ă-măs′tĭ-gōt) [″ + mastix, lash]
paramastitis (păr″ă-măs-tī′tĭs) [″ + mastos, breast, + itis, inflammation]
paramastoid (păr″ă-măs′toyd) [″ + ″ + eidos, form, shape]
paramedian (păr″ă-mē′dē-ăn) [″ +

L. medianus, median]
paramedian incision
paramedic (păr″ă-mĕd′ĭk) [Gr. para, alongside, past, beyond, + L. medicus, doctor]
paramedical
paramedical personnel
paramenia (păr″ă-mē′nē-ă) [″ + meniaia, menses]
paramesial (păr″ă-mē′sē-ăl) [″ + mesos, middle]
parameter (păr-ăm′ĕ-tĕr) [″ + metron, measure]
paramethadione (păr″ă-mĕth″ă-dī′ōn)
paramethasone acetate (păr″ă-mĕth′ă-sōn)
parametric (păr″ă-mĕt′rĭk) [Gr. para, alongside, past, beyond, + metra, uterus]
parametritic (păr″ă-mē-trĭt′ĭk)
parametritis (păr″ă-mē-trī′tĭs) [″ + metra, uterus, + itis, inflammation]
parametrium (păr-ă-mē′trē-ŭm) [″ + metra, uterus]
paramimia (păr″ă-mĭm′ē-ă) [″ + mimeisthai, to imitate]
paramnesia (păr″ăm-nē′zē-ă) [″ + amnesia, loss of memory]
paramolar (păr″ă-mō′lăr)
paramorphia (păr″ă-mor′fē-ă) [″ + morphe, form]
paramucin (păr″ă-mū′sĭn)
paramusia (păr″ă-mū′zē-ă) [″ + mousa, music]
paramyloidosis (păr-ăm″ĭ-loy-dō′sĭs) [″ + Gr. amylon, starch, + Gr. eidos, form, shape, + osis, condition]
paramyoclonus multiplex (păr-ă-mī-ŏk′lō-nŭs mŭl′tĭ-plĕks) [″ + mys, muscle, + klonos, tumult]
paramyosinogen (păr″ă-mī″ō-sĭn′ō-jĕn) [Gr. para, alongside, past, beyond, + myosin, protein globin of muscle, + gennan, to produce]
paramyotonia (păr″ă-mī″ō-tō′nē-ă) [″ + mys, muscle, + tonos, act

of stretching, tension, tone]
p. ataxia
p. congenita
p., symptomatic
paramyotonus (păr″ă-mī-ŏt′ō-nŭs) [″ + ″ + *tonos,* act of stretching, tension, tone]
paramyxoviruses
paranalgesia (păr″ăn-ăl-jē′sē-ă) [″ + *an-,* not, + *algos,* pain]
paranasal (păr″ă-nā′săl) [″ + L. *nasalis,* pert. to nose]
paranasal sinuses
paraneoplastic syndromes
paranephric (păr″ă-nĕf′rĭk) [″ + *nephros,* kidney]
paranephritis (păr″ă-nĕ-frī′tĭs) [″ + ″ + *itis,* inflammation]
paranephros (păr-ă-nĕf′rŏs)
paranesthesia (păr″ăn-ĕs-thē′zē-ă) [″ + *an-,* not, + *aisthesis,* feeling, perception]
paraneural (păr″ă-nū′răl) [″ + *neuron,* nerve]
paranoia (păr″ă-noy′ă) [Gr. *para,* alongside, past, beyond, + *nous,* mind]
p., litigious
paranoiac (păr-ă-noy′ăk)
paranoid (păr′ă-noyd) [″ + *nous,* mind, + *eidos,* form, shape]
paranoid ideation
paranoid reaction type
paranomia (păr″ă-nō′mē-ă) [″ + *onoma,* name]
paranormal
paranuclear (păr″ă-nū′klē-ăr)
paranucleate (păr″ă-nū′klē-āt)
paranucleolus (păr″ă-nū-klē′ō-lŭs)
paranucleus (păr″ă-nū′klē-ŭs) [Gr. *para,* alongside, past, beyond, + L. *nucleus,* a kernel]
paraomphalic (păr″ă-ŏm-făl′ĭk) [″ + *omphalos,* navel]
paraoperative (păr″ă-ŏp′ĕr-ă-tĭv) [″ + L. *operari,* to work]
paraosteoarthropathy (păr″ă-ŏs″tē-ō-ăr-thrŏp′ăth-ē) [″ + *os-*

teon, bone, + *arthron,* joint, + *pathos,* disease, suffering]
parapancreatic (păr″ă-păn″krē-ăt′ĭk) [″ + *pan,* all, + *kreas,* flesh]
paraparesis (păr″ă-păr-ē′sĭs, -păr′ĕ-sĭs) [″ + *parienai,* let fall]
parapedesis (păr″ă-pĕd-ē′sĭs) [″ + *pedesis,* leaping]
parapeptone (păr″ă-pĕp′tōn) [″ + *peptein,* to digest]
paraperitoneal (păr″ă-pĕr″ĭ-tō-nē′ăl) [″ + *peritonaion,* stretched around or over]
parapestis (păr″ă-pĕs′tĭs) [″ + L. *pestis,* plague]
paraphasia (păr-ă-fā′zē-ă) [″ + *aphasis,* speech loss]
paraphemia (păr″ă-fē′mē-ă) [″ + *pheme,* speech]
paraphia (păr-ă′fē-ă) [″ + *haphe,* touch]
paraphilia [″ + *philein,* to love]
paraphimosis (păr″ă-fĭ-mō′sĭs) [″ + *phimoun,* to muzzle, + *osis,* condition]
paraphimosis oculi
paraphobia (păr″ă-fō′bē-ă) [″ + *phobos,* fear]
paraphonia (păr″ă-fō′nē-ă) [″ + *phone,* voice]
p. puberum
paraphora (păr-ăf′ō-ră) [Gr., a wandering]
paraphrasia (păr-ă-frā′zē-ă) [Gr. *para,* alongside, past, beyond, + *phrasis,* diction]
paraphrenitis (păr″ă-frē-nī′tĭs) [″ + *phren,* diaphragm, + *itis,* inflammation]
paraphronia (păr″ă-frō′nē-ă)
paraphyseal (păr″ă-fĭz′ē-ăl)
paraphysis (pă-răf′ĭ-sĭs) [Gr., offshoot]
paraplasm (păr′ă-plăzm) [″ + LL. *plasma,* form, mold]
paraplastic (păr″ă-plăs′tĭk) [″ + *plastikos,* formed]
paraplectic (păr″ă-plĕk′tĭk) [Gr. *paraplektikos,* striking at the side]

paraplegia (păr-ă-plē′jē-ă) [Gr. paraplegia, stroke on one side]
  p., alcoholic
  p., ataxic
  p., cerebral
  p., congenital spastic
  p. dolorosa
  p., infantile spastic
  p., peripheral
  p., Pott's
  p., senile
  p., spastic
  p., spastic, primary
  p., superior
  p., tetanoid
paraplegic (păr-ă-plē′jĭk) [Gr. paraplegia, stroke on one side]
paraplegiform (păr″ă-plĕj′ĭ-form)
[″ + L. forma, form]
parapleuritis (păr″ă-plū-rī′tĭs) [Gr.
para, alongside, past, beyond, +
pleura, side, + itis, inflammation]
parapoplexy (păr-ăp′ō-plĕk″sē)
[″ + apoplessein, to cripple by a
stroke]
parapraxia (păr-ă-prăk′sē-ă) [″ +
praxis, doing]
paraproctitis (păr″ă-prŏk-tī′tĭs) [Gr.
para, alongside, past, beyond, +
proktos, anus, + itis, inflammation]
paraproctium (păr″ă-prŏk′shē-ŭm)
[″ + proktos, anus]
paraprostatitis (păr″ă-prŏs″tă-tī′tĭs)
[″ + prostates, prostate, +
itis, inflammation]
paraprotein (păr″ă-prō′tē-ĭn)
paraproteinemia
parapsia, parapsis (păr-ăp′sē-ă, -sĭs)
[″ + hapsis, touch]
parapsoriasis (păr″ă-sō-rī′ă-sĭs)
[″ + psoriasis, an itching]
  p. en plaque
  p. lichenoides chronica
parapsychology (păr″ă-sī-kŏl′ō-jē)
paraquat (păr′ă-kwăt)
pararectal (păr″ă-rĕk′tăl) [″ + L.
rectum, straight]
parareflexia (păr″ă-rē-flĕk′sē-ă)

pararenal (păr″ă-rē′năl) [″ + L.
ren, kidney]
pararhotacism (păr″ă-rō′tă-sĭzm)
[″ + rho, Gr. letter R, +
-ismos, condition]
pararrhythmia (păr″ă-rĭth′mē-ă)
[″ + a-, not, + rhythmos,
rhythm]
pararthria (păr-ăr′thrē-ă) [″ +
arthron, articulation]
parasacral (păr″ă-sā′krăl) [″ + L.
sacrum, sacred]
parasalpingitis (păr″ă-săl-pĭn-jī′tĭs)
[″ + salpinx, tube, + itis, in-
flammation]
parasecretion (păr″ă-sē-krē′shŭn)
[″ + L. secretio, separation]
parasexuality (păr″ă-sĕks″ū-ăl′ĭ-tē)
[″ + L. sexus, sex]
parasigmatism (păr″ă-sĭg′mă-tĭzm)
[″ + sigma, Gr. letter S, +
-ismos, condition]
parasinoidal (păr″ă-sī-noy′dăl) [″ +
L. sinus, a curve]
parasite (păr′ă-sīt) [″ + sitos, food]
  p., accidental
  p., external
  p., facultative
  p., incidental
  p., intermittent
  p., internal
  p., malarial
  p., obligate
  p., occasional
  p., periodic
  p., permanent
  p., specific
  p., temporary
parasitemia (păr″ă-sī-tē′mē-ă) [″ +
″ + haima, blood]
parasitic (păr″ă-sĭt′ĭk) [Gr. para, alongside, past, beyond, + sitos, food]
parasitic disease drug service
parasiticide (păr″ă-sĭt′ĭ-sīd) [″ + ″
+ L. caedere, to kill]
parasitism (păr′ă-sĭt″ĭzm) [″ + ″
+ -ismos, condition]
parasitize (păr′ă-sĭt-īz″, -sĭt-īz″)

parasitogenic (păr″ă-sī″tō-jĕn′ĭk) [″ + ″ + *gennan*, to produce]
parasitologist (păr″ă-sī-tŏl′ō-jĭst) [″ + ″ + *logos*, word, reason]
parasitology (păr″ă-sī-tŏl′ō-jē) [″ + ″ + *logos*, word, reason]
parasitophobia (păr″ă-sī″tō-fō′bē-ă) [″ + ″ + *phobos*, fear]
parasitosis (păr″ă-sī-tō′sĭs) [″ + ″ + *osis*, condition]
parasitotropic (păr″ă-sī″tō-trŏp′ĭk) [″ + ″ + *tropos*, turning]
parasitotropism (păr″ă-sī-tŏt′rō-pĭzm) [″ + ″ + ″ + *-ismos*, condition]
parasitotropy (păr″ă-sī-tŏt′rō-pē)
parasomnias (păr″ă-sŏm′nē-ăz) [″ + *somnus*, sleep]
paraspadia (păr-ă-spā′dē-ă) [Gr. *paraspadein*, to draw aside]
paraspasm (păr′ă-spăzm) [L. *paraspasmus*]
parasteatosis (păr″ă-stē″ă-tō′sĭs) [Gr. *para*, alongside, past, beyond, + *steatos*, fat, + *osis*, condition]
parasternal (păr-ă-stĕrn′ăl) [″ + *sternon*, chest]
parasternal line
parasternal region
parasthenia (păr″ăs-thē′nē-ă) [″ + *sthenos*, strength]
parastruma (păr″ă-stroo′mă) [″ + L. *struma*, goiter]
parasympathetic (păr″ă-sĭm″pă-thĕt′ĭk) [″ + *sympathetikos*, sympathetic nerve]
parasympathetic nervous system
parasympathicotonia (păr″ă-sĭm-păth″ĭk-ō-tō′nē-ă) [″ + *sympathetikos*, sympathetic nerve, + *tonos*, act of stretching, tension, tone]
parasympatholytic (păr″ă-sĭm″pă-thō-lĭt′ĭk) [″ + ″ + *lytikos*, dissolving]
parasympathomimetic (păr″ă-sĭm″pă-thō-mĭm-ĕt′ĭk) [″ + ″ + *mimetikos*, imitative]
parasynapsis (păr″ă-sĭ-năp′sĭs) [″ + *synapsis*, conjunction]
parasynovitis (păr″ă-sĭn″ō-vī′tĭs) [″ + *syn*, with, + *oon*, egg, + *itis*, inflammation]
parasystole (păr-ă-sĭs′tō-lē) [″ + *systole*, contraction]
paratarsium (păr-ă-tăr′sē-ŭm) [″ + *tarsos*, flat of the foot, flat surface, edge of eyelid]
paratenon (păr″ă-tĕn′ŏn) [″ + *tenon*, tendon]
paratereseomania (păr″ă-tĕr-ē″sē-ō-mă′nē-ă) [Gr. *parateresis*, observation, + *mania*, madness]
parathion (păr″ă-thī′ŏn)
parathion poisoning
parathormone (păr″ă-thor′mōn) [Gr. *para*, alongside, past, beyond, + *thyreos*, shield, + *eidos*, form, shape, + *hormaein*, to excite]
parathymia (păr″ă-thī′mē-ă) [″ + *thymos*, mind, spirit]
parathyroid (păr-ă-thī′royd) [″ + *thyreos*, shield, + *eidos*, form, shape]
parathyroidectomy (păr″ă-thī-royd-ĕk′tō-mē) [″ + ″ + ″ + *ektome*, excision]
parathyroid injection
parathyroprivia (păr″ă-thī″rō-prī′vē-ă) [″ + ″ + L. *privus*, deprived of]
parathyroprivic (păr″ă-thī″rō-prĭv′ĭk)
parathyrotropic (păr″ă-thī-rō-trŏp′ĭk) [″ + ″ + ″ + *tropikos*, turning]
paratonsillar (păr″ă-tŏn′sĭl-ăr) [″ + L. *tonsillaris*, pert. to tonsil]
paratope (păr′ă-tōp) [″ + *topos*, a place]
paratrichosis (păr″ă-trī-kō′sĭs) [″ + *trichosis*, being hairy]
paratripsis (păr″ă-trĭp′sĭs) [″ + *tribein*, to rub]
paratrophic (păr″ă-trō′fĭk) [″ + *trophe*, nourishment]
paratrophy (păr-ăt′rō-fē) [″ + *trophe*, nourishment]

paratyphlitis (păr″ă-tĭf-lī′tĭs) [″ +
typhlos, blind, + itis, inflammation]
paratyphoid (păr-ă-tī′foyd) [″ +
typhos, fever, + eidos, form,
shape]
paratyphoid fever
paratypic (păr″ă-tĭp′ĭk) [″ + typos,
type]
paraumbilical (păr″ă-ŭm-bĭl′ĭk-ăl)
[″ + L. umbilicus, navel]
paraurethral (păr″ă-ū-rē′thrăl) [″ +
ourethra, urethra]
parauterine (păr″ă-ū′tĕr-īn) [″ +
L. uterus womb]
paravaccinia (păr″ă-văk-sĭn′ē-ă)
paravaginal (păr″ă-văj′ĭn-ăl) [″ +
vagina, sheath]
paravaginitis (păr″ă-văj-ĭn-ī′tĭs) [″ +
″ + itis, inflammation]
paravenous (păr″ă-vē′nŭs) [″ + L.
vena, vein]
paravertebral (păr″ă-vĕr′tĕ-brăl)
[″ + L. vertebralis, pert. to verte-
brae]
paravertebral anesthesia
paravesical (păr″ă-vĕs′ĭk-ăl) [″ +
L. vesica, bladder]
paravitaminosis (păr″ă-vī″tă-mĭ-
nō′sĭs)
paraxial (păr-ăk′sē-ăl) [″ + L.
axis, axis]
paraxon (păr-ăk′sŏn) [″ + axon,
axis]
parazoon (păr″ă-zō′ŏn) [″ +
zoon, animal]
parched [ME. parchen]
Paré, Ambroise (păr-ā′) [Fr. surgeon,
1510–1590]
parectasia, parectasis (păr″ĕk-
tā′sē-ă, -tă-sĭs) [″ + ektasis,
stretching]
parectropia (păr″ĕk-trō′pē-ă) [″ +
Gr. ek, out, + trope, a turn]
paregoric (păr-ĕ-gor′ĭk) [L. paregor-
icus, soothing]
paregoric poisoning
parelectronomic (păr″ē-lĕk″trō-
nŏm′ĭk) [Gr. para, alongside, past,

beyond, + elektron, amber, +
nomos, law]
parencephalia (păr″ĕn-sĕ-fā′lē-ă)
[″ + enkephalos, brain]
parencephalocele (păr″ĕn-sĕf′ă-lō-
sēl) [″ + ″ + kele, tumor,
swelling]
parencephalous (păr″ĕn-sĕf′ă-lŭs)
[″ + enkephalos, brain]
parenchyma (păr-ĕn′kĭ-mă) [Gr. par-
enkheim, to pour in beside]
p. testis
parenchymatitis (păr″ĕn-kĭm″ă-tī′tĭs)
[″ + itis, inflammation]
parenchymatous (păr″ĕn-kĭm′ă-tŭs)
parent [L. parens]
parenteral (păr-ĕn′tĕr-ăl) [Gr. para,
alongside, past, beyond, + enteron, intestine]
parenteral digestion
parenteral nutrition
parenting
p., surrogate
parepididymus (păr″ĕp-ĭ-dĭd′ĭ-mĭs)
parepithymia (păr″ĕp-ĭ-thī′mē-ă)
[″ + epithymia, desire]
paresis (păr′ē-sĭs, pă-rē′sĭs) [Gr. parienai, let fall]
p., juvenile
paresthesia (păr″ĕs-thē′zē-ă) [″ +
aisthesis, feeling, perception]
p., Berger's
paretic (pă-rĕt′ĭk, pă-rē′tĭk) [Gr. parienai, to let fall]
Parfuran
pargyline hydrochloride (păr′gĭ-lēn)
paridrosis (păr″ĭ-drō′sĭs) [″ + hidrosis, sweat]
paries (pā′rē-ĕs) [L., a wall]
parietal (pă-rī′ĕ-tăl) [L. parietalis]
parietal bone
parietal cells
parietal lobe
parietes (pă-rī′ĕ-tēs) [L.]
parietofrontal (pă-rī″ĕ-tō-frŏn′tăl)
parietography (pă-rī″ĕ-tŏg′ră-fē)
[″ + Gr. graphein, to write]
parieto-occipital (pă-rī″ĕ-tō-ŏk-

sīp′ĭ-tăl)

parietosplanchnic (pă-rī″ĕ-tō-splănk′nĭk)

parietosquamosal (pă-rī″ĕ-tō-skwă-mō′săl)

parietotemporal (pă-rī″ĕ-tō-tĕm′pō-răl)

parietovisceral (pă-rī″ĕ-tō-vĭs′ĕr-ăl)

Parinaud, Henri (pă-rĭ-nō′) [Fr. ophthalmologist, 1844–1905]

  P.'s oculoglandular syndrome

  P.'s ophthalmoplegia syndrome

pari passu (păr′ē-păs′ū) [L., with equal speed]

parity (păr′ĭ-tē) [L. par, equal; parere, to beget, produce]

Parkinson, James [Brit. physician, 1755–1824]

  P.'s disease

  P.'s facies

  P.'s mask

parkinsonian (păr″kĭn-sōn′ē-ăn)

parkinsonism (păr′kĭn-sŏn-ĭzm″)

Parlodel

Parnate

paroccipital (păr-ŏk-sĭp′ĭt-ăl) [Gr. para, alongside, past, beyond, + L. occiput, occiput]

parodontitis (păr″ō-dŏn-tī′tĭs) [″ + odous, tooth, + itis, inflammation]

parodontium (păr″ō-dŏn′shē-ŭm)

parodynia (păr-ō-dĭn′ē-ă) [L. parere, to beget, produce, + Gr. odyne, pain]

  p. perversa

parolivary (păr-ŏl′ĭ-vă″rē) [Gr. para, alongside, past, beyond, + L. oliva, olive]

parolivary bodies

paromomycin sulfate (păr′ō-mō-mī″sĭn)

paromphalocele (păr″ŏm-făl′ō-sēl″) [″ + omphalos, navel, + kele, tumor, swelling]

paroniria (păr-ō-nī′rē-ă) [″ + on-eiros, dream]

  p. ambulans

  p. salax

paronychia (păr-ō-nĭk′ē-ă) [″ + onyx, nail]

  p. tendinosa

paronychomycosis (păr″ō-nĭk″ō-mī-kō′sĭs) [″ + ″ + mykes, fungus, + osis, condition]

paronychosis (păr-ō-nī-kō′sĭs)

paroophoritis (păr″ō-ŏf-ō-rī′tĭs) [″ + L. oophoron, ovary, + Gr. itis, inflammation]

paroophoron (păr-ō-ŏf′ō-rŏn) [″ + NL. oophoron, ovary]

parophthalmia (păr-ŏf-thăl′mē-ă) [″ + ophthalmos, eye]

parophthalmoncus (păr″ŏf-thăl-mŏn′kŭs) [″ + ″ + onkos, bulk, mass]

parorchidium (păr-or-kĭd′ē-ŭm) [″ + orchis, testicle]

parorchis (păr-or′kĭs) [″ + orchis, testicle]

parorexia (păr-ō-rĕk′sē-ă) [″ + orexis, appetite]

parosmia (păr-ŏz′mē-ă) [″ + osme, odor]

parosphresia, parosphresis (păr″ŏs-frē′ zē-ă, -sĭs) [″ + osphresis, smell]

parosteal (păr-ŏs′tē-ăl)

parosteitis, parostitis (păr-ŏs-tē-ī′tĭs, -tī′tĭs) [Gr. para, alongside, past, beyond, + osteon, bone, + itis, inflammation]

parosteosis, parostosis (păr″ŏs-tē-ō′sĭs, -tō′sĭs) [″ + osteon, bone, + osis, condition]

parotic (pă-rŏt′ĭk) [″ + ous, ear]

parotid (pă-rŏt′ĭd)

parotid duct

parotidectomy (pă-rŏt″ĭ-dĕk′tō-mē) [″ + ous, ear, + ektome, excision]

parotid gland

parotiditis (pă-rŏt″ĭ-dī′tĭs) [″ + ″ + itis, inflammation]

parotidoscirrhus (pă-rŏt″ĭd-ō-skīr′ŭs) [″ + ″ + skirrhos, hardness]

parotitis (pă″rō-tī′tĭs) [″ + ous,

ear, + *itis*, inflammation]
parous (pă'rŭs) [L. *pario*, to bear]
parovarian (păr-ō-vā'rē-ăn) [" +
NL. *ovarium*, ovary]
parovariotomy (păr"ō-vā"rē-ŏt'ō-
mē) [" + " + Gr. *tome*, a cutting, slice]
parovaritis (păr"ō-vă-rī'tĭs) [" +
NL. *ovarium*, ovary, + Gr. *itis*, in-
flammation]
parovarium (păr"ō-vā'rē-ŭm)
paroxysm (păr'ŏk-sĭzm) [Gr. *paroxysmos*, irritation]
paroxysmal (păr"ŏk-sĭz'măl)
paroxysmal cold hemoglobinuria
parricide (păr'ĭ-sīd) [L. *parricidium*]
Parrot, Jules Marie (păr-ō') [Fr. physician, 1839–1883]
    P.'s disease
    P.'s nodes
    P.'s pseudoparalysis
    P.'s sign
    P.'s ulcer
parrot fever
Parry's disease (păr'ēz) [Caleb H.
Parry, Brit. physician, 1755–1822]
pars (părz) [L.]
    p. basilaris ossis occipitalis
    p. buccalis hypophyseos
    p. caeca oculi
    p. caeca retinae
    p. cephalica et cervicalis systematis
      autonomici
    p. ciliaris retinae
    p. distalis adenohypophyseos
    p. flaccida membranae tympani
    p. intermedia adenohypophyseos
    p. iridica retinae
    p. mastoidea ossis temporalis
    p. membranacea urethrae mascu-
      linae
    p. nervosa hypophyseos
    p. optica hypothalami
    p. optica retinae
    p. petrosa ossis temporalis
    p. plana corporis ciliaris
    p. radiata lobuli corticalis renis
    p. spongiosa urethrae masculinae

    p. squamosa ossis temporalis
    p. tensa membranae tympani
    p. tuberalis adenohypophyseos
    p. tympanica ossis temporalis
pars planitis (părs plă-nī'tĭs)
part. aeq. [L.] *partes aequales*, in equal
parts
partes (păr'tēs)
parthenogenesis (păr"thĕn-ō-jĕn'ĕ-
sĭs) [Gr. *parthenos*, virgin, + genesis, generation, birth]
parthenophobia (păr"thē-nō-fō'bē-ă)
[" + *phobos*, fear]
particle [L. *particula*]
    p., alpha
    p., beta
    p., Dane
    p., elementary
    p., elementary, of the mitochondria
particulate (păr-tĭk'ū-lāt)
parts per million
parturient (păr-tū'rē-ĕnt) [L. *parturiens*,
in labor]
parturifacient (păr-tū-rĭ-fā'shĕnt)
[" + *facere*, to make]
parturiometer (păr"tū-rē-ŏm'ĕ-tĕr)
[" + Gr. *metron*, measure]
parturiphobia [" + Gr. *phobos*,
fear]
parturition (păr-tū-rĭsh'ŭn) [L. *parturi-
tio*]
part. vic. [L.] *partibus vicibus*, in divided
doses
parulis (păr-ū'lĭs) [Gr. *para*, alongside,
past, beyond, + *oulon*, gum]
parumbilical (păr"ŭm-bĭl'ĭ-kăl) [" +
L. *umbilicus*, navel]
paruria (păr-ū'rē-ă) [Gr. *para*, alongside, past, beyond, + *ouron*,
urine]
parvicellular (păr-vĭ-sĕl'ū-lăr) [L.
parvus, small, + *cellula*, little box]
parvoline (păr'vō-lĭn)
parvovirus (păr"vō-vī'rŭs) [" +
virus, poison]
parvule (păr'vŭl) [L. *parvulus*, very
small]
PAS, PASA *para-aminosalicylic acid*

pascal
Paschen bodies (pă'shĕn) [Enrique Paschen, Ger. pathologist, 1860–1936]
passage (păs'ăj) [ME., to pass]
passion (păsh'ŭn) [L. *passio*, suffering]
passional (păsh'ŭn-ăl)
passive (păs'ĭv) [L. *passivus*, capable of suffering]
passive congestion
passive exercise
passive hyperemia
passive motion
passive movement
passive smoking
passivism (păs'ĭ-vĭzm) [" + Gr. -*ismos*, condition]
passivity (păs-sĭv'ĭ-tē) [L. *passivus*, capable of suffering]
paste
Pasteur, Louis (păs-stĕr') [Fr. chemist and bacteriologist, 1822–1895]
　　P. effect
　　P. treatment
Pasteurella (păs-tĕr-ĕl'ă) [Louis Pasteur]
　　P. multocida
pasteurellosis (păs"tĕr-ĕ-lō'sĭs)
pasteurization (păs"tūr-ĭ-zā'shŭn) [Louis Pasteur]
pastille (păs-tĕl', -tĭl') [L. *pastillus*, a little roll]
past-pointing
PAT *paroxysmal atrial tachycardia*
patagia (pă-tā'jē-ă) [L.]
patagium (pă-tā'jē-ŭm) [L.]
patch (păch) [ME. *pacche*]
　　p., cotton wool
　　p., herald
　　p., Hutchinson's
　　p., mucous
　　p., opaline
　　p., Peyer's
　　p., salmon
　　p., smoker's
　　p., soldier's
patch test
patefaction (păt"ĕ-făk'shŭn) [L. *pate-*

facere, to lay open]
patella (pă-tĕl'ă) [L., a small pan]
　　p., bipartite
　　p., floating
　　p., fracture of
　　p., rider's painful
　　p., slipping
patellapexy (pă-tĕl'ă-pĕk"sē) [L. *patella*, a small pan, + Gr. *pexis*, fixation]
patellar (pă-tĕl'ăr)
patellar ligament
patellar reflex
patellectomy (păt"ĕ-lĕk'tō-mē) [" + Gr. *ektome*, excision]
patelliform (pă-tĕl'ĭ-form) [" + *forma*, shape]
patellofemoral (pă-tĕl"ō-fĕm'ō-răl)
patellometer (păt"ĕ-lŏm'ĕ-tĕr) [" + Gr. *metron*, measure]
patency (pā'tĕn-sē) [L. *patens*, open]
patent (păt'ĕnt, pā'tĕnt)
patent ductus arteriosus
patent medicine
paternal (pă-tĕr'năl) [L. *paternis*, fatherly]
paternity test
path
　　p., condyle
　　p., incisor
　　p. of closure
path-, patho- [Gr. *pathema*, disease]
pathema (pă-thē'mă) [Gr.]
pathergasia (păth"ĕr-gā'zē-ă) [Gr. *pathos*, disease, suffering, + *ergasia*, work]
pathergia (pă-thĕr'jē-ă)
pathergy (păth'ĕr-jē)
pathetic (pă-thĕt'ĭk) [L. *patheticus*]
pathetism (păth'ĕ-tĭzm) [Gr. *pathein*, to suffer, + -*ismos*, condition]
pathfinder [AS. *paeth*, road, + *findan*, to locate]
-pathic (pă'thĭk) [Gr. *pathos*, disease, suffering]
Pathilon
patho- (păth'ō) [Gr. *pathos*, disease, suffering]

pathoamine (păth″ō-ăm′ĭn)
pathoanatomy (păth″ō-ă-năt′ō-mē)
pathobiology (păth″ō-bī-ŏl′ō-jē)
Pathocil
pathoclisis (păth″ō-klĭs′ĭs)
pathocrine (păth′ō-krĭn, -krēn, -krĭn)
[Gr. *pathos*, disease, suffering, + *krinein*, to secrete]
pathodixia [″ + Gr. *deiknunia*, to show]
pathodontia (păth″ō-dŏn′shē-ă) [″ + *odous* tooth]
pathoformic (păth″ō-for′mĭk) [″ + L. *forma*, form]
pathogen (păth′ō-jĕn) [″ + *gennan*, to produce]
pathogenesis (păth″ō-jĕn′ĕ-sĭs)
pathogenetic, pathogenic (păth″ō-jĕn-ĕt′ĭk, -jĕn′ĭk)
pathogenicity (păth″ō-jĕ-nĭs′ĭ-tē) [″ + *gennan*, to produce]
pathogeny (păth-ŏj′ĕn-ē)
pathognomonic (păth″ŏg-nō-mŏn′ĭk) [Gr. *pathognomonikos*, skilled in diagnosing]
pathognomy (păth-ŏg′nō-mē) [Gr. *pathos*, disease, suffering, + *gnome*, a means of knowing]
pathognostic (păth″ŏg-nŏs′tĭk) [″ + *gnosis*, knowledge]
pathography (păth-ŏg′ră-fē) [″ + *graphein*, to write]
pathologic, pathological (păth-ō-lŏj′ĭk, -ĭ-kăl) [Gr. *pathos*, disease, suffering, + *logos*, word, reason]
pathological reaction to alcohol
pathologist (pă-thŏl′ō-jĭst) [″ + *logos*, word, reason]
pathology (pă-thŏl′ō-jē)
   p., anatomic
   p., cellular
   p., chemical
   p., clinical
   p., comparative
   p., dental
   p., experimental
   p., functional
   p., geographical

   p., humoral
   p., medical
   p., molecular
   p., oral
   p., special
   p., surgical
pathomimesis (păth″ō-mĭm-ē′sĭs) [Gr. *pathos*, disease, suffering, + *mimesis*, imitation]
pathomimicry (păth″ō-mĭm′ĭ-krē)
pathomorphism (păth″ō-mor′fĭzm) [″ + *morphe*, form, + *-ismos*, condition]
pathonomia (păth-ō-nō′mē-ă) [″ + *nomos*, law]
pathophilia (păth″ō-fĭl′ē-ă) [″ + *philein*, to love]
pathophobia (păth-ō-fō′bē-ă) [″ + *phobos*, fear]
pathophoric (păth″ō-for′ĭk) [″ + *phoros*, carrying]
pathophysiology (păth″ō-fĭz″ē-ŏl′ō-jē) [″ + *physis*, nature, + *logos*, word, reason]
pathopoiesis (păth″ō-poy-ē′sĭs) [″ + *poiesis*, production]
pathopsychology (păth″ō-sī-kŏl′ō-jē) [″ + *psyche*, soul, + *logos*, word, reason]
pathotropism (pă-thŏt′rō-pĭzm) [″ + *trope*, a turn, + *-ismos*, condition]
pathway
   p., afferent
   p., biosynthetic
   p., central
   p., conduction
   p., efferent
   p., Embden-Myerhof
   p., metabolic
   p., motor
   p. of incidence
   p., pentose phosphate
   p., sensory
patient (pā′shĕnt) [L. *patiens*]
patient advocate
patient-controlled analgesia
patient day
patient delay

patient dumping
patient mix
patricide (păt′rĭ-sīd) [L. *patricidium*]
Patrick's test (păt′rĭks) [Hugh T. Patrick, U.S. neurologist, 1860–1938]
patrilineal (păt-rĕ-lĭn′ē-ăl) [L. *pater*, father, + *linea*, line]
patten (păt′ĕn) [Fr. *patin*, wooden shoe]
pattern
　p., occlusal
　p., wear
patterning
patulous (păt′ū-lŭs) [L. *patulus*]
paucisynaptic (paw″sĭ-sĭn-ăp′tĭk) [L. *paucus*, few, + Gr. *synapsis*, point of contact]
Paul-Bunnell test [John R. Paul, U.S. physician, 1891–1971; Walls W. Bunnell, U.S. physician, b. 1902]
pause [ME.]
　p., compensatory
Pavabid
pavementing
Pavlik harness
Pavlov, Ivan Patrovich (păv′lŏv) [Russian physiologist, 1849–1936]
pavor (pā′vor) [L.]
　p. diurnus
　p. nocturnus
Pavulon
P.B. *Pharmacopoeia Britannica*
Pb [L.] *plumbum*, lead
PBI *protein-bound iodine*
P.B.W. *posterior bitewing*
PBZ *pyribenzamine*
p.c. [L.] *post cibum*, after a meal
PCG *phonocardiogram*
pCO₂
PCV *packed cell volume*
Pd *palladium*
p.d. *prism diopter; pupilla diameter; pupillary distance*
PDR *Physicians' Desk Reference*
peanut oil
pearl [ME. *perle*]
　p.'s, enamel
　p., epithelial
　p., gouty

　p., Laënnec's
peau d'orange (pō″dō-rănj′) [Fr., orange skin]
peccant (pĕk′ănt) [L. *peccans*, sinning]
peccatiphobia (pĕk″ăt-ĭ-fō′bē-ă) [L. *peccata*, sins, + Gr. *phobos*, fear]
pecten (pĕk′tĕn) [L., comb]
　p. ossis pubis
pectenosis (pĕk″tĕ-nō′sĭs) [″ + Gr. *osis*, condition]
pectic acid (pĕk′tĭk) [Gr. *pektos*, congealed]
pectin (pĕk′tĭn) [Gr. *pektos*, congealed]
pectinase (pĕk′tĭ-nās)
pectinate (pĕk′tĭ-nāt) [L. *pecten*, comb]
pectineal (pĕk-tĭn′ē-ăl)
pectineal line
pectineus (pĕk-tĭn-ē′ŭs) [L. *pecten*, comb]
pectiniform (pĕk-tĭn′ĭ-form) [″ + *forma*, shape]
pectization (pĕk-tĭ-zā′shŭn) [Gr. *pektos*, congealed]
pectora (pĕk′tor-ă) [L.]
pectoral (pĕk′tō-răl) [L. *pectoralis*]
pectoralgia (pĕk″tō-răl′jē-ă) [″ + Gr. *algos*, pain]
pectoralis (pĕk″tō-rā′lĭs) [L.]
　p. major
　p. minor
pectoriloquy (pĕk″tō-rĭl′ō-kwē) [L. *pectoralis*, chest, + *loqui*, to speak]
　p., aphonic
　p., whispering
pectorophony (pĕk″tō-rŏf′ō-nē) [″ + Gr. *phone*, voice]
pectose (pĕk′tōs) [Gr. *pektos*, congealed]
pectunculus (pĕk-tŭn′kū-lŭs) [L., little comb]
pectus (pĕk′tŭs) [L.]
　p. carinatum
　p. excavatum
　p. recurvatum
pedal (pĕd′l) [L. *pedalis*]
pedarthrocace (pē″dăr-thrŏk′ă-sē) [Gr. *pais*, child, + *arthron*, joint, + *kakos*, bad]

pedatrophia

pedatrophy (pē-dăt′rō-fē) [Gr. *pais*, child, + *atrophia*, want of nourishment]

pederast (pĕd′ĕr-ăst) [Gr. *paiderastes*, a lover of boys]

pederasty (pĕd′ĕr-ăs″tē)

pedes (pē′dēz)

pedesis (pē-dē′sĭs) [Gr., leaping]

pedi- (pĕd′ĭ) [L. *pedalis*]

pedia- [Gr. *pais*, child]

Pediaflor

pedialgia (pĕd-ē-ăl′jē-ă, pē-dē-) [Gr. *pedion*, foot, + *algos*, pain]

Pediamycin

pediatric (pē-dē-ăt′rĭk) [Gr. *pais*, child, + *iatreia*, treatment]

pediatrician (pē-dē-ă-trĭsh′ăn) [″ + *iatrikos*, healing]

Pediatric Nurse Practitioner

pediatrics (pē-dē-ăt′rĭks) [Gr. *pais*, child, + *iatreia*, treatment]

pediatrist (pē″dē-ăt′rĭst) [″ + *iatrikos*, healing]

pediatry (pĕd′ē-ăt′rē, pē′dē-ăt″rē)

pedicel (pĕd′ĭ-sĕl)

pedicellation (pĕd″ĭ-sĕl-ā′shŭn) [L. *pediculus*, a little foot, stalk]

pedicle (pĕd′ĭ-kl)

pedicle flap

pedicterus (pē-dĭk′tĕr-ŭs) [Gr. *pais*, child, + *ikteros*, jaundice]

pedicular (pē-dĭk′ū-lar) [L. *pediculus*, a louse, a little foot]

pediculate (pē-dĭk′ū-lāt) [L. *pediculus*, a little foot]

pediculation (pē-dĭk″ū-lā′shŭn) [L. *pediculatio*]

pediculicide (pē-dĭk′ū-lĭ-sīd) [L. *pediculus*, a louse, + *caedere*, to kill]

Pediculidae

pediculophobia (pē-dĭk″ū-lō-fō′bē-ă) [″ + Gr. *phobein*, to fear]

pediculosis (pē-dĭk″ū-lō′sĭs) [″ + Gr. *osis*, condition]

   p. capitis
   p. corporis
   p. palpebrarum

   p. pubis
   p. vestimenti

pediculous (pē-dĭk′ū-lŭs)

Pediculus (pē-dĭk′ū-lŭs)

   P. humanus capitis
   P. humanus corporis

pediculus (pē-dĭk′ū-lŭs) [L.]

pedicure (pĕd′ĭ-kūr) [L. *pes*, foot, + *cura*, care]

pediform (pĕd′ĭ-form) [″ + *forma*, shape]

pedigree

pediluvium (pĕd-ĭ-lū′vē-ŭm) [″ + *luere*, to wash]

pedionalgia (pē″dē-ō-năl′jē-ă) [Gr. *pedion*, metatarsus, + *algos*, pain]

pediophobia (pē″dē-ō-fō′bē-ă) [Gr. *pais*, child, + *phobos*, fear]

pediphalanx (pĕd″ĭ-fā′lănks) [L. *pes*, foot, + Gr. *phalanx*, line of battle]

pedobaromacrometer (pē″dō-băr″ō-mă-krŏm′ĕt-ĕr) [″ + *baros*, weight, + *makros*, long, + *metron*, measure]

pedodontia, pedodontics (pē″dō-dŏn′shē-ă, -tĭks) [Gr. *pais*, child, + *odous*, tooth]

pedodontist (pē″dō-dŏn′tĭst)

pedodynamometer (pĕd″ō-dī-nă-mŏm′ĕ-tĕr) [L. *pes*, foot, + Gr. *dynamis*, power, + *metron*, measure]

pedograph (pĕd′ō-grăf) [″ + Gr. *graphein*, to write]

pedologist (pē-dŏl′ō-jĭst) [Gr. *pais*, child, + *logos*, word, reason]

pedology (pē-dŏl′ō-jē)

pedometer (pē-dŏm′ĕt-ĕr) [Gr. *pais*, child, + *metron*, measure]; (pĕd-ŏm′ĕt-ĕr) [L. *pes*, foot, + Gr. *metron*, measure]

pedomorphism (pē″dō-mor′fĭzm) [Gr. *pais*, child, + *morphe*, form, + *-ismos*, condition]

pedophilia (pē″dō-fĭl′ē-ă) [″ + *philein*, to love]

peduncle (pē-dŭn′kl) [L. *pedunculus*, a little foot]

p., cerebellar, inferior
p., cerebellar, middle
p., cerebellar, superior
p., cerebral
p., mamillary
p. of flocculus
p. of superior olive
p., olfactory
p., pineal
p., thalamic

peduncular (pē-dŭn'kū-lăr) [L. *pedunculus*, a little foot]

pedunculate, pedunculated (pē-dŭn'kū-lāt, -ĕd)

pedunculotomy (pĕ-dŭng″kū-lŏt'ō-mē) [″ + Gr. *tome*, a cutting, slice]

pedunculus (pĕ-dŭng'kū-lŭs) [L.]

peeling [ME. *pelen*, to peel]

peenash (pē'năsh) [Indian]

PEEP *positive end-expiratory pressure*

peer (pēr) [ME.]

peer review

peg, rete

Peganone

pejorative (pī-jor'ă-tĭv, pē″jă-rā'tĭv) [L. *pejor*, worse]

PEL *permissible exposure limits*

pelade (pĕl-ăd') [Fr., to remove hair]

pelage (pĕl'ĭj) [Fr.]

Pel-Ebstein fever [Pieter K. Pel, Dutch physician, 1852–1919; Wilhelm Ebstein, Ger. physician, 1836–1912]

Pelger-Huët anomaly (pĕl″jĕr hū'ĕt) [Karel Pelger, Dutch physician, 1885–1931; G. J. Huet, Dutch physician, b. 1879]

pelioma (pē-lē-ō'mă) [Gr.]

peliosis (pē-lē-ō'sĭs) [Gr.]

pellagra (pĕl-ă'gră, pĕ-lăg'ră) [L. *pellis*, skin, + Gr. *agra*, rough]
    p. sine pellagra

pellagrazein (pĕl-ă-gră'zē-ĭn)

pellagrin (pĕ-lā'grĭn, -lăg'rĭn)

pellagroid (pĕ-lăg'royd, -lăg'royd) [L. *pellis*, skin, + Gr. *agra*, rough, + *eidos*, form, shape]

pellagrous (pĕ-lā'grŭs, -lăg'rŭs)

pellant (pĕl'ănt) [L. *pellere*, to drive]

Pellegrini's disease, Pellegrini-Stieda disease (pĕl″ă-grē'nē-stē'dă) [Augusto Pellegrini, It. surgeon; Alfred Stieda, Ger. surgeon, 1869–1945]

pellet (pĕl'ĕt) [Fr. *pelote*, a ball]
    p., cotton
    p., foil

pellicle (pĕl'ĭ-kl) [L. *pellicula*, a little skin]
    p., salivary

pellotine (pĕl'ō-tēn)

pellucid (pĕl-lū'sĭd) [L. *pellucidus*]

pellucid zone

pelotherapy (pē″lō-thĕr'ă-pē) [Gr. *pelos*, mud, + *therapeia*, treatment]

pelvic (pĕl'vĭk) [L. *pelvis*, basin]

pelvic bone

pelvic diameter

pelvicephalography (pĕl″vē-sĕf″ă-lŏg'ră-fē) [″ + Gr. *kephale*, head, + *graphein*, to write]

pelvicephalometry (pĕl″vē-sĕf″ă-lŏm'ĕ-trē) [″ + ″ + *metron*, measure]

pelvic girdle

pelvic inflammatory disease

pelvic inlet

pelvic outlet

pelvic relaxation

pelvifixation (pĕl″vē-fĭk-sā'shŭn) [″ + *fixatio*, fixation]

pelvilithotomy (pĕl″vĭ-lĭ-thŏt'ō-mē) [″ + Gr. *lithos*, stone, + *tome*, a cutting, slice]

pelvimeter (pĕl-vĭm'ĕ-tĕr) [″ + Gr. *metron*, measure]

pelvimetry (pĕl-vĭm'ĕt-rē)

pelviolithotomy (pĕl″vē-ō-lĭ-thŏt'ō-mē) [L. *pelvis*, basin, + Gr. *lithos*, stone, + *tome*, a cutting, slice]

pelvioplasty (pĕl'vē-ō-plăs″tē) [″ + Gr. *plassein*, to form]

pelvioscopy (pĕl″vē-ŏs'kō-pē) [L. *pelvis*, basin, + Gr. *skopein*, to examine]

pelviotomy (pĕl-vē-ŏt'ō-mē) [″ + Gr. *tome*, a cutting, slice]

pelviperitonitis (pĕl"vĭ-pĕr-ĭ-tō-nī'tĭs) [" + Gr. *peritonaion*, stretched around or over, + *itis*, inflammation]

pelvirectal (pĕl"vē-rĕk'tăl) [" + *rectum*, straight]

pelvis (pĕl'vĭs) [L., basin]
   p. aequabiliter justo major
   p. aequabiliter justo minor
   p., android
   p., anthropoid
   p., assimilation
   p., beaked
   p., brachypellic
   p., brim of
   p., contracted
   p., cordate
   p., coxalgic
   p., dolichopellic
   p., dwarf
   p., elastic
   p., extrarenal
   p., false
   p. fissa
   p., fissured
   p., flat
   p., frozen
   p., funnel-shaped
   p., giant
   p., gynecoid
   p., halisteretic
   p., infantile
   p., justo major
   p., justo minor
   p., juvenile
   p., Kilian's
   p., kyphoscoliotic
   p., kyphotic
   p., large
   p., lordotic
   p. major
   p., malacosteon
   p., masculine
   p., mesatipellic
   p. minor
   p., Naegele's
   p. nana
   p. obtecta

   p., osteomalacic
   p., Otto
   p. plana
   p., platypellic
   p., Prague
   p., pseudo-osteomalacic
   p., rachitic
   p., reduced
   p., renal
   p., reniform
   p., Robert's
   p., Rokitansky
   p., rostrate
   p. rotunda
   p., round
   p., rubber
   p., scoliotic
   p., simple flat
   p., small
   p. spinosa
   p., split
   p., spondylolisthetic
   p. spuria
   p., triangular
   p., triradiate
   p., true

pelvitherm (pĕl'vĭ-thĕrm) [L. *pelvis*, basin, + Gr. *therme*, heat]

pelvoscopy (pĕl-vŏs'kō-pē) [" + Gr. *skopein*, to examine]

pelvospondylitis (pĕl"vō-spŏn"dĭ-lī'tĭs) [" + Gr. *spondylos*, vertebra, + *itis*, inflammation]
   p. ossificans

pemoline (pĕm'ō-lēn)

pemphigoid (pĕm'fĭ-goyd) [Gr. *pemphigodes*, breaking out in blisters]
   p., benign mucosal
   p., bullous
   p., cicatricial

pemphigus (pĕm'fĭ-gŭs) [Gr. *pemphix*, a blister]
   p. acutus
   p., benign familial
   p. circinatus
   p., erythematous
   p. foliaceus
   p. neonatorum

p., ocular
p. vegetans, Hallopeau type
p. vegetans, Neumann type
p. vulgaris
Pen A/N
Penapar VK
pendular (pĕn′dū-lĕr) [L. *pendulus*]
pendulous (pĕn′dū-lŭs)
penetrance
penetrate (pĕn′ĕ-trāt) [L. *penetrare*]
penetrating (pĕn′ĕ-trāt-ĭng)
penetrating power
penetrating wound
penetration (pĕn″ĕ-trā′shŭn) [L. *penetrare*, to go within]
penetrometer (pĕn″ĕ-trŏm′ĕ-tĕr) [″ + Gr. *metron*, measure]
-penia (pĕ′nē-ă) [Gr. *penia*, lack]
penicillamine (pĕn″ĭ-sĭl′ă-mēn)
penicillic acid
penicillin (pĕn-ĭ-sĭl′ĭn)
p., beta-lactamase resistant
p. G benzathine
p. V potassium
penicillinase (pĕn-ĭ-sĭl′ĭ-nās)
penicillinase-producing Neisseria gonococcus
penicilliosis (pĕn″ĭ-sĭl″ē-ō′sĭs) [L. *penicillum*, brush, + *osis*, condition]
Penicillium (pĕn″ĭ-sĭl′ē-ŭm) [L. *penicillum*, brush]
penicilloyl-polylysine (pĕn″ĭ-sĭl′oyl-pŏl″ĕ-lī′sēn)
penicillus (pĕn″ĭ-sĭl′ŭs) [L., paint brush]
penile (pē′nĭl, -nīl) [L. *penis*, penis]
penile prosthesis
penile reflex
penile ring
penis (pē′nĭs) [L.]
p. captivus
p., clubbed
p., double
p. lunatus
p. palmatus
p., webbed
penischisis (pĕ-nĭs′kĭ-sĭs) [L. *penis*, penis, + Gr. *schisis*, cleavage]
penitis (pĕ-nī′tĭs) [″ + Gr. *itis*, inflammation]

pennate (pĕn′āt) [L. *penna*, feather]
penniform (pĕn′ĭ-form) [″ + *forma*, shape]
pennyroyal (pĕn″ē-roy′ăl)
pennyweight
penoscrotal (pē″nō-skrō′tăl)
pension neurosis
pent-, penta- [Gr. *pente*, five]
pentabasic (pĕn″tă-bā′sĭk)
pentachlorophenol
pentad (pĕn′tăd) [Gr. *pente*, five]
pentadactyl (pĕn″tă-dăk′tĭl) [″ + *daktylos*, finger]
pentaerythritol tetranitrate (pĕn″tă-ĕ-rĭth′rĭ-tŏl)
pentagastrin (pĕn″tă-găs′trĭn)
pentalogy (pĕn-tăl′ō-jē)
pentamethylenediamine (pĕn″tă-mĕth″ĭl-ēn-dī′ă-mēn)
pentamidine (pĕn-tăm′ĭ-dēn)
pentane (pĕn′tān)
pentapeptide (pĕn″tă-pĕp′tīd)
pentaploid (pĕn″tă-ployd) [″ + *ploos*, a fold, + *eidos*, form, shape]
pentastomiasis (pĕn″tă-stō-mī′ă-sĭs)
pentatomic (pĕn″tă-tŏm′ĭk) [″ + *atomos*, indivisible]
pentavalent (pĕn″tă-vā′lĕnt, -tăv′ă-lĕnt) [Gr. *pente*, five, + L. *valens*, having power]
pentazocine (pĕn-tăz′ō-sēn)
Pentids
pentobarbital (pĕn″tō-băr′bĭ-tăl)
p. sodium
pentosazon (pĕn″tō-sā′zŏn)
pentose (pĕn′tōs) [Gr. *pente*, five]
pentosemia (pĕn″tō-sē′mē-ă)
pentoside (pĕn′tō-sīd)
pentostam
pentosuria (pĕn″tō-sū′rē-ă)
Pentothal Sodium
pentoxide (pĕn-tŏk′sīd)
Pen-Vee-K
peonin (pē′ō-nĭn)
peotillomania (pē″ō-tĭl″ō-mā′nē-ă) [Gr. *peos*, penis, + *tillein*, to pull, + *mania*, madness]
peotomy (pē-ŏt′ō-mē) [″ + *tome*,

a cutting, slice]

pepo (pē'pō) [L., pumpkin]

pepper (pĕp'ĕr) [ME. peper]

peppermint spirit

pepsic (pĕp'sĭk) [Gr. peptein, to digest]

pepsin (pĕp'sĭn) [Gr. pepsis, digestion]

pepsinogen (pĕp-sĭn'ō-jĕn) [" + gennan, to produce]

pepsinuria (pĕp"sĭ-nū'rē-ă) [" + ouron, urine]

peptic (pĕp'tĭk) [Gr. peptikos]

peptic ulcer

peptidase

peptide (pĕp'tĭd) [Gr. peptein, to digest]

peptidoglycan

peptidolytic (pĕp"tĭ-dō-lĭt'ĭk) [" + lytikos, dissolving]

peptinotoxin (pĕp"tĭn-ō-tŏk'sĭn) [" + toxikon, poison]

peptization (pĕp"tĭ-zā'shŭn) [Gr. peptein, to digest]

Pepto-Bismol

Peptococcus (pĕp"tō-kŏk'ŭs)

peptogenic, peptogenous (pĕp-tō-jĕn'ĭk, -tŏj'ĕn-ŭs) [" + gennan, to produce]

peptoid (pĕp'toyd) [" + eidos, form, shape]

peptolysis (pĕp-tŏl'ĭ-sĭs) [Gr. peptein, to digest, + lysis, dissolution]

peptolytic (pĕp-tō-lĭt'ĭk)

peptone (pĕp'tōn) [Gr. pepton, digesting]

peptonemia (pĕp"tō-nē'mē-ă) [" + haima, blood]

peptonization (pĕp"tō-nĭ-zā'shŭn) [Gr. pepton, digesting]

peptonize

peptonolysis (pĕp"tō-nŏl'ĭ-sĭs) [Gr. pepton, digesting, + lysis, dissolution]

peptonuria (pĕp"tō-nū'rē-ă) [" + ouron, urine]

Peptostreptococcus (pĕp"tō-strĕp"tō-kŏk'ŭs)

peptotoxin (pĕp"tō-tŏk'sĭn) [" + toxikon, poison]

per, per- [L. per, through]

peracephalus (pĕr"ă-sĕf'ă-lŭs) [" + Gr. a-, not, + kephale, head]

peracid (pĕr-ăs'ĭd)

peracidity (pĕr"ă-sĭd'ĭt-ē) [L. per, through, + acidus, sour]

peracute (pĕr"ă-kūt') [" + acutus, keen]

per anum (pĕr ā'nŭm) [L.]

perarticulation (pĕr"ăr-tĭk"ū-lā'shŭn) [L. per, through, + articulatio, joint]

peratodynia (pĕr"ăt-ō-dĭn'ē-ă) [Gr. peran, to pierce, + odyne, pain]

percent

percentile (pĕr-sĕn'tĭl)

percept (pĕr'sĕpt)

perception (pĕr-sĕp'shŭn) [L. percepitio, perceive]

    p., depth

    p., extrasensory

    p., stereognostic

perceptivity (pĕr-sĕp-tĭv'ĭ-tē)

percolate (pĕr'kō-lāt) [L. percolare, to strain through]

percolation (pĕr"kō-lā'shŭn) [L. percolatio]

percolator (pĕr'kō-lā"tor)

per contiguum (pĕr kŏn-tĭg'ū-ŭm) [L.]

per continuum (pĕr kŏn-tĭn'ū-ŭm) [L.]

percuss (pĕr-kŭs') [L. percutere]

percussible (pĕr-kŭs'ĭ-b'l)

percussion (pĕr-kŭsh'ŭn) [L. percussio, a striking]

    p., auscultatory

    p., bimanual

    p., deep

    p., direct

    p., finger

    p., immediate

    p., indirect

    p., mediate

    p., palpation

    p., threshold

percussor (pĕr-kŭs'or) [L., striker]

percutaneous (pĕr"kū-tā'nē-ŭs) [L. per, through, + cutis, skin]

percutaneous transluminal coronary angioplasty

percutaneous ultrasonic lithotriptor

per diem cost

perencephaly (pĕr″ĕn-sĕf′ă-lē) [Gr. *pera*, pouch, + *enkephalos*, brain]
perfectionism (pĕr-fĕk′shŭn-ĭzm)
perflation (pĕr-flā′shŭn) [L. *perflatio*]
perforans (pĕr′fō-răns) [L.]
perforate (pĕr′fō-rāt) [L. *perforatus*, pierced with holes]
perforation (pĕr″fō-rā′shŭn)
   p., Bezold's
   p., tooth
perforation of stomach or intestine
perforator (pĕr′fō-rā-tor) [L., a piercing device]
   p., tympanum
perforatorium (pĕr″fō-ră-tō′rē-ŭm)
performance
perfrication (pĕr-frĭ-kā′shŭn) [L. *perfricare*, to rub]
perfrigeration (pĕr-frĭj″ĕr-ā′shŭn) [L. *per*, through, + *frigere*, to be cold]
perfusate (pĕr-fū′zāt)
perfusion (pĕr-fū′zhŭn) [L. *perfundere*, to pour through]
perfusionist
Pergonal
perhydrocyclopentanophen- anthrene (pĕr-hī″drō-sī″klō-pĕn-tăn″ō-phĕn-ăn′thrēn)
periacinal, periacinous (pĕr″ē-ăs′ĭ-năl, -nŭs) [Gr. *peri*, around, + L. *acinus*, grape]
Periactin
periadenitis (pĕr″ē-ă″dĕ-nī′tĭs) [″ + *aden*, gland, + *itis*, inflammation]
   p. mucosa necrotica recurrens
perialienitis (pĕr″ē-ă″lē-ĕn-ī′tĭs) [″ + L. *alienus*, foreign, + Gr. *itis*, inflammation]
periamygdalitis (pĕr″ē-ăm-ĭg″dăl-ī′tĭs) [″ + *amygdale*, tonsil, + *itis*, inflammation]
perianal (pĕr″ē-ā′năl) [″ + L. *anus*, anus]
periangiitis (pĕr″ē-ăn″jē-ī′tĭs) [″ + *angeion*, vessel, + *itis*, inflammation]
periangiocholitis (pĕr″ē-ăn″jē-ō-kō-lī′tĭs) [″ + ″ + *chole*, bile, +

itis, inflammation]
periaortic (pĕr″ē-ā-or′tĭk) [″ + *aorte*, aorta]
periaortitis (pĕr″ē-ā-or-tī′tĭs) [″ + *aorte*, aorta, + *itis*, inflammation]
periapex (pĕr″ē-ā′pĕks) [″ + L. *apex*, tip]
periapical (pĕr″ē-ăp′ĭ-kăl) [″ + L. *apex*, tip]
periappendicitis (pĕr″ē-ă-pĕn″dĭ-sī′tĭs) [″ + L. *appendix*, appendage, + Gr. *itis*, inflammation]
   p. decidualis
periappendicular (pĕr″ē-ăp″ĕn-dĭk′ū-lăr) [″ + L. *appendix*, appendage]
periarterial (pĕr″ē-ăr-tē′rē-ăl) [″ + *arteria*, artery]
periarteritis (pĕr″ē-ăr-tĕr-ī′tĭs) [″ + ″ + *itis*, inflammation]
   p. gummosa
   p. nodosa
periarthric (pĕr″ē-ăr′thrĭk) [″ + *arthron*, joint]
periarthritis (pĕr″ē-ăr-thrī′tĭs) [″ + ″ + *itis*, inflammation]
periarticular (pĕr″ē-ăr-tĭk′ū-lăr) [Gr. *peri*, around, + L. *articulus*, a joint]
periatrial (pĕr″ē-ā′trē-ăl) [″ + L. *atrium*, corridor]
periauricular
periaxial (pĕr-ē-ăk′sē-ăl) [″ + *axon*, axis]
periaxillary (pĕr″ē-ăk′sĭl-ĕ″rē) [″ + L. *axilla*, armpit]
periaxonal (pĕr″ē-ăk′sō-năl) [″ + *axon*, axis]
periblast (pĕr′ĭ-blăst) [″ + *blastos*, germ]
peribronchial (pĕr″ĭ-brŏng′kē-ăl) [″ + *bronchos*, windpipe]
peribronchiolar (pĕr″ĭ-brŏng-kē′ō-lăr) [″ + L. *bronchiolus*, bronchiole]
peribronchiolitis (pĕr″ĭ-brŏng″kē-ō-lī′tĭs) [″ + ″ + *itis*, inflammation]
peribronchitis (pĕr″ĭ-brŏng-kī′tĭs) [″ + *bronchos*, windpipe, +

itis, inflammation]

peribulbar (pĕr"ĭ-bŭl'băr) [" + L. *bulbus,* bulbous root]

peribursal (pĕr"ĭ-bĕr'săl) [" + *bursa,* leather sack]

pericanalicular (pĕr"ĭ-kăn"ă-lĭk'ū-lăr) [" + L. *canaliculus,* small canal]

pericardiac, pericardial (pĕr-ĭ-kăr'dē-ăk, -ăl) [" + *kardia,* heart]

pericardial rub

pericardicentesis, pericardiocentesis (pĕr"ĭ-kăr"dĭ-sĕn-tē'sĭs, -kăr"dē-ō-sĕn-tē'sĭs) [" + " + *kentesis,* puncture]

pericardiectomy (pĕr"ĭ-kăr-dē-ĕk'tō-mē) [" + " + *ektome,* excision]

pericardiolysis (pĕr"ĭ-kăr"dē-ŏl'ĭ-sĭs) [" + " + *lysis,* dissolution]

pericardiomediastinitis (pĕr"ĭ-kăr"dē-ō-mē-dē-ăs"tĭ-nī'tĭs) [" + " + L. *mediastinum,* + Gr. *itis,* inflammation]

pericardiopexy [" + " + *pexis,* fixation]

pericardiophrenic (pĕr-ĭ-kăr"dē-ō-frĕn'ĭk) [" + *kardia,* heart, + *phren,* diaphragm]

pericardiopleural (pĕr"ĭ-kăr"dē-ō-ploo'răl) [" + " + *pleura,* rib]

pericardiorrhaphy (pĕr"ĭ-kăr"dē-or'ă-fē) [" + " + *rhaphe,* seam]

pericardiostomy (pĕr"ĭ-kăr"dē-ŏs'tō-mē) [" + *kardia,* heart, + *stoma,* mouth, opening]

pericardiosymphysis (pĕr"ĭ-kăr"dē-ō-sĭm'fĭ-sĭs) [" + " + *symphysis,* a joining]

pericardiotomy (pĕr"ĭ-kăr-dē-ŏt'ō-mē) [" + " + *tome,* a cutting, slice]

pericarditic (pĕr"ĭ-kăr-dĭt'ĭk)

pericarditis (pĕr-ĭ-kăr-dī'tĭs) [" + *kardia,* heart, + *itis,* inflammation]

  p., acute fibrinous
  p., acute nonspecific
  p., adhesive
  p., constrictive

  p., external
  p., fibrinous
  p., hemorrhagic
  p., idiopathic
  p., ischemic
  p., neoplastic
  p. obliterans
  p., serofibrinous
  p., uremic

pericardium (pĕr"ĭ-kăr'dē-ŭm) [Gr. *peri,* around, + *kardia,* heart]

  p., adherent
  p., bread-and-butter
  p. externum
  p., fibrous
  p. internum
  p., parietal
  p., serous
  p., shaggy
  p., visceral

pericardotomy (pĕr"ĭ-kăr-dŏt'ō-mē) [Gr. *peri,* around, + *kardia,* heart, + *tome,* a cutting, slice]

pericecal (pĕr"ĭ-sē'kăl) [" + L. *caecum,* blind]

pericecitis (pĕr"ĭ-sē-sī'tĭs) [" + " + Gr. *itis,* inflammation]

pericellular (pĕr"ĭ-sĕl'ū-lăr) [" + L. *cellula,* cell]

pericemental (pĕr"ĭ-sē-mĕn'tăl) [" + L. *caementum,* cement]

pericementitis (pĕr"ĭ-sē-mĕn-tī'tĭs) [" + " + Gr. *itis,* inflammation]

  p., apical

pericementoclasia (pĕr"ĭ-sē-mĕn"tō-klā'zē-ă) [" + " + Gr. *klasis,* a breaking]

pericementum (pĕr"ĭ-sē-mĕn'tŭm)

pericentral (pĕr"ĭ-sĕn'trăl) [" + *kentron,* center]

pericholangitis (pĕr"ĭ-kō-lăn-jī'tĭs) [Gr. *peri,* around, + *chole,* bile, + *angeion,* vessel, + *itis,* inflammation]

pericholecystitis (pĕr"ĭ-kō-lē-sĭs-tī'tĭs) [" + " + *kystis,* a sac, + *itis,* inflammation]

perichondral, perichondrial (pĕr-ĭ-kŏn'drăl, -drē-ăl) [" + chondros, cartilage]

perichondritis (pĕr-ĭ-kŏn-drī'tĭs) [" + " + itis, inflammation]

perichondrium (pĕr-ĭ-kŏn'drē-ŭm) [" + chondros, cartilage]

perichondroma (pĕr"ĭ-kŏn-drō'mă) [" + " + oma, tumor]

perichord (pĕr'ĭ-kord) [" + chorde, cord]

perichordal (pĕr-ĭ-kor'dăl) [" + chorde, cord]

perichorioidal, perichoroidal (pĕr" ĭ-kō-rē-oy'dăl, -roy'dăl) [" + chorioeides, skinlike]

pericolic (pĕr-ĭ-kō'lĭk) [" + kolon, colon]

pericolitis (pĕr"ĭ-kō-lī'tĭs) [" + " + itis, inflammation]

pericolonitis (pĕr"ĭ-kō-lŏn-ī'tĭs)

pericolpitis (pĕr"ĭ-kŏl-pī'tĭs) [Gr. peri, around, + kolpos, vagina, + itis, inflammation]

periconchal (pĕr-ĭ-kŏng'kăl) [" + konche, concha]

pericorneal (pĕr"ĭ-kor'nē-ăl) [" + L. cornu, horn]

pericoronal (pĕr"ĭ-kor'ō-năl) [" + korone, crown]

pericoronitis (pĕr"ĭ-kor"ō-nī'tĭs) [" + " + itis, inflammation]

pericranial (pĕr"ĭ-krā-nē-ăl) [" + kranion, skull]

pericranitis (pĕr"ĭ-krā-nī'tĭs) [" + " + itis, inflammation]

pericranium (pĕr"ĭ-krā'nē-ŭm) p. internum

pericystic (pĕr"ĭ-sĭs'tĭk) [" + kystis, bladder]

pericystitis (pĕr"ĭ-sĭs-tī'tĭs) [" + " + itis, inflammation]

pericystium (pĕr"ĭ-sĭs'tē-ŭm) [" + kystis, bladder]

pericyte (pĕr'ĭ-sīt) [" + kytos, cell]

pericytial (pĕr-ĭ-sĭsh'ăl) [" + kytos, cell]

peridectomy (pĕr"ĭ-dĕk'tō-mē) [" + ektome, excision]

peridendritic (pĕr"ĭ-dĕn-drīt'ĭk) [" + dendron, a tree]

peridens (pĕr'ĭ-dĕns) [" + L. dens, tooth]

peridental (pĕr"ĭ-dĕn'tăl) [" + L. dens, tooth]

peridentitis [" + " + itis, inflammation]

peridentium (pĕr"ĭ-dĕn'shē-ŭm) [" + L. dens, tooth]

periderm [" + derma, skin]

peridesmitis (pĕr"ĭ-dĕz-mī'tĭs) [" + desmion, band, + itis, inflammation]

peridesmium (pĕr"ĭ-dĕz'mē-ŭm)

perididymis (pĕr"ĭ-dĭd'ĭ-mĭs) [" + didymos, testicle]

perididymitis (pĕr"ĭ-dĭd"ĭ-mī'tĭs) [" + " + itis, inflammation]

peridiverticulitis (pĕr"ĭ-dī"vĕr-tĭk"ū-lī'tĭs) [" + L. diverticulare, to turn aside, + Gr. itis, inflammation]

periductal (pĕr-ĭ-dŭk'tăl) [" + L. ductus, a passage]

periduodenitis (pĕr"ĭ-dū"ō-dē-nī'tĭs) [" + L. duodeni, twelve, + Gr. itis, inflammation]

peridural (pĕr"ĭ-dū'răl) [" + L. durus, hard]

periencephalitis (pĕr"ē-ĕn-sĕf"ă-lī'tĭs) [" + enkephalos, brain, + itis, inflammation]

periencephalomeningitis (pĕr"ē-ĕn-sĕf"ă-lō-mĕn"ĭn-jī'tĭs) [" + " + meninx, membrane, + itis, inflammation]

periendothelioma (pĕr"ē-ĕn"dō-thē"lē-ō'mă) [" + endon, within, + thele, nipple, + oma, tumor]

perienteric (pĕr"ē-ĕn-tĕr'ĭk) [Gr. peri, around, + enteron, intestine]

perienteritis (pĕr"ē-ĕn"tĕr-ī'tĭs) [" + " + itis, inflammation]

perienteron (pĕr"ē-ĕn'tĕr-ŏn) [" + enteron, intestine]

periependymal (pĕr"ē-ĕp-ĕn'dĭ-măl) [" + ependyma, an upper garment]

periesophagitis (pĕr″ē-ē-sŏf″ă-jī′tĭs) [″ + oisophagos, gullet, + itis, inflammation]

perifistular (pĕr-ĭ-fĭs′tū-lĕr) [″ + L. fistula, pipe]

perifocal (pĕr″ĭ-fō′kăl) [″ + L. focus, hearth]

perifollicular (pĕr″ĭ-fŏl-lĭk′ū-lăr) [″ + L. folliculus, a little sac]

perifolliculitis (pĕr″ĭ-fō-lĭk″ū-lī′tĭs) [″ + ″ + Gr. itis, inflammation]

perigangliitis (pĕr″ĭ-găng″lē-ī′tĭs) [″ + ganglion, knot, + itis, inflammation]

periganglionic (pĕr″ĭ-găng″glē-ŏn′ĭk) [″ + ganglion, knot]

perigastric (pĕr″ĭ-găs′trĭk) [″ + gaster, belly]

perigastritis (pĕr″ĭ-găs-trī′tĭs) [″ + ″ + itis, inflammation]

perigemmal (pĕr″ĭ-jĕm′ăl) [″ + L. gemma, bud]

periglandulitis (pĕr″ĭ-glăn″dū-lī′tĭs) [″ + L. glandula, small gland, + Gr. itis, inflammation]

periglottic (pĕr″ĭ-glŏt′ĭk) [″ + glotta, tongue]

perihepatic (pĕr″ĭ-hĕ-păt′ĭk) [″ + hepar, liver]

perihepatitis (pĕr″ĭ-hĕp-ă-tī′tĭs) [″ + ″ + itis, inflammation]

perihernial (pĕr″ĭ-hĕr′nē-ăl) [″ + L. hernia, rupture]

perijejunitis (pĕr″ĭ-jē-jū-nī′tĭs) [″ + L. jejunum, empty, + Gr. itis, inflammation]

perikaryon (pĕr″ĭ-kăr′ē-ŏn) [″ + karyon, nucleus]

perikeratic (pĕr″ĭ-kĕr-ă′tĭk) [″ + keras, horn]

perikymata (pĕr″ĭ-kī′mă-tă) [″ + kyma, wave]

perilabyrinthitis (pĕr″ĭ-lăb″ĭr-ĭn-thī′tĭs) [″ + labyrinthos, a maze of canals, + itis, inflammation]

perilaryngeal (pĕr″ĭ-lă-rĭn′jē-ăl) [″ + larynx, larynx]

perilaryngitis (pĕr″ĭ-lăr″ĭn-jī′tĭs) [″ + ″ + itis, inflammation]

perilenticular (pĕr″ĭ-lĕn-tĭk′ū-lăr) [″ + L. lenticularis, pert. to a lens]

periligamentous (pĕr″ĭ-lĭg″ă-mĕn′tŭs) [″ + L. ligamentum, a band]

perilymph, perilympha (pĕr′ĭ-lĭmf, pĕr″ĭ-lĭm′fă) [″ + L. lympha, serum]

perilymphangeal (pĕr″ĭ-lĭm-făn′jē-ăl) [″ + ″ + Gr. angeion, vessel]

perilymphangitis (pĕr″ĭ-lĭmf-ăn-jī′tĭs) [″ + ″ + angeion, vessel, + itis, inflammation]

perimastitis (pĕr″ĭ-măs-tī′tĭs) [″ + mastos, breast, + itis, inflammation]

perimeningitis (pĕr″ĭ-mĕn″ĭn-jī′tĭs) [″ + meninx, membrane, + itis, inflammation]

perimeter (pĕr-ĭm′ĕt-ĕr) [″ + metron, measure]

perimetric (pĕr″ĭ-mĕt′rĭk) [″ + metron, measure; ″ + metra, uterus]

perimetritic (pĕr″ĭ-mē-trĭt′ĭk) [″ + metra, uterus, + itis, inflammation]

perimetritis (pĕr″ĭ-mē-trī′tĭs) [″ + ″ + itis, inflammation]

perimetrium (pĕr-ĭ-mē′trē-ŭm)

perimetry (pĕr-ĭm′ĕ-trē) [″ + metron, measure]

perimyelis (pĕr″ĭ-mī′ĕ-lĭs) [″ + myelos, marrow]

perimyelitis (pĕr″ĭ-mī″ĕ-lī′tĭs) [″ + ″ + itis, inflammation]

perimyelography (pĕr″ĭ-mī″ĕ-lŏg′ră-fē) [″ + ″ + graphein, to write]

perimyoendocarditis (pĕr″ĭ-mī″ō-ĕn″dō-kăr-dī′tĭs) [″ + mys, muscle, + endon, within, + kardia, heart, + itis, inflammation]

perimyositis (pĕr″ĭ-mī″ō-sī′tĭs) [″ + ″ + itis, inflammation]

perimysia (pĕr″ĭ-mĭs′ē-ă)

perimysial (pĕr-ĭ-mĭs′ē-ăl)

perimysiitis (pĕr″ĭ-mĭs″ē-ī′tĭs) [″ + mys, muscle, + itis, inflammation]

perimysium (pĕr″ĭ-mĭs′ē-ŭm)
p. externum

perinatal (pĕr″ĭ-nā′tăl) [″ + L. *natalis*, birth]
perinatology
perineal (pĕr″ĭ-nē′ăl) [Gr. *perinaion*, perineum]
perineal body
perineal fascia
perineal hernia
perineal section
perineo- [Gr. *perinaion*]
perineocele (pĕr″ĭ-nē′ō-sēl) [Gr. *perinaion*, perineum, + *kele*, tumor, swelling]
perineocolporectomyomectomy (pĕr″ĭ-nē-ō-kŏl″pō-rĕk″tō-mī″ō-mĕk′tō-mē) [″ + *kolpos*, vagina, + L. *rectus*, straight, + Gr. *mys*, muscle, + *oma*, tumor, + *ektome*, excision]
perineometer (pĕr″ĭ-nē-ŏm′ĕ-ter) [Gr. *perinaion*, perineum, + *metron*, measure]
perineoplasty (pĕr″ĭ-nē′ō-plăs″tē) [″ + *plassein*, to form]
perineorrhaphy (pĕr″ĭ-nē-or′ă-fē) [″ + *rhaphe*, seam]
  p., anterior
  p., colpo-
  p., posterior
perineoscrotal (pĕr″ĭ-nē-ō-skrō′tăl) [″ + L. *scrotum*, a bag]
perineotomy (pĕr″ĭ-nē-ŏt′ō-mē) [″ + *tome*, a cutting, slice]
perineovaginal (pĕr″ĭ-nē″ō-văj′ĭn-ăl) [″ + L. *vagina*, sheath]
perinephrial (pĕr″ĭ-nĕf′rĭ-ăl)
perinephric (pĕr″ĭ-nĕf′rĭk) [Gr. *peri*, around, + *nephros*, kidney]
perinephric abscess
perinephritis (pĕr″ĭ-nĕ-frī′tĭs) [″ + ″ + *itis*, inflammation]
perinephrium (pĕr″ĭ-nĕf′rē-ŭm)
perineum (pĕr″ĭ-nē′ŭm) [Gr. *perinaion*]
perineum, tears of the
perineural (pĕr″ĭ-nū′răl) [Gr. *peri*, around, + *neuron*, nerve]
perineurial (pĕr″ĭ-nū′rē-ăl) [″ + *neuron*, sinew]

perineuritis (pĕr″ĭ-nū-rī′tĭs) [″ + ″ + *itis*, inflammation]
perineurium (pĕr″ĭ-nū′rē-ŭm) [″ + *neuron*, sinew]
perinuclear (pĕr″ĭ-nū′klē-ăr) [″ + L. *nucleus*, a kernel]
periocular (pĕr″ē-ŏk′ū-lăr) [″ + L. *oculus*, eye]
period [L. *periodus*]
  p., absolute refractory
  p., childbearing
  p., critical
  p., effective refractory
  p., ejection
  p., fertile
  p., gestation
  p., incubation
  p., isoelectric
  p., isometric
  p., latency
  p., latent
  p., menstrual
  p., missed
  p., monthly
  p., neonatal
  p., patent
  p., postsphygmic
  p., presphygmic
  p., puerperal
  p., relative refractory
  p., safe
  p., silent
  p., sphygmic
  p., Wenckebach
periodic (pĕr-ē-ŏd′ĭk) [Gr. *periodikos*]
periodicity (pĕr″ē-ō-dĭs′ĭ-tē)
periodic law
periodic table
periodontal (pĕr″ē-ō-dŏn′tăl) [Gr. *peri*, around, + *odous*, tooth]
periodontal abscess
periodontal disease
periodontal ligament
periodontal pocket
periodontia (pĕr″ē-ō-dŏn′shē-ă) [Gr. *peri*, around, + *odous*, tooth]
periodontics (pĕr″ē-ō-dŏn′tĭks) [″ + *odous*, tooth]

periodontitis (pĕr″ē-ō-dŏn-tī′tĭs)
[″ + ″ + itis, inflammation]
  p., apical
periodontium (pĕr-ē-ō-dŏn′shē-ŭm)
periodontoclasia (pĕr″ē-ō-dŏn″tō-
klā′zē-ă) [″ + odous, tooth, +
klasis, breaking]
periodontology (pĕr″ē-ō-dŏn-tŏl′ō-
jē) [″ + ″ + logos, word, rea-
son]
periodontosis (pĕr″ē-ō-dŏn-tō′sĭs)
[″ + ″ + osis, condition]
periodoscope (pĕr″ē-ŏd′ō-skōp) [LL.
periodus, interval of time, + skopein, to examine]
periomphalic (pĕr″ē-ŏm-făl′ĭk) [Gr.
peri, around, + omphalos, navel]
periontogenic [″ + on, existing,
+ gennan, to produce]
perionychia (pĕr″ē-ō-nĭk′ē-ă) [″ +
onyx, nail]
perionychium (pĕr″ē-ō-nĭk′ē-ŭm)
perionyx (pĕr″ē-ō′nĭks) [″ + onyx,
nail]
perionyxis (pĕr″ē-ō-nĭk′sĭs)
perioophoritis (pĕr″ē-ō-ŏf″ō-rī′tĭs)
[″ + NL. oophoron, ovary, +
Gr. itis, inflammation]
perioophorosalpingitis (pĕr″ē-ō-
ŏf″ō-rō-săl″pĭn-jī′tĭs) [″ + ″ +
salpinx, tube, + itis, inflammation]
perioothecitis (pĕr″ē-ō″ō-thē-sī′tĭs)
[″ + oon, egg, + theke, box,
+ itis, inflammation]
perioothecosalpingitis (pĕr″ē-ō″ō-
thē″kō-săl-pĭn-jī′tĭs) [″ + ″ + ″
+ salpinx, tube, + itis, inflam-
mation]
perioperative
periophthalmic (pĕr″ē-ŏf-thăl′mĭk)
[″ + ophthalmos, eye]
perioptometry (pĕr″ē-ŏp-tŏm′ĕ-trē)
[″ + optos, visible, + metron,
measure]
perioral (pĕr″ē-or′ăl) [″ + L. oralis,
mouth]
periorbita (pĕr″ē-or′bĭ-tă) [″ + L.
orbita, orbit]

periorbital (pĕr″ē-or′bĭ-tăl)
periorbititis (pĕr″ē-or″bĭ-tī′tĭs) [″ +
L. orbita, orbit, + Gr. itis, inflam-
mation]
periorchitis (pĕr″ē-or-kī′tĭs) [″ +
orchis, testicle, + itis, inflammation]
  p. hemorrhagica
periosteal (pĕr-ē-ŏs′tē-ăl) [″ + osteon, bone]
periosteitis (pĕr″ē-ŏs″tē-ī′tĭs) [″ +
″ + itis, inflammation]
periosteoedema (pĕr″ē-ŏs″tē-ō-ē-
dē′mă) [Gr. peri, around, + osteon, bone, + oidema, swelling]
periosteoma (pĕr″ē-ŏs-tē-ō′mă)
[″ + ″ + oma, tumor]
periosteomyelitis (pĕr″ē-ŏs″tē-ō-
mī″ĕ-lī′tĭs) [″ + ″ + myelos,
marrow, + itis, inflammation]
periosteophyte (pĕr″ē-ŏs′tē-ō-fīt)
[″ + osteon, bone, + phyton,
growth]
periosteorrhaphy (pĕr″ē-ŏs″tē-or′ă-
fē) [″ + ″ + rhaphe, seam]
periosteosis (pĕr″ē-ŏs″tē-ō′sĭs) [″ +
″ + osis, condition]
periosteotome (pĕr″ē-ŏs′tē-ō-tōm)
[″ + osteon, bone, + tome, a
cutting, slice]
periosteotomy (pĕr″ē-ŏs-tē-ŏt′ō-mē)
periosteous (pĕr″ē-ŏs′tē-ŭs) [″ +
osteon, bone]
periosteum (pĕr-ē-ŏs′tē-ŭm) [Gr. per-
iosteon]
  p., alveolar
  p. externum
  p. internum
periostitis (pĕr″ē-ŏs-tī′tĭs) [″ + itis,
inflammation]
  p., albuminous
  p., alveolar
  p., dental
  p., diffuse
  p., hemorrhagic
periostoma (pĕr″ē-ŏs-tō′mă) [Gr. peri,
around + osteon, bone, +
oma, tumor]
periostomedullitis (pĕr″ē-ŏs″tō-mĕd-

ū-lī'tĭs) [" + " + L. *medulla,*
marrow, + Gr. *itis,* inflammation]
periostosis (pĕr"ē-ŏs-tō'sĭs) [" + "
+ *osis,* condition]
periostosteitis (pĕr"ē-ŏs-tŏs"tē-ī'tĭs)
[" + " + *osteon,* bone, +
itis, inflammation]
periostotome (pĕr"ē-ŏs'tō-tōm)
[" + " + *tome,* a cutting, slice]
periostotomy (pĕ"ē-ŏs-tŏt'ō-mē)
[" + " + *tome,* a cutting, slice]
periotic (pĕr-ē-ō'tĭk) [" + *ous,* ear]
periotic bone
periovaritis (pĕr"ē-ō"vă-rī'tĭs) [" +
NL. *ovarium,* ovary, + Gr. *itis,* in-
flammation]
periovular (pĕr"ē-ō'vū-lăr) [" + L.
ovulum, little egg]
peripachymeningitis (pĕr"ĭ-pak"ē-
mĕn"ĭn-jī'tĭs) [" + *pachys,* thick,
+ *meninx,* membrane, + *itis,* in-
flammation]
peripancreatitis (pĕr"ĭ-păn"krē-ă-
tī'tĭs) [" + *pankreas,* pancreas,
+ *itis,* inflammation]
peripapillary (pĕr"ĭ-păp'ĭ-lĕr"ē)
[" + L. *papilla,* nipple]
peripatetic (pĕr"ĭ-pă-tĕt'ĭk) [L. *peripa-
teticus,* to walk about while teaching]
peripenial (pĕr"ĭ-pē'nē-ăl) [Gr. *peri,*
around, + L. *penis,* penis]
periphacitis (pĕr-ĭ-fă-sī'tĭs) [" +
phakos, lens, + *itis,* inflammation]
periphakus (pĕr"ĭ-fă'kŭs)
peripharyngeal (pĕr"ĭ-fă-rĭn'jē-ăl)
[" + *pharynx,* throat]
peripherad (pĕr-ĭf'ĕr-ăd) [" +
pherein, to bear, + L. *ad,* to]
peripheral (pĕr-ĭf'ĕr-ăl)
peripheral nervous system
peripheral vascular disease
peripheraphose (pĕr-ĭf'ĕr-ă-fōs)
peripherocentral (pĕ-rĭf"ĕr-ō-sĕn'
trăl) [" + *pherein,* to bear, +
kentron, center]
peripherophose (per-ĭf'ĕr-ō-fōs)
periphery (pĕr-ĭf'ē-rē) [Gr. *peripher-
eia*]

periphlebitis (pĕr"ĭ-flĕ-bī'tĭs) [Gr. *peri,*
around, + *phleps,* blood vessel,
vein, + *itis,* inflammation]
periphoria (pĕr-ĭ-fō'rē-ă) [" +
phoros, bearing]
periphrastic (pĕr"ĭ-frăs'tĭk) [Gr. *per-
iphrastikos*]
periphrenitis (pĕr"ĭ-frē-nī'tĭs) [Gr. *peri,*
around + *phren,* diaphragm, +
itis, inflammation]
Periplaneta (pĕr"ĭ-plă-nē'tă)
    P. americana
    P. australasiae
periplasmic vesicles
periplast (pĕr'ĭ-plăst) [" + *plassein,* to form]
peripleural (pĕr"ĭ-plū'răl) [" +
pleura, rib]
peripleuritis (pĕr-ĭ-plū-rī'tĭs) [" + "
+ *itis,* inflammation]
peripolar (pĕr"ĭ-pō'lăr) [" + L.
polus, pole]
peripolesis (pĕr"ĭ-pō-lē'sĭs) [Gr., a
going about]
periporitis (pĕr"ĭ-por-ī'tĭs) [Gr. *peri,*
around, + L. *porus,* pore, +
Gr. *itis*]
periportal (pĕr"ĭ-por'tăl) [" + L.
porta, gate]
periproctic (pĕr"ĭ-prŏk'tĭk) [" +
proktos, anus]
periproctitis (pĕr"ĭ-prŏk-tī'tĭs) [" +
" + *itis,* inflammation]
periprostatic (pĕr"ĭ-prŏs-tăt'ĭk) [" +
prostates, prostate]
periprostatitis (pĕr"ĭ-prŏs-tă-tī'tĭs)
[" + " + *itis,* inflammation]
peripylephlebitis (pĕr"ĭ-pī"lē-flĕ-
bī'tĭs) [" + *pyle,* gate, +
phlebos, blood vessel, vein, + *itis,*
inflammation]
peripyloric (pĕr"ĭ-pī-lor'ĭk) [" +
pyloros, gatekeeper]
periradicular
perirectal (pĕr"ĭ-rĕk'tăl) [" + L.
rectus, straight]
perirectitis (pĕr"ĭ-rĕk-tī'tĭs) [" + "
+ Gr. *itis,* inflammation]

perirenal (pĕr″ĭ-rē′năl) [″ + L. ren, kidney]

perirhinal (pĕr″ĭ-rī′năl) [″ + rhis, nose]

perirhizoclasia (pĕr″ĭ-rī″zō-klā′zē-ă) [″ + rhiza, root, + klasis, destruction]

perisalpingitis (pĕr″ĭ-săl″pĭn-jī′tĭs) [″ + salpinx, tube, + itis, inflammation]

perisalpingoovaritis (pĕr″ĭ-săl-pĭn″ gō-o″văr-ī′tĭs) [″ + ″ + NL. ovarium, ovary, + Gr. itis, inflammation]

perisalpinx (pĕr″ĭ-săl′pĭnks) [″ + salpinx, tube]

perisclerium (pĕr″ĭ-sklē′rē-ŭm) [″ + skleros, hard]

periscopic (pĕr″ĭ-skŏp′ĭk) [″ + skopein, to examine]

perish (pĕr′ĭsh) [ME. perisshen]

perisigmoiditis (pĕr″ĭ-sĭg″moy-dī′tĭs) [Gr. peri, around, + sigma, Gr. letter S, + eidos, form, shape, + itis, inflammation]

perisinuous

perisinusitis (pĕr″ĭ-sī″nŭ-sī′tĭs) [″ + L. sinus, cavity, + Gr. itis, inflammation]

perispermatitis (pĕr″ĭ-spĕr″mă-tī′tĭs) [″ + sperma, seed, + itis, inflammation]
 p. serosa

perisplanchnic (pĕr″ĭ-splănk′nĭk) [″ + splanchnon, viscus]

perisplanchnitis (pĕr″ĭ-splănk-nī′tĭs) [″ + ″ + itis, inflammation]

perisplenic (pĕr″ĭ-splĕn′ĭk) [″ + splen, spleen]

perisplenitis (pĕr″ĭ-splĕ-nī′tĭs) [″ + ″ + itis, inflammation]
 p. cartilaginea

perispondylic (pĕr″ĭ-spŏn-dĭl′ĭk) [Gr. peri, around, + spondylos, vertebra]

perispondylitis (pĕr″ĭ-spŏn-dĭl-ī′tĭs) [″ + ″ + itis, inflammation]

perissodactylous (pĕr-ĭs″sō-dăk′tĭ-lŭs) [Gr. perissos, odd, + daktylos, finger]

peristalsis (pĕr-ĭ-stăl′sĭs) [Gr. peri, around, + stalsis, contraction]
 p., mass
 p., reverse

peristaltic (pĕr″ĭ-stăl′tĭk)

peristaphyline (pĕr″ĭ-stăf′ĭ-lĭn) [″ + staphyle, uvula]

peristasis (pĕr-rĭs′tă-sĭs) [″ + stasis, standing still]

peristomatous (pĕr″ĭ-stŏm′ă-tŭs) [″ + stoma, mouth, opening]

peristome (pĕr′ĭ-stōm) [″ + stoma, mouth, opening]

peristrumitis (pĕr″ĭ-stroo-mī′tĭs) [″ + L. struma, goiter, + itis, inflammation]

peristrumous (pĕr″ĭ-stroo′mŭs) [″ + struma, goiter]

perisynovial (pĕr″ĭ-sĭ-nō′vē-ăl) [Gr. peri, around, + L. synovia, joint fluid]

perisystole (pĕr″ĭ-sĭs′tō-lē) [″ + systole, contraction]

peritectomy (pĕr″ĭ-tĕk′tō-mē) [″ + ektome, excision]

peritendineum (pĕr″ĭ-tĕn-dĭn′ē-ŭm) [″ + L. tendo, tendon]

peritendinitis, peritenonitis (pĕr″ĭ-tĕn″dĭ-nī′tĭs, -tĕn″ō-nī′tĭs) [″ + ″ + Gr. itis, inflammation]
 p. calcarea
 p. serosa

peritenon (pĕr″ĭ-tē′nŏn) [″ + tenon, tendon]

perithelioma (pĕr″ĭ-thē-lē-ō′mă) [″ + thele, nipple, + oma, tumor]

perithelium (pĕr″ĭ-thē′lē-ŭm)
 p., Eberth's

perithoracic (pĕr″ĭ-thō-răs′ĭk) [″ + thorax, chest]

perithyroiditis (pĕr″ĭ-thī-roy-dī′tĭs) [″ + thyreos, shield, + eidos, form, shape, + itis, inflammation]

peritomy (pĕr-ĭt′ō-mē) [″ + tome, a cutting, slice]

peritoneal (pĕr″ĭ-tō-nē′ăl) [Gr. *peritonaion*, stretched around or over]
peritoneal cavity
peritoneal dialysis
    p.d., continuous ambulatory
peritoneal fluid
peritonealgia (pĕr″ĭ-tō″nē-ăl′jē-ă) [″ + *algos*, pain]
peritonealize
peritoneocentesis (pĕr″ĭ-tō″nē-ō-sĕn-tē′sĭs) [Gr. *peritonaion*, stretched around or over, + *kentesis*, puncture]
peritoneoclysis (pĕr″ĭ-tō″nē-ō-klī′sĭs) [″ + *klysis*, a washing]
peritoneopathy (pĕr″ĭ-tō-nē-ōp′-ăth-ē) [″ + *pathos*, disease, suffering]
peritoneopericardial (pĕr″ĭ-tō-nē″ō-pĕr″ĭ-kăr′dē-ăl) [″ + *peri*, around, + *kardia*, heart]
peritoneopexy (pĕr″ĭ-tō′nē-ō-pĕks″ē) [Gr. *peritonaion*, stretched around or over, + *pexis*, fixation]
peritoneoplasty (per″ĭ-tō′nē-ō-plăs″tē) [″ + *plassein*, to form]
peritoneoscope (pĕr″ĭ-tō′nē-ō-skōp″) [Gr. *peritonaion*, stretched around or over, + *skopein*, to examine]
peritoneoscopy (pĕr″ĭ-tō″nē-ŏs′kō-pē)
peritoneotomy (pĕr″ĭ-tō″nē-ŏt′ō-mē)
peritoneum (pĕr″ĭ-tō-nē′ŭm) [LL., Gr. *peritonaion*, stretched around or over]
    p., parietal
    p., visceral
peritonism (pĕr′ĭ-tō-nĭzm) [Gr. *peritonaion*, stretched around or over, + *-ismos*, condition]
peritonitic (pĕr″ĭ-tō-nĭt′ĭk) [″ + *itis*, inflammation]
peritonitis (pĕr″ĭ-tō-nī′tĭs) [″ + *itis*, inflammation]
    p., acute diffuse
    p., adhesive
    p., aseptic
    p., benign paroxysmal
    p., bile

    p., chemical
    p., chronic
    p., circumscribed
    p. deformans
    p., diaphragmatic
    p., diffuse
    p. encapsulans
    p., fibrocaseous
    p., gas
    p., generalized
    p., localized
    p. meconium
    p., pelvic
    p., periodic
    p., primary
    p., puerperal
    p., secondary
    p., septic
    p., serous
    p., silent
    p., talc
    p., traumatic
    p., tuberculous
peritonize (pĕr′ĭ-tō-nīz) [Gr. *peritonaion*, stretched around or over]
peritonsillar (pĕr″ĭ-tŏn′sĭ-lăr) [Gr. *peri*, around, + L. *tonsilla*, tonsil]
peritonsillitis (pĕr″ĭ-tŏn″sĭ-lī′tĭs) [″ + ″ + Gr. *itis*, inflammation]
peritracheal (pĕr″ĭ-trā′kē-ăl) [″ + *tracheia*, trachea]
Peritrate
Peritricha (pĕr-ĭt′rĭ-kă) [Gr. *peri*, around, + *thrix*, hair]
peritrichal, peritrichic (pĕ-rĭt′rĭ-kăl, pĕr″ē-trĭk′ĭk) [″ + *thrix*, hair]
peritrichous (pĕ-rĭt′rĭk-ŭs) [″ + *thrix*, hair]
peritrochanteric (pĕr″ĭ-trō″kăn-tĕr′ĭk) [″ + *trokhanter*, runner]
perityphlic (pĕr″ĭ-tĭf′lĭk) [″ + *typhlon*, cecum]
perityphlitis (pĕr″ĭ-tĭf-lī′tĭs) [″ + ″ + *itis*, inflammation]
periumbilical (pĕr″ē-ŭm-bĭl′ĭ-kăl) [″ + L. *umbilicus*, a pit]
periungual (pĕr″ē-ŭng′gwăl) [″ + L. *unguis*, nail]

periureteral (pĕr″ē-ū-rē′tĕr-ăl) [″ + oureter, ureter]

periureteritis (pĕr″ē-ū-rē″tĕr-ī′tĭs) [″ + ″ + itis, inflammation]

periurethral (pĕr″ē-ū-rē′thrăl) [″ + ourethra, urethra]

periurethritis (pĕr″ē-ū″rē-thrī′tĭs) [″ + ″ + itis, inflammation]

periuterine (pĕr″ē-ū′tĕr-ĭn) [″ + L. uterus, womb]

periuvular (pĕr″ē-ū′vū-lăr) [″ + L. uvula, little grape]

perivaginal (pĕr″ĭ-văj′ĭ-năl) [″ + L. vagina, sheath]

perivaginitis (pĕr″ĭ-văj″ĭ-nī′tĭs) [″ + ″ + Gr. itis, inflammation]

perivascular (pĕr″ĭ-văs′kū-lăr) [″ + L. vasculus, a little vessel]

perivasculitis (pĕr″ĭ-văs″kū-lī′tĭs) [″ + ″ + Gr. itis, inflammation]

perivenous (pĕr″ĭ-vē′nŭs) [″ + L. vena, vein]

perivertebral (pĕr″ĭ-vĕr′tĕ-brăl) [″ + L. vertebra, vertebra]

perivesical (pĕr″ĭ-vĕs′ĭ-kăl) [″ + L. vesia, bladder]

perivesiculitis (pĕr″ĭ-vĕ-sĭk″ū-lī′tĭs) [″ + vesicula, a tiny bladder, + Gr. itis, inflammation]

perivisceral (pĕr″ĭ-vĭs′ĕr-ăl) [″ + L. viscera, internal organs]

perivisceritis (pĕr″ĭ-vĭs″ĕr-ī′tĭs) [″ + ″ + Gr. itis, inflammation]

perivitelline (pĕr″ĭ-vī-tĕl′ēn) [″ + L. vitellus, yolk]

perixenitis (pĕr″ĭ-zĕ-nī′tĭs) [″ + xenos, strange, + itis, inflammation]

perle (pĕrl) [Fr., pearl]

perlèche (pĕr-lĕsh′) [Fr.]

perlingual (pĕr-lĭng′gwăl) [L. per, through, + lingua, tongue]

permanent (pĕr′mă-nĕnt) [″ + manere, to remain]

permanent teeth

permanganate (pĕr-măn′gă-nāt)

Permapen

permeability (pĕr″mē-ă-bĭl′ĭ-tē) [LL.

permeabilis]
p., capillary

permeable (pĕr′mē-ă-bl)

permeation (pĕr″mē-ā′shŭn) [L. permeare, permeate]

permissible exposure limits

Permitil

permutation (pĕr″mū-tā′shŭn) [L. per, completely, + mutare, to change]

perniciosiform (pĕr-nĭsh″ē-ō′sĭ-form) [L. perniciosus, destructive, + forma, form]

pernicious (pĕr-nĭsh′ŭs) [L. perniciosus, destructive]

pernicious anemia

pernicious trend

pernio (pĕr′nē-ō) [L.]

pero- [Gr. peros, maimed]

perobrachius (pē″rō-brā′kē-ŭs) [″ + brachion, arm]

perocephalus (pē″rō-sĕf′ă-lŭs) [″ + kephale, head]

perochirus (pē″rō-kī′rŭs) [″ + cheir, hand]

perocormus (pē″rō-kor′mŭs) [″ + kormos, trunk]

perodactylia (pē″rō-dăk-tĭl′ē-ă) [″ + daktylos, finger]

perodactylus (pē″rō-dăk′tĭ-lŭs) [″ + daktylos, finger]

peromelia (pē″rō-mē′lē-ă) [″ + melos, limb]

peromelus (pē-rŏm′ĕ-lŭs) [″ + melos, limb]

perone (pĕr-ō′nē) [Gr. perone, pin]

peroneal (pĕr″ō-nē′ăl) [Gr. perone, pin]

peroneal sign

peroneo- [Gr. perone, pin]

peroneotibial (pĕr″ō-nē″ō-tĭb′ē-ăl) [″ + L. tibia, shinbone]

peroneus (pĕr″ō-nē′ŭs) [Gr. perone, pin]

peronia (pē-rō′nē-ă) [Gr. peros, maimed]

peropus (pē′rō-pŭs) [″ + pous, foot]

peroral (pĕr-or′ăl) [L. per, through, +

oris, mouth]

per os [L.]

perosomus (pĕ″rō-sō′mŭs) [Gr. *peros*, maimed, + *soma*, body]

perosplanchnia (pĕ″rō-splănk′nē-ă) [″ + *splanchnon*, viscus]

perosseous (pĕr-ŏs′ē-ŭs) [L. *per*, through, + *os*, bone]

peroxidase (pĕr-ŏk′sĭ-dās) [″ + *oxys*, acid, + *-ase*, enzyme]

peroxide (pĕr-ŏk′sīd)

peroxisome (pĕ-rŏks′ĭ-sōm)

perphenazine (pĕr-fĕn′ă-zēn)

perplication (pĕr-plĭ-kā′shŭn) [″ + *plicare*, to fold]

per primam intentionem (pĕr prī′măm ĭn-tĕn-shē-ō′nĕm) [L.]

per rectum (pĕr rĕk′tŭm) [L.]

PERRLA *pupils equal, regular, react to light and accommodation*

Persadox

persalt (pĕr′sawlt)

Persantine

per secundam intentionem (pĕr sē-kŭn′dăm ĭn-tĕn-shē-ō′nĕm) [L.]

perseveration (pĕr-sĕv′ĕr-ā′shŭn) [L. *perseverare*, to persist]

person

persona (pĕr-sō′nă) [L., mask]

personal [L. *personalis*]

personality [LL. *personalitas*]

   p., alternating

   p., antisocial

   p., borderline

   p., compulsive

   p., double

   p., dual

   p., extroverted

   p., histrionic

   p., inadequate

   p., introverted

   p., multiple

   p., neurotic

   p., obsessive-compulsive

   p., paranoid

   p., passive-aggressive

   p., psychopathic

   p., schizoid

persons in need of supervision

perspiration (pĕr″spīr-ā′shŭn) [L. *perspirare*, breathe through]

   p., insensible

   p., sensible

perspire (pĕr-spīr′) [L. *perspirare*, breathe through]

persuasion (pĕr-swā′zhŭn)

persulfate (pĕr-sŭl′fāt)

per tertiam intentionem (pĕr tĕr′shē-ăm ĭn-tĕn-shē-ō′nĕm) [L.]

Perthes' disease (pĕr′tēz) [Georg C. Perthes, Ger. surgeon, 1869–1927]

Pertofrane

per tubam (pĕr tū′băm) [L.]

perturbation (pĕr″tĕr-bā′shŭn) [L. *perturbare*, thoroughly disordered]

pertussis (pĕr-tŭs′ĭs) [L. *per*, through, + *tussis*, cough]

pertussis immune globulin

pertussis vaccine

pertussoid (pĕr-tŭs′oyd) [L. *per*, through, + *tussis*, cough, + Gr. *eidos*, form, shape]

per vaginam (pĕr vă-jī′năm) [L.]

perversion (pĕr-vĕr′zhŭn) [L. *perversus*, perverted]

   p., sexual

pervert (pĕr-vĕrt′; pĕr′vĕrt) [L. *pervertere*, to turn the wrong way]

per vias naturales (pĕr vē′ăs năt″ū-rā′lēz) [L.]

pervious (pĕr′vē-ŭs) [L. *pervius*]

pes (pĕs) [L.]

   p. abductus

   p. adductus

   p. anserinus

   p. cavus

   p. contortus

   p. equinovalgus

   p. equinovarus

   p. equinus

   p. gigas

   p. hippocampi

   p., infraorbital

   p. planus

   p. valgus

   p. varus

pessary (pĕs'ă-rē) [L. *pessarium*]
- p., cup
- p., diaphragm
- p., Gariel's
- p., Hodge's
- p., lever
- p., Menge's
- p., ring
- p., stem

pessimism [L. *pessimus*, worst]
- p., therapeutic

pest (pĕst) [L. *pestis*, plague]

pesticemia (pĕs"tĭ-sē'mē-ă) [" + Gr. *haima*, blood]

pesticide (pĕs'tĭ-sīd) [" + *cida* fr. *caedere*, to kill]

pesticide residue

pestiferous (pĕs-tĭf'ĕr-ŭs) [L. *pestiferus*]

pestilence (pĕs'tĭl-ĕns) [L. *pestilentia*]

pestilential (pĕs-tĭ-lĕn'shăl)

pestis (pĕs'tĭs) [L.]
- p. ambulans
- p. fulminans
- p. major
- p. minor
- p. siderans
- p. variolosa

pestle (pĕs'l) [L. *pistillum*]

PET *positron emission tomography*

petechiae (pē-tē'kē-ē) [It. *petecchia*, skin spot]

petechial (pē-tē'kē-ăl)

pethidine hydrochloride (pĕth'ĭ-dĭn)

petiole (pĕt'ē-ōl) [LL. *petiolus*]

petiolus (pĕ-tī'ō-lŭs) [LL.]
- p. epiglottidis

Petit, François Pourfour du (pĕt-ē') [Fr. anatomist and surgeon, 1664–1741]
- P.'s canal
- P.'s sinuses

Petit, Jean Louis (pĕt-ē') [Fr. surgeon, 1674–1750]
- P.'s ligament
- P.'s triangle

petit mal (pĕt-ē' măl') [Fr., little illness]

Petri dish (pē'trē) [Julius Petri, Ger. bacteriologist, 1852–1921]

petrifaction (pĕt-rĭ-făk'shŭn) [L. *petra*, stone, + *facere*, to make]

petrified (pĕt'rĭ-fĭd)

petrify (pĕt'rĭ-fī)

pétrissage (pā"trē-săzh') [Fr.]

petro- [L. *petra*, stone]

petrolatoma (pĕt"rō-lă-tō'mă) [L. *petrolatum*, petroleum]

petrolatum (pĕt"rō-lā'tŭm) [L.]
- p., liquid
- p., white

petroleum (pĕ-trō'lē-ŭm) [L. *petra*, stone, + *oleum*, oil]

petromastoid (pĕt"rō-măs'toyd)

petro-occipital (pĕt"rō-ŏk-sĭp'ĭ-tăl) [" + *occipitalis*, occipital]

petropharyngeus (pĕt"rō-făr-rĭn'jē-ŭs) [" + Gr. *pharynx*, throat]

petrosa (pē-trō'să) [L. *petrosus*, stony]

petrosal (pĕt-rō'săl) [L. *petrosus*, stony]

petrosalpingostaphylinus (pĕt"rō-săl-pĭng"gō-stăf"ĭ-lī'nŭs) [L. *petra*, stone, + Gr. *salpinx*, tube, + *staphyle*, uvula]

petrositis (pĕt"rō-sī'tĭs) [" + Gr. *itis*, inflammation]

petrosomastoid (pē-trō"sō-măs'toyd) [" + Gr. *mastos*, breast, + *eidos*, form, shape]

petrosphenoid (pĕt"rō-sfē'noyd) [" + Gr. *sphen*, wedge, + *eidos*, form, shape]

petrosquamous (pĕt"rō-skwā'mŭs) [" + *squamosus*, scaly]

petrostaphylinus (pĕt"rō-stăf"ĭ-lī'nŭs) [" + Gr. *staphyle*, uvula]

petrous (pĕt'rŭs) [L. *petrosus*]

petrous ganglion

Peutz-Jeghers syndrome (pūtz-jā'kĕrs) [J. L. A. Peutz, 20th-cent. Dutch physician; H. Jeghers, U.S. physician, b. 1904]

pexin (pĕk'sĭn)

-pexy [Gr. *pexis*, fixation]

Peyer's patch (pī'ĕrz) [Johann Conrad Peyer, Swiss anatomist, 1653–1712]

peyote (pā-ō'tē)

Peyronie's disease (pā-rō-nēz')

[François de la Peyronie, Fr. surgeon, 1678–1747]

Pfeiffer, Emil (fī'fĕr) [Ger. physician, 1846–1921]
P.'s disease

Pfeiffer, Richard F. (fī'fĕr) [Ger. bacteriologist, 1858–1945]
P.'s bacillus
P.'s phenomenon

PG *prostaglandin*

pg *picogram*

PGA *pteroylglutamic acid*

Ph. *Pharmacopoeia; phenyl*

pH *potential of hydrogen*

phacitis (fă-sī'tĭs) [Gr. *phakos*, lens, + *itis*, inflammation]

phaco- [Gr. *phakos*]

phacoanaphylaxis (făk"ō-ăn"ă-fĭ-lăk'sĭs) [" + *ana*, excessive, + *phylaxis*, guard]

phacocele (făk'ō-sēl) [" + *kele*, tumor, swelling]

phacocyst (făk'ō-sĭst) [Gr. *phakos*, lens, + *kystis*, a sac]

phacocystectomy (făk"ō-sĭs-tĕk'tō-mē) [" + " + *ektome*, excision]

phacocystitis (făk"ō-sĭs-fī'tĭs) [" + " + *itis*, inflammation]

phacoemulsification (făk"ō-ē-mŭl'sĭ-fĭ-kā"shŭn)

phacoerysis (făk"ō-ĕr-ē'sĭs) [" + *eresis*, removal]

phacoglaucoma (făk"ō-glaw-kō'mă) [" + *glaukos*, gleaming, gray, + *oma*, tumor]

phacohymenitis (făk"ō-hī"mĕn-ī'tĭs) [" + *hymen*, membrane, + *itis*, inflammation]

phacoid (făk'oyd) [" + *eidos*, form, shape]

phacoiditis (făk"oy-dī'tĭs) [" + " + *itis*, inflammation]

phacoidoscope (fă-koyd'ō-skōp) [" + " + *skopein*, to examine]

phacolysis (făk-ŏl'ĭ-sĭs) [" + *lysis*, dissolution]

phacoma (fă-kō'mă) [" + *oma*, tumor]

phacomalacia (făk"ō-mă-lā'shē-ă) [" + *malakia*, softening]

phacomatosis (fă"kō-mă-tō'sĭs) [" + *oma*, tumor, + *osis*, condition]

phacometachoresis (făk"ō-mĕt"ă-kō-rē'sĭs) [" + *metachoresis*, displacement]

phacometer (făk-ŏm'ĕ-tĕr) [Gr. *phakos*, lens, + *metron*, measure]

phacoplanesis (făk"ō-plăn-ē'sĭs) [" + *planesis*, wandering]

phacosclerosis (făk"ō-sklĕr-ō'sĭs) [" + *sklerosis*, a hardening]

phacoscope (făk'ō-skōp) [" + *skopein*, to examine]

phacoscotasmus (făk"ō-skō-tăs'mŭs) [" + *skotasmos*, clouding]

phacotoxic (făk"ō-tŏk'sĭk) [" + *toxikon*, poison]

Phaedra complex [Wife of King Theseus of Athens]

phag-, phago- [Gr. *phagein*, to eat]

phage (fāj) [Gr. *phagein*, to eat]

phagedena (făj-ē-dē'nă) [Gr. *phagedaina*]
p., sloughing

phagedenic (făj-ē-dĕn'ĭk)

phage typing

phagocyte (făg'ō-sīt) [Gr. *phagein*, to eat, + *kytos*, cell]

phagocytic (făg"ō-sīt'ĭk)

phagocytic index

phagocytize (făg'ō-sīt"īz)

phagocytoblast (făg"ō-sī'tō-blăst) [" + " + *blastos*, germ]

phagocytolysis (făg"ō-sī-tŏl'ĭ-sĭs) [" + *kytos*, cell, + *lysis*, dissolution]

phagocytolytic (făg"ō-sī"tō-lĭt'ĭk)

phagocytose (făg"ō-sī'tōs) [" + *kytos*, cell]

phagocytosis (făg"ō-sī-tō'sĭs) [" + " + *osis*, condition]
p., induced
p., spontaneous

phagodynamometer (făg"ō-dī"nă-mŏm'ĕ-tĕr) [" + *dynamis*, power, + *metron*, measure]

phagokaryosis (făg"ō-kăr"ē-ō'sĭs) [" + karyon, nucleus, + osis, condition]

phagolysis (făg-ŏl'ĭ-sĭs) [" + lysis, dissolution]

phagolysosome (făg"ō-lī'sō-sōm) [" + lysis, dissolution, + soma, body]

phagomania (făg"ō-mā'nē-ă) [" + mania, madness]

phagophobia (făg"ō-fō'bē-ă)[" + phobos, fear]

phagopyrism (făg"ō-pī'rĭzm) [" + pyr, fever, + -ismos, condition]

phagosome (făg'ō-sōm) [" + soma, body]

phagotherapy (făg"ō-thĕr'ă-pē) [" + therapeia, treatment]

phagotype (făg'ō-tīp) [" + typos, mark]

phakitis (făk-ī'tĭs) [Gr. phakos, lens, + itis, inflammation]

phakolysis (făk-ŏl'ĭ-sĭs) [" + lysis, dissolution]

phakoma (fă-kō'mă) [" + oma, tumor]

phalacrosis (făl-ă-krō'sĭs) [Gr. phalakrosis]

phalacrotic (făl-ă-krŏt'ĭk)

phalacrous (făl-ăk'rŭs)

phalangeal (fă-lăn'jē-ăl) [Gr. phalanx, line of battle]

phalangeal cells, inner

phalangeal cells, outer

phalangectomy (făl-ăn-jĕk'tō-mē) [" + ektome, excision]

phalanges (fă-lăn'jēz)

phalangette (făl"ăn-jĕt')
  p., drop

phalangitis (făl"ăn-jī'tĭs) [Gr. phalanx, line of battle, + itis, inflammation]

phalanx (făl'ănks) [Gr., closely knit row]
  p., distal
  p., metacarpal
  p., metatarsal
  p., middle
  p., proximal
  p., terminal

  p., ungual

phallalgia (făl-ăl'jē-ă) [Gr. phallos, penis, + algos, pain]

phallectomy (făl-ĕk'tō-mē) [" + ektome, excision]

phallic (făl'ĭk)

phalliform (făl'ĭ-form) [" + L. forma, form]

phallitis (făl-ī'tĭs) [" + itis, inflammation]

phallocampsis (făl-ō-kămp'sĭs) [" + kampsis, a bending]

phallocrypsis (făl"ō-krĭp'sĭs) [" + krypsis, hiding]

phallodynia (făl-ō-dĭn'ē-ă) [" + odyne, pain]

phalloid (făl'oyd) [" + eidos, form, shape]

phalloidin (fă-loyd'ĭn)

phalloncus (făl-ŏn'kŭs) [" + onkos, bulk, mass]

phalloplasty (făl'ō-plăs"tē) [" + plassein, to form]

phallorrhagia (făl-ō-rā'jē-ă) [" + rhegnynai, to burst forth]

phallus (făl'ŭs) [Gr. phallos, penis]

phanero-, phaner- [Gr. phaneros, visible]

phanerogenic (făn"ĕr-ō-jĕn'ĭk) [" + gennan, to produce]

phaneromania (făn"ĕr-ō-mā'nē-ă) [" + mania, madness]

phanerosis (făn"ĕr-ō'sĭs) [Gr.]

phanic (făn'ĭk) [Gr. phainein, to show]

phantasia (făn-tā'zē-ă) [Gr.]

phantasm (făn'tăzm) [Gr. phantasma]

phantasmology (făn"tăz-mŏl'ō-jē) [" + logos, word, reason]

phantasy (făn'tă-sē) [Gr. phantasia, imagination]

phantogeusia (făn-tō-gū'sē-ă) [" + geusis, taste]

phantom (făn'tŭm) [Gr. phantasma, an appearance]

phantom corpuscle

phantom limb

phantom tumor

phantom vision

phantosmia (făn-tŏs'mē-ă) [" + osme, smell]
pharmacal (făr'mă-kăl) [Gr. pharmakon, drug]
pharmaceutical (făr-mă-sū'tĭ-kăl) [Gr. pharmakeutikos]
pharmaceutical chemistry
pharmaceutics (făr-mă-sū'tĭks)
pharmacist (făr'mă-sĭst) [Gr. pharmakon, drug]
pharmaco- [Gr. pharmakon, drug]
pharmacochemistry (făr"mă-kō-kĕm'ĭs-trē) [" + chemeia, chemistry]
pharmacodiagnosis (făr"mă-kō-dī"ăg-nō'sĭs) [" + dia, through, + gnosis, knowledge]
pharmacodynamics (făr"mă-kō-dī-nam'ĭks) [" + dynamis, power]
pharmacoendocrinology (făr"mă-kō-ĕn"dō-krī-nŏl'ō-jē) [" + endon, within, + krinein, to secrete, + logos, word, reason]
pharmacogenetics (făr"mă-kō-jĕn-ĕt'ĭks) [" + genesis, generation, birth]
pharmacognosy (făr"mă-kŏg'nō-sē) [" + gnosis, knowledge]
pharmacography (făr"mă-kŏg'ră-fē) [" + graphein, to write]
pharmacokinetics (făr"mă-kō-kĭ-nĕt'ĭks)
pharmacologist (făr"mă-kŏl'ō-jĭst)
pharmacology (făr"mă-kŏl'ō-jē) [" + logos, word, reason]
pharmacomania (făr"mă-kō-mā'nē-ă) [" + mania, madness]
pharmacopedia (făr"mă-kō-pē'dē-ă) [" + paideia, education]
pharmacopeia (făr"mă-kō-pē'ă) [Gr. pharmakopoeia, preparation of drugs]
Pharmacopeia, United States
pharmacophilia (făr"mă-kō-fĭl'ē-ă) [Gr. pharmakon, drug, + philos, love]
pharmacophobia (făr"mă-kō-fō'bē-ă) [" + phobos, fear]
pharmacophore (făr'mă-kō-for)

[" + phoros, bearing]
pharmacopsychosis (făr"mă-kō-sī-kō'sĭs) [" + psyche, soul, + osis, condition]
pharmacotherapy (făr"mă-kō-thĕr'ă-pē) [" + therapeia, treatment]
pharmacy (făr'mă-sē) [Gr. pharmakon, drug]
Pharm.D. Doctor of Pharmacy
pharyngalgia (făr"ĭn-găl'jē-ă) [Gr. pharynx, throat, + algos, pain]
pharyngeal (făr-ĭn'jē-ăl) [L. pharyngeus]
pharyngeal bursa
pharyngeal hypophysis
pharyngeal reflex
pharyngeal tonsil
pharyngectomy (făr-ĭn-jĕk'tō-mē) [" + ektome, excision]
pharyngemphraxis (făr"ĭn-jĕm-frăk'sĭs) [" + emphraxis, stoppage]
pharyngismus (făr"ĭn-jĭz'mŭs) [" + -ismos, condition]
pharyngitis (făr"ĭn-jī'tĭs) [" + itis, inflammation]
    p., acute
    p., atrophic
    p., chronic
    p., croupous
    p., diphtheritic
    p., follicular
    p., gangrenous
    p., granular
    p. herpetica
    p., hypertrophic
    p., membranous
    p. sicca
    p. ulcerosa
pharyngo- [Gr. pharynx, throat]
pharyngoamygdalitis (fă-rĭn"gō-ă-mĭg"dăl-ī'tĭs) [" + amygdale, tonsil, + itis, inflammation]
pharyngocele (făr-ĭn'gō-sēl) [" + kele, tumor, swelling]
pharyngoceratosis (fă-rĭng"gō-sĕr"ă-tō'sĭs) [" + keras, horn, + osis, condition]
pharyngoconjunctival fever, acute

pharyngodynia (făr-ĭn″gō-dĭn′ē-ă) [″ + odyne, pain]

pharyngoepiglottic, pharyngoepiglottidean (fă-rĭng″gō-ĕp″ĭ-glŏt′ĭk, -glō-tĭd′ē-ăn) [″ + epi, upon, + glottis, tongue]

pharyngoesophageal (fă-rĭng″gō-ē-sŏf′ă-jē″ăl) [″ + oisophagos, gullet]

pharyngoglossal (fă-rĭng″gō-glŏs′ăl) [″ + glossa, tongue]

pharyngography

pharyngokeratosis (făr-ĭn″gō-kĕr″ă-tō′sĭs) [″ + keras, horn, + osis, condition]

pharyngolaryngeal (fă-rĭng″gō-lă-rĭn′jē-ăl) [″ + larynx, larynx]

pharyngolaryngitis (făr-ĭn″gō-lăr-ĭn-jī′tĭs) [″ + ″ + itis, inflammation]

pharyngolith (făr-ĭn′gō-lĭth) [″ + lithos, stone]

pharyngology (făr″ĭn-gŏl′ō-jē) [″ + logos, word, reason]

pharyngolysis (făr″ĭn-gŏl′ĭ-sĭs) [″ + lysis, dissolution]

pharyngomaxillary (fă-rĭng″gō-măk′sĭ-lĕr″ē) [″ + L. maxilla, jawbone]

pharyngomycosis (făr-ĭn″gō-mī-kō′sĭs) [″ + mykes, fungus, + osis, condition]

pharyngonasal (fă-rĭng″gō-nā′săl) [″ + L. nasus, nose]

pharyngo-oral (fă-rĭng″gō-or′ăl) [″ + L. os, mouth]

pharyngopalatine (fă-rĭng″gō-păl′ă-tĭn) [″ + L. palatum, palate]

pharyngoparalysis (făr-ĭn″gō-păr-ăl′ĭ-sĭs) [″ + paralyein, to loosen, disable]

pharyngopathy (făr″ĭn-gŏp′ă-thē) [″ + pathos, disease, suffering]

pharyngoperistole (făr-ĭn″gō-pĕr-ĭs′tō-lē) [″ + peristole, contracture]

pharyngoplasty (făr-ĭn′gō-plăs″tē) [″ + plassein, to form]

pharyngoplegia (făr-ĭn″gō-plē′jē-ă) [″ + plege, a stroke]

pharyngorhinitis (făr-ĭn″gō-rī-nī′tĭs) [″ + rhis, nose, + itis, inflammation]

pharyngorhinoscopy (făr-ĭn″gō-rī-nŏs′ko-pē) [″ + ″ + skopein, to examine]

pharyngorrhea (făr″ĭn-gō-rē′ă) [″ + rhein, to flow]

pharyngoscleroma (făr-ĭng″gō-sklē-rō′mă) [″ + skleroma, induration]

pharyngoscope (făr-ĭn′gō-skōp) [″ + skopein, to examine]

pharyngoscopy (făr″ĭn-gŏs′kō-pē)

pharyngospasm (făr-ĭn′gō-spăzm) [″ + spasmos, a convulsion]

pharyngostenosis (fă-rĭng″gō-stē-nō′sĭs) [″ + stenosis, act of narrowing]

pharyngotherapy (făr-ĭn″gō-thĕr′ă-pē) [″ + therapeia, treatment]

pharyngotome (făr-ĭn′gō-tōm) [″ + tome, a cutting, slice]

pharyngotomy (făr-ĭn-gŏt′ō-mē)

pharyngotonsillitis (fă-rĭng″gō-tŏn″sĭ-lī′tĭs) [″ + L. tonsilla, almond, + Gr. itis, inflammation]

pharyngoxerosis (fă-rĭng″gō-zē-rō′sĭs) [″ + xerosis, dryness]

pharynx (făr′ĭnks) [Gr.]

phase (fāz) [Gr. phasis, appearance]
　p., continuous
　p., disperse

phasic (fā′sĭk)

phatnorrhagia (făt″nō-rā′jē-ă) [″ + rhegnynai, to burst forth]

Ph.D. Doctor of Philosophy

phenacaine hydrochloride (fĕn′ă-kān)

phenacemide (fĕ-năs′ē-mīd)

phenacetin (fĕ-năs′ē-tĭn)

phenakistoscope (fē″nă-kĭs′tō-skōp) [Gr. phenakistos, deceiver, + skopein, to view]

phenanthrene (fē-năn′thrēn)

Phenaphen

phenate (fē′nāt)

phenazopyridine hydrochloride

(fĕn"ă-zō-pēr'ĭ-dēn)
phencyclidine hydrochloride
phenelzine sulfate (fĕn'ĕl-zēn)
Phenergan
phenethicillin potassium (fĕ-nĕth"ĭ-sĭl'ĭn)
phenformin hydrochloride (fĕn-for'mĭn)
phengophobia (fĕn"gō-fō'bē-ă) [Gr. phengos, light, + phobos, fear]
phenic acid (fē'nĭk)
phenindione (fĕn"ĭn-dī'ōn)
pheniramine maleate (fĕn-ĭr'ă-mēn)
phenmetrazine hydrochloride (fĕn-mĕt'ră-zēn)
phenobarbital (fē"nō-băr'bĭ-tăl)
   p., sodium
phenocopy (fē'nō-kŏp"ē) [Gr. phainein, to show, + copy]
phenol (fē'nōl)
   p. red
Phenolax
phenolemia (fē"nō-lē'mē-ă) [phenol + Gr. haima, blood]
phenology (fē-nŏl'ō-jē) [Gr. phainesthai, to appear, + logos, word, reason]
phenolphthalein (fē"nŏl-thăl'ē-ĭn, fē"nōl-thăl'ēn)
phenol poisoning
phenolsulfonphthalein (fē"nōl-sŭl"fōn-thăl'ē-ĭn)
phenoluria (fē"nŏl-ū'rē-ă)
phenomenology (fē-nŏm"ē-nŏl'ō-jē) [Gr. phainomenon, appearing, + logos, word, reason]
phenomenon (fē-nŏm'ē-nōn) [Gr. phainomenon, appearing]
   p., Bell's
phenothiazine (fē"nō-thī'ă-zēn)
phenotype (fē'nō-tīp) [Gr. phainein, to show, + typos, type]
phenoxybenzamine hydrochloride (fē-nŏk"sē-bĕn'ză-mēn)
phenozygous (fē-nŏz'ĭ-gŭs) [" + zygon, yoke]
phenprocoumon (fĕn-prō'koo-mōn)
phensuximide (fĕn-sŭk'sĭ-mīd)
phentermine (fĕn'tĕr-mēn)

phentolamine hydrochloride (fĕn-tŏl'ă-mēn)
Phenurone
phenyl (fĕn'ĭl, fē'nĭl)
phenylalanine (fĕn"ĭl-ăl'ă-nīn)
phenylamine
phenylbutazone (fĕn"ĭl-bū'tă-zōn)
phenylephrine hydrochloride
phenylethyl alcohol
phenylhydrazine (fĕn"ĭl-hī'dră-zēn)
phenylketonuria (fĕn"ĭl-kē"tō-nū'rē-ă)
phenylmercuric acetate (fĕn"ĭl-mĕr-kū'rĭk)
phenylmercuric nitrate
phenylpropanolamine hydrochloride (fĕn"ĭl-prō"pă-nōl'ă-mēn)
phenylpyruvic acid (fĕn"ĭl-pī-roo'vĭk)
phenylpyruvic acid oligophrenia
phenylthiocarbamide (fĕn"ĭl-thī"ō-kăr'bă-mīd)
phenylthiourea (fĕn"ĭl-thī"ō-ū-rē'ă)
phenytoin (fĕn'ĭ-tō-ĭn)
pheochrome (fē'ō-krōm) [Gr. phaios, dusky, + chroma, color]
pheochromoblast (fē"ō-krō'mō-blăst) [" + blastos, germ]
pheochromoblastoma (fē"ō-krō"mō-blăs-tō'mă) [" + " + oma, tumor]
pheochromocyte (fē"ō-krō'mō-sīt) [" + " + kytos, cell]
pheochromocytoma (fē-ō-krō"mō-sī-tō'mă) [" + " + " + oma, tumor]
pheomelanins (fē-ō-mĕl'ă-nīn) [" + Gr. melas, black]
pheromone (fĕr'ō-mōn)
Ph.G. German Pharmacopeia; Graduate in Pharmacy
phial (fī'ăl) [Gr. phiale, a bowl]
Philadelphia chromosome
-philia (fĭl'ē-ă) [Gr. philein, to love]
philiater (fĭ-lī'ă-tĕr) [" + iatreia, healing]
philoneism (fĭ-lō'nē-ĭzm) [Gr. philein, to love, + neos, new, + -ismos, condition]
philoprogenitive (fĭl"lō-prō-jĕn'ĭ-tĭv)

[" + pro, for, + gennan, to produce]

philter, philtre [Gr. *philtron*]

philtrum

phimosis (fĭ-mō′sĭs) [Gr., a muzzling]
p. vaginalis

pHisoHex (fī′sō-hĕks)

phlebalgia (flĕ-băl′jē-ă) [Gr. *phlebos*, blood vessel, vein, + *algos*, pain]

phlebangioma (flĕb″ăn-jē-ō′mă) [" + *angeion*, vessel, + *oma*, tumor]

phlebarteriectasia (flĕb″ăr-tē″rē-ĕk-tā′zē-ă) [" + *arteria*, artery, + *ektasis*, dilatation]

phlebarteriodialysis (flĕb″ar-tē″rē-ō-dĭ-ăl′ĭ-sĭs) [" + " + *dia*, through, + *lysis*, dissolution]

phlebectasia, phlebectasis (flĕb-ĕk-tā′zē-ă, -ĕk′tă-sĭs) [" + *ektasis*, dilatation]

phlebectomy (flĕb-ĕk′tō-mē) [" + *ektome*, excision]

phlebectopia (flĕb″ĕk-tō′pē-ă) [" + *ek*, out, + *topos*, place]

phlebemphraxis (flĕb″ĕm-frăk′sĭs) [" + *emphraxis*, stoppage]

phlebismus (flĕb-ĭz′mŭs) [" + *-ismos*, condition]

phlebitis (flĕ-bī′tĭs) [" + *itis*, inflammation]
p., adhesive
p., migrating
p. nodularis necrotisans
p., obliterative
p., plastic
p., proliferative
p., puerperal
p., sclerosing
p., sinus
p., suppurative

phlebo- [Gr. *phleps*, *phlebos*]

phlebogram (flĕb′ō-grăm) [Gr. *phlebos*, blood vessel, vein, + *gramma*, letter, piece of writing]

phlebograph (flĕb′ō-grăf)

phlebography (flĕ-bŏg′ră-fē) [" + *graphein*, to write]

phleboid (flĕb′oyd) [" + *eidos*, form, shape]

phlebolith, phlebolite (flĕb′ō-lĭth, -lĭt) [" + *lithos*, a stone]

phlebolithiasis (flĕb″ō-lĭ-thī′ă-sĭs) [" + *lithiasis*, forming stones]

phlebology (flĕb-ŏl′ō-jē) [" + *logos*, word, reason]

phlebomanometer (flĕb″ō-mă-nŏm′ĕ-tĕr) [" + *manos*, thin, + *metron*, measure]

phlebometritis (flĕb″ō-mē-trī′tĭs) [" + *metra*, uterus, + *itis*, inflammation]

phlebomyomatosis (flĕb″ō-mī″ō-mă-tō′sĭs) [" + *mys*, muscle, + *oma*, tumor, + *osis*, condition]

phlebopexy (flĕb′ō-pĕk″sē) [" + *peksis*, fixation]

phlebophlebostomy (flĕb″ō-flĕ-bŏs′tō-mē) [" + *phlebos*, blood vessel, vein, + *stoma*, mouth, opening]

phleboplasty (flĕb′ō-plăs″tē) [" + *plassein*, to form]

phleborrhagia (flĕb″ō-rā′jē-ă) [" + *rhegnynai*, to burst forth]

phleborrhaphy (flĕb-or′ă-fē) [" + *rhaphe*, seam]

phleborrhexis (flĕb″ō-rĕk′sĭs) [" + *rhexis*, rupture]

phlebosclerosis (flĕb″ō-sklē-rō′sĭs) [" + *sklerosis*, a hardening]

phlebostasia, phlebostasis (flĕb-ō-stā′zē-ă, -ŏs′tă-sĭs) [" + *stasis*, standing still]

phlebostenosis (flĕb″ō-stĕ-nō′sĭs) [" + *stenosis*, act of narrowing]

phlebothrombosis (flĕb″ō-thrŏm-bō′sĭs) [" + *thrombos*, a clot]

phlebotome (flĕb′ō-tōm) [" + *tome*, a cutting, slice]

phlebotomist (flĕ-bŏt′ō-mĭst) [" + *tome*, a cutting, slice]

phlebotomize (flĕ-bŏt′ō-mīz)

Phlebotomus (flĕ-bŏt′ō-mŭs) [" + *tome*, a cutting, slice]
P. argentipes
P. chinensis
P. papatasii

P. sergenti

P. verrucarum

phlebotomus fever (flĕ-bŏt′ō-mŭs)

phlebotomy (flĕ-bŏt′ō-mē) [″ + *tome*, a cutting, slice]

    p., bloodless

phlegm (flĕm) [Gr. *phlegma*]

phlegmasia (flĕg-mā′zē-ă) [Gr. *phlegmasia*]

    p. alba dolens

    p., cellulitic

    p. malabarica

phlegmatic (flĕg-măt′ĭk) [Gr. *phlegmatikos*]

phlegmon (flĕg′mŏn) [Gr. *phlegmone*, inflammation]

    p., bronze

    p., diffuse

    p., gas

    p., Holz

phlegmonous (flĕg′mŏn-ŭs)

phlogistic (flō-jĭs′tĭk) [Gr. *phlogistos*]

phlogogenic, phlogogenous (flō-gō-jĕn′ĭk, -gŏj′ĕn-ŭs) [Gr. *phlogosis*, inflammation, + *gennan*, to produce]

phlorhizin (flō-rī′zĭn)

phlyctena (flĭk-tē′nă) [Gr. *phlyktaina*]

phlyctenar (flĭk′tĕ-năr)

phlyctenoid (flĭk′tĕ-noyd) [″ + *eidos*, form, shape]

phlyctenosis (flĭk″tĕ-nō′sĭs) [″ + *osis*, condition]

phlyctenula (flĭk-tĕn′ū-lă) [L.]

phlyctenular (flĭk-tĕn′ū-lăr)

phlyctenule (flĭk′tĕn-ūl) [Gr. *phlyktaina*, a blister; L. *phlyctenula*]

phlyctenulosis (flĭk-tĕn-ū-lō′sĭs) [″ + *osis*, condition]

phobia (fō′bē-ă) [Gr. *phobos*, fear]

phobic (fō′bĭk) [Gr. *phobos*, fear]

phobic desensitization

phobophobia (fō″bō-fō′bē-ă) [″ + *phobos*, fear]

phocomelia (fō″kō-mē′lē-ă) [Gr. *phoke*, seal, + *melos*, limb]

phocomelus (fō-kŏm′ĕ-lŭs)

phonacoscope (fō-năk′ō-skōp) [Gr.

phone, voice, + *skopein*, to examine]

phonacoscopy (fō-nă-kŏs′kō-pē)

phonal (fō′năl) [Gr. *phone*, voice]

phonasthenia (fōn-ăs-thē′nē-ă) [″ + *asthenia*, weakness]

phonation (fō-nā′shŭn)

phonatory (fō′nă-tō″rē) [Gr. *phone*, voice]

phonautograph (fōn-aw′tō-grăf) [″ + *autos*, self, + *graphein*, to write]

phone, -phone (fōn) [Gr. *phone*, voice]

phoneme (fō′nēm) [Gr. *phonema*, an utterance]

phonendoscope (fō-nĕn′dō-skōp) [Gr. *phone*, voice, + *endon*, within, + *skopein*, to examine]

phonendoskiascope (fō-nĕn″dō-skī′ă-skōp) [″ + ″ + *skia*, shadow, + *skopein*, to examine]

phonetics (fō-nĕt′ĭks) [Gr. *phonetikos*, spoken]

phoniatrics (fō″nē-ăt′rĭks) [Gr. *phone*, voice, + *iatrikos*, treatment]

phonic (fō′nĭk)

phonism (fō′nĭzm) [″ + *-ismos*, condition]

phono- [Gr. *phone*, voice]

phonocardiogram (fō″nō-kăr′dē-ō-grăm) [″ + *kardia*, heart, + *gramma*, letter, piece of writing]

phonocardiography (fō″nō-kăr″dē-ŏg′ră-fē) [″ + ″ + *graphein*, to write]

phonocatheter (fō″nō-kăth′ĕ-tĕr) [″ + *katheter*, something inserted]

phonogram (fō′nō-grăm) [″ + *gramma*, letter, piece of writing]

phonograph (fō′nō-grăf) [″ + *graphein*, to write]

phonology (fō-nŏl′ō-jē) [″ + *logos*, word, reason]

phonomania (fōn″ō-mā′nē-ă) [Gr. *phonos*, murder, + *mania*, madness]

phonomassage (fō″nō-mă-sahzh′)

[Gr. *phone*, voice, + *massein*, to knead]

phonometer (fō-nŏm'ĕ-tĕr) [" + *metron*, measure]

phonomyoclonus (fō"nō-mī-ŏk'lō-nŭs) [" + *mys*, muscle, + *klonos*, a contraction]

phonomyogram (fō"nō-mī'ō-grăm) [" + " + *gramma*, letter, piece of writing]

phonomyography (fō"nō-mī-ŏg'ră-fē) [" + " + *graphein*, to write]

phonopathy (fō-nŏp'ă-thē) [" + *pathos*, disease, suffering]

phonophobia (fō"nō-fō'bē-ă) [" + *phobos*, fear]

phonophotography

phonopsia (fō-nŏp'sē-ă) [" + *opsis*, sight, appearance, vision]

phonoreceptor

phonorenogram (fō"nō-rē'nō-grăm) [" + L. *ren*, kidney, + Gr. *gramma*, letter, piece of writing]

phonoscope (fō'nō-skōp) [" + *skopein*, to examine]

phonoscopy (fō-nŏs'kō-pē)

-phoresis (fō-rē'sĭs) [Gr. *phoresis*, being borne]

-phoria [Gr. *phoresis*, being borne]

Phormia (for'mē-ă)

phorotone (fō'rō-tōn) [Gr. *phora*, motion, + *tonos*, act of stretching, tension, tone]

phorozoon (fō"rō-zō'ŏn) [Gr. *phoros*, fruitful, + *zoon*, animal]

phose (fōz) [Gr. *phos*, light]

phosgene (fŏs'jēn) [" + *genes*, born]

phosphagen (fŏs'fă-jĕn)

Phosphaljel

phosphatase (fŏs'fă-tās)
    p., acid
    p., alkaline

phosphate (fŏs'fāt) [Gr. *phosphas*]
    p., acid
    p., calcium
    p., creatine

    p., normal
    p., triple

phosphate-bond energy

phosphatemia (fŏs"fă-tē'mē-ă) [Gr. *phosphas*, phosphate, + *haima*, blood]

phosphatide (fŏs'fă-tīd)

phosphatoptosis (fŏs"fă-tŏp-tō'sĭs) [" + *ptosis*, fall, falling]

phosphaturia (fŏs"fă-tū'rē-ă) [" + *ouron*, urine]

phosphene (fŏs'fēn) [Gr. *phos*, light, + *phainein*, to show]
    p., accommodation

phosphide (fŏs'fīd) [" + *phorein*, to carry]

phosphite (fŏs'fīt)

phosphoamidase (fŏs"fō-ăm'ĭ-dās)

phosphocreatine (fŏs"fō-krē'ă-tĭn)

phosphofructokinase (fŏs"fō-frŭk"tō-kī'nās)

Phospholine Iodide

phospholipase (fŏs"fō-lĭp'ās)

phospholipid (fŏs"fō-lĭp'ĭd) [Gr. *phos*, light, + *phorein*, to carry, + *lipos*, fat]

phospholipin (fŏs"fō-lĭp'ĭn)

phosphonecrosis (fŏs"fō-nĕ-krō'sĭs) [" + *phorein*, to carry, + *nekrosis*, state of death]

phosphonuclease (fŏs"fō-nū'klē-ās)

phosphopenia (fŏs"fō-pē'nĕ-ă) [" + *phorein*, to carry, + *penia*, lack]

phosphoprotein (fŏs"fō-prō'tē-ĭn) [" + " + *protos*, first]

phosphor
    p., rare earth

phosphorated (fŏs'fō-rā"tĕd) [" + *phorein*, to carry]

phosphorescence (fŏs-fō-rĕs'ĕns)

phosphorhidrosis (fŏs"for-hĭd-rō'sĭs) [" + *phorein*, to carry, + *hidrosis*, sweating]

phosphoribosyltransferase (fŏs"fō-rī"bō-sĭl-trăns'fĕr-ās)

phosphoric acid (fŏs-for'ĭk)

phosphoridrosis (fŏs'for-ĭd-rō'sĭs)

[" + *phorein*, to carry, + *hi-drosis*, sweat]

phosphorism (fŏs'for-ĭzm) [" + " + *-ismos*, condition]

phosphorolysis (fŏs"fō-rŏl'ĭ-sĭs)

phosphorous acid (fŏs-fō'rŭs, fŏs'for-ŭs) [" + *phoros*, carrying]

phosphoruria (fŏs"for-ū'rē-ă) [" + *phorein*, to carry, + *ouron*, urine]

phosphorus (fŏs'fō-rŭs) [Gr. *phos*, light, + *phoros*, carrying]

phosphorus poisoning

phosphoryl (fŏs'for-ĭl)

phosphorylase (fŏs-for'ĭ-lās)

phosphorylation (fŏs"for-ĭ-lā'shŭn)

phosphuria (fŏs-fū'rē-ă) [Gr. *phos*, light, + *phoros*, a bearer, + *ouron*, urine]

phot (fŏt) [Gr. *photos*, light]

photalgia (fō-tăl'jē-ă) [Gr. *photos*, light, + *algos*, pain]

photaugiaphobia (fō-taw"jē-ă-fō'bē-ă) [Gr. *photaugeia*, glare, + *phobos*, fear]

photechy (fō'tĕk-ē) [Gr. *photos*, light, + *echo*, echo]

photesthesis (fō"tĕs-thē'sĭs) [" + *aisthesis*, feeling, perception]

photic (fō'tĭk)

photic driving

photic epilepsy

photic sneezing

photism (fō'tĭzm) [" + *-ismos*, condition]

photo- [Gr. *photos*]

photoactinic (fō"tō-ăk-tĭn'ĭk)

photoallergic contact dermatitis

photoallergy (fō"tō-ăl'ĕr-jē) [" + *allos*, other, + *ergon*, work]

photobacterium (fō"tō-băk-tē'rē-ŭm)

photobiology (fō"tō-bī-ŏl'ō-jē) [" + *bios*, life, + *logos*, word, reason]

photobiotic (fō"tō-bī-ŏt'ĭk) [" + *bios*, life]

photocatalysis (fō"tō-kă-tăl'ĭ-sĭs) [" + *katalyein*, to dissolve]

photoceptor (fō"tō-sĕp'tor) [" + L. *ceptor*, a receiver]

photochemistry (fō"tō-kĕm'ĭs-trē)

[" + *chemeia*, chemistry]

photochromic glass

photochromogen [" + *chroma*, color, + *gennan*, to produce]

photocoagulation

photodermatitis (fō"tō-dĕr-mă-tī'tĭs) [" + *dermatos*, skin, + *itis*, inflammation]

photodynamic (fō"tō-dī-năm'ĭk) [" + *dynamis*, force]

photodynamic action

photodynia (fō"tō-dĭn'ē-ă) [" + *odyne*, pain]

photodysphoria (fō"tō-dĭs-for'ē-ă) [" + *dysphoria*, distress]

photoelectricity (fō"tō-ē-lĕk-trĭ'sĭ-tē) [" + *elektron*, amber]

photoelectron (fō"tō-ē-lĕk'trŏn) [" + *elektron*, amber]

photoerythema (fō"tō-ĕr"ĭ-thē'mă) [" + *erythema*, redness]

photofluorography (fō"tō-flū"ĕr-ŏg'ră-fē)

photogastroscope (fō"tō-găs'trō-skōp) [" + *gaster*, belly, + *skopein*, to view]

photogene (fō"tō-jēn) [" + *gennan*, to produce]

photogenic, photogenous (fō"tō-jĕn'ĭk, -tŏj'ĕn-ŭs)

photogenic epilepsy

photographic radiometer

photohemotachometer (fō"tō-hĕm"ō-tăk-ŏm'ĕ-tĕr) [" + *haima*, blood, + *tachys*, swift, + *metron*, measure]

photokinetic (fō"tō-kĭn-ĕt'ĭk) [" + *kinetikos*, motion]

photokymograph (fō"tō-kī'mō-grăf) [" + *kyma*, wave, + *graphein*, to write]

photolabile

photoluminescence (fō"tō-lū-mĭ-nĕs'ĕns) [" + L. *lumen*, light]

photolysis (fō-tŏl'ĭ-sĭs) [" + *lysis*, dissolution]

photolyte (fō'tō-līt)

photolytic (fō"tō-lĭt'ĭk)

photomania (fō"tō-mā'nē-ă) [" +

mania, madness]
photometer (fō-tŏm'ĕt-ĕr) [" + *metron*, measure]
photometry (fō-tŏm'ĕ-trē)
photomicrograph (fō"tō-mī'krō-grăf) [" + *mikros*, small, + *graphein*, to write]
photomotor
photon (fō'tŏn) [Gr. *photos*, light]
photonosus (fō-tŏn'ō-sŭs) [" + *nosos*, disease]
photo-ophthalmia, photophthalmia (fō"tō-ŏf-thăl'mē-ă, fō"tŏf-thăl'mē-ă) [" + *ophthalmos*, eye]
photopathy (fō-tŏp'ă-thē) [" + *pathos*, disease, suffering]
photoperceptive (fō"tō-pĕr-sĕp'tĭv) [" + *percipere*, to receive]
photoperiod (fō"tō-pēr'ē-ŏd) [" + *periodus*, period]
photoperiodism (fō"tō-pēr'ē-ō-dĭzm) [" + " + Gr. *-ismos*, condition]
photophilic (fō-tō-fil'ĭk) [" + *philein*, to love]
photophobia (fō"tō-fō'bē-ă) [" + *phobos*, fear]
photophone (fō'tō-fōn) [" + *phone*, voice]
photopia
photopic (fō-tŏp'ĭk)
photopsia, photopsy (fō-tŏp'sē-ă, fō-tŏp'sē) [Gr. *photos*, light, + *opsis*, sight, appearance, vision]
photopsin (fō-tŏp'sĭn)
photoptarmosis (fō"tō-tăr-mō'sĭs) [" + *ptarmosis*, sneezing]
photoptometer (fō-tō-tŏp'tŏm'ĕ-tĕr) [" + *opsis*, sight, appearance, vision, + *metron*, measure]
photoptometry (fō"tŏp-tŏm'ĕ-trē)
photoradiometer (fō"tō-rā"dē-ŏm'ĕ-tĕr) [" + L. *radius*, ray, + Gr. *metron*, measure]
photoreaction (fō"tō-rē-ăk'shŭn) [" + LL. *reactus*, reacted]
photoreactivation (fō"tō-rē-ăk"tĭ-vā'shŭn)
photoreception (fō"tō-rē-sĕp'shŭn) [" + L. *recipere*, to receive]

photoreceptive (fō"tō-rē-sĕp'tĭv) [" + *receptor*, a receiver]
photoreceptor (fō"tō-rē-sĕp'tor)
photoretinitis (fō"tō-rĕt"ĭ-nī'tĭs) [Gr. *photos*, light, + L. *retina*, retina, + Gr. *itis*, inflammation]
photoscan
photoscope (fō'tō-skōp) [" + *skopein*, to examine]
photoscopy (fō-tŏs'kō-pē)
photosensitivity [" + L. *sensitivus*, feeling]
photosensitization (fō"tō-sĕn"sī-tĭ-zā'shŭn)
photosensitizer (fō"tō-sĕn"sī-tī'zĕr)
photostable (fō'tō-stā"b'l) [" + L. *stabilis*, stable]
photosynthesis (fō"tō-sĭn'thĕ-sĭs) [" + *synthesis*, placing together]
phototaxis (fō"tō-tăk'sĭs) [Gr. *photos*, light, + *taxis*, arrangement]
phototherapy (fō"tō-thĕr'ă-pē) [" + *therapeia*, treatment]
photothermal (fō"tō-thĕr'măl) [" + *therme*, heat]
photothermal radiation
phototimer
phototonus (fō-tŏt'ō-nŭs) [" + *tonos*, act of stretching, tension, tone]
phototopia (fō"tō-tō'pē-ă)
phototoxic (fō"tō-tŏk'sĭk) [" + *toxikon*, poison]
phototoxis (fō"tō-tŏk'sĭs)
phototrophic (fō"tō-trŏf'ĭk) [" + *trophe*, nutrition]
phototropism (fō-tŏt'rō-pĭzm) [" + *tropos*, turning, + *-ismos*, condition]
photuria (fō-tū'rē-ă) [" + *ouron*, urine]
phren (frĕn, frēn) [Gr.]
phrenalgia (frĕ-năl'jē-ă) [Gr. *phren*, mind, + *algos*, pain; *phren*, diaphragm, + *algos*, pain]
phrenectomy (frĕ-nĕk'tō-mē) [Gr. *phren*, diaphragm, + *ektome*, excision]
phrenemphraxis (frĕn"ĕm-frăk'sĭs) [" + *emphraxis*, stoppage]

phrenetic (frĕn-ĕt'ĭk) [Gr. *phren*, mind]
phrenic (frĕn'ĭk) [Gr. *phren*, diaphragm, mind]
phrenic avulsion
phrenicectomy (frĕn-ĭ-sĕk'tō-mē [" + *ektome*, excision]
phreniclasia (frĕn"ĭ-klā'zē-ă) [" + *klasis*, destruction]
phrenic nerve
phrenicoexeresis (frĕn"ĭ-kō-ĕk-sĕr'ĕ-sĭs) [" + *exairesis*, taking out]
phreniconeurectomy (frĕn"ĭ-kō-nū-rĕk'tō-mē) [" + *neuron*, nerve, + *ektome*, excision]
phrenicotomy (frĕn"ĭ-kŏt'ō-mē) [" + *tome*, a cutting, slice]
phrenicotripsy (frĕn"ĭ-kō-trĭp'sē) [" + *tripsis*, a rubbing, friction]
phrenitis (frē-nī'tĭs) [" + *itis*, inflammation]
phreno- [Gr. *phren*, mind; L. *phrenicus*, diaphragm]
phrenocolic (frĕn"ō-kŏl'ĭk) [Gr. *phren*, diaphragm, + *kolon*, colon]
phrenocolopexy (frĕn"ō-kō'lō-pĕk"sē) [" + *kolon*, colon, + *pexis*, fixation]
phrenodynia (frĕn"ō-dĭn'ē-ă) [" + *odyne*, pain]
phrenogastric (frĕn"ō-găs'trĭk) [" + *gaster*, belly]
phrenoglottic (frĕn"ō-glŏt'ĭk) [" + *glottis*, tongue]
phrenograph (frĕn'ō-grăf) [" + *graphein*, to write]
phrenohepatic (frĕn"ō-hĕ-păt'ĭk) [" + *hepar*, liver]
phrenologist (frē-nŏl'ō-jĭst) [Gr. *phren*, mind, + *logos*, word, reason]
phrenology (frē-nŏl'ō-jē) [" + *logos*, word, reason]
phrenopericarditis (frē"nō-pĕr"ĭ-kar-dī'tĭs) [Gr. *phren*, diaphragm, + *peri*, around, + *kardia*, heart, + *itis*, inflammation]
phrenoplegia (frĕn-ō-plē'jē-ă) [Gr. *phren*, mind, + *plege*, stroke; *phren*, diaphragm, + Gr. *plege*, stroke]

phrenoptosis (frĕn"ŏp-tō'sĭs) [Gr. *phren*, diaphragm, + *ptosis*, fall, falling]
phrenosin (frĕn'ō-sĭn)
phrenospasm (frĕn'ō-spăzm) [" + *spasmos*, a convulsion]
phrenosplenic (frĕn"ō-splĕn'ĭk) [" + *splen*, spleen]
phrenotropic (frĕn"ō-trōp'ĭk) [Gr. *phren*, mind, + *tropikos*, turning]
phrictopathic (frĭk-tō-păth'ĭk) [Gr. *phriktos*, shuddering, + *pathos*, disease, suffering]
phronesis (frō-nē'sĭs) [Gr.]
phrynoderma (frĭn-ō-dĕr'mă) [Gr. *phryne*, toad, + *derma*, skin]
phthalylsulfathiazole (thăl"ĭl-sŭl"fă-thī'ă-zōl)
phthiriasis (thĭr-ī'ă-sĭs) [Gr. *phtheiriasis*]
phthiriophobia (thĭr"ē-ō-fō'bē-ă) [Gr. *phtheir*, louse, + *phobos*, fear]
Phthirus (thĭr'ŭs) [Gr. *phtheir*, louse]
    P. pubis
phthisic (tĭz'ĭk) [*phthisikos*]
phthisical (tĭz-ĭ-kăl)
phthisis (tī'sĭs) [Gr., a wasting]
    p., abdominal
    p., black
    p. bulbi
    p., fibroid
    p., grinders
    p., miner's
    p., pulmonary
    p., stonecutter's
phycobilin (fī"kō-bĭl'ĭn)
phycochrome (fī'kō-krōm) [Gr. *phykos*, seaweed, + *chroma*, color]
phycocyanin (fī"kō-sī'ăn-ĭn)
phycoerythrin (fī"kō-ĕr'ĭ-thrĭn)
phycology (fī-kŏl'ō-jē) [Gr. *phykos*, seaweed, + *logos*, word, reason]
Phycomycetes (fī"kō-mī-sē'tēz) [" + *mykes*, fungus]
phycomycosis (fī"kō-mī-kō'sĭs) [" + " + *osis*, condition]
phylactic (fĭ-lăk'tĭk) [Gr. *phylaktikos*, preservative]
phylaxis (fĭ-lăk'sĭs) [Gr., protection]
phyletic (fĭ-lĕt'ĭk) [Gr. *phyletikos*]

phyllo- [Gr. *phyllon,* leaf]
phylloquinone (fĭl″ō-kwĭn′ōn)
phylogenesis (fī″lō-jĕn′ĕ-sĭs) [Gr. *phyle,* tribe, + *genesis,* generation, birth]
phylogenetic (fī″lō-jĕ-nĕt′ĭk)
phylogeny (fī-lŏj′ĕ-nē)
phylum (fī′lŭm) [Gr. *phylon,* tribe]
phyma (fī′mă) [Gr., a growth]
phymatoid (fī′mă-toyd) [″ + *eidos,* form, shape]
phymatorrhysin (fī″mă-tō-rī′sĭn)
phymatosis (fī-mă-tō′sĭs) [Gr. *phyma,* a growth, + *osis,* condition]
physaliform, physalliform (fĭ-săl′ĭ-form) [Gr. *physallis,* bubble, + L. *forma,* shape]
physaliphore (fĭ-săl′ĭ-for) [″ + *phorein,* to carry]
physaliphorous (fĭs″ă-lĭf′ō-rŭs)
physalis (fĭs′ă-lĭs) [Gr. *physallis,* bubble]
Physaloptera (fĭs″ă-lŏp′tĕr-ă) [″ + *pteron,* wing]
  P. caucasica
physiatrics (fĭz″ē-ăt′rĭks) [Gr. *physis,* nature, + *iatrikos,* treatment]
physiatrist (fĭz″ē-ăt′rĭst)
physic (fĭz′ĭk) [Gr. *physikos,* natural]
physical (fĭz′ĭ-kăl)
physical activity and exercise
physical examination
physical fitness
physical sign
physical therapist
physical therapy
physician (fĭ-zĭsh′ŭn) [O. Fr. *physicien*]
  p., attending
  p., family
  p., primary care
  p., resident
physician accountability
physician's assistant
Physicians' Desk Reference
physician shortage area
physicist (fĭz′ĭ-sĭst) [L. *physics,* natural sciences]
physico- [Gr. *physikos*]
physicochemical (fĭz″ĭ-kō-kĕm′ĭ-kăl) [″ + *chemeia,* chemistry]

physics (fĭz′ĭks) [Gr. *physis,* nature]
physio- [Gr. *physis*]
physiochemical (fĭz″ē-ō-kĕm′ĭ-kăl) [Gr. *physis,* nature, + *chemeia,* chemistry]
physiocogenic (fĭz″ē-ō-kō-jĕn′ĭk) [″ + *gennan,* to produce]
physiocopyrexia (fĭz″ē-ō-kō″pī-rĕk′sē-ă) [″ + *pyressein,* feverish]
physiognomy (fĭz″ē-ŏg′nō-mē) [Gr. *physis,* nature, + *gnomon,* a judge]
physiognosis (fĭz″ē-ŏg-nō′sĭs) [″ + *gnosis,* knowledge]
physiological (fĭz″ē-ō-lŏj′ĭ-kăl) [Gr. *physis,* nature, + *logos,* word, reason]
physiological salt solution
physiological tooth movement
physiologicoanatomical (fĭz″ē-ō-lŏj″ĭ-kō-ăn″ă-tŏm′ĭ-kăl) [″ + ″ + *anatome,* dissection]
physiologist (fĭz″ē-ŏl′ō-jĭst)
physiology (fĭz″ē-ŏl′ō-jē) [Gr. *physis,* nature, + *logos,* word, reason]
  p., cell
  p., comparative
  p., general
  p., pathologic
  p., special
physiomedical (fĭz″ē-ō-mĕd′ĭ-kăl) [″ + L. *medicina,* medicine]
physiopathologic (fĭz″ē-ō-păth″ō-lŏj′ĭk) [″ + *pathos,* disease, suffering, + *logos,* word, reason]
physiotherapy (fĭz″ē-ō-thĕr′ă-pē) [″ + *therapeia,* treatment]
physique (fĭ-zēk′) [Fr.]
physis (fī′sĭs) [Gr. *phyein,* to generate]
physo- [Gr. *physa,* air]
physocele (fī′sō-sēl) [Gr. *physa,* air, + *kele,* tumor, swelling]
physocephaly (fī″sō-sĕf′ă-lē) [″ + *kephale,* head]
physohematometra (fī″sō-hĕm″ă-tō-mē′tră) [″ + *haima,* blood, + *metra,* uterus]
physohydrometra (fī″sō-hī″drō-mē′tră) [″ + *hydor,* water, +

metra, uterus]

physometra (fĭ″sō-mē′tră) [″ + *metra*, uterus]

physopyosalpinx (fĭ″sō-pī″ō-săl′pĭnks) [″ + *pyon*, pus, + *salpinx*, tube]

physostigmine salicylate (fĭ″sō-stĭg′mēn săl-ĭs′ĭl-āt)

phytalbumose (fĭ-tăl′bū-mōs) [Gr. *phyton*, plant, + L. *albumen*, white of egg]

phytase (fĭ′tās) [″ + *ase*, enzyme]

phytin (fĭ′tĭn)

phyto-, phyt- [Gr. *phyton*]

phytoagglutinin (fĭ″tō-ă-gloo′tĭ-nĭn) [Gr. *phyton*, plant, + L. *agglutinans*, gluing]

phytoalexins

phytobezoar (fĭ″tō-bē′zor) [″ + Arabic *bazahr*, protecting against poison]

phytochemistry (fĭ″tō-kĕm′ĭs-trē) [″ + *chemeia*, chemistry]

phytocholesterol (fĭ″tō-kō-lĕs′tĕr-ōl) [″ + *chole*, bile, + *stereos*, solid]

phytogenesis (fĭ″tō-jĕn′ĕ-sĭs) [″ + *genesis*, generation, birth]

phytogenous (fĭ-tŏj′ĕ-nŭs) [″ + *gennan*, to produce]

phytohemagglutinin (fĭ″tō-hĕm-ă-glŭ′tĭ-nĭn) [″ + *haima*, blood, + L. *agglutinare*, to glue to]

phytoid (fĭ′toyd) [″ + *eidos*, form, shape]

phytomenadione (fĭ″tō-mĕn″ă-dī′ōn)

phytonadione (fĭ″tō-nă-dī′ōn)

phytoparasite (fĭ″tō-păr′ă-sīt) [Gr. *phyton*, plant, + *parasitos*, fellow guest]

phytopathogenic (fĭ″tō-păth″ō-jĕn′ĭk) [″ + *pathos*, disease, suffering + *gennan*, to produce]

phytopathology (fĭ″tō-pă-thŏl′ō-jē) [″ + ″ + *logos*, word, reason]

phytophagous (fĭ-tŏf′ă-gŭs) [″ + *phagein*, to eat]

phytopharmacology (fĭ″tō-făr″mă-kŏl′ō-jē) [″ + *pharmakon*, drug, + *logos*, word, reason]

phytophotodermatitis (fĭ″tō-fō″tō-dĕr″mă-tī′tĭs) [″ + *photos*, light, + *derma*, skin, + *itis*, inflammation]

phytoplankton (fĭ″tō-plănk′tŏn) [″ + *planktos*, wandering]

phytoplasm (fĭ′tō-plăzm) [″ + LL. *plasma*, form, mold]

phytoprecipitin (fĭ″tō-prē-sĭp′ĭ-tĭn)

phytosis (fĭ-tō′sĭs) [″ + *osis*, condition]

phytosterol (fĭ″tō-stē′rŏl)

phytotoxic (fĭ″tō-tŏk′sĭk)

phytotoxin (fĭ″tō-tŏk′sĭn) [Gr. *phyton*, plant, + *toxikon*, poison]

pl

pia (pē′ă) [L.]

pia-arachnitis (pē″ă-ăr″ăk-nī′tĭs)

pia-arachnoid

Piaget, Jean [Swiss philosopher and psychologist, 1896 – 1980]

pial (pī′ăl)

pia mater (pē′ă mā′tĕr) [L. *pia*, soft, + *mater*, mother]

pian (pē-ăn′) [Fr.]

pianists' cramp

piarachnitis (pī″ăr-ăk-nī′tĭs) [L. *pia*, tender, + Gr. *arachne*, spider, + *itis*, inflammation]

piarachnoid (pī″ăr-ăk′noyd) [″ + ″ + *eidos*, form, shape]

pica (pī′kă) [L., magpie]

piceous (pī′sē-ŭs) [L. *piceus*, pitch]

Pick, Arnold [Czechoslovakian physician, 1851 – 1924]
P.'s disease

Pick, Friedel [Czechoslovakian physician, 1867 – 1926]
P.'s disease

Pick, Ludwig [Ger. physician, 1868 – 1944]
P.'s cells
P.'s disease

pick

pickling

pickwickian syndrome

pico- [It. *pico*, small]
picogram
picornaviruses (pī-kor″nă-vī'rŭ-sĕs) [″ + RNA, ribonucleic acid, + L. *virus*, virus]
picrate (pĭk'rāt)
picric acid
picro-, picr- [Gr. *pikros*, bitter]
picrocarmine (păk″rō-kăr'mĭn)
picroformal (pĭk″rō-for'măl)
picrotoxin (pĭk″rō-tŏk'sĭn) [″ + *toxikon*, poison]
pictograph (pĭk'tō-grăf)
PID *pelvic inflammatory disease*
piebald skin (pī'băld) [ME. *pie*, magpie, + *ballede*, bald]
piedra (pē-ā'dră) [Sp., stone]
Pierre Robin syndrome [Pierre Robin, Fr. pediatrician, 1867–1950]
piesesthesia (pī-ē″zĕs-thē'zē-ă) [Gr. *piesis*, pressure, + *aisthesis*, feeling, perception]
piesimeter, piesometer (pī″ĕ-sĭm'ĕ-tĕr, -sŏm'ĕ-tĕr) [″ + *metron*, measure]
piezochemistry (pī-ē'zō-kĕm″ĭs-trē) [Gr. *piezein*, to squeeze, + *chemeia*, chemistry]
piezoelectricity [″ + *elektron*, amber]
piezogenic pedal papules (pī-ē'zō-jĕn″ĭk) [″ + *gennan*, to produce]
piezometer (pī″ē-zŏm'ĕ-tĕr) [″ + *metron*, measure]
PIF *proliferation inhibiting factor*
pigeon breast
pigeon-breeder's disease
pigeon-toed
pigment (pĭg'mĕnt) [L. *pigmentum*, paint]
   p.'s, bile
   p., blood
   p., endogenous
   p., exogenous
   p., hematogenous
   p., hepatogenous
   p., respiratory
   p., skin

   p., urinary
   p., uveal
pigmentary (pĭg'mĕn-tĕr″ē) [L. *pigmentum*, paint]
pigmentation (pĭg″mĕn-tā'shŭn)
   p., hematogenous
pigmented (pĭg'mĕnt-ĕd)
pigmentolysin (pĭg″mĕn-tŏl'ĭ-sĭn) [″ + Gr. *lysis*, dissolution]
pigmentophage (pĭg-mĕn'tō-fāj) [″ + Gr. *phagein*, to eat]
pigmentophore (pĭg-mĕn'tō-for) [″ + Gr. *phorein*, to carry]
pigmentum nigrum (pĭg-mĕn'tŭm nī'grŭm) [L., black paint]
piitis (pī-ī'tĭs) [L. *pia*, tender, + Gr. *itis*, inflammation]
pil. [L.] *pilula*, pill, or *pilulae*, pills
pila (pī'lă) [L., pillar]
pilar, pilary (pī'lăr, pĭl'ă-rē) [L. *pilaris*]
pilaster (pī-lăs'tĕr) [L. *pilastrum*, small pillar]
pile [L. *pila*, a ball, a pillar]
   p., sentinel
pileous (pī'lē-ŭs) [L. *pilus*, hair]
piles (pīls) [L. *pila*, a mass]
pileum (pī'lē-ŭm) [L., a cap]
pileus (pī'lē-ŭs) [L., a cap]
pili (pī'lē)
   p. annulata
   p. incarnati
   p. tactiles
   p. torti
piliation (pī-lē-ā'shŭn) [L. *pilus*, hair]
piliform (pī'lĭ-form) [″ + *forma*, shape]
pilimiction (pī″lĭ-mĭk'shŭn) [″ + *mictio*, micturition]
pill (pĭl) [L. *pilula*, small mass]
   p., morning-after
pillar (pĭl'ĕr) [L. *pila*, a column]
   p.'s, anterior, of fornix
   p.'s of Corti
   p.'s of diaphragm
   p.'s of fauces
pillar cells
pillet (pĭl'ĕt)
pillion (pĭl'yŭn) [L. *pellis*, skin]

pilo- [L. *pilus*]

pilobezoar (pī"lō-bē'zor) [" + Arabic *bazahr*, protecting against poison]

pilocarpine hydrochloride (pī"lō-kǎr'pīn)

pilocarpine nitrate

pilocystic (pī"lō-sĭs'tĭk) [L. *pilus*, hair, + Gr. *kystis*, bladder]

piloerection

pilojection [" + *jacere*, to throw]

pilomatrixoma

pilomotor (pī"lō-mō'tor) [" + *motor*, mover]

pilomotor nerve

pilomotor reflex

pilonidal (pī"lō-nī'dǎl) [" + *nidus*, nest]

pilonidal cyst

pilonidal fistula

pilonidal sinus

pilose (pī'lōs) [L. *pilosus*]

pilosebaceous (pī"lō-sē-bā'shŭs) [" + *sebaceus*, fatty]

pilosis (pī-lō'sĭs) [L. *pilosus*, hairy, + Gr. *osis*, condition]

pilosity (pī-lŏs'ĭ-tē)

pilous (pī'lŭs) [L. *pilus*, hair]

Piltz's reflex (pĭlts'ĕz) [Jan Piltz, Polish neurologist, 1870–1931]

pilula (pĭl'ū-lǎ) [L., pill]

pilular (pĭl'ū-lar)

pilule (pĭl'ūl) [L. *pilula*]

pilus (pī'lŭs) [L.]
    p. cuniculatus
    p. incarnatus
    p. tortus

pimel- [Gr. *pimele*, fat]

pimelitis (pĭm-ĕl-ī'tĭs) [Gr. *pimele*, fat, + *itis*, inflammation]

pimeloma (pĭm"ĕ-lō'mǎ) [" + *oma*, tumor]

pimelopterygium (pĭm"ĕ-lō-tĕ-rĭj'ē-ŭm) [" + *pterygion*, wing]

pimelorrhea (pĭm"ĕl-or-ē'ǎ) [" + *rhein*, to flow]

pimelorthopnea (pĭm"ĕl-or"thŏp'nē-ǎ) [" + *orthos*, straight, + *pnoia*, breath]

pimelosis (pĭm"ĕ-lō'sĭs) [" + *osis*, condition]

pimeluria (pĭm"ĕl-ū'rē-ǎ) [" + *ouron*, urine]

pimple (pĭm'pl) [ME. *pinple*]

pin
    p., endodontic
    p., self-threading
    p., Steinmann

pincement (pǎns-mŏn') [Fr.]

pinch

pinch meter

pindolol (pĭn'dō-lōl)

pineal (pĭn'ē-ǎl) [Fr., pine cone]

pineal body (gland)

pinealectomy (pĭn"ē-ǎl-ĕk'tō-mē) [L. *pineus*, of the pine, + Gr. *ektome*, excision]

pineal gland

pinealism (pĭn'ē-ǎl-ĭzm) [" + Gr. *-ismos*, condition]

pinealoblastoma (pĭn"ē-ǎ-lō-blǎs-tō'mǎ) [" + Gr. *blastos*, germ, + *oma*, tumor]

pinealocyte (pĭn'ē-ǎ-lō-sīt") [" + Gr. *kytos*, cell]

pinealoma (pĭn"ē-ǎ-lō'mǎ) [" + Gr. *oma*, tumor]

pinealopathy (pĭn"ē-ǎ-lŏp'ǎ-thē) [" + Gr. *pathos*, disease, suffering]

Pinel, Philippe (pē-nĕl') [Fr. psychologist, 1745–1826]

pineoblastoma (pĭn"ē-ō-blǎs-tō'mǎ) [L. *pineus*, of the pine, + Gr. *blastos*, germ, + *oma*, tumor]

pine tar

ping-ponging

pinguecula (pĭn-gwĕk'ū-lǎ) [L. *pinguiculus*, fatty]

pinhole (pĭn'hōl) [AS. *pinn*, pin, + *hol*, hole]

pinhole os

pinhole pupil

piniform (pĭn'ĭ-form) [L. *pinea*, pine cone, + *forma*, shape]

pink disease

pinkeye [D. *pinck oog*]

pinna (pĭn′ă) [L., feather]
   p. nasi
pinnal (pĭn′ăl)
pinocyte (pī′nō-sīt) [Gr. *pinein*, to drink,
   + *kytos*, cell]
pinocytosis (pī″nō-sī-tō′sĭs) [″ + ″
   + *osis*, condition]
pinosome (pī′nō-, pĭn′ō-sōm) [″ +
   soma, body]
PINS *persons in need of supervision*
Pins' sign [Emil Pins, Aust. physician,
   1845–1913]
pint (pīnt) [ME. *pinte*]
pinta (pēn′tă) [Sp., paint]
pintid (pĭn′tĭd)
pinus (pī′nŭs) [L., pine]
pinworm
pioepithelium (pī″ō-ĕp″ĭ-thē′lē-ŭm)
   [Gr. *pion*, fat, + *epi*, upon, +
   thele, nipple]
pionemia (pī″ō-nē′mē-ă) [″ +
   haima, blood]
pion therapy
piorthopnea (pī″or-thŏp-nē′ă) [″ +
   orthos, straight, + *pnoia*, breath]
Piper (pī′pĕr) [L.]
piperacetazine (pĭp″ĕr-ă-sĕt′ă-zēn)
piperazine (pī-pĕr′ă-zēn)
piperoxan (pī″pĕr-ŏks′ăn)
pipet, pipette (pī-pĕt′) [Fr. *pipette*, tiny
   pipe]
pipobroman (pī″pō-brō′măn)
piptonychia (pĭp″tō-nĭk′ē-ă) [Gr. *pip-
tein*, to fall, + *onyx*, nails]
piriform (pĭr′ĭ-form) [L. *pirum*, pear,
   + *forma*, shape]
Pirogoff's amputation (pĭr″ō-gŏfs′)
   [Nicolai I. Pirogoff, Russ. surgeon
   1810–1881]
Pirquet's test (pĕr-kāz′) [Clemens P.
   Pirquet, Aust. pediatrician, 1874–
   1929]
piscicide (pĭs′ĭ-sīd) [L. *piscis*, fish, +
   caedere, to kill]
pisiform (pī′sĭ-form) [L. *pisum*, pea, +
   forma, shape]
pit (pĭt) [ME. *pitt*, hole]
   p., anal

   p., auditory
   p., costal
   p., gastric
   p., lens
   p., nasal
   p. of stomach
   p., olfactory
   p., primitive
pitch (pĭch) [ME. *picchen*, to fix]
pitchblende (pĭch′blĕnd)
pith (pĭth)
pithecoid (pĭth′ē-koyd) [Gr. *pithekos*,
   ape, + *eidos*, form, shape]
pithiatic (pĭth-ē-ăt′ĭk) [Gr. *peithein*, to
   persuade, + *iatrikos*, healing]
pithiatism (pĭth-ī′ă-tĭzm) [″ + *iatos*,
   curable, + *-ismos*, condition]
pithiatric (pĭth″ē-ăt′rĭk) [″ + *iatreia*, healing]
pithiatry (pĭth-ī′ă-trē) [″ + *iatreia*,
   healing]
pithing (pĭth′ĭng) [ME. *pithe*]
pithode (pī′thōd) [Gr. *pithose*, wine
   cask, + *eidos*, form, shape]
Pitocin
Pitres' sections (pē-trēs′) [Jean A.
   Pitres, Fr. physician, 1848–1927]
Pitressin (pĭt-rĕs′ĭn)
Pitressin Tannate (synthetic)
pitting (pĭt′ĭng) [ME. *pitt*, hole]
pitting edema
pituicyte (pī-tū′ĭ-sīt) [L. *pituita*, phlegm,
   + Gr. *kytos*, cell]
pituita (pī-tū′ĭ-tă) [L., phlegm]
pituitarism (pī-tū′ĭ-tă-rĭzm) [″ +
   Gr. *-ismos*, condition]
pituitarium (pī-tū″ĭ-tăr′ē-ŭm) [L.]
pituitary (pī-tū′ĭ-tār″ē) [L. *pituitarius*,
   phlegm]
   p., anterior
   p., posterior
   p., whole
pituitary gland
pituitary (injection), posterior
pituitous (pī-tū′ĭ-tŭs)
Pituitrin (pī-tū′ĭ-trĭn)
pityriasis (pĭt″ĭ-rī′ă-sĭs) [Gr. *pityron*,
   bran, + *-iasis*, state or condi-

tion of]
  p. alba
  p. amiantacea
  p. capitis
  p. lichenoides, acute
  p. linguae
  p. nigra
  p. rosea
  p. rubra pilaris
  p. versicolor
pityroid (pĭt′ĭ-royd) [Gr. *pityron*, bran, + *eidos*, form, shape]
pivot (pĭv′ŭt)
pix (pĭks) [L.]
PJC *premature junctional contraction*
PK *psychokinesis*
pK *negative logarithm of the ionization constant*
PKU *phenylketonuria*
placebo (plă-sē′bō) [L., I shall please]
placenta (plă-sĕn′tă) [L., a flat cake]
  p., abruption of
  p., accessory
  p. accreta
  p., adherent
  p., annular
  p., battledore
  p., bidiscoidal
  p., bilobate
  p., bipartite
  p., chorioallantoic
  p., circinate
  p. circumvallata
  p., cirsoid
  p., cordiform
  p., deciduate
  p., dimidiate
  p., discoid
  p., double
  p., duplex
  p., endotheliochorial
  p., epitheliochorial
  p. fenestrata
  p., fetal
  p., fundal
  p., hemochorial
  p., hemoendothelial
  p., horseshoe

  p., incarcerated
  p., increta
  p., lateral
  p., maternal
  p., membranous
  p., multilobate
  p., nondeciduate
  p. percreta
  p. previa
  p. previa partialis
  p. reflexa
  p., reniform
  p., retained
  p. spuria
  p., succenturiate
  p., trilobate
  p., tripartite
  p., triple
  p. uterina
  p., velamentous
  p., villous
  p., zonary
placental (plă-sĕn′tăl) [L. *placenta*, a flat cake]
placental souffle
placentation (plă″sĕn-tā′shŭn)
placentitis (plă″sĕn-tī′tĭs) [″ + Gr. *itis*, inflammation]
placentography (plă″sĕn-tŏg′ră-fē) [″ + Gr. *graphein*, to write]
  p., indirect
placentoid (plă-sĕn′toyd) [″ + Gr. *eidos*, form, shape]
placentolysin (plă″sĕn-tŏl′ĭ-sĭn) [″ + Gr. *lysis*, dissolution]
placentoma (plă″sĕn-tō′mă) [″ + Gr. *oma*, tumor]
placentotherapy (plă-sĕn″tō-thĕr′ă-pē) [″ + Gr. *therapeia*, treatment]
Placido's disk (plă-sē′dōz) [Antonio Placido, Portuguese ophthalmologist, 1848–1916]
Placidyl
placing reflex
placode (plăk′ōd) [Gr. *plax*, plate, + *eidos*, form, shape]
  p., auditory
  p., lens

p., olfactory
placoid (plăk'oyd) [" + *eidos*, form, shape]
pladaroma (plăd-ă-rō'mă) [Gr. *pladaros*, damp, + *oma*, tumor]
pladarosis (plăd-ă-rō'sĭs) [" + *osis*, condition]
plagiocephalic (plă-jē"ō-sĕ-făl'ĭk) [Gr. *plagios*, oblique, + *kephale*, head]
plagiocephalism (plă"jē-ō-sĕf'ă-lĭzm)
plagiocephaly (plă"jē-ō-sĕf'ă-lē)
plague (plāg) [ME., calamity]
    p., ambulatory
    p., black
    p., bubonic
    p., glandular
    p., hemorrhagic
    p., larval
    p., murine
    p., pneumonic
    p., septicemic
    p., sylvatic
    p., white
plague vaccine
plan
    p., medical care
    p., nursing care
planaria (plă-năr'ē-ă)
planchet (plăn'chĕt)
plane (plān) [L. *planus*]
    p.'s, Addison's
    p., Aeby's
    p., alveolocondylar
    p., axiolabiolingual
    p., axiomesiodistal
    p., Baer's
    p., bite
    p., coccygeal
    p., coronal
    p., datum
    p., Daubenton's
    p.'s, focal
    p., Frankfort horizontal
    p., frontal
    p., Hodge's
    p., horizontal
    p.'s, inclined, of pelvis

p., intertubercular
p., Listing's
p., Meckel's
p., median
p., midsagittal
p., Morton's
p., occlusal
p.'s of pelvis
p. of refraction
p. of regard
p.'s, parallel, of pelvis
p., sagittal
p., subcostal
p., transverse
p., vertical
p., visual
planigram (plă'nĭ-grăm) [L. *planus*, plane, + Gr. *gramma*, letter, piece of writing]
planigraphy (plă-nĭg'ră-fē) [" + Gr. *graphein*, to write]
planimeter (plă-nĭm'ĕ-tĕr) [" + Gr. *metron*, measure]
planing (plā'nĭng)
plankton (plănk'tŏn) [Gr. *planktos*, wandering]
Planned Parenthood
planning
planocellular (plă"nō-sĕl'ū-lăr) [L. *planus*, plane, + *cellula*, cell]
planoconcave (plă"nō-kŏn'kāv) [" + *concavus*, hollow]
planoconvex (plă"nō-kŏn'vĕks) [" + L. *convexus*, arched]
planography (plă-nŏg'ră-fē) [" + Gr. *graphein*, to write]
planomania (plă"nō-mā'nē-ă) [Gr. *plane*, wandering, + Gr. *mania*, madness]
Planorbis (plăn-or'bĭs)
planotopokinesia (plă"nō-tŏp"ō-kĭ-nē'zē-ă) [" + *topos*, place, + *kinesis*, motion]
plant (plănt) [L. *planta*, shoot for planting]
planta pedis (plăn'tă pē'dŭs) [L.]
plantago seed (plăn-tă'gō)
plantalgia (plăn-tăl'jē-ă) [L. *planta*,

sole of the foot, + Gr. *algos*, pain]
plantar (plăn'tăr)
plantar arch
plantar flexion
plantar grasp reflex
plantaris (plăn-tăr'ĭs) [L.]
plantar reflex
plantar wart
plantation (plăn-tā'shŭn) [L. *plantare*, to plant]
plantigrade [L. *planta*, sole of the foot, + *gradi*, to walk]
planula (plăn'ū-lă)
planum (plā'nŭm) [L.]
　　p., nuchal
　　p., occipital
　　p., orbital
　　p., popliteal
　　p., sternal
　　p., temporal
planuria (plā-nū'rē-ă) [Gr. *plane*, wandering, + *ouron*, urine]
plaque (plăk) [Fr., a plate]
　　p., atheromatous
　　p., bacterial
　　p., dental
　　p., Hollenhorst
　　p., mucous
Plaquenil Sulfate
plasm (plăzm) [LL. *plasma*, form, mold]
plasma (plăz'mă) [LL. *plasma*, form, mold]
　　p., antihemophilic factor
　　p., blood
　　p., fresh frozen
　　p., hyperimmune
　　p., lymph
　　p., normal human
plasmablast (plăz'mă-blăst) [LL. *plasma*, form, mold, + Gr. *blastos*, germ]
plasmacyte (plăz'mă-sīt) [" + Gr. *kytos*, cell]
plasmacytoma (plăz"mă-sī'tō'mă) [" + " + *oma*, tumor]
plasmacytosis (plăz"mă-sī-tō'sĭs) [" + " + *osis*, condition]
plasma exchange therapy

plasmagel (plăz'mă-jĕl") [" + L. *gelare*, to congeal]
plasmagene (plăz'mă-jēn") [" + Gr. *gennan*, to produce]
plasmalemma (plăz"mă-lĕm'ă) [" + Gr. *lemma*, husk]
Plasmanate
plasmapheresis (plăz"mă-fĕr-ē'sĭs) [" + Gr. *aphairesis*, separation]
plasma protein fraction
plasmasome (plăz'mă-sōm) [" + Gr. *soma*, body]
Plasmatein
plasmatherapy (plăz"mă-thĕr'ă-pē) [" + Gr. *therapeia*, service]
plasmatic (plăz-măt'ĭk)
plasmatogamy (plăz"mă-tŏg'ă-mē) [" + Gr. *gamos*, marriage]
plasmatorrhexis (plăz"mă-tō-rĕk'sĭs) [" + Gr. *rhexis*, rupture]
plasma volume extender
plasmic (plăz'mĭk) [LL. *plasma*, form, mold]
plasmid
plasmin (plăz'mĭn)
plasminogen (plăz-mĭn'ō-jĕn)
plasmocyte (plăz'mō-sīt) [" + Gr. *kytos*, cell]
plasmocytoma (plăz"mō-sī-tō'mă) [" + " + *oma*, tumor]
plasmodesma (plăz"mō-dĕz'mă)
plasmodesmata (plăz"mō-dĕz'mă-tă) [" + Gr. *desmos*, bond]
plasmodial (plăz-mō'dē-ăl)
plasmodicidal (plăz"mō-dĭ-sī'dăl) [" + *eidos*, form, shape, + L. *cida* fr. *caedere*, to kill]
Plasmodium (plăz-mō'dē-ŭm)
　　P. falciparum
　　P. malariae
　　P. ovale
　　P. vivax
plasmodium (plăz-mō'dē-ŭm) [LL. *plasma*, form, mold, + Gr. *eidos*, form, shape]
plasmogamy (plăs-mŏg'ă-mē) [" + Gr. *gamos*, marriage]
plasmogen (plăz'mō-jĕn) [" + Gr.

gennan, to produce]
plasmology (plăz-mŏl'ō-jē) [" +
Gr. *logos,* word, reason]
plasmolysis (plăz-mŏl'ĭ-sĭs) [" +
Gr. *lysis,* dissolution]
plasmolyzable (plăz"mō-līz'ă-b'l)
plasmolyze (plăz'mō-līz)
plasmoma (plăz-mō'mă) [" + Gr.
oma, tumor]
plasmon (plăz'mŏn)
plasmoptysis (plăz-mŏp'tĭ-sĭs) [" +
Gr. *ptyein,* to spit]
plasmorrhexis (plăz"mō-rĕk'sĭs)
[" + Gr. *rhexis,* rupture]
plasmoschisis (plăz-mŏs'kĭ-sĭs) [" +
Gr. *schisis,* cleavage]
plasmotomy (plăz-mŏt'ō-mē) [" +
Gr. *tome,* a cutting, slice]
plasson (plăs'sŏn) [Gr. *plasson,*
forming]
plastein (plăs'tē-ĭn)
plaster [Gr. *emplastron*]
  p., adhesive
  p., blistering
  p., mustard
  p. of paris
  p., porous
  p., resin
  p., salicylic acid
  p., warming
plaster cast
plastic (plăs'tĭk) [Gr. *plastikos,* fit for
molding]
plastic bronchitis
plasticity (plăs-tĭs'ĭ-tē)
plastic surgery
plastid (plăs'tĭd) [Gr. *plastos,* formed]
plastogamy (plăs-tŏg'ă-mē) [" +
gamos, marriage]
plastron [Fr., breastplate]
-plasty [Gr. *plastos,* formed]
plate (plāt) [Gr. *plate,* flat]
  p., approximation
  p., auditory
  p., axial
  p., bite
  p., blood
  p., bone

  p., cortical
  p., deck
  p., dental
  p., dorsal
  p., end
  p., epiphyseal
  p., equatorial
  p., floor
  p., foot
  p., medullary
  p., muscle
  p., neural
  p., palate
  p., polar
  p., roof
  p., tarsal
  p., tympanic
  p., ventral
plateau
  p., ventricular
platelet (plāt'lĕt) [Gr. *plate,* flat]
platelet concentrate
plateletpheresis
plating
platinic (plă-tĭn'ĭk)
Platinol
platinosis
platinous (plăt'ĭ-nŭs)
platinum (plăt'ĭ-nŭm) [Sp. *platina*]
platy- [Gr. *platys,* broad]
platybasia (plăt"ē-bā'sē-ă)
platycelous (plăt-ē-sē'lŭs) [Gr. *platys,*
broad, + *koilos,* hollow]
platycephalic, **platycephalous**
(plăt"ē-sē-făl'ĭk, -sĕf'ă-lŭs) [" +
kephale, head]
platycephaly (plăt"ē-sĕf'ă-lē)
platycnemia (plăt-ĭk-nē'mē-ă) [" +
kneme, leg]
platycnemic (plăt"ĭk-nē'mĭk)
platycnemism (plăt"ĭk'nē-mĭzm)
platycoria, platycoriasis (plăt"ē-
kor-ē'ă, -kor-ī'ă-sĭs) [" + *kore,*
pupil]
platycoriasis (plăt"ē-kor-ī'ă-sĭs)
platycrania (plăt"ē-krā'nē-ă) [" +
kranion, skull]
platyglossal (plăt"ē-glŏs'ăl) [Gr.

platys, broad, + *glossa*, tongue]
platyhelminth (plăt″ē-hĕl′mĭnth)
Platyhelminthes (plăt″ē-hĕl-mĭn′thēz)
[″ + *helmins*, worm]
platyhieric (plăt″ē-hī-ĕr-ĭk) [″ +
hieron, sacrum]
platymeric (plăt″ē-mē′rĭk) [″ +
meros, thigh]
platymorphia (plăt″ē-mor′fē-ă) [″ +
morphe, form]
platyopia (plăt″ē-ō′pē-ă) [″ +
ops, face]
platyopic (plăt″ē-ŏp′ĭk)
platypellic, platypelvic (plăt″ē-
pĕl′ĭk, -vĭk) [″ + *pella*, a basin]
platypnea (plă″tĭp′nē-ă) [″ +
pnoia, breath]
platypodia (plăt″ē-pō′dē-ă) [″ +
pous, foot]
platyrrhine (plăt′ĭr-īn) [″ + *rhis*,
nose]
platysmal reflex (plăt-tĭz′măl rē′flĕks)
platysma myoides (plă-tĭz′mă
mī-oy′dēz) [Gr. *platysma*, plate, +
mys, muscle, + *eidos*, form, shape]
platyspondylia (plăt″ē-spŏn-dĭl′ē-ă)
platyspondylisis (plăt″ĭ-spŏn-dĭl′ĭ-sĭs)
[Gr. *platys*, flat, + *spondylos*, ver-
tebra]
platystencephaly (plăt″ĭ-stĕn-sĕf′ă-
lē) [″ + *kephale*, head]
play
pleasure principle
pledget (plĕj′ĕt) [origin uncertain]
plegaphonia (plĕg″ă-fō′nē-ă) [Gr.
plege, stroke, + *a-*, not, +
phone, voice]
-plegia (plē′jē-ă) [Gr. *plege*, stroke]
Plegine
pleio-, pleo-, plio- [Gr. *pleion, pleon*,
more]
pleiotropia (plī″ō-trō′pē-ă) [Gr.
pleion, more, + *trope*, turn]
pleiotropism (plī-ŏt′rō-pĭzm) [″ +
″ + *-ismos*, condition]
pleochroic (plē″ō-krō′ĭk) [Gr. *pleon*,
more, + *chroia*, color]
pleochroism (plē-ŏk′rō-ĭzm) [″ + ″

+ *-ismos*, condition]
pleochromatic (plē″ō-krō-măt′ĭk)
[″ + *chroma*, color]
pleocytosis (plē″ō-sī-tō′sĭs) [″ +
kytos, cell, + *osis*, condition]
pleomastia, pleomazia (plē″ō-
măs′tē-ă, -mā′zē-ă) [Gr. *pleon*, more,
+ *mastos, mazos*, breast]
pleomorphic (plē-ō-mor′fĭk) [″ +
morphe, form]
pleomorphism (plē-ō-mor′fĭzm) [″ +
″ + *-ismos*, condition]
pleomorphous (plē-ō-mor′fŭs)
pleonasm (plē′ō-năzm) [Gr. *pleon-
asmos*, exaggeration]
pleonexia (plē″ō-nĕk′sē-ă) [Gr.]
pleonosteosis (plē″ŏn-ŏs″tē-ō′sĭs)
[Gr. *pleon*, more, + *osteon*, bone,
+ *osis*, condition]
p., Leri's
pleoptics (plē-ŏp′tĭks) [″ + *optikos*,
sight]
plerocercoid
plerosis (plē-rō′sĭs) [Gr. *plerosis*, filling
up]
plesiomorphism (plē″sē-ō-mor′fĭzm)
[Gr. *plesios*, close, + *morphe*,
form, + *-ismos*, condition]
plesiomorphous (plē″sē-ō-mor′fŭs)
[″ + *morphe*, form]
plesiopia (plē″sē-ō′pē-ă) [″ +
ops, eye]
plessesthesia (plĕs″ĕs-thē′zē-ă) [Gr.
plessein, to strike, + *aisthesis*, feeling, perception]
plessimeter (plĕs-sĭm′ĕ-tĕr) [″ +
metron, measure]
plessor (plĕs′or) [Gr. *plessein*, to strike]
plethora (plĕth′ō-ră) [Gr. *plethore*, full-
ness]
plethoric (plē-thor′ĭk, plĕth′ō-rĭk)
plethysmograph (plē-thĭz′mō-grăf)
[Gr. *plethysmos*, to increase, +
graphein, to write]
plethysmography (plĕth″ĭz-mŏg′ră-fē)
pleur-, pleuro- [Gr. *pleura*, rib, side]
pleura (ploo′ră) [Gr., side]
p., costal

p. diaphragmatica
p., mediastinal
p., parietal
p. pericardiaca
p. phrenica
p. pulmonalis
p., visceral

pleuracentesis (ploor"ă-sĕn-tē'sĭs) [Gr. *pleura*, side, + *kentesis*, puncture]

pleuracotomy (ploor"ă-kŏt'ō-mē) [" + *tome*, a cutting, slice]

pleural (ploo'răl) [Gr. *pleura*, side]

pleural cavity

pleural fibrosis

pleuralgia (ploo-răl'jē-ă) [" + *algos*, pain]

pleurapophysis (ploo-ră-pŏf'ĭ-sĭs) [" + *apo*, from, + *physis*, a growth]

pleurectomy (ploo-rĕk'tō-mē) [" + *ektome*, excision]

pleurisy (ploo'rĭs-ē) [Gr. *pleuritis*]
p., acute
p., adhesive
p., diaphragmatic
p., dry
p., encysted
p., fibrinous
p., hemorrhagic
p., interlobar
p., plastic
p., pulmonary
p., purulent
p., sacculated
p., serofibrinous
p., serous
p., suppurative
p., tuberculous
p., typhoid
p., visceral
p., wet
p. with effusion

pleuritic (ploo-rĭt'ĭk) [Gr. *pleuritis*, pleurisy]

pleuritis (ploo-rī'tĭs) [Gr.]

pleuritogenous (ploor"ĭ-tŏj'ĕ-nŭs) [" + *gennan*, to produce]

pleurocele (ploo'rō-sēl) [Gr. *pleura*, side, + *kele*, tumor, swelling]

pleurocentesis (ploo"rō-sĕn-tē'sĭs) [" + *kentesis*, a piercing]

pleurocentrum (ploo"rō-sĕn'trŭm) [" + *kentron*, center]

pleurocholecystitis (ploo"rō-kō"lē-sĭst-ī'tĭs) [" + *chole*, bile, + *kystis*, bladder, + *itis*, inflammation]

pleuroclysis (ploo-rŏk'lĭ-sĭs) [" + *klysis*, a washing]

pleurodesis (ploo"rō-dē'sĭs) [" + *desis*, binding]

pleurodynia (ploo"rō-dĭn'ē-ă) [" + *odyne*, pain]
p., epidemic

pleurogenic (ploo"rō-jĕn'ĭk) [" + *gennan*, to produce]

pleurogenous (ploo-rŏj'ĕn-ŭs)

pleurography (ploo-rŏg'ră-fē) [" + *graphein*, to write]

pleurohepatitis (ploo"rō-hĕp"ă-tī'tĭs) [" + *hepatos*, liver, + *itis*, inflammation]

pleurolith (ploo'rō-lĭth) [" + *lithos*, stone]

pleurolysis (ploo-rŏl'ĭ-sĭs) [" + *lysis*, dissolution]

pleuromelus (ploor"ō-mē'lŭs) [" + *melos*, limb]

pleuroparietopexy (ploo"rō-păr-ī'ĕt-ō-pĕk"sē) [" + L. *parietalis*, wall, + Gr. *pexis*, fixation]

pleuropericardial (ploor"ō-pĕr-ī-kăr'dē-ăl) [" + *peri*, around, + *kardia*, heart]

pleuropericarditis (ploo"rō-pĕr"ī-kăr-dī'tĭs) [" + " + *itis*, inflammation]

pleuroperitoneal (ploo"rō-pĕr"ī-tō-nē'ăl) [" + *peritonaion*, stretched around or over]

pleuroperitoneal cavity

pleuropneumonia (ploo"rō-nū-mō'nē-ă) [" + *pneumon*, lung]

pleuropneumonia-like organisms

pleuropneumonolysis (ploo"rō-nū"mōn-ŏl'ĭ-sĭs) [Gr. *pleura*, side, + *pneumon*, lung, + *lysis*, dissolution]

pleuropulmonary (ploor"ō-pŭl'mō-nĕr"ē) [" + L. *pulmo*, lung]

pleurorrhea (ploor"ō-rē'ă) [" + *rhein*, to flow]

pleuroscopy (ploo-rŏs'kō-pē) [" + *skopein*, to examine]

pleurosoma (ploor"ō-sō'mă) [" + *soma*, body]

pleurothotonos (ploo"rō-thŏt'ō-nŏs) [Gr. *pleurothen*, from the side, + *tonos*, act of stretching, tension, tone]

pleurotomy (ploo-rŏt'ō-mē) [Gr. *pleura*, side, + *tome*, a cutting, slice]

pleurotyphoid (ploo"rō-tī'foyd) [" + *typhos*, fever, + *eidos*, form, shape]

pleurovisceral (ploo"rō-vĭs'ĕr-ăl) [" + L. *viscera*, viscera]

plexal (plĕk'săl) [L. *plexus*, a braid]

plexectomy (plĕk-sĕk'tō-mē) [" + Gr. *ektome*, excision]

plexiform (plĕk'sĭ-form) [" + *forma*, shape]

pleximeter (plĕks-ĭm'ĕ-tĕr) [Gr. *plexis*, stroke, + *metron*, measure]

plexitis (plĕk-sī'tĭs) [L. *plexus*, a braid, + Gr. *itis*, inflammation]

plexometer (plĕk-sŏm'ĕ-tĕr)

plexor (plĕks'or)

plexus (plĕks'ŭs) [L., a braid]
    p., autonomic
    p., cavernous
    p., enteric
    p., myenteric
    p., nerve
    p., pampiniform
    p., prevertebral

pliability (plī"ă-bĭl'ĭ-tē) [O. Fr. *pliant*, bend, + L. *abilis*, able]

plica (plī'kă) [L.]
    p., circular
    p., epiglottic
    p., lacrimal
    p., palmate
    p. polonica

    p., semilunar, of colon
    p., semilunar, of conjunctiva
    p., synovial
    p., transverse, of rectum

plicamycin

plicate (plī'kāt) [L. *plicatus*]

plication (plĭ-kā'shŭn) [L. *plicare*, to fold]
    p. of stomach

plicotomy (plĭ-kŏt'ō-mē) [" + Gr. *tome*, a cutting, slice]

plinth [Gr. *plinthos*, tile]

ploidy (ploy'dē) [Gr. *ploos*, a fold, + *eidos*, form, shape]

plombage (plŏm-băzh') [Fr. *plomber*, to plug]

plototoxin (plō"tō-tŏk'sĭn)

plug (plŭg) [MD. *plugge*]
    p., Dittrich's
    p., epithelial
    p., mucous
    p., Traube's
    p., vaginal

plugger
    p., automatic
    p., back-action
    p., foot

plumbic (plŭm'bĭk) [L. *plumbicus*, leaden]

plumbism (plŭm'bĭzm) [L. *plumbum*, lead, + Gr. *-ismos*, condition]

plumbum (plŭm'bŭm) [L.]

Plummer-Vinson syndrome (plŭm'ĕr-vĭn'sŏn) [Henry S. Plummer, U.S. physician, 1874–1937; Porter P. Vinson, U.S. surgeon, 1890–1959]

plumose (plū'mōs) [L. *plumosus*]

plumper (plŭm'pĕr) [Middle Low Ger. *plump*, to fill]

pluri- [L. *plus*, more]

pluriceptor (ploo"rĭ-sĕp'tor) [L. *plus*, more, + *ceptor*, a receiver]

pluridyscrinia (ploo"rĭ-dĭs-krĭn'ē-ă) [" + Gr. *dys*, bad, difficult, painful, disordered, + *krinein*, to secrete]

pluriglandular (ploo"rĭ-glănd'ū-lăr) [" + *glandula*, gland]

plurigravida (ploo"rĭ-grăv'ĭ-dă) [" +

gravida, pregnant]

plurilocular (ploo″rĭ-lŏk′ū-lăr) [″ + *loculus,* a cell]

plurinuclear (ploor″ĭ-nū′klē-ăr) [″ + *nucleus,* kernel]

pluripara (ploo-rĭp′ă-ră) [″ + *parere,* to beget, produce]

pluriparity (ploo″rĭ-păr′ĭ-tē)

pluripotent, pluripotential (ploo-rĭp′ō-tĕnt, ploor″ĭ-pō-tĕn′shăl) [″ + *potentia,* power]

pluripotentiality (ploor″ĭ-pō-tĕn″shē-ăl′ĭ-tē)

pluriresistant (ploor″ĭ-rē-zĭs′tănt) [″ + *resistens,* standing back]

plutomania (ploo″tō-mā′nē-ă) [Gr. *ploutos,* wealth, + *mania,* madness]

plutonium (ploo-tō′nē-ŭm) [Named after the planet Pluto]

Pm *promethium*

PMS *premenstrual syndrome*

PMSG *pregnant mare serum gonadotrophin*

PMT *premenstrual tension*

PNC *premature nodal contraction or complex*

pneo- (nē′ō) [Gr. *pnein,* to breathe]

pneocardiac reflex (nē″ō-kăr′dē-ăk) [Gr. *pnein,* to breathe, + *kardia,* heart]

pneodynamics (nē″ō-dĭ-năm′ĭks) [″ + *dynamis,* force]

pneogram (nē′ō-grăm) [″ + *gramma,* letter, piece of writing]

pneograph (nē′ō-grăf) [″ + *graphein,* to write]

pneometer (nē-ŏm′ĕ-tĕr) [Gr. *pnein,* to breathe, + *metron,* measure]

pneopneic reflex (nē-ŏp-nē′ĭk) [″ + *pnein,* to breathe]

pneoscope (nē′ō-skōp) [″ + *skopein,* to examine]

pneum-, pneuma-, pneumato- [Gr. *pneuma, pneumatos,* air, breath]

pneumarthrogram (nū-măr′thrō-grăm) [Gr. *pneuma,* air, + *arthron,* joint, + *gramma,* letter,

piece of writing]

pneumarthrography (nū″măr-thrŏg′ră-fē) [″ + ″ + *graphein,* to write]

pneumarthrosis (nū-măr-thrō′sĭs) [″ + ″ + *osis,* condition]

pneumascope (nū′mă-skōp) [″ + *skopein,* to examine]

pneumatic (nū-măt′ĭk) [Gr. *pneumatikos,* pert. to air]

pneumatics (nū-măt′ĭks)

pneumatinuria (nū″măt-ĭn-ū′rē-ă) [″ + *ouron,* urine]

pneumatization (nū″mă-tĭ-zā′shŭn)

pneumatized (nū′mă-tīzd)

pneumatocardia (nū″măt-ō-kăr′dē-ă) [″ + *kardia,* heart]

pneumatocele (nū-măt′ō-sēl) [″ + *kele,* tumor, swelling]

   p., extracranial

   p., intracranial

pneumatodyspnea (nū″măt-ō-dĭsp′nē-ă) [″ + *dys,* bad, difficult, painful, disordered, + *pneia,* breath]

pneumatogram (nū-măt′ō-grăm) [″ + *gramma,* letter, piece of writing]

pneumatograph (nū-măt′ō-grăf) [″ + *graphein,* to write]

pneumatology (nū″mă-tŏl′ō-jē) [″ + *logos,* word, reason]

pneumatometer (nū″măt-ŏm′ĕ-tĕr) [″ + *metron,* measure]

pneumatometry (nū″măt-ŏm′ĕ-trē)

pneumatorrhachis (nū″măt-or′ă-kĭs) [″ + *rhachis,* spine]

pneumatoscope (nū-măt′ō-skōp) [″ + *skopein,* to inspect]

pneumatosis (nū″mă-tō′sĭs) [Gr. *pneumatosis*]

   p. abdominis

   p. cystoides intestinalis

pneumatotherapy (nū″măt-ō-thĕr′ă-pē) [Gr. *pneumatos,* air, + *therapeia,* treatment]

pneumatothorax (nū″măt-ō-thō′răks) [″ + *thorax,* chest]

pneumaturia (nū″măt-ū′rē-ă) [Gr.

pneuma, air,　+　*ouron,* urine]

pneumatype (nū′mă-tīp) [″　+　*typos,* type]

pneumectomy (nū-mĕk′tō-mē) [Gr. *pneumon,* lung,　+　*ektome,* excision]

pneumo-, pneumono- [Gr. *pneumon,* lung]

pneumoangiography (nū″mō-ăn″jē-ŏg′ră-fē) [Gr. *pneumon,* lung,　+　*angeion,* vessel,　+　*graphein,* to write]

pneumoarthrography (nū″mō-ăr-thrŏg′ră-fē) [″　+　*arthron,* joint,　+　*graphein,* to write]

pneumobulbar (nū″mō-bŭl′băr) [″　+　L. *bulbus,* bulbous root]

pneumocardial (nū″mō-kăr′dē-ăl) [″　+　*kardia,* heart]

pneumocele (nū′mō-sēl)

pneumocentesis (nū″mō-sĕn-tē′sĭs) [″　+　*kentesis,* a piercing]

pneumocephalus (nū″mō-sĕf′ă-lŭs) [Gr. *pneuma,* air,　+　*kephale,* head]

pneumocholecystitis (nū″mō-kō″lē-sĭs-tī′tĭs) [″　+　*chole,* bile,　+　*kystis,* bladder,　+　*itis,* inflammation]

pneumococcal (nū″mō-kŏk′ăl) [″　+　*kokkos,* berry]

pneumococcal vaccine, polyvalent

pneumococcemia (nū″mō-kŏk-sē′mē-ă)

pneumococci (nū″mō-kŏk′sī)

pneumococcidal (nū″mō-kŏk-sī′dăl) [″　+　″　+　L. *cida,* fr. *caedere, to kill*]

pneumococcolysis (nū″mō-kŏk-ŏl′ĭ-sĭs) [″　+　*kokkos,* berry,　+　*lysis,* dissolution]

pneumococcus (nū″mō-kŏk′ŭs) [″　+　*kokkos,* berry]

pneumocolon (nū″mō-kō′lŏn) [″　+　*kolon,* colon]

pneumoconiosis (nū″mō-kō″nē-ō′sĭs) [″　+　*konis,* dust,　+　*osis,* condition]

pneumocranium (nū″mō-krā′nē-ŭm) [″　+　*kranion,* skull]

Pneumocystis carinii (nū″mō-sĭs′tĭs kă′rī-nē-ē)

pneumocystis pneumonia

pneumocystography (nū″mō-sĭs-tŏg′ră-fē) [Gr. *pneuma,* air,　+　*kystis,* bladder,　+　*graphein,* to write]

pneumocystosis (nū″mō-sĭs-tō′sĭs)

pneumoderma (nū″mō-dĕr′mă) [″　+　*derma,* skin]

pneumodynamics (nū″mō-dī-năm′ĭks) [″　+　*dynamis,* force]

pneumoempyema (nū″mō-ĕm-pī-ē′mă) [″　+　*en,* in　+　*pyon,* pus]

pneumoencephalitis (nū″mō-ĕn-sĕf″ă-lī′tĭs) [″　+　*enkephalos,* brain,　+　*itis,* inflammation]

pneumoencephalogram (nū″mō-ĕn-sĕf′ă-lō-grăm) [″　+　″　+　*gramma,* letter, piece of writing]

pneumoencephalography (nū″mō-ĕn-sĕf″ă-lŏg′ră-fē) [″　+　″　+　*graphein,* to write]

pneumoenteritis (nū″mō-ĕn″tĕr-ī′tĭs) [″　+　*enteron,* intestine,　+　*itis,* inflammation]

pneumofasciogram (nū″mō-făs′ē-ō-grăm) [″　+　L. *fascia,* a band,　+　Gr. *gramma,* letter, piece of writing]

pneumogalactocele (nū″mō-găl-ăk′tō-sēl) [″　+　*gala,* milk,　+　*kele,* tumor, swelling]

pneumogastric (nū″mō-găs′trĭk) [Gr. *pneumon,* lung,　+　*gaster,* stomach]

pneumogastric nerve

pneumogastrography (nū″mō-găs-trŏg′ră-fē) [Gr. *pneuma,* air,　+　″　+　*graphein,* to write]

pneumogram (nū′mō-grăm) [″　+　*gramma,* letter, piece of writing]

pneumograph (nū′mō-grăf) [″　+　*graphein,* to write]

pneumography (nū-mŏg′ră-fē)
p., pelvic

pneumohemia (nū″mō-hē′mē-ă) [″　+　*haima,* blood]

pneumohemopericardium (nū"mō-hēm"ō-pĕr-ĭ-kăr'dē-ŭm) [Gr. *pneumon*, lung, + *haima*, blood, + *peri*, around, + *kardia*, heart]

pneumohemorrhagica (nū"mō-hēm-ō-rā'jĭ-kă) [" + " + *rhegnynai*, to burst forth]

pneumohemothorax (nū"mō-hēm"ō-thō'răks) [" + " + *thorax*, chest]

pneumohydrometra (nū"mō-hī"drō-mē'tră) [" + *hydor*, water, + *metra*, uterus]

pneumohydropericardium (nū"mō-hī"drō-pĕr-ĭ-kăr'dē-ŭm) [" + *hydor*, water, + *peri*, around, + *kardia*, heart]

pneumohydrothorax (nū"mō-hī"drō-thō'răks) [" + " + *thorax*, chest]

pneumohypoderma (nū"mō-hī"pō-der'mă) [" + *hypo*, under, beneath, below, + *derma*, skin]

pneumokidney (nū"mō-kĭd'nē) [" + ME. *kidenei*, kidney]

pneumolith (nū'mō-lĭth) [" + *lithos*, stone]

pneumolithiasis (nū"mō-lĭth-ī'ăs-ĭs) [Gr. *pneumon*, lung, + " + -*iasis*, state or condition of]

pneumology (nū-mŏl'ō-jē) [" + *logos*, word, reason]

pneumolysin (nū-mŏl'ĭ-sĭn)

pneumolysis (nū-mŏl'ĭs-ĭs) [" + *lysis*, dissolution]

pneumomalacia (nū"mō-mă'lā'shē-ă) [" + *malakia*, a softening]

pneumomassage (nū"mō-mă-săzh') [Gr. *pneuma*, air, + *massein*, to knead]

pneumomediastinum (nū"mō-mē"dē-ăs-tī'nŭm) [" + L. *mediastinum*, in the middle]

pneumomelanosis (nū"mō-mĕl-ăn-ō'sĭs) [Gr. *pneumon*, lung, + *melano*, black, + *osis*, condition]

pneumometer (nū-mŏm'ĕt-ĕr) [Gr. *pneuma*, air, + *metron*, measure]

pneumomycosis (nū"mō-mī-kō'sĭs) [Gr. *pneumon*, lung, + *mykes*, fungus, + *osis*, condition]

pneumomyelography (nū"mō-mī-ĕl-ŏg'ră-fē) [Gr. *pneuma*, air + *myelos*, marrow, + *graphein*, to write]

pneumonectasia, pneumonectasis (nū"mōn-ĕk-tā'zē-ă, -ĕk'tă-sĭs) [" + *ektasis*, dilatation]

pneumonectomy (nū"mōn-ĕk'tō-mē) [Gr. *pneumon*, lung, + *ektome*, excision]

pneumonia (nū-mō'nē-ă) [Gr.]
- p., abortive
- p., acute lobar
- p. alba
- p., anthrax
- p., apex, apical
- p., aspiration
- p., atypical
- p., bronchial
- p., caseous
- p., catarrhal
- p., central
- p., congenital aspiration
- p., contusion
- p., croupous
- p., deglutition
- p., desquamative interstitial
- p., double
- p., Eaton agent
- p., embolic
- p., eosinophilic
- p., fibrinous
- p., fibrous
- p., Friedländer's
- p., gangrenous
- p., giant cell
- p., hypostatic
- p., influenza
- p., interstitial
- p., interstitial plasma cell
- p., intrauterine
- p., Legionella
- p., lipid
- p., lobar
- p., migratory

p., pneumocystis
p., primary atypical
p., secondary
p., staphylococcal
p., streptococcal
p., terminal
p., traumatic
p., tuberculous
p., tularemic
p., typhoid
p., varicella
p., viral
p., woolsorter's
pneumonic (nū-mŏn'ĭk) [Gr. *pneumon*, lung]
pneumonitis (nū"mō-nī'tĭs) [" + *itis*, inflammation]
p., hypersensitivity
pneumono- [Gr. *pneumon*, lung]
pneumonocele (nū-mŏn'ō-sēl) [" + *kele*, tumor, swelling]
pneumonocentesis (nū-mō"nō-sĕn-tē'sĭs) [" + *kentesis*, a piercing]
pneumonoconiosis (nū-mō"nō-kō"nē-ō'sĭs) [" + *konis*, dust, + *osis*, condition]
pneumonograph (nū-mŏn'ō-grăf) [" + *graphein*, to write]
pneumonography (nū"mŏn-ŏg'ră-fē)
pneumonolysis (nū"mŏn-ŏl'ĭs-ĭs) [" + *lysis*, dissolution]
p., extrapleural
p., intrapleural
pneumonomelanosis (nū"mō-nō-mĕl"ăn-ō'sĭs) [" + *melano*, black, + *osis*, condition]
pneumonomycosis (nū-mŏn"ō-mī-kō'sĭs) [" + *mykes*, fungus, + *osis*, condition]
pneumonopathy (nū"mō-nŏp'ăth-ē) [" + *pathos*, disease, suffering]
pneumonoperitonitis (nū"mō-nō-pĕr"ĭ-tō-nī'tĭs) [" + *peritonaion*, stretched around or over, + *itis*, inflammation]
pneumonopexy (nū-mō"nō-pĕk'sē) [" + *pexis*, fixation]
pneumonopleuritis (nū-mō"nō-ploo-

rī'tĭs) [Gr. *pneumon*, lung, + *pleura*, side, + *itis*, inflammation]
pneumonorrhaphy (nū"mō-nor'ă-fē) [" + *rhaphe*, seam]
pneumonosis (nū-mō-nō'sĭs) [" + *osis*, condition]
pneumonotherapy
pneumonotomy (nū-mō-nŏt'ō-mē) [" + *tome*, a cutting, slice]
pneumopathy (nū-mŏp'ă-thē) [" + *pathos*, disease, suffering]
pneumopericardium (nū"mō-pĕr-ĭ-kăr'dē-ŭm) [Gr. *pneuma*, air, + *peri*, around, + *kardia*, heart]
pneumoperitoneography
pneumoperitoneum (nū"mō-pĕr-ĭ-tō-nē'ŭm) [" + *peritonaion*, stretched around or over]
pneumoperitonitis (nū"mō-pĕr-ĭ-tō-nī'tĭs) [" + *peritonaion*, stretched around or over, + *itis*, inflammation]
pneumopexy (nū'mō-pĕks"ē) [Gr. *pneumon*, lung, + *pexis*, fixation]
pneumopleuritis (nū"mō-ploo-rī'tĭs) [" + *pleura*, a side, + *itis*, inflammation]
pneumopleuroparietopexy (nū"mō-ploo"rō-pă-rī'ĕt-ō-pĕk"sē) [" + " + L. *paries*, wall, + Gr. *pexis*, fixation]
pneumopyelography (nū"mō-pī-ĕ-lŏg'ră-fē) [Gr. *pneuma*, air, + *pyelos*, pelvis, + *graphein*, to write]
pneumopyopericardium (nū"mō-pī"ō-pĕr-ĭ-kar'dē-ŭm) [" + *pyon*, pus, + *peri*, around, + *kardia*, heart]
pneumopyothorax (nū"mō-pī"ō-thō'răks) [" + " + *thorax*, chest]
pneumoradiography (nū"mō-rā-dē-ŏg'ră-fē) [" + L. *radius*, ray, + Gr. *graphein*, to write]
pneumoretroperitoneum (nū"mō-rĕt"rō-pĕr"ĭ-tō-nē'ŭm) [" + L. *retro*, backwards, + Gr. *peritonaion*,

stretched around or over]

pneumorrhachis (nū″mō-rā′kĭs) [Gr. *pneumon*, lung, + *rhachis*, spine]

pneumorrhagia (nū″mō-rā′jē-ă) [Gr. *pneumon*, lung, + *rhegnynai*, to burst forth]

pneumoserothorax (nū″mō-sē-rō-thō′răks) [Gr. *pneuma*, air, + L. *serum*, whey, + Gr. *thorax*, chest]

pneumosilicosis (nū″mō-sĭl″ĭ-kō′sĭs) [Gr. *pneumon*, lung, + L. *silex*, flint, + Gr. *osis*, condition]

pneumotachograph (nū″mō-tăk′ō-grăf) [Gr. *pneuma*, air, + *tachys*, swift, + *graphein*, to write]

pneumotachometer (nū″mō-tăk-ŏm′ĕ-tĕr) [″ + *tachos*, speed, + *metron*, measure]

pneumotaxic (nū″mō-tăk′sĭk) [″ + *taxis*, arrangement]

pneumotherapy (nū-mō-thĕr′ă-pē) [Gr. *pneumon*, lung, + *therapeia*, treatment; Gr. *pneuma*, air, + *therapeia*, treatment]

pneumothermomassage (nū″mō-thĕr″mō-măs-ăzh′) [Gr. *pneuma*, air, + *therme*, heat, + *massein*, to knead]

pneumothorax (nū-mō-thō′răks) [″ + *thorax*, chest]
    p., artificial
    p., extrapleural
    p., open
    p., spontaneous
    p., tension
    p., therapeutic
    p., valvular

pneumotomy (nū-mŏt′ō-mē) [Gr. *pneumon*, lung, + *tome*, a cutting, slice]

pneumotoxin (nū″mō-tŏks′ĭn) [″ + *toxikon*, poison]

pneumotyphus (nū″mō-tī′fŭs) [″ + *typhos*, fever]

pneumouria (nū″mō-ū′rē-ă) [Gr. *pneuma*, air, + *ouron*, urine]

pneumoventricle (nū″mō-vĕn′trĭ-kl) [″ + L. *ventriculus*, little belly]

pneumoventriculography (nū″mō-vĕn-trĭk″ū-lŏg′ră-fē) [″ + ″ + Gr. *graphein*, to write]

pneusis (nū′sĭs) [Gr. *pnein*, to breathe]

pnigophobia (nī″gō-fō′bē-ă) [Gr. *pnigos*, choking, + *phobos*, fear]

Po *polonium*

Po₂ *partial pressure of oxygen*

p.o. [L.] *per os*, by mouth

pock (pŏk) [AS. *poc*, pustule]

pocket (pŏk′ĕt) [ME. *poket*, pouch]
    p., gingival
    p., pseudo-

pocketing

pockmarked

poculum diogenis (pŏk′ū-lŭm dī-ŏj′ĕ-nĭs) [L. *poculum*, cup, + Diogenes, Gr. philosopher, 412–323 B.C.]

podagra (pō-dăg′ră) [Gr. *podos*, foot, + *agra*, seizure]

podalgia (pō-dăl′jē-ă) [″ + *algos*, pain]

podalic (pō-dăl′ĭk) [Gr. *podos*, foot]

podalic version

podarthritis (pŏd″ăr-thrī′tĭs) [″ + *arthron*, joint, + *itis*, inflammation]

podedema (pŏd″ē-dē′mă) [″ + *oidema*, swelling]

podencephalus (pŏd″ĕn-sĕf′ă-lŭs) [″ + *enkephalos*, brain]

podiatrist (pō-dī′ă-trĭst″) [″ + *iatreia*, treatment]

podiatry (pō-dī′ă-trē)

podium (pō′dē-ŭm) [Gr. *podos*, foot]

podo-, pod- [Gr. *pous*, *podos*, foot]

podobromidrosis (pŏd″ō-brō″mĭ-drō′sĭs) [″ + *bromos*, stench, + *hidros*, sweat]

podocyte (pŏd′ō-sīt) [″ + *kytos*, cell]

pododynamometer (pŏd″ō-dī″nă-mŏm′ĕ-ter) [″ + *dynamis*, force, + *metron*, measure]

pododynia (pŏd″ō-dĭn′ē-ă) [″ + *odyne*, pain]

podogram (pŏd′ō-grăm) [″ + *gramma*, letter, piece of writing]

podograph (pŏd′ō-grăf) [″ + *gra-*

phein, to write]

podology (pŏd-ŏl′ō-jē) [″ + *logos*, word, reason]

podophyllum (pŏd-ō-fĭl′ŭm) [″ + *phyllon*, leaf]

podophyllum resin (pŏd″ō-fĭl′ŭm)

pogoniasis (pō″gō-nī′ă-sĭs) [Gr. *pogon*, beard, + *-iasis*, state or condition of]

pogonion (pō-gō′nē-ŏn)

-poietic [Gr.]

poikiloblast (poy′kĭ-lō-blăst″) [Gr. *poikilos*, varied, + *blastos*, germ]

poikilocyte (poy′kĭl-ō-sīt) [″ + *kytos*, cell]

poikilocytosis (poy″kĭl-ō-sī-tō′sĭs) [″ + ″ + *osis*, condition]

poikilodentosis (poy″kī-lō-dĕn-tō′sĭs) [″ + L. *dens*, tooth, + Gr. *osis*, condition]

poikiloderma (poy-kĭl-ō-dĕr′mă) [″ + *derma*, skin]
   p. atrophicans vasculare
   p. of Civatte

poikilonymy (poy″kī-lŏn′ĭ-mē) [″ + *onoma*, name]

poikilotherm (poy-kĭl′ō-thĕrm) [″ + *therme*, heat]

poikilothermal, poikilothermic (poy″kī-lō-thĕr′măl, -mĭk)

poikilothermy (poy″kī-lō-thĕr′mē)

poikilothrombocyte (poy-kĭl″ō-thrŏm′bō-sīt) [″ + *thrombos*, clot, + *kytos*, cell]

point (poynt) [O.Fr., a prick, a dot]
   p., absorbent
   p., auricular
   p., Boas'
   p., boiling
   p., Broca's
   p.'s, Capuron's
   p.'s, cardinal
   p., cold rigor
   p., contact
   p., convergence
   p.'s, corresponding
   p., craniometric
   p., critical, of gases

   p., critical, of liquids
   p.'s, deaf, of ear
   p., dew
   p.'s, disparate
   p., Erb's
   p., external orbital
   p., far
   p., fixation
   p., flash
   p., focal
   p., freezing
   p., fusion
   p., Guéneau de Mussy's
   p., gutta-percha
   p., Halle's
   p., hot
   p.'s, hysterogenic
   p., ice
   p.'s, identical retinal
   p., isoelectric
   p., isoionic
   p., jugal
   p., lacrimal
   p., Lanz's
   p., Lian's
   p., malar
   p., maximum occipital
   p., McBurney's
   p., median mandibular
   p., melting
   p., mental
   p., metopic
   p., motor
   p., Munro's
   p., nasal
   p., near
   p.'s, nodal
   p., occipital
   p. of maximal impulse
   p. of regard
   p.'s, painful
   p., preauricular
   p.'s, pressure
   p.'s, principal
   p., spinal
   p., subnasal
   p., supra-auricular
   p., supranasal

p., supraorbital
p., thermal death
p., trigger
p., triple
p.'s, Trousseau's apophysiary
p.'s, Valleix's
p., vital
p., Voillemier's
pointillage (pwăn"tĭ-yăzh') [Fr.]
pointing
poise (poyz) [J. M. Poiseuille]
Poiseuille's law (pwă-zŭ'yĕz) [Jean Marie Poiseuille, Fr. physiologist, 1799–1869]
Poiseuille's space
poison (poy'zn) [L. *potio*, a poisonous draft]
p., cellular
p., pesticidal
poison control center
poisoning [L. *potio*, a poisonous draft]
p., arsenic
p., blood
p., convulsive
p., corrosive
p., fish
p., food
p., lead
p., mercury
p., mushroom
p., potato
p., unknown substances
poison ivy
poison ivy dermatitis
poison oak
poisonous (poy'zŏn-ŭs) [L. *potio*, a poisonous draft]
poisonous plants
poison sumac
poker back
pokeroot (pōk'root)
pokeroot poisoning
polar [L. *polaris*]
polarimeter (pō"lăr-ĭm'ĕ-tĕr) [" + Gr. *metron*, measure]
polarimetry (pō"lăr-ĭm'ĕ-trē)
polariscope (pō-lăr'ĭ-skōp) [L. *polaris*, pole, + Gr. *skopein*, to examine]

polariscopy (pō"lăr-ĭs'kō-pē)
polarity (pō-lăr'ĭ-tē)
polarization (pō"lăr-ĭ-zā'shŭn) [L. *polaris*, pole]
polarizer (pō'lă-rīz"ĕr)
poldine methylsulfate (pŏl'dēn)
pole (pōl) [L. *polus*]
p., animal
p., frontal
p., germinal
p., occipital
p.'s of eye
p.'s of kidney
p.'s of testicle
p., pelvic
p., placental, of chorion
p., temporal
p., vegetal
policlinic (pŏl"ĭ-klĭn'ĭk) [Gr. *polis*, city, + *kline*, bed]
polio *poliomyelitis, acute anterior*
polio- [Gr. *polios*, gray]
polioclastic (pŏl"ē-ō-klăs'tĭk) [" + *klastos*, breaking]
polioencephalitis (pŏl"ē-ō-ĕn-sĕf"ă-lī'tĭs) [" + *enkephalos*, brain, + *itis*, inflammation]
p., anterior superior
p. hemorrhagica
p., posterior
polioencephalomeningomyelitis (pŏl"ē-ō-ĕn-sĕf"ăl-ō-mĕn-ĭn"gō-mī-ĕl-ī'tĭs) [" + " + *meninx*, membrane, + *myelos*, marrow, + *itis* inflammation]
polioencephalomyelitis (pŏl"ē-ō-ĕn-sĕf"ăl-ō-mī"ĕl-ī'tĭs)
polioencephalopathy (pŏl"ē-ō-ĕn-sĕf"ăl-ŏp'ă-thē) [Gr. *polios*, gray, + *enkephalos*, brain, + *pathos*, disease, suffering]
poliomyelencephalitis (pŏl"ē-ō-mī"ĕl-ĕn-sĕf"ăl-ī'tĭs) [" + *myelos*, marrow, + *enkephalos*, brain, + *itis*, inflammation]
poliomyelitis (pŏl"ē-ō-mī"ĕl-ī'tĭs) [" + " + *itis*, inflammation]
p., abortive

p., acute anterior
p., anterior
p., ascending
p., bulbar
p., chronic anterior
p., nonparalytic
p., paralytic
poliomyelopathy (pōl″ē-ō-mī″ĕl-ŏp′ȧ-thē) [Gr. *polios*, gray, + *myelos*, marrow, + *pathos*, disease, suffering]
polioplasm (pōl′ē-ō-plăzm) [″ + LL. *plasma*, form, mold]
poliosis (pŏl″ē-ō′sĭs) [″ + *osis*, condition]
poliovirus (pō″lē-ō-vī′rŭs)
poliovirus vaccine, inactivated
poliovirus vaccine, live oral
polishing (pŏl′ĭsh-ĭng)
Politzer bag (pŏl′ĭt-zĕr) [Adam Politzer, Hungarian otologist, 1835–1920]
politzerization (pŏl″ĭt-sĕr-ĭ-zā′shŭn)
pollakiuria (pŏl″ȧ-kē-ū′rē-ȧ) [Gr. *pollakis*, often, + *ouron*, urine]
pollen (pŏl′ĕn) [L., dust]
pollenogenic (pŏl″ĕn-ō-jĕn′ĭk) [″ + Gr. *gennan*, to produce]
pollenosis (pŏl″ĕn-ō′sĭs) [″ + Gr. *osis*, condition]
pollex (pŏl′ĕks) [L.]
p. extensus
p. flexus
p. valgus
p. varus
pollicization (pŏl″ĭs-ĭ-zā′shŭn) [L. *pollex*, thumb]
pollinosis (pŏl-ĭn-ō′sĭs) [L. *pollen*, dust, + Gr. *osis*, condition]
pollodic (pŏl-lō′dĭk) [Gr. *polloi*, many, + *hodos*, way]
pollution (pū-loo′shŭn) [ME. *polluten*]
p., noise
polocyte (pō′lō-sīt) [Gr. *polos*, pole, + *kytos*, cell]
polonium (pō-lō′nē-ŭm) [L. *Polonia*, Poland]
poltophagy (pŏl-tŏf′ȧ-jē) [Gr. *poltos*, porridge, + *phagein*, to eat]
polus (pō′lŭs) [L.]
poly (pŏl′ē) *polymorphonuclear leukocyte*
poly- [Gr. *polys*, many]
polyacid (pŏl″ē-ăs′ĭd)
polyadenitis (pŏl″ē-ăd″ĕ-nī′tĭs) [″ + Gr. *aden*, gland, + *itis*, inflammation]
polyadenomatosis (pŏl″ē-ăd″ĕ-nō-mȧ-tō′sĭs) [″ + ″ + *oma*, tumor, + *osis*, condition]
polyadenopathy (pŏl″ē-ăd″ĕ-nŏp′ȧ-thē) [″ + ″ + *pathos*, disease, suffering]
polyadenous (pŏl″ē-ăd′ĕ-nŭs)
polyalgesia (pŏl″ē-ăl-jē′zē-ȧ) [″ + *algesis*, sense of pain]
polyandry (pŏl′ē-ăn′drē) [Gr. *polyandria*]
polyangitis (pŏl″ē-ăn″jē-ī′tĭs) [Gr. *polys*, many, + *angeion*, vessel, + *itis*, inflammation]
polyarteritis (nodosa) (pŏl″ē-ăr″tĕr-ī′tĭs) [″ + *arteria*, artery, + *itis*, inflammation]
polyarthric (pŏl″ē-ăr″thrĭk) [″ + *arthron*, joint]
polyarthritis (pŏl-ē-ăr-thrī′tĭs) [″ + ″ + *itis*, inflammation]
p., chronic villous
p. rheumatica, acute
polyarticular (pŏl″ē-ăr-tĭk′ū-lăr) [″ + L. *articulus*, a joint]
polyatomic (pŏl″ē-ȧ-tŏm′ĭk) [″ + *atomon*, atom]
polyavitaminosis (pŏl″ē-ȧ-vī″tȧ-mĭn-ō′sĭs) [″ + *a-*, not, + L. *vita*, life, + *amine* + Gr. *osis*, condition]
polybasic (pŏl″ē-bā′sĭk) [Gr. *polys*, many, + *basis*, base]
polyblast (pŏl′ē-blăst) [″ + *blastos*, a germ]
polyblennia (pŏl″ē-blĕ′nē-ȧ) [″ + *blennos*, mucus]
polycarbophil (pŏl″ē-kăr′bō-fĭl)
polycentric (pŏl″ē-sĕn′trĭk) [″ +

kentron, center]

polycheiria (pŏl″ē-kī′rē-ă) [″ + *cheir,* hand]

polychemotherapy (pŏl″ē-kē″mō-thĕr′ă-pē) [″ + *chemeia,* chemistry, + *therapeia,* treatment]

polychlorinated biphenyls

polycholia (pŏl″ē-kō′lē-ă) [″ + *chole,* bile]

polychondritis (pŏl″ē-kŏn-drī′tĭs) [″ + *chondros,* cartilage, + *itis,* inflammation]

p., chronic atrophic relapsing

polychrest (pŏl′ē-krĕst) [″ + *chrestos,* useful]

polychromasia (pŏl″ē-krō-mā′zē-ă) [″ + *chroma,* color]

polychromatic (pŏl″ē-krō-măt′ĭk)

polychromatocyte (pŏl″ē-krō-măt′ō-sīt) [″ + ″ + *kytos,* cell]

polychromatophil(e) (pŏl″ē-krō-măt′ō-fĭl) [Gr. *polys,* many, + *chroma,* color, + *philein,* to love]

polychromatophilia (pŏl″ē-krō-măt″ō-fĭl′ē-ă)

polychromophilia (pŏl″ē-krō-mō-fĭl′ē-ă) [″ + ″ + *philos,* love]

polychylia (pŏl″ē-kī′lē-ă) [″ + *chylos,* juice]

Polycillin-N

polyclinic (pŏl″ē-klĭn′ĭk) [″ + *kline,* bed]

polyclonal (pŏl″ē-klōn′ăl)

polyclonia (pŏl″ē-klō′nē-ă) [″ + *klonos,* tumult]

polycoria (pŏl″ē-kō′rē-ă) [″ + *kore,* pupil]

polycrotic (pŏl″ē-krŏt′ĭk) [″ + *krotos,* beat]

polycrotism (pŏl-ĭk′rō-tĭzm) [″ + ″ + *-ismos,* condition]

polycyesis (pŏl″ē-sī-ē′sĭs) [″ + *kyesis,* pregnancy]

polycystic (pŏl″ē-sĭs′tĭk) [″ + *kystis,* cyst]

polycystic ovary syndrome

polycythemia (pŏl″ē-sī-thē′mē-ă) [″ + *kytos,* cell, + *haima,* blood]

p., compensatory
p., myelopathic
p., primary
p., relative
p. rubra; p. rubra vera
p., secondary
p., splenomegalic
p. vera

polycytotropic

polydactylism (pŏl″ē-dăk′tĭ-lĭzm) [Gr. *polys,* many, + *daktylos,* finger, + *-ismos,* condition]

polydactyly (pŏl″ē-dăk′tĭ-lē) [″ + *daktylos,* finger]

polydentia (pŏl″ē-dĕn′shē-ă) [″ + L. *dens,* tooth]

polydipsia (pŏl″ē-dĭp′sē-ă) [″ + *dipsa,* thirst]

polydysplasia (pŏl″ē-dĭs-plā′zē-ă) [″ + *dys,* bad, difficult, painful, disordered, + *plassein,* to form]

polydystrophic (pŏl″ē-dĭs-trō′fĭk)

polydystrophy (pŏl″ē-dĭs′trō-fē) [″ + ″ + *trophe,* nourishment]

polyemia (pŏl″ē-ē′mē-ă) [″ + *haima,* blood]

polyendocrine (pŏl″ē-ĕn′dō-krĭn, -krĭn) [″ + *endon,* within, + *krinein,* to secrete]

polyendocrine deficiency syndromes

polyene (pŏl-ē′ēn)

polyergic (pŏl″ē-ĕr′jĭk) [″ + *ergon,* work]

polyesthesia (pŏl″ē-ĕs-thē′zē-ă) [″ + *aisthesis,* feeling, perception]

polyesthetic (pŏl″ē-ĕs-thĕt′ĭk)

polyestrous (pŏl″ē-ĕs′trŭs) [″ + *oistros,* mad desire]

polyethylene (pŏl″ē-ĕth′ĭ-lēn)
p. glycol 400
p. glycol 4000
p. glycol electrolyte for gastrointestinal lavage solution

polygalactia (pŏl″ē-gă-lăk′shē-ă) [Gr. *polys,* many, + *gala,* milk]

polygalacturonase (pŏl″ē-gă-lăk-tū′rō-nās)

polygamy (pō-lĭg′ă-mē) [″ + gamos, marriage]

polyganglionic (pŏl″ē-găng″glē-ŏn′ĭk) [″ + ganglion, ganglion]

polygastria (pŏl″ē-găs′trē-ă) [″ + gaster, stomach]

polygen (pŏl′ē-jĕn)

polygenic (pŏl″ē-jĕn′ĭk) [″ + gennan, to produce]

polyglandular (pŏl″ē-glăn′dŭ-lar) [″ + L. glandula, a little kernel]

polyglycolic acid

polygnathus (pō-lĭg′nă-thŭs) [″ + gnathos, jaw]

polygram (pŏl′ē-grăm) [″ + gramma, letter, piece of writing]

polygraph (pŏl′ē-grăf) [″ + graphein, to write]

polygyny

polygyria (pŏl″ē-jī′rē-ă) [″ + gyros, circle]

polyhedral (pŏl″ē-hē′drăl) [Gr. polys, many, + hedra, base]

polyhemia (pŏl″ē-hē′mē-ă) [″ + haima, blood]

polyhidrosis (pŏl″ē-hī-drō′sĭs) [″ + hidrosis, sweat]

polyhistor (pŏl″ē-hĭs′tŭr) [″ + histor, learned]

polyhybrid (pŏl″ē-hī′brĭd) [″ + L. hybrida, mongrel]

polyhydramnios (pŏl″ē-hī-drăm′nē-ŏs) [″ + hydor, water, + amnion, amnion]

polyhydric (pŏl″ē-hī′drĭk)

polyhydruria (pŏl″ē-hī-droo′rē-ă) [″ + ″ + ouron, urine]

polyhypermenorrhea (pŏl″ē-hī′pĕr-mĕn″ō-rē′ă) [″ + hyper, over, above, excessive, + men, month, + rhein, to flow]

polyhypomenorrhea (pŏl″ē-hī″pō-mĕn″ō-rē′ă) [″ + hypo, under, beneath, below, + men, month, + rhein, to flow]

Poly I:C

polyidrosis (pŏl″ē-ĭd-rō′sĭs) [″ + hidrosis, sweat]

polyinfection (pŏl″ē-ĭn-fĕk′shŭn) [″ + ME. infecten, infect]

polykaryocyte (pŏl″ē-kăr′ē-ō-sīt) [″ + karyon, nucleus, + kytos, cell]

polyleptic (pŏl″ē-lĕp′tĭk) [″ + lepsis, a seizure]

polylysine (pŏl″ē-lī′sīn)

polymastia (pŏl″ē-măs′tē-ă) [Gr. polys, many, + mastos, breast]

polymastigote (pŏl″ē-măs′tĭ-gōt) [″ + mastix, whip]

polymath

polymazia [″ + mazos, breast]

polymelia (pŏl″ē-mē′lē-ă) [″ + melos, limb]

polymelus (pō-lĭm′ē-lŭs) [″ + melos, limb]

polymenia (pŏl″ē-mē′nē-ă) [″ + men, month]

polymenorrhea (pŏl″ē-mĕn-ō-rē′ă) [″ + ″ + rhein, to flow]

polymer (pŏl′ĭ-mĕr) [″ + meros, a part]

polymerase (pŏl-ĭm′ĕr-ās)

polymer fume fever

polymeria (pŏl-ĭ-mē′rē-ă)

polymeric (pŏl″ĭ-mĕr′ĭk)

polymerid (pō-lĭm′ĕr-ĭd)

polymerism (pŏl′ĭ-mĕr″ĭzm, pō-lĭm′ĕr-ĭzm) [″ + meros, part, + -ismos, condition]

polymerization (pŏl″ĭ-mĕr″ĭ-zā′shŭn)

polymerize (pŏl′ĭ-mĕr-īz)

polymicrobial (pŏl″ē-mī-krō′bē-ăl) [Gr. polys, many, + mikros, small, + bios, life]

polymicrobic infections

polymicrogyria (pŏl″ē-mī″krō-jī′rē-ă) [″ + ″ + gyros, convolution]

polymitus (pō-lĭm′ĭ-tŭs) [″ + mitos, thread]

polymorph (pŏl′ē-morf) [″ + morphe, form]

polymorphic

polymorphism [″ + morphe, form, + -ismos, condition]

polymorphocellular (pŏl″ē-mor″fō-sĕl′ū-lăr) [″ + ″ + L. cellula, a small chamber]

polymorphonuclear (pŏl″ē-mor″fō-nū′klē-ăr) [″ + ″ + L. *nucleus,* a kernel]

polymorphonuclear leukocyte

polymorphous (pŏl″ē-mor′fŭs)

Polymox

polymyalgia arteritica (pŏl″ē-mī-ăl′jē-ă) [″ + *mys,* muscle, + *algos,* pain]

polymyalgia rheumatica

polymyoclonus (pŏl″ē-mī-ŏk′lō-nŭs) [″ + ″ + *klonos,* tumult]

polymyopathy (pŏl″ē-mī-ŏp′ă-thē) [″ + ″ + *pathos,* disease, suffering]

polymyositis (pŏl″ē-mī″ō-sī′tĭs) [″ + ″ + *itis,* inflammation]

polymyxin (pŏl″ē-mĭks′ĭn)
  p. B
  p. B sulfate

polynesic (pŏl″ē-nē′sĭk) [″ + *nesos,* island]

polyneural (pŏl″ē-nū′răl) [″ + *neuron,* nerve, sinew]

polyneuralgia (pŏl″ē-nū-răl′jē-ă) [″ + ″ + *algos,* pain]

polyneuritic (pŏl″ē-nū-rīt′ĭk) [″ + ″ + *itis,* inflammation]

polyneuritis (pŏl″ē-nū-rī′tĭs) [″ + ″ + *itis,* inflammation]
  p., acute idiopathic
  p., Jamaica ginger
  p., metabolic
  p., toxic

polyneuromyositis (pŏl″ē-nū″rō-mī″ō-sī′tĭs) [″ + ″ + *mys,* muscle, + *itis,* inflammation]

polyneuropathy (pŏl″ē-nū-rŏp′ă-thē) [Gr. *polys,* many, + *neuron,* nerve, sinew, + *pathos,* disease, suffering]
  p., amyloid
  p., buckthorn
  p., erythredema
  p., porphyric
  p., progressive hypertrophic

polyneuroradiculitis (pŏl″ē-nū″rō-ră-

dĭk″ū-lī′tĭs) [″ + ″ + *radix,* root, + *itis,* inflammation]

polynuclear (pŏl″ē-nū′klē-ăr) [″ + L. *nucleus,* a kernel]

polynucleate (pŏl″ē-nū′klē-āt)

polynucleotidase (pŏl″ē-nū″klē-ō′tĭ-dās)

polynucleotide (pŏl″ē-nū′klē-ō-tīd)

polyodontia (pŏl″ē-ō-dŏn′shē-ă) [″ + *odous,* tooth]

polyomavirus (pŏl″ē-ō-mă-vī′rŭs)

polyonychia (pŏl″ē-ō-nĭk′ē-ă) [″ + *onyx,* nail]

polyopia, polyopsia (pŏl″ē-ō′pē-ă, -ŏp′sē-ă) [″ + *opsis,* sight, appearance, vision]

polyorchidism (pŏl″ē-or′kĭ-dĭzm) [″ + *orchis,* testicle, + *-ismos,* condition]

polyorchis (pŏl″ē-or′kĭs)

polyorchism (pŏl″ē-or′kĭzm) [″ + *orchis,* testicle, + *-ismos,* condition]

polyostotic (pŏl″ē-ŏs-tŏt′ĭk) [″ + *osteon,* bone]

polyotia (pŏl″ē-ō′shē-ă) [″ + *ous,* ear]

polyovulatory (pŏl″ē-ŏv′ū-lă-tō″rē) [″ + L. *ovulum,* little egg]

polyoxyl stearate (pŏl″ē-ŏks′ĭl)

polyp (pŏl′ĭp) [Gr. *polypous,* many footed]
  p., adenomatous
  p., bleeding
  p., cardiac
  p., cervical
  p., choanal
  p., fibrinous
  p., fleshy
  p., gelatinous
  p., Hopmann's
  p., hydatid
  p., juvenile
  p., laryngeal
  p., lymphoid
  p., mucous
  p., nasal
  p., placental
  p., retention

p., vascular

polypapilloma (pŏl"ē-păp"ĭ-lō'mă)
[Gr. *polys*, many + L. *papilla*, nipple, + Gr. *oma*, tumor]

polyparesis (pŏl"ē-pă-rē'sĭs) ["
parienai, let fall]

polypathia (pŏl"ē-păth'ē-ă) ["
+ *pathos*, disease, suffering]

polypectomy (pŏl"ĭ-pĕk'tō-mē) ["
+ *pous*, foot, + *ektome*, excision]

polypeptidase (pŏl"ē-pĕp'tĭ-dās)

polypeptide (pŏl"ē-pĕp'tīd) ["
+ *peptein*, to digest]

polypeptidemia (pŏl"ē-pĕp"tĭ-dē'mē-
ă) [" + " + *haima*, blood]

polypeptidorrhachia (pŏl"ē-pĕp"tĭ-
dō-ră'kē-ă) [" + " + *rhachis*,
spine]

polyphagia (pŏl"ē-fā'jē-ă) [Gr. *polys*,
many, + *phagein*, to eat]

polyphalangism (pŏl"ē-fă-lăn'jĭzm)
[" + *phalanx*, line of battle, +
-ismos, condition]

polypharmacy (pŏl"ē-făr'mă-sē)
[" + *pharmakon*, drug]

polyphenoloxidase (pŏl"ē-fē"nŏl-
ŏk'sĭ-dās)

polyphobia (pŏl"ē-fō'bē-ă) [Gr. *polys*,
many, + *phobos*, fear]

polyphrasia (pŏl"ē-frā'zē-ă) ["
phrasis, diction]

polyphyletic (pŏl"ē-fī-lĕt'ĭk) ["
phyle, tribe]

polyphyodont (pŏl"ē-fī'ō-dŏnt) ["
phyein, to produce, + *odous*,
tooth]

polypiform (pō-lĭp'ĭ-form) ["
pous, foot, + L. *forma*, form]

polyplastic (pŏl"ē-plăs'tĭk) ["
plastos, formed]

polyplegia (pŏl"ē-plē'jē-ă) ["
plege, stroke]

polyploid (pŏl'ē-ployd)

polyploidy (pŏl'ē-ploy"dē)

polypnea (pŏl"ĭp-nē'ă) ["
pnoia, breath]

polypodia (pŏl"ē-pō'dē-ă) ["
pous, foot]

polypoid (pŏl'ē-poyd) ["
" + *eidos*, form, shape]

polyporous (pŏl-ĭp'ō-rŭs) ["
poros, passage]

polyposia (pŏl"ē-pō'zē-ă) [" + "
+ *posis*, drinking]

polyposis (pŏl"ē-pō'sĭs) ["
pous, foot, + *osis*, condition]
p. coli
p., familial
p. ventriculi

polypotome (pŏl-ĭp'ō-tōm) [" + "
+ *tome*, a cutting, slice]

polypotrite (pō-lĭp'ō-trīt) [" + "
+ L. *terere*, to crush]

polypsychotropia (pŏl"ē-sī-kō-
trō'pē-ă)

polyptychial (pŏl"ē-tī'kē-ăl) ["
ptyche, fold]

polypus (pŏl'ĭ-pŭs) [L.]

polyradiculitis (pŏl"ē-ră-dĭk'ū-lī'tĭs)
[" + L. *radix*, root, + Gr. *itis*,
inflammation]

polyradiculoneuritis (pŏl"ē-ră-dĭk"ū-
lō-nū-rī'tĭs) [" + " + Gr.
neuron, nerve, + *itis*, inflammation]

polyradiculoneuropathy (pŏl"ē-ră-
dĭk"ū-lō-nū-rŏp'ă-thē) [" + " +
" + *pathos*, disease, suffering]

polyribosome (pŏl"ē-rī'bō-sōm)

polyrrhea, polyrrhoea (pŏl"ē-rē'ă)
[" + *rhein*, to flow]

polysaccharide (pŏl"ē-săk'ă-rīd)
[" + Sanskrit *sarkara*, sugar]
p.'s, immune

polysaccharose (pŏl"ē-săk'ă-rōs)

polyscelia (pŏl"ē-sē'lē-ă) ["
skelos, leg]

polyscelus (pō-lĭs'ē-lŭs)

polyserositis (pŏl"ē-sē-rō-sī'tĭs) ["
L. *serum*, whey, + *itis*, inflammation]
p., familial paroxysmal

polysialia (pŏl"ē-sī-ā'lē-ă) ["
sialon, saliva]

polysinusitis, polysinuitis (pŏl"ē-
sī"nŭs-ī'tĭs, -nū-ī'tĭs) [" + L. *sinus*, a
hollow, + Gr. *itis*, inflammation]

polysomaty (pŏl″ē-sō′mă-tē) [″ + soma, body]

polysome

polysomia (pŏl″ē-sō′mē-ă) [″ + soma, body]

polysorbates (pŏl″ē-sor′bāts)

polyspermia (pŏl″ē-spĕr′mē-ă) [Gr. polys, many, + sperma, seed]

polyspermism (pŏl″ē-spĕrm′ĭzm)

polyspermy (pŏl″ē-spĕr′mē)

polystichia (pŏl″ē-stĭk′ē-ă) [″ + stichos, a row]

polystomatous (pŏl″ē-stō′mă-tŭs) [″ + stoma, mouth, opening]

polystyrene (pŏl″ē-stī′rēn)

polysynaptic (pŏl″ē-sĭ-năp′tĭk) [″ + synapsis, point of contact]

polysyndactyly (pŏl″ē-sĭn-dăk′tĭl-ē) [″ + syn, together, + daktylos, finger]

polytendinitis (pŏl″ē-tĕn″dĭ-nī′tĭs) [″ + L. tendo, tendon, + Gr. itis, inflammation]

polytene (pŏl′ē-tēn) [″ + tainia, band]

polyteny (pŏl″ē-tē′nē) [″ + tainia, band]

polythelia (pŏl″ē-thē′lē-ă) [″ + thele, nipple, + -ismos, condition]

polythelism (pŏl″ē-thē′lĭzm)

polythiazide (pŏl″ē-thī′ă-zīd)

polytocous (pō-lĭt′ō-kŭs) [″ + tokos, birth]

polytrichia (pŏl″ē-trĭk′ē-ă) [″ + thrix, hair]

polytrichosis (pŏl″ē-trĭ-kō′sĭs) [″ + osis, condition]

polytrophia (pŏl″ē-trō′fē-ă) [″ + trophe, nourishment]

polytrophy (pō-lĭt′rō-fē)

polytropic (pŏl″ē-trŏp′ĭk) [″ + trope, a turning]

polyunguia (pŏl″ē-ŭng′gwē-ă) [″ + L. unguis, nail]

polyunsaturated

polyuria (pŏl″ē-ū′rē-ă) [″ + ouron, urine]

polyvalent (pŏl″ē-vă′lĕnt, pō-lĭv′ă-lĕnt) [″ + L. valere, to be strong]

polyvalent serum

polyvalent vaccine

polyvinyl alcohol (pŏl″ē-vī′nĭl)

polyvinyl chloride

polyvinylpyrrolidone (pŏl″ē-vī″nĭl-pĕr-rŏl′ĭ-dōn)

pomade (pō-mād′) [Fr. pommade]

pomatum (pō-mā′tŭm)

Pompe's disease

pompholyx

pomphus (pŏm′fŭs) [L.]

POMR problem-oriented medical record

pomum (pō′mŭm) [L.]
p. adami

ponderal (pŏn′dĕr-ăl) [L. pondus, weight]

ponderal index

Pondimin

ponograph (pō′nō-grăf) [Gr. ponos, pain, fatigue, + graphein, to write]

ponophobia (pō″nō-fō′bē-ă) [″ + phobos, fear]

pons (pŏnz) [L., bridge]
p. cerebelli
p. hepatis
p. varolii [Costanzo Varolio, It. anatomist, 1544–1575]

Ponstel

pontic (pŏn′tĭk) [L. pons, pontis, bridge]

ponticulus (pŏn-tĭk′ū-lŭs) [L., little bridge]

pontile (pŏn′tēl)

pontile hemiplegia

pontile nuclei

pontine (pŏn′tēn)

pontobulbar (pŏn″tō-bŭl′bar)

Pontocaine

Pontocaine Hydrochloride (pŏn′tō-kān)

pool
p., abdominal
p., gene
p., metabolic
p., vaginal

poples (pŏp′lēz) [L., ham of the knee]

popliteal (pŏp″lĭt-ē′ăl, pŏp-lĭt′ē-ăl) [L.

poples, ham of the knee]
popliteus (pŏp-lĭt′ē-ŭs, -lĭt-ē′ŭs)
poppy
population dynamics
population of world
POR *problem-oriented record*
poradenitis (por″ăd-ĕ-nī′tĭs) [Gr.
poros, passage, + *aden,* gland,
+ *itis,* inflammation]
porcelain (por′sĕ-lĭn)
porcelaneous, porcelanous (por″sĕ-
lā′nē-ŭs, -sĕl′ăn-ŭs) [Fr. *porcelaine*]
porcine (por′sīn) [L. *porcus,* pig]
pore (por) [Gr. *poros,* passage]
    p., alveolar
    p., gustatory
    p., taste
porencephalia, porencephaly (por″
ĕn-sĕf-ă′lē-ă, por″ĕn-sĕf′ă-lē)
[″ + *enkephalos,* brain]
porencephalitis (por″ĕn-sĕf″ă-lī′tĭs)
[″ + ″ + *itis,* inflammation]
porencephalous
pori
poriomania [Gr. *poreia,* walking, +
mania, madness]
porion (pō′rē-ŏn) [Gr. *poros,* passage]
pornography (por-nŏg′ră-fē) [Gr.
porne, prostitute, + *graphein,* to
write]
porocele (pō′rō-sēl) [Gr. *poros,* passage, + *kele,* tumor, swelling]
porocephaliasis, porocephalosis
(pō″rō-sĕf″ă-lī′ă-sĭs, -lō′sĭs) [″ + *kephale,* head, + *-iasis,* state or
condition of]
Porocephalus (pō″rō-sĕf′ă-lŭs)
porokeratosis (pō″rō-kĕr″ă-tō′sĭs)
[″ + *keras,* horn, + *osis,* con-
dition]
poroma (pō-rō′mă) [Gr.]
    p., cerebral
    p., eccrine
porosis (pō-rō′sĭs) [Gr. *poros,* passage,
+ *osis,* condition]
porosity (pō-rŏs′ĭ-tē) [Gr. *poros,* pas-
sage]
porotomy (pō-rŏt′ō-mē) [″ +

tome, a cutting, slice]
porous (pō′rŭs)
porphin (por′fĭn)
porphobilinogen (por″fō-bī-lĭn′ō-jĕn)
porphyria (por-fī′rē-ă, por-fĭr′ē-ă) [Gr.
porphyra, purple]
    p., acute intermittent
    p., congenital erythropoietic
    p. cutanea tarda hereditaria
    p. erythropoietica
    p. hepatica
    p., South African genetic
    p., variegate
porphyrin (por′fĭ-rĭn) [Gr. *porphyra,*
purple]
porphyrinuria (por″fĭ-rĭ-nū′rē-ă) [″ +
ouron, urine]
porphyrization (por″fĭr-ĭ-zā′shŭn)
porphyruria (por″fĭr-ū′rē-ă) [″ +
ouron, urine]
Porro's operation (por′ōz) [Eduardo
Porro, It. obstetrician, 1842–1902]
porta [L., gate]
    p. hepatis
    p. lienis
    p. pulmonis
    p. renis
portacaval (por″tă-kā′văl)
portacaval shunt
portal [L. *porta,* gate]
    p., intestinal
    p. of entry
portal circulation
portal hypertension
portal system
portal vein
portio (por′shē-ō) [L.]
    p. dura
    p. intermedia
    p. vaginalis
portogram (por′tō-grăm) [L. *porta,*
gate, + Gr. *gramma,* letter, piece
of writing]
portography (por-tŏg′ră-fē) [″ +
Gr. *graphein,* to write]
    p., portal
    p., splenic
portosystemic (por″tō-sĭs-tĕm′ĭk)

Portuguese man-of-war
port-wine mark, stain
porus (pō'rŭs) [L.]
    p. acusticus externus
    p. acusticus internus
    p. gustatorious
    p. lactiferous
    p. opticus
    p. sudoriferus
position (pō-zīsh'ŭn) [L. *positio*]
    p., anatomic
    p., Bonnet's
    p., Bozeman's
    p., Brickner
    p., centric
    p., decubitus
    p., dorsal
    p., dorsal elevated
    p., dorsal recumbent
    p., dorsosacral
    p., Edebohls'
    p., Elliot's
    p., English
    p., Fowler's
    p., genucubital
    p., genupectoral
    p., horizontal
    p., horizontal abdominal
    p., jackknife
    p., knee-chest
    p., knee-elbow
    p., laterosemiprone
    p., left lateral recumbent
    p., lithotomy
    p., Noble's
    p., obstetrical
    p., orthograde
    p., orthopneic
    p., PA
    p., physiologic rest
    p., prone
    p., reclining
    p., rest
    p., Rose's
    p., side, semiprone
    p., Simon's
    p., Sims'
    p., Trendelenburg

    p., unilateral recumbent
    p., Walcher
positioner (pō-zīsh'ŭn-ĕr)
positive (pŏz'ĭ-tĭv) [L. *positivus*, to put,
    place]
positive end-expiratory pressure
positron (pŏz'ĭ-trŏn)
positron emission tomography
posological (pŏ"sō-lŏj'ĭ-kăl) [Gr.
    posos, how much, + *logos*, word,
    reason]
posology (pō-sŏl'ō-jē)
possessed
possession (pō-zĕsh'ŭn) [ME. *posses-
sen*]
    p., demoniacal
Possum (pŏs'ŭm) [patient operated se-
lector *mechanism*]
post
post- [L.]
postabortal (pōst"ă-bor'tăl) [L. *post*,
    behind, after, + *abortus*, abortion]
postacetabular (pōst"ăs-ĕ-tăb'ū-lăr)
    [" + *acetabulum*, a little saucer for
    vinegar]
postadolescent (pōst"ăd-ō-lĕs'ĕnt)
    [" + *adolescens*, to grow up]
postanal (pōst-ā'năl) [" + *anus*,
    anus]
postanesthetic (pōst"ăn-ĕs-thĕt'ĭk)
    [" + *an-*, not, + *aisthesis*, feel-
ing, perception]
postapoplectic (pōst"ăp-ō-plĕk'tĭk)
    [" + Gr. *apoplessein*, to cripple by
    a stroke]
postaxial (pōst-ăk'sē-ăl) [" + Gr.
    axon, axis]
postbrachial (pōst-brā'kē-ăl) [" +
    brachiolis, arm]
postcapillary (pōst-kăp'ĭl-lā-rē)
postcardial (pōst-kăr'dē-ăl) [" +
    Gr. *kardia*, heart]
postcardiotomy (pōst-kăr"dē-ŏt'ō-
mē) [" + " + *tome*, a cutting,
slice]
postcaval
postcentral (pōst-sĕn'trăl) [" +
    Gr. *kentron*, center]

postcibal (pōst-sī'băl) [" + cibum, food]

postclavicular (pōst"klă-vĭk'ū-lăr) [" + clavicula, a little key]

postclimacteric (pōst"klī-măk-tĕr'ĭk, -măk'tĕr-ĭk) [" + Gr. klimakter, rung of a ladder]

postcoital (pōst-kō'ĭt-ăl) [" + coitio, a coming together]

postconnubial (pōst"kŏn-ū'bē-ăl) [" + connubium, marriage]

postconvulsive (pōst"kŏn-vŭl'sĭv) [" + convulsus, pull violently]

postdiastolic (pōst"dī-ăs-tŏl'ĭk) [" + diastole, expansion]

postdicrotic (pōst"dī-krŏt'ĭk) [" + Gr. dikrotos, beating double]

postdicrotic wave

postdiphtheritic (pōst"dĭf-thĕr-ĭt'ĭk)

postencephalitis (pōst"ĕn-sĕf-ă-lī'tĭs) [" + enkephalos, brain, + itis, inflammation]

postepileptic (pōst"ĕp-ĭ-lĕp'tĭk) [" + Gr. epi, upon, + lepsis, a seizure]

posterior (pŏs-tē'rē-or) [L. posterus, behind]

posterior central gyrus

posterior drawer sign

posterior pituitary injection

postero- (pŏs'tĕr-ō) [L.]

posteroanterior (pŏs"tĕr-ō-ăn-tēr'ē-or) [L. posterus, behind, + anterior, anterior]

posteroexternal (pŏs"tĕr-ō-ĕks-tĕr'năl) [" + externus, outer]

posteroinferior (pŏs"tĕr-ō-ĭn-fĕr'ē-or) [" + inferus, below]

posterointernal [" + internus, inner]

posterolateral [" + lateralis, side]

posteromedial (pŏs"tĕr-ō-mē'dē-ăl) [" + medius, middle]

posteromedian

posteroparietal (pŏs"tĕr-ō-pă-rī'ĕ-tăl) [" + paries, a wall]

posterosuperior (pŏs"tĕr-ō-sū-pē'rē-or) [" + superior, upper]

posterotemporal (pŏs"tĕr-ō-tĕm'pō-răl) [" + temporalis, temporal]

postesophageal (pōst"ē-sŏf"ă-jē'ăl) [L. post, behind, after, + Gr. oisophagos, gullet]

postethmoid (pōst-ĕth'moyd) [" + Gr. ethmos, sieve, + eidos, form, shape]

postfebrile (pōst-fē'brĭl) [" + febris, fever]

postganglionic (pōst"găn-glē-ŏn'ĭk) [" + Gr. ganglion, knot]

postganglionic fiber

postganglionic neuron

posthemiplegic (pōst"hĕm-ĭ-plē'jĭk) [" + Gr. hemi, half, + plege, a stroke]

posthemorrhagic (pōst-hĕm"ō-răj'ĭk) [" + Gr. haima, blood, + rhegnynai, to burst forth]

posthepatitic (pōst"hĕp-ă-tĭt'ĭk) [" + Gr. hepar, liver, + itis, inflammation]

posthetomy (pŏs-thĕt'ō-mē) [Gr. posthe, foreskin, + tome, a cutting, slice]

posthioplasty (pŏs'thē-ō-plăs"tē) [" + plastos, formed]

posthitis (pŏs-thī'tĭs) [" + itis, inflammation]

posthumous (pŏs'tū-mŭs) [L. postumus, last]

posthypnotic (pōst"hĭp-nŏt'ĭk) [L. post, behind, after, + Gr. hypnos, sleep]

posthypnotic suggestion

postictal (pōst-ĭk'tăl) [" + ictus, a blow or stroke]

posticteric (pōst"ĭk-tĕr'ĭk) [" + Gr. ikteros, jaundice]

postmalarial (pōst"mă-lā'rē-ăl) [" + It. malaria, bad air]

postmature (pōst"mă-tūr') [" + maturus, ripe]

postmaturity (pōst"mă-tū'rĭ-tē) [" + maturus, ripe]

postmediastinal (pōst"mē-dē-ăs'tĭ-năl) [" + mediastinum, in the middle]

postmenopausal (pōst"mĕn-ōpaw'zăl) [" + Gr. *men,* month, + *pausis,* cessation]

post mortem, postmortem [L.]

postmortem examination

postnasal (pōst-nā'zăl) [L. *post,* behind, after, + *nasus,* nose]

postnatal [" + *natus,* birth]

postnecrotic (pōst″nĕ-krŏt'ĭk) [" + Gr. *nekrotikos,* dead]

postneuritic (pōst″nū-rĭt'ĭk) [" + *neuron,* nerve, + *itis,* inflammation]

postocular (pōst-ŏk'ū-lar) [" + *oculus,* eye]

postocular neuritis

postolivary (pōst-ŏl'ĭ-vă-rē) [" + *oliva,* olive]

postoperative care [" + *operatus,* work]

postoperculum (pōst-ō-pŭr'kū-lŭm) [" + *operculum,* a covering]

postoral (pōst-or'ăl)[" + *os,* mouth]

postorbital (pōst-or'bĭ-tăl) [" + *orbita,* track]

postpalatine (pōst-păl'ă-tīn) [" + *palatum,* palate]

postpallium (pōst-păl'ē-ŭm) [" + *pallium,* cloak]

postpaludal (pōst-păl'ū-dăl) [" + *palus,* swamp]

postparalytic (pōst″păr-ă-lĭt'ĭk) [" + *paralytikos]*

post partum, postpartum (pōst-păr'tŭm) [L. *post,* behind, after, + *partus,* birth]

postpartum blues

postpartum depression

postpartum hemorrhage

postpartum pituitary necrosis

postpartum psychosis

postpharyngeal (pōst-fă-rĭn'jē-ăl) [L. *post,* behind, after, + Gr. *pharynx,* throat]

postpneumonic (pōst″nū-mŏn'ĭk) [" + *pneumon,* lung]

postpoliomyelitis muscular atrophy

postpontile (pōst-pŏn'tĭl) [" + *pons,* bridge]

postprandial (pōst-prăn'dē-ăl)

postpubertal (pōst-pū'bĕr-tăl) [" + *pubertas,* puberty]

postpuberty (pōst-pū'bĕr-tē)

postpubescent (pōst″pū-bĕs'ĕnt) [" + *pubescens,* becoming hairy]

postpyramidal (pōst-pī-răm'ĭd-ăl)

postpyramidal nucleus

postradiation (pōst″rā-dē-ā'shŭn)

postsacral (pōst-sā'krăl) [" + *sacrum,* sacred]

postscapular (pōst-skăp'ū-lăr) [" + *scapula,* shoulder blade]

postscarlatinal (pōst″skăr-lă-tē'năl) [" + *scarlatina,* scarlet fever]

postsphygmic (pōst-sfĭg'mĭk) [" + Gr. *sphygmos,* pulse]

postsplenic (pōst-splĕn'ĭk) [" + Gr. *splen,* spleen]

poststenotic (pōst″stĕ-nŏt'ĭk) [" + Gr. *stenosis,* act of narrowing]

postsynaptic (pōst″sĭ-năp'tĭk) [" + Gr. *synapsis,* point of contact]

post-tarsal (pōst-tăr'săl) [" + Gr. *tarsos,* flat of the foot, flat surface, edge of eyelid]

post-term infant

post-tibial (pōst-tĭb'ē-ăl) [" + *tibia,* shinbone]

post-transfusion syndrome

post-traumatic (pōst″traw-măt'ĭk) [" + *traumatikos,* traumatic]

post-traumatic stress syndrome

postulate (pŏs'tū-lāt) [L. *postulare,* to request]

postural (pŏs'tū-răl) [L. *postura,* position]

postural drainage

postural hypotension

posture (pŏs'tŭr) [L. *postura]*
    p., coiled
    p., dorsal rigid
    p., orthopnea
    p., orthotonos
    p., prone
    p., semireclining

postuterine (pōst-ū'tĕr-īn) [L. *post,* behind, after, + *uterus,* womb]

postvaccinal (pōst-văk'sĭ-năl) [" + *vaccinus,* pert. to cows]

postviral fatigue syndrome
potable (pō'tǎ-bl) [LL. *potabilis*]
Potain's apparatus (pō-tānz') [Pierre
C. E. Potain, Fr. physician, 1825–
1901]
Potain's sign
potamophobia (pŏt"ǎ-mō-fō'bē-ǎ)
[Gr. *potamos*, river, + *phobos*,
fear]
potash (pŏt'ǎsh) [Obsolete Dutch, *po-
tasschan*]
    p., caustic
    p., sulfurated
potassemia (pŏt-ǎ-sē'mē-ǎ) [NL. *potassa*, potash, + Gr. *haima*,
blood]
potassic (pō-tǎs'ĭk)
potassium (pō-tǎs'ē-ŭm) [NL. *potassa*,
potash]
    p. acetate
    p. alum
    p. aminosalicylate
    p. arsenite solution
    p. bicarbonate
    p. bitartrate
    p. bromide
    p. carbonate
    p. chlorate
    p. chloride
    p. chromate
    p. citrate
    p. cyanide
    p. gluconate
    p. guaiacolsulfonate
    p. hydroxide
    p. iodide
    p. nitrite
    p. permanganate
    p. phosphate, dibasic
    p. sodium tartrate
    p. sulfate
    p. tartrate
potassium chlorate poisoning
potassium chromate poisoning
potassium hydroxide poisoning
potbelly
potency (pō'tĕn-sē) [L. *potentia*,
power]

potent (pō'tĕnt) [L. *potens*, powerful]
potentia coeundi (pō-tĕn'shē-ǎ kō-ē-
ŭn'dĭ) [L.]
potential
    p., action
    p., after
    p., demarcation
    p., injury
    p., membrane
    p., resting
    p., spike
potentiate (pō-tĕn'shē-āt)
potentiation (pō-tĕn"shē-ā'shŭn)
potentiometer (pō-tĕn"shē-ŏm'ĕ-tĕr)
potion (pō'shŭn) [L. *potio*, draft]
Pott's disease [Percivall Pott, Brit. surgeon, 1713–1788]
Pott's fracture
pouch (powch) [ME. *pouche*]
    p., abdominovesical
    p., branchial
    p., Broca's
    p., Heidenhain
    p., laryngeal
    p. of Douglas
    p., Pavlov
    p., pharyngeal
    p., Prussak's
    p., Rathke's
    p., rectouterine
    p., rectovesical
poudrage (pū-drǎzh') [Fr.]
poultice (pōl'tĭs) [L. *pultes*, thick paste]
pound (pownd) [L. *pondus*, weight]
    p., avoirdupois
    p., foot-
    p., troy
Poupart's ligament (pū-pǎrz') [Fran-
çois Poupart, Fr. anatomist, 1616–
1708]
poverty
poverty of thought
povidone (pō'vĭ-dōn)
povidone-iodine
powder [ME. *poudre*]
power [ME. *power*]
pox (pŏks) [ME. *pokkes*, pits]
poxvirus (pŏks'vī-rŭs)

p.p. [L.] *punctum proximum,* near point of accommodation
ppb *parts per billion*
P.P.D. *purified protein derivative*
P.P.F. *pellagra preventive factor*
PPLO *pleuropneumonia-like organisms*
ppm *parts per million*
ppt *parts per trillion; precipitate; pre-pared*
Pr. *presbyopia; praseodymium*
p.r. [L.] *punctum remotum,* far point of visual accommodation
practical nurse
practice (prăk′tĭs) [Gr. *praktike,* business]
practitioner (prăk-tĭsh′ŭn-ĕr)
praecox (prē′kŏks) [L.]
praevia, praevius (prē′vē-ă, prē′vē-ŭs) [L.]
pragmatagnosia (prăg″măt-ăg-nō′zē-ă) [Gr. *pragma,* object, + *agnosia,* lack of recognition]
pragmatamnesia (prăg″măt-ăm-nē′zē-ă) [″ + *amnesia,* forgetfulness]
  p., visual
pragmatic (prăg-măt′ĭk) [Gr. *pragma,* a thing done]
pragmatism (prăg′mă-tĭzm) [″ + *-ismos,* condition]
pragmatist (prăg′mă-tĭst)
pralidoxime chloride (prăl″ĭ-dŏks′ēm)
pramoxine hydrochloride (prăm-ŏk′sēn)
prandial (prăn′dē-ăl) [L. *prandium,* breakfast]
Prantal
praseodymium (prā″sē-ō-dĭm′ē-ŭm) [Gr. *prasios,* leek-green, + *didymium*]
Prausnitz-Küstner reaction (prows′nĭts-kĭst′nĕr) [Carl W. Prausnitz, Ger. hygienist, b. 1876; Heinz Küstner, Ger. gynecologist, b. 1897]
praxinoscope (prăk-sĭn′ō-skōp) [Gr. *praxis,* action, + *skopein,* to examine]

praxiology (prăk″sē-ŏl′ō-jē) [″ + *logos,* word, reason]
praxis (prăk′sĭs) [Gr., action]
-praxis [Gr., action]
Prayer of Maimonides [Rabbi Moses ben Maimon, Jewish philosopher and physician, 1135–1204]
prazepam (prā′zē-păm)
praziquantel
prazosin hydrochloride
pre- [L. *prae,* before, in front of]
preadmission certification
preagonal (prē-ăg′ō-năl) [L. *prae,* before, in front of, + Gr. *agonia,* agony]
prealbuminuric (prē″ăl-bū″mĭn-ū′rĭk) [″ + *albumen,* white of egg]
preanal (prē-ā′năl) [″ + *anus,* anus]
preanesthesia (prē″ăn-ĕs-thē′zē-ă)
preanesthetic (prē″ăn-ĕs-thĕt′ĭk) [″ + Gr. *anaisthesia,* lack of sensation]
preantiseptic (prē″ăn-tĭ-sĕp′tĭk) [″ + Gr. *anti,* against, + *sepsis,* decay]
preaortic (prē″ā-or′tĭk) [″ + Gr. *aorte,* aorta]
preataxic (prē-ă-tăk′sĭk) [″ + Gr. *ataxia,* lack of order]
preauricular (prē″aw-rĭk′ū-lăr) [″ + *auricula,* little ear]
preaxial (prē-ăk′sē-ăl) [″ + Gr. *axon,* axis]
precancer (prē′kăn-sĕr) [″ + *cancer,* crab]
precancerous (prē-kăn′sĕr-ŭs) [″ + *cancer,* crab]
precapillary [″ + *capillaris,* hairlike]
precava (prē-kā′vă) [″ + *cavus,* hollow]
precentral (prē-sĕn′trăl) [″ + Gr. *kentron,* center]
precentral convolution
prechordal (prē-kor′dăl) [″ + Gr. *chorde,* cord]
precipitable (prē-sĭp′ĭ-tă-b′l)
precipitant (prē-sĭp′ĭ-tănt) [L. *praecipi-*

tare, to cast down]
precipitate (prē-sĭp′ĭ-tāt)
precipitation (prē-sĭp″ĭ-tā′shŭn) [L. *praecipitatio*]
precipitation test
precipitin (prē-sĭp′ĭ-tĭn)
precipitinogen (prē-sĭp″ĭ-tĭn′ō-jĕn)
precipitinoid (prĕ-sĭp′ĭt-ĭn-oyd)
precipitin test
precipitophore (prē-sĭp′ĭt-ō-for″)
precipitum (prē-sĭp′ĭ-tŭm)
preclinical (prē-klĭn′ĭ-kăl) [L. *prae*, before, in front of, + Gr. *klinike*, medical treatment in bed]
preclinical dental training
preclinical technique
preclival (prē-klī′văl) [″ + *clivus*, slope]
precocious (prē-kō′shŭs) [L. *praecox*, ripening early]
precocity (prē-kŏs′ĭ-tē)
   p., sexual
precognition (prē″kŏg-nĭsh′ŭn) [L. *prae*, before, in front of, + *cognoscere*, to know]
precoital (prē-kō′ĭ-tăl) [″ + *coitio*, a going together]
precoma (prē-kō′mă) [″ + Gr. *koma*, deep sleep]
preconscious (prē-kŏn′shŭs) [″ + *conscius*, aware]
preconvulsive (prē″kŏn-vŭl′sĭv) [″ + *convulsio*, pulling together]
precordia (prē-kor′dē-ă) [L. *praecordia*]
precordial (prē-kor′dē-ăl)
precordialgia (prē″kor-dē-ăl′jē-ă) [L. *praecordia*, precordia, + Gr. *algos*, pain]
precordium (prē-kor′dē-ŭm)
precornu (prē-kor′nū) [L. *prae*, before, in front of, + *cornu*, horn]
precostal (prē-kŏs′tăl) [″ + Gr. *costa*, rib]
precritical (prē-krĭt′ĭ-kăl) [″ + Gr. *kritikos*, critical]
precuneus (prē-kū′nē-ŭs) [″ + *cuneus*, wedge]

precursor
predentin
prediabetes (prē-dī″ă-bē′tēz) [″ + Gr. *diabetes*, passing through]
prediastole (prē″dī-ăs′tō-lē) [″ + Gr. *diastellein*, to expand]
prediastolic (prē″dī-ă-stŏl′ĭk) [″ + Gr. *diastole*, expansion]
predicrotic (prē″dī-krŏt′ĭk) [″ + Gr. *dikrotos*, beating double]
prediction rules
predigestion (prē″dī-jĕs′chŭn)[″ + *digestio*, carrying apart]
predisposing (prē″dĭs-pōz′ĭng) [″ + *disponere*, to dispose]
predisposition (prē″dĭs-pō-zĭsh′ŭn)
prednisolone (prĕd-nĭs′ō-lōn)
prednisone (prĕd′nĭ-sōn)
predormition (prē-dor-mĭ′shŭn) [″ + *dormire*, to sleep]
preeclampsia (prē″ē-klămp′sē-ă) [″ + Gr. *ek*, out, + *lampein*, to flash]
preeruptive (prē″ē-rŭp′tĭv) [″ + *eruptio*, a breaking out]
pre-excitation (prē-ĕk″sī-tā′shŭn) [″ + *excitare*, to arouse]
preexisting condition
preferred provider organization
Prefrin Liquifilm
prefrontal (prē-frŏn′tăl)[″ + *frons*, front]
preganglionic (prē″găng-lē-ŏn′ĭk) [″ + Gr. *ganglion*, knot]
preganglionic fiber
preganglionic neuron
pregenital (prē-jĕn′ĭ-tăl) [″ + *genitalia*, genitals]
pregnancy (prĕg′năn-sē) [L. *praegnans*]
   p., abdominal
   p., ampullar
   p., bigeminal
   p., cervical
   p., cornual
   p., ectopic
   p., extrauterine
   p., false

p., heterotopic
p., hydatid
p., interstitial
p., intraligamentary
p., intramural
p., mask of
p., membranous
p., mesenteric
p., molar
p., multiple
p., mural
p., ovarian
p., phantom
p., postdate
p., tubal
p., tuboabdominal
p., tuboligamentary
p., tubo-ovarian
p., uteroabdominal
pregnancy, coitus during
pregnancy-specific β_1 glycoprotein
pregnancy test
pregnane (prĕg'nān)
pregnanediol (prĕg"nān-dī'ŏl)
pregnanetriol (prĕg"nān-trī'ŏl)
pregnant (prĕg'nănt) [L. praegnans]
pregnene (prĕg'nēn)
pregneninolone (prĕg"nēn-īn'ō-lōn)
pregnenolone (prĕg-nĕn'ō-lōn)
Pregnyl
pregravidic (prē-gră-vĭd'ĭk) [L. prae, before, in front of, + gravida, pregnant]
prehallux (prē-hăl'ŭks) [" + hallux, the great toe]
prehemiplegic (prē"hĕm-ĭ-plē'jĭk) [" + Gr. hemi, half, + plege, a stroke]
prehensile (prē-hĕn'sĭl) [L. prehendere, to seize]
prehension (prē-hĕn'shŭn) [L. prehensio]
prehormone
prehyoid (prē-hī'oyd) [L. prae, before, in front of, + Gr. hyoeides, U-shaped]
prehypophysis (prē"hī-pŏf'ĭ-sĭs) [" + Gr. hypophysis, an under-growth]
preictal (prē-ĭk'tăl) [" + ictus, stroke]
preicteric (prē-ĭk-tĕr'ĭk) [" + ikteros, jaundice]
preimmunization (prē-ĭm"ū-nĭ-zā'shŭn) [" + immunis, safe]
preinvasive (prē"ĭn-vā'sĭv) [" + in, into, + vadere, to go]
Preiser's disease (prī'zĕrz) [Georg K.F. Preiser, Ger. orthopedic surgeon, 1879-1913]
preleukemia
preload
Preludin
premaniacal (prē"mă-nī'ă-kăl) [L. prae, before, in front of, + Gr. mania, madness]
Premarin
premature (prē-mă-chūr') [L. praematurus, ripening early]
premature beat
premature ejaculation
premature infant
premature labor
prematurity
premaxilla (prē"măk-sĭl'ă) [L. prae, before, in front of, + maxilla, jawbone]
premaxillary (prē-măk'sĭ-lĕr"ē)
premedication (prē"mĕd-ĭ-kā'shŭn) [" + medicari, to heal]
premenarchal (prē"mĕ-năr'kăl) [" + Gr. men, mouth, + arche, beginning]
premenstrual (prē-mĕn'stroo-ăl) [" + menstruare, to discharge the menses]
premenstrual tension syndrome
premenstruum (prē-mĕn'stroo-ŭm) [" + menstruus, menstral fluid]
premolar (prē-mō'lĕr) [" + moles, a mass]
premonition (prĕm'ĕ-, prē-mĕ-nĭsh'ŭn) [L. praemonere, to warn beforehand]
premonitory (prē-mŏn'ĭ-tō-rē) [LL. praemonitorius]
premonocyte (prē-mŏn'ō-sīt) [L. prae,

before, in front of, + Gr. *monos*, alone, + *kytos*, cell]

premorbid (prē-mor'bĭd) [" + *morbidus*, sick]

premunition (prē"mū-nĭsh'ŭn) [" + *munitio*, a fortification]

premyeloblast (prē-mī'ĕ-lō-blăst) [" + Gr. *myelos*, marrow, + *blastos*, germ]

premyelocyte (prē-mī'ĕl-ō-sīt) [" + " + *kytos*, cell]

prenarcosis (prē-năr-kō'sĭs) [" + Gr. *narkosis*, action of benumbing]

prenares (prē-nā'rēz) [" + *naris*, nostril]

prenatal (prē-nā'tl) [" + *natalis*, birth]

prenatal care

prenatal diagnosis

preneoplastic (prē"nē-ō-plăs'tĭk) [" + *neos*, new, + *plassein*, to form]

preoperative care (prē-ŏp'er-ă-tĭv) [" + *operatus*, work]

preoptic area

preoral (prē-ō'răl) [L. *prae*, before, in front of, + *os*, mouth]

prep (prĕp) [*prepare; preparation*]

prepalatal (prē-păl'ă-tăl) [L. *prae*, before, in front of, + *palatum*, plate]

preparalytic (prē"păr-ă-lĭt'ĭk) [" + Gr. *paralytikos*]

preparation (prĕp-ă-rā'shŭn) [L. *prae-paratio*]

  p., corrosion

  p., heart-lung

  p.'s, rectal

prepatellar (prē"pă-tĕl'ăr) [L. *prae*, before, in front of, + *patella*, a small pan]

prepatellar bursitis

prepatent

prepatent period

preperception (prē"pĕr-sĕp'shŭn) [" + *percepitio*, to perceive]

preperitoneal (prē"pĕr-ĭ-tō-nē'ăl) [" + Gr. *peritonaion*, stretched around or over]

preplacental (prē"plă-sĕn'tăl) [" + *placenta*, a flat cake]

prepotent (prē-pō'tĕnt) [" + *potentia*, power]

preprandial (prē-prăn'dē-ăl) [" + *prandium*, breakfast]

prepuberal, prepubertal (prē-pū'bĕr-ăl, -tăl) [" + *pubertas*, puberty]

prepubescent (prē"pū-bĕs'ĕnt) [" + *pubescens*, becoming hairy]

prepuce (prē'pūs) [L. *praeputium*, prepuce]

  p. of clitoris

preputial (prē-pū'shăl)

preputial glands

preputiotomy (prē-pū"shē-ŏt'ō-mē) [" + Gr. *tome*, a cutting, slice]

preputium (prē-pū'shē-ŭm)

  p. clitoridis

  p. penis

prepyloric (prē"pī-lor'ĭk)

prerectal (prē-rĕk'tăl) [L. *prae*, before, in front of, + *rectus*, straight]

prerenal (prē-rē'năl) [" + *ren*, kidney]

preretinal (prē-rĕt'ĭ-năl) [" + *retina*, retina]

presacral (prē-sā'krăl) [" + *sacrum*, sacred]

presbyacusia, presbyacousia (prĕz"bē-ă-kū'sē-ă) [Gr. *presbys*, old, + *akousis*, hearing]

presbyatrics, presbyatry (prĕz-bē-ăt'rĭks, prĕz'bē-ăt-rē) [" + *iatridos*, healing]

presbycardia (prĕz-bĭ-kăr'dē-ă) [" + *kardia*, heart]

presbycusis, presbykousis (prĕz-bĭ-kū'sĭs) [" + *akousis*, hearing]

presbyope (prĕs'bē-ōp) [" + *ops*, eye]

presbyopia (prĕz-bē-ō'pē-ă) [" + *ops*, eye]

presbyopic (prĕs"bē-ŏp'ĭk)

presbytiatrics (prĕz"bĭ-tē-ăt'rĭks) [" + *iatrikos*, healing]

prescribe (prē-skrīb') [L. *praescriptio*,

prescription]
prescribing nurses
prescription (prē-skrĭp'shŭn) [L. *prae-scriptio*]
  p., shotgun
prescription drug
prescription writing
presenile (prē-sē'nĭl) [L. *prae*, before, in front of, + *senilis*, old]
presenium (prē-sē'nē-ŭm) [" + *senium*, old age]
presentation (prē"zĕn-tā'shŭn) [L. *praesentatio*]
  p., breech
  p., brow
  p., cephalic
  p., compound
  p., face
  p., footling
  p., funic; p., funis
  p., longitudinal
  p., oblique
  p., pelvic
  p., placental
  p., shoulder
  p., transverse
  p., vertex
preservative (prē-zĕr'vă-tĭv) [L. *prae*, before, in front of, + *servare*, to keep]
presomite (prē-sō'mīt) [" + Gr. *soma*, body]
presphenoid (prē-sfē'noyd) [" + Gr. *sphen*, wedge, + *eidos*, form, shape]
presphygmic (prē-sfĭg'mĭk) [" + Gr. *sphygmos*, pulse]
prespinal (prē-spī'năl) [" + *spina*, thorn]
prespondylolisthesis (prē-spŏn"dĭl-ō-lĭs-thē'sĭs) [" + Gr. *spondylos*, vertebra, + *olisthanein*, to slip]
pressor (prĕs'or) [O. Fr. *presser*, to press]
pressor base
pressoreceptive (prĕs"ō-rē-sĕp'tĭv)
pressoreceptor (prĕs"ō-rē-sĕp'tor)
pressor nerves

pressor reflex
pressosensitive (prĕs"ō-sĕn'sĭ-tĭv)
pressure (prĕsh'ŭr) [L. *pressura*]
  p., after-
  p., arterial
  p., atmospheric
  p., back
  p., biting
  p., blood
  p., capillary
  p., central venous
  p., cerebrospinal
  p., diastolic
  p., effective osmotic
  p., end-diastolic
  p., endocardiac
  p., hydrostatic
  p., intra-abdominal
  p., intracranial
  p., intraocular
  p., intrathoracic
  p., intraventricular
  p., negative
  p., occlusal
  p., oncotic
  p., osmotic
  p., partial
  p., positive
  p., positive end-expiratory
  p., preload filling
  p., pulse
  p., solution
  p., static
  p., systolic
  p., venous
  p., wedge
pressure of speech
pressure palsy
pressure paralysis
pressure points
pressure sore
presternum (prē-stĕr'nŭm) [L. *prae*, before, in front of, + Gr. *sternon*, chest]
presuppurative (prē-sŭp'ū-rā"tĭv) [" + *sub*, under, + *puris*, pus]
presylvian fissure (prē-sĭl'vē-ăn)
presymptomatic (prē"sĭmp-tō-măt'ĭk)

presynaptic (prē"sĭ-nǎp'tĭk) [" + Gr. *synapsis*, point of contact]

presystole (prē-sĭs'tō-lē) [L. *prae*, before, in front of, + Gr. *systole*, contraction]

presystolic (prē-sĭs-tŏl'ĭk)

pretarsal (prē-tăr'săl) [" + Gr. *tarsos*, flat of the foot, flat surface, edge of eyelid]

preterm

pretibial (prē-tĭb'ē-ăl) [" + *tibia*, shinbone]

pretibial fever

pretympanic (prē"tĭm-păn'ĭk) [" + *tympanon*, drum]

preurethritis (prē"ū-rē-thrī'tĭs) [" + Gr. *ourethra*, urethra, + *itis*, inflammation]

prevalence (prĕv'ă-lĕns) [L. *praevalens*, prevail]

preventive (prē-vĕn'tĭv) [ME. *preventen*, to anticipate]

preventive dentistry

preventive medicine

preventive nursing

prevertebral (prē-vĕr'tē-brăl) [L. *prae*, before, in front of, + *vertebra*, vertebra]

prevertebral ganglia

prevertiginous (prē-vĕr-tĭj'ĭ-nŭs) [" + *vertigo*, a turning round]

prevesical (prē-vĕs'ĭ-kl) [" + *vesica*, bladder]

previa, praevia (prē'vē-ă) [L.]

previable

prevocational evaluation

prezonular

prezygotic (prē-zī-gŏt'ĭk) [" + *zygotos*, yoked]

priapism (prī'ă-pĭzm) [LL. *priapismus*] p., stuttering

priapitis (prī-ă-pī'tĭs) [Gr. *priapos*, phallus, + *itis*, inflammation]

priapus (prī'ă-pŭs) [Gr. *priapos*]

prickle cell (prĭk'l)

prickly heat

prilocaine hydrochloride (prĭl'ō-kān)

primal scene

primaquine phosphate (prĭm'ă-kwĭn)

primary (prī'mă-rē) [L. *primarius*, principal]

primary amputation

primary bubo

primary care

primary cell

primary hemorrhage

primary lesion

primary nursing

primary physician

primary radiation

primary sore

primate (prī'māt) [L. *primus*, first]

Primatene Mist

Primates (prī-mā'tēz)

prime (prīm) [L. *primus*, first]

primidone (prĭm'ĭ-dōn)

primigravida (prī-mĭ-grăv'ĭ-dă) [" + *gravida*, pregnant]

primipara (prī-mĭp'ă-ră) [" + *parere*, to beget, produce]

primiparity (prī"mĭ-păr'ĭ-tē)

primiparous (prī-mĭp'ă-rŭs)

primitiae (prī-mĭsh'ē-ē) [L. *primus*, first]

primitive (prĭm'ĭ-tĭv) [L. *primitivus*]

primitive groove

primitive streak

primordial (prī-mor'dē-ăl) [L. *primordialis*]

primordium (prī-mor'dē-ŭm) [L., origin]

primum non nocere (prī"mŭm nŏn nō'sĕ-ră) [L.]

princeps (prĭn'sĕps) [L., chief]

principal (prĭn'sĭ-păl)

principal fibers of the periodontal ligament

principle (prĭn'sĭ-pl) [L. *principium*, foundation]

    p., active

    p., antianemic

    p., antidiuretic

    p.'s, gastrointestinal

    p., oxytocic

    p., pleasure

    p., proximate

    p., purpura-producing

    p., reality

Prinzmetal's angina [Myron Prinzmetal, U.S. cardiologist, b. 1908]
prion
Priscoline Hydrochloride
prism (prĭzm) [Gr. *prisma*]
    p., enamel
    p., Maddox
    p., Nicol
    p., Risley's rotary
prismatic (prĭz-măt'ĭk)
prismoid (prĭz'moyd) [" + *eidos*, form, shape]
prismoptometer (prĭz-mŏp-tŏm'ĕ-tĕr) [" + *opsis*, sight, appearance, vision, + *metron*, measure]
privacy
private patient
private practice
privileged communication
Privine Hydrochloride
p.r.n. [L.] *pro re nata*, as circumstance may require; as necessary
pro- [L., Gr. *pro*, before]
proaccelerin
proactinomycin (prō-ăk"tĭ-nō-mī'sĭn)
proactivator (prō-ăk'tĭ-vā"tor)
proagglutinoid (prō"ă-gloo'tĭ-noyd)
proal (prō'ăl) [Gr. *pro*, before]
proamnion (prō-ăm'nē-ŏn) [Gr. *pro*, before, + *amnion*, amnion]
proantithrombin (prō"ăn-tĭ-thrŏm'bĭn)
proatlas (prō-ăt'lăs) [" + *atlas*, a support]
probability
proband [L. *probare*, to test]
probang (prō'băng)
Pro-Banthine
probationary (prō-bā'shŭn-ăr-ē) [L. *probatio*, probation]
probationer (prō-bā'shŭn-ĕr)
probe (prōb) [L. *probare*, to test]
    p., dental
    p., periodontal
probenecid
problem-oriented medical record
problem-oriented record
probucol (prō'bū-kŏl)
procainamide hydrochloride

procaine hydrochloride (prō'kān)
Procan
procarbazine hydrochloride (prō-kăr'bă-zēn)
procarboxypeptidase (prō"kăr-bŏk"sē-pĕp'tĭ-dās)
procaryote (prō-kăr'ē-ōt) [Gr. *pro*, before, + *karyon*, nucleus]
procatarctic (prō"kă-tărk'tĭk) [" + *katarchein*, to begin]
procatarxis (prō"kă-tărk'sĭs)
procedure (prō-sē'dūr) [L. *procedere*, to proceed]
procelous (prō-sē'lŭs) [Gr. *pro*, before, + *koilos*, hollow]
procentriole (prō-sĕn'trē-ōl)
procephalic (pro"sē-făl'ĭk) [" + *kephale*, head]
procercoid (prō-sĕr'koyd)
procerus muscle
process (prŏs'ĕs) [L. *processus*, going before]
    p., acromion
    p., alar
    p., alveolar
    p., articular, of vertebra
    p., basilar
    p., caudate
    p., ciliary
    p., clinoid
    p., condyloid
    p., coracoid
    p., coronoid
    p., ensiform
    p., ethmoidal
    p., falciform
    p., frontal
    p., frontonasal
    p., frontosphenoidal
    p., head
    p., infraorbital
    p., jugular
    p., lacrimal
    p., lenticular
    p., malar
    p., mandibular
    p., mastoid
    p., maxillary

p., nursing
p., odontoid
p., olecranon
p., orbital
p., palatine
p., postglenoid
p., pterygoid
p., spinous, of vertebrae
p., styloid
p., transverse
p., uncinate, of ethmoid bone
p., vermiform
p., vocal
p., xiphoid
p., zygomatic

processus (prō-sĕs'ŭs) [L.]
p. cochleariformis
p. retromandibularis
p. uncinatus

procheilon (prō-kī'lŏn) [Gr. pro, before, + cheilon, lip]

prochlorperazine (prō"klor-pĕr'ă-zēn)

prochondral (prō-kŏn'drăl) [" + chondros, cartilage]

prochordal (prō-kor'dăl) [" + chorde, cord]

procidentia (prō"sī-dĕn'shē-ă) [L.]

procollagen (prō-kŏl'ă-jĕn) [" + kolla, glue, + gennan, to produce]

proconvertin (prō"kŏn-vĕr'tĭn)

procreate [L. procreare]

procreation (prō"krē-ā'shŭn)

procreative (prō'krē-ā"tĭv)

proctagra (prŏk-tăg'ră) [Gr. proktos, anus, + agra, seizure]

proctalgia (prŏk-tăl'jē-ă) [" + algos, pain]
p. fugax

proctatresia (prŏk"tă-trē'zē-ă) [" + atresis, imperforation]

proctectasia (prŏk"tĕk-tā'sē-ă) [" + ektasis, dilatation]

proctectomy (prŏk-tĕk'tō-mē) [" + ektome, excision]

proctenclisis (prŏk"tĕn-klī'sĭs) [" + enkleiein, to shut in]

procteurynter (prŏk'tū-rĭn"tĕr) [" +

eurynein, to widen]

proctitis [" + itis, inflammation]
p., diphtheritic
p., dysenteric
p., gonorrheal
p., traumatic

procto-, proct- [Gr. proktos, anus]

proctocele (prŏk'tō-sēl) [" + kele, tumor, swelling]

proctoclysis (prŏk-tŏk'lĭ-sĭs) [" + klysis, a washing]

proctococcypexia, proctococcypexy (prŏk"tō-kŏk-sī-pĕk'sē-ă, -kŏk'sī-pĕk"sē) [" + kokkyx, coccyx, + pexis, fixation]

proctocolitis (prŏk"tō-kō-lī'tĭs) [" + kolon, colon, + itis, inflammation]

proctocolonoscopy (prŏk"tō-kō"lŏn-ŏs'kō-pē) [" + " + skopein, to examine]

Proctocort

proctocystoplasty (prŏk"tō-sĭs'tō-plăs"tē) [Gr. proktos, anus, + kystis, bladder, + plastos, formed]

proctocystotomy (prŏk"tō-sĭs-tŏt'ō-mē) [" + kystis, bladder, + tome, a cutting, slice]

proctodeum (prŏk-tō-dē'ŭm) [" + hodaios, a way]

proctodynia (prŏk"tō-dĭn'ē-ă) [" + odyne, pain]

proctologic (prŏk"tō-lŏj'ĭk) [" + logos, word, reason]

proctologist (prŏk-tŏl'ō-jĭst) [" + logos, word, reason]

proctology (prŏk-tŏl'ō-jē)

proctoparalysis (prŏk"tō-păr-ăl'ĭ-sĭs) [" + paralyein, to loosen, disable]

proctoperineoplasty (prŏk"tō-pĕr"ĭ-nē'ō-plăs"tē) [" + perinaion, perineum, + plassein, to form]

proctoperineorrhaphy (prŏk"tō-pĕr"ĭ-nē-or'ă-fē) [" + " + rhaphe, seam]

proctopexia, proctopexy (prŏk-tō-ĕk'sē-ă, prŏk'tō-pĕk"sē) [" + pexis, fixation]

proctophobia (prŏk"tō-fō'bē-ă)

[" + *phobos*, fear]
proctoplasty (prŏk'tō-plăs"tē) [" + *plastos*, formed]
proctoplegia (prŏk"tō-plē'jē-ă) [" + *plege*, a stroke]
proctopolypus (prŏk"tō-pŏl'ĭ-pŭs) [" + *polys*, many, + *pous*, foot]
proctoptosis (prŏk"tŏp-tō'sĭs) [" + *ptosis*, fall, falling]
proctorrhagia (prŏk"tō-rā'jē-ă) [" + *rhegnynai*, to burst forth]
proctorrhaphy (prŏk-tor'ă-fē) [" + *rhaphe*, seam]
proctorrhea (prŏk-tōr-ē'ă) [" + *rhein*, to flow]
proctoscope [" + *skopein*, to examine]
proctoscopy (prŏk-tŏs'kō-pē)
proctosigmoidectomy (prŏk"tō-sĭg"moy-dĕk'tō-mē) [" + *sigma*, Gr. letter S, + *eidos*, form, shape, + *ektome*, excision]
proctosigmoiditis (prŏk"tō-sĭg"moyd-ī'tĭs) [" + " + *eidos*, form, shape, + *itis*, inflammation]
proctosigmoidoscopy (prŏk"tō-sĭg-moyd-ŏs'kō-pē)
proctospasm [" + *spasmos*, a convulsion]
proctostasis (prŏk"tō-stā'sĭs) [" + *stasis*, standing still]
proctostenosis (prŏk"tō-stĕn-ō'sĭs) [" + *stenosis*, act of narrowing]
proctostomy (prŏk-tŏs'tō-mē) [" + *stoma*, mouth, opening]
proctotome (prŏk'tō-tōm) [" + *tome*, a cutting, slice]
proctotomy (prŏk-tŏt'ō-mē)
proctotoreusis (prŏk"tō-tō-roo'sĭs) [" + *toreusis*, boring]
proctotresia (prŏk-tō-trē'sē-ă) [" + *tresis*, a perforation]
proctovalvotomy (prŏk"tō-văl-vŏt'ō-mē) [" + L. *valva*, leaf of a folding door, + Gr. *tome*, a cutting, slice]
procumbent [L. *procumbens*, lying down]

procursive (prō-kŭr'sĭv) [L. *procursivus*]
procurvation (prō"kŭr-vā'shŭn) [L. *procurvare*, to bend forward]
procyclidine hydrochloride (prō-sī'klĭ-dēn)
prodromal (prō-drō'măl) [Gr. *prodromos*, running before]
prodromal rash
prodrome
prodromic (prō-drō'mĭk)
prodrug
product (prŏd'ŭkt) [L. *productum*]
production (prō-dŭk'shŭn)
productive (prō-dŭk'tĭv)
productive inflammation
proencephalus (prō"ĕn-sĕf'ă-lŭs) [Gr. *pro*, before, + *enkephalos*, brain]
proenzyme (prō-ĕn'zīm) [" + *en*, in, + *zyme*, a leaven]
proerythroblast (prō"ē-rĭth'rō-blăst) [" + *erythros*, red, + *blastos*, germ]
proestrus (prō-ĕs'trŭs)
proferment [Gr. *pro*, before, + L. *fermentum*, leaven]
professional (prō-fĕsh'ŭn-ăl) [ME. *profession*, sacred vow]
professional liability
Professional Standards Review Organization
profibrinolysin (prō"fĭ-brĭ-nō-lī'sĭn) [Gr. *pro*, before, + L. *fibra*, fiber, + Gr. *lysis*, dissolution]
profile (prō'fĭl) [L. *pro*, forward, + *filare*, to draw a line]
profluvium (prō-floo'vē-ŭm) [L.]
 p. lactis
 p. seminis
profondometer (prō"fŏn-dŏm'ĕ-tĕr) [L. *profundus*, deep, + Gr. *metron*, a measure]
profunda [L.]
profundus (prō-fŭn'dŭs) [L.]
progastrin (prō-găs'trĭn)
progenitor (prō-jĕn'ĭ-tor) [L.]
progeny (prŏj'ĕ-nē) [ME. *progenie*]
progeria (prō-jē'rē-ă) [Gr. *pro*, before, + *geras*, old age]

progestational (prō"jĕs-tā'shŭn-ăl)
progestational agent
progesterone (prō-jĕs'tĕr-ōn)
progestin (prō-jĕs'tĭn)
progestogen (prō-jĕs'tō-jĕn)
proglossis (prō-glŏs'ĭs) [Gr.]
proglottid
proglottis (prō-glŏt'tĭs) [Gr. *pro*, before, + *glottis*, tongue]
Proglycem
prognathic (prŏg-nă'thĭk) [" + *gnathos*, jaw]
prognathism (prŏg'nă-thĭzm) [" + *gnathos*, jaw + -*ismos*, condition]
prognathous (prŏg'nă-thŭs)
prognose (prŏg-nōs')
prognosis (prŏg-nō'sĭs) [Gr., foreknowledge]
prognostic
prognosticate (prŏg-nŏs'tĭ-kāt) [Gr. *prognostikon*, knowing before]
prognostician (prŏg"nŏs-tĭsh'ăn)
progonoma (prō"gō-nō'mă) [Gr. *pro*, before, + *gonos*, offspring, procreation, + *oma*, tumor]
progranulocyte (prō-grăn'ū-lō-sīt) [" + L. *granula*, granule, + Gr. *kytos*, cell]
progravid (prō-grăv'ĭd) [" + L. *gravidus*, pregnant]
progression (prō-grĕsh'ŭn) [L. *progressus*]
progressive (prō-grĕs'ĭv)
progressive muscular atrophy
progressive ossifying myositis
progressive resistive exercise
progress notes
prohormone (prō-hor'mōn)
proinsulin
projectile vomiting
projection (prō'jĕk'shŭn) [Gr. *pro*, before, + *jacere*, to throw]
prokaryon (prō-kăr'ē-ŏn) [" + *karyon*, nucleus]
prokaryote (prō-kăr'ē-ōt) [" + *karyon*, nucleus]
Proklar
prolabium (prō-lā'bē-ŭm) [" + la-

bium, lip]
prolactin (prō-lăk'tĭn) [" + *lac*, milk]
prolamin(e) (prō-lăm'ĭn, prō'lă-mĭn)
prolapse (prō-lăps') [L. *prolapsus*]
  p. of anus
  p. of cord
  p. of iris
  p. of rectum
  p. of uterus
prolapsus [L.]
prolepsis [Gr. *pro*, before, + *lepsis*, a seizure]
proleptic
proleukocyte (prō-lū'kō-sīt) [" + *leukos*, white, + *kytos*, cell]
proliferate (prō-lĭf'ĕr-āt) [L. *proles*, offspring, + *ferre*, to bear]
proliferation (prō-lĭf"ĕr-ā'shŭn)
proliferous
proliferous cyst
prolific [L. *prolificus*]
prolinase
proline (prō'lēn)
Prolixin Enanthate
Proloid
Proloprim
prolymphocyte (prō"lĭmf'ō-sīt) [" + L. *lympha*, lymph, + Gr. *kytos*, cell]
Promapar
promazine hydrochloride (prō'mă-zēn)
promegakaryocyte (prō-mĕg"ă-kăr'ē-ō-sīt) [" + *megas*, big, + *karyon*, nucleus, + *kytos*, cell]
promegaloblast (prō-mĕg'ă-lō-blast") [" + " + *blastos*, germ]
prometaphase (prō-mĕt'ă-fāz) [" + *meta*, change, + *phasis*, appearance]
promethazine hydrochloride (prō-mĕth'ă-zēn)
promethium (prō-mē'thē-ŭm)
promine
prominence (prŏm'ĭ-nĕns) [L. *prominens*, project]
prominentia (prŏm"ĭ-nĕn'shē-ă) [L.]
  p. laryngea
  p. spiralis

promonocyte (prō-mŏn'ō-sīt) [Gr. *pro*, before, + *monos*, single, + *kytos*, cell]

promontory (prŏm'ŏn-tor"ē) [L. *promontorium*]
  p. of sacrum
  p. of tympanic cavity

promoter (prō-mō'tĕr)

promyelocyte (prō-mī'ĕl-ō-sīt) [Gr. *pro*, before, + *myelos*, marrow, + *kytos*, cell]

pronate (prō'nāt)

pronation (prō-nā'shŭn) [L. *pronus*, prone]

pronator

pronator syndrome

pronaus, pronaeus (prō-nā'ŭs) [Gr. *pro*, before, + *naos*, temple]

prone (prōn) [ME.]

pronephric (prō-nĕf'rĭk) [Gr. *pro*, before, + *nephros*, kidney]

pronephric duct

pronephric tubules

pronephros, pronephron (prō-nĕf'rŏs, -rŏn)

Pronestyl

prong (prŏng)

pronograde (prō'nō-grād) [L. *pronus*, prone, + *gradus*, a step]

pronometer (prō-nŏm'ĕ-tĕr) [" + Gr. *metron*, measure]

pronormoblast (prō-nor'mō-blăst) [Gr. *pro*, before, + L. *norma*, rule, + Gr. *blastos*, germ]

pronucleus (prō-nū'klē-ŭs) [Gr. *pro*, before, + *nucleus*, little kernel]

prootic (prō-ŏt'ĭk, -ō'tĭk) [" + *ous*, ear]

propagation (prŏp-ă-gā'shŭn) [L.]

propagative (prŏp'ă-gā"tĭv)

propalinal (prō-păl'ĭ-năl) [Gr. *pro*, before, + *palin*, back]

propane (prō'pān)

propantheline bromide (prō-păn'thĕ-lēn)

proparacaine hydrochloride (prō-păr'ă-kān)

propepsin (prō-pĕp'sĭn)

propeptone (prō-pĕp'tōn) [" + *peptein*, to digest]

propeptonuria (prō"pĕp-tō-nū'rē-ă) [" + " + *ouron*, urine]

properdin (prō-pĕrd'ĭn)

prophase (prō'fāz) [" + *phasis*, appearance]

prophylactic (prō-fĭ-lăk'tĭk) [Gr. *prophylaktikos*, guarding]

prophylaxis (prō-fĭ-lăk'sĭs, prō-fĭl-ăks'ĭs) [Gr. *prophylassein*, to guard against]
  p., oral

propiolactone (prō"pē-ō-lăk'tōn)

propiomazine hydrochloride (prō"pē-ō-mā'zēn)

propionic acid

proplasmacyte (prō-plăz'mă-sīt) [Gr. *pro*, before, + LL. *plasma*, form, mold, + Gr. *kytos*, cell]

proplastid (prō-plăs'tĭd)

Proplex

propolis [Gr. *pro*, before, + *polis*, city]

propositus (prō-pŏz'ĭ-tŭs) [L. *proponere*, to put on view]

propoxycaine hydrochloride (prō-pŏk'sē-kān)

propoxyphene hydrochloride (prō-pŏk'sē-fēn)

propranolol hydrochloride

proprietary medicine (prō-prī'ĕ-tar"ē) [L. *proprietarius*, pert. to property]

proprioception (prō"prē-ō-sĕp'shŭn) [L. *proprius*, one's own, + *capio*, to take]

proprioceptive (prō"prē-ō-sĕp'tĭv)

proprioceptive impulses

proprioceptive sense

proprioceptor (prō"prē-ō-sĕp'tor) [" + *ceptor*, a receiver]

propriospinal (prō"prē-ō-spī'năl) [" + *spina*, thorn]

proptometer (prŏp-tŏm'ĕ-tĕr) [Gr. *proptosis*, to fall forward, + *metron*, a measure]

proptosis (prŏp-tō'sĭs)

propulsion (prō-pŭl'shŭn) [L. *propulsus*, driven forward]

propyl (prō'pĭl)

proplyene glycol (prŏp'ĭ-lēn)

propylhexedrine (prō"pĭl-hĕk'sĕ-drēn)

propyliodone (prō"pĭl-ī'ō-dōn)

propylparaben (prō"pĭl-păr'ă-bĕn)

propylthiouracil (prō"pĭl-thī"ō-ū'ră-sĭl)

pro re nata (prō rē nā'tă) [L.]

prorrhaphy (prō'ră-fē) [Gr. *pro*, before, + *rhaphe*, seam]

prorsad (pror'săd)

prorubricyte (prō-roo'brĭ-sīt)

prosecretin (prō"sē-krē'tĭn) [" + *secretio*, separation]

prosection (prō-sĕk'shŭn) [" + L. *sectio*, a cutting]

prosector (prō-sĕk'tor) [L.]

prosencephalon (prŏs"ĕn-sĕf'ă-lŏn) [Gr. *proso*, before, + *enkephalos*, brain]

proso- [Gr. *proso*, forward]

prosodemic (prŏs"ō-dĕm'ĭk) [" + *demos*, people]

prosody (prŏs'ă-dē) [L. *prosodia*, accent of a syllable]

prosopagnosia (prŏs"ō-păg-nō'sē-ă) [Gr. *prosopon*, face, + *a-*, not, + *gnosis*, recognition]

prosopalgia (prŏs"ō-păl'jē-ă) [" + *algos*, pain]

prosopectasia (prŏs"ō-pĕk-tā'zē-ă) [" + *ektasis*, dilatation]

prosopic (prō'sŏp'ĭk)

prosoplasia (prŏs"ō-plā'sē-ă) [Gr. *proso*, forward, + *plassein*, to form]

prosopoanoschisis (prŏs"ō-pō"ă-nŏs'kĭ-sĭs) [Gr. *prosopon*, face, + *ana*, up, + *schisis*, cleavage]

prosopodiplegia (prŏs"ō-pō-dĭ-plē'jē-ă) [" + *dis*, twice, double, + *plege*, a stroke]

prosopodynia (prŏs"ō-pō-dĭn'ē-ă) [" + *odyne*, pain]

prosoponeuralgia (prŏs"ō-pō-nū-răl'jē-ă) [" + *neuron*, sinew, + *algos*, pain]

prosopopagus (prŏs"ō-pŏp'ă-gŭs) [" + *pagos*, a thing fixed]

prosopoplegia (prŏs"ō-pō-plē'jē-ă) [" + *plege*, stroke]

prosoposchisis (prŏs-ō-pŏs'kĭ-sĭs) [Gr. *prosopon*, face, + *schisis*, cleavage]

prosopospasm (prŏs'ō-pō-spăzm) [" + *spasmos*, a convulsion]

prosopothoracopagus (prŏs"ō-pō-thō"ră-kŏp'ă-gŭs) [" + *thorax*, chest, + *pagos*, a thing fixed]

prosopotocia (prŏs"ō-pō-tō'shē-ă) [" + *tokos*, birth]

prosopus varus (prŏs'ō-pūs vā'rŭs) [Gr. *prosopon*, face, + L. *varus*, crooked]

prospective study

prostaglandins (prŏs"tă-glănd-īns)

Prostaphlin

prostatalgia (prŏs-tă-tăl'jē-ă) [Gr. *prostates*, prostate, + *algos*, pain]

prostate (prŏs'tāt) [Gr. *prostates*]

prostatectomy (prŏs"tă-tĕk'tō-mē) [Gr. *prostates*, prostate, + *ektome*, excision]

prostathelcosis (prŏs"tă-thĕl-kō'sĭs) [" + *helkosis*, ulceration]

prostatic (prŏs-tăt'ĭk) [Gr. *prostates*, prostate]

prostatic calculus

prostatic plexus

prostatic syncope

prostatic urethra

prostatism (prŏs'tă-tĭzm) [" + *-ismos*, condition]

prostatitis (prŏs"tă-tī'tĭs) [" + *itis*, inflammation]
   p., acute
   p., chronic
   p., chronic bacterial

prostatocystitis (prŏs"tă-tō-sĭs-tī'tĭs) [Gr. *prostates*, prostate, + *kystis*, bladder, + *itis*, inflammation]

prostatocystotomy (prŏs"tă-tō-sĭs-tŏt'ō-mē) [" + " + *tome*, a cutting, slice]

prostatodynia (prŏs"tă-tō-dĭn'ē-ă)

[" + odyne, pain]
prostatography (prŏs"tă-tŏg'ră-fē)
[" + graphein, to write]
prostatolith (prŏs-tăt'ō-lĭth) [" +
lithos, stone]
prostatolithotomy (prŏs-tăt"ō-lĭ-
thŏt'ō-mē) [" + " + tome, a
cutting, slice]
prostatomegaly (prŏs"tă-tō-mĕg'ă-
lē) [" + megas, large]
prostatomy, prostatotomy (prŏs-
tăt'ō-mē, prŏs"tă-tŏt'ō-mē) [" +
tome, a cutting, slice]
prostatomyomectomy (prŏs"tă-tō-
mī"ō-mĕk'tō-mē) [" + mys, muscle,
+ ektome, excision]
prostatorrhea (prŏs"tă-tō-rē'ă) [" +
rhein, to flow]
prostatosis (prŏs"tă-tō'sĭs) [" +
osis, condition]
prostatovesiculectomy (prŏs"tă-tō-
vē-sĭk"ū-lĕk'tō-mē) [Gr. prostates, prostate, + L. vesiculus, a little sac,
+ Gr. ektome, excision]
prostatovesiculitis (prŏs"tă-tō-vē-
sĭk"ū-lī'tĭs) [" + " + Gr. itis,
inflammation]
prosternation (prō"stĕr-nā'shŭn) [Gr.
pro, before, + sternon, chest]
prostheon (prŏs'thē-ŏn) [Gr. prosthios,
foremost]
prosthesis (prŏs'thē-sĭs) [Gr. prosthesis, an addition]
  p., dental
  p., maxillofacial
  p., penile
prosthetic group (prŏs-thĕt'ĭk)
prosthetics (prŏs-thĕt'ĭks)
prosthetist (prŏs'thē-tĭst)
prosthetosclerokeratoplasty
  (prŏs"thē-tō-sklĕ"rō-kĕr'ă-tō-plăs"tē)
prosthion (prŏs'thē-ŏn) [Gr. prosthios,
foremost]
prosthodontics (prŏs"thō-dŏn'tĭks)
[" + odous, tooth]
prosthodontist (prŏs"thō-dŏn'tĭst)
prosthokeratoplasty (prŏs"thō-
kĕr'ă-tō-plăs"tē) [" + keras, horn,

+ plassein, to form]
Prostigmin
Prostin E₂
Prostin F₂ Alpha
Prostin/15M
prostitute (prŏs'tĭ-tūt) [L. prostituere, to
prostitute]
prostitution (prŏs"tĭ-tū'shŭn)
prostrate (prŏs'trāt) [Gr. pro, before,
+ L. sternere, stretch out]
prostrated
prostration (prŏs-trā'shŭn)
  p., heat
  p., nervous
protactinium (prō"tăk-tĭn'ē-ŭm)
protal (prō'tăl) [Gr. protos, first]
protamine (prō'tă-mēn)
  p. insulin
  p. sulfate
protanope (prō'tă-nōp) [Gr. protos,
first, + an-, not, + opsis,
sight, appearance, vision]
protanopia (prō-tăn-ō'pē-ă) [" +
" + opsis, sight, appearance, vi-
sion]
protean (prō'tē-ăn) [Gr. Proteus, a god
who could change his form]
protease (prō'tē-ās) [Gr. protos, first,
+ -ase, enzyme]
protective (prō-tĕk'tĭv) [L. protectus,
shielding]
protective isolation
proteidogenous (prō"tē-ĭd-ŏj'ĕn-ŭs)
protein (prō'tē-ĭn, prō'tēn) [Gr. protos,
first]
  p., Bence Jones
  p.'s, blood
  p., carrier
  p.'s, complete
  p.'s, conjugated
  p., C-reactive
  p., denatured
  p., derived
  p.'s, immune
  p., incomplete
  p., native
  p.'s, plasma
  p.'s, serum

p.'s, simple
proteinaceous (prō″tē-ĭn-ā′shŭs)
proteinase (prō′tē-ĭn-ās) [Gr. *protos,*
first, + *lase,* enzyme]
protein balance
protein C
protein-calorie malnutrition
proteinemia (prō″tē-ĭn-ē′mē-ă) [″ +
haima, blood]
protein hydrolysate injection
proteinic (prō″tē-ĭn′ĭk)
protein-losing enteropathy
proteinogenous (prō″tē-ĭn-ŏj′ĕn-ŭs)
[″ + *gennan,* to produce]
proteinophobia (prō″tē-ĭn-ō-fō′bē-ă)
[″ + *phobos,* fear]
proteinosis (prō″tē-ĭn-ō′sĭs) [″ +
osis, condition]
　　p., lipoid; p., lipid
　　p., pulmonary alveolar
protein sensitization
protein sparer
proteinuria (prō″tē-ĭn-ū′rē-ă) [″ +
ouron, urine]
　　p., orthostatic
　　p., postural
Protenate
proteoclastic (prō″tē-ō-klăs′tĭk) [Gr.
protos, first, + *klasis,* a breaking]
proteolipid (prō″tē-ō-lĭp′ĭd)
proteolysin (prō″tē-ŏl′ĭ-sĭn) [″ +
lysis, dissolution]
proteolysis (prō″tē-ŏl′ĭ-sĭs)
proteolytic (prō″tē-ō-lĭt′ĭk)
proteometabolism (prō″tē-ō-mĕ-
tăb′ō-lizm) [″ + *metabole,* change,
+ *-ismos,* condition]
proteopepsis (prō″tē-ō-pĕp′sĭs)
[″ + *peptein,* to digest]
proteopeptic (prō″tē-ō-pĕp′tĭk) [″ +
peptein, to digest]
proteopexic (prō-tē-ō-pĕks′ĭk) [″ +
pexis, fixation]
proteopexy (prō″tē-ō-pĕks′ē)
proteose (prō′tē-ōs) [Gr. *protos,* first]
　　p., primary
　　p., secondary
proteosuria (prō″tē-ōs-ū′rē-ă) [″ +

ouron, urine]
proteuria (prō″tē-ū′rē-ă)
Proteus (prō′tē-ŭs) [Gr. *Proteus,* a god
who could change his form]
　　P. mirabilis
　　P. morganii
　　P. vulgaris
prothrombin
prothrombinase
prothrombinemia (prō-thrŏm″bĭn-
ē′mē-ă) [Gr. *pro,* before, +
thrombos, clot, + *haima,* blood]
prothrombinogenic (prō-thrŏm″bĭ-
nō-jĕn′ĭk) [″ + ″ + *gennan,* to
produce]
prothrombinopenia (prō-thrŏm″bĭ-
nō-pē′nē-ă) [″ + ″ + *penia,*
lack]
prothrombin time
protide (prō′tĭd)
protist (prō′tĭst)
Protista (prō-tĭs′tă) [LL., simplest orga-
nisms]
protistologist (prō-tĭs-tŏl′ō-jĭst) [″ +
logos, word, reason]
protistology (prō-tĭs-tŏl′ō-jē)
protium (prō-tē-ŭm)
proto- [Gr. *protos,* first]
protobiology (prō″tō-bī-ŏl′ō-jē)
[″ + *bios,* life, + *logos,* word,
reason]
protoblast (prō′tō-blăst) [″ +
blastos, germ]
protoblastic (prō′tō-blăs′tĭk)
protocol (prō′tō-kŏl) [Gr. *protokollon,*
first notes glued to manuscript]
protodiastole (prō″tō-dĭ-ăs′tō-lē) [Gr.
protos, first, + *diastole,* expan-
sion]
protoduodenum (prō″tō-dū-ō-
dē′nŭm) [″ + L. *duodeni,* twelve]
protogaster (prō″tō-găs′tĕr) [″ +
gaster, belly]
protoleukocyte (prō″tō-lū′kō-sīt)
[″ + *leukos,* white, + *kytos,*
cell]
Protomastigida (prō″tō-măst-ĭj′ĭ-dă)
[″ + *mastix,* whip, + *eidos,*

form, shape]
proton (prō'tŏn) [Gr. *protos*, first]
protoneuron (prō"tō-nū'rŏn) [" + *neuron*, nerve]
Protopam Chloride
protopathic [" + *pathos*, disease, suffering]
protoplasia (prō-tō-plā'zē-ă) [" + *plassein*, to form]
protoplasm (prō'tō-plăzm) [" + LL. *plasma*, form, mold]
protoplasmic (prō-tō-plăz'mĭk)
protoplast (prō'tō-plăst) [" + *plassein*, to form]
protoporphyria (prō"tō-por-fīr'ē-ă)
protoporphyrin (prō"tō-por'fĭ-rĭn)
protoporphyrinuria (prō"tō-por"fĭ-rĭn-ū'rē-ă)
protoproteose (prō"tō-prō'tē-ōz)
protospasm (prō'tō-spăzm) [Gr. *protos*, first, + *spasmos*, a convulsion]
prototroph (prō'tō-trōf)
prototrophic (prō"tō-trō'fĭk) [" + *trophe*, nourishment]
prototype (prō"tō-tīp)
protovertebra (prō"tō-věr'tě-bră) [" + L. *vertebra*, vertebra]
protoxide (prō-tŏk'sīd)
Protozoa [" + *zoon*, animal]
protozoa
protozoacide (prō-tō-zō'ă-sīd) [" + *zoon*, animal, + L. *caedere*, to kill]
protozoal (prō"tō-zō'ăl)
protozoal diseases
protozoan (prō"tō-zō'ăn) [" + *zoon*, animal]
protozoiasis (prō"tō-zō-ī'ă-sĭs) [" + " + *-iasis*, state or condition of]
protozoology (prō"tō-zō-ŏl'ō-jē) [Gr. *protos*, first, + *zoon*, animal, + *logos*, word, reason]
protozoon
protozoophage (prō"tō-zō'ō-fāj) [" + *zoon*, animal, + *phagein*, to eat]
protraction (prō-trăk'shŭn) [" + L. *protractus*, dragged out]

protractor (prō-trăk'tor) [L. *protractus*, dragged out]
protriptyline hydrochloride (prō-trĭp'tĭ-lēn)
protrude [L. *protrudere*]
protrusion (prō-troo'zhŭn)
protuberance (prō-tū'bĕr-ăns) [Gr. *pro*, before, + L. *tuber*, bulge]
protuberantia (prō-tū"bĕr-ăn'shē-ă)
proud flesh
Provera
provertebra (prō-věr'tě-bră)
provirus (prō-vī'rŭs)
provisional (prō-vĭzh'ŭn-ăl) [L. *provisio*, provision]
provitamin (prō-vī'tă-mĭn) [L. *pro*, before, + *vita*, life, + *amine*] p. A
proximad (prŏk'sĭm-ăd) [L. *proximus*, next, + *ad*, toward]
proximal (prŏk'sĭm-ăl)
proximalis (prŏk"sĭ-mā'lĭs)
proximate (prŏk'sĭm-āt)
proximoataxia (prŏk"sĭ-mō-ă-tăk'sē-ă) [" + Gr. *ataxia*, lack of order]
proximobuccal (prŏk"sĭ-mō-bŭk'ăl) [" + *bucca*, cheek]
proximolabial (prŏk"sĭ-mō-lā'bē-ăl) [" + *labialis*, pert. to the lips]
proximolingual (prŏk"sĭ-mō-lĭng'gwăl) [" + *lingua*, tongue]
prozone
prozymogen (prō-zī'mō-jĕn) [Gr. *pro*, before, + *zyme*, leaven, + *gennan*, to produce]
prune (proon) [L. *pruna*]
prune-belly defect
pruriginous (proo-rĭj'ĭ-nŭs) [L. *prurigo*, itch]
prurigo (proo-rī'gō) [L., the itch]
    p. agria
    p. estivalis
    p., Hebra's
    p. mitis
    p. nodularis
    p., pregnancy
    p., simple acute
    p. simplex

pruritogenic (proo″rĭ-tō-jĕn′ĭk) [L. *pruritus*, itching, + *gennan*, to produce]

pruritus (proo-rī′tŭs) [L., itching]
  p. ani
  p., emperor of
  p., essential
  p. estivalis
  p. hiemalis
  p. senilis
  p., symptomatic
  p. vulvae

Prussak's space (proo′săks) [Alexander Prussak, Russ. otologist, 1839–1897]

prussic acid (prŭs′ĭk)

psalterium (săl-tē′rē-ŭm) [Gr. *psalterion*, harp]

psammoma (săm-ō′mă) [Gr. *psammos*, sand, + *oma*, tumor]

psammoma bodies

psammosarcoma (săm″ō-săr-kō′mă) [″ + *sarx*, flesh, + *oma*, tumor]

psammotherapy (săm″ō-thĕr′ă-pē) [″ + *therapeia*, treatment]

psammous (săm′ŭs)

pselaphesia, pselaphesis (sĕl-ă-fē′zē-ă, -sĭs) [Gr. *pselaphesis*, touch]

psellism, psellismus (sĕl′ĭzm, sĕl-ĭz′mŭs) [Gr. *psellisma*, stammer]
  p. mercurialis

pseudacousma (soo″dă-kooz′mă) [Gr. *pseudes*, false, + *akousma*, a thing heard]

pseudacusis (soo″dă-kū′sĭs)

pseudagraphia (soo″dă-grăf′ē-ă) [″ + *a-*, not, + *graphein*, to write]

pseudarthritis (soo″dăr-thrī′tĭs) [″ + *arthron*, joint, + *itis*, inflammation]

pseudarthrosis (soo″dăr-thrō′sĭs) [″ + *arthron*, joint, + *osis*, condition]

pseudencephalus (soo″dĕn-sĕf′ă-lŭs) [″ + *enkephalos*, brain]

pseudesthesia (soo″dĕs-thē′zē-ă) [″ + *aisthesis*, feeling, perception]

pseudo- (soo′dō) [Gr. *pseudes*, false]

pseudoacanthosis nigricans (soo″dō-ăk″ăn-thō′sĭs) [″ + *akantha*, thorn, + *osis*, condition]

pseudoacephalus (soo″dō-ă-sĕf′ă-lŭs) [″ + *a-*, not, + *kephale*, head]

pseudoagglutination (soo″dō-ă-glū″tĭ-nā′ shŭn)

pseudoagraphia

pseudoalbinism (soo″dō-ăl′bĭ-nĭzm) [″ + L. *albus*, white, + Gr. *-ismos*, condition]

pseudoalleles (soo″dō-ă-lēlz′) [″ + *allelon*, of one another]

pseudoanemia (soo″dō-ă-nē′mē-ă) [″ + *an-*, not, + *haima*, blood]

pseudoangina (soo″dō-ăn′jĭ-nă, -ăn-jī′nă) [″ + L. *angina*, a choking]

pseudoaneurysm (soo″dō-ăn′ū-rĭzm) [″ + *aneurysma*, a widening]

pseudoankylosis (soo″dō-ăng″kĭ-lō′sĭs) [″ + *ankyle*, stiff joint, + *osis*, condition]

pseudoapoplexy (soo″dō-ăp′ŏ-plĕk″sē)

pseudoataxia (soo″dō-ă-tăk′sē-ă) [″ + *ataxia*, lack of order]

pseudoblepsia, pseudoblepsis (soo″dō-blĕp′sē-ă, -sĭs) [″ + *blepsis*, sight]

pseudobulbar paralysis (soo″dō-bŭl′bĕr) [″ + *bolbos*, a swollen end]

pseudocartilaginous (soo″dō-kăr″tĭ-lăj′ĭ-nŭs) [″ + L. *cartilago*, gristle]

pseudocast (soo′dō-kăst) [″ + ME. *casten*, to carry]

pseudocele (soo′dō-sēl) [″ + *koilos*, hollow]

pseudochancre (soo″dō-shăng′kĕr) [″ + Fr. *chancre*, ulcer]

pseudocholesteatoma (soo″dō-kō″lĕs-tē-ă-tō′mă) [″ + *chole*, bile, + *steatos*, fat, + *oma*, tumor]

pseudocholinesterase (soo″dō-kō″lĭn-ĕs′tĕr-ās)

pseudochorea (soo″dō-kō-rē′ă)

[" + *choreia,* dance]

pseudochromesthesia (soo"dō-krō"
mĕs-thē'zē-ă) [" + *chroma,* color,
+ *aisthesis,* feeling, perception]

pseudochromidrosis (soo"dō-krō"
mĭd-rō'sĭs) [" + " +
hidros, sweat, + *osis,* condition]

pseudocirrhosis (soo"dō-sĭr-ō'sĭs)
[" + *kirrhos,* orange yellow, +
osis, condition]

pseudocoele (soo'dō-sēl) [" +
koilos, hollow]

pseudocolloid (soo"dō-kŏl'oyd)
[" + *kollodes,* glutinous]
p. of lips

pseudocoloboma (soo"dō-kŏl-ō-
bō'mă) [" + *koloboma,* a mutila-
tion]

pseudocoma

pseudocoxalgia (soo"dō-kŏk-săl'jē-
ă) [" + L. *coxa,* hip, + Gr.
algos, pain]

pseudocrisis (soo-dō-krī'sĭs) [" +
krisis, turning point]

pseudocroup (soo-dō-kroop')

pseudocyesis (soo"dō-sī-ē'sĭs) [" +
kyesis, pregnancy]

pseudocylindroid (soo"dō-sī-lĭn'
droyd) [" + *kylindros,* cylinder,
+ *eidos,* form, shape]

pseudocyst (soo'dō-sĭst) [" +
kystis, bladder]

pseudodementia (soo"dō-dē-mĕn'
shē-ă) [" + L. *demens,* mad]

pseudodiphtheria (soo"dō-dĭf-thē'rē-
ă) [" + *diphthera,* membrane]

pseudoedema (soo"dō-ē-dē'mă)
[" + *oidema,* a swelling]

pseudoemphysema (soo"dō-ĕm-fĭ'
zē'mă) [" + *emphysema,* an infla-
tion]

pseudoencephalitis (soo"dō-ĕn-
sĕf"ă-lī'tĭs) [" + *enkephalos,* brain,
+ *itis,* inflammation]

pseudoephedrine hydrochloride
(soo"dō-ē-fĕd'rĭn)

pseudoerysipelas (soo"dō-ĕr-ĭ-sĭp'ĕ-
lăs) [" + *erythros,* red, +

pella, skin]

pseudoesthesia (soo"dō-ĕs-thē'zē-ă)
[" + *aisthesis,* feeling, perception]

pseudofracture (soo"dō-frăk'chŭr)

pseudoganglion (soo"dō-găn'glē-ŏn)
[" + *ganglion,* knot]

pseudogeusesthesia (soo"dō-gūs"
ĕs-thē'zē-ă) [" + *geusis,* taste,
+ *aisthesis,* feeling, perception]

pseudogeusia (soo"dō-gū'sē-ă)

pseudoglioma (soo"dō-glī-ō'mă)
[" + *glia,* glue, + *oma,* tumor]

pseudoglobulin (soo"dō-glŏb'ū-lĭn)
[" + L. *globulus,* little globe]

pseudoglottis (soo"dō-glŏt'ĭs) [" +
glottis, tongue]

pseudogout (soo'dō-gowt")

pseudogynecomastia (soo"dō-jĭn"ĕ-
kō-măs'tē-ă) [Gr. *pseudes,* false, +
gyne, woman, + *mastos,* breast]

pseudohematuria (soo"dō-hē"mă-
tū'rē-ă) [" + *haima,* blood, +
ouron, urine]

pseudohemophilia (soo"dō-hē"mō-
fĭl'ē-ă) [" + " + *philos,* love]

pseudohemoptysis (soo"dō-hē-
mŏp'tĭ-sĭs) [" + *haima,* blood, +
ptyein, to spit]

pseudohermaphrodite (soo"dō-hĕr-
măf'rō-dīt)

pseudohermaphroditism (soo"dō-
hĕr-măf'rō-dīt"ĭzm) [" + *Hermaphroditos,* mythical two-sexed god,
+ *-ismos,* condition]
p., female
p., male

pseudohernia (soo"dō-hĕr'nē-ă)
[" + L. *hernia,* rupture]

pseudohypertrophic (soo"dō-hī-pĕr-
trō'fĭk) [" + *hyper,* over, above,
excessive, + *trophe,* nourishment]

pseudohypertrophy (soo"dō-hī-
pĕr'trō-fē)

pseudohypoparathyroidism (soo"
dō-hī"pō-păr"ă-thī'royd-ĭzm)

pseudoicterus (soo"dō-ĭk'tĕr-ŭs)
[" + *ikteros,* jaundice]

pseudoisochromatic (soo"dō-ī"sō-krō-măt'ĭk) [" + isos, equal, + chroma, color]

pseudojaundice (soo"dō-jawn'dĭs) [" + Fr. jaune, yellow]

pseudologia (soo-dō-lō'jē-ă) [" + logos, word, reason]
  p. fantastica

pseudomania (soo-dō-mā'nē-ă) [" + mania, madness]

pseudomasturbation (soo"dō-măs-tŭr-bā'shŭn) [" + L. manus, hand, + stuprare, to rape]

pseudomelanosis (soo"dō-mĕl-ă-nō'sĭs) [" + melas, black, + osis, condition]

pseudomembrane (soo"dō-mĕm'brān) [" + L. membrana, membrane]

pseudomembranous (soo"dō-mĕm'bră-nŭs)

pseudomeningitis (soo"dō-mĕn-ĭn-jī'tĭs) [" + meninx, membrane, + itis, inflammation]

pseudomenstruation (soo"dō-mĕn"strū-ā'shŭn) [" + L. menstruare, menstruate]

pseudomnesia (soo"dŏm-nē'zē-ă) [" + mnesis, memory]

Pseudomonas (soo-dō-mō'năs) [" + monas, single]
  P. aeruginosa
  P. mallei
  P. pseudomallei

pseudomucin (soo-dō-mū'sĭn) [" + L. mucus, mucus]

pseudomyopia (soo"dō-mī-ō'pē-ă) [" + myein, to shut, + ops, eye]

pseudomyxoma (soo"dō-mĭk-sō'mă) [" + myxa, mucus, + oma, tumor]
  p. peritonei

pseudoneoplasm (soo-dō-nē'ō-plăsm) [" + neos, new, + LL. plasma, form, mold]

pseudoneuritis (soo"dō-nū-rī'tĭs) [" + neuron, nerve, + itis, inflammation]

pseudoneuroma (soo"dō-nū-rō'mă) ["

+ " + oma, tumor]

pseudonucleolus (soo"dō-nū"klē-ōl'ŭs) [" + L. nucleus, a nut]

pseudopapilledema (soo"dō-păp"ĭ-lĕ-dē'mă) [" + papilla, nipple, + oidema, swelling]

pseudoparalysis (soo"dō-pă-răl'ĭ-sĭs) [" + paralyein, to loosen, disable]

pseudoparaplegia (soo"dō-păr-ă-plē'jē-ă) [" + " + plege, a stroke]

pseudoparasite (soo"dō-păr'ă-sīt) [" + " + sitos, food]

pseudoparesis (soo"dō-păr-ē'sĭs, -păr'ē-sĭs) [" + parienai, let fall]

pseudopelade (soo"dō-pē'lād) [" + Fr. pelade, to remove hair]

Pseudophyllidea (soo"dō-fĭ-lĭd'ē-ă)

pseudoplegia (soo"dō-plē'jē-ă) [" + plege, a stroke]

pseudopod (soo'dō-pŏd) [" + pous, foot]

pseudopodium (soo"dō-pō'dē-ŭm)

pseudopolyp (soo"dō-pŏl'ĭp) [" + polys, many, + pous, foot]

pseudopolyposis (soo"dō-pŏl"ĭ-pō'sĭs) [" + " + " + osis, condition]

pseudopregnancy (soo"dō-prĕg'năn-sē) [Gr. pseudes, false, + L. praegnans, with child]

pseudo-pseudohypoparathyroidism (soo"dō-soo"dō-hī"pō-păr"ă-thī'royd-ĭzm) [" + pseudes, false, + hypo, under, beneath, below, + para, alongside, past, beyond, + thyreos, shield, + eidos, form, shape + -ismos, condition]

pseudopsia (soo-dŏp'sē-ă) [" + opsis, sight, appearance, vision]

pseudopterygium (soo"dō-tĕr-ĭj'ē-ŭm) [" + pterygion, wing]

pseudoptosis (soo-dō-tō'sĭs) [" + ptosis, fall, falling]

pseudorabies (soo"dō-rā'bēz) [" + L. rabere, to rage]

pseudoreaction (soo"dō-rē-ăk'shŭn)

pseudorickets (soo"dō-rĭk'ĕts)

pseudoscarlatina (soo"dō-skăr-lă-tē'nă)

pseudosclerosis (soo"dō-sklē-rō'sĭs) [" + *sklerosis*, a hardening]
   p., Westphal-Strümpell

pseudosmia (soo-dŏz'mē-ă) [" + *osme*, smell]

pseudostoma (soo-dŏs'tō-mă) [" + *stoma*, mouth, opening]

pseudostratified (soo-dō-străt'ĭ-fĭd) [" + L. *stratificare*, to arrange in layers]

pseudostratified epithelium

pseudosyphilis (soo"dō-sĭf'ĭ-lĭs)

pseudotabes (soo"dō-tā'bēz) [Gr. *pseudes*, false, + L. *tabes*, wasting disease]

pseudotetanus (soo"dō-tĕt'ă-nŭs) [" + *tetanos*, rigid, stretched]

pseudotruncus arteriosus (soo"dō-trŭnk'ŭs ăr-tē"rē-ō'sŭs)

pseudotuberculosis (soo"dō-tū-ber"kū-lō'sĭs) [" + L. *tuberculus*, tubercle, + Gr. *osis*, condition]

pseudotumor cerebri (soo"dō-tū'mor sĕr'ĕ-brī)

pseudotympany (soo"dō-tĭm'pă-nē) [" + *tympanon*, drum]

pseudoxanthoma (soo"dō-zăn-thō'mă) [" + *xanthos*, yellow, + *oma*, tumor]
   p. elasticum

p.s.i. *pounds per square inch*

psilocin (sī'lō-sĭn)

psilocybin (sī"lō-sī'bĭn)

psi phenomena

psittacosis (sĭt-ă-kō'sĭs) [Gr. *psittakos*, parrot, + *osis*, condition]

psoas (sō'ăs) [Gr. *psoa*]

psoas abscess

psoitis (sō-ī'tĭs) [Gr. *psoa*, muscle of the loin, + *itis*, inflammation]

psomophagia (sō"mō-fā'jē-ă) [Gr. *psomos*, morsel, + *phagein*, to eat]

psora (sō'ră) [Gr., itch]

psoralen

psorelcosis (sō"rĕl-kō'sĭs) [" + *helkosis*, ulceration]

psorenteritis (sō"rĕn-tĕr-ī'tĭs) [" + *enteron*, intestine, + *itis*, inflammation]

psoriasis (sō-rī'ă-sĭs) [Gr., an itching]
   p. annularis
   p. arthropica
   p. buccalis
   p., elephantine
   p., guttate
   p., nummular
   p., pustular
   p., rupioid
   p. universalis

psorophthalmia (sō"rŏf-thăl'mē-ă) [Gr.]

psorous (sō'rŭs) [Gr. *psoros*]

P.S.P. *phenolsulfonphthalein*

PSRO *Professional Standards Review Organization*

psych-, psycho- [Gr. *psyche*, mind]

psychagogy (sī"kă-gō'jē) [Gr. *psyche*, soul, mind, + *agein*, to lead]

psychalgia (sī-kăl'jē-ă) [" + *algos*, pain]

psychanopsia (sī-kăn-ŏp'sē-ă) [" + *an-*, not, + *opsis*, sight, appearance, vision]

psychataxia (sī"kă-tăk'sē-ă) [" + *ataxia*, lack of order]

psychauditory (sĭk-aw'dĭ-tor-ē) [" + L. *auditorius*, hearing]

psyche (sī'kē) [Gr. *psyche*, soul, mind]

psychedelic (sī"kĕ-dĕl'ĭk) [" + *delos*, manifest]

psychiatric (sī-kē-ă'trĭk) [" + *iatrikos*, healing]

psychiatrist (sī-kī'ă-trĭst)

psychiatry (sī-kī'ă-trē)
   p., descriptive
   p., dynamic
   p., forensic
   p., orthomolecular

psychic (sī'kĭk) [Gr. *psychikos*]

psychic blindness

psychic contagion

psychic deafness

psychic determinism

psychic force

psychoactive (sī″kō-ăk′tĭv) [″ + L. actio, action]

psychoanaleptic (sī″kō-ăn″ă-lĕp′tĭk) [″ + analepsis, a taking up]

psychoanalysis (sī″kō-ă-năl′ĭ-sĭs) [″ + analyein, to dissolve]

psychoanalyst (sī″kō-ăn′ă-lĭst) [Gr. psyche, mind, + analyein, to dissolve]

psychobiology (sī″kō-bī-ŏl′ō-jē) [″ + bios, life, + logos, word, reason]
p., objective

psychocatharsis (sī″kō-kă-thăr′sĭs) [″ + katharsis, to cleanse, purify]

psychochrome (sī′kō-krōm) [″ + chroma, color]

psychochromesthesia (sī″kō-krōm″ ĕs-thē′zē-ă) [″ + ″ + aisthesis, feeling, perception]

psychocoma (sī″kō-kō′mă) [″ + koma, deep sleep]

psychocortical (sī″kō-kor′tĭ-kăl) [″ + L. cortex, rind]

psychodiagnosis (sī″kō-dī″ăg-nō′sĭs) [″ + diagignoskein, to discern]

psychodiagnostics (sī″kō-dī″ăg-nŏs′tĭks)

Psychodidae (sī″kŏd′ĭ-dē)

psychodometry (sī″kō-dŏm′ĕ-trē) [″ + hodos, way, + metron, measure]

psychodrama (sī″kō-drăm′ă) [″ + L. drama, drama]

psychodynamics (sī″kō-dī-năm′ĭks) [″ + dynamis, power]

psychoepilepsy (sī″kō-ĕp″ĭ-lĕp′sē) [″ + epilepsia, to seize]

psychogalvanic reflex

psychogalvanometer (sī″kō-găl″vă-nŏm′ĕ-tĕr) [″ + galvanism + Gr. metron, measure]

psychogenesis (sī″kō-jĕn′ĕ-sĭs) [″ + genesis, generation, birth]

psychogenetic (sī″kō-jĕn-ĕt′ĭk)

psychogenic (sī-kō-jĕn′ĭk) [″ + gennan, to produce]

psychogeusic (sī″kō-gū′sĭk) [″ + geusis, taste]

psychogram (sī′kō-grăm) [Gr. psyche, mind, + gramma, letter, piece of writing]

psychograph (sī′kō-grăf) [″ + graphein, to write]

psychokinesis (sī″kō-kī-nē′sĭs) [″ + kinesis, motion]

psycholagny (sī″kō-lăg′nē) [″ + lagneia, lust]

psycholepsy (sī″kō-lĕp′sē) [″ + lepsis, seizure]

psycholeptic (sī″kō-lĕp′tĭk)

psycholinguistics (sī″kō-lĭng-gwĭs′tĭks)

psychological (sī″kō-lŏj′ĭ-kăl) [″ + logos, word, reason]

psychologist (sī-kŏl′ō-jĭst)

psychology (sī-kŏl′ō-jē) [″ + logos, word, reason]
p., abnormal
p., analytic
p., animal
p., applied
p., clinical
p., criminal
p., dynamic
p., experimental
p., genetic
p., gestalt
p., individual
p., physiologic
p., social

psychometrician (sī″kō-mĕ-trĭsh′ăn) [Gr. psyche, mind, + metron, measure]

psychometry (sī-kŏm′ĕ-trē) [″ + metron, measure]

psychomotor (sī″kō-mō′tor) [″ + L. motor, a mover]

psychomotor and physical development of infant

psychomotor epilepsy

psychomotor retardation

psychoneurosis (sī″kō-nū-rō′sĭs) [″ + neuron, sinew, + osis, condition]
p., anxiety reaction
p., conversion reaction

p., depressive reaction
p., dissociated reaction
p., obsessive-compulsive reaction
p., phobic reaction
psychoneurotic (sī″kō-nū-rŏt′ĭk) [Gr.
psyche, mind, + *neuron*, sinew]
psychoparesis (sī″kō-pă-rē′sĭs,
-păr′ĕ-sĭs) [″ + *parienai*, let fall]
psychopath (sī′kō-păth) [″ +
pathos, disease, suffering]
psychopathia
psychopathic (sī″kō-păth′ĭk)
psychopathology (sī″kō-păth-ŏl′ō-jē)
[″ + *pathos*, disease, suffering
+ *logos*, word, reason]
psychopathy (sī-kŏp′ă-thē)
psychopharmacology (sī″kō-făr″mă-
kŏl′ō-jē)
psychophysical (sī″kō-fĭz′ĭ-kăl) [″ +
physikos, natural]
psychophysics (sī″kō-fĭz′ĭks)
psychophysiologic (sī″kō-fĭz-ē-ō-
lŏ′jĭk)
psychophysiologic disorders
psychophysiology (sī″kō-fĭz″ē-
ŏl′ō-jē)
psychoplegic (sī″kō-plē′jĭk) [″ +
plege, a stroke]
**psychoprophylactic preparation
for childbirth**
psychoprophylaxis (sī″kō-prō″fĭ-
lăk′sĭs)
psychorhythmia (sī″kō-rĭth′mē-ă)
[″ + *rhythmos*, rhythm]
psychorrhea (sī″kō-rē′ă) [″ +
rhein, to flow]
psychosensory (sī″kō-sĕn′sō-rē)
[″ + L. *sensorius*, organ of sensa-
tion]
psychosexual (sī″kō-sĕks′ū-ăl) [Gr.
psyche, soul, mind, + L. *sexus*, sex]
psychosexual development
psychosexual disorders
psychosine (sī′kō-sēn)
psychosis (sī-kō′sĭs) [″ + *osis*, con-
dition]
p., alcoholic
p., depressive

p., drug
p., exhaustion
p., functional
p., gestational
p., involutional
p., Korsakoff's
p., manic-depressive
p., organic
p., polyneuritic
p., postinfectious
p., postpartum
p., puerperal
p., senile
p., situational
p., toxic
p., traumatic
psychosocial (sī″kō-sō′shăl)
psychosomatic (sī″kō-sō-măt′ĭk) [Gr.
psyche, mind, + *soma*, body]
psychosomatic medicine
psychosurgery (sī″kō-sur′jĕr-ē) [″ +
L. *chirurgia*, surgery]
psychotechnics (sī″kō-tĕk′nĭks) [″ +
techne, art]
psychotherapeutic drugs
psychotherapy (sī-kō-thĕr′ă-pē) [Gr.
psyche, mind, + *therapeia*, treat-
ment]
psychotic (sī-kŏt′ĭk)
psychotogenic (sī-kŏt″ō-jĕn′ĭk) [″ +
gennan, to produce]
psychotomimetic (sī-kŏt″ō-mī-mĕ′tĭk)
[″ + *mimetikos*, imitative]
psychotropic drugs [″ + *trope*, a
turning]
psychroalgia (sī″krō-ăl′jē-ă) [Gr.
psychros, cold, + *algos*, pain]
psychroesthesia (sī″krō-ĕs-thē′zē-ă)
[″ + *aisthesis*, feeling, perception]
psychrometer (sī-krŏm′ĕ-tĕr) [″ +
metron, measure]
psychrophilic (sī-krō-fĭl′ĭk) [″ +
philein, to love]
psychrophobia (sī-krō-fō′bē-ă) [″ +
phobos, fear]
psychrophore (sī′krō-for) [″ +
phorein, to carry]
psychrotherapy (sī″krō-thĕr′ă-pē)

[" + *therapeia*, treatment]
psyllium seed (sĭl′ē-ŭm)
PT *prothrombin time*
Pt *platinum*
pt *pint*
PTA *plasma thromboplastin antecedent*
ptarmic (tăr′mĭk) [Gr. *ptarmikos*, causing to sneeze]
ptarmus (tar′mŭs)
PTC *plasma thromboplastin component; phenylthiocarbamide*
PTCA *percutaneous transluminal coronary angioplasty*
pterion (tē′rē-ŏn) [Gr. *pteron*, wing]
pternalgia (tĕr-năl′jē-ă) [Gr. *pterna*, heel, + *algos*, pain]
pteroylglutamic acid
pterygium (tĕr-ĭj′ē-ŭm) [Gr. *pterygion*, little wing]
  p. colli
  p., progressive
  p., stationary
pterygoid (tĕr′ĭ-goyd) [Gr. *pterygoeides*, winglike]
pterygoid process
pterygomandibular (tĕr″ĭ-gō-măn-dĭb′ū-lăr) [" + L. *mandibula*, lower jawbone]
pterygomaxillary (tĕr″ĭ-gō-măk′sĭ-lĕr″ē) [" + L. *maxillaris*, upper jaw]
pterygopalatine (tĕr″ĭ-gō-păl′ă-tīn) [" + L. *palatinus*, palate]
PTH *parathyroid hormone*
ptilosis (tĭ-lō′sĭs) [Gr.]
ptomaine (tō′mān, tō-mān′) [Gr. *ptoma*, dead body]
ptosed (tōst)
ptosis (tō′sĭs) [Gr., fall, falling]
  p., abdominal
  p., morning
  p., waking
ptotic (tŏt′ĭk)
ptyalagogue (tĭ-ăl′ă-gŏg) [Gr. *ptyalon*, saliva, + *agogos*, leading]
ptyalectasis (tĭ″ă-lĕk′tă-sĭs) [" + *ektasis*, dilation]
ptyalin (tĭ′ă-lĭn)
ptyalism (tĭ′ă-lĭzm) [" + *-ismos*, condition]

ptyalith (tĭ′ă-lĭth) [" + *lithos*, stone]
ptyalocele (tĭ-ăl′ō-sēl) [" + *kele*, tumor, swelling]
ptyalogenic (tĭ″ăl-ō-jĕn′ĭk) [Gr. *ptyalon*, saliva, + *gennan*, to produce]
ptyalogogue (tĭ″ăl′ō-gŏg) [" + *agogos*, leading]
ptyalography (tĭ-ăl-ŏg′ră-fē) [" + *graphein*, to write]
ptyalolith (tĭ′ă-lō-lĭth) [" + *lithos*, stone]
ptyalolithiasis (tĭ″ă-lō-lĭ-thī′ă-sĭs)
ptyalolithotomy (tĭ″ăl-ō-lĭ-thŏt′ō-mē) [Gr. *ptyalon*, saliva, + *lithos*, stone, + *tome*, a cutting, slice]
ptyaloreaction (tĭ″ă-lō-rē-ăk′shŭn)
ptyalorrhea (tĭ″ă-lō-rē′ă) [" + *rhein*, to flow]
ptyocrinous (tĭ-ŏk′rĭ-nŭs)
ptysis (tĭ′sĭs) [Gr.]
Pu *plutonium*
pubarche (pū-băr′kē) [L. *puber*, grown up, + Gr. *arche*, beginning]
puber (pū′bĕr) [L., grown up]
puberal (pū′bĕr-ăl) [L. *pubertas*, puberty]
pubertal
pubertas (pū′bĕr-tăs) [L.]
  p. praecox
puberty (pū′bĕr-tē)
  p., onset of
  p., precocious
pubes (pū′bēz) [L., grown up]
pubescence (pū-bĕs′ĕns) [L. *pubescens*, becoming hairy]
pubescent (pū-bĕs′ĕnt)
pubetrotomy (pū″bĕ-trŏt′ō-mē) [NL. *(os) pubis*, bone of the groin, + Gr. *etron*, belly, + *tome*, a cutting, slice]
pubic (pū′bĭk) [L. *pubes*, pubic hair]
pubic bone
pubic hair
pubio-, pubo- [L. *pubes*, pubic hair]
pubiotomy (pū-bē-ŏt′ō-mē) [L. *pubes*, pubic region, + *tome*, a cutting, slice]

pubis (pū'bĭs) [NL. *(os) pubis*, bone of the groin]

public health

Public Health Service Act

pubococcygeal (pū"bō-kŏk-sĭj'ē-ăl) [" + Gr. *kokkyx*, coccyx]

pubofemoral (pū"bō-fĕm'or-ăl) [" + *femur*, thigh bone]

puboprostatic (pū"bō-prŏs-tăt'ĭk) [" + Gr. *prostates*, prostate]

puborectal (pū"bō-rĕk'tăl) [" + *rectus*, straight]

pubovaginal device

pubovesical (pū"bō-vĕs'ĭ-kl) [" + *vesia*, bladder]

pudenda (pū-dĕn'dă) [L.]

pudendagra (pū"dĕn-dăg'ră) [" + Gr. *agra*, seizure]

pudendal (pū-dĕn'dăl) [L. *pudenda*, external genitals]

pudendum (pū-dĕn'dŭm) [L.]
   p. feminum
   p. muliebre

pudic (pū'dĭk) [L. *pudicus*, modest]

puerile (pyūr'ăl) [L. *puerilis*]

puerilism (pū'ĕr-ĭl-ĭzm) [" + Gr. *-ismos*, condition]

puerpera (pū-ĕr'pĕr-ă) [L. *puer*, child, + *parere*, to beget, produce]

puerperal (pū-ĕr'pĕr-ăl) [L. *puerperalis*]

puerperal eclampsia

puerperal fever

puerperalism (pū-ĕr'pĕr-ăl-ĭzm) [L. *puer*, child, + *parere*, to beget, produce, + Gr. *-ismos*, condition]

puerperal period

puerperal sepsis

puerperant (pū-ĕr'pĕr-ănt)

puerperium (pū"ĕr-pē'rē-ŭm) [L.]

puerperous (pū-ĕr'pĕr-ŭs) [" + *parere*, to beget, produce]

PUFA *polyunsaturated fatty acids*

puff

Pulex (pū'lĕks) [L., flea]
   P. irritans

pulicatio (pū"lĭ-kā'tē-ō)

Pulicidae (pū-lĭs'ĭ-dē)

pulicide (pū'lĭ-sīd) [L. *pulex*, flea, + *caedere*, to kill]

pullulate (pŭl"ū-lāt) [L. *pullulare*, to sprout]

pullulation (pŭl"ū-lā'shŭn)

pulmo- (pŭl'mō-, pool'mō-) [L. *pulmo*, lung]

pulmoaortic (pŭl"mō-ā-or'tĭk) [" + Gr. *aorte*, aorta]

pulmometer (pŭl-mŏm'ĕ-tĕr) [" + Gr. *metron*, measure]

pulmometry (pŭl-mŏm'ĕ-trē)

pulmonary (pŭl'mō-nĕ-rē) [L. *pulmonarius*]

pulmonary alveolar proteinosis

pulmonary arterial webs

pulmonary artery

pulmonary artery wedge pressure

pulmonary circulation

pulmonary edema

pulmonary embolism

pulmonary emphysema

pulmonary function tests

pulmonary insufficiency

pulmonary mucociliary clearance

pulmonary stenosis

pulmonary surfactant

pulmonary valve

pulmonary vein

pulmonectomy (pŭl"mō-nĕk'tō-mē) [L. *pulmonis*, lung, + Gr. *ektome*, excision]

pulmonic (pŭl-mŏn'ĭk)

pulmonitis (pŭl-mō-nī'tĭs) [" + Gr. *itis*, inflammation]

pulmotor (pŭl'mō-tor) [" + *motor*, mover]

pulp [L. *pulpa*, flesh]
   p., coronal
   p., dead
   p., dental
   p., digital
   p., enamel
   p., exposed
   p., nonvital
   p., putrescent
   p., radicular
   p., red

p., splenic
p., vertebral
p., vital
p., white
pulpa (pŭl'pă) [L., flesh]
pulpal (pŭl'păl)
pulpalgia (pŭl-păl'jē-ă) [" + Gr. algos, pain]
pulp amputation
pulp capping
pulpectomy (pŭl-pĕk'tō-mē) [" + Gr. ektome, excision]
pulpefaction (pŭl-pī-făk'shŭn) [L. pulpa, pulp, + facere, to make]
pulp extirpation
pulpitis (pŭl-pī'tĭs) [" + itis, inflammation]
pulpotomy (pŭl-pŏt'ō-mē) [" + Gr. tome, a cutting, slice]
pulpy (pŭl'pē)
pulsate (pŭl'sāt) [L. pulsare]
pulsatile (pŭl'să-tĭl)
pulsation (pŭl-sā'shŭn) [L. pulsatio, a beating]
pulse (pŭls) [L. pulsus, beating]
    p., abdominal
    p., accelerated
    p., alternating
    p., anacrotic
    p., anadicrotic
    p., apical
    p., asymmetrical radial
    p., bigeminal
    p., bounding
    p., brachial
    p., capillary
    p., carotid
    p., catacrotic
    p., catadicrotic
    p., central
    p., collapsing
    p., Corrigan's
    p., coupled
    p., deficit
    p., dicrotic
    p., dorsalis pedis
    p., entoptic
    p., febrile

p., femoral
p., filiform
p., formicant
p., full
p., hard
p., hepatic
p., high-tension
p., incident
p., intermediate
p., intermittent
p., irregular
p., jerky
p., jugular
p., Kussmaul's
p., long
p., low-tension
p., monocrotic
p., nail
p., paradoxical
p., peripheral
p., pistol-shot
p., plateau
p., popliteal
p., Quincke's
p., radial
p., rapid
p., regular
p., respiratory
p., Riegel's
p., running
p., senile
p., short
p., slow
p., soft
p., tense
p., thready
p., tremulous
p., tricrotic
p., trigeminal
p., triphammer
p., undulating
p., unequal
p., vagus
p., venous
p., vermicular
p., waterhammer
p., wiry
pulse generator

pulseless disease
pulse pressure
pulse wave
pulsimeter (pŭl-sĭm′ĕt-ĕr) [L. *pulsus*, a beat, + Gr. *metron*, measure]
pulsing electromagnetic field
pulsion (pŭl′shŭn)
    p., lateral
pulsus (pŭl′sŭs) [L.]
    p. alternans
    p., bigeminus
    p. celer
    p. differens
    p. paradoxus
    p. parvus et tardus
    p. tardus
pultaceous (pŭl-tā′shŭs) [L. *pultaceus*]
pulv. [L.] *pulvis*, powder
pulverization (pŭl″vĕr-ĭ-zā′shŭn) [L. *pulvis*, powder]
pulverulent (pŭl-vĕr′ū-lĕnt)
pulvinar (pŭl-vī′năr) [L., cushioned seat]
pulvinate (pŭl′vĭ-nāt) [L. *pulvinus*, cushion]
pulvis [L.]
pumice (pŭm′ĭs)
pump [ME. *pumpe*]
    p., air
    p., blood
    p., breast
    p., dental
    p., sodium
    p., stomach
pump-oxygenator
puna (poo′nă)
punch
punchdrunk
punched out
puncta (pŭnk′tă) [L.]
punctate (pŭnk′tāt) [L. *punctum*, point]
punctate keratoses
punctate pits
punctate rash
punctiform (pŭnk′tĭ-form) [″ + *forma*, shape]
punctio (pŭnk′shē-ō) [L. *punctura*, prick]
punctograph (pŭnk′tō-grăf) [″ + Gr. *graphein*, to write]

punctum (pŭnk′tŭm) [L.]
    p. caecum
    puncta dolorosa
    p. lacrimale
    p. nasale inferius
    p. proximum
    p. remotum
    p. saliens
    puncta vasculosa
puncture (pŭnk′chŭr) [L. *punctura*, prick]
    p., cisternal
    p., diabetic
    p., exploratory
    p., lumbar
    p., Quincke's
    p., spinal
    p., sternal
    p., ventricular
puncture wound
pungency (pŭn′jĕn-sē) [L. *pungens*, prick]
pungent (pŭn′jĕnt)
P.U.O. *pyrexia of unknown origin*
pupa (pū′pă) [L., girl]
pupil (pū′pĭl) [L. *pupilla*]
    p., Adie's
    p., Argyll Robertson
    p., artificial
    p., bounding
    p., Bumke's
    p., cat's-eye
    p., cornpicker's
    p., fixed
    p., Hutchinson's
    p., keyhole
    p., Marcus Gunn
    p., occlusion of
    p., pinhole
    p., stiff
    p., tonic
pupilla (pū-pĭl′ă) [L., pupil]
pupillary (pū′pĭ-lĕr-ē) [L. *pupilla*, pupil]
pupillary reflex
pupillometer (pū-pĭl-ŏm′ĕ-tĕr) [″ + Gr. *metron*, measure]
pupillometry (pū-pĭl-lŏm′ĕ-trē) [″ + *metron*, measure]
pupillomotor reflex

pupilloplegia   (pū″pĭ-lō-plē′jē-ă)
[″ + plege, stroke]
pupilloscopy (pū-pĭl-ŏs′kō-pē) [″ +
Gr. skopein, to examine]
pupillostatometer   (pū″pĭl-ō-stă-
tŏm′ĕ-tĕr) [″ + Gr. statos, placed,
+ metron, measure]
pure (pūr) [ME.]
pure line
purgation (pŭr-gā′shŭn) [L. purgatio]
purgative (pŭr′gă-tĭv) [L. purgativus]
     p., cholagogue
     p., drastic
     p., saline
purgative enema
purge (pŭrj) [L. purgare, to cleanse]
puriform (pū′rĭ-form) [L. pus, pus,   +
forma, shape]
purinase (pū′rĭ-nās)
purine (pū′rēn″) [L. purum, pure,   +
uricus, uric acid]
     p., endogenous
     p., exogenous
purine base
purine-free diet
purine-low diet
purinemia (pū″rĭ-nē′mē-ă) [purine,   +
Gr. haima, blood]
Purinethol
Purkinje, Johannes E. von (pŭr-kĭn′jē)
     [Bohemian anatomist and physiologist,
     1787–1869]
     P. cells
     P. fibers
     P. figures
     P. network
     P. phenomenon
     P.-Sanson images [Louis J. Sanson,
          Fr. physician, 1790–1841]
     P. vesicle
purohepatitis (pū″rō-hĕp″ă-tī′tĭs) [L.
pus, pus + Gr. hepar, liver, +
itis, inflammation]
puromucous (pū″rō-mū′kŭs) [″   +
mucus, mucus]
purple
     p., visual
purposeful movement

purpura (pŭr′pū-ră) [L., purple]
     p., allergic
     p., anaphylactoid
     p. annularis telangiectodes
     p., fibrinolytic
     p. fulminans
     p., hemorrhagic
     p., Henoch
     p., idiopathic thrombocytopenic
     p. nervosa
     p., nonthrombocytopenic
     p. rheumatica
     p., Schönlein-Henoch
     p., senile
     p. simplex
     p., thrombocytopenic
     p., thrombopenic
     p., thrombotic thrombocytopenic
purpureaglycosides   A   and   B
     (pŭr-pū″rē-ă-glĭ′kō-sīds)
purpuric (pŭr-pū′rĭk) [L. purpura, purple]
purpurin (pŭr′pū-rĭn)
purpurinuria (pŭr″pū-rĭn-ū′rē-ă) [″   +
Gr. ouron, urine]
purpuru
purring thrill
purulence (pŭr′ū-lĕntz) [L. purulentus,
full of pus]
purulency (pŭr′ū-lĕn″sē)
purulent (pŭr′ū-lĕnt) [L. purulentus, full
of pus]
puruloid (pŭr′ū-loyd) [L. pus, pus,   +
Gr. eidos, form, shape]
pus (pŭs) [L.]
     p., blue
     p., cheesy
     p., ichorous
pus cells
pustula (pŭs′tū-lă) [L., blister]
pustulant (pŭs′tū-lănt) [L. pustula, blis-
ter]
pustular (pŭs′tū-lĕr)
pustulation (pŭs″tū-lā′shŭn)
pustule (pŭs′tŭl) [L. pustula, blister]
pustulocrustaceous   (pŭs″tū-lō-krŭs-
tā′shŭs) [″   +   crusta, shell, crust]
pustulosis (pŭs″tū-lō′sĭs) [″   +   Gr.
osis, condition]

putamen (pū'tă-mĕn) [L., shell]
Putnam-Dana syndrome (pŭt'năm-dā'nă) [James J. Putnam, U.S. neurologist, 1846–1918; Charles L. Dana, U.S. neurologist, 1852–1935]
putrefaction (pū"trĕ-făk'shŭn) [L. putrefactio]
putrefactive (pū"trĕ-făk'tĭv) [L. putrefacere, to putrefy]
putrefy (pū'trĕ-fī) [L. putrefacere, to putrefy]
putrescence (pū-trĕs'ĕns) [L. putrescens, grow rotten]
putrescine (pū-trĕs'ĭn)
putrid (pū'trĭd) [L. putridus]
PUVA therapy [psoralen + ultraviolet A]
PVC polyvinyl chloride; premature ventricular contraction
PVP polyvinylpyrrolidone
PVP-iodine povidone-iodine
pyarthrosis (pī"ăr-thrō'sĭs) [Gr. pyon, pus, + arthron, joint, + osis, condition]
pycnemia (pĭk-nē'mē-ă) [Gr. pyknos, thick, + haima, blood]
pycno- (pĭk'nō) [Gr. pyknos, thick]
pyecchysis (pī-ĕk'ĭ-sĭs) [Gr. pyon, pus, + ek, out, + chein, to pour]
pyelectasia, pyelectasis (pī"ĕ-lĕk-tā'zē-ă, -lĕk'tăs-ĭs) [Gr. pyelos, pelvis, + ektasis, dilatation]
pyelitic (pī"ĕ-lĭt'ĭk)
pyelitis (pī"ĕ-lī'tĭs) [Gr. pyelos, pelvis, + itis, inflammation]
    p., calculous
    p. cystica
pyelo- [Gr. pyelos, pelvis]
pyelocaliectasis (pī"ĕ-lō-kăl"ĕ-ĕk'tă-sĭs) [" + kalyx, cup of a flower, + ektasis, dilation]
pyelocystitis (pī"ĕ-lō-sĭs-tī'tĭs) [" + kystis, bladder, + itis, inflammation]
pyelocystostomosis (pī"ĕ-lō-sĭs"tō-stō-mō'sĭs) [" + " + stoma, mouth, opening, + osis, condition]
pyelogram (pī'ĕ-lō-grăm) [Gr. pyelos,

pelvis, + gramma, letter, piece of writing]
    p., intravenous
pyelography (pī"ĕ-lŏg'ră-fē) [" + graphein, to write]
pyelolithotomy (pī"ĕ-lō-lĭth-ŏt'ō-mē) [" + lithos, stone, + tome, a cutting, slice]
pyelonephritis (pī"ĕ-lō-nĕ-frī'tĭs) [" + nephros, kidney, + itis, inflammation]
pyelonephrosis (pī"ĕ-lō-nĕ-frō'sĭs) [" + " + osis, condition]
pyelopathy (pī"ĕ-lŏp'ăth-ē) [" + pathos, disease, suffering]
pyeloplasty (pī'ĕ-lō-plăs"tē) [" + plastos, formed]
pyeloplication (pī"ĕ-lō-plĭ-kā'shŭn) [" + L. plicare, to fold]
pyeloscopy (pī"ĕl-ŏs'kō-pē) [" + skopein, to examine]
pyelostomy (pī"ĕ-lŏs'tō-mē) [" + stoma, mouth, opening]
pyelotomy (pī"ĕ-lŏt'ō-mē) [" + tome, a cutting, slice]
pyemesis (pī-ĕm'ĭ-sĭs) [Gr. pyon, pus, + emein, to vomit]
pyemia (pī-ē'mē-ă) [" + haima, blood]
    p., arterial
    p., cryptogenic
    p., metastatic
    p., portal
pyemic (pī-ē'mĭk) [Gr. pyon, pus, + haima, blood]
Pyemotes (pī-ĕ-mō'tēz)
    P. ventricosus
pyencephalus (pī"ĕn-sĕf'ă-lŭs) [" + enkephalos, brain]
pyesis (pī-ē'sĭs)
pygal (pī'găl) [Gr. pyge, rump]
pygalgia (pī-găl'jē-ă) [" + algos, pain]
pygmalionism (pĭg-mā'lē-ŏn-ĭzm) [named for Pygmalion, a sculptor and king in Gr. mythology, who fell in love with a figure he carved]
pygmy (pĭg'mē)

pygo- [Gr. *pyge*, rump]

pygoamorphus (pī″gō-ă-mor′fŭs) [″ + *a-*, not, + *morphe*, form]

pygodidymus (pī″gō-dĭd′ĭ-mŭs) [″ + *didymos*, twin]

pygomelus (pī-gŏm′ĕ-lŭs) [″ + *melos*, limb]

pyknemia

pyknic (pĭk′nĭk) [Gr. *pyknos*, thick]

pykno- [Gr. *pyknos*, thick]

pyknocardia (pĭk-nō-kăr′dē-ă) [″ + *kardia*, heart]

pyknocyte (pĭk′nō-sīt) [″ + *kytos*, cell]

pyknodysostosis (pĭk″nō-dĭs″ŏs-tō′sĭs) [″ + *dys*, bad, difficult, painful, disordered, + *osteon*, bone, + *osis*, condition]

pyknometer (pĭk-nŏm′ĕ-tĕr) [″ + *metron*, measure]

pyknomorphous (pĭk″nō-morf′ŭs) [″ + *morphe*, form]

pyknophrasia (pĭk″nō-frā′zē-ă) [″ + *phrasis*, diction]

pyknosis (pĭk-nō′sĭs) [″ + *osis*, condition]

pyle- [Gr. *pyle*, gate]

pylemphraxis (pī″lĕm-frăk′sĭs) [″ + *emphraxis*, stoppage]

pylephlebectasia, pylephlebectasis (pī″lē-flē-bĕk-tā′zē-ă, -bĕk′tă-sĭs) [″ + *phleps*, blood vessel, vein, + *ektasis*, dilatation]

pylephlebitis (pī″lē-flē-bī′tĭs) [″ + ″ + *itis*, inflammation]
   p., adhesive
   p. obturans

pylethrombophlebitis (pī″lē-thrŏm″bō-flē-bī′tĭs) [″ + *thrombos*, clot, + *phleps*, blood vessel, vein, + *itis*, inflammation]

pylethrombosis (pī″lē-thrŏm-bō′sĭs) [Gr. *pyle*, gate, + *thrombos*, clot, + *osis*, condition]

pylon (pī′lŏn)

pyloralgia (pī″lō-răl′jē-ă) [Gr. *pyloros*, gatekeeper, + *algos*, pain]

pylorectomy (pī″lō-rĕk′tō-mē) [″ + *ektome*, excision]

pyloric (pī-lor′ĭk) [Gr. *pyloros*, gatekeeper]

pyloric antrum

pyloric canal

pyloric cap

pyloric gland

pyloric obstruction and dilatation

pyloric orifice

pyloric stenosis

pyloristenosis (pī-lor″ĭ-stĕn-ō′sĭs) [Gr. *pyloros*, gatekeeper, + *stenosis*, act of narrowing]

pyloritis (pī″lō-rī′tĭs) [″ + *itis*, inflammation]

pyloro- [Gr. *pyloros*, gatekeeper]

pylorodiosis (pī-lō″rō-dī-ō′sĭs) [″ + *diosis*, pushing under]

pyloroduodenitis (pī-lor″ō-dū″ō-dē-nī′tĭs) [″ + L. *duodeni*, twelve, + Gr. *itis*, inflammation]

pylorogastrectomy (pī-lor″ō-găs-trĕk′tō-mē) [″ + *gaster*, belly, + *ektome*, excision]

pyloromyotomy (pī-lor″ō-mī-ŏt′ō-mē) [″ + *mys*, muscle, + *tome*, a cutting, slice]

pyloroplasty (pī-lor′ō-plăs″tē) [″ + *plassein*, to form]
   p., Finney
   p., Heineke-Mikulicz

pyloroscopy (pī-lō-rŏs′kō-pē) [Gr. *pyloros*, gatekeeper, + *skopein*, to examine]

pylorospasm (pī-lor′ō-spăzm) [″ + *spasmos*, a convulsion]

pylorostenosis (pī-lor″ō-stĕn-ō′sĭs) [″ + *stenosis*, act of narrowing]

pylorostomy (pī-lor-ŏs′tō-mē) [″ + *stoma*, mouth, opening]

pylorotomy (pī-lor-ŏt′ō-mē) [″ + *tome*, a cutting, slice]

pylorus (pī-lor′ŭs) [Gr. *pyloros*, gatekeeper]

pyo-, py- [Gr. *pyon*, pus]

pyocele (pī′ō-sēl) [Gr. *pyon*, pus, + *kele*, tumor, swelling]

pyocelia (pī″ō-sē′lē-ă) [″ + *koilia*,

cavity, belly]

pyocephalus (pī″ō-sĕf′ă-lŭs) [″ + kephale, head]
p., circumscribed
p., external
p., internal

pyochezia (pī″ō-kē′zē-ă) [Gr. pyon, pus, + chezein, to go to stool]

pyococcus (pī″ō-kŏk′ŭs) [″ + kokkos, berry]

pyocolpocele (pī″ō-kŏl′pō-sēl) [″ + kolpos, vagina, + kele, tumor, swelling]

pyocolpos (pī″ō-kŭl′pōs)

pyoculture (pī′ō-kŭl″chūr) [″ + L. cultura, tillage]

pyocyanic (pī″ō-sī-ăn′ĭk) [″ + kyanos, dark blue]

pyocyst (pī′ō-sĭst) [″ + kystis, sac]

pyoderma (pī-ō-dĕr′mă) [″ + derma, skin]
p. gangrenosum

pyodermatitis (pī″ō-dĕr″mă-tī′tĭs) [″ + ″ + itis, inflammation]

pyodermatosis (pī″ō-dĕr″mă-tō′sĭs) [″ + ″ + osis, condition]

pyodermia (pī″ō-dĕr′mē-ă)

pyofecia (pī″ō-fē′sē-ă) [Gr. pyon, pus, + L. faeces, refuse]

pyogenesis (pī″ō-jĕn′ĕ-sĭs) [″ + genesis, generation, birth]

pyogenic (pī-ō-jĕn′ĭk) [″ + gennan, to produce]

pyogenic microorganisms

pyohemia (pī″ō-hē′mē-ă) [″ + haima, blood]

pyohemothorax (pī″ō-hē″mō-thō′rāks) [″ + haima, blood, + thorax, chest]

pyoid (pī′oyd) [″ + eidos, form, shape]

pyolabyrinthitis (pī″ō-lăb″ĭ-rĭn-thī′tĭs) [″ + labyrinthos, maze, + itis, inflammation]

pyometra (pī″ō-mē′tră) [″ + metra, uterus]

pyometritis (pī″ō-mē-trī′tĭs) [″ + ″ + itis, inflammation]

pyonephritis (pī″ō-nĕf-rī′tĭs) [″ + nephros, kidney, + itis, inflammation]

pyonephrolithiasis (pī″ō-nĕf″rō-lĭth-ī′ă-sĭs) [″ + ″ + lithos, stone, + -iasis, state or condition of]

pyonephrosis (pī″ō-nĕf-rō′sĭs) [″ + ″ + osis, condition]

pyoovarium (pī″ō-ō-vā′rē-ŭm) [″ + NL. ovarium, ovary]

Pyopen

pyopericarditis (pī″ō-pĕr″ĭ-kăr-dī′tĭs) [″ + peri, around, + kardia, heart, + itis, inflammation]

pyopericardium (pī″ō-pĕr″ĭ-kăr′dē-ŭm)

pyoperitoneum (pī″ō-pĕr″ĭ-tō-nē′ŭm) [Gr. pyon, pus, + peritonaion, stretched around or over]

pyoperitonitis (pī″ō-pĕr″ĭ-tō-nī′tĭs) [″ + ″ + itis, inflammation]

pyophthalmia (pī″ŏf-thăl′mē-ă) [″ + ophthalmos, eye]

pyophthalmitis (pī″ŏf-thăl-mī′tĭs) [″ + ″ + itis, inflammation]

pyophylactic (pī″ō-fī-lăk′tĭk) [″ + phylaxis, guard]

pyophylactic membrane

pyophysometra (pī″ō-fī″sō-mē′tră) [″ + physa, air, + metra, uterus]

pyoplania (pī″ō-plă′nē-ă) [″ + planos, wandering]

pyopneumocholecystitis (pī″ō-nū″mō-kō-lē-sĭs-tī′tĭs) [″ + pneuma, air, + chole, bile, + kystis, sac, + itis, inflammation]

pyopneumocyst (pī″ō-nū′mō-sĭst) [″ + ″ + kystis, bladder]

pyopneumohepatitis (pī″ō-nū″mō-hĕp″ă-tī′tĭs) [″ + pneuma, air, + hepar, liver, + itis, inflammation]

pyopneumopericardium (pī″ō-nū″mō-pĕr″ĭ-kăr′dē-ŭm) [″ + ″ + peri, around, + kardia, heart]

pyopneumoperitoneum (pī″ō-nū″mō-pĕr″ĭ-tō-nē′ŭm) [″ + ″ + peritonaion, stretched around or over]

pyopneumoperitonitis (pī″ō-nū″mō-pĕr″ĭ-tō-nī′tĭs) [″ + ″ + ″ +

itis, inflammation]

pyopneumothorax (pī″ō-nū″mō-thō′răks) [″ + ″ + *thorax*, chest]

pyopoiesis (pī″ō-poy-ē′sĭs) [″ + *poiein*, to make]

pyopoietic (pī″ō-poy-ĕt′ĭk)

pyoptysis (pī-ŏp′tĭ-sĭs) [″ + *ptysis*, spitting]

pyopyelectasis (pī″ō-pī″ĕ-lĕk′tă-sĭs) [″ + *pyelos*, pelvis, + *ektasis*, dilation]

pyorrhagia (pī-or-ă′jē-ă) [″ + *rhegnynai*, to burst forth]

pyorrhea (pī″ō-rē′ă) [″ + *rhein*, to flow]
   p. alveolaris

pyosalpingitis (pī″ō-săl″pĭn-jī′tĭs) [Gr. *pyon*, pus, + *salpinx*, tube, + *itis*, inflammation]

pyosalpingo-oophoritis (pī″ō-săl-pĭn″gō-ō″ŏf-ō-rī′tĭs) [″ + ″ + NL. *oophoron*, ovary, + Gr. *itis*, inflammation]

pyosalpinx (pī″ō-săl′pĭnks)

pyosemia (pī″ō-sē′mē-ă) [Gr. *pyon*, pus, + L. *semen*, seed]

pyostatic (pī″ō-stăt′ĭk) [″ + *statikos*, standing]

pyothorax (pī″ō-thō′răks) [″ + *thorax*, chest]

pyotorrhea (pī″ō-tō-rē′ă) [″ + *ous*, ear, + *rhein*, to flow]

pyotoxinemia (pī″ō-tŏk″sī-nē′mē-ă) [″ + *toxikon*, poison, + *haima*, blood]

pyoturia (pī″ō-tū′rē-ă) [″ + *ouron*, urine]

pyourachus (pī″ō-ū′ră-kŭs) [″ + *ourachos*, fetal urinary canal]

pyoureter (pī″ō-ū-rē′tĕr) [″ + *oureter*, ureter]

pyovesiculosis (pī″ō-vĕ-sĭk″ū-lō′sĭs) [″ + L. *vesiculus*, a small vessel, + Gr. *osis*, condition]

pyoxanthin(e) (pī″ō-zăn′thĭn) [″ + *xanthos*, yellow]

pyramid (pĭr′ă-mĭd) [Gr. *pyramis*, a

pyramid]
   p., malpighian
   p. of cerebellum
   p. of light
   p. of medulla
   p. of temporal bone
   p. of thyroid
   p. of tympanum
   p., renal

pyramidal (pĭ-răm′ĭ-dăl) [L. *pyramidalis*]

pyramidal cell

pyramidalis (pĭ-răm″ĭ-dăl′ĭs) [L.]
   p. auriculae

pyramidal tract

pyramidotomy (pĕr″ăm-ĭ-dŏt′ō-mē) [Gr. *pyramis*, a pyramid, + *tome*, a cutting, slice]

pyramis (pĭr′ă-mĭs) [Gr., a pyramid]

pyran (pī′răn)

pyranose (pī′ră-nōs)

pyrantel pamoate (pī-răn′tĕl)

pyrazinamide (pī″ră-zĭn′ă-mīd)

pyrectic (pī-rĕk′tĭk)

pyrenemia (pī″rĕ-nē′mē-ă) [Gr. *pyren*, fruit stone, + *haima*, blood]

pyretherapy (pī″rĕ-thĕr′ă-pē) [Gr. *pyr*, fever, + *therapeia*, treatment]

pyrethrins (pī-rē′thrĭnz)

pyretic (pī-rĕt′ĭk) [Gr. *pyretos*, fever]

pyretic therapy

pyreticosis (pī-rĕt″ĭ-kō′sĭs) [″ + *osis*, condition]

pyreto- (pī-rĕt′ō) [Gr. *pyretos*, fever]

pyretogen (pī-rĕt′ō-jĕn) [″ + *gennan*, to produce]

pyretogenesia, **pyretogenesis** (pi″rĕ-tō-jĕn-ē′zē-ă, -jĕn′ĕ-sĭs) [″ + *enesis*, generation, birth]

pyretogenic (pī″rĕt-ō-jĕn′ĭk)

pyretogenic bacteria

pyretogenic stage

pyretogenous (pī″rĕ-tŏj′ĕn-ŭs)

pyretolysis (pī″rĕ-tŏl′ĭ-sĭs) [″ + *lysis*, dissolution]

pyretotherapy (pī″rĕ-tō-thĕr′ă-pē) [″ + *therapeia*, treatment]

pyretotyphosis (pī″rĕ-tō-tĭ-fō′sĭs) [″

+ typhosis, delirium]

pyrexia (pī-rĕk'sē-ă) [Gr. pyressein, to be feverish]

pyrexial (pī-rĕk'sē-ăl)

pyrexin (pī'rĕks'ĭn)

Pyribenzamine Hydrochloride

pyridine (pĕr'ĭ-dēn)

Pyridium

pyridostigmine bromide (pĕr"ĭ-dō-stĭg'mĕn)

pyridoxal 5-phosphate

pyridoxamine (pĭr"ĭ-dŏks'ă-mĭn)

4-pyridoxic acid (pĭr"ĭ-dŏks'ĭk)

pyridoxine hydrochloride (pĭ-rĭ-dŏks'ēn)

pyriform (pĭr'ĭ-form) [L. pirum, pear, + forma, shape]

pyrilamine maleate (pĕr-ĭl'ă-mēn)

pyrimethamine (pĕr"ĭ-mĕth'ă-mēn)

pyrimidine (pĭ-rĭm'ĭd-ĭn)

pyrithiamine (pĭr"ĭ-thī'ă-mĭn)

pyro- (pī'rō) [Gr. pyr, fire]

pyrogallol (pī"rō-găl'ŏl)

pyrogen (pī'rō-jĕn) [Gr. pyr, fire, + gennan, to produce]
p., leukocytic

pyrogenic (pī"rō-jĕn'ĭk) [Gr. pyr, fire, + gennan, to produce]

pyroglobulinemia (pī"rō-glŏb"ū-lĭ-nē'mē-ă) [" + globulus, globule, + haima, blood]

pyrolagnia (pī"rō-lăg'nē-ă) [" + lagneia, lust]

pyrolysis (pī-rŏl'ĭ-sĭs) [" + lysis, dissolution]

pyromania (pī"rō-mā'nē-ă) [" + mania, madness]

pyrometer (pī-rŏm'ĕ-tĕr) [" + metron, measure]

pyronine (pī'rō-nĭn)

pyronyxis (pī"rō-nĭk'sĭs) [" + nyxis, a piercing]

pyrophobia (pī"rō-fō'bē-ă) [" + phobos, fear]

pyrophosphatase (pī"rō-fŏs'fă-tās)

pyrophosphate (pī"rō-fŏs'fāt)

pyroptothymia (pī"rŏp-tō-thī'mē-ă) [" + ptoein, to scare, + thymos, mind, spirit]

pyropuncture (pī"rō-pŭnk'chŭr) [" + L. punctura, prick]

pyrosis (pī-rō'sĭs) [Gr. pyrosis, burning]

pyrotic (pī-rŏt'ĭk) [Gr. pyrotikos]

pyrotoxin (pī"rō-tŏk'sĭn) [Gr. pyr, fire, + toxikon, poison]

pyroxylin (pī-rŏk'sĭ-lĭn)

pyrrobutamine phosphate (pĕr"rō-bū'tă-mēn)

pyrrol cells

pyrrole (pĕr'ŏl)

pyrrolidine (pĭ-rŏl'ĭ-dĭn)

pyruvate (pī'roo-vāt)

pyruvic acid (pī-roo'vĭk)

pyrvinium pamoate (pĭr-vĭn'ē-ŭm)

pythogenesis (pī"thō-jĕn'ē-sĭs) [Gr. pythein, to rot, + genesis, generation, birth]

pyuria (pī-ū'rē-ă) [Gr. pyon, pus, + ouron, urine]

PZI protamine zinc insulin

Q

Q *quantity; coulomb*
Q angle
Qco_2
q.d. [L.] *quaque die,* every day
Q disk
Q fever
q.h. [L.] *quaque hora,* every hour
q.i.d. [L.] *quater in die,* four times a day
q.l. [L.] *quantum libet,* as much as one pleases
Q law
Qo_2
q.q.h. [L.] *quaque quarta hora,* every four hours
QRS complex
QRST complex
q.s. [L.] *quantum sufficit,* as much as suffices
qt *quart*
Q-T segment
Quaalude
quack (kwăk) [D. *kwaksalven,* to peddle salve]
quad. *quadriceps; quadrilateral; quadrant; quadriplegia*
quadrangular (kwŏd-răng'ū-lĕr) [L. *quadri,* four, + *angulus,* angle]
quadrangular lobe
quadrangular membrane
quadrant (kwŏd'rănt) [L. *quadrans,* a fourth]
    q., dental
quadrantanopia (kwŏd"rănt-ă-nō'pē-ă) [" + Gr. *an-,* not, + *opsis,* sight, appearance, vision]
quadrantanopsia (kwŏd"rănt-ăn-ŏp'sē-ă) [" + " + *opsis,* sight, appearance, vision]
quadrate (kwŏd'rāt) [L. *quadratus,* squared]
quadrate lobe

quadrate lobule
quadri-, quadr- [L. *quattuor,* four]
quadribasic (kwŏd"rī-bā'sĭk)
quadriceps (kwŏd'rī-sĕps) [" + *caput,* head]
quadriceps femoris
quadricepsplasty (kwŏd"rī-sĕps'plăs-tē) [" + " + Gr. *plassein,* to form]
quadriceps reflex
quadricuspid (kwŏd"rī-kŭs'pĭd) [" + *cuspis,* point]
quadridigitate (kwŏd"rī-dĭj'ĭ-tāt)
quadrigemina (kwŏd"rī-jĕm'ĭn-ă) [" + *geminus,* twin]
quadrigeminal (kwŏd"rī-jĕm'ĭn-ăl)
quadrigeminum (kwŏd"rī-jĕm'ĭ-nŭm)
quadrigeminus (kwŏd"rī-jĕm'ĭ-nŭs)
quadrilateral (kwŏd"rī-lăt'ĕr-ăl) [" + *latus,* side]
quadrilocular (kwŏd"rī-lŏk'ū-lăr) [" + *loculus,* a small space]
quadripara (kwŏd-rĭp'ă-ră) [" + *parere,* to beget, produce]
quadripartite (kwŏd"rī-păr'tīt) [" + *partire,* to divide]
quadriplegia (kwŏd"rī-plē'jē-ă) [" + Gr. *plege,* stroke]
quadripolar (kwŏd"rī-pō'lăr)
quadrisect (kwŏd"rī-sĕkt) [" + *sectio,* a cutting]
quadrisection (kwŏd"rī-sĕk'shŭn)
quadritubercular (kwŏd"rī-tū-bĕr'kū-lĕr) [" + *tuberculum,* a little swelling]
quadrivalent (kwŏd"rī-vā'lĕnt) [" + *valens,* powerful]
quadruped (kwŏd'roo-pĕd") [" + *pes,* foot]
quadrupedal reflex (kwŏd-roop'ĕd-ăl)

quadruplet (kwŏd'roo-plĕt, kwŏ-droo'plĕt) [L. *quadruplus,* fourfold]
quale (kwā'lē) [L. *qualis,* of what kind]
qualimeter (kwŏl-ĭm'ĕt-ĕr) [" + Gr. *metron,* measure]
qualitative (kwŏl'ĭ-tā"tĭv) [L. *qualitativus*]
qualitative analysis
quality (kwŏl'ĭ-tē) [L. *qualitas,* quality]
quality assurance
quality of life
quanta (kwŏn'tă) [L.]
quantimeter (kwŏn-tĭm'ĕt-ĕr) [L. *quantus,* how great, + Gr. *metron,* measure]
quanti-Pirquet (kwŏn"tĭ-pēr-kă') [Clemens Pirquet, Austrian physician, 1874–1929]
quantitative (kwŏn"tĭ-tā'tĭv) [LL. *quantitativus*]
quantitative analysis
quantity (kwŏn'tĭ-tē) [L. *quantitas,* quantity]
quantivalence
quantum (kwŏn'tŭm) [L., how much]
quantum libet (kwŏn'tŭm lĭ'bĕt) [L.]
quantum sufficit (kwŏn'tŭm sŭf'fĭ sĭt) [L.]
quantum theory
quarantine (kwor'ăn-tēn") [It. *quarantina,* 40 days]
quart (kwort) [L. *quartus,* a fourth]
quartan (kwor'tăn) [L. *quartana,* of the fourth]
    q., double
    q., triple
quartile (kwor'tĭl) [L. *quartus,* a fourth]
quartipara (kwor-tĭp'ă-ră) [" + *parere,* to beget, produce]
quartisect (kwor'tĭ-sĕkt) [" + *sectio,* a cutting]
quartz (kwărts) [Ger. *quarz*]
quartz applicator
quartz glass
Quarzan
quassation (kwă-sā'shŭn) [L. *quassatio*]
quassia (kwŏsh'ă, kwŏsh'ē-ă) [*Quassi,* Surinam inhabitant who discovered its medicinal value]
Quatelet index
quater in die (kwŏ'tĕr ĭn dē'ă) [L.]
quaternary (kwŏ-tĕr'nă-rē) [L. *quaternarius,* of four]
Queckenstedt's sign (kwĕk'ĕn-stĕts) [Hans Queckenstedt, Ger. physician, 1887–1918]
quenching (kwĕnch'ĭng)
    q., fluorescence
querulent (kwĕr'ū-lĕnt) [L. *querulus,* complaining]
Quervain's disease (kār'vănz) [Fritz de Quervain, Swiss surgeon, 1868–1940]
Questran
quick (kwĭk) [ME. *quicke,* alive]
quickening (kwĭk'ĕn-ĭng)
quicklime
quicksilver [ME. *quicke,* alive, + *silver,* silver]
Quick's test (kwĭks) [Armand J. Quick, U.S. physician, b. 1894]
quinacrine hydrochloride
Quinaglute
Quincke's disease (kwĭnk'ēz) [Heinrich I. Quincke, Ger. physician, 1842–1922]
Quincke's pulse
Quincke's puncture
Quine
quinestrol (kwĭn-ĕs'trŏl)
quinethazone (kwĭn-ĕth'ă-zōn)
quingestanol acetate (kwĭn-jĕs'tă-nŏl)
quinic acid
Quinidex
quinidine sulfate (kwĭn'ĭ-dēn)
quinine (kwī'nīn", kwī-nēn') [Sp. *quina*]
    q. bisulfate
    q. dihydrochloride
    q. hydrochloride
    q. sulfate
    q. tannate
quinine and urea hydrochloride
quininism (kwī'nīn-ĭzm, kwī-nēn'ĭzm) [Sp. *quina,* quinine, + Gr. *-ismos,* condition]

quinoline (kwĭn′ō-lēn″)

quinone (kwĭn′ōn)

quinqu- [L. *quinque*]

Quinquaud's disease (kăn-kōz′) [Charles E. Quinquaud, Fr. physician, 1841 – 1894]

quinquetubercular (kwĭn″kwē-tū-bĕr′kū-lăr)

quinquevalent (kwĭng″kwĕ-vā′lĕnt)

quinquina (kwĭn-kwĭ′nă, kĭn-kē′nă)

quinsy (kwĭn′zē) [ME. *quinesye*, sore throat]

quintan (kwĭn′tăn) [L. *quintanus*, of a fifth]

quinti- [L. *quintus*, fifth]

quintipara (kwĭn-tĭp′ă-ră) [″ + *parere*, to beget, produce]

quintuplet (kwĭn′tū-plĕt, kwĭn-tŭp′lĕt) [LL. *quintuplex*, fivefold]

quotidian (kwō-tĭd′ē-ăn) [L. *quotidianus*, daily]

quotidian fever

quotient (kwō′shĕnt) [L. *quotiens*, how many times]

    q., achievement

    q., intelligence

    q., respiratory

q.v. [L.] *quantum vis*, as much as you please; [L.] *quod vide*, which see

Q wave

R

R *respiration; right; roentgen; a radical*
R— *part of a molecule*
—R *Rinne negative*
+R *Rinne positive*
℞ *[L.] recipe, take*
RA *rheumatoid arthritis; right atrium*
Ra *radium*
rabbetting (răb'ĕt-ĭng) [Fr. *raboter*, to plane]
rabbit fever
rabbitpox
rabiate (rā'bē-āt) [L. *rabies*, rage]
rabic (răb'ĭk)
rabicidal (răb-ĭ-sī'dăl) [L. *rabies*, rage, + *cida* fr. *caedere*, to kill]
rabid (răb'ĭd)
rabies (rā'bēz) [L. *rabere*, to rage]
rabies immune globulin
rabies virus group
rabiform (rā'bĭ-form) [" + *forma*, shape]
race (rās) [Fr.]
racemase (rā'sē-mās)
racemate (rā'sē-māt)
racemic (rā-sē'mĭk)
racemization (rā"sē-mĭ-zā'shŭn)
racemose (răs'ĕ-mōs) [L. *racemosus*, full of clusters]
rachi-, rachio- [Gr. *rhachis*, spine]
rachial (rā'kē-ăl) [Gr. *rhachis*, spine]
rachialbuminimeter (rā"kē-ăl-bū"mĭn-ĭm'ĕt-ĕr) [" + L. *albumen*, white of egg, + Gr. *metron*, measure]
rachialbuminimetry (rā"kē-ăl-bū"mĭn-ĭm'ĕt-rē)
rachialgia (rā-kē-ăl'jē-ă) [" + *algos*, pain]
rachianalgesia (rā"kē-ăn-ăl-jē'zē-ă) [" + *analgesia*, lack of pain]
rachianesthesia (rā"kē-ăn-ĕs-thē'zē-ă) [" + *an-*, negative, + *aisth-esis*, feeling, perception]
rachicele (rā'kĭ-sēl) [" + *kele*, tumor, swelling]
rachicentesis (rā"kĭ-sĕn-tē'sĭs) [" + *kentesis*, puncture]
rachidial (ră-kĭd'ē-ăl)
rachidian (ră-kĭd'ē-ăn)
rachigraph (rā'kĭ-grăf) [" + *gra-phein*, to write]
rachilysis (ră-kĭl'ĭ-sĭs [" + *lysis*, dis-solution]
rachiocampsis (rā-kē-ō-kămp'sĭs) [" + *kampsis*, a bending]
rachiocentesis (rā"kē-ō-sĕn-tē'sĭs) [" + *kentesis*, puncture]
rachiochysis (rā-kē-ŏk'ĭ-sĭs) [" + *chysis*, a pouring]
rachiodynia (rā-kē-ō-dĭn'ē-ă) [" + *odyne*, pain]
rachiometer (rā-kē-ŏm'ĕ-tĕr) [" + *metron*, measure]
rachiomyelitis (rā"kē-ō-mī"ĕ-lī'tĭs) [" + *myelos*, marrow, + *itis*, inflammation]
rachiopagus (rā"kē-ŏp'ă-gŭs) [" + *pagos*, thing fixed]
rachiopathy (rā"kē-ŏp'ă-thē) [" + *pathos*, disease, suffering]
rachioplegia (rā-kē-ō-plē'jē-ă) [" + *plege*, a stroke]
rachioscoliosis (rā"kē-ō-skō"lē-ō'sĭs) [" + *skoliosis*, crookedness]
rachiotome (rā'kē-ō-tōm") [" + *tome*, a cutting, slice]
rachiotomy (rā"kē-ŏt'ō-mē)
rachis (rā'kĭs) [Gr. *rhachis*]
rachischisis (ră-kĭs'kĭ-sĭs) [" + *schisis*, cleavage]
   r., posterior
rachitic (ră-kĭt'ĭk) [" + *itis*, inflam-

matory]
r. fetalis annularis
r. fetalis micromelica
rachitism (răk'ĭ-tĭzm)
rachitogenic (ră-kĭt"ō-jĕn'ĭk) [" + genesis, generation, birth]
rachitome (răk'ĭ-tōm") [" + tome, a cutting, slice]
rachitomy (ră-kĭt'ō-mē) [" + tome, a cutting, slice]
raclage (ră-klŏzh') [Fr.]
rad radiation absorbed dose
radectomy (ră-dĕk'tō-mē) [L. radix, root, + Gr. ektome, excision]
radiability (rā"dē-ă-bĭl'ĭ-tē) [L. radius, ray, + habilitas, able]
radiad (rā'dē-ăd) [L. radialis, radial, + ad, toward]
radial (rā'dē-ăl)
radialis (rā"dē-ā'lĭs) [L.]
radial reflex
radian (rā'dē-ăn)
radiant (rā'dē-ănt) [L. radians, radiate]
radiate (rā'dē-āt) [L. radiare, to emit rays]
radiatio (rā-dē-ā'shē-ō) [L.]
radiation (rā-dē-ā'shŭn) [L. radiatio, to radiate]
　　r., acoustic
　　r., auditory
　　r., corpuscular
　　r., electromagnetic
　　r., heterogeneous
　　r., homogeneous
　　r., infrared
　　r., interstitial
　　r., ionizing
　　r., irritative
　　r., occipitothalamic
　　r. of corpus callosum
　　r., optic
　　r., photochemical
　　r., pyramidal
　　r.'s, solar
　　r., striatomesencephalic
　　r., striatosubthalamic
　　r., striatothalamic
　　r., thalamic
　　r., ultraviolet
　　r., visible
radiation absorbed dose
radiation injury, ionizing
radiation sickness
radiation syndrome
radiation therapy
radiator (rā'dē-ā"tor) [LL. radiatus, furnished with rays]
　　r., infrared
radical (răd'ĭ-kăl) [LL. radicalis, having roots]
　　r., acid
　　r., alcohol
　　r., color
　　r., free
radical treatment
radices (răd'ĭ-sēz) [L.]
radiciform
radicle (răd'ĭ-kl) [L. radicula, little root]
radicotomy (răd"ĭ-kŏt'ō-mē) [L. radix, root, + Gr. tome, a cutting, slice]
radicula (ră-dĭk'ū-lă) [L.]
radiculalgia (ră-dĭk"ū-lăl'jē-ă) [L. radix, root, + Gr. algos, pain]
radicular (ră-dĭk'ū-lăr) [L. radix, root]
radiculectomy (ră-dĭk"ū-lĕk'tō-mē) [" + Gr. ektome, excision]
radiculitis (ră-dĭk"ū-lī'tĭs) [L. radicula, little root, + Gr. itis, inflammation]
radiculoganglionitis (ră-dĭk"ū-lō-găng"glē-ō-nī'tĭs) [" + Gr. ganglion, knot, + itis, inflammation]
radiculomedullary (ră-dĭk"ū-lō-mĕd'ū-lĕr"ē) [" + medullaris, marrow]
radiculomeningomyelitis (ră-dĭk"ū-lō-mĕ-nĭn"gō-mī-ĕl-ī'tĭs) [" + Gr. meninx, membrane, + myelos, marrow, + itis, inflammation]
radiculomyelopathy (ră-dĭk"ū-lō-mī"ĕ-lŏp'ă-thē) [" + Gr. myelos, marrow, + pathos, disease, suffering]
radiculoneuritis (ră-dĭk"ū-lō"nū-rī'tĭs) [L. radicula, little root, + Gr. neuron, sinew, + itis, inflammation]
radiculoneuropathy (ră-dĭk"ū-lō-nū-rŏp'ă-thē) [" + " + pathos,

disease, suffering]
radiculopathy (ră-dĭk"ū-lŏp'ă-thē)
[" + Gr. *pathos*, disease, suffering]
radiectomy (rā"dē-ĕk'tō-mē) [L. *radix*,
root, + Gr. *ektome*, excision]
radiferous (ră-dĭf'ĕr-ŭs)
radii (rā'dē-ī) [L.]
radio- [L. *radius*, ray]
radioactinium (rā"dē-ō-ăk-tĭn'ē-ŭm)
radioactive (rā"dē-ō-ăk'tĭv) [L. *radius*,
ray, + *activus*, acting]
radioactive decay
radioactive patient
radioactive tracer
radioactivity (rā"dē-ō-ăk"tĭv'ĭ-tē)
   r., artificial
   r., induced
   r., natural
radioallergosorbent test (rā"dē-ō-
ăl"ĕr-gō-sor'bĕnt)
radioanaphylaxis (rā"dē-ō-ăn"ă-fĭ-
lăk'sĭs) [" + Gr. *ana*, away from,
+ *phylaxis*, guard]
radioautogram (rā"dē-ō-aw'tō-grăm)
[" + Gr. *autos*, self, +
gramma, letter, piece of writing]
radioautograph (rā"dē-ō-aw'tō-grăf)
[" + " + *graphein*, to write]
radioautography (rā"dē-ō-aw-tŏg'ră-
fē)
radiobicipital (rā"dē-ō-bī-sĭp'ĭ-tăl)
radiobiology (rā"dē-ō-bī-ŏl'ō-jē)
radiocalcium (rā"dē-ō-kăl'sē-ŭm)
radiocarbon (rā"dē-ō-kăr'bŏn)
radiocardiogram (rā"dē-ō-kăr'dē-ō-
grăm) [L. *radius*, ray, + Gr. *kardia*,
heart, + *gramma*, letter, piece of
writing]
radiocardiography (rā"dē-ō-kăr"dē-
ŏg'ră-fē) [" + " + *graphein*, to
write]
radiocarpal (rā"dē-ō-kăr'păl) [" +
Gr. *karpos*, wrist]
radiochemistry [" + Gr. *chemeia*,
chemistry]
radiochroism (rā"dē-ō-krō'ĭzm) [" +
Gr. *chroa*, color]
radiochrometer (rā"dē-ō-krŏm'ē-tĕr)

[" + Gr. *chroma*, color, +
metron, measure]
radiocinematograph (rā"dē-ō-sĭn"ē-
măt'ō-grăf) [" + Gr. *kinema*, motion, + *graphein*, to write]
radiocurable (rā"dē-ō-kūr'ă-bl)
radiocystitis (rā"dē-ō-sĭs-tī'tĭs) [" +
Gr. *kystis*, bladder, + *itis*, inflamma-
tion]
radiode (rā'dē-ōd) [" + Gr. *hodos*,
way]
radiodense
radiodermatitis (rā"dē-ō-dĕr"mă-tī'tĭs)
[" + Gr. *derma*, skin, +
osis, condition]
radiodiagnosis (rā"dē-ō-dī"ăg-nō'sĭs)
[" + Gr. *dia*, through, +
gnosis, knowledge]
radiodigital (rā"dē-ō-dĭg'ĭ-tăl)
radiodontia (rā"dē-ō-dŏn'shē-ă)
[" + Gr. *odous*, tooth]
radioecology (rā"dē-ō-ē-kŏl'ō-jē)
[" + Gr. *oikos*, house, + *logos*,
word, reason]
radioelectrocardiogram (rā"dē-ō-
ē-lĕk"trō-kăr'dē-ō-grăm)
radioelectrocardiography (rā"dē-ō-
ē-lĕk"trō-kăr"dē-ŏg'ră-fē) [L. *radius*,
ray, + Gr. *elektron*, amber,
+ *kardia*, heart, + *graphein*,
to write]
radioelement (rā"dē-ō-ĕl'ĕ-mĕnt)
[" + *elementum*, a rudiment]
radioencephalogram (rā"dē-ō-ĕn-
sĕf'ă-lō-grăm") [" + Gr. *enkephalos*, brain, + *gramma*, letter,
piece of writing]
radioencephalography (rā"dē-ō-
ĕn-sĕf"ă-lŏg'ră-fē) [" + " +
graphein, to write]
radioepidermitis (rā"dē-ō-ĕp"ĭ-dĕr-
mī'tĭs) [" + Gr. *epi*, upon, +
derma, skin, + *itis*, inflammation]
radioepitheliitis (rā"dē-ō-ĕp"ĭ-thē-lē-
ī'tĭs) [" + " + *thele*, nipple,
+ *itis*, inflammation]
**radiofrequency electrophrenic res-
piration**

radiogenesis (rā″dē-ō-jĕn′ĕ-sĭs) [″ +
Gr. *genesis*, generation, birth]
radiogenic (rā″dē-ō-jĕn′ĭk) [″ +
gennan, to produce]
radiogold (rā′dē-ō-gōld)
radiogram (rā′dē-ō-grăm) [″ +
Gr. *gramma*, letter, piece of writing]
radiograph (rā′dē-ō-grăf) [″ +
Gr. *graphein*, to write]
   r., bitewing
   r., dental
   r., lateral cephalometric
   r., panoramic
   r., periapical
radiography (rā-dē-ŏg′rȧ-fē)
radiohumeral (rā″dē-ō-hū′mĕr-ăl)
[″ + *humerus*, upper arm]
radioimmunity (rā″dē-ō-ĭ-mū′nĭ-tē)
[″ + *immunitas*, immunity]
radioimmunoassay (rā″dē-ō-ĭm″ū-
nō-ăs′ā)
radioimmunodiffusion (rā″dē-ō-ĭm″ū-
nō-dĭf-fū′zhŭn) [″ + ″ +
dis, apart, + *fundere*, to pour]
radioimmunoelectrophoresis
(rā″dē-ō-ĭm″ū-nō-ē-lĕk″trō-fō-rē′sĭs) [″
+ ″ + Gr. *elektron*, amber, +
phoresis, bearing]
radioiodine (rā″dē-ō-ī′ō-dīn)
radioiron (rā″dē-ō-ī′ĕrn)
radioisotope (rā″dē-ō-ī′sō-tōp)
radiolead (rā″dē-ō-lĕd′)
radiolesion (rā″dē-ō-lē′zhŭn)
radioligand (rā″dē-ō-lī′gănd, răd″dē-
ō-lĭg′ănd)
radiological emergency assistance
radiologic technologist
radiologist (rā-dē-ŏl′ō-jĭst) [L. *radius*,
ray, + Gr. *logos*, word, reason]
radiology (rā-dē-ŏl′ō-jē)
radiolucency (rā″dē-ō-lū′sĕn-sē)
[″ + *lucere*, to shine]
radiolucent (rā″dē-ō-lū′sĕnt) [″ +
lucere, to shine]
radiolus (rā-dē′ō-lŭs) [L., a little ray]
radiometer (rā-dē-ŏm′ĕ-tĕr) [″ +
Gr. *metron*, measure]
radiomicrometer (rā″dē-ō-mī-krŏm′ĕ-

tĕr) [″ + Gr. *mikros*, small, +
metron, measure]
radiomimetic (rā″dē-ō-mĭm-ĕt′ĭk)
[″ + Gr. *mimetikos*, imitation]
radiomuscular (rā″dē-ō-mŭs′kū-lăr)
radiomutation
radion (rā′dē-ŏn) [″ + Gr. *on*,
being]
radionecrosis (rā″dē-ō-nĕ-krō′sĭs)
[″ + Gr. *nekrosis*, state of death]
radioneuritis (rā″dē-ō-nū-rī′tĭs) [″ +
Gr. *neuron*, sinew, + *itis*, inflam-
mation]
radionitrogen (rā″dē-ō-nī′trō-jĕn)
radionuclide (rā″dē-ō-nū′klĭd)
radiopacity (rā″dē-ō-păs′ĭ-tē)
radiopaque (rā-dē-ō-pāk′) [″ +
opacus, dark]
radioparency (rā″dē-ō-păr′ĕn-sē)
radioparent (rā″dē-ō-păr′ĕnt) [″ +
parere, to be visible, appear, show]
radiopathology (rā″dē-ō-pă-thŏl′ō-
jē) [″ + Gr. *pathos*, disease, suffering, + *logos*, word, reason]
radiopelvimetry (rā″dē-ō-pĕl-vĭm′ĕt-
rē) [″ + *pelvis*, basin, + Gr.
metron, measure]
radiopharmaceuticals (rā″dē-ō-
fărm″ȧ-sū′tĭ-kăls)
radiophobia (rā″dē-ō-fō′bē-ȧ) [″ +
Gr. *phobos*, fear]
radiophosphorus (rā″dē-ō-fŏs′fō-rŭs)
radiopotassium (rā″dē-ō-pō-
tăs′ē-ŭm)
radiopotentiation (rā″dē-ō-pō-
tĕn″shē-ā′shŭn) [″ + *potentia*,
power]
radiopraxis (rā″dē-ō-prăk′sĭs) [″ +
Gr. *praxis*, practice]
radioprotective drugs
radiopulmonography (rā″dē-ō-
pŭl″mō-nŏg′rȧ-fē) [″ + *pulmo*,
lung, + Gr. *graphein*, to write]
radioreaction (rā″dē-ō-rē-ăk′shŭn)
radioreceptor (rā″dē-ō-rē-sĕp′tor)
radioresistant
radioresponsive (rā″dē-ō-rē-spŏn′sĭv)
radioscopy (rā-dē-ŏs′kō-pē) [L. *radius*,

ray, + Gr. *skopein*, to examine]
radiosensibility
radiosensitivity (rā″dē-ō-sĕn″sī-tĭv′ĭ-tē)
radiosodium (rā″dē-ō-sō′dē-ŭm)
radiostrontium (rā″dē-ō-strŏn′shē-ŭm)
radiosulfur (rā″dē-ō-sŭl′fŭr)
radiosurgery (rā″dē-ō-sŭr′jĕr-ē) [″ + Gr. *cheirurgia*, handwork]
radiotelemetry (rā″dē-ō-tĕl-ĕm′ĕ-trē) [″ + Gr. *tele*, distant, + *metron*, measure]
radiotherapeutics (rā″dē-ō-thĕr″ă-pū′tĭks)
radiotherapist (rā″dē-ō-thĕr′ă-pĭst) [″ + Gr. *therapeia*, treatment]
radiotherapy (rā″dē-ō-thĕr′ă-pē)
radiothermy (rā″dē-ō-thĕr′mē) [″ + Gr. *therme*, heat]
radiothorium (rā″dē-ō-thō′rē-ŭm)
radiotoxemia (rā″dē-ō-tŏk-sē′mē-ă) [″ + Gr. *toxikon*, poison, + *haima*, blood]
radiotransparent (rā″dē-ō-trăns-păr′ĕnt) [″ + *trans*, across, + *parere*, to be visible, appear, show]
radiotropic (rā″dē-ō-trŏp′ĭk) [″ + Gr. *tropos*, turning]
radioulnar (rā″dē-ō-ŭl′năr) [″ + *ulna*, arm]
radium (rā′dē-ŭm) [L. *radius*, ray]
radium needles
radium therapy [″ + Gr. *therapeia*, treatment]
radius [L., ray]
    r., fracture of
radix (rā′dĭks) [L., root]
radon (rā′dŏn) [L. *radius*, ray]
raffinose (răf′ĭ-nōs)
rage (rāj′) [ME.]
    r., sham
ragsorters' disease
ragweed
Raillietina (rāl-yĕ′tĭ-nă)
    R. demerariensis
railway sickness
Raimiste's phenomenon

raised (rāzd) [ME. *reisen*, to rise]
rale (răl) [Fr., rattle]
    r., amphoric
    r., atelectatic
    r., bronchiectatic
    r., bubbling
    r., cavernous
    r., clicking
    r., coarse
    r., consonating
    r., crackling
    r., crepitant
    r., dry
    r., gurgling
    r., moist
    r. redux
    r., sibilant
    r., sonorous
    r., subcrepitant
    r., vesicular
ramal (rā′măl) [L. *ramus*, branch]
rami (rā′mī) [L.]
ramicotomy (răm″ī-kŏt′ō-mē) [L. *ramus*, branch, + Gr. *tome*, a cutting, slice]
ramification (răm″ī-fī-kā′shŭn) [L. *ramificare*, to make branches]
ramify (răm′ī-fī)
ramisection (răm′ī-sĕk″shŭn) [L. *ramus*, branch, + *sectio*, a cutting]
ramisectomy (răm-ĭs-ĕk′tō-mē) [″ + Gr. *ektome*, excision]
ramitis (răm-ī′tĭs) [″ + Gr. *itis*, inflammation]
ramollissement (rā″mŏl-ēs-mŏn′) [Fr.]
ramose (rā′mōs) [L. *ramus*, branch]
ramulus [L.]
ramus (rā′mŭs) [L., branch]
    r., anterior
    r., bronchial
    r. communicans
    r., mandibular
    r., meningeal
    r., posterior
rancid (răn′sĭd) [L. *rancidus*, stink]
rancidify (răn-sĭd′ĭ-fī)
rancidity (răn-sĭd′ĭ-tē)
random controlled trial

randomization
random sample
range [ME., series]
range of accommodation
range of motion
range-of-motion exercise
ranine (rā'nīn) [L. *rana*, a frog]
ranula (răn'ū-là) [L., little frog]
   r., pancreatic
Ranvier's nodes (rŏn-vē-āz') [Louis A. Ranvier, Fr. pathologist, 1835–1922]
rape (rāp) [L. *rapere*, to seize]
   r., date
   r., marital
   r., prison
   r., statutory
rape counseling
rapeseed [L. *rapa*, turnip]
raphania (ră-fā'nē-à) [Gr. *rhaphanos*, radish]
raphe (rā'fē) [Gr. *rhaphe*]
   r., abdominal
   r., buccal
   r. of penis
   r. of scrotum
   r. of tongue
   r., palatine
   r., perineal
   r., pterygomandibular
rapport (ră-por') [Fr. *rapporter*, to bring back]
raptus (răp'tŭs) [L.]
rarefaction (rār"ĕ-făk'shŭn) [L. *rarefacere*, to make thin]
   r. of bone
rarefy (rār'ĕ-fī)
rarefying osteitis
RAS *reticular activating system*
rash (răsh) [O. Fr. *rasche*]
   r., butterfly
   r., cable
   r., diaper
   r., drug
   r., ecchymotic
   r., gum
   r., heat
   r., hemorrhagic
   r., macular

   r., maculopapular
   r., mulberry
   r., nettle
   r., red
   r., rose
   r., serum
   r., sunburnlike
   r., tooth
   r., wandering
rasion (rā'zhŭn) [L. *rasio*]
raspatory (răs'pă-tō"rē) [L. *raspatorium*]
RAST *radioallergosorbent test*
Rastafarian cult
rasura (ră-sū'ră) [L. *rasura*, a scraping]
rat [ME]
rat-bite fever
rate (rāt) [L. *rata*, calculated]
   r., attack
   r., basal metabolic
   r., birth
   r., case
   r., case fatality
   r., death
   r., DMF
   r., dose
   r., erythrocyte sedimentation
   r., false-negative
   r., false-positive
   r., glomerular filtration
   r., growth
   r., heart
   r., morbidity
   r., mortality
   r., periodontal disease
   r., pulse
   r., respiration
   r., sedimentation
Rathke's pouch (răth'kĕz) [Martin H. Rathke, Ger. anatomist, 1793–1860]
ratio (rā'shē-ō) [L., computation]
   r., A/G
   r., albumin-globulin
   r., arm
   r., body-weight
   r., cardiothoracic
   r., curative
   r., dextrose-nitrogen

r., lecithin-sphingomyelin
r., odds
r., sex
r., therapeutic
ration (rǎ'shŭn)
rational (rǎsh'ŭn-ǎl) [L. *rationalis*, reason]
rationale (rǎsh"ŭn-ǎl') [L.]
rationalization (rǎsh"ŭn-ǎl-ĭ-zā'shŭn)
rattle (rǎt'l) [ME. *ratelen*, to rattle]
r., death
rattlesnake
raucous (raw'kŭs) [L. *raucus*, hoarse]
Raudixin
Rauscher leukemia virus [Frank J. Rauscher, U.S. virologist, b. 1931]
Rauwiloid
rauwolfia serpentina (raw-wŭlf'ē-ǎ) [Leonhard Rauwolf, Ger. botanist, 1535–1596]
rave (rāv) [ME. *raven*, to be delirious]
raving
ray (rā) [L. *radius*, ray]
r., actinic
r., alpha
r., antirachitic
r., bactericidal
r.'s, Becquerel's
r.'s, beta
r.'s, border
r.'s, cathode
r.'s, characteristic
r., chemical
r.'s, cosmic
r.'s, delta
r., erythema-producing
r.'s, fluorescent roentgen
r.'s, gamma
r.'s, grenz
r.'s, hard
r.'s, heat
r.'s, hertzian
r.'s, infrared
r., luminous
r.'s, medullary
r.'s, Millikan
r.'s, monochromatic
r.'s, pigment-producing

r.'s, positive
r., primary
r.'s, roentgen
r.'s, scattered
r.'s, Schumann
r.'s, secondary
r.'s, ultraviolet
r.'s, x
Raynaud's disease (rā-nōz') [Maurice Raynaud, Fr. physician, 1834–1881]
Raynaud's phenomenon
rayon, purified
Rb *rubidium*
RBBB *right bundle branch block*
RBC, rbc *red blood cell; red blood count*
R.B.E. *relative biological effectiveness*
R.C.D. *relative cardiac dullness*
R.C.P. *Royal College of Physicians*
R.C.S. *Royal College of Surgeons*
R.D.A. *right dorsoanterior*
R.D.P. *right dorsoposterior*
RDS *respiratory distress syndrome*
R.E. *radium emanation; right eye; reticuloendothelium*
Re *rhenium*
re- [L., back, again]
reabsorb (rē"ǎb-sorb')
reabsorption (rē"ǎb-sorp'shŭn)
reacher
react (rē-ǎkt') [L. *re*, again, + *agere*, to act]
reactant (rē-ǎk'tǎnt)
reaction (rē-ǎk'shŭn) [LL. *reactus*, reacted]
r., alarm
r., allergic
r., anamnestic
r., anaphylactic
r., antigen-antibody
r., anxiety
r., Arias-Stella
r., biuret
r., chain
r., complement-fixation
r., consensual
r., conversion
r., cross
r., defense

r., delayed
r., dissociative
r., false-negative
r., false-positive
r., hemianopic
r., hemiopic pupillary
r., immune
r., leukemic or leukemoid
r., local
r., myasthenic
r., neutral
r. of degeneration
r., ophthalmic
r., Prausnitz-Küstner
r., quellung
r., transfusion
r., wheal and flare

reaction time
reactivate
reactive depression
reactivation (rē-ăk″tĭ-vā′shŭn)
reactivity (rē″ăk-tĭv′ĭ-tē)
reading
r., lip
read-only memory
reagent (rē-ā′jĕnt) [L. reagere, to react]
reagin (rē′ă-jĭn)
reaginic (rē′ă-jĭn-ĭk)
reality principle (rē-ăl′ĭ-tē)
reality testing
reality therapy
reamer (rē′mĕr)
reanastomosis, surgical
reanimate (rē-ăn′ĭ-māt) [L. re, again, + animare, fill with life]
reapers' keratitis (rēp′ĕrs kĕr-ă-tī′tĭs)
reasonable care
reasonable charge
reasonable cost
reattachment (rē″ă-tăch′mĕnt)
rebase (rē-bās′)
rebound [ME. rebounden, to leap back]
rebound phenomenon
recalcification (rē″kăl-sĭ-fĭ-kā′shŭn) [L. re, again, + calx, lime, + facere, to make]
recall [″ + AS. ceallian, to call]

recanalization
recapitulation theory (rē″kă-pĭt-ū-lā′shŭn) [″ + capitulum, a section]
receiver (rē-sēv′ĕr) [″ + capere, to take]
receptaculum (rē″sĕp-tăk′ū-lŭm) [L.]
r. chyli
receptor (rē-sĕp′tor) [L., a receiver]
r., adrenergic
r., auditory
r., cell
r., cholinergic
r., contact
r., cutaneous
r., distance
r., drug
r.'s, gravity
r.'s, olfactory
r.'s, optic
r.'s, proprioceptive
r.'s, rotary
r., sensory
r.'s, stretch
r.'s, taste
r.'s, temperature
r.'s, touch
r., universal
receptosome
recess (rē′sĕs) [L. recessus, receded]
r., cochlear
r., elliptical
r., epitympanic
r., infundibular
r., lateral, of fourth ventricle
r., nasopalatine
r., omental
r., optic
r., pharyngeal
r., pineal
r., piriform
r., sphenoethmoidal
r., spherical
r., suprapineal
r., tympanic membrane
r., umbilical
recession (rē-sĕsh′ŭn) [L. recessus, recess]
recessive

recessive gene
recessus (rē-sĕs'ŭs) [L.]
recidivation (rē-sĭd"ĭ-vā'shŭn) [L. *reci-divus*, falling back]
recidivism
recidivist
recidivity
recipe (rĕs'ĭ-pē) [L., take]
recipient (rĭ-sĭp'ē-ĕnt) [L. *recipiens*, receiving]
recipiomotor (rĭ-sĭp"ē-ō-mō'tor) [" + *motor*, mover]
reciprocal (rĭ-sĭp'rō-kăl) [L. *reciprocus*, alternate]
reciprocal inhibition
reciprocation (rĭ-sĭp"rō-kā'shŭn) [L. *reciprocare*, to move backward and forward]
reciprocity
Recklinghausen, Friedrich D. von (rĕk'lĭng-how"zĕn) [Ger. pathologist, 1833 – 1910]
   R.'s canals
   R.'s disease
   R.'s tumor
reclination (rĕk"lĭ-nā'shŭn) [L. *reclinatio*, lean back]
recline (rē-klīn') [L. *reclinare*]
Reclus' disease (rā-klooz') [Paul Reclus, Fr. surgeon, 1847 – 1914]
recombinant DNA
recombinant TPA
recombination (rē"kŏm-bĭ-nā'shŭn)
recomposition [L. *re*, again, + *composer*, to place together]
recompression [" + LL. *compressare*, press together]
recon (rē'kŏn)
reconstitution (rē"kŏn-stĭ-tū'shŭn)
record (rĕk'ord)
   r., functional chew-in
   r., interocclusal
recover (rĭ-kŭv'ĕr) [O. Fr. *recoverer*]
recovery (rĭ-kŭv'ĕr-ē)
recovery room
recrement (rĕk'rē-mĕnt) [L. *recrementum*, sifted again]
recrudescence (rē"kroo-dĕs'ĕns) [L.

recrudescere, to get worse]
recrudescent (rē"kroo-dĕs'ĕnt)
recruitment (rĭ-kroot'mĕnt) [O. Fr. *recrute*, new growth]
recruitment of end organs
rectal (rĕk'tăl) [L. *rectus*, straight]
rectal alimentation
rectal anesthesia
rectal crisis
rectal feeding
rectalgia (rĕk-tăl'jē-ă) [L. *rectus*, straight, + Gr. *algos*, pain]
rectal reflex
rectectomy (rĕk-tĕk'tō-mē) [" + Gr. *ektome*, excision]
rectification (rĕk"tĭ-fĭ-kā'shŭn) [" + *facere*, to make]
rectified (rĕk'tĭ-fīd)
rectifier (rĕk'tĭ-fī"ĕr) [L. *rectum*, straight, + *-ficare*, to make]
rectitis (rĕk-tī'tĭs) [" + Gr. *itis*, inflammation]
recto- [L. *rectus*, straight]
rectoabdominal (rĕk"tō-ăb-dŏm'ĭ-năl) [" + *abdomen*, belly]
rectocele (rĕk'tō-sēl) [" + Gr. *kele*, tumor, swelling]
rectoclysis (rĕk-tŏk'lĭ-sĭs) [" + Gr. *klysis*, a washing]
rectococcygeal (rĕk-tō-kŏk-sĭj'ē-ăl) [" + Gr. *kokkyx*, coccyx]
rectococcypexia (rĕk"tō-kŏk-sī-pĕks' sē-ă) [" + " + pexis, fixation]
rectocolitis (rĕk"tō-kō-lī'tĭs) [" + Gr. *kolon*, colon, + *itis*, inflammation]
rectocystotomy (rĕk"tō-sĭs-tŏt'ō-mē) [" + Gr. *kystis*, bladder, + *tome*, a cutting, slice]
rectolabial (rĕk"tō-lā'bē-ăl) [" + *labium*, lip]
rectoperineorrhaphy (rĕk"tō-pĕr"ĭ-nē-or'ă-fē)
rectopexy (rĕk'tō-pĕk-sē) [" + Gr. *pexis*, fixation]
rectophobia (rĕk"tō-fō'bē-ă) [" + Gr. *phobos*, fear]
rectoplasty (rĕk'tō-plăs"tē) [" +

Gr. *plassein*, to form]

rectorrhaphy (rĕk-tor'ă-fē) [L. *rectus*, straight, + Gr. *rhaphe*, seam]

rectoscope (rĕk'tō-skōp) [" + Gr. *skopein*, to examine]

rectoscopy (rĕk-tŏs'kō-pē)

rectosigmoid (rĕk"tō-sĭg'moyd) [" + Gr. *sigma*, letter S, + *eidos*, form, shape]

rectosigmoidectomy (rĕk"tō-sĭg"moy-dĕk'tō-mē) [" + " + *ektome*, excision]

rectostenosis (rĕk"tō-stĕn-ō'sĭs) [" + Gr. *stenosis*, act of narrowing]

rectostomy (rĕk-tŏs'tō-mē) [" + Gr. *stoma*, mouth, opening]

rectotomy (rĕk-tŏt'ō-mē) [" + Gr. *tome*, a cutting, slice]

rectourethral (rĕk"tō-ū-rē'thrăl) [" + Gr. *ourethra*, urethra]

rectouterine (rĕk"tō-ū'tĕr-ĭn) [" + *uterus*, womb]

rectovaginal (rĕk"tō-văj'ĭ-năl) [" + *vagina*, sheath]

rectovesical (rĕk"tō-vĕs'ĭ-kăl) [" + *vesica*, bladder]

rectovestibular (rĕk"tō-vĕs-tĭb'ū-lăr) [" + *vestibulum*, vestibule]

rectovulvar (rĕk"tō-vŭl'văr) [" + *vulva*, covering]

rectum (rĕk'tŭm) [L., straight]

rectus (rĕk'tŭs) [L.]

rectus muscles

recumbency (rĭ-kŭm'bĕn-sē) [L. *recumbens*, lying down]

recumbent
  r., dorsal
  r., lateral
  r., ventral

recuperation (rĭ-kū"pĕr-ā'shŭn) [L. *recuperare*, to recover]

recurrence (rĭ-kŭr'ĕns) [L. *re*, again, + *currere*, to run]

recurrent (rĭ-kŭr'ĕnt) [L. *recurrens*, returning]

recurvation (rī"kŭr-vă'shŭn) [L. *recurvus*, bent back]

recurve (rē-kŭrv')

red (rĕd) [AS. *read*]
  r., Congo
  r., cresol
  r., methyl
  r., neutral
  r., phenol
  r., scarlet
  r., vital

red blindness

red blood cell
  r.b.c., spiculed

red cross

redia (rē'dē-ă) [Francesco Redi, It. naturalist, 1626–1698]

redifferentiation (rē"dĭf-ĕr-ĕn"shē-ā'shŭn)

red. in pulv. [L.] *reductus in pulverum*, let it be reduced to powder

redintegration (rĕd-ĭn"tĕ-grā'shŭn) [L. *redintegratio*]

Redisol

red lead

red nucleus

red-out (rĕd'owt)

redox

red precipitate

redressement (rĕ-drĕs-mŏn') [Fr.]

reduce (rĭ-dūs') [L. *re*, again, + *ducere*, to lead]

reducible (rĭ-dūs'ĭ-bl)

reducing agent

reductant (rĭ-dŭk'tănt)

reductase (rĭ-dŭk'tās) [" + *ducere*, to lead, + *ase*, enzyme]

reduction (rĭ-dŭk'shŭn) [L. *reductio*, leading back]
  r. of fractures, closed
  r. of fractures, open

reduction division

redundant (rĭ-dŭn'dĕnt) [L. *redundare*, to overflow]

reduplicated (rĭ-dū'plĭ-kā"tĕd) [L. *re*, again, + *duplicare*, to double]

reduplication (rĭ-dū"plĭ-kā'shŭn)

Reduviidae (rē"dū-vī'ĭ-dē)

Reduvius (rē-dū'vē-ŭs)
  R. personatus

Reed-Sternberg cells [Dorothy Reed,

U.S. pathologist, 1874–1964; Karl
Sternberg, Aust. pathologist, 1872–
1935]

re-education (rē"ĕd-ū-kā'shŭn) [L. *re,*
again, + *educare,* to educate]

reef (rēf)

re-entry (rē-ĕn'trē)

refection (rē-fĕk'shŭn) [L. *reficere,* to re-
fresh]

reference man

reference woman

referred pain

refine (rē-fīn') [L. *re,* again, + ME.
fin, finished]

reflection (rĭ-flĕk'shŭn) [L. *reflexio,* a
bending back]

reflector (rĭ-flĕk'tor) [L. *re,* again, +
flectere, to bend]

reflex (rē'flĕks) [L. *reflexus,* to bend,
turn]
  r., abdominal
  r., abdominocardiac
  r.'s, accommodation
  r., Achilles
  r., acquired
  r., after-discharge of
  r.'s, allied
  r., anal
  r., ankle
  r's, antagonistic
  r., auditory
  r., autonomic
  r., autonomic, true
  r., axon
  r., Babinski's
  r., Bainbridge
  r., biceps
  r., Brain's
  r., carotid sinus
  r., cat's eye
  r.'s, Chaddock's
  r., chain
  r., chin
  r., ciliary
  r., ciliospinal
  r., clasp-knife
  r., conditioned
  r., conjunctival

r., consensual
r., convulsive
r., corneal
r., cough
r., cranial
r., cremasteric
r., crossed
r., crossed extension
r., deep
r., delayed
r., digital
r., diving
r., elbow
r., elementary
r., embrace
r., extensor thrust
r., flexor withdrawal
r., gag
r., gastrocolic
r., gastroileal
r., grasp
r., Grünfelder's
r., Hering-Breuer
r., Hoffmann's
r., hung-up
r., inborn
r., indirect
r.'s, inhibition of
r., intersegmental
r., intestinal
r., intrasegmental
r.'s, irradiation of
r., jaw
r., kinetic
r., knee-jerk
r., labyrinthine
r., light
r., local
r., long
r., lung
r., Magnus-de Kleijn
r., mass
r., Mayer's
r., Mendel-Bekhterev
r., monosynaptic
r., Moro
r., myenteric
r., myotatic

r., near
r., neck-righting
r., nociceptive
r., optical righting
r., palatal
r., palmar grasp
r., palm-chin
r. (response), parachute
r., patellar
r., pathologic
r., pharyngeal
r., pilomotor
r., placing
r., plantar
r., plantar grasp
r., postural
r., pressor
r.'s, proprioceptive
r., psychogalvanic
r., pupillary
r., quadriceps
r., quadrupedal extensor
r., red
r., righting
r., rooting
r., Rossolimo's
r.'s, sexual
r., short
r., somatic
r., spinal
r., startle
r., static
r.'s, statokinetic
r., stepping
r., stretch
r., sucking
r., superficial
r., swallowing
r., tendon
r., tonic neck
r., tonic neck, asymmetrical
r., triceps
r., triceps surae
r., unconditioned
r., vascular
r., vasomotor
r., visceral
r., visceromotor

reflex action
reflex arc
reflex center
reflexogenic (rĭ-flĕks″ō-jĕn′ĭk) [L. re-flexus, to bend, turn, + Gr. gen-nan, to produce]
reflexogenous (rĭ″flĕks-ŏj′ĕ-nŭs)
reflexograph (rĭ-flĕks′ō-grăf) [″ + Gr. graphein, to write]
reflexology (rē″flĕk-sŏl′ō-jē) [″ + Gr. logos, word, reason]
reflexometer (rē″flĕks-ŏm′ĕ-tĕr) [″ + Gr. metron, measure]
reflexophil (rē-flĕks′ō-fĭl) [″ + Gr. philein, to love]
reflexotherapy (rē-flĕks″ō-thĕr′ă-pē) [″ + Gr. therapeia, treatment]
reflux (rē′flŭks) [L. re, back, + fluxus, flow]
    r., hepatojugular
    r., vesicoureteral
refract (rĭ-frăkt′) [L. refractus, broken off]
refracta dosi (rē-frăk′tă dō′sē) [L.]
refraction (rĭ-frăk′shŭn) [LL. refractio, break back]
    r., angle of
    r., coefficient of
    r., double
    r., dynamic
    r., errors of
    r., index of
    r., ocular
    r. of eye
    r., static
refractionist (rĭ-frăk′shŭn-ĭst) [LL. re-fractio, break back]
refractive (rĭ-frăk′tĭv) [L. refractus, bro-ken off]
refractive power
refractivity (rē″frăk-tĭv′ĭ-tē)
refractometer (rē-frăk-tŏm′ĕt-ĕr) [″ + Gr. metron, measure]
refractometry (rē″frăk-tŏm′ĕ-trē)
refractory (rē-frăk′tō-rē) [L. refrac-tarius]
refractory period, relative
refracture (rē-frăk′chūr) [L. refractus,

broken off]
refrangible (rē-frăn'jĭ-bl) [L. *re*, again,
+ ME. *frangible*, breakable]
refresh (rĭ-frĕsh') [O. Fr. *refreschir*, to
renew]
refrigerant (rĭ-frĭj'ĕr-ănt) [L. *refrigerans*,
making cold]
refrigerant gases
refrigeration (rĭ-frĭj"ĕr-ā'shŭn) [L. *refri-
geratio*, make cold]
refrigeration anesthesia
refringent
Refsum's disease (rĕf'soomz) [S. Refsum, Norwegian physician, b. 1907]
refusion (rē-fū'zhŭn) [L. *refusus*, poured
back]
regainer (rē-gān'ĕr)
regel [Ger.]
    r. kleine
regeneration (rē-jĕn"ĕr-ā'shŭn) [L. *re*,
again, + *generare*, to produce]
regimen (rĕj'ĭ-mĕn) [L., rule]
regio (rē'jē-ō) [L.]
region (rē'jŭn) [L. *regio*, direction, terri-
tory]
regional (rē'jŭn-ăl)
register [LL. *regesta*, list]
registered nurse
registrant (rĕj'ĭs-trănt) [L. *registrans*,
registering]
registrar (rĕj'ĭs-trär) [O. Fr. *registreur*]
registration [L. *registratio*]
registry (rĕj'ĭs-trē) [LL. *regesta*, list]
Reglan
Regonol
regression (rĭ-grĕsh'ŭn) [L. *regressio*, a
going back]
    r., filial
regressive (rĭ-grĕs'ĭv)
regressive resistive exercise
regular (rĕg'ū-lăr) [L. *regula*, rule]
regulation
regulation development
regulative
regulator
regurgitant (rē-gŭr'jĭ-tănt) [L. *re*, again,
+ *gurgitare*, to flood]
regurgitation (rē-gŭr"jĭ-tā'shŭn)

r., aortic
r., cardiac
r., duodenal
r., functional
r., mitral
r., pulmonic
r., tricuspid
r., valvular
rehabilitation (rē"hă-bĭl"ĭ-tā'shŭn) [L.
rehabilitare]
    r., cardiac
rehabilitee (rē"hă-bĭl'ĭ-tē)
rehalation (rē"hă-lā'shŭn) [L. *re*, again,
+ *halare*, to breathe]
rehydration (rē"hī-drā'shŭn) [" +
Gr. *hydor*, water]
Reichert's cartilage (rī'kĕrts) [Karl B.
Reichert, Ger. anatomist, 1811–
1884]
Reid's base line (rēdz) [Robert W.
Reid, Scottish anatomist, 1851–1938]
Reil's island (rīlz) [Johann C. Reil, Ger.
anatomist, 1759–1813]
reimplantation (rē"ĭm-plăn-tā'shŭn) [L.
re, again, + *in*, into, + *plantare*, to plant]
reinfection (rē"ĭn-fĕk'shŭn) [" +
ME. *infecten*, infect]
reinforcement (rē"ĭn-fors'mĕnt) [" +
inforce, enforce]
reinforcement of reflex
reinforcer (rē"ĭn-fors'ĕr)
reinfusion (rē"ĭn-fū'zhŭn) [" + *infusio*, to pour in]
reinnervation (rē"ĭn-ĕr-vā'shŭn)
[" + *in*, into, + *nervus*, nerve]
reinoculation (rē"ĭn-ŏk"ū-lā'shŭn)
[" + *in*, into, + *oculus*, bud]
reintegration
reinversion (rē"ĭn-vĕr'shŭn) [" +
in, into, + *versio*, turning]
Reissner's membrane (rīs'nĕrz) [Er-
nest Reissner, Ger. anatomist, 1824–
1878]
Reiter's syndrome (rī'tĕrz) [Hans
Reiter, Ger. bacteriologist, 1881–
1969]
rejection [L. *rejicere*, to throw back]

r., acute
r., chronic
r., hyperacute
rejuvenation (rĭ-jū"vĕ-nā'shŭn) [L. re, again, + juvenis, young]
rejuvenescence (rĭ-jū"vĕ-nĕs'ĕns) [" + juvenescere, to become young]
Rela
relapse (rē-lăps') [L. relapsus]
relapsing
relapsing fever
relation (rĭ-lā'shŭn) [L. relatio, a carrying back]
r., jaw
r., occlusal jaw
r., unstrained jaw
relative biological effect
relative risk
relax [L. relaxare, to loosen]
relaxant (rĭ-lăk'sănt)
r., muscle
relaxation (rē-lăk-sā'shŭn)
r., general
r., local
r., pelvic
relaxation response
relaxed movement
relaxin (rĭ-lăk'sĭn)
releasing hormone
relief (rĭ-lēf') [ME.]
relieve [L. relevare, to raise]
reline (rē-līn')
REM rapid eye movements
rem roentgen equivalent (in) man
Remak's axis cylinder (ră'măk) [Robert Remak, Ger. neurologist, 1815–1865]
Remak's band
Remak's fibers
Remak's ganglion
Remak's sign [Ernest Julius Remak, Ger. neurologist, 1849–1911]
remedial (rĭ-mē'dē-ăl) [L. remedialis]
remedy (rĕm'ĕd-ē) [L. remedium, medicine]
r., local
r., systemic

remineralization (rē-mĭn"ĕr-ăl-ĭ-zā'shŭn)
remission (rĭ-mĭsh'ŭn) [L. remissio, remit]
remittance (rē-mĭt'ĕns)
remittent (rē-mĭt'ĕnt) [L. remittere, to send back]
remittent fever
remnant
remnant radiation
remodeling
r., temporomandibular joint
Remsed
ren (rĕn) [L.]
r. amyloidens
r. mobilis
r. unguliformis
renal (rē'năl) [LL. renalis, kidney]
renal clearance test
renal failure, acute
renal insufficiency
renal papillary necrosis
renal pelvis
renal scanning
renal transplantation
renal tubule
Rendu-Osler-Weber disease (rŏn-dū'ōs'lĕr-wĕb'ĕr) [Henri L. M. Rendu, Fr. physician, 1844–1902; Sir William Osler, Canadian-born physician, 1849–1919; Frederick P. Weber, Brit. physician, 1863–1962]
Renese
reniculus (rē-nĭk'ū-lŭs) [L.]
renifleur (rā-nĭ-flŭr') [Fr.]
reniform (rĕn'ĭ-form) [L. ren, kidney, + forma, shape]
renin (rĕn'ĭn)
renin substrate
renipelvic (rĕn"ĭ-pĕl'vĭk) [" + pelvis, basin]
reniportal (rĕn"ĭ-por'tăl)[" + porta, gate]
renipuncture (rĕn"ĭ-pŭnk'chūr) [" + punctura, prick]
rennet (rĕn'ĕt) [ME.]
rennin (rĕn'ĭn)
renninogen (rĕn-ĭn'ō-jĕn) [ME. rennet, rennet, + Gr. gennan, to produce]

renocutaneous (rē″nō-kū-tā′nē-ŭs) [″ + cutis, skin]
renogastric (rē″nō-găs′trĭk) [L. ren, kidney, + Gr. gaster, belly]
renogram (rē′nō-grăm) [″ + Gr. gramma, letter, piece of writing]
renography (rē-nŏg′ră-fē) [″ + Gr. graphein, to write]
renointestinal (rē″nō-ĭn-tĕs′tĭn-ăl) [″ + intestinum, intestine]
renopathy (rē-nŏp′ă-thē) [″ + Gr. pathos, disease, suffering]
renoprival (rē″nō-prī′văl)
Renoquid
renotrophic (rē″nō-trŏf′ĭk) [″ + Gr. trophe, nourishment]
renotropic (rē″nō-trŏp′ĭk) [″ + trope, a turn]
Renshaw cells (rĕn′shaw) [B. Renshaw, U.S. neurophysiologist, 1911–1948]
reovirus (rē″ō-vī′rŭs) [respiratory enteric orphan virus]
rep. [L.] repetatur, let it be repeated
repair (rī-păr′) [L. reparare, to prepare again]
  r., plastic
repellent [L. repellere, to drive back]
repercolation (rē″pĕr-kō-lā′shŭn) [L. re, again, + percolare, to filter]
repercussion (rē-pĕr-kŭsh′ŭn) [L. repercussio, rebound]
repercussive (rē″pĕr-kŭs′ĭv)
replacement
replantation [L. re, again, + planto, to plant]
repletion (rē-plē′shŭn) [L. repletio, a filling up]
replication (rĕp″lĭ-kā′shŭn)
replicon (rĕp′lĭ-kŏn)
repolarization
report
reportable diseases
reposition (rē″pō-zĭsh′ŭn) [L. repositio, a replacing]
repositioning (rē″pō-zĭsh′ŭn-ĭng)
  r., jaw
  r., muscle
repositor

r., inversion
r., uterine
repression (rē-prĕsh′ŭn) [L. repressus, press back]
  r., coordinate
  r., enzyme
repressor (rē-prĕs′or) [L. repressus, press back]
reproduction (rē-prō-dŭk′shŭn) [L. re, again, + productio, production]
  r., asexual
  r., cytogenic
  r., sexual
  r., somatic
reproductive (rē″prō-dŭk′tĭv)
repullulation (rē-pŭl″ū-lā′shŭn) [″ + pullulare, to sprout]
repulsion (rĭ-pŭl′shŭn) [L. repulsio, a thrusting back]
required services
RES reticuloendothelial system
rescinnamine (rē-sĭn′ă-mēn)
research (rĭ-sĕrch′, rē′sĕrch) [O. Fr. recerche, research]
  r., clinical
  r., laboratory
  r., medical
resect (rē-sĕkt′) [L. resectus, cut off]
resectable (rē-sĕk′tă-bl)
resection (rē-sĕk′shŭn) [L. resectio, a cutting off]
  r., gastric
  r., transurethral
  r., wedge
  r., window
resectoscope (rē-sĕk′tō-skōp) [L. resectus, cut off, + Gr. skopein, to examine]
resectoscopy (rē″sĕk-tŏs′kō-pē)
reserpine (rĭ-sĕr′pēn)
reserve (rē-zĕrv′) [L. reservare, to keep back]
  r., alkali
  r., cardiac
reserve air
reservoir (rĕz′ĕr-vwor) [Fr.]
reservoir of infectious agents
residency

resident
residual (rĭ-zĭd′ū-ăl) [L. *residuum*, residue]
residual function
residual urine
residue (rĕz′ĭ-dū)
residue diet, high-
residue diet, low-
residue-free diet
residuum (rē-zĭd′ū-ŭm) [L.]
resilience (rē-zĭl′ē-ĕns) [L. *resiliens*, leaping back]
resilient (rē-zĭl′ē-ĕnt)
resin (rĕz′ĭn) [L. *resina*, fr. Gr. *rhetine*, resin of the pine]
   r., ion-exchange
resinoid (rĕz′ĭ-noyd) [″ + Gr. *eidos*, form, shape]
resinous (rĕz′ĭ-nŭs)
res ipsa loquitur [L.]
resistance (rĭ-zĭs′tăns) [L. *resistens*, standing back]
   r., peripheral
resistance transfer factor
resolution (rĕz-ō-lū′shŭn) [L. *resolutio*, a relaxing]
resolve (rē-zŏlv′) [L. *resolvere*, to release]
resolvent (rĭ-zŏl′vĕnt) [ME. *resolven*, releasing]
resonance (rĕz′ō-năns) [L. *resonantia*, resound]
   r., amphoric
   r., bandbox
   r., bell-metal
   r., cracked-pot
   r., normal
   r., skodaic
   r., tympanic
   r., tympanitic
   r., vesicular
   r., vocal
   r., whispering
resonant (rĕz′ō-nănt)
resonating [L. *resonantia*, resound]
resonating cavities
resonator (rĕz′ō-nā″tĕr)
resorb (rē-sorb′, rē-zorb′) [L. *resorbere*, to suck in]

resorbent (rē-sor′bĕnt) [L. *resorbens*, sucking in]
resorcin (rĕ-zor′sĭn)
resorcinol (rĕ-zor′sĭ-nŏl)
resorcinolphthalein (rē-zor″sĭ-nŏl-thăl′ē-ĭn)
resorption (rē-sorp′shŭn) [L. *resorbere*, to suck in]
respirable (rē-spīr′ă-bl, rĕs′pĕr-ă-bl) [L. *respirare*, breathe again]
respiration (rĕs-pīr-ā′shŭn) [L. *respiratio*, breathing]
   r., abdominal
   r., absent
   r., accelerated
   r., aerobic
   r., amphoric
   r., anaerobic
   r., apneustic
   r., artificial
   r., Biot's
   r., cell
   r., Cheyne-Stokes
   r., cogwheel
   r., costal
   r., decreased
   r., diaphragmatic
   r., direct
   r., electrophrenic
   r., external
   r., fetal
   r., forced
   r., internal
   r., interrupted
   r., intrauterine
   r., Kussmaul's
   r., labored
   r., muscles of
   r., paradoxical
   r., periodic
   r., placental
   r., slow
   r., stertorous
   r., stridulous
   r., thoracic
   r., tissue
respirator (rĕs′pĭ-rā″tor) [L. *respirare*,

to breathe]
respiratory (rĕs-pīr′ă-tō-rē, rĕs′pĭ-ră-tō″rē) [L. *respiratio,* breathing]
respiratory anemometer
respiratory arrest
respiratory center
respiratory distress syndrome of the premature infant
respiratory failure, acute
respiratory failure, chronic
respiratory insufficiency
respiratory myoclonus
respiratory quotient
respiratory syncytial virus
respiratory system
respiratory therapist
respiratory therapy
respirometer (rĕs″pīr-ŏm′ĕt-ĕr) [L. *respirare,* to breathe, + Gr. *metron,* a measure]
response [L. *respondere,* to reply]
   r., anamnestic
   r., conditioned
   r., galvanic skin
   r., immune
   r., inflammatory
   r., reticulocyte
   r., triple
   r., unconditioned
rest (rĕst) [AS. *raest*]
restenosis (rē″stĕ-nō′sĭs) [L. *re,* again, + Gr. *stenosis,* act of narrowing]
restiform (rĕs′tĭ-form) [L. *restis,* rope, + *forma,* shape]
restiform body
resting
resting cell
resting pan splint
resting potential
restitutio ad integrum (rĕs″tĭ-tū′shē-ō ăd ĭn-tĕ′grŭm) [L.]
restitution (rĕs″tĭ-tū′shŭn) [L. *restitutio*]
restless legs
restoration (rĕs″tō-rā′shŭn) [L. *restaurare,* to fix]
   r., temporary
restorative (rĭ-stor′ă-tĭv) [L. *restaurare,* to fix]

restraint (rĭ-strănt′) [O. Fr. *restrainte*]
   r. in bed
   r., mechanical
   r., medicinal
   r. of lower extremities
resuscitation (rĭ-sŭs″ĭ-tā′shŭn) [L. *resuscitatio*]
   r., cardiopulmonary
   r., heart-lung
   r., oral
resuscitator (rĭ-sŭs′ĭ-tā″tor) [L. *resuscitare,* to revive]
ret *roentgen equivalent therapy*
retainer (rĭ-tān′ĕr)
retardate (rĭ-tăr′dāt) [L. *retardare,* to delay]
retardation (rē″tăr-dā′shŭn) [L. *retardare,* to delay]
   r., mental
retch (rĕch) [AS. *hraecan,* to cough up phlegm]
retching (rĕch′ĭng)
rete (rē′tē) [L.]
   r., arterial; r. arteriosum
   r., articular
   r. cutaneum
   r., malpighian
   r. mirabile
   r. olecrani
   r. ovarii
   r. patellae
   r. subpapillare
   r. testis
   r. venosum
   r., vertebral
retention (rĭ-tĕn′shŭn) [L. *retentio,* a holding back]
retention cyst
retention defect
retention enema
retention of urine
retention with overflow
retia (rē′shē-ă) [L.]
retial (rē′shē-ăl)
reticula (rē-tĭk′ū-lă) [L.]
reticular (rĭ-tĭk′ū-lăr) [L. *reticula,* net]
reticular activating system
reticular cells

reticular fibers
reticular formation
reticular layer
reticular membrane
reticular tissue
reticulate (rē-tĭk′ū-lāt)
reticulated (rē-tĭk′ū-lā″tĕd) [L. *reticula*, net]
reticulate substance
reticulation (rē-tĭk″ū-lā′shŭn)
reticulin (rē-tĭk′ū-lĭn) [L. *reticula*, net]
reticulocyte (rĕ-tĭk′ū-lō-sīt) [″ + Gr. *kytos*, cell]
reticulocytopenia (rē-tĭk″ū-lō-sī″tō-pē′nē-ă) [″ + ″ + *penia*, lack]
reticulocytosis (rē-tĭk″ū-lō-sī-tō′sĭs) [″ + ″ + *osis*, condition]
reticuloendothelial (rē-tĭk″ū-lō-ĕn″dō-thē′lē-ăl) [″ + Gr. *endon*, within, + *thele*, nipple]
reticuloendothelial cell
reticuloendothelial system
reticuloendothelioma (rē-tĭk″ū-lō-ĕn″dō-thē-lē-ō′mă) [″ + ″ + *oma*, tumor]
reticuloendotheliosis (rē-tĭk″ū-lō-ĕn″dō-thē-lē-ō′sĭs) [″ + ″ + *thele*, nipple, + *osis*, condition]
reticuloendothelium (rē-tĭk″ū-lō-ĕn″dō-thē′lē-ŭm)
reticulohistiocytoma (rē-tĭk″ū-lō-hĭs″tē-ō-sī-tō′mă) [L. *reticula*, net, + Gr. *histion*, little web, + *kytos*, cell, + *oma*, tumor]
reticulohistiocytosis (rē-tĭk″ū-lō-hĭs″tē-ō-sī-tō′sĭs) [″ + ″ + ″ + *osis*, condition]
reticuloid (rē-tĭk′ū-loyd) [″ + Gr. *eidos*, form, shape]
reticuloma (rē-tĭk″ū-lō′mă) [″ + Gr. *oma*, tumor]
reticulopenia (rē-tĭk″ū-lō-pē′nē-ă) [″ + Gr. *penia*, lack]
reticulopodium (rē-tĭk″ū-lō-pō′dē-ŭm)
reticulosarcoma (rē-tĭk″ū-lō-săr-kō′mă) [″ + Gr. *sarx*, flesh, + *oma*, tumor]
reticulosis (rē-tĭk-ū-lō′sĭs) [″ + Gr.

osis, condition]
   r., familial histiocytic
reticulum (rĕ-tĭk′ū-lŭm) [L., a little net]
   r., endoplasmic
   r. of nucleus
   r., sarcoplasmic
   r., stellate
retiform (rĕt′ĭ-form) [L. *rete*, net, + *forma*, shape]
Retin-A
retina (rĕt′ĭ-nă) [L.]
   r., coarctate
   r., detachment of
   r., shot-silk
   r., tigroid
retinaculum (rĕt″ĭ-năk′ū-lŭm) [L., halter]
   r. cutis
   r. extensor, of ankle
   r., extensor, of wrist
   r., flexor, of ankle
   r., flexor, of hand
   r., flexor, of wrist
   r. mammae
   r. of hip joint
   r., patellar
   r., peroneal
   r. tendinum
retinal (rĕt′ĭ-năl) [L. *retina*, retina]
retinal break
retinal correspondence
retinal detachment
retine (rĕt′ĕn)
retinene (rĕt′ĭ-nēn)
retinitis (rĕt-ĭ-nī′tĭs) [L. *retina*, retina, + Gr. *itis*, inflammation]
   r., actinic
   r., albuminuric
   r., apoplectic
   r., circinate
   r., circumpapillar
   r., diabetic
   r., disciform
   r., exogenous purulent
   r., external exudative
   r., exudative
   r., hemorrhagic
   r., metastatic
   r. of prematurity

r. pigmentosa
r. proliferans
r. punctata albescens
r., punctate
r., solar
r., stellate
r., suppurative
r., syphilitic

retinoblastoma (rĕt″ĭ-nō-blăs-tō′mă) [L. *retina*, retina, + Gr. *blastos*, germ, + *oma*, tumor]

retinochoroid (rĕt″ĭ-nō-kō′royd) [″ + Gr. *chorioeides*, skinlike]

retinochoroiditis (rĕt″ĭ-nō-kō-royd-ī′tĭs) [″ + ″ + *itis*, inflammation]
r. juxtapapillaris

retinocystoma (rĕt″ĭ-nō-sĭs-tō′mă) [″ + Gr. *kysis*, sac, + *oma*, tumor]

retinodialysis (rĕt″ĭ-nō-dī-ăl′ĭ-sĭs) [″ + Gr. *dia*, through, + *lysis*, dissolution]

retinoid (rĕt′ĭ-noyd) [″ + Gr. *eidos*, form, shape; Gr. *rhetine*, resin, + *eidos*, form, shape]

retinol (rĕt′ĭ-nŏl)

retinopapillitis (rĕt″ĭ-nō-pă″pĭl-ī′tĭs) [L. *retina*, retina, + *papilla*, nipple, + Gr. *itis*, inflammation]

retinopathy (rĕt″ĭn-ŏp′ă-thē) [″ + Gr. *pathos*, disease, suffering]
r., arteriosclerotic
r., circinate
r., diabetic
r., hypertensive
r., solar
r., syphilitic

retinoschisis (rĕt″ĭ-nŏs′kĭ-sĭs) [″ + Gr. *schisis*, cleavage]

retinoscope (rĕt′ĭ-nō-skōp) [″ + Gr. *skopein*, to examine]

retinoscopy (rĕt″ĭn-ŏs′kō-pē)

retinosis (rĕt″ĭ-nō′sĭs) [″ + Gr. *osis*, condition]

retisolution (rĕt″ĭ-sō-lū′shŭn) [L. *rete*, net, + *solutio*, dissolution]

retispersion (rĕt″ĭ-spĕr′zhŭn) [″ + *spersio*, a scattering]

retoperithelium (rē″tō-pĕr″ĭ-thē′lē-ŭm) [L. *rete*, net, + Gr. *peri*, around, + *thele*, nipple]

retort (rē-tort′) [L. *retortus*, bent back]

retothelium (rē″tō-thē′lē-ŭm) [L. *rete*, net, + Gr. *thele*, nipple]

retract (rī-trăkt′) [L. *retractus*]

retractile (rī-trăkt′ĭl) [L. *retractilis*]

retraction (rī-trăk′shŭn)
r., clot
r., uterine

retraction ring

retractor

retrad (rē′trăd) [L. *retro*, backward]

retreat (rī-trēt′) [ME. *retret*, draw back]

retrenchment [Fr. *retrenchier*, to cut back]

retrieval (rī-trē′văl)

retro- [L.]

retroaction (rĕt″rō-ăk′shŭn)

retroauricular (rĕt″rō-aw-rĭk′ū-lăr) [L. *retro*, behind, + *auricula*, ear]

retrobuccal (rĕt″rō-bŭk′ăl) [L. *retro*, back, + *bucca*, cheek]

retrobulbar (rĕt″rō-bŭl′băr) [L. *retro*, behind, + Gr. *bulbus*, bulb]

retrocecal (rĕt″rō-sē′kăl) [L. *retro*, back, + *caecum*, cecum]

retrocedent (rĕt″rō-sē′dĕnt) [L. *retrocedere*]

retrocervical (rĕt″rō-sĕr′vī-kăl) [L. *retro*, back, + *cervix*, neck]

retrocession (rĕt″rō-sĕsh′ŭn) [L. *retrocessio*, going back]

retroclusion (rĕt″rō-kloo′zhŭn) [″ + *claudere*, to close]

retrocolic (rĕt″rō-kŏl′ĭk) [L. *retro*, back, + Gr. *kolon*, colon]

retrocollic (rĕt″rō-kŏl′ĭk) [″ + *collum*, neck]

retrocollic spasm

retrocollis (rĕt″rō-kŏl′ĭs)

retrocursive (rĕt″rō-kŭr′sĭv) [L. *retro*, back, + *curro*, to run]

retrodeviation (rĕt″rō-dē″vē-ā′shŭn) [″ + *deviare*, to turn aside]

retrodisplacement (rĕt″rō-dĭs-plăs′mĕnt) [″ + Fr. *desplacer*, displace]

672   retroesophageal

retroesophageal (rĕt″rō-ē-sŏf″ă-jē′ăl) [L. *retro*, behind, + Gr. *oisophagos*, gullet]
retrofilling (rĕt″rō-fĭl′ĭng)
retroflexed (rĕt′rō-flĕkst″) [L. *retro*, backward, + *flexus*, bent]
retroflexion (rĕt″rō-flĕk′shŭn)
retroflexion of uterus
retrogasserian (rĕt″rō-găs-sē′rē-ăn)
retrognathia (rĕt″rō-năth′ē-ă) [L. *retro*, back, + Gr. *gnathos*, jaw]
retrognathism (rĕt″rō-năth′ĭzm) [″ + Gr. *gnathos*, jaw]
retrograde (rĕt′rō-grād) [L. *retro*, backward, + *gradi*, to step]
retrograde amnesia
retrograde aortography
retrograde flow
retrograde pyelography
retrography (rĕt″rŏg′ră-fē) [″ + Gr. *graphein*, to write]
retrogression (rĕt″rō-grĕsh′ŭn) [L. *retrogressus*, go backward]
retroinfection (rĕt″rō-ĭn-fĕk′shŭn) [L. *retro*, backward, + *infectio*, infection]
retroinsular (rĕt″rō-ĭn′sū-lăr) [″ + *insula*, island]
retroiridian (rĕt″rō-ī-rĭd′ē-ăn) [L. *retro*, behind, + Gr. *iridos*, colored circle]
retrojection (rĕt″rō-jĕk′shŭn) [″ + *jacio*, throw]
retrolabyrinthine (rĕt″rō-lăb″ĭ-rĭn′thĭn) [L. *retro*, behind + Gr. *labyrinthos*, a maze]
retrolental
retrolental fibroplasia
retrolenticular (rĕt″rō-lĕn-tĭk′ū-lăr) [″ + *lenticularis*, pert. to a lens]
retrolingual (rĕt″rō-lĭng′gwăl) [L. *retro*, behind, + *lingua*, tongue]
retromammary (rĕt″rō-măm′mă-rē) [″ + *mamma*, breast]
retromandibular (rĕt″rō-măn-dĭb′ū-lăr) [″ + *mandibulum*, jaw]
retromastoid (rĕt″rō-măs′toyd) [″ + Gr. *mastos*, breast, +

eidos, form, shape]
retromorphosis (rĕt″rō-mor′fō-sĭs) [″ + Gr. *morphe*, form, + *osis*, condition]
retronasal (rĕt″rō-nā′zăl) [L. *retro*, back, + *nasus*, nose]
retroocular (rĕt″rō-ŏk′ū-lar) [L. *retro*, behind, + *oculus*, eye]
retroparotid (rĕt″rō-pă-rŏt′ĭd) [″ + Gr. *para*, alongside, past, beyond, + *ous*, ear]
retroperitoneal (rĕt″rō-pĕr″ĭ-tō-nē′ăl) [″ + Gr. *peritonaion*, stretched around or over]
retroperitoneal fibrosis
retroperitoneum (rĕt″rō-pĕr-ĭ-tō-nē′ŭm)
retroperitonitis (rĕt″rō-pĕr″ĭ-tō-nī′tĭs)
retropharyngeal (rĕt″rō-făr-ĭn′jē-ăl) [″ + Gr. *pharynx*, throat]
retropharyngitis (rĕt″rō-făr″ĭn-jī′tĭs) [″ + ″ + *itis*, inflammation]
retropharynx (rĕt″rō-făr′ĭnks) [″ + Gr. *pharynx*, throat]
retroplacental (rĕt″rō-plă-sĕn′tăl) [″ + *placenta*, a flat cake]
retroplasia (rĕt″rō-plā′zē-ă) [″ + Gr. *plassein*, to form]
retroposed (rĕt-rō-pōsd′) [L. *retro*, backward, + *positus*, placed]
retroposition (rĕt″rō-pō-zĭsh′ŭn)
retropulsion (rĕt″rō-pŭl′shŭn) [″ + *pulsio*, a thrusting]
retrospective study
retrospondylolisthesis (rĕt″rō-spŏn″dĭ-lō-lĭs-thē′sĭs) [L. *retro*, behind + Gr. *spondylos*, vertebra, + *olisthesis*, a slipping]
retrosternal (rĕt″rō-stĕr′năl) [″ + Gr. *sternon*, chest]
retrosternal pulse
retrotarsal (rĕt″rō-tăr′săl) [″ + Gr. *tarsos*, flat of the foot, flat surface, edge of eyelid]
retrouterine (rĕt″rō-ū′tĕr-ĭn) [L. *retro*, backward, + *uterus*, womb]
retroversioflexion (rĕt″rō-vĕr″sē-ō-flĕk′shŭn) [″ + *versio*, a turning,

+   *flexio,* flexion]
retroversion (rĕt″rō-vĕr′shŭn) [L. *retro,*
    back,   +   *versio,* a turning]
retroversion of uterus
Retrovir
retroviruses (rĕt″r-vī′rŭs-ĕs)
retrude (rĭ-trood′) [L. *re,* back,   +
    trudere, to shove]
retrusion (rĭ-troo′shŭn)
Retzius, lines of (rĕt′zē-ŭs) [Magnus
    Gustav Retzius, Swedish anatomist,
    1842–1919]
Retzius, space of (rĕt′zē-ŭs) [Anders
    Adolf Retzius, Swedish anatomist,
    1796–1860]
Retzius, veins of [A. A. Retzius]
reunient (rē-ūn′yĕnt)   [L.   *re,*
    again,   +   *unire,* to unite]
Reuss, August R. von (roys) Austrian
    ophthalmologist, 1841–1924
    R.'s color charts
revaccination (rē″văk-sĭ-nā′shŭn)
revascularization   (rē-văs″kū-lăr-ĭ-
    zā′shŭn)
revellent (rē-vĕl′ĕnt) [L. *re,* back,   +
    vellere, to draw]
reverberation (rĭ″vĕr-bĕr-ā′shŭn) [L.
    reverberare, to cause to rebound]
Reverdin's   needle   (rā-vĕr-dănz′)
    [Jacques L. Reverdin, Swiss surgeon,
    1842–1929]
reversal (rĭ-vĕr′săl) [L. *reversus,* revert]
    r., sex
reversible (rĭ-vĕr′sĭ-bl)
reversion (rĭ-vĕr′zhŭn)
revertant
review of systems
revivescence (rē″vī-vĕs′ĕns)
revivification (rē-vĭv″ĭ-fĭ-kā′shŭn) [L. *re,*
    again,   +   *vivere,* to live,   +   *fa-
    cere,* to make]
revulsant (rĭ-vŭl′sănt) [L. *revulsio,* pulling
    back]
revulsion (rĭ-vŭl′shŭn)
revulsive (rĭ-vŭl′sĭv)
reward
rewarming
Reye's syndrome (rīz) [R. D. K. Reye,

Australian pathologist, 1912–1977]
RF, Rf *rheumatoid factor*
R.F.A.   *right frontoanterior*
R factor *resistance transfer factor*
R.F.P.   *right frontoposterior*
R.F.T.   *right frontotransverse*
RH *releasing hormone*
Rh *rhodium; Rhesus*
Rhabditis (răb-dĭ′tĭs) [Gr. *rhabdos,* rod]
rhabdo- [Gr. *rhabdos,* rod]
rhabdoid (răb′doyd) [″   +   *eidos,*
    form, shape]
rhabdomyoblastoma   (răb″dō-mī″ō-
    blăs-tō′mă) [″   +   *mys,* muscle,   +
    blastos, germ,   +   *oma,* tumor]
rhabdomyolysis   (răb″dō-mī-ŏl′ĭ-sĭs)
    [″   +   ″   +   *lysis,* dissolution]
rhabdomyoma   (răb″dō-mī-ō′mă)
    [″   +   ″   +   *oma,* tumor]
rhabdomyosarcoma   (răb″dō-mī″ō-
    săr-kō′mă) [″   +   ″   +   *sarx,*
    flesh,   +   *oma,* tumor]
rhabdophobia (răb-dō-fō′bē-ă) [″   +
    phobos, fear]
rhabdosarcoma   (răb″dō-săr-kō′mă)
    [″   +   *sarx,* flesh,   +   *oma,*
    tumor]
rhabdovirus (răb″dō-vī′rŭs) [″   +
    L. *virus,* poison]
rhachialgia (rā″kē-ăl′jē-ă) [Gr. *rhachis,*
    spine,   +   *algos,* pain]
rhachiocampsis   (rā″kē-ō-kămp′sĭs)
    [″   +   *kampsis,* a bending]
rhachioplegia (rā″kē-ō-plē′jē-ă) [″   +
    plege, stroke]
rhachioscoliosis (rā″kē-ō-skō″lē-ō′sĭs)
    [″   +   *skoliosis,* crookedness]
rhachis (rā′kĭs) [Gr.]
rhachischisis (ră-kĭs′kĭ-sĭs) [″   +
    schisis, cleavage]
rhachitis (ră-kī′tĭs) [″   +   *itis,* inflam-
    mation]
rhacoma (ră-kō′mă) [Gr. *rhakoma,*
    rags]
rhagades (răg′ă-dēz) [Gr., tears]
rhagadiform   (ră-găd′ĭ-form)   [Gr.
    rhagas, tear,   +   L. *forma,* shape]
-rhage, -rhagia [Gr. *rhegnynai,* to

burst forth]

Rh antiserum

rhaphania (ră-fā'nē-ă) [Gr. *raphanos*, radish]

rhaphe (ră'fē) [Gr.]

-rhaphy [Gr. *rhaphe*]

Rh blood group

-rhea [Gr. *rhein*, to flow]

rhegma (rĕg'mă) [Gr. *rhegma*, a tear]

rhegmatogenous (rĕg"mă-tŏj'ĕ-nŭs) [" + *gennan*, to produce]

rhenium (rē'nē-ŭm)

rheo- [Gr. *rheos*, current]

rheobase (rē'ō-bās) [" + *basis*, base]

rheobasic (rē"ō-bā'sĭk)

rheology (rē-ŏl'ō-jē) [" + *logos*, word, reason]

Rheomacrodex

rheometer (rē-ŏm'ĕt-ĕr) [" + *metron*, measure]

rheostat (rē'ō-stăt) [" + *statos*, standing]

rheostosis (rē-ŏs-tō'sĭs) [" + *osteon*, bone]

rheotachygraphy (rē"ō-tă-kĭg'ră-fē) [" + *tachys*, swift, + *graphein*, to write]

rheotaxis (rē"ō-tăk'sĭs) [" + *taxis*, arrangement]

rheotropism (rē-ŏt'rō-pĭzm) [" + *trope*, a turn, + *-ismos*, condition]

rheum, rheuma (room, room'ă) [Gr. *rheuma*, discharge]

rheumatic (roo-măt'ĭk) [Gr. *rheumatikos*]

rheumatic fever

rheumatid (roo'mă-tĭd)

rheumatism (roo'mă-tĭzm) [Gr. *rheumatismos*]

    r., acute articular

    r., chronic

    r., gonorrheal

    r., muscular

    r., palindromic

    r., psychogenic

    r., soft tissue

rheumatismal (roo"mă-tĭz'măl)

rheumatoid (roo'mă-toyd) [Gr. *rheuma*, discharge, + *eidos*, form, shape]

rheumatoid arthritis

rheumatoid factor

rheumatologist (roo"mă-tŏl'ō-jĭst)

rheumatology (roo"mă-tŏl'ō-jē)

rhexis (rĕk'sĭs) [Gr., rupture]

Rh factor

Rh genes

rhigosis (rī-gō'sĭs) [Gr., shivering]

Rh immune globulin

rhinal (rī'năl) [Gr. *rhis*, nose]

rhinalgia (rī-năl'jē-ă) [" + *algos*, pain]

rhinedema (rī"nĕ-dē'mă) [" + *oidema*, swelling]

rhinencephalon (rī-nĕn-sĕf'ă-lŏn) [" + *enkephalos*, brain]

rhinencephalus (rī"nĕn-sĕf'ă-lŭs) [" + *enkephalos*, brain]

rhinesthesia (rī-nĕs-thē'zē-ă) [" + *aisthesis*, feeling, perception]

rhineurynter (rīn"ū-rĭn'tĕr) [" + *eurynein*, to dilate]

rhinion (rĭn'ē-ŏn) [Gr.]

rhinism (rī'nĭzm) [Gr. *rhis*, nose, + *-ismos*, condition]

rhinitis (rī-nī'tĭs) [" + *itis*, inflammation]

    r., acute

    r., allergic

    r., atrophic

    r. caseosa

    r., chronic hyperplastic

    r., chronic hypertrophic

    r., fibrinous

    r., hypertrophic

    r., membranous

    r., perennial

    r., periodic

    r., pseudomembranous

    r., purulent

    r., vasomotor

rhino- [Gr. *rhis*]

rhinoanemometer (rī"nō-ăn"ĕ-mŏm'ĕ-tĕr)

rhinoantritis (rī"nō-ăn-trī'tĭs) [" +

antron, cavity, + *itis*, inflammation]
rhinobyon (rī-nō'bē-ŏn) [" +
byein, to plug]
rhinocanthectomy (rī″nō-kăn-thĕk'tō-
mē) [Gr. *rhis*, nose, + *kanthos*,
corner of the eye, + *ektome*, exci-
sion]
rhinocele (rī'nō-sēl) [" + *koilia*,
cavity, belly]
rhinocephalus (rī″nō-sĕf'ă-lŭs) [" +
kephale, head]
rhinocephaly (rī″nō-sĕf'ă-lē) [" +
kephale, head]
rhinocheiloplasty (rī″nō-kī'lō-plăs″tē)
[" + *cheilos*, lip, + *plastos*,
formed]
rhinocleisis (rī-nō-klī'sīs) [Gr. *rhis*, nose,
+ *kleisis*, closure]
rhinodacryolith (rī″nō-dăk're-ō-līth) ["
+ *dakryon*, tear, + *lithos*, stone]
rhinodynia (rī″nō-dĭn'ē-ă) [" +
odyne, pain]
Rhinoestrus (rī-nĕs'trŭs)
  R. purpureus
rhinogenous (rī-nŏj'ĕn-ŭs) [" +
gennan, to produce]
rhinokyphosis (rī″nō-kī-fō'sīs) [" +
kyphos, hump, + *osis*, condition]
rhinolalia (rī″nō-lā'lē-ă) [" + *lalia*,
chatter, prattle]
  r. aperta
  r. clausa
rhinolaryngitis (rī″nō-lăr″ĭn-jī'tīs) [" +
larynx, larynx, + *itis*, inflammation]
rhinolith (rī'nō-līth) [" + *lithos*,
stone]
rhinolithiasis (rī″nō-līth-ī'ă-sīs)
rhinologist (rī-nŏl'ō-jĭst) [" + *logos*,
word, reason]
rhinology (rī-nŏl'ō-jē)
rhinomanometer (rī″nō-măn-ŏm'ĕt-
ĕr) [Gr. *rhis*, nose, + *manos*, thin,
+ *metron*, measure]
rhinomanometry (rī″nō-mă-nŏm'ĕ-
trē)
rhinometer (rī-nŏm'ĕt-ĕr)
rhinomiosis (rī″nō-mī-ō'sīs) [" +
meiosis, a lessening]

rhinommectomy (rī″nŏm-mĕk'tō-mē)
[" + *omma*, eye, + *ektome*,
excision]
rhinomycosis (rī″nō-mī-kō'sīs) [" +
mykes, fungus, + *osis*, condition]
rhinonecrosis (rī″nō-nĕ-krō'sīs) [" +
nekrosis, state of death]
rhinopathy (rī-nŏp'ă-thē) [" +
pathos, disease, suffering]
rhinopharyngeal (rī″nō-fă-rīn'jē-ăl)
rhinopharyngitis (rī″nō-făr-ĭn-jī'tīs)
[" + *pharynx*, throat, + *itis*,
inflammation]
rhinopharyngocele (rī″nō-făr-īn'gō-
sēl) [" + " + *kele*, tumor,
swelling]
rhinopharyngolith (rī″nō-făr-īn'gō-
līth) [" + " + *lithos*, stone]
rhinopharynx (rī″nō-făr'īnks)
rhinophonia (rī″nō-fō'nē-ă) [" +
phone, voice]
rhinophycomycosis (rī″nō-fī″kō-mī-
kō'sīs) [" + *phykos*, seaweed, +
mykes, fungus, + *osis*, condition]
rhinophyma (rī-nō-fī'mă) [" +
phyma, growth]
rhinoplasty (rī'nō-plăs″tē) [" +
plastos, formed]
rhinopneumonitis (rī″nō-nū″mō-nī'tīs)
[Gr. *rhis*, nose, + *pneumon*, lung,
+ *itis*, inflammation]
rhinopolypus (rī″nō-pŏl'ī-pŭs) [" +
polys, many, + *pous*, foot]
rhinorrhagia (rī″nō-rā'jē-ă) [" +
rhegnynai, to burst forth]
rhinorrhea (rī″nō-rē'ă) [" + *rhein*,
to flow]
  r., cerebrospinal
  r., gustatory
rhinosalpingitis (rī″nō-săl″pīn-jī'tīs)
[" + *salpinx*, tube, + *itis*, in-
flammation]
rhinoscleroma (rī″nō-sklē-rō'mă)
[" + *skleros*, hard, + *oma*,
tumor]
rhinoscope (rī'nō-skōp) [" + *skopein*, to examine]
rhinoscopic (rī″nō-skōp'īk)

rhinoscopy (rĭ-nŏs′kō-pē)
r., anterior
r., posterior
rhinosporidiosis (rī″nō-spō-rĭd″ē-ō′sĭs) [″ + sporidion, little seed, + osis, condition]
Rhinosporidium (rī″nō-spō-rĭd′ē-ŭm)
R. seeberi
rhinostenosis (rī″nō-stĕn-ō-′sĭs) [″ + stenosis, act of narrowing]
rhinotomy (rī-nŏt′ō-mē) [″ + tome, a cutting, slice]
rhinotracheitis (rī″nō-trā″kē-ī′tĭs) [″ + tracheia, rough, + itis, inflammation]
rhinovaccination (rī″nō-văk-sĭn-ā′shŭn) [″ + L. vaccinus, pert. to cows]
rhinovirus (rī″nō-vī′rŭs)
Rhipicephalus (rī″pĭ-sĕf′ă-lŭs) [Gr. rhipis, fan, + kephale, head]
rhitidectomy (rĭt″ĭ-dĕk′tō-mē) [Gr. rhytis, wrinkle, + ektome, excision]
rhitidosis (rĭt-ĭ-dō′sĭs) [Gr. rhytidosis]
rhizo- [Gr. rhiza]
rhizodontropy (rī″zō-dŏn′trō-pē) [Gr. rhiza, root, + odous, tooth, + trope, a turning]
rhizodontrypy (rī″zō-dŏn′trĭ-pē) [″ + ″ + trype, a hole]
rhizoid (rī′zoyd) [″ + eidos, form, shape]
rhizome (rī′zōm) [Gr. rhizoma, mass of roots]
rhizomelic (rī″zō-mĕl′ĭk) [Gr. rhiza, root, + melos, limb]
rhizomeningomyelitis (rī″zō-mĕ-nĭn″gō-mī″ĕ-lī′tĭs) [″ + meninx, membrane, + myelos, marrow, + itis, inflammation]
Rhizopoda (rī-zŏp′ō-dă) [″ + pous, foot]
rhizotomy (rī-zŏt′ō-mē) [″ + tome, a cutting, slice]
r., anterior
r., posterior
Rh₀(D) immune globulin
rhodium (rō′dē-ŭm)
rhodo- (rō′dō) [Gr. rhodon, rose]

rhodogenesis (rō″dō-jĕn′ē-sĭs) [″ + genesis, generation, birth]
rhodophane (rō′dō-făn) [″ + phainein, to show]
rhodophylaxis (rō″dō-fĭ-lăk′sĭs) [″ + phylaxis, guard]
rhodopsin (rō-dŏp′sĭn) [″ + opsis, sight, appearance, vision]
RhoGAM
rhombencephalon (rŏm″bĕn-sĕf′ă-lŏn) [Gr. rhombos, rhomb, + enkephalos, brain]
rhombocele (rŏm′bō-sēl) [″ + koilos, a hollow]
rhomboid (rŏm′boyd) [″ + eidos, form, shape]
rhomboideus (rŏm-boyd′ē-ŭs) [L.]
rhomboid fossa
rhombomere (rŏm′bō-mēr) [Gr. rhombos, rhomb, + meros, a part]
rhoncal, rhonchial (rŏng′kăl, rŏng′kē-ăl) [Gr. rhonchos, a snore]
rhonchi
rhonchus (rŏng′kŭs)
rhopheocytosis (rō″fē-ō-sī-tō′sĭs) [Gr. rhophein, gulp down, + kytos, cell, + osis, condition]
rhotacism (rō′tă-sĭzm) [Gr. rhotakizein, to overuse letter ''r'']
rhubarb (roo′bărb) [ME. rubarbe]
Rhus (rŭs) [L.]
rhypophobia (rī″pō-fō′bē-ă) [Gr. rhypos, filth, + phobos, fear]
rhythm (rĭth′ŭm) [Gr. rhythmos, measured motion]
r., alpha
r., atrioventricular
r., beta
r., bigeminal
r., biological
r., cantering
r., cardiac
r., circadian
r., coupled
r., delta
r., diurnal
r., ectopic

r., escape
r., gallop
r., gamma
r., idioventricular
r., nodal
r., normal sinus
r., nyctohemeral
r., pendulum
r., sinus
r., theta
r., tic-tac
r., ventricular
rhythmic [Gr. *rhythmos*]
rhythmicity (rĭth-mĭs'ĭ-tē)
rhytidectomy (rĭt″ĭ-dĕk'tō-mē) [Gr. *rhytis*, wrinkle, + *ektome*, excision]
rhytidoplasty (rĭt'ĭ-dō-plăs″tē) [" + *plassein*, to form]
rhytidosis (rĭt″ĭ-dō'sĭs) [" + *osis*, condition]
RIA *radioimmunoassay*
rib (rĭb) [AS. *ribb*]
r., abdominal
r.'s, asternal
r., bicipital
r., cervical
r.'s, false
r.'s, floating
r., lumbar
r., slipping
r.'s, sternal
r.'s, true
r., vertebral
r.'s, vertebrocostal
r., vertebrosternal
ribbon (rĭb'ŭn)
riboflavin (rī″bō-flā'vĭn)
ribonuclease (rī″bō-nū'klē-ās)
ribonucleic acid (rī″bō-nū″klē'ĭk)
ribonucleoprotein (rī″bō-nū″klē-ō-prō'tē-ĭn)
ribonucleotide (rī″bō-nū″klē-ō-tīd)
ribose (rī'bōs)
ribosome (rī'bō-sōm)
ribosyl (rī'bō-sĭl)
rice, polished
ricin (rī'sĭn)
ricinine (rĭs'ĭn-ĕn, -ĭn)

ricinoleic acid
rickets (rĭk'ĕts)
r., adult
r., late
r., renal
r., vitamin D-resistant
Rickettsia (rĭ-kĕt'sē-ă) [Howard T. Ricketts, U.S. pathologist, 1871–1910]
R. typhi
rickettsia (rĭ-kĕt'sē-ă)
rickettsial disease
rickettsialpox (rĭ-kĕt'sē-ăl-pŏks″)
rickettsicidal (rĭ-kĕt″sĭ-sī'dăl)
rickettsiosis (rĭ-kĕt″sē-ō'sĭs)
rickettsiostatic (rĭ-kĕt″sē-ō-stăt'ĭk)
riders' bone
riders' sprain
ridge (rĭj) [ME. *rigge*]
r., alveolar
r., carotid
r., dental
r., dermal
r., epicondylic
r., gastrocnemial
r., genital
r., gluteal
r., interosseous
r., interureteric
r., mammary
r., mesonephric
r., pronator
r., pterygoid
r., superciliary
r., supracondylar
r., tentorial
r., trapezoid
r., urogenital
r., wolffian
ridgel (rĭj'ĕl)
Riedel's lobe (rē'dĕlz) [Bernhard M. C. L. Riedel, Ger. surgeon, 1846–1916]
Rifadin
rifampin (rĭf'ăm-pĭn)
rifamycin (rĭf″ă-mī'sĭn)
Riga-Fede's disease (rē'gă fā'dāz) [Antonio Riga, It. physician, 1832–1919; Francesco Fede, It. physician, 1832–1913]

Riggs' disease   [John M. Riggs, U.S. dentist, 1810–1885]
right   (rīt) [AS. *riht*]
right-handedness
right to know law
rigid   (rĭ'jĭd) [L. *rigidus*]
rigidity   (rĭ-jĭd'ĭ-tē)
   r., cadaveric
   r., cerebellar
   r., clasp-knife
   r., cogwheel
   r., decerebrate
rigor   (rĭg'or) [L. *rigor*, stiffness]
   r. mortis
rim
   r., bite
   r., occlusion
rima   (rī'mă) [L., a slit]
   r. cornealis
   r. glottidis
   r. oris
   r. palpebrarum
   r. pudendi
   r. respiratoria
   r. vestibuli
   r. vocalis
Rimactane
rimose   (rī'mōs, rī-mōs') [L. *rimosus*]
rimula   (rĭm'ū-lă) [L.]
rind   (rīnd) [AS.]
ring   (rĭng) [AS. *hring*]
   r.'s, abdominal
   r., Albl's
   r., Bandl's
   r., benzene
   r., Cannon's
   r., ciliary
   r., conjunctival
   r., constriction
   r., femoral
   r., inguinal, abdominal
   r., inguinal, deep
   r., inguinal, subcutaneous
   r., inguinal, superficial
   r., Kayser-Fleischer
   r., lymphoid
   r., pathologic retraction
   r., physiologic retraction

   r., Schatzki
   r., Schwalbe's
   r., tympanic
   r., umbilical
   r., vascular
   r., Waldeyer's
Ringer, Sydney   (rĭng'ĕr) [Brit. physiologist, 1835–1910]
   R.'s injection, lactated
   R.'s irrigation
ringworm   (rĭng'wŭrm)
Rinne test   (rĭn'nē) [Heinrich A. Rinne, Ger. otologist, 1819–1868]
Riolan's arch   (rē"ō-lănz') [Jean Riolan, Fr. anatomist, 1577–1657]
Riolan's bouquet
Riolan's muscle
Riopan
ripa   (rī'pă) [L., bank]
Ripault's sign   (rē-pōz') [Louis H. A. Ripault, Fr. physician, 1807–1856]
ripening
risk-benefit analysis
risk factors
risorius   (rĭ-sŏ'rē-ŭs) [L., laughing]
ristocetin   (rĭs"tō-sē'tĭn)
risus   (rī'sŭs) [L.]
   r. sardonicus
Ritalin Hydrochloride
Ritter's disease   (rĭt'ĕrz) [Gottfried Ritter von Rittershain, Ger. physician, 1820–1883]
ritual   (rĭch'ū-ăl)
ritualistic surgery
rivalry   (rī'văl-rē)
   r., binocular
   r., retinal
   r., sibling
rivalry strife
Rivinus' canals   (rē-vē'nŭs) [August Quirinus Rivinus, Ger. anatomist, 1652–1723]
Rivinus' gland
Rivinus' incisure
Rivinus' ligament
rivus lacrimalis   (rī'vŭs) [L. *rivus*, little stream, + *lacrima*, tear]
riziform   (rĭz'ĭ-form) [Fr. *riz*, rice, +

L. *forma,* form]
R.L.E. *right lower extremity*
RLF *retrolental fibroplasia*
R.L.L. *right lower lobe*
RLQ *right lower quadrant*
R.M.A. *Registered Medical Assistant; right mentoanterior presentation*
R.M.P. *right mentoposterior presentation*
R.M.T. *right mentotransverse*
R.N. *registered nurse*
Rn *radon*
RNA *ribonucleic acid*
RNase *ribonuclease*
R.O.A. *right occipitoanterior*
Robaxin
Robert's pelvis (rō'bărts) [Heinrich L. F. Robert, Ger. gynecologist, 1814–1874]
Robertson's pupil
Robicillin VK
Robimycin
Robinul
Robitussin
Rocaltrol
Rochelle salt (rō-shĕl')
rocker knife
rocking
Rocky Mountain spotted fever
rod (rŏd) [AS. *rodd,* club]
   r., Corti's
   r.'s, enamel
   r., retinal
rodent
rodenticide (rō-dĕn'tĭ-sīd) [L. *rodens,* gnawing, + *caedere,* to kill]
rodent ulcer [" + *ulcus,* ulcer]
rodonalgia (rō-dō-năl'jē-ă) [Gr. *rhodon,* rose, + *algos,* pain]
rods and cones
Roentgen, Wilhelm Konrad (rĕnt'gĕn) [Ger. physicist, 1845–1923]
roentgen (rĕnt'gĕn)
roentgenkymogram (rĕnt"gĕn-kī'mō-grăm) [*roentgen* + Gr. *kyme,* wave, + *gramma,* letter, piece of writing]

roentgenkymograph (rĕnt"gĕn-kī'mō-grăf) [" + " + *graphein,* to write]
roentgenkymography (rĕnt"gĕn-kī-mŏg'ră-fē)
roentgenocinematography (rĕnt" gĕn-ō-sīn"ĕ-mă-tŏg'ră-fē) [" + Gr. *kinema,* motion, + *graphein,* to write]
roentgenogram (rĕnt-gĕn'ō-grăm, rĕnt'gĕn-ō-grăm")
roentgenography (rĕnt"gĕn-ŏg'ră-fē) [*roentgen* + Gr. *graphein,* to write]
   r., body section
   r., mucosal relief
   r., serial
   r., spot-film
roentgenologist (rĕnt"gĕn-ŏl'ō-jĭst) [" + Gr. *logos,* word, reason]
roentgenology (rĕnt"gĕn-ŏl'ō-jē)
roentgenometer (rĕnt"gĕ-nŏm'ĕ-tĕr) [" + Gr. *metron,* measure]
roentgenoscope (rĕnt-gĕn'ō-skōp) [" + Gr. *skopein,* to examine]
roentgenoscopy (rĕnt"gĕ-nŏs'kō-pē)
roentgenotherapy, roentgentherapy (rĕnt"gĕn-ō-thĕr'ăp-ē) [*roentgen* + Gr. *therapeia,* treatment]
roentgen ray
roeteln, roetheln (rĕt'ĕln) [Ger.]
Roger's disease (rō-zhăz') [Henri L. Roger, Fr. physician, 1809–1891]
Rokitansky's disease (rō"kĭ-tăn'skēz) [Karl Freiherr von Rokitansky, Austrian pathologist, 1804–1878]
Rolaids
Rolando's area (rō-lăn'dōz) [Luigi Rolando, It. anatomist, 1773–1831]
Rolando's fissure
role (rōl) [O. Fr. *rolle,* roll of paper on which a part is written]
   r., gender
role model
role playing
rolfing [Ida Rolf, U.S. physiotherapist, 1897–1979]
rolitetracycline (rō"lē-tĕt"ră-sī'klēn)

roll
   r., cotton
   r., ilial
   r., scleral
roller (rōl′ĕr) [O. Fr., roll]
ROM *read-only memory; rupture of membranes*
R.O.M. *range of motion*
roman numerals
romanopexy (rō-măn′ō-pĕk″sē) [L. *romanum*, the sigmoid, + Gr. *pexis*, fixation]
romanoscope (rō-măn′ō-skōp) [″ + Gr. *skopein*, to examine]
rombergism (rŏm′bĕrg-ĭzm)
Romberg's sign (rŏm′bĕrgs) [Maritz Heinrich Romberg, Ger. physician, 1795–1873]
Rondomycin
rongeur (rŏn-zhŭr′) [Fr., to gnaw]
Roniacol
roof nucleus
room [AS. *rum*]
   r., clean
   r., dark-
   r., delivery
   r., dust-free
   r., intensive therapy
   r., labor
   r., operating
   r., postdelivery
   r., recovery
rooming-in
root (rūt) [AS. *rot*]
   r., anterior
   r., dorsal
   r., motor
   r., posterior
   r., sensory
   r., ventral
root arteries
root canal
rooting reflex
root resorption of teeth
root sheath
root zone
R.O.P. *right occipitoposterior*
Rorschach test (ror′shăk) [Hermann Rorschach, Swiss pyschiatrist, 1884–1922]
rosa (rō′ză) [L.]
rosacea (rō-zā′sē-ă) [L. *rosaceus*, rosy]
rosaniline (rō-zăn′ĭ-lĭn)
rosary (rō′ză-rē)
   r., rachitic
Rose, Frank A (rōz) [Brit. surgeon]
   R.'s position
rose bengal sodium I 131
rose fever
Rosenbach, Ottomar (rō′zĕn-bŏk) [Ger. physician, 1851–1907]
   R.'s sign
   R.'s test
Rosenmüller, Johann Christian (rō′zĕn-mĭl″ĕr) [Ger. anatomist, 1771–1820]
   R.'s body
   R.'s cavity
roseo- [L. *roseus*, rosy]
roseola (rō-zē′ō-lă, rō″zē-ō′lă) [L. *roseus*, rosy]
   r. idiopathica
   r. infantum
   r. symptomatica
roseolous (rō-zē′ō-lŭs) [L. *roseus*, rosy]
rosette [Fr., small rose]
rose water
rose water ointment
rosin (rŏz′ĭn) [L. *resina*]
Ross' bodies [Edward Halford Ross, Brit. pathologist, 1875–1928]
Rossolimo's reflex (rŏs″ō-lē′mōz) [Gregoriy I. Rossolimo, Russian neurologist, 1860–1928]
rostellum (rŏs-tĕl′lŭm) [L., little beak]
rostral (rŏs′trăl) [L. *rostralis*]
rostrate (rŏs′trāt) [L. *rostratus*, beaked]
rostriform (rŏs′trĭ-form) [″ + *forma*, shape]
rostrum (rŏs′trŭm) [L., beak]
rosulate (rŏs′ū-lāt) [L. *rosulatus*, like a rose]
R.O.T. *right occipitotransverse*
rot (rŏt) [ME. *roten*]
   r., jungle
rotameter (rō-tăm′ĕ-tĕr)

rotate (rō-tāt) [L. *rotare*, to turn]
rotating tourniquet
rotation (rō-tā'shŭn) [L. *rotatio*, a turning]
   r., fetal
   r., optical
   r., tooth
rotator (rō-tā'tor)
rotaviruses (rō'tă-vī"rŭs-ĕs) [L. *rota*, wheel, + *virus*, poison]
röteln, rötheln (rĕt'ĕln) [Ger. *rot*, red]
rotenone (rō'tĕn-nōn)
Roth's spots [Moritz Roth, Swiss physician and pathologist, 1849 – 1914]
rotoxamine tartrate (rō-tŏks'ă-mēn)
Rouget's cells (roo-zhāz') [Charles M. B. Rouget, Fr. physiologist, 1824 – 1904]
rough (rŭf)
roughage (rŭf'ĭj) [AS. *ruh*, rough]
rouleau (roo-lō') [Fr., roll]
round (rownd) [O. Fr. *ronde*]
round ligament
roundworm
Roux-en-Y
Roven's IMDC [Milton D. Roven, contemporary U.S. podiatrist]
Royal Free disease [After Royal Free Hospital, London, from which cases were reported in 1955]
RPF *renal plasma flow*
rpm *revolutions per minute*
RPS *renal pressor substance*
R.Q. *respiratory quotient*
-rrhagia (rā'jē-ă) [Gr. *rhegnynai*, to burst forth]
rRNA *ribosomal RNA*
R.S.A. *right sacroanterior*
R.Sc.A. *right scapuloanterior*
R.Sc.P. *right scapuloposterior*
R.S.P. *right sacroposterior*
R.S.T. *right sacrotransverse*
R.S.V. *Rous sarcoma virus*
R.T. *radiation therapy; reading test; registered technologist*
R.T.(N.) *registered technologist — nuclear medicine*
R.T.(R.) *registered technologist radio-*

grapher
R.T.(T.) *registered technologist — radiation therapy*
R.U. *rat unit*
Ru *ruthenium*
rub
   r., pericardial
   r., pleural friction
rubber dam
rubefacient (roo"bĕ-fā'shĕnt) [L. *rubefaciens*, making red]
rubella (roo-bĕl'lă) [L. *rubellus*, reddish]
rubella titer
rubella virus vaccine, live
rubeola (roo-bē'ō-lă, roo"bē-ō'lă) [L. *rubeolus*, reddish]
rubeosis iridis
ruber (roo'bĕr) [L.]
rubescent (roo-bĕs'ĕnt) [L. *rubescere*, to grow red]
rubidium (roo-bĭd'ē-ŭm) [L. *rubidus*, red]
rubiginous (roo-bĭj'ĭ-nŭs) [L. *rubiginosus*]
rubigo (roo-bī'gō) [L., rust]
Rubin's test (roo'bĭns) [Isidor Clinton Rubin, U.S. physician, 1883 – 1958]
Rubner's test (roob'nĕrz) [Max Rubner, Ger. physiologist, 1854 – 1932]
rubor (roo'bor) [L.]
Rubramin PC
rubriblast (roo'brĭ-blăst) [L. *rubrica*, red, + Gr. *blastos*, germ]
rubric (roo'brĭk) [L. *ruber*, red]
rubricyte (roo'brĭ-sīt) [L. *ruber*, red, + Gr. *kytos*, cell]
rubrospinal (roo"brō-spī'năl) [" + *spina*, thorn]
rubrothalamic (roo"brō-thăl-lăm'ĭk) [" + Gr. *thalamos*, chamber]
rubrum (roo'brŭm) [L., red]
   r. scarlatinum
ructus (rŭk'tŭs) [L.]
rudiment (roo'dĭ-mĕnt) [L. *rudimentum*, beginning]
rudimentary (roo"dĭ-mĕn'tă-rē)
rudimentum (roo"dĭ-mĕn'tŭm) [L., be-

ginning]

Ruffini's corpuscles (roo-fē'nēz) [Angelo Ruffini, It. anatomist, 1864 – 1929]

rufous (roo'fŭs) [L. *rufus*, red]

ruga (roo'gă) [L.]
    rugae of vagina

Ruggeri's reflex [Ruggero Ruggeri, It. physician, d. 1905]

rugine (roo-zhēn')

rugose, rugous (roo'gōs, -gŭs) [L. *rugosus*, wrinkled]

rugosity (rū-gòs'ĭ-tē) [L. *rugositas*]

R.U.L.   *right upper lobe*

rule (rool) [ME. *riule*]
    r. of nines

rum fits

ruminant (roo'mĭ-nănt)

rumination (roo"mĭ-nā'shŭn) [L. *ruminatio*]

rump (rŭmp) [ME. *rumpe*]

Rumpf's symptom (roompfs) [Heinrich Theodor Rumpf, Ger. physician, 1851 – 1923]

run [AS. *rinnan*, run]

runaround, runround

runners' high

rupia (roo'pē-ă) [Gr. *rhypos*, filth]

rupioid (roo'pē-oyd) [" + *eidos*, form, shape]

rupophobia (roo"pō-fō'bē-ă) [" + *phobos*, fear]

rupture (rŭp'chŭr) [L. *ruptura*, breaking]

r. of membranes
r. of perineum
r. of tubes
r. of uterus

RUQ   *right upper quadrant*

rush

Russell bodies (rŭs'ĕl) [William Russell, Brit. physician, 1852 – 1940]

Russell's viper venom (rŭs'ĕlz) [Patrick Russell, Irish physician who worked in India, 1727 – 1805]

Russian bath

Rust's disease (rŭsts) [Johann N. Rust, Ger. surgeon, 1775 – 1840]

rusts

rusty (rŭst'ē) [AS. *rustig*]

rut (rŭt) [O. Fr. *ruit*, roaring of deer]

rut-formation

ruthenium (roo-thē'nē-ŭm)

rutherford [Ernest Rutherford, Brit. physicist, 1871 – 1937]

rutidosis (roo"tĭ-dō'sĭs) [Gr. *rhytis*, wrinkle]

rutilism (roo'tĭl-ĭzm) [L. *rutilis*, red, + Gr. *-ismos*, condition]

rutin (roo'tĭn)

RV   *residual volume; right ventricle*

℞ [L.] *recipe*, take

rye (rī) [AS. *ryge*]

rytidosis (rĭt"ĭ-dō'sĭs) [Gr. *rhytis*, a wrinkle, + *osis*, condition]

S

σ   *sigma; standard deviation*
Σ   *capital of Greek letter sigma; summation*
S   [L.] *signa*, mark; [L.] *signetur*, let it be written; *smooth; spherical; spherical lens; subject; sulfur*
s   *semis*, half; [L.] *sinister*, left
s̄, s   [L.] *sine*, without
S1, S2, etc.   first sacral nerve, second sacral nerve
S₁, S₂
S₃
S₄
S-A, SA, S.A.   sinoatrial
saber shin
Sabin vaccine   [Albert B. Sabin, U.S. virologist, b. 1906]
sabulous   (săb'ū-lŭs) [L. *sabulosus*, sand]
saburra   (să-bŭr'ră) [NL., sand]
sac   (săk) [L. *saccus*, sack, bag]
    s., air
    s., allantoic
    s., alveolar
    s., amniotic
    s., chorionic
    s., conjunctival
    s., dental
    s., endolymphatic
    s., heart
    s., hernial
    s., lacrimal
    s., lesser peritoneal
    s., vitelline
    s., yolk
saccades   (să-kāds') [Fr. *saccade*, jerk]
saccadic   (să-kăd'ĭk) [Fr. *saccade*, jerk]
saccate   (săk'āt) [NL. *saccatus*, baglike]
saccharase   (săk'ă-rās) [Sanskrit *sarkara*, sugar]
saccharated   (săk'ă-rāt"ĕd)
saccharic acid

saccharide   (săk'ă-rīd)
sacchariferous   (săk"ă-rĭf'ĕr-ŭs) [Sanskrit *sarkara*, sugar, + L. *ferre*, to carry]
saccharification   (săk"ăr-ĭ-fĭ-kā'shŭn) [" + L. *facere*, to make]
saccharin   (săk'ă-rĭn)
saccharine   (săk'ă-rĭn, -rīn) [L. *saccharum*, sugar]
saccharo-   [Sanskrit *sarkara*, sugar]
saccharogalactorrhea   (săk"ă-rō-gă-lăk"tō-rē'ă) [" + Gr. *gala*, milk, + *rhein*, to flow]
saccharolytic   (săk"ă-rō-lĭt'ĭk) [" + Gr. *lysis*, dissolution]
Saccharomyces   (săk"ă-rō-mī'sēz) [Sanskrit *sarkara*, sugar, + Gr. *mykes*, fungus]
saccharomycosis   (săk"ă-rō-mī-kō'sĭs) [" + " + *osis*, condition]
saccharorrhea   (săk"ă-rō-rē'ă) [" + Gr. *rhein*, to flow]
saccharose   (săk'ă-rōs)
saccharosuria   (săk"ă-rō-sū'rē-ă) [Sanskrit *sarkara*, sugar, + Gr. *ouron*, urine]
saccharum   (săk'ă-rŭm) [L.]
    s. album
    s. canadense
    s. candidum
    s. lactis
    s. ustum
saccharuria   (săk"ă-roo'rē-ă) [Sanskrit *sarkara*, sugar, + Gr. *ouron*, urine]
sacciform   (săk'sĭ-form) [L. *saccus*, sack, bag, + *forma*, shape]
saccular   (săk'ū-lăr) [NL. *sacculus*, small bag]
sacculated   (săk'ū-lāt"ĕd) [NL. *sacculus*, small bag]
sacculation   (săk"ū-lā'shŭn)

saccule (săk'ūl) [NL. *sacculus,* small bag]
s., laryngeal
sacculocochlear (săk"ū-lō-kŏk'lē-ăr)
[" + Gr. *kokhlos,* land snail]
sacculus (săk'ū-lŭs) [NL., small bag]
s. laryngis
saccus (săk'ŭs) [L., sack, bag]
s. endolymphaticus
s. lacrimalis
sacrad (sā'krăd) [L. *sacrum,* sacred,
+ *ad,* toward]
sacral (sā'krăl) [L. *sacralis*]
sacral bone
sacral canal
sacral flexure
sacralgia (sā-krăl'jē-ă) [L. *sacrum,*
sacred, + Gr. *algos,* pain]
sacral index
sacralization (sā"krăl-ĭ-zā'shŭn)
sacral nerves
sacral plexus
sacral vertebra
sacrectomy (sā-krĕk'tō-mē) [L. *sacrum,*
sacred, + Gr. *ektome,* excision]
sacro- (sā'krō) [L. *sacrum,* sacred]
sacroanterior (sā"krō-ăn-tē'rē-or)
[" + *anterior,* before]
sacrococcygeal (sā"krō-kŏk-sĭj'ē-ăl)
[" + Gr. *kokkyx,* coccyx]
sacrococcygeus (săk"rō-kŏk-sĭj'ē-ŭs)
sacrocoxalgia (sā"krō-kŏks-ăl'jē-ă)
[" + *coxa,* hip, + Gr. *algos,*
pain]
sacrocoxitis (sā"krō-kŏks-ī'tĭs) [" +
" + Gr. *itis,* inflammation]
sacrodynia (sā"krō-dĭn'ē-ă) [" +
odyne, pain]
sacroiliac (sā"krō-ĭl'ē-ăk) [" +
iliacus, hipbone]
sacroiliac joint
sacroiliitis (sā"krō-ĭl"ē-ī'tĭs) [" + "
+ Gr. *itis,* inflammation]
sacrolisthesis (sā"krō-lĭs-thē'sĭs) [" +
Gr. *olisthesis,* a slipping]
sacrolumbar (sā"krō-lŭm'băr) [" +
lumbus, loin]
sacrolumbar angle
sacroposterior (sā"krō-pŏs-tē'rē-or)
[" + *posterus,* behind]

sacrosciatic (sā"krō-sī-ăt'ĭk) [" +
sciaticus, hipjoint]
sacrospinal (sā"krō-spī'năl) [" +
spina, thorn]
sacrospinalis [" + *spina,* thorn]
sacrotomy (sā-krŏt'ō-mē) [" + Gr.
tome, a cutting, slice]
sacrouterine (sā"krō-ū'tĕr-ĭn) [" +
uterus, womb]
sacrovertebral (sā"krō-vĕr'tĕ-brăl)
[" + *vertebra,* vertebra]
sacrovertebral angle
sacrum (sā'krŭm) [L., sacred]
sactosalpinx (săk"tō-săl'pĭnks) [Gr.
saktos, stuffed, + *salpinx,* tube]
SAD *seasonal affective disorder*
saddle
saddle area
saddle back
saddle block anesthesia
saddle joint
saddle nose
sadism (sā'dĭzm, săd'ĭzm) [Comte Don-
atien Alphonse François de Sade, Mar-
quis de Sade, 1740 – 1814]
sadist (sā'dĭst, săd'ĭst)
sadness
sadomasochism (sā"dō-măs'ĕ-kĭzm,
săd"ō-măs'ĕ-kĭzm)
sadomasochist (sā"dō-măs'ĕ-kĭst)
Saemisch's ulcer (sā'mĭsh-ĕs) [Edwin
Theodor Saemisch, Ger. ophthalmologist, 1833 – 1909]
safelight
safe sex
sagittal (săj'ĭ-tăl) [L. *sagittalis*]
sagittalis (săj"ĭ-tā'lĭs) [L.]
sagittal plane
sagittal sinus
sagittal sulcus
sagittal suture
sago (sā'gō) [Malay *sagu*]
**St. Joseph's Cough Syrup for Chil-
dren**
Saint Vitus' dance
sal (săl) [L.]
s. ammoniac
s. soda
salaam convulsion (sŭ-lŏm') [Arabic

salam, peace]
salacious (să-lā'shŭs) [L. *salax*, lustful]
salicylamide (săl"ĭ-sĭl-ăm'ĭd)
salicylanilide (săl"ĭ-sĭl-ăn'ĭ-lĭd)
salicylate (săl"ĭ-sĭl'āt, săl-ĭs'ĭl-āt)
s., methyl
s., sodium
salicylated (săl-ĭs'ĭl-āt-ĕd)
salicylate poisoning
salicylazosulfapyridine (săl"ĭ-sĭl"ă-zō-sŭl" fă-pĭr'ĭ-dēn)
salicylic acid (săl"ĭ-sĭl'ĭk)
salicylism (săl'ĭ-sĭl"ĭzm)
salicylsulfonic acid test
salicyluric acid (săl"ĭ-sĭ-lū'rĭk)
salifiable (săl"ĭ-fī'ă-bl) [L. *sal*, salt, + *fieri*, to be made]
salify (săl'ĭ-fī) [" + *fieri*, to be made]
salimeter (săl-ĭm'ĕ-tĕr) [" + Gr. *metron*, a measure]
saline (sā'lĭn, sā'lēn) [L. *salinus*, of salt]
s., hypertonic
s., hypotonic
saline cathartic
saline enema
saline solution
salinometer (săl"ĭ-nŏm'ĕ-tĕr) [L. *salinus*, of salt, + *metron*, measure]
saliva (să-lī'vă) [L., spittle]
s., artificial
salivant (săl'ĭ-vănt) [L. *saliva*, spittle]
salivary (săl'ĭ-vĕr-ē) [L. *salivarius*, slimy]
salivary corpuscles
salivary digestion
salivary glands
salivation (săl"ĭ-vā'shŭn) [LL. *salivatio*, to spit out]
salivatory (săl'ĭ-vă-tor"ē)
salivolithiasis (să-lī"vō-lĭ-thī'ă-sĭs) [L. *saliva*, spittle, + Gr. *lithos*, stone, + *-iasis*, state or condition of]
Salk vaccine (sŏlk) [Jonas E. Salk, U.S. microbiologist, b. 1914]
sallow (săl'ō) [AS. *salo*]
salmin(e) (săl'mēn, -mĭn) [L. *salmo*, salmon]
Salmonella (săl"mō-nĕl'ă) [NL.] [Daniel E. Salmon, U.S. pathologist, 1850–

1914]
S. choleraesuis
S. enteritidis
S. paratyphi
S. schottmülleri
S. typhimurium
S. typhi
salmonellosis (săl-mō-nĕ-lō'sĭs)
salmon patch
salpingectomy (săl"pĭn-jĕk'tō-mē) [Gr. *salpinx*, tube, + *ektome*, excision]
salpingemphraxis (săl"pĭn-jĕm-frăk'sĭs) [" + *emphraxis*, a stoppage]
salpingian (săl-pĭn'jē-ăn)
salpingion (săl-pĭn'jē-ŏn)
salpingitis (săl"pĭn-jī'tĭs) [Gr. *salpinx*, tube, + *itis*, inflammation]
s., eustachian
s., gonococcal
salpingo- [Gr. *salpinx*, tube]
salpingocatheterism (săl-pĭng"gō-kăth'ĕt-ĕr-ĭzm) [" + *katheter*, something inserted, + *-ismos*, condition]
salpingocele (săl-pĭng'gō-sēl) [" + *kele*, tumor, swelling]
salpingocyesis (săl-pĭng"ō-sī-ē'sĭs) [" + *kyesis*, pregnancy]
salpingography (săl"pĭng-gŏg'ră-fē) [" + *graphein*, to write]
salpingolithiasis (săl-pĭng"gō-lĭ-thī'ă-sĭs) [" + *lithos*, stone, + *-iasis*, state or condition of]
salpingolysis (săl"pĭng-gŏl'ĭ-sĭs) [" + *lysis*, dissolution]
salpingo-oophorectomy (săl-pĭng"gō-ō"ŏf-ō-rĕk'tō-mē) [" + NL. *oophoron*, ovary, + Gr. *ektome*, excision]
salpingo-oophoritis (săl-pĭng"ō-ō"ŏf-ō-rī'tĭs) [" + " + Gr. *itis*, inflammation]
salpingo-oophorocele (săl-pĭng"gō-ō-ŏf'or-ō-sēl) [Gr. *salpinx*, tube, + NL. *oophoron*, ovary, + Gr. *kele*, tumor, swelling]
salpingo-oothecitis (săl-pĭng"gō-ō"ō-thē-sī'tĭs) [" + *ootheke*, ovary, + *itis*, inflammation]

salpingo-oothecocele (săl-pĭng"gō-ŏ"ŏ-thē'kō-sēl) [" + " + *kele*, tumor, swelling]

salpingo-ovariectomy (săl-pĭng"gō-ŏ"văr-ē-ĕk'tō-mē) [" + NL. *ovarium*, ovary, + Gr. *ektome*, excision]

salpingoperitonitis (săl-pĭng"gō-pĕr"ĭ-tō-nī'tĭs) [" + *peritonaion*, stretched around or over, + *itis*, inflammation]

salpingopexy (săl-pĭng'ō-pĕk"sē) [" + *pexis*, fixation]

salpingopharyngeal (săl-pĭng"gō-fă-rĭn'jē-ăl) [" + *pharynx*, throat]

salpingopharyngeus (săl-pĭng"gō-făr-ĭn'jē-ŭs) [" + *pharynx*, throat]

salpingoplasty (săl-pĭng'gō-plăs"tē) [" + *plassein*, to form]

salpingorrhaphy (săl"pĭng-gor'ă-fē) [" + *rhaphe*, seam]

salpingosalpingostomy (săl-pĭng"gō-săl"pĭng-gŏs'tō-mē) [" + *salpinx*, tube, + *stoma*, mouth, opening]

salpingoscope (săl-pĭng'gō-skōp") [" + *skopein*, to examine]

salpingostenochoria (săl-pĭng"gō-stĕn"ō-kor'ē-ă) [" + *stenos*, narrow, + *choreia*, dance]

salpingostomatomy (săl-pĭng"gō-stō-măt'ō-mē) [" + *stoma*, mouth, opening, + *tome*, a cutting, slice]

salpingostomy (săl-pĭng-ŏs'tō-mē)

salpingotomy (săl-pĭng-ŏt'ō-mē) [" + *tome*, a cutting, slice]

salpingo-ureterostomy (săl-pĭng"gō-ūr-ēt"ĕr-ŏs'tō-mē) [" + *oureter*, ureter, + *stoma*, mouth, opening]

salpingysterocyesis (săl"pĭng-jĭs"tĕr-ō-sī-ē'sĭs) [" + *hystera*, womb, + *kyesis*, pregnancy]

salpinx (săl'pĭnks) [Gr., tube]

salt [AS. *sealt*]
   s., acid
   s., basic
   s., bile
   s., buffer

   s., double
   s., epsom
   s., Glauber's
   s., haloid
   s., iodized
   s., neutral
   s., Rochelle
   s., rock
   s., smelling

saltation (săl-tā'shŭn) [L. *saltatio*, leaping]

saltatory (săl'tă-tō"rē)

saltatory conduction

saltatory spasm

salt-free diet

salt glow

salting out

salt-losing syndrome

saltpeter, saltpetre (sawlt-pē'tĕr) [L. *sal*, salt, + *petra*, rock]
   s., Chile

salt-poor diet

salts

salt solution, normal

salt solution, physiological

salubrious (să-lū'brē-ŭs) [L. *salubris*, healthful]

saluresis (săl"ū-rē'sĭs) [L. *sal*, salt, + Gr. *ouresis*, urination]

saluretic (săl"ū-rĕt'ĭk)

Saluron

salutary (săl'ū-tā"rē) [L. *salutaris*, health]

Salvarsan (săl'văr-săn) [L. *salvus*, safe, + Gr. *arsen*, arsenic]

salve (săv) [AS. *sealf*]

Samaritans

samarium (să-mā'rē-ŭm)

sample
   s., biased

sampling
   s., random

sanative (săn'ă-tĭv) [L. *sanare*, to cure]

sanatorium (săn"ă-tō'rē-ŭm) [L. *sanatorius*, healing]

sanatory (săn'ă-tō"rē)

sand (sănd) [AS.]
   s., auditory

s., brain
sandflies
sandfly fever
Sandhoff's disease
Sandril
Sandwith's bald tongue (sănd′wĭths) [Fleming M. Sandwith, Br. physician, 1777–1843]
sane (sān) [L. *sanus*, healthy]
Sanfilippo's disease [S. J. Sanfilippo, contemporary U.S. pediatrician]
sanguicolous (săng-gwĭk′ō-lŭs) [L. *sanguis*, blood, + *colere*, to dwell]
sanguifacient (săng-gwĭ-fā′shĕnt) [″ + *facere*, to make]
sanguiferous (săng-gwĭf′ĕr-ŭs) [″ + *ferre*, to carry]
sanguification (săng″gwĭ-fĭ-kā′shŭn) [″ + *facere*, to make]
sanguimotor, **sanguimotory** (săng″gwĭ-mō′tor, -tō-rē) [″ + *motor*, a mover]
sanguine (săng′gwĭn) [L. *sanguineus*, bloody]
sanguineous (săng-gwĭn′ē-ŭs) [L. *sanguineus*, bloody]
sanguinolent (săng-gwĭn′ō-lĕnt) [L. *sanguinolentus*, bloody]
sanguinopoietic (săng″gwĭn-ō-poy-ĕt′ĭk) [L. *sanguis*, blood, + *poiein*, to form]
sanguinopurulent (săng″gwĭ-nō-pū′rū-lĕnt) [″ + *purulentus*, full of pus]
sanguinous (săng′gwĭ-nŭs) [L. *sanguineus*, bloody]
sanguirenal (săng″gwĭ-rē′năl) [L. *sanguis*, blood, + *ren*, kidney]
sanguis (săng′gwĭs) [L.]
sanguisuga (săng-gwĭ-sū′gă) [″ + *sugere*, to suck]
sanguivorous (săng-gwĭv′ō-rŭs) [″ + *vovare*, to eat]
sanies (sā′nē-ēz) [L., thin, fetid pus]
saniopurulent (sā″nē-ō-pūr′ū-lĕnt) [L. *sanies*, thin, fetid pus, + *purulentus*, full of pus]
sanioserous (sā″nē-ō-sē′rŭs) [″ +

serum, whey]
sanitarian (săn″ĭ-tā′rē-ăn) [L. *sanitas*, health]
sanitarium (săn-ĭ-tā′rē-ŭm) [L. *sanitas*, health]
sanitary (săn′ĭ-tā″rē) [L. *sanitas*, health]
sanitary napkin
sanitation (săn″ĭ-tā′shŭn) [L. *sanitas*, health]
sanitization (săn″ĭ-tĭ-zā′shŭn) [L. *sanitas*, health]
sanitize (săn′ĭ-tīz)
sanitizer
sanity (săn′ĭ-tē)
San Joaquin valley fever
SA node
Sanorex
Sansert
santonin (săn′tō-nĭn)
sap (săp) [AS. *saep*]
s., cell
s., nuclear
saphena (să-fē′nă) [Gr. *saphenes*, manifest]
saphenectomy (săf″ĕ-nĕk′tō-mē) [″ + *ektome*, excision]
saphenous (să′fĕ-nŭs)
saphenous nerve
saphenous opening
saphenous veins
sapid (săp′ĭd) [L. *sapidus*, tasty]
sapo (sā′pō) [L.]
saponaceous (sā″pō-nā′shŭs) [NL. *saponaceus*, soapy]
saponatus (sā″pō-nā′tŭs) [L.]
saponification (să-pŏn″ĭ-fĭ-kā′shŭn) [L. *sapo*, soap, + *facere*, to make]
saponification number
saponify (să-pŏn′ĭ-fī)
saponin (săp′ō-nĭn) [Fr. *saponine*, soap]
sapophore (săp′ō-for) [L. *sapor*, taste, + Gr. *phoros*, bearing]
saporific (săp″ō-rĭf′ĭk) [NL. *saporificus*, producing taste]
sapphism (săf′ĭzm) [Sappho, Gr. poetess, 7th-century B.C.]
sapro- [Gr. *sapros*, putrid]
saprobes (să′prōbs) [Gr. *sapros*, pu-

trid, + *bios*, life]

saprogen (săp'rō-jĕn) [" + *gennan*, to produce]

saprogenic (săp"rō-jĕn'ĭk)

saprophilous (săp-rŏf'ĭl-ŭs) [Gr. *sapros*, putrid, + *philein*, to love]

saprophyte (săp'rō-fīt) [" + *phyton*, plant]

saprophytic (săp"rō-fĭt'ĭk)

saprozoic (săp"rō-zō'ĭk) [" + *zoon*, animal]

sarapus (săr'ă-pŭs) [Gr. *sarapous*]

Sarcina (săr'sĭ-nă) [L., bundle]

sarcina (săr'sĭ-nă)

sarcitis (săr-sī'tĭs) [Gr. *sarx*, flesh, + *itis*, inflammation]

sarco- [Gr. *sarx*, flesh]

sarcoadenoma (săr"kō-ăd"ĕn-ō'mă) [" + *aden*, gland, + *oma*, tumor]

sarcobiont (săr"kō-bī'ŏnt) [" + *bioun*, to live]

sarcoblast (săr'kō-blăst) [" + *blastos*, a germ]

sarcocarcinoma (săr"kō-kăr"sĭn-ō'mă) [" + *karkinos*, crab, + *oma*, tumor]

sarcocele (săr'kō-sēl) [" + *kele*, tumor, swelling]

sarcocyst (săr'kō-sĭst) [" + *kystis*, bladder]

Sarcocystis (săr"kō-sĭs'tĭs) [" + *kystis*, bladder]
  S. lindemanni

Sarcodina (săr-kō-dī'nă) [" + *eidos*, form, shape]

sarcogenic (săr"kō-jĕn'ĭk) [" + *gennan*, to produce]

sarcoid (săr'koyd) [" + *eidos*, form, shape]
  s., Boeck's

sarcoidosis (săr"koyd-ō'sĭs) [" + " + *osis*, condition]

sarcolemma (săr"kō-lĕm'ă) [" + *lemma*, husk]

sarcology (săr-kŏl'ō-jē) [" + *logos*, word, reason]

sarcolysis (săr-kŏl'ĭ-sĭs) [" + *lysis*, dissolution]

sarcolytic (săr"kō-lĭt'ĭk)

sarcoma (săr-kō'mă) [" + *oma*, tumor]
  s., alveolar soft part
  s., botryoid
  s., chondro-
  s., endometrial
  s., Ewing's
  s., fibro-
  s., giant cell
  s., Kaposi's
  s., lipo-
  s., lymphangio-
  s., myeloid
  s., myxo-
  s., osteogenic
  s., reticulum cell
  s., rhabdomyo-
  s., spindle cell

sarcomatoid (sar-kō'mă-toyd) [Gr. *sarx*, flesh, + *oma*, tumor, + *eidos*, form, shape]

sarcomatosis (săr"kō-mă-tō'sĭs) [" + " + *osis*, condition]

sarcomatous (sar-kō'mă-tŭs)

sarcomere (săr-kō-mēr) [" + *meros*, a part]

sarcomphalocele (săr"kŏm-făl'ō-sēl) [" + *omphalos*, umbilicus, + *kele*, tumor, swelling]

sarcomyces (săr"kō-mī'sēz) [" + *mykes*, fungus]

Sarcophagidae (săr"kō-făj'ĭ-dē) [Gr. *sarx*, flesh, + *phagein*, to eat]

sarcophagy (săr-kŏf'ă-jē)

sarcoplasm (săr'kō-plăzm) [" + LL. *plasma*, form, mold]

sarcoplasmic (săr"kō-plăz'mĭk)

sarcopoietic (săr"kō-poy-ĕt'ĭk) [" + *poiein*, to form]

Sarcoptes (săr-kŏp'tēz)

Sarcoptidae (săr-kŏp'tĭ-dē)

sarcosis (săr-kō'sĭs) [" + *osis*, condition]

sarcosome (săr'kō-sōm) [" + *soma*, body]

Sarcosporidia (săr"kō-spō-rĭd'ē-ă) [" + *sporos*, seed]

sarcosporidiosis (săr"kō-spō-rĭd"ē-

ō'sĭs) [" + " + osis, condition]
sarcostosis (săr"kŏs-tō'sĭs) [" + osteon, bone, + osis, condition]
sarcostyle (săr'kō-stĭl) [" + stylos, a column]
sarcotic (săr-kŏt'ĭk) [Gr. sarx, flesh]
sarcotubules (săr"kō-tū'būlz)
sarcous (săr'kŭs) [Gr. sarko, flesh]
sardonic laugh
sarin (GB)
sartorius (săr-tō'rē-ŭs) [L. sartor, tailor]
SAS-500
sat. saturated
satellite (săt'ĕl-ĭt) [L. satelles, attendant]
   s., bacterial
satellite cells
satellitosis (săt"ĕl-ĭ-tō'sĭs) [" + Gr. osis, condition]
satiety (sā-tī'ĕt-ē) [L. satietas, enough]
saturated (săt'ū-rā"tĕd) [L. saturare, to fill]
saturated compound
saturated hydrocarbon
saturated solution
saturation (săt"ū-rā'shŭn)
   s., oxygen
saturation index
saturation time
Saturday night paralysis
saturnine (săt'ŭr-nīn) [L. saturnus, lead]
saturnine breath
saturnine gout
saturnism (săt'ŭr-nīzm) [" + Gr. -ismos, condition]
satyriasis (săt-ĭ-rī'ă-sīs) [LL.]
satyromania (săt"ĭ-rō-mā'nē-ă)
saucerization (saw"sĕr-ĭ-zā'shŭn)
sauna
savory (sā'vō-rē) [O. Fr. savoure, tasty]
saw [AS. sagu]
saxifragant (săks-ĭf'ră-gănt) [L. saxum, rock, + frangere, to break]
saxitoxin (săk"sĭ-tŏk'sĭn)
Sayre's jacket (sārz) [Lewis Albert Sayre, U.S. surgeon, 1820–1900]
Sb antimony
SbCl₃ antimony trichloride
Sb₂O₅ antimonic oxide; antimony pentoxide

Sb₄O₆ antimonious oxide
Sc scandium
s.c. subcutaneously
scab (skăb) [ME. scabbe]
scabicide (skā'bĭ-sīd)
scabies (skā'bē-ēz, -bēz) [L. scabies, itch]
   s., Norwegian
scabietic (skā"bē-ĕt'ĭk) [L. scabies, itch]
scabieticide (skā"bē-ĕt'ĭ-sīd) [" + caedere, to kill]
scabiphobia (skă"bĭ-fō'bē-ă) [" + Gr. phobos, fear]
scabrities (skā-brĭsh'ē-ēz) [L. scaber, rough]
   s. unguium
scala (skā'lă) [L. scala, staircase]
   s. media
   s. tympani
   s. vestibuli
scald (skŏld) [ME. scalden, to burn with hot liquid]
scalded skin syndrome
scale (skāl) [O. Fr. escale, husk; ME. scole, balance; L. scala, staircase]
   s., absolute
   s., Baumé
   s., Celsius
   s., centigrade
   s., Fahrenheit
   s., French
   s., Kelvin
   s. of contrast
scalene (skā-lēn') [Gr. skalenos, uneven]
   s. tubercle
scalenectomy (skā"lĕ-nĕk'tō-mē) [" + ektome, excision]
scaleniotomy (skā-lēn"ē-ŏt'ō-mē) [" + tome, a cutting, slice]
scalenotomy (skā"lĕ-nŏt'ō-mē) [" + tome, a cutting, slice]
scalenus (skā-lē'nŭs) [L., uneven]
scalenus syndrome
scaler (skā'lĕr) [O. Fr. escale, husk]
scaling (skāl'ĭng) [O. Fr. escale, husk]
scall (skawl) [Norse skalli, baldhead]
scalp (skălp) [ME., sheath]
scalpel (skăl'pĕl) [L. scalpellum, knife]

scalpriform (skăl′prĭ-form) [L. *scalprum*, knife, + *forma*, shape]
scalprum (skăl′prŭm) [L., knife]
scalp tourniquet
scaly (skā′lē) [O. Fr. *escale*, husk]
scan
scandium [L. *Scandia*, Scandinavia]
scanning
   s., radioisotope
scanning electron microscope
scanning speech
scanty (skăn′tē) [ME. from O. Norse, *skamt*, short]
scapha (skā′fă) [NL., skiff]
scapho- [Gr. *skaphe*, skiff]
scaphocephalic (skăf″ō-sĕf-ăl′ĭk) [″ + *kephale*, head]
scaphocephalism (skăf″ō-sĕf′ăl-ĭzm) [″ + ″ + -*ismos*, condition]
scaphocephalous (skăf″ō-sĕf′ă-lŭs) [″ + *kephale*, head]
scaphocephaly (skăf″ō-sĕf′ă-lē) [″ + *kephale*, head]
scaphohydrocephaly (skăf″ō-hī″drō-sĕf′ă-lē) [″ + *hydor*, water, + *kephale*, head]
scaphoid (skăf′oyd) [″ + *eidos*, form, shape]
scaphoid fossa
scaphoiditis (skăf″oyd-ī′tĭs) [″ + ″ + *itis*, inflammation]
scapula [L., shoulder blade]
   s., winged
scapulalgia (skăp-ū-lăl′jē-ă) [L. *scapula*, shoulder blade, + Gr. *algos*, pain]
scapular (skăp′ū-lăr)
scapular reflex
scapulary (skăp′ū-lă-rē)
scapulectomy (skăp″ū-lĕk′tō-mē) [L. *scapula*, shoulder blade, + Gr. *ektome*, excision]
scapulo- [L. *scapula*, shoulder blade]
scapuloclavicular (skăp″ū-lō-klă-vĭk′ū-lar) [″ + *clavicula*, little key]
scapulodynia (skăp″ū-lō-dĭn′ē-ă) [″ + *odyne*, pain]
scapulohumeral (skăp″ū-lō-hū′mĕr-ăl) [″ + *humerus*, upper arm]

scapulohumeral reflex
scapulopexy (skăp″ū-lō-pĕk′sē) [″ + Gr. *pexis*, fixation]
scapulothoracic (skăp″ū-lō-thō-răs′ĭk) [″ + Gr. *thorax*, chest]
scapus (skā′pŭs) [L. *scapus*, stalk]
   s. penis
   s. pili
scar (skăr) [Gr. *eskhara*, scab]
   s., cicatricial
   s., keloid
   s., painful
scarabiasis (skăr″ă-bī′ă-sĭs) [L. *scarabaeus*, beetle, + Gr. -*iasis*, state or condition of]
scarification (skăr″ĭ-fĭ-kā′shŭn) [Gr. *skariphismos*, scratching up]
scarificator (skăr′ĭf-ĭ-kā″tor)
scarifier
scarlatina (skăr″lă-tē′nă) [NL., red]
   s. anginosa
   s. hemorrhagica
   s. maligna
scarlatinal (skăr″lă-tē′năl)
scarlatinella (skăr-lăt″ĭ-nĕl′ă) [L.]
scarlatiniform (skăr-lă-tĭn′ĭ-form) [L. *scarlatina*, red, + *forma*, shape]
scarlatinoid (skăr-lăt′ĭ-noyd) [″ + Gr. *eidos*, form, shape]
scarlet fever [L. *scarlatum*, red]
scarlet rash
scarlet red
Scarpa's fascia (skăr′păs) [Antonio Scarpa, It. anatomist, 1747 – 1832]
Scarpa's fluid
Scarpa's foramina
Scarpa's ganglion
Scarpa's membrane
Scarpa's triangle
SCAT *sheep cell agglutination test*
scatemia (skă-tē′mē-ă) [Gr. *skato-*, dung, + *haima*, blood]
scato- [Gr. *skato-*, dung]
scatologic (skăt″ō-lŏj′ĭk)
scatology (skă-tŏl′ō-jē) [″ + *logos*, word, reason]
scatoma (skă-tō′mă) [″ + *oma*, tumor]
scatophagy (skă-tŏf′ă-jē) [″ +

phagein, to eat]
scatoscopy (skă-tŏs'kō-pē) [" + *skopein*, to examine]
scatter (skăt'ĕr)
s., back-
scattered radiation
scattergram (skăt'ĕr-grăm)
scavenger cell (skăv'ĕn-jer) [ME. *skawager*, toll collector]
Sc.D. *Doctor of Science*
scent (sĕnt)
Schafer's method of artificial respiration [Sir Edward A. Sharpey-Schafer, Brit. physiologist, 1850–1935]
Schäffer's reflex (shā'fĕrs) [Max Schäffer, Ger. neurologist, 1852–1923]
Schatzki ring [Richard Schatzki, U.S. radiologist, b. 1901]
Scheie's syndrome [H. G. Scheie, U.S. ophthalmologist, b. 1909]
schema (skē'mă) [Gr., shape]
schematic (skē-măt'ĭk) [NL. *schematicus*, shape, figure]
scheroma (shē-rō'mă)
Schick test (shĭk) [Béla Schick, U.S. pediatrician, 1877–1967]
Schick test control
Schilder's disease (shĭl'dĕrs) [Paul Ferdinand Schilder, Austrian-U.S. neurologist, 1886–1940]
Schiller's test (shĭl'ĕrs) [Walter Schiller, Austrian-U.S. pathologist, 1887–1960]
Schilling's classification [Victor Schilling, Ger. hematologist, 1883–1960]
Schilling test [Robert F. Schilling, U.S. hematologist, b. 1919]
schindylesis (skĭn"dĭ-lē'sĭs) [Gr. *schindylesis*, a splitting]
Schirmer's test [Rudolph Schirmer, Ger. ophthalmologist, 1831–1896]
schisto- (skĭs'tō) [Gr. *schistos*, divided]
schistocelia (skĭs"tō-sē'lē-ă) [" + *koilia*, cavity, belly]
schistocephalus (skĭs"tō-sĕf'ă-lŭs) [" + *kephale*, head]

schistocormia (skĭs"tō-kor'mē-ă) [" + *kormos*, trunk]
schistocystis (skĭs"tō-sĭs'tĭs) [" + *kystis*, bladder]
schistocyte (skĭs'tō-sīt) [" + *kytos*, cell]
schistocytosis (skĭs"tō-sī-tō'sĭs) [" + p.tō-sī-tō'sĭs) [" +
schistoglossia (skĭs"tō-glŏs'ē-ă) [" + *glossa*, tongue].
schistomelus (skĭs-tŏm'ĕ-lŭs) [" + *melos*, limb]
schistoprosopia (skĭs"tō-prō-sō'pē-ă) [" + *prosopon*, face]
schistorachis (skĭs-tor'ă-kĭs) [" + *rhachis*, spine]
Schistosoma (skĭs"tō-sō'mă) [" + *soma*, body]
  S. haematobium
  S. japonicum
  S. mansoni
schistosome dermatitis (skĭs'tō-sōm)
schistosomia (skĭs"tō-sō'mē-ă) [" + *soma*, body]
schistosomiasis (skĭs"tō-sō-mī'ăs-ĭs) [Gr. *schistos*, divided, + *soma*, body, + *-iasis*, state or condition of]
schistosomicide (skĭs"tō-sō'mĭ-sīd) [" + " + L. *caedere*, to kill]
schistosternia (skĭs"tō-stĕr'nē-ă) [" + *sternon*, chest]
schistothorax (skĭs"tō-thō'răks) [" + *thorax*, chest]
schistotrachelus (skĭs"tō-tră-kē'lŭs)
schizamnion (skĭz-ăm'nē-ŏn) [Gr. *schizein*, to split, + *amnion*, lamb]
schizaxon (skĭz-ăk'sŏn) [" + *axon*, axle]
schizencephaly (skĭz"ĕn-sĕf'ă-lē) [" + *enkephalos*, brain]
schizo- (skĭz'ō) [Gr. *schizein*, to split]
schizoblepharia (skĭz"ō-blĕf'ă-rē"ă) [" + *blepharon*, eyelid]
schizocyte (skĭz'ō-sīt) [" + *kytos*, cell]
schizocytosis (skĭz"ō-sī-tō'sĭs) [" + " + *osis*, condition]

schizogenesis (skīz″ō-jĕn′ĕs-īs) [″ + *genesis*, generation, birth]

schizogony (skīz-ŏg′ō-nē) [″ + *gone*, seed]

schizogyria (skīz″ō-jī′rē-ă) [″ + *gyros*, a circle]

schizoid (skīz′oyd) [″ + *eidos*, form, shape]

schizoid personality disorder

schizomycete (skīz″ō-mī-sēt′) [″ + *mykes*, fungus]

Schizomycetes (skīz″ō-mī-sē′tēz) [″ + *mykes*, fungus]

schizont (skīz′ŏnt) [″ + *ontos*, being]

schizonticide (skī-zŏn′tĭ-sīd) [″ + ″ + L. *caedere*, to kill]

schizonychia (skīz″ō-nĭk′ē-ă) [″ + *onyx*, nail]

schizophasia (skīz″ō-fā′zē-ă) [″ + *phasis*, utterance]

schizophrenia (schizophrenic disorders)
   s., catatonic
   s., disorganized
   s., paranoid
   s., undifferentiated

schizophrenic (skīz″ō-frĕn′ĭk) [Gr. *schizein*, to split, + *phren*, mind]

schizoprosopia (skīz″ō-prō-sō′pē-ă) [″ + *prosopon*, face]

schizotonia (skīz″ō-tō′nē-ă) [″ + *tonos*, act of stretching, tension, tone]

schizotrichia (skīz″ō-trĭk′ē-ă) [″ + *thrix*, hair]

schizozoite (skīz″ō-zō′ĭt) [″ + *zoon*, animal]

Schlatter-Osgood disease (shlăt′ĕr-ŏz′good)

Schlemm, canal of (shlĕm) [Friedrich S. Schlemm, Ger. anatomist, 1795–1858]

Schmorl's disease [Christian G. Schmorl, Ger. pathologist, 1861–1932]

Schmorl's nodules

schneiderian membrane (shnī-dē′rē-ăn) [Conrad Victor Schneider, Ger. physician, 1610–1680]

Schönlein's disease (shān′līnz) [Johann Lukas Schönlein, Ger. physician, 1793–1864]

Schönlein-Henoch purpura

school phobia

Schüffner's dots (shĭf′nĕrz) [Wilhelm P. A. Schüffner, Ger. pathologist, 1867–1949]

Schüller's disease

Schultz reaction [Werner Schultz, Ger. physician, 1878–1947]

Schultze's bundle (shooltz′ĕs) [Max Johann Schultze, Ger. biologist, 1825–1874]

Schultze's cells

Schultze's granule masses

Schwabach test (shvä′băk) [Dagobert Schwabach, Ger. otologist, 1846–1920]

Schwalbe's ring (shvăl′bĕz) [Gustav A. Schwalbe, Ger. anatomist, 1844–1917]

Schwann's cells (shvŏnz) [Theodor Schwann, Ger. anatomist, 1810–1882]

schwannoma (shwŏn-nō′mă)

schwannosis (shwŏn-nō′sĭs)

Schwann's sheath

Schwann's white substance

sciage (sē-äzh′) [Fr., a sawing]

sciatic (sī-ăt′ĭk) [L. *sciaticus*]

sciatica (sī-ăt′ĭ-kă) [L.]

sciatic nerve

sciatic nerve, small

science (sī′ĕns) [L. *scientia*, knowledge]
   s.'s, life

scieropia (sī-ĕr-ō′pē-ă) [Gr. *skieros*, shadow, + *opsis*, sight, appearance, vision]

scintigram (sĭn′tĭ-grăm)

scintillascope (sĭn-tĭl′ă-skōp) [L. *scintilla*, spark, + Gr. *skopein*, to examine]

scintillation (sĭn″tĭ-lā′shŭn) [L. *scintillatio*]

scintiphotography (sĭn″tĭ-fō-tŏg′ră-fē)

scintiscan (sĭn′tĭ-skăn)
scintiscanner (sĭn″tĭ-skăn′ĕr)
scirrho- [Gr. *skirrhos*, hard]
scirrhoid (skĭr′oyd) [″ + *eidos*, form, shape]
scirrhoma (skĭr-ō′mă) [″ + *oma*, tumor]
scirrhosarca (skĭr″ō-săr′kă) [″ + *sarx*, flesh]
scirrhous (skĭr′ŭs) [NL. *scirrhosus*, hard]
scirrhus (skĭr′ŭs) [Gr. *skirrhos*, hard tumor]
scission (sĭzh′ŭn) [L. *scindere*, to split]
scissor gait
scissor leg
scissors (sĭz′ors) [LL. *cisorium*]
scissura (sĭ-sū′ră) [L., to split]
sclera (sklĕr′ă) [Gr. *skleros*, hard]
   s., blue
scleradenitis (sklĕ″răd-ĕn-ī′tĭs) [″ + *aden*, gland, + *itis*, inflammation]
scleral (sklĕr′ăl) [Gr. *skleros*, hard]
scleratogenous (sklĕ″ră-tŏj′ĕ-nŭs)
sclerectasia (sklĕ″rĕk-tā′zē-ă) [″ + *ektasis*, dilatation]
sclerectoiridectomy (sklĕ-rĕk″tō-ĭr″ĭ-dĕk′tō-mē) [″ + *iris*, bend, turn, + *ektome*, excision]
sclerectoiridodialysis (sklĕ-rĕk″tō-ĭr″ĭd-ō-dī-ăl′ĭ-sĭs) [″ + ″ + *dia*, through, + *lysis*, dissolution]
sclerectomy (sklĕ-rĕk′tō-mē) [″ + *ektome*, excision]
scleredema (sklĕr″ĕ-dē′mă) [″ + *oidema*, swelling]
   s. adultorum
   s., Buschke's
   s. neonatorum
sclerema (sklĕ-rē′mă) [Gr. *skleros*, hard]
   s. adiposum
   s. adultorum
   s. neonatorum
sclerencephalia (sklĕ″rĕn-sĕ-fă′lē-ă) [″ + *enkephalos*, brain]
scleriasis (sklĕ-rī′ă-sĭs) [Gr. *skleriasis*]
scleriritomy (sklĕ-rĭ-rĭt′ō-mē) [″ + *iris*, bend, turn, + *tome*, a cutting, slice]

scleritis (sklĕ-rī′tĭs) [″ + *itis*, inflammation]
   s., annular
   s., anterior
   s., posterior
scleroblastema (sklĕ″rō-blăs-tē′mă) [Gr. *skleros*, hard, + *blastema*, sprout]
scleroblastemic (sklĕ″rō-blăs-tĕm′ĭk)
sclerocataracta (sklĕ″rō-kăt-ă-răk′tă) [″ + L. *cataracta*, waterfall]
sclerochoroiditis (sklĕ″rō-kō″royd-ī′tĭs) [″ + *chorioeides*, skinlike, + *itis*, inflammation]
   s., posterior
scleroconjunctival (sklĕ″rō-kŏn″jŭnk-tī′văl) [″ + L. *conjunctivus*, to bind together]
sclerocornea (sklĕ″rō-kor′nē-ă) [″ + L. *corneus*, horny]
sclerodactylia (sklĕr″ō-dăk-tĭl′ē-ă) [″ + *daktylos*, finger]
scleroderma (sklĕr″ă-dĕr′mă) [Gr. *skleros*, hard, + *derma*, skin]
   s., circumscribed
   s. neonatorum
sclerodermatitis (sklĕ″rō-dĕr-mă-tī′tĭs) [Gr. *skleros*, hard, + *derma*, skin, + *itis*, inflammation]
sclerodermatous (sklĕ″rō-dĕr′mă-tŭs) [″ + *derma*, skin]
sclerogenic (sklĕ″rō-jĕn′ĭk) [″ + *gennan*, to produce]
sclerogenous (sklĕ-rŏj′ĕ-nŭs) [″ + *gennan*, to produce]
scleroid (sklĕ′royd) [″ + *eidos*, form, shape]
scleroiritis (sklĕ″rō-ī-rī′tĭs) [″ + *iris*, bend, turn, + *itis*, inflammation]
sclerokeratitis (sklĕr″ō-kĕr-ă-tī′tĭs) [″ + *keras*, horn, + *itis*, inflammation]
sclerokeratoiritis (sklĕ″rō-kĕr″ă-tō-ī-rī′tĭs) [″ + ″ + *iris*, bend, turn, + *itis*, inflammation]
sclerokeratosis (sklĕr″ō-kĕr″ă-tō′sĭs) [″ + ″ + *osis*, condition]

scleroma (sklĕ-rō'mă) [" + oma, tumor]

scleromalacia (sklĕ"rō-mă-lā'shē-ă) [Gr. skleros, hard, + malakia, softening]

s. perforans

scleromere (sklĕr'ō-mēr) [" + meros, a part]

scleromyxedema (sklĕr"ō-mĭks"ĕ-dē'mă) [" + myxa, mucus, + oidema, swelling]

scleronychia (sklĕ"rō-nĭk'ē-ă) [" + onyx, nail]

scleronyxis (sklĕ-rō-nĭk'sĭs) [Gr. skleros, hard, + nyxis, a piercing]

sclero-oophoritis (sklĕ"rō-ō-ŏf"ō-rī'tĭs) [" + NL. oophoron, ovary, + Gr. itis, inflammation]

sclerophthalmia (sklĕ"rŏf-thăl'mē-ă) [" + ophthalmos, eye]

scleroplasty (sklĕ'rō-plăs"tē) [" + plassein, to form]

scleroprotein (sklĕ"rō-prō'tē-ĭn) [" + protos, first]

sclerosal (sklĕ-rō'săl)

sclerosant (sklĕ-rō'sănt) [Gr. skleros, hard]

sclerose (sklĕ-rōs') [Gr. skleros, hard]

sclerosed (sklĕ-rōsd', sklē'rōsd) [Gr. skleros, hard]

sclerosing (sklĕ-rōs'ĭng)

sclerosis (sklĕ-rō'sĭs) [Gr. sklerosis, a hardening]

s., Alzheimer's
s., amyotrophic lateral
s., annular
s., arterial
s., arteriolar
s., diffuse
s., disseminated
s., hyperplastic
s., insular
s., intimal
s., lateral
s., lobar
s., medial
s., multiple
s., neural

s., renal
s., tuberous
s., vascular
s., venous

scleroskeleton (sklĕr"ō-skĕl'ĕ-tŏn) [Gr. skleros, hard, + skeleton, a dried-up body]

sclerostenosis (sklĕr"ō-stĕ-nō'sĭs) [" + stenosis, act of narrowing]

s. cutanea

sclerostomy (sklĕ-rŏs'tō-mē) [" + stoma, mouth, opening]

sclerotherapy (sklĕr"ō-thĕr'ă-pē) [" + therapeia, treatment]

sclerothrix (sklĕr'ō-thrĭks) [" + thrix, hair]

sclerotic (sklĕ-rŏt'ĭk) [L. scleroticus, hard]

sclerotica (sklĕ-rŏt'ĭ-kă) [L. scleroticus, hard]

sclerotic acid

sclerotic dentin

scleroticectomy (sklĕ-rŏt"ĭ-sĕk'tō-mē) [" + Gr. ektome, excision]

scleroticochoroiditis (sklĕ-rŏt"ĭ-kō-kō"roy-dī'tĭs) [" + Gr. chorioeides, skinlike, + itis, inflammation]

scleroticonyxis (sklĕ-rŏt"ĭ-kō-nĭk'sĭs) [" + Gr. nyxis, a piercing]

scleroticopuncture (sklĕ-rŏt"ĭ-kō-pŭnk'tŭr) [" + punctura, prick]

scleroticotomy (sklĕ-rŏt"ĭ-kŏt'ō-mē) [" + Gr. tome, a cutting, slice]

sclerotic teeth

sclerotitis (sklĕr-ō-tī'tĭs) [Gr. skleros, hard, + itis, inflammation]

sclerotium (sklĕ-rō'shē-ŭm)

sclerotome (sklĕr'ō-tōm) [" + tome, a cutting, slice]

sclerotomy (sklĕ-rŏt'ō-mē)

s., anterior
s., posterior

sclerotrichia (sklĕ-rō-trĭk'ē-ă) [Gr. sclerosis, hard, + thrix, hair]

sclerous (sklĕr'ŭs)

scobinate (skō'bĭn-āt) [L. scobina, rasp]

scoleciasis (skō-lĕ-sī'ă-sĭs) [Gr. skolex, worm, + -iasis, state or condition of]

scoleciform (skō-lĕs'ĭ-form) [" + L. *forma*, form]

scolecoid (skō'lĕ-koyd) [" + *eidos*, form, shape]

scolecology (skō"lĕ-kŏl'ō-jē) [" + *logos*, word, reason]

scolex (skō'lĕks) [Gr. *skolex*, worm]

scoliokyphosis (skō"lē-ō-kī-fō'sīs) [Gr. *skolios*, twisted, + *kyphosis*, humpback]

scoliometer (skō"lē-ŏm'ĕt-ĕr) [" + *metron*, measure]

scoliorachitic (skō"lē-ō-rǎ-kĭt'ĭk) [" + *rhachis*, spine]

scoliosiometry (skō"lē-ō-sē-ŏm'ĕ-trē) [" + *metron*, measure]

scoliosis (skō"lē-ō'sīs) [Gr. *skoliosis*, crookedness]
　　s., cicatricial
　　s., congenital
　　s., coxitic
　　s., empyematic
　　s., habit
　　s., inflammatory
　　s., ischiatic
　　s., myopathic
　　s., ocular
　　s., osteopathic
　　s., paralytic
　　s., rachitic
　　s., rheumatic
　　s., sciatic
　　s., static

scoliosometry (skō"lē-ō-sŏm'ĕt-rē) [" + *metron*, measure]

scoliotic (skō-lē-ŏt'ĭk)

scoliotone (skō'lē-ō-tōn) [Gr. *skolios*, twisted, + *tonos*, act of stretching, tension, tone]

scombrine (skŏm'brĭn)

scombroid

scombroid poisoning

scoop (skoop) [ME., a ladle]
　　s., bone
　　s., bullet
　　s., cataract
　　s., ear
　　s., lithotomy

　　s., mastoid
　　s., renal

scoparius (skō-pā'rē-ŭs)

-scope [Gr. *skopein*, to examine]

scopolamine hydrobromide (skō-pŏl'ǎ-mēn hī"drō-brō'mĭd)

scopometer (skō-pŏm'ĕ-tĕr) [Gr. *skopein*, to examine, + *metron*, measure]

scopophilia (skō"pō-fĭl'ē-ǎ) [" + *philein*, to love]

scopophobia (skō"pō-fō'bē-ǎ) [" + *phobos*, fear]

scopophobiac (skō"pō-fō'bē-ǎk)

-scopy [Gr. *skopein*, to examine]

scoracratia (skor"ǎ-krā'shē-ǎ) [Gr. *skor*, dung, + *akratia*, lack of control]

scorbutic (skor-bū'tĭk) [NL. *scorbuticus*, scurvy]

scorbutigenic (skor-bū"tĭ-jĕn'ĭk) [LL. *scorbutus*, scurvy, + Gr. *gennan*, to produce]

scorbutus (skor-bū'tŭs) [LL., scurvy]

scordinema (skor-dĭ-nē'mǎ) [Gr. *skordinema*, yawning]

score (skor)
　　s., Apgar

scoretemia (skor-ē-tē'mē-ǎ) [Gr. *skor*, dung, + *haima*, blood]

scorpion (skor'pē-ŏn) [Gr. *skorpios*, to cut off]

scorpion sting

scoto- (skō'tō) [Gr. *skotos*, darkness]

scotochromogen (skō"tō-krō'mō-jĕn) [" + *chroma*, color, + *gennan*, to produce]

scotodinia (skō"tō-dĭn'ē-ǎ) [" + *dinos*, whirling]

scotogram, scotograph (skō'tō-grăm, -grăf) [" + *gramma*, letter, piece of writing; " + *graphein*, to write]

scotoma (skō-tō'mǎ) [Gr. *skotoma*, to darken]
　　s., absolute
　　s., annular
　　s., arcuate

s., central
s., centrocecal
s., color
s., eclipse
s., flittering
s., negative
s., peripheral
s., physiological
s., positive
s., relative
s., ring
s., scintillating
scotomagraph (skō-tō'mă-grăf) [Gr. *skotoma*, to darken, + *graphein*, to write]
scotomata (skō-tō'mă-tă) [Gr.]
scotomatous (skō-tŏm'ă-tŭs) [Gr. *skotoma*, to darken]
scotometer (skō-tŏm'ĕt-ĕr) [" + *metron*, a measure]
scotometry (skō-tŏm'ĕ-trē)
scotomization (skō"tō-mĭ-zā'shŭn) [Gr. *skotoma*, to darken]
scotophilia (skō"tō-fĭl'ē-ă) [" + *philein*, to love]
scotophobia (skō"tō-fō'bē-ă) [" + *phobos*, fear]
scotopia (skō-tō'pē-ă) [" + *ops*, eye]
scotopic (skō-tŏp'ĭk)
scotopic vision
scotopsin (skō-tŏp'sīn)
scotoscopy (skō-tŏs'kō-pē) [Gr. *skotos*, darkness, + *skopein*, to examine]
scout film
scr. *scruple*
scratch (skrăch) [ME. *cracchen*, to scratch]
scratch test
screatus (skrē-ā'tŭs) [L., a hawking]
screen [O. Fr. *escren*]
s., Bjerrum [P. J. Bjerrum, Danish ophthalmologist, 1827–1872]
s., fluorescent
s., intensifying
s., tangent
screening
s., multiphasic

Scribner shunt [Belding Scribner, U.S. physician, b. 1921]
scrobiculate (skrō-bĭk'ū-lāt) [L. *scrobiculus*, little trench]
scrobiculus (skrō-bĭk'ū-lŭs) [L., little trench]
s. cordis
scrofula (skrŏf'ū-lă) [L., breeding sow]
scrofulid(e) (skrŏf'ū-lĭd, -lĭd)
scrofuloderma (skrŏf"ū-lō-dĕr'mă) [L. *scrofula*, breeding sow, + Gr. *derma*, skin]
scrofulosis (skrŏf"ū-lō'sĭs) [" + Gr. *osis*, condition]
scrofulous (skrŏf'ū-lŭs) [L. *scrofula*, breeding sow]
scrotal (skrō'tăl) [L. *scrotum*, a bag]
scrotal reflex
scrotectomy (skrō-tĕk'tō-mē) [" + Gr. *ektome*, excision]
scrotitis [" + Gr. *itis*, inflammation]
scrotocele (skrō'tō-sēl) [" + Gr. *kele*, tumor, swelling]
scrotoplasty (skrō'tō-plăs"tē) [" + Gr. *plassein*, to form]
scrotum (skrō'tŭm) [L., a bag]
scrubbing [MD. *schrubben*]
scrub nurse
scrub typhus
scruple (skrū'pl) [L. *scrupulus*, small, sharp stone]
Scultetus bandage (skŭl-tē'tŭs) [Johann Schultes (Scultetus), Ger. surgeon, 1595–1645]
Scultetus position
scum (skŭm) [ME. *scume*]
scurf [AS. *scurf*]
scurvy (skŭr'vē) [L. *scorbutus*]
s., infantile
scute (skūt) [L. *scutum*, shield]
scutiform (skū'tĭ-form) [" + *forma*, shape]
scutular (skū'tū-lăr) [L. *scutulum*, a little shield]
scutulum (skū'tū-lŭm) [L., a little shield]
scutum (skū'tŭm) [L., shield]
scybalous (sĭb'ă-lŭs) [Gr. *skybalon*, dung]

scybalum (sĭb'ă-lŭm)
scypho- [Gr. *skyphos*, cup]
scyphoid (sī'foyd) [" + *eidos*, form, shape]
S.D. *skin dose; standard deviation*
SDA *specific dynamic action;* [L.] *sacro-dextra anterior*
S.E. *standard error*
Se *selenium*
seabather's eruption
seal
 s., border
 s., posterior palatal
 s., velopharyngeal
sealant
 s., dental
 s., pit and fissure
seal finger
searcher (sĕrch'ĕr) [ME. *serchen*]
seasickness [AS. *sae*, sea, + *seocness*, illness]
seasonal affective disorder
seat
 s., basal
 s., rest
Seattle foot [after the city Seattle, Washington, U.S., where it was developed]
seatworm
sebaceous (sĕ-bā'shŭs) [L. *sebaceus*, made of tallow]
sebaceous cyst
sebaceous gland
sebastomania (sĕ-băs"tō-mā'nē-ă) [Gr. *sebastos*, reverend, + *mania*, madness]
sebiferous (sĕ-bĭf'ĕr-ŭs) [L. *sebum*, tallow, + *ferre*, to carry]
sebiparous (sĕ-bĭp'ă-rŭs) [" + *parere*, to beget, produce]
sebolite, sebolith (sĕb'ō-līt, -lĭth) [" + Gr. *lithos*, a stone]
seborrhagia (sĕb"ō-rā'jē-ă) [" + Gr. *rhegnynai*, to burst forth]
seborrhea (sĕb-or-ē'ă) [" + Gr. *rhein*, to flow]
 s. capiti
 s. congestiva

 s. corporis
 s. faciei
 s. furfuracea
 s. nigricans
 s. oleosa
 s. sicca
seborrheic (sĕb"ō-rē'ĭk) [L. *sebum*, tallow, + Gr. *rhein*, to flow]
seborrheid (sĕb"ō-rē'ĭd) [" + Gr. *rhein*, to flow]
seborrhoic (sĕb"ō-rō'ĭk)
sebum (sē'bŭm) [L., tallow]
 s. palpebrale
secernent (sē-sĕr'nĕnt) [L. *secernens*, secreting]
seclusion of pupil
seclusio pupillae siderosis bulbi
secobarbital
 s. sodium
secodont (sē'kō-dŏnt) [L. *secare*, to cut, + Gr. *odous*, tooth]
Seconal
Seconal Sodium
secondary
secondary areola
secondary care
secondary gain
secondary hemorrhage
secondary nursing care
secondary radiation
second cranial nerve
second intention
second sight
second stage of labor
second wind
secreta (sē-krē'tă) [L.]
secretagogue (sē-krē'tă-gŏg) [L. *secretum*, secretion, + Gr. *agogos*, leading]
secrete (sē-krēt') [L. *secretio*, separation]
secretin (sē-krē'tĭn)
secretinase (sē-krē'tĭ-năs)
secretion [L. *secretio*, separation]
 s., apocrine
 s., external
 s., holocrine
 s., internal

s., merocrine
s., paralytic
secretogogue (sē-krē′tō-gŏg) [L. se-cretio, separation, + Gr. agogos, leading]
secretoinhibitory (sē-krē″tō-ĭn-hĭb′ĭ-tō″rē)
secretomotor (sē-krē″tō-mō′tor)
secretor (sē-krē′tor) [L. secretio, separation]
secretory (sē-krē′tō-rē, sē′krē-tō″rē)
secretory capillaries
secretory fibers
sectarian (sĕk-tā′rē-ăn) [L. sectus, having cut]
sectile (sĕk′tĭl) [L. sectilis]
sectio (sĕk′shē-ō) [L., a cutting]
section [L. sectio, a cutting]
    s., abdominal
    s., cesarean
    s., cesarean, postmortem
    s., coronal
    s., frontal
    s., frozen
    s., midsagittal
    s., paraffin
    s., perineal
    s., Pitres'
    s., sagittal
    s., serial
    s., vaginal
sectioning [L. sectio, a cutting]
    s., ultrathin
sector (sĕk′tor) [L., cutter]
sectorial (sĕk-tō′rē-ăl)
secundigravida (sē-kŭn″dĭ-grăv′ĭd-ă) [L. secundus, second, + gravida, pregnant]
secundina (sē″kŭn-dī′nă) [L. from secundinus, following]
secundines (sĕk′ŭn-dĭnz, sĭ-kŭn′dĭnz) [LL. secundinae]
secundipara (sē″kŭn-dĭp′ă-ră) [L. secundus, second, + parere, to beget, produce]
secundiparity (sē-kŭn″dĭ-păr′ĭ-tē)
secundum artem (sē-kŭn′dŭm ăr′tĕm) [L.]

S.E.D. skin erythema dose
sedation (sē-dā′shŭn) [L. sedatio, from sedare, to calm]
sedative (sĕd′ă-tĭv) [L. sedativus, calming]
    s., cardiac
    s., nervous
sedentary (sĕd′ĕn-tā′rē) [L. sedentarius]
sedentary living
sediment (sĕd′ĭ-mĕnt) [L. sedimentum, a settling]
    s., urinary
sedimentation (sĕd″ĭ-mĕn-tā′shŭn)
sedimentation rate
sedimentator (sĕd″ĭ-mĕn-tā′tor)
seed (sēd) [AS. saed]
Seessel's pouch (zā′sĕlz) [Albert Seessel, U.S. embryologist and neurologist, 1850–1910]
segment (sĕg′mĕnt) [L. segmentum, a portion]
    s., bronchopulmonary
    s.'s, hepatic
    s., interannular
    s., mesodermal
    s.'s, uterine
segmental (sĕg-mĕn′tăl)
segmental reflex
segmental static reactions
segmentation (sĕg″mĕn-tā′shŭn) [L. segmentum, a portion]
    s., rhythmic
segmenter
segmentum (sĕg-mĕn′tŭm) [L.]
segregation [L. segregare, to separate]
segregator
Séguin's signal symptom (sā-gănz′) [Edouard Séguin, 1812–1880]
SeHCAT
Seidlitz powder (sĕd′lĭts, sīd′lĭtz) [Seidlitz, village in Bohemia]
seisesthesia (sīz″ĕs-thē′zē-ă) [Gr. seisis, concussion, + aisthesis, feeling, perception]
seismesthesia (sīz″mĕs-thē′zē-ă)[Gr. seismos, a shaking, + aisthesis,

feeling, perception]
seizure (sē'zhūr) [O. Fr. *seisir*, to take
possession of]
   s., absence
   s., convulsive
   s., grand mal
   s., jacksonian
   s., petit mal
Seldinger technique
selection [L. *selectus*, having chosen]
   s., artificial
   s., natural
   s., sexual
selenium (sē-lē'nē-ŭm) [Gr. *selene*,
moon]
   s. sulfide
selenoid cells
selenomethionine Se 75 injection
   (sĕl"ĕn-ō-mĕ-thī'ō-nēn)
self
self-acceptance
self-conscious
self-defeating personality disorder
self-differentiation
self-digestion
self-hypnosis
self-infection
self-limited disease
self-tolerance
sellar (sĕl'ăr)
sella turcica (sĕl'ă tŭr'sĭ-kă) [NL., Turkish saddle]
Selsun
Selsun Blue
seltzer water
semantics (sē-măn'tĭks) [Gr. *seman-
tikos*, significant]
semeiography (sē"mē-ŏg'ră-fē) [Gr.
semeion, sign, + *graphein*, to
write]
semeiology (sē"mī-ŏl'ō-jē) [" +
logos, word, reason]
semeiotics (sē"mī-ŏt'ĭks)
semelincident (sĕm"ĕl-ĭn'sĭ-dĕnt) [L.
semel, once, + *incidens*, falling
upon]
semen (sē'mĕn) [L., seed]
   s., frozen

semenarche (sē'mĕn-ăr"kē) [" +
arche, beginning]
semenuria (sē"mĕn-ū'rē-ă) [L. *semen*,
seed, + Gr. *ouron*, urine]
semi- [L. *semis*, half]
semicanal (sĕm"ē-kăn-ăl') [" +
canalis, channel]
semicanalis (sĕm"ē-kă-nā'lĭs) [L., semi-
canal]
   s. musculi tensoris tympani
   s. tubae auditivae
semicartilaginous (sĕm"ē-kăr"tĭ-lăj'ĭ-
nŭs) [" + *cartilago*, gristle]
semicircular (sĕm"ē-sŭr'kū-lăr) [" +
circulus, a ring]
semicircular canals
semicoma (sĕm"ē-kō'mă) [" + Gr.
koma, deep sleep]
semicomatose (sĕm"ē-kō'măt-ōs)
semicrista (sĕm"ē-krĭs'tă) [L.]
   s. incisiva
semidecussation (sĕm"ē-dē"kŭs-
sā'shŭn) [" + *decussare*, to make
an X]
semierection (sĕm"ē-ē-rĕk'shŭn)
[" + *erigere*, to erect]
semiflexion (sĕm"ē-flĕk'shŭn) [" +
flexio, bending]
semi-Fowler's position
semilunar (sĕm"ē-lū'năr) [L. *semis*, half,
+ *luna*, moon]
semilunar bone
semilunar cartilages
semilunar cusps
semilunare (sĕm"ē-lū-nā'rē) [L.]
semilunar ganglion
semilunar line
semilunar lobe
semilunar notch
semilunar valves
semiluxation (sĕm"ē-lŭk-sā'shŭn)
[" + *luxatio*, dislocation]
semimembranous (sĕm"ē-mĕm'bră-
nŭs) [" + L. *membrana*, membrane]
semimembranosus (sĕm"ē-mĕm"
brăn-ō'sŭs) [L.]
seminal (sĕm'ĭ-năl) [L. *seminalis*]
seminal duct

seminal emission
seminal fluid
seminal vesicle
semination (sĕm-ĭ-nā′shŭn) [L. *semina-tio*, a begetting]
  s., artificial
seminiferous (sĕm-ĭn-ĭf′ĕr-ŭs) [L. *semen*, seed, + *ferre*, to produce]
seminoma (sĕm″ĭ-nō′mă) [″ + Gr. *oma*, tumor]
seminormal (sĕm″ē-nor′măl) [L. *semis*, half, + *norma*, rule]
seminormal solution
seminose (sĕm′ĭ-nōs)
seminuria (sē″mĭn-ū′rē-ă) [L. *semen*, seed, + Gr. *ouron*, urine]
semiology (sē″mē-ŏl′ō-jē) [Gr. *semeion*, sign, + *logos*, word, reason]
semiorbicular (sĕm″ē-or-bĭk′ū-lăr) [L. *semis*, half, + *orbiculus*, a small circle]
semiotic (sē″mē-ŏt′ĭk) [Gr. *semeiotikos*]
semiotics (sē″mē-ŏt′ĭks)
semipenniform (sĕm″ē-pĕn′ĭ-form) [L. *semis*, half, + *penna*, feather, + *forma*, shape]
semipermeable (sĕm″ē-per′mē-ă-bl) [″ + *per*, through, + *meare*, to pass]
semipronation (sĕm″ē-prō-nā′shŭn) [″ + *pronus*, prone]
semiprone (sĕm-ē-prōn′) [″ + *pronus*, prone]
semirecumbent (sĕm″ē-rĭ-kŭm′bĕnt) [″ + *recumbere*, to lie down]
semis (sē′mĭs) [L.]
semisideratio,   semisideration (sĕm″ē-sĭd-ĕr-ā′shē-ō, -ā′shŭn) [″ + *sideratio*, a blight]
semisopor (sĕm″ē-sō′por) [″ + *sopor*, deep sleep]
semispinalis (sĕm″ē-spī-nāl′ĭs) [L.]
semisulcus (sĕm″ē-sŭl′kŭs) [L. *semis*, half, + *sulcus*, groove]
semisupination (sĕm″ē-sū-pĭn-ā′shŭn) [″ + *supinus*, lying on the back]
semisupine (sĕm″ē-sū′pīn) [″ + *su-*

pinus, lying on the back]
semisynthetic (sĕm″ē-sĭn-thĕt′ĭk) [″ + Gr. *synthetikos*, synthetic]
semitendinosus (sĕm″ē-tĕn″dĭn-ō′sŭs) [L.]
semitendinous (sĕm″ē-tĕn′dĭ-nŭs) [L. *semis*, half, + *tendinosus*, tendinous]
senescence (sē-nĕs′ĕns) [L. *senescens*, growing old]
Sengstaken-Blakemore   tube (sĕngz′tā-kĕn-blāk′mor) [Robert W. Sengstaken, U.S. neurosurgeon, b. 1923; Arthur H. Blakemore, U.S. surgeon, 1897–1970]
senile (sē′nĭl, sĕn′ĭl) [L. *senilis*, old]
senilism (sē′nĭl-ĭzm, -nĭl-ĭzm) [″ + Gr. *-ismos*, condition]
senility (sē-nĭl′ĭ-tē) [L. *senilis*, old]
  s., premature
  s., psychosis of
senium (sē′nē-ŭm) [L.]
senna (sĕn′ă) [Arabic *sana*]
sennosides (sĕn′ō-sīdz)
senopia (sĕn-ō′pē-ă, sē-nō′-) [L. *senilis*, old, + Gr. *ops*, eye]
sensation (sĕn-sā′shŭn) [L. *sensatio*]
  s., cincture
  s., cutaneous
  s., delayed
  s., epigastric
  s., external
  s., girdle
  s., gnostic
  s., internal
  s., palmesthetic
  s., primary
  s., proprioceptive
  s., referred
  s., reflex
  s., somesthetic
  s., subjective
  s., tactile
sense (sĕns) [L. *sensus*, feeling, sensation, understanding]
  s., color
  s., kinesthetic
  s., light

s., muscular
s., posture
s., pressure
s., proprioception
s., sixth
s., space
s.'s, special
s., static
s., stereognostic
s., temperature
s., time
s., tone
s., visceral
sensibility (sĕn″sĭ-bĭl′ĭ-tē) [L. *sensibilitas*]
s., deep
s., mesoblastic
s., palmesthetic
sensibilization (sĕn″sĭ-bĭl-īz-ā′shŭn)
sensible (sĕn′sĭ-bl) [L. *sensibilis*, capable of being perceived]
sensiferous (sĕn-sĭf′ĕr-ŭs) [L. *sensus*, feeling, sensation, understanding, + *ferre*, to bear]
sensigenous (sĕn-sĭj′ĕn-ŭs) [" + Gr. *gennan*, to produce]
sensimeter (sĕn-sĭm′ĕ-tĕr) [" + Gr. *metron*, measure]
sensitinogen (sĕn″sĭ-tĭn′ō-jĕn) [" + Gr. *gennan*, to produce]
sensitive (sĕn′sĭ-tĭv) [L. *sensitivus*, of sensation]
sensitivity
sensitivity tests, antimicrobial
sensitivity training
sensitization (sĕn″sĭ-tĭ-zā′shŭn)
s., active
s., autoerythrocyte
s., passive
s., protein
sensitized (sĕn′sĭ-tīzd)
sensitized vaccine
sensitizer (sĕn′sĭ-tī″zĕr) [L. *sensitivus*, of sensation]
sensitometer (sĕn″sĭ-tŏm′ĕt-ĕr) [" + Gr. *metron*, a measure]
sensomobile (sĕn″sō-mō′bĭl) [L. *sensus*, feeling, sensation, understanding, + *mobilis*, mobile]
sensomobility (sĕn″sō-mō-bĭl′ĭ-tē) [" + *mobilitas*, mobility]
sensomotor
sensorial (sĕn-sō′rē-ăl) [L. *sensorialis*]
sensoriglandular (sĕn″sō-rē-glănd′dū-lăr) [L. *sensus*, feeling, sensation, understanding, + *glandula*, little acorn]
sensorimetabolism (sĕn″sō-rē-mĕ-tăb′ō-lĭzm) [" + Gr. *metabole*, change, + *-ismos*, condition]
sensorimotor (sĕn″sō-rē-mō′tor) [L. *sensus*, feeling, sensation, understanding, + *motus*, moving]
sensorimuscular (sĕn″sō-rē-mŭs′kū-lăr) [" + *muscularis*, muscular]
sensorineural (sĕn″sō-rē-nū′ral) [" + *neuralis*, neural]
sensorium (sĕn-sor′ē-ŭm) [L., organ of sensation]
sensorivasomotor (sĕn″sō-rē-văs″ō-mō′tor) [L. *sensus*, feeling, sensation, understanding, + *vas*, vessel, + *motor*, a mover]
sensory (sĕn′sō-rē) [L. *sensorius*]
sensory amusia
sensory aphasia
sensory area
s.a., somesthetic
sensory deprivation
sensory ending
sensory epilepsy
sensory integration
sensory nerve
sensory unit
sensual (sĕn′shū-ăl) [L. *sensus*, feeling, sensation, understanding]
sensualism (sĕn′shū-ăl-īzm)
sensuous (sĕn′shū-ŭs) [L. *sensus*, feeling, sensation, understanding]
sentient (sĕn′shē-ĕnt) [L. *sentiens*, perceive]
sentiment (sĕn′tĭ-mĕnt) [L. *sentio*, to feel]
sentinel gland
sentinel node
separation

separator [LL. *separator*]
separatorium (sĕp″ă-rā-tō′rē-ŭm) [L.]
sepsis (sĕp′sĭs) [Gr., putrefaction]
 s., puerperal
septa (sĕp′tă) [L. *saeptum*, a partition]
septal (sĕp′tăl) [L. *saeptum*, a partition]
septan (sĕp′tăn) [L. *septem*, seven]
septate (sĕp′tāt) [L. *saeptum*, a partition]
septectomy (sĕp-tĕk′tō-mē) [″ + Gr. *ektome*, excision]
septemia (sĕp-tē′mē-ă)
septic (sĕp′tĭk) [Gr. *septikos*, putrefying]
septicemia (sĕp-tĭ-sē′mē-ă) [″ + *haima*, blood]
 s., bronchopulmonary
 s., cryptogenic
 s., fungal
 s., puerperal
septicemic (sĕp-tĭ-sē′mĭk)
septic fever
septicophlebitis (sĕp″tĭ-kō-flĕ-bī′tĭs) [Gr. *septikos*, putrefying, + *phleps*, blood vessel, vein, + *itis*, inflammation]
septicopyemia (sĕp″tĭ-kō-pī-ē′mē-ă) [″ + *pyon*, pus, + *haima*, blood]
septic shock
septic sore throat
septigravida (sĕp″tĭ-grăv′ĭ-dă) [L. *septem*, seven, + *gravida*, pregnant]
septimetritis (sĕp″tĭ-mē-trī′tĭs) [Gr. *septos*, putrid, + *metra*, uterus, + *itis*, inflammation]
septipara (sĕp-tĭp′ă-ră) [L. *septem*, seven, + *parere*, to beget, produce]
septivalent (sĕp-tĭ-vā′lĕnt, -tĭv′ă-lĕnt) [″ + *valere*, to be strong]
septomarginal (sĕp″tō-măr′jĭ-năl) [L. *saeptum*, a partition, + *marginalis*, border]
septometer (sĕp-tŏm′ĕ-ter) [L. *saeptum*, a partition, + Gr. *metron*, measure; Gr. *sepsis*, decay, + *metron*, measure]
septonasal (sĕp-tō-nā′zăl) [L. *saep-*

tum, a partition, + *nasus*, nose]
septoplasty (sĕp″tō-plăs′tē) [″ + Gr. *plassein*, to form]
septostomy (sĕp-tŏs′tō-mē) [″ + Gr. *stoma*, mouth, opening]
septotome (sĕp′tō-tōm) [″ + Gr. *tome*, a cutting, slice]
septotomy (sĕp-tŏt′ō-mē) [″ + Gr. *tome*, a cutting, slice]
septula (sĕp-tū′lă) [L.]
 s. testis
septulum (sĕp′tū-lŭm) [L.]
septum (sĕp′tŭm) [L. *saeptum*, a partition]
 s., atrial
 s. atriorum cordis
 s., atrioventricular
 s., crural
 s., femoral
 s., interatrial
 s., interdental
 s., intermuscular
 s., interradicular
 s., interventricular
 s., lingual
 s. lucidum
 s., mediastinal
 s., nasal
 s., orbital
 s. pectiniforme
 s. pellucidum
 s. primum
 s., rectovaginal
 s., rectovesical
 s. scroti
 s., ventricular
septuplet (sĕp-tŭp′lĕt) [L. *septuplus*, sevenfold]
sequel (sē′kwĕl) [L. *sequela*, sequel]
sequela (sē-kwē′lă) [L., sequel]
sequence (sē′kwĕns) [L.]
sequester (sē-kwĕs′tĕr) [L. *sequestrare*, to separate]
sequestra (sē-kwĕs′tră) [L.]
sequestral (sē-kwĕs′trăl)
sequestration (sē″kwĕs-trā′shŭn) [L. *sequestratio*, a separation]
 s., pulmonary

sequestrectomy (sē"kwĕs-trĕk'tō-mē) [" + Gr. *ektome*, excision]

sequestrotomy (sē"kwĕs-trŏt'ō-mē) [" + Gr. *tome*, a cutting, slice]

sequestrum (sē-kwĕs'trŭm) [L., something set aside]

sera (sē'rä) [L.]

seralbumin (sĕr-ăl-bū'mĭn) [L. *serum*, whey, + *albumen*, white of egg]

Serax

serendipity (sĕr"ĕn-dĭp'ĭ-tē)

serial (sē'rē-ăl) [L. *series*, row, chain]

serial sevens test

sericeps (sĕr'ĭ-sĕps) [L. *sericus*, silken, + *caput*, head]

series (sĕr'ēz) [L. *series*, row, chain]
   s., aliphatic
   s., aromatic
   s., erythrocytic
   s., fatty
   s., granulocytic
   s., homologous
   s., leukocytic
   s., monocytic
   s., thrombocytic

serine

seriscission (sĕr-ĭ-sĕsh'ŭn) [L. *sericum*, silk, + *scindere*, to cut]

sero- [L.]

seroalbuminuria (sē"rō-ăl-bū"mĭn-ū'rē-ă) [L. *serum*, whey, + *albumen*, white of egg, + Gr. *ouron*, urine]

serocolitis (sē"rō-kō-lī'tĭs) [" + Gr. *kolon*, colon, + *itis*, inflammation]

seroconversion

seroculture (sē'rō-kŭl-chūr) [L. *serum*, whey, + *cultura*, tillage]

serocystic (sē"rō-sĭs'tĭk) [" + Gr. *kystis*, bladder, sac]

serodermatosis (sē"rō-der-mă-tō'sĭs) [" + Gr. *derma*, skin, + *osis*, condition]

serodiagnosis (sē"rō-dī-ăg-nō'sĭs) [" + Gr. *dia*, through, + *gnosis*, knowledge]

seroenteritis (sē"rō-ĕn-tĕr-ī'tĭs) [" + Gr. *enteron*, intestine, + *itis*, inflammation]

seroepidemiology (sē-rō-ĕp"ĭ-dē-mē-ŏl'ō-jē) [" + *epi*, upon, + *demos*, people, + *logos*, word, reason]

serofast (sē'rō-făst")

serofibrinous (sē"rō-fī'brĭn-ŭs) [" + *fibra*, fiber]

serofibrous (sē"rō-fī'brŭs) [" + *fibra*, fiber]

seroflocculation (sē"rō-flŏk"ū-lā'shŭn) [" + *flocculus*, little tuft]

serohepatitis (sē"rō-hĕp-ă-tī'tĭs) [" + Gr. *hepar*, liver, + *itis*, inflammation]

seroimmunity (sē"rō-ĭ-mū'nĭ-tē) [" + *immunitas*, immunity]

serolipase (sē"rō-lĭp'ās) [" + Gr. *lipos*, fat, + *ase*, enzyme]

serologic, serological (sē-rō-lŏj'ĭk, -ăl) [" + Gr. *logos*, word, reason]

serologist (sē-rŏl'ō-jĭst) [" + Gr. *logos*, word, reason]

serology (sē-rŏl'ō-jē) [" + Gr. *logos*, word, reason]

serolysin (sē-rŏl'ĭs-ĭn) [" + Gr. *lysis*, dissolution]

seroma (sĕr-ō'mă) [" + Gr. *oma*, tumor]

seromembranous (sē"rō-mĕm'brăn-ŭs) [" + *membrana*, membrane]

seromucous (sē"rō-mū'kŭs) [" + *mucus*, mucus]

seromuscular (sē"rō-mŭs'kū-lăr) [" + *muscularis*, muscular]

seronegative (sē"rō-nĕg'ă-tĭv)

seroperitoneum (sē"rō-pĕr"ĭ-tō-nē'ŭm) [" + Gr. *peritonaion*, stretched around or over]

seropositive (sē"rō-pŏz'ĭ-tĭv)

seroprevention

seroprognosis (sē"rō-prŏg-nō'sĭs) [" + Gr. *pro*, before, + *gnosis*, knowledge]

seroprophylaxis (sē"rō-prō-fĭ-lăks'ĭs) [" + Gr. *prophylatikos*, guarding]

seropurulent (sē"rō-pūr'ŭ-lĕnt) [" + *purulentus*, full of pus]

seropus (sē″rō-pŭs′) [″ + pus, pus]
seroreaction (sē″rō-rē-ăk′shŭn) [″ + re, back, + actio, action]
seroresistance (sē″rō-rē-zĭs′tăns)
seroresistant (sē″rō-rē-zĭs′tănt)
serosa (sē-rō′sǎ) [L. serum, whey]
serosamucin (sē-rō″sǎ-mū′sĭn) [L. serosus, serous, + mucus, mucus]
serosanguineous (sē″rō-săn-gwĭn′ē-ŭs) [L. serum, whey, + sanguineus, bloody]
seroserous (sē″rō-sē′rŭs) [L. serosus, serous, + serum, whey]
serositis (sē″rō-sī′tĭs) [″ + Gr. itis, inflammation]
serosity (sē-rŏs′ĭ-tē) [Fr. serosite]
serosynovial (sē″rō-sĭ-nō′vē-ăl) [L. serum, whey, + synovia, joint fluid]
serosynovitis (sē″rō-sĭn″ō-vī′tĭs) [″ + synovia, joint fluid, + Gr. itis, inflammation]
serotherapy (sē″rō-thĕr′ǎ-pē) [″ + Gr. therapeia, treatment]
serotonin (sĕr″ō-tōn′ĭn)
serotype (sē′rō-tīp)
serous (sĕr′ŭs) [L. serosus]
serous cavity
serous cell
serous effusion
serous exudate
serous fluids
serous glands
serous inflammation
serous membrane
serovaccination
serovar
serozymogenic (sē″rō-zī″mō-jĕn′ĭk) [L. serum, whey, + Gr. zyme, ferment, + gennan, to produce]
serpiginous (sĕr-pĭj′ĭ-nŭs) [L. serpere, to creep]
serrate (sĕr′āt) [L. serratus, toothed]
Serratia (sĕr-ā′shē-ǎ) [Serafino Serrati, 18th-century It. physicist]
     S. marcescens
serration (sĕr-ā′shŭn) [L. serratio, a notching]
serratus muscle

serrefine (sār-fēn′) [Fr.]
serrenoeud (sār-nŭd′) [Fr. serrer, to squeeze, + noeud, knot]
serrulate (sĕr′ū-lāt) [L. serrulatus]
Sertoli's cells (sĕr-tō′lēz) [Enrico Sertoli, It. histologist, 1842 – 1910]
serum (sē′rŭm) [L., whey]
     s. albumin
     s., anticrotalus
     s., antidiphtheritic
     s., antilymphocytic
     s., antimeningococcal
     s., antipneumococcal
     s., antitetanic
     s., antitoxic
     s., antityphoid
     s., bactericidal
     s., bacteriolytic
     s., blood
     s., convalescent
     s., foreign
     s., immune
     s., polyvalent
     s., pooled
     s., pregnancy
     s., pregnant mare's
serumal (sĕ-roo′mǎl) [L. serum, whey]
serum-fast
serum glutamic-oxaloacetic transaminase
serum glutamic pyruvic transaminase
serum protein
serum rash
serum sickness
servomechanism (sŭr″vō-mĕk′ǎ-nīzm)
SES socioeconomic status
sesame oil
sesamoid (sĕs′ǎ-moyd) [L. sesamoides]
sesamoid bone
sesamoid cartilage
sesamoiditis (sĕs″ǎ-moy-dī′tĭs) [″ + Gr. itis, inflammation]
sesqui- [L.]
sesquihora (sĕs″kwī-hō′rǎ) [L.]
sesquioxide (sĕs″kwē-ŏk′sĭd)
sessile (sĕs′l) [L. sessilis, low]
set

seta (sē'tă) [L., bristle]
setaceous (sē-tā'shŭs) [L. *setaceus*]
Setchenow's inhibitory centers (sĕtch'en-ŏfs) [Ivan M. Setchenow, Russian neurologist, 1829–1905]
setiferous (sē-tĭf'ĕr-ŭs) [L. *seta*, bristle, + *ferre*, to bear]
setigerous (sē-tĭj'ĕr-ŭs) [" + *gerere*, to carry]
seton (sē"tŏn) [L. *seta*, bristle]
setose (sē'tōs)
set point weight
setup
seventh cranial nerve
seven-year itch
sevum (sē'vŭm) [L.]
sewer gas
sex [L. *sexus*]
    s., chromosomal
    s., morphological
    s., nuclear
    s., psychological
sex chromatin
sex chromosomes
sex clinic
sex determination
sexdigital (sĕks-dĭj'ĭ-tăl) [L. *sex*, six, + *digitus*, finger, toe]
sexduction (sĕks-dŭk'shŭn)
sexism
sexivalent (sĕks"ĭ-vă'lĕnt, -ĭv'ăl-ĕnt) [" + *valere*, to be strong]
sex-limited
sex-linked
sexology [L. *sexus*, sex, + Gr. *logos*, word, reason]
sex ratio
sex surrogate
sextan (sĕks'tăn) [L. *sextanus*, of the sixth]
sextigravida (sĕks"tĭ-grăv'ĭd-ă) [L. *sextus*, six, + *gravida*, a pregnant woman]
sextipara (sĕks-tĭp'ă-ră) [" + *parere*, to beget, produce]
sextuplet (sĕks-tŭp'lĕt) [L. *sextus*, six]
sexual (sĕks'ū-ăl) [L. *sexualis*]
sexual dysfunction

sexual health
sexual intercourse
    s.i., homosexual
sexuality (sĕks-ū-ăl'ĭ-tē) [L. *sexus*, sex]
sexually transmitted disease
sexual reassignment
sexual reflex
Sézary cell [A. Sézary, Fr. dermatologist, 1880–1956]
Sézary syndrome
SGA *small for gestational age*
S.G.O. *Surgeon-General's Office*
SGOT *serum glutamic-oxaloacetic transaminase*
SGPT *serum glutamic pyruvic transaminase*
SH *serum hepatitis*
shadow [AS. *sceaduwe*]
shadow-casting
shadowgram, shadowgraph [" + Gr. *gramma*, letter, piece of writing; " + Gr. *graphein*, to write]
shaft [AS. *sceaft*]
    s., hair
shakes (shāks) [AS. *sceacen*]
shaking
shaking palsy
shaman (shā'mŭn, shŏ'-) [Russ., ascetic]
shamanism (shā'mŭn-ĭsm, shŏ'-)
shank (shăngk) [AS. *sceanca*]
shape (shāp) [AS. *sceapan*]
sharkskin
Sharpey's intercrossing fibers (shăr'pēz) [William Sharpey, Scot. physiologist, 1802–1880]
Sharpey's perforating fibers
shear (shēr)
sheath (shēth) [AS. *sceath*]
    s., arachnoid
    s., axon
    s., carotid
    s., crural
    s., dentinal
    s., dural
    s., femoral
    s., lamellar
    s., medullary
    s., myelin

s., nerve
s. of Henle
s. of Key and Retzius, connective tissue
s. of Neumann
s. of Schwann
s. of Schweigger-Seidel
s., pial
s., root
s., synovial
s., tendon
shedding [ME. *sheden,* shed]
Sheehan's syndrome
sheep cell agglutination test
sheet (shēt) [AS. *sciete,* cloth]
s., draw
s., lift
shelf
s., dental
shelf-life
shell
shellac (shě-lăk')
shell shock
Shenton's line (shěn'tŏnz) [Thomas Shenton, Brit. radiologist, 1872–1955]
shield (shēld) [AS. *scild,* shield]
s., embryonic
s., gonadal
s., nipple
s., phallic
shift [AS. *sciftan,* to arrange]
s., chloride
s. to the left
s. to the right
Shiga's bacillus (shē'gǎs) [Kiyoshi Shiga, Japanese physician, 1870–1957]
Shigella (shǐ-gěl'lǎ) [Kiyoshi Shiga]
S. boydii
S. dysenteriae
S. flexneri
S. sonnei
shigellosis (shǐ"gěl-lō'sǐs) [*Shigella* + *osis,* condition]
shin (shǐn) [AS. *scinu,* shin]
s., saber
shingles (shǐng'lz) [L. *cingulus,* a girdle]

shinsplints
shin spots
Shirodkar operation [Shirodkar, contemporary Indian physician]
shiver (shǐv'ěr) [ME. *chiveren*]
shock (shŏk) [ME. *schokke*]
s., anaphylactic
s., anesthesia
s., cardiogenic
s., deferred
s., electric
s., endotoxin
s., epigastric
s., hemorrhagic
s., hypovolemic
s., insulin
s., mental
s., peptone
s., psychic
s., secondary
s., septic
s., serum
s., spinal
s., surgical
s. syndrome, toxic
s., traumatic
shock therapy
shoemakers' cramp
Shohl's solution
short bowel syndrome
shortsightedness (short-sīt'ěd-něs)
shot
shotgun prescription
shoulder (shōl'děr) [AS. *sculdor*]
s., dislocation of
shoulder blade
shoulder girdle
shoulder joint
show (shō) [AS. *scewian,* to look at]
Shrapnell's membrane (shrăp'něls) [Henry J. Shrapnell, Brit. anatomist, 1761–1841]
shreds (shrĕds) [AS. *screade*]
shrink [from *headshrinker*]
shudder [ME. *shuddren*]
shunt (shŭnt) [ME. *shunten,* to avoid]
s., arteriovenous
s., cardiovascular

s., dialysis
s., left-to-right
s., LeVeen
s., portacaval
s., postcaval
s., reversed
s., right-to-left
Shy-Drager syndrome [G. M. Shy, U.S. neurologist, 1919–1967; G. A. Drager, U.S. physician, 1917–1967]
SI Système International
Si silicon
siagonantritis (sī″ăg-ōn-ăn-trī′tĭs) [Gr. siagon, jawbone, + antron, cavity, + itis, inflammation]
sial(o)- (sī′ă-lō) [Gr. sialon, saliva]
sialaden (sī-ăl′ă-dĕn) [″ + aden, gland]
sialadenitis (sī″ăl-ăd″ĕ-nī′tĭs) [″ + ″ + itis, inflammation]
sialadenoncus (sī″ăl-ăd″ĕ-nŏng′kŭs) [″ + ″ + onkos, bulk, mass]
sialagogue (sī-ăl′ă-gŏg) [″ + agogos, leading]
sialaporia (sī″ăl-ă-pō′rē-ă) [″ + aporia, lack]
sialectasia, sialectasis (sī″ăl-ĕk-tā′sē-ă, sī″a-lĕk′tă-sĭs) [″ + ektasis, dilatation]
sialemesis (sī″ăl-ĕm′ĕs-ĭs) [″ + emein, to vomit]
sialic (sī-ăl′ĭk)
sialine (sī′ă-lĭn) [Gr. sialon, saliva]
sialism, sialismus (sī′ăl-ĭzm, sī-ăl-ĭz′mŭs) [″ + -ismos, condition]
sialitis (sī″ă-lī′tĭs) [″ + itis, inflammation]
sialoadenitis (sī″ă-lō-ăd″ĕ-nī′tĭs) [″ + aden, gland, + itis, inflammation]
sialoadenotomy (sī″ă-lō-ăd″ĕ-nŏt′ō-mē) [″ + ″ + tome, a cutting, slice]
sialoaerophagy (sī″ă-lō-ĕr″ŏf′ă-jē) [″ + aer, air, + phagein, to eat]
sialoangiectasis (sī″ă-lō-ăn″jē-ĕk′tă-sĭs) [Gr. sialon, saliva, + angeion,

vessel, + ektasis, dilatation]
sialoangiography (sī″ă-lō-ăn″jē-ŏg′ră-fē) [″ + ″ + graphein, to write]
sialoangitis, sialoangiitis (sī″ă-lō-ăn-jī′tĭs, -ăn″jē-ī′tĭs) [″ + ″ + itis, inflammation]
sialocele (sī′ă-lō-sēl) [″ + kele, tumor, swelling]
sialodochitis (sī″ă-lō-dō-kī′tĭs) [″ + doche, receptacle, + itis, inflammation]
    s. fibrinosa
sialodochoplasty (sī″ă-lō-dō″kō-plăs″tē) [″ + ″ + plassein, to form]
sialoductitis (sī″ă-lō-dŭk-tī′tĭs) [″ + L. ductus, duct, + Gr. itis, inflammation]
sialogenous (sī″ă-lŏj′ĕ-nŭs) [″ + gennan, to produce]
sialogogic (sī″ă-lō-gŏj′ĭk)
sialogogue (sī-ăl′ō-gŏg) [″ + agogos, leading]
sialogram (sī-ăl′ō-grăm) [″ + gramma, letter, piece of writing]
sialography (sī″ă-lŏg′ră-fē) [″ + graphein, to write]
sialolith (sī-ăl′ō-lĭth) [″ + lithos, stone]
sialolithiasis (sī″ă-lō-lĭ-thī′ă-sĭs)
sialolithotomy (sī″ă-lō-lĭ-thŏt′ō-mē) [Gr. sialon, saliva, + lithos, stone, + tome, a cutting, slice]
sialoncus (sī″ă-lŏng′kŭs) [″ + onkos, bulk, mass]
sialoporia (sī″ă-lō-pō′rē-ă) [″ + aporia, lack]
sialorrhea (sī″ă-lō-rē′ă) [″ + rhein, to flow]
sialoschesis (sī″ă-lŏs′kĕ-sĭs) [″ + schesis, suppression]
sialosemeiology (sī″ă-lō-sē″mī-ŏl′ō-jē) [″ + semeion, sign, + logos, word, reason]
sialosis (sī-ă-lō′sĭs) [″ + osis, condition]
sialostenosis (sī″ă-lō-stĕ-nō′sĭs) [″ + stenosis, act of narrowing]

sialosyrinx (sī″ă-lō-sīr′ĭnks) [″ +
syrinx, a pipe]
sialotic (sī″ă-lŏt′ĭk) [Gr. sialon, saliva]
Siamese twins (sī-ă-mēz′) [After
Chang and Eng, 1811–1874, joined
Chinese twins born in Siam]
sib [AS. sibb, kin]
sibilant (sĭb′ĭ-lănt) [L. sibilans, hissing]
sibilation
sibilismus
 s. aurium
sibilus (sĭb′ĭ-lŭs) [L. sibilans, hissing]
sibling (sĭb′lĭng) [AS. sibb, kin, +
-ling, having the quality of]
 s., half
sibship
siccant (sĭk′ănt) [L. siccus, dry]
siccative (sĭk′ă-tĭv) [L. siccativus, drying]
sicchasia (sĭ-kă′shē-ă) [Gr. sikchasia,
loathing]
siccolabile (sĭk″ō-lā′bĭl) [L. siccus, dry,
 + labilis, unstable]
siccostabile (sĭk″ō-stā′bĭl) [″ + stabilis, stable]
siccus (sĭk′ŭs) [L.]
sick (sĭk) [AS seoc, ill]
sickle cell
sickle cell anemia
sickle cell crisis
sicklemia (sĭk-lē′mē-ă) [AS. sicol, sickle,
 + Gr. haima, blood]
sickling
sickness [AS. seoc, ill]
 s., balloon
 s., bleeding
 s., car
 s., falling
 s., green
 s., morning
 s., motion
 s., mountain
 s., sea
 s., serum
 s., sleeping
sick sinus syndrome
SICU surgical intensive care unit
S.I.D. Society for Investigative Dermatology

side (sīd) [AS. side]
side effect
side position
sideration (sĭd-ĕr-ā′shŭn) [L. siderari, to
be struck by a star]
siderism, siderismus (sĭd′ĕr-ĭzm,
sĭd-ĕr-ĭz′mŭs) [Gr. sideros, iron, +
-ismos, condition]
sidero- (sĭd′ĕr-ō) [Gr. sideros, iron]
sideroblast (sĭd′ĕr-ō-blăst″) [″ +
blastos, germ]
siderocyte (sĭd′ĕr-ō-sīt) [″ + kytos,
cell]
sideroderma (sĭd″ĕr-ō-dĕr′mă) [″ +
derma, skin]
siderodromophobia (sĭd″ĕr-ō-drō″
mō-fō′bē-ă) [″ + dromos, a way,
 + phobos, fear]
siderofibrosis (sĭd″ĕr-ō-fī-brō′sĭs)
[″ + L. fibra, fiber, + Gr. osis,
condition]
siderogenous (sĭd″ĕr-ŏj′ĕ-nŭs) [″ +
gennan, to produce]
sideropenia (sĭd″ĕr-ō-pē′nē-ă) [″ +
penia, lack]
sideropenic (sĭd″ĕr-ō-pē′nĭk)
siderophil (sĭd′ĕr-ō-fĭl)
siderophilin (sī′dĭr-ŏf″ĭ-lĭn)
siderophilous (sĭd″ĕr-ŏf′ĭ-lŭs) [″ +
philein, to love]
siderophone (sĭd′ĕr-ō-fōn)
siderophore (sĭd′ĕr-ō-for) [″ +
phoros, bearing]
sideroscope (sĭd′ĕr-ō-skōp) [″ +
skopein, to examine]
siderosis (sĭd″ĕr-ō′sĭs) [″ + osis,
condition]
 s., hepatic
 s., urinary
siderosome (sĭd″ĕr-ō-sōm′) [″ +
soma, body]
siderotic (sĭd″ĕr-ŏt′ĭk)
SIDS sudden infant death syndrome
SIECUS Sex Information and Education
Council of the U.S.
siemens (sē′mĕnz)
Siemens' syndrome [H.W. Siemens,
Ger. physician, b. 1891]

sieve (sĭv)
  s., molecular
sig. [L.] *signa*, label it
Sigault's operation (sē-gōz') [Jean René Sigault, Fr. obstetrician, b. 1740]
sigh [AS. *sican*]
sight (sīt) [AS. *sihth*]
  s., blind
  s., day
  s., far
  s., near
  s., night
  s., old
  s., second
sigma (sĭg'mă)
sigmatism (sĭg'mă-tĭzm) [Gr. *sigma*, letter S, + *-ismos*, condition]
sigmoid (sĭg'moyd) [Gr. *sigmoeides*]
sigmoidectomy (sĭg"moyd-ĕk'tō-mē) [" + *ektome*, excision]
sigmoid flexure
sigmoiditis (sĭg"moyd-ī'tĭs) [" + *itis*, inflammation]
sigmoidopexy (sig-moy'dō-pĕk"sē) [" + *pexis*, fixation]
sigmoidoproctostomy (sĭg-moy"dō-prŏk-tŏs'tō-mē) [Gr. *sigmoeides*, shaped like Gr. letter S, + *proktos*, anus, + *stoma*, mouth, opening]
sigmoidorectostomy (sĭg-moy"dō-rĕk-tŏs'tō-mē) [" + L. *rectus*, straight, + Gr. *stoma*, mouth, opening]
sigmoidoscope (sĭg-moy'dō-skōp) [" + *skopein*, to examine]
  s., flexible
sigmoidoscopy (sĭg"moy-dŏs'kō-pē) [" + *skopein*, to examine]
sigmoidosigmoidostomy (sĭg-moy"dō-sĭg-moy-dŏs'tō-mē) [" + *sigmoeides*, sigmoid, + *stoma*, mouth, opening]
sigmoidostomy (sĭg-moyd-ŏs'tō-mē) [" + *stoma*, mouth, opening]
sigmoidotomy (sĭg-moyd-ŏt'ō-mē) [" + *tome*, a cutting, slice]
sigmoidovesical (sĭg-moy"dō-vĕs'ĭ-kăl) [" + L. *vesica*, bladder]

sign (sīn) [L. *signum*]
  s., objective
  s., physical
  s.'s, vital
signa (sĭg'nă) [L.]
signal
signature (sĭg'nă-tūr) [L. *signatura*, to mark]
significance, statistical
significant (sĭg-nĭf'ĭ-kănt)
significant others
signing
sign language
Silain
Silastic
silent
silent disease
silent period
silica (sĭl'ĭ-kă) [L. *silex*, flint]
silicate (sĭl'ĭ-kāt) [L. *silicus*, flintlike]
siliceous, silicious (sĭ-lĭsh'ŭs)
silicic (sĭl-ĭs'ĭk)
silicoanthracosis (sĭl"ĭ-kō-ăn"thră-kō'sĭs) [L. *silex*, flint, + Gr. *anthrax*, coal, + *osis*, condition]
silicofluoride (sĭl"ĭ-kō-floo'ō-rīd)
silicon (sĭl'ĭ-kŏn) [L. *silex*, flint]
silicone (sĭl'ĭ-kōn")
  s., injectable
silicosiderosis (sĭl"ĭ-kō-sĭd"ĕr-ō'sĭs) [" + Gr. *sideros*, iron, + *osis*, condition]
silicosis (sĭl-ĭ-kō'sĭs) [" + Gr. *osis*, condition]
silicotic (sĭl-ĭ-kŏt'ĭk)
silicotuberculosis (sĭl"ĭ-kō-tū-bĕr-kū-lō'sĭs) [" + *tuberculum*, a little swelling, + Gr. *osis*, condition]
siliqua olivae (sĭl'ĭ-kwē ŏl'ĭ-vē) [L.]
siliquose (sĭl'ĭ-kwōs) [L. *siliqua*, pod]
siliquose cataract
siliquose desquamation
silo-filler's disease
Silvadene
silver (sĭl'vĕr) [AS. *siolfor*]
  s. amalgam
  s. chloride
  s., colloidal

s. halide
s. nitrate
s. nitrate, toughened
s. picrate
s. protein
s. sulfadiazine
silver fork deformity
silver nitrate poisoning
Silvester's method [Henry Robert Silvester, Brit. physician, 1829–1908]
simesthesia (sĭm-ĕs-thē′zē-ă) [Gr. *aisthesis*, feeling, perception]
simethicone (sĭ-mĕth′ĭ-kōn)
simian crease
similia similibus curantur (sĭ-mĭl′ē-ă sĭmĭl′ĭ-bŭs kū-răn′tūr) [L., likes are cured by likes]
similimum (sĭ-mĭl′ĭ-mŭm) [L., most like]
Simmonds' disease (sĭm′mŏnds) [Morris Simmonds, Ger. physician, 1855–1925]
Simon's position (zē′mŏns) [Gustav Simon, Ger. surgeon, 1824–1876]
simple (sĭm′pl) [L. *simplex*]
simple fracture
simple inflammation
simple reflex
Sims' position (sĭmz) [J. Marion Sims, U.S. gynecologist, 1813–1883]
simul (sĭ′mŭl, sĭm′ŭl) [L.]
simulation (sĭm-ū-lā′shŭn) [L. *simulatio*, imitation]
simulator (sĭm″ū-lā′tor)
Simulium (sĭ-mū′lē-ŭm)
S. damnosum
S. venustum
Sinapis (sĭn-ā′pĭs) [Gr. *sinapi*, mustard]
sinapism (sĭn′ă-pĭzm) [Gr. *sinapismos*]
sincipital (sĭn-sĭp′ĭ-tăl) [L. *sinciput*, half a head]
sinciput (sĭn′sĭp-ŭt) [L., half a head]
Sinemet
Sinequan
sinew (sĭn′ū) [AS. *sinu*]
s., weeping
sing. [L.] *singulorum*, of each
singer's node
singleton

singultation (sĭng″gŭl-tā′shŭn) [L. *singultus*, a hiccup]
singultus (sĭng-gŭl′tŭs) [L.]
sinister (sĭn-ĭs′tĕr) [L.]
sinistrad (sĭn′ĭs-trăd) [L. *sinister*, left, + *ad*, toward]
sinistral (sĭn′ĭs-trăl) [L.]
sinistrality (sĭn″ĭs-trăl′ĭ-tē)
sinistraural (sĭn-ĭs-traw′răl) [″ + *auris*, ear]
sinistro- (sĭn′ĭs-trō) [L. *sinister*, left]
sinistrocardia (sĭn″ĭs-trō-kăr′dē-ă) [″ + Gr. *kardia*, heart]
sinistrocerebral (sĭn″ĭs-trō-sĕr′ĕ-brăl) [″ + *cerebrum*, brain]
sinistrocular (sĭn-ĭs-trŏk′ū-lar) [″ + *oculus*, eye]
sinistrocularity (sĭn″ĭs-trŏk″ū-lăr′ĭ-tē)
sinistrogyration (sĭn″ĭs-trō-jī-rā′shŭn) [″ + Gr. *gyros*, a circle]
sinistromanual (sĭn″ĭs-trō-măn′ū-ăl) [″ + *manus*, hand]
sinistropedal (sĭn-ĭs-trŏp′ĕd-ăl) [″ + *pes*, foot]
sinistrotorsion (sĭn″ĭs-trō-tor′shŭn) [″ + *torsio*, a twisting]
sinistrous (sĭn′ĭs-trŭs)
sinoatrial (sĭn″ō-ā′trē-ăl)
sinoatrial node
sinoauricular (sī″nō-aw-rĭk′ū-lar)
sinobronchitis (sī″nō-brŏng-kī′tĭs) [L. *sinus*, curve, + Gr. *bronchos*, windpipe, + *itis*, inflammation]
sinogram (sī′nō-grăm″) [L. *sinus*, curve, + Gr. *gramma*, letter, piece of writing]
sinter (sĭn′tĕr)
sinuitis (sī-nū-ī′tĭs) [″ + Gr. *itis*, inflammation]
sinuotomy (sĭn-ū-ŏt′ō-mē) [″ + Gr. *tome*, a cutting, slice]
sinuous (sĭn′ū-ŭs) [L. *sinuosus*, winding]
sinus (sī′nŭs) [L., curve, hollow]
s.'s, accessory nasal
s., anal
s., aortic
s., basilar
s., carotid

s. cavernosus
s., cerebral
s., circular
s., coccygeal
s., coronary, of heart
s.'s, cranial
s., dermal
s., draining
s.'s, ethmoidal
s., frontal
s., genitourinary
s., hair
s., inferior longitudinal
s., inferior petrosal
s., inferior sagittal
s.'s, intercavernous
s., lateral
s.'s, lymph
s., marginal
s., maxillary
s., occipital
s. of the pulmonary trunk
s. of spleen
s. of Valsalva
s. of venal canal; s. venarum cavarum
s.'s, paranasal
s., pilonidal
s.'s, pleural
s. pocularis
s. prostaticus
s. rectus
s., renal
s., rhomboid
s., sigmoid
s.'s, sphenoidal
s., sphenoparietal
s., straight
s., superior longitudinal
s., superior petrosal
s., superior sagittal
s., tarsal
s., tentorial
s., terminal
s., transverse
s.'s, transverse, of the dura mater
s., transverse, of the pericardium
s., tympanic

s., urogenital
s., uterine
s.'s, uteroplacental
s., venous
s.'s, venous, of the dura mater
s., venous, of sclera
sinus arrhythmia
sinusitis (sī-nŭs-ī'tĭs) [L. sinus, curve, hollow, + Gr. itis, inflammation]
    s., acute catarrhal
    s., acute suppurative
    s., chronic hyperplastic
    s., chronic hypertrophic
sinusoid (sī'nŭs-oyd) [" + Gr. eidos, form, shape]
sinusoidal (sī-nŭs-oyd'ăl)
sinusoidal current
sinusoidalization (sī"nŭ-soy"dăl-ī-zā'shŭn) [L. sinus, hollow, curve, + Gr. eidos, form, shape]
sinusotomy (sī-nŭs-ŏt'ō-mē) [" + Gr. tome, a cutting, slice]
sinus rhythm
SiO₂ silicon dioxide
Sioux alarm
siphon (sī'fŭn) [Gr. siphon, tube]
siphonage (sī'fŭn-ĭj)
Siphonaptera (sī"fō-năp'tĕr-ă) [" + apteros, wingless]
siphonoma (sī-fōn-ō'mă) [" + oma, tumor]
Sipple syndrome [John H. Sipple, U.S. physician, b. 1930]
Sippy diet (sĭp'ē) [Bertram W. Sippy, U.S. physician, 1866–1924]
sirenomelia (sī"rĕn-ŏm-ē'lē-ă) [Gr. seiren, mermaid, + melos, limb]
siriasis (sī-rī'ă-sĭs) [Gr. seirian, to be hot]
sister
Sister Mary Joseph nodule
site [L. situs, place]
    s., active
    s., binding
    s., receptor
sitieirgia (sĭt-ē-ĭr'jē-ă) [Gr. sition, food, + eirgein, to shut out]
sitio-, sito- [Gr. sition, sitos, food]
sitophobia (sī"tō-fō'bē-ă) [" +

phobos, fear]
sitosterols (sī-tŏs'tĕr-ŏls)
sitotaxis (sī"tō-tăk'sĭs) [" + *taxis,*
arrangement]
sitotherapy (sī"tō-thĕr'ă-pē) [" +
therapeia, treatment]
sitotoxin (sī"tō-tŏk'sĭn) [" + *toxikon,* poison]
sitotoxism (sī"tō-tŏks'ĭzm) [" +
" + *-ismos,* condition]
sitotropism (sī-tŏt'rō-pĭzm) [" +
tropos, a turning, + *-ismos,* condi-
tion]
situation
situs (sī'tŭs) [L.]
s. inversus viscerum
s. perversus
sitz bath (sĭtz)
SI units *International System of Units*
sixth cranial nerve
Sjögren's syndrome
SK-65
SK-Apap
skateboard
skatol(e) (skăt'ōl) [Gr. *skatos,* dung]
skatoxyl (skă-tŏk'sĭl)
SK-Bamate
SK-Chlorothiazide
SK-Dexamethasone
skein (skān)
skelalgia (skĕ-lăl'jē-ă) [Gr. *skelis,* leg,
+ *algos,* pain]
skeletal (skĕl'ĕ-tăl) [Gr. *skeleton,* a
dried-up body]
skeletal muscle
skeletal survey
skeletal traction
skeletization (skĕl"ĕt-ī-zā'shŭn)
skeleto- [Gr. *skeleton,* a dried-up
body]
skeletogenous (skĕl-ĕ-tŏj'ĕ-nŭs)
[" + *gennan,* to produce]
skeletology (skĕl"ĕ-tŏl'ō-jē) [" +
logos, word, reason]
skeleton (skĕl'ĕt-ŏn) [Gr., a dried-up
body]
s., appendicular
s., axial

s., cartilaginous
Skene's glands (skēns) [Alexander J.
C. Skene, U.S. gynecologist, 1838–
1900]
skenitis (skē-nī'tĭs) [*Skene* + Gr.
itis, inflammation]
skeocytosis (skē"ō-sī-tō'sĭs) [Gr.
skaios, left, + *kytos,* cell, +
osis, condition]
SK-Erythromycin
skew (skyū) [ME. *skewen,* to escape]
skew deviation
skia- (skī'ă) [Gr., shadow]
skiascopy
skin (skĭn) [Old Norse *skinn*]
s., alligator
s., deciduous
s., elastic
s., glossy
s., hidebound
s., loose
s., parchment
s., piebald
s., scarf
s., true
skin cancer
skinfold thickness
skin graft
skin-marking
Skinner box (skĭn'ĕr) [Burrhus F. Skinner, U.S. psychologist, b. 1904]
skin rash
skin test
sklero- [Gr.]
SK-Lygen
skodaic (skō-dā'ĭk)
Skoda's rales (skō'dăs) [Josef Skoda,
Austrian physician, 1805–1881]
Skoda's resonance
SK-Penicillin VK
SK-Phenobarbital
SK-Potassium Chloride
SK-Pramine
SK-Prednisone
SK-Probenecid
SK-Quinidine Sulfate
SK-Tetracycline
SK-Tolbutamide

skull (skŭl) [ME. *skulle*, bowl]
  s., fracture of
skullcap
slant
slave
SLE *systemic lupus erythematosus*
sleep (slēp) [AS. *slaep*]
  s., hypnotic
  s., NREM
  s., pathological
  s., REM
  s., twilight
sleep drunkenness
sleeping sickness
sleepwalking
slide
slime mold
slimy (slī'mē) [AS. *slim*, smooth]
sling (slĭng) [AS. *slingan*, to wind]
  s., clove-hitch
  s., counterbalanced
  s., cravat
  s., folded cravat
  s., open
  s., St. John's
  s., simple figure-of-eight roller arm
  s., swathe arm or cravat
  s., triangular
  s., triangular, reversed
slit [ME. *slitte*]
  s., vestibular
slit lamp
slope
  s., lower ridge
Slo-Phyllin
slough (slŭf) [ME. *slughe*, a skin]
sloughing (slŭf'ĭng)
slow (slō) [AS. *slaw*, dull]
Slow K
**slow-reacting aubstance of ana-
  phylaxis**
slows (slōz)
slow virus infection
sludge (slŭjh)
sludged blood
slurry (slŭr'ē) [ME. *slory*]
Sm *samarium*
SMA-12

small-for-gestational age
smallpox (smawl'pŏks) [AS. *smael*, tiny,
  + *poc*, pustule]
smallpox vaccine
smear (smēr) [AS. *smerian*, to anoint]
  s., blood
  s., Pap; s., Papanicolaou
smegma (smĕg'mă) [Gr. *smegma*,
  soap]
  s. clitordis
  s. embryonum
  s. praeputii
smegmatic (smĕg-măt'ĭk)
smegmolith (smĕg'mō-lĭth) [Gr.
  smegma, soap, + *lithos*, a stone]
smell (smĕl) [ME. *smellen*, to reek]
Smith's fracture [Robert W. Smith, Irish
  physician, 1807–1873]
Smith-Petersen nail [Marius N. Smith-
  Petersen, U.S. orthopedic surgeon,
  1886–1953]
Smith-Strang disease
smog [blend of *smoke* and *fog*]
smoke inhalation
smokeless tobacco
smoke poisoning
smoker's cancer
smoking, passive
SMON *subacute myelo-optic neuropathy*
smooth muscle
smudging (smŭj'ĭng)
Sn [L.] *stannum*, tin
snail [ME.]
snake [ME.]
  s., poisonous
snake bite
snap
  s., closing
  s., opening
snapping finger
snapping hip
snare (snār) [AS. *sneare*, noose]
sneeze (snēz) [AS. *fneosan*, to pant]
sneeze reflex, solar
Snellen's chart (snĕl'ĕns) [Herman
  Snellen, Dutch ophthalmologist, 1834–
  1908]

Snellen's reflex
Snellen's test
snore (snor) [AS. *snora*]
snoring rale (snor'ĭng răl)
snow, carbon dioxide
snow blindness
SNS *Society of Neurological Surgeons*
snuff
snuffbox, anatomical
snuffles (snŭf'ls) [D. *snuffelen*, to snuff]
SOAP *subjective, objective, assessment, plan*
soap (sōp) [AS. *sape*]
   s., green
   s., soft medicinal
soap liniment
soapsuds enema
SOB *short of breath*
sob [ME. *sobben*, to catch breath]
socialization (sō"shă-lĭ-zā'shŭn)
social phobias
socioacusis (sō"sē-ō-ă-kū'sĭs) [L. *socius*, companion,   +   Gr. *akoustikos*, hearing]
sociobiology (sō"sē-ō-bī-ŏl'ō-jē) ["   +   Gr. *bios*, life,   +   *logos*, word, reason]
socioeconomic status
sociology (sō-sē-ŏl'ō-jē) ["   +   *logos*, word, reason]
sociomedical
sociometry (sō"sē-ŏm'ĕ-trē) ["   +   Gr. *metron*, measure]
sociopath (sō'sē-ō-păth) ["   +   Gr. *pathos*, disease, suffering]
sociopathic personality
sociopathy (sō"sē-ŏp'ă-thē) ["   +   Gr. *pathos*, disease, suffering]
socket (sŏk'ĕt) [ME. *soket*, a spearhead]
   s., alveolar
   s., dry
   s., tooth
soda (sō'dă) [Medieval L., barilla, from which soda is made]
   s., baking
   s., caustic
   s. lime
Soda Mint

soda water
Sodestrin
sodic (sō'dĭk)
sodium (sō'dē-ŭm) [LL.]
   s. acetate
   s. alginate
   s., amobarbital
   s. ascorbate
   s. benzoate
   s. bicarbonate
   s. carbonate
   s., carboxymethylcellulose
   s. chloride
   s. citrate
   s. fluoride
   s. hydroxide
   s. hypochlorite [solution]
   s. iodide
   s. lactate [injection]
   s. lauryl sulfate
   s. monofluorophosphate
   s., morrhuate [injection]
   s. nitrite
   s. nitroprusside
   s. phosphate, dibasic
   s. phosphate P 32 [solution]
   s. polystyrene sulfonate
   s. propionate
   s. salicylate
   s. sulfate
   s. thiosulfate
sodium fluoride poisoning
Sodium Versenate
sodokosis (sŏd-ō-kō'sĭs) [Jap. *sodoku*, rat poison   +   Gr. *osis*, condition]
sodoku (sŏ-dō'koo)
sodomist, sodomite (sŏd'ō-mĭst, -mīt) [LL. *Sodoma*, Sodom]
sodomy (sŏd'ō-mē) [LL. *Sodoma*, Sodom]
Soemmering's bone (sĕm'ĕr-ĭngz) [Samuel T. von Soemmering, Ger. anatomist, 1755–1830]
Soemmering's foramen
Soemmering's ring
Soemmering's spot
soft (sŏft) [AS. *softe*]
soft diet

soft palate
soft sore
softening (sŏf'ĕn-ĭng) [AS.]
   s., anemic
   s., colliquative
   s., gray
   s., hemorrhagic
   s., mucoid
   s. of bones
   s. of brain
   s. of heart
   s. of stomach
   s., red
   s., white
sol (sŏl, sōl) [Gr. *sole*, salt water]
sol. *solution*
solace
Solanaceae (sŏl"ă-nā'sē-ē)
solanaceous (sŏl"ă-nā'shŭs)
solanine (sō'lă-nēn)
solar (sō'lăr) [L. *solaris*]
solarium (sō-lā'rē-ŭm) [L. *solarium*, terrace]
solar plexus
solar therapy
solation (sō-lā'shŭn)
solder (sŏd'ĕr)
   s., building
   s., gold
   s., hard
   s., soft
soldering
sole (sōl) [AS. *sole*]
solenoid (sŏl'lĕ-noyd)
sole reflex
soleus (sō'lĕ-ŭs) [L. *solea*, sole of foot]
Solfoton
Solganal
solid (sŏl'ĭd) [L. *solidus*]
solipsism (sŏl'ĭp-sĭzm) [L. *solus*, alone, + *ipse*, self]
solitary (sŏl'ĭ-tăr-ē) [L. *solitarius*, aloneness]
solitary lymph nodules
solo practitioner
solubility (sŏl"ū-bĭl'ĭ-tē) [LL. *solubilis*, to loosen, dissolve]
soluble (sŏl'ū-bl)

Solu-Cortef
Solu-Medrol
solum tympani (sō'lŭm tĭm'pă-nē) [L.]
solute (sŏl'ūt) [L. *solutus*, to loosen, dissolve]
solutio (sō-lū'shē-ō) [L. *solutus*, to loosen, dissolve]
solution (sō-lū'shŭn) [L. *solutus*, to loosen, dissolve]
   s., aqueous
   s., buffer
   s., colloidal
   s., contrast
   s., hyperbaric
   s., hypertonic
   s., hypotonic
   s., iodine
   s., isobaric
   s., isohydric
   s., isosmotic
   s., isotonic
   s., Locke-Ringer's
   s., molar
   s., normal
   s., normal saline
   s., ophthalmic
   s., physiological saline
   s., repair
   s., Ringer's
   s., saline
   s., saturated
   s., sclerosing
   s., seminormal
   s., standard
   s., supersaturation
   s., test
   s., Tyrode's
   s., volumetric
solv. [L.] *solve*, dissolve
solvate (sŏl'vāt)
solvation (sŏl'vā'shŭn)
solvent (sŏl'vĕnt) [L. *solvens*]
solvolysis (sŏl-vŏl'ĭ-sĭs)
Soma
soma (sō'mă) [Gr. *soma*, body]
soman
somasthenia (sŏm"ăs-thē'nē-ă) [" + *astheneia*, weakness]

somat(o)- (sō'mă-tō) [Gr. *soma*, body]
somatasthenia (sō"mat-ăs-thē'nē-ă)
somatesthesia (sō"măt-ĕs-thē'zĕ-ă)
[" + *aisthesis*, feeling, perception]
somatic (sō-măt'ĭk) [Gr. *soma*, body]
somaticosplanchnic (sō-măt"ĭ-kō-
splănk'nĭk) [" + *splanchnikos*, pert.
to the viscera]
somaticovisceral (sō-măt"ĭ-kō-vĭs'ĕr-
ăl) [" + L. *viscera*, body organs]
somatist (sō'mă-tĭst) [Gr. *soma*, body]
somatization (sō"mă-tĭ-zā'shŭn)
somatization disorder
somatoceptors (sō-măt"ō-sĕp'tors)
somatochrome (sō-măt'ō-krōm)
[" + *chroma*, color]
somatocrinin
somatoform disorders
somatogenic (sō"mă-tō-jĕn'ĭk) [" +
gennan, to produce]
somatology (sō"mă-tŏl'ō-jē) [" +
logos, word, reason]
somatome (sō'mă-tōm) [" + *tome*,
a cutting, slice]
somatomedin
somatomegaly (sō"mă-tō-mĕg'ă-lē)
[" + *megas*, large]
somatometry (sō"mă-tŏm'ĕ-trē)
[" + *metron*, measure]
somatopagus (sō"mă-tŏp'ă-gŭs)
[" + *pagos*, thing fixed]
somatopathic (sō"mă-tō-păth'ĭk)
[" + *pathos*, disease, suffering]
somatoplasm (sō-măt'ō-plăzm) [Gr.
soma, body, + LL. *plasma*, form,
mold]
somatopleural (sō"mă-tō-ploor'ăl)
somatopleure (sō-măt'ō-ploor) [" +
pleura, side]
somatopsychic (sō"măt-ō-sī'kĭk)
[" + *psyche*, mind]
somatopsychosis (sō"mă-tō-sī-kō'sĭs)
[" + " + *osis*, condition]
somatoschisis (sō"mă-tŏs'kĭ-sĭs) [" +
schistos, divided]
somatoscopy (sō-mă-tŏs'kō-pē)
[" + *skopein*, to examine]
somatosexual (sō"mă-tō-sĕks'ū-ăl)

[" + L. *sexus*, sex]
somatostatin (sō-măt'ō-stăt"ĭn)
somatotonia (sō"mă-tō-tō'nē-ă)
[" + L. *tonus*, tension, pitch, tone]
somatotopic (sō"mă-tō-tŏp'ĭk) [" +
topos, place]
somatrophic (sō"m̃a-tō-trŏf'ĭk) [" +
tropos, a turning]
somatotrophin (sō"mă-tō-trō'fĭn)
[" + *trophe*, nourishment]
somatotropic (sō"mă-tō-trŏp'ĭk)
[" + *trope*, a turn]
somatotropin (sō"măt-ō-trō'pĭn)
[" + *tropos*, a turning]
somatotype (sō-măt'ō-tīp)
Sombulex
somesthesia (sŏm-ĕs-thē'sē-ă) [" +
aisthesis, feeling, perception]
somesthetic (sō-mĕs-thĕt'ĭk)
somesthetic area
somesthetic path
somite (sō'mīt) [Gr. *soma*, body]
somnambulance (sŏm-năm'bū-lăns)
[L. *somnus*, sleep, + *ambulare*, to
walk]
somnambule
somnambulism (sŏm-năm'bū-lĭzm) [L.
somnus, sleep, + *ambulare*, to
walk]
somnambulist (sŏm-năm'bū-lĭst)
somnifacient (sŏm-nĭ-fā'shĕnt) [" +
facere, to make]
somniferous (sŏm-nĭf'ĕr-ŭs) [" +
ferre, to bear]
somnific (sŏm-nĭf'ĭk)
somniloquence (sŏm-nĭl'ō-kwĕns)
[" + *loqui*, to speak]
somniloquism (sŏm-nĭl'ō-kwĭzm)
[" + " + *-ismos*, condition]
somniloquist (sŏm-nĭl'ō-kwĭst) [" +
loqui, to speak]
somniloquy (sŏm-nĭl'ō-kwē) [" +
loqui, to speak]
somnipathist (sŏm-nĭp'ă-thĭst) [" +
Gr. *pathos*, disease, suffering]
somnipathy (sŏm-nĭp'ă-thē) [" +
Gr. *pathos*, disease, suffering]
somnocinematograph (sŏm"nō-sĭn-

ĕ-măt'ō-grăf) [" + Gr. *kinema*,
motion, + *graphein*, to write]
somnolence (sŏm'nō-lĕns) [L. *somnolentia*, sleepiness]
somnolent (sŏm"nō-lĕnt) [L. *somno-
lentus*]
somnolentia (sŏm"nō-lĕn'shē-ă) [L.]
somnolism (sŏm'nō-lĭzm) [" +
-ismos, condition]
Somogyi phenomenon [Michael Somogyi, U.S. biochemist, 1883 – 1971]
Somophyllin-CRT
sone (sōn) [L. *sonus*, sound]
sonicate (sŏn'ĭ-kāt) [L. *sonus*, sound]
sonication (sŏn"ĭ-kā'shŭn)
sonic boom (sŏn'ĭk) [L. *sonus*, sound]
sonitus (sŏn'ĭ-tŭs) [L.]
sonogram (sō'nō-grăm) [L. *sonus*,
sound, + Gr. *gramma*, letter,
piece of writing]
sonographer
　s., diagnostic medical
sonography (sō-nŏg'ră-fē) [" +
Gr. *graphein*, to write]
sonolucent (sō"nō-loo'sĕnt)
sonometer (sō-nŏm'ĕ-tĕr) [" +
Gr. *metron*, a measure]
sonorous (sō-nō'rŭs) [L.]
sonorous rale
sophistication (sō-fĭs"tĭ-kā'shŭn) [Gr.
sophistikos, deceitful]
sophomania (sŏf"ō-mā'nē-ă) [Gr.
sophos, wise, + *mania*, madness]
sopor (sō'por) [L.]
soporiferous (sŏp"ō-rĭf'ĕr-ŭs) [" +
ferre, to bring]
soporific (sŏp-ō-rĭf'ĭk) [" + *facere*,
to make]
soporose, soporous (sō'por-ōs, -ŭs)
[L.]
sorbefacient (sor"bē-fā'shĕnt) [L. *sorbere*, to suck up, + *facere*, to
make]
sorbitol
sorcery
sordes (sor'dēz) [L. *sordere*, to be dirty]
sore (sor) [AS. *sar*, sore]
　s., bed

s., canker
s., cold
s., Delhi
s., desert
s., hard
s., Oriental
s., pressure
s., soft venereal
s., tropical
s., venereal
sore throat
　s.t., diphtheritic
　s.t., quinsy
　s.t., septic
soroche (sō-rō'chă) [Sp.]
sororiation (sō-ror-ē-ā'shŭn) [L. *soror-
iare*, to increase together]
sorption (sorp'shŭn) [L. *sorbere*, to suck
in]
s.o.s. [L.] *si opus sit*, if necessary or required
sotalol hydrochloride (sō'tă-lŏl)
soterenol hydrochloride (sō'tĕr'ĕ-
nōl)
soufflé (soo-flā') [Fr. *souffler*, to puff]
　s., cardiac
　s., fetal
　s., funic
　s., placental
　s., splenic
　s., uterine
sound (sownd) [L. *sonus*, sound]
　s., anasarcous
　s., blowing
　s., bottle
　s.'s, breath
　s., bronchial
　s.'s, bronchovesicular
　s., cracked-pot
　s., ejection
　s., fetal heart
　s., friction
　s.'s, heart
　s.'s, Korotkoff's
　s., percussion
　s.'s, physiological
　s., respiratory
　s., succussion

s., to-and-fro
s., tracheal
s., tubular
s., urethral
s., vesicular
s., white
Souques' phenomenon [A. A. Souques, Fr. neurologist, 1860–1944]
source-skin distance
soybean oil
sp. [L.] *spiritus,* spirit; *species*
spa (spä) [Spa, a Belgium resort town]
space (spās) [L. *spatium,* space]
s., anatomical dead
s., axillary
s., circumlental
s., dead
s., epidural
s., intercostal
s., interfascial
s., interpleural
s., interproximal
s., interradicular
s., intervillous
s., lymph
s., Meckel's
s., mediastinal
s., medullary
s., Nuel's
s.'s of Fontana
s., palmar
s.'s, parasinoidal
s., perforated
s.'s, perivascular
s., personal
s., physiological dead
s., plantar
s., pneumatic
s., popliteal
s., prezonular
s., Prussak's
s., retroperitoneal
s., retropharyngeal
s.'s, subarachnoid
s., subdural
s., subphrenic
s., suprasternal
s., Tenon's

s., thenar
s., tissue
s.'s, zonular
space maintainer
space medicine
space sickness
spallation (spawl-lā'shŭn)
span
Spanish fly
sparer (spär'ĕr) [AS. *sparian,* to refrain]
s., protein
sparganosis (spär"gă-nō'sĭs)
Sparganum (spär'gă-nŭm) [Gr. *sparganon,* swathing band]
S. mansoni
S. mansonoides
S. proliferum
sparge (spärj) [L. *spargere,* to scatter]
spargosis (spär-gō'sĭs) [Gr. *spargosis,* swelling]
Sparine
spark coil
spark gap
s.g., quenched
spasm (spăzm) [Gr. *spasmos,* a convulsion]
s., Bell's
s., bronchial
s., choreiform
s., clonic
s., habit
s., nodding
s. of esophagus
s., saltatory
s., tetanic
s., tonic
s., torsion
s., toxic
s., winking
spasmatic (spăz-măt'ĭk) [Gr. *spasmos,* a convulsion]
spasmatic asthma
spasmatic croup
spasmatic stricture
spasmodic (spăz-mŏd'ĭk) [Gr. *spasmos,* a convulsion]
spasmogen (spăz'mō-jĕn) [" + *gennan,* to produce]

spasmology (spăz-mŏl′ō-jē) [″ + *logos*, word, reason]

spasmolygmus (spăz-mō-lĭg′mŭs) [″ + *lygmos*, a sob]

spasmolysin (spăz-mŏl′ĭ-sĭn)

spasmolytic (spăz-mō-lĭt′ĭk) [″ + *lysis*, dissolution]

spasmophemia (spăz-mō-fē′mē-ă) [″ + *pheme*, speech]

spasmophilia (spăz-mō-fĭl′ē-ă) [″ + *philein*, to love]

spasmous (spăz′mŭs) [Gr. *spasmos*, a convulsion]

spasmus (spăz′mŭs) [Gr. *spasmos*, a convulsion]

   s. agitans
   s. bronchialis
   s. caninus
   s. coordinatus
   s. cynicus
   s. Dubini
   s. glottidis
   s. nictitans
   s. nutans

spastic (spăs′tĭk) [Gr. *spastikos*, drawing]

spastic colon

spastic gait

spastic hemiplegia

spasticity (spăs-tĭs′ĭ-tē)

spastic paralysis

spastic paraplegia

spatial (spā′shăl)

spatial discrimination

spatium (spā′shē-ŭm) [L.]

spatula (spăch′ū-lă) [L. *spatula*, blade]

   s., eye
   s., nasal

spatulate (spăch′ŭ-lāt)

spay, spaying (spā, spā′ĭng) [Gael. *spoth*, castrate]

SPCA *Society for the Prevention of Cruelty to Animals*

specialist (spĕsh′ăl-ĭst) [L. *specialis*]

specialization (spĕsh″ăl-ĭ-zā′shŭn)

specialty (spĕsh′ăl-tē)

speciation (spē″sē-ā′shŭn) [L. *species*, a kind]

species (spē′shēz) [L. *species*, a kind]

species-specific

species type

specific (spĕ-sĭf′ĭk) [L. *specificus*, pert. to a kind]

specific dynamic action

specific gravity

specificity (spē-sĭ-fĭs′ĭ-tē)

   s., diagnostic

specillum (spē-sĭl′lŭm) [L. *specere*, to look]

specimen (spĕs′ĭ-mĕn) [L. *specere*, to look]

spectacles (spĕk′tăk-lz) [L. *spectare*, to see]

spectinomycin hydrochloride, sterile

spectral (spĕk′trăl) [L. *spectrum*, image]

spectro- [L. *spectrum*, image]

spectrocolorimeter (spĕk-trō-kŭl-or-ĭm′ĕ-tĕr) [″ + *color*, color, + Gr. *metron*, measure]

spectrofluorometer (spĕk″trō-floo″or-ŏm′ĕ-tĕr)

spectrograph (spĕk′trō-grăf) [″ + Gr. *graphein*, to write]

   s., mass

spectrometer (spĕk-trŏm′ĕt-ĕr) [″ + Gr. *metron*, measure]

spectrometry (spĕk-trŏm′ĕ-trē) [″ + Gr. *metron*, measure]

spectrophotometer (spĕk″trō-fō-tŏm′ĕt-ĕr) [″ + Gr. *photos*, light, + *metron*, measure]

spectrophotometry (spĕk″trō-fō-tŏm′ĕt-rē)

spectropolarimeter (spĕk″trō-pō″lăr-ĭm′ĕ-tĕr) [″ + *polaris*, pole, + *metron*, measure]

spectropyrheliometer (spĕk″trō-pĭr-hē-lē-ŏm′ĕ-tĕr) [″ + Gr. *pyr*, fire, + *helios*, sun, + *metron*, measure]

spectroscope (spĕk′trō-skōp) [″ + Gr. *skopein*, to examine]

spectroscopic (spĕk″trō-skŏp′ĭk)

spectroscopy (spĕk-trŏs′kō-pē)

spectrum (spĕk′trŭm) [L., image]

s., absorption
s., broad
s., chromatic
s., invisible
s., visible
s., visible electromagnetic
spectrum emission
speculum (spĕk'ū-lŭm) [L., a mirror]
s., ear
s., eye
s., vaginal
speech [AS. spaec]
s., aphonic
s., ataxic
s., clipped
s., echo
s., esophageal
s., explosive
s., interjectional
s., mirror
s., scamping
s., scanning
s., slurring
s., staccato
speech abnormalities
speech pathologist
speech synthesizer
speech therapy
sperm (spĕrm) [Gr. sperma, seed]
sperma (spĕr'mă) [Gr.]
spermacrasia (spĕr"măk-rā'zē-ă) [Gr. sperma, seed, + akrasia, bad mixture]
spermagglutination
spermatemphraxis (spĕr"măt-ĕm-frăk'sĭs) [" + emphraxis, stoppage]
spermatic (spĕr-măt'ĭk) [Gr. sperma, seed]
spermatic arteries
spermatic cord
spermatic duct
spermaticidal (spĕrm"ăt-ĭ-sīd'ăl) [Gr. sperma, seed, + L. cida fr. caedere, to kill]
spermatic vein
spermatid (spĕr'mă-tĭd)
spermatin (spĕr'mă-tĭn)
spermatism (spĕr'mă-tĭzm) [" +

-ismos, condition]
spermatitis (spĕr"mă-tī'tĭs) [" + itis, inflammation]
spermato- [Gr. sperma, spermatos, seed]
spermatoblast (spĕr-măt'ō-blăst) [" + blastos, germ]
spermatocele (spĕr-măt'ō-sēl) [" + kele, tumor, swelling]
spermatocidal (spĕr"mă-tō-sī'dăl) [" + L. cida fr. caedere, to kill]
spermatocyst (spĕr-măt'ō-sĭst) [" + kystis, bladder]
spermatocystectomy (spĕr"măt-ō-sĭs-tĕk'tō-mē) [" + " + ektome, excision]
spermatocystitis (spĕr"măt-ō-sĭs-tī'tĭs) [" + " + itis, inflammation]
spermatocystotomy (spĕr"mă-tō-sĭs-tŏt'ō-mē) [" + " + tome, a cutting, slice]
spermatocytal (spĕr"mă-tō-sī'tăl) [" + kytos, cell]
spermatocyte (spĕr-măt'ō-sīt) [" + kytos, cell]
s., primary
s., secondary
spermatocytogenesis (spĕr"mă-tō-sī"tō-jĕn'ĕ-sĭs) [" + " + genesis, generation, birth]
spermatogenesis (spĕr"măt-ō-jĕn'ĕ-sĭs) [" + genesis, generation, birth]
spermatogenic, spermatogenous (spĕr"mă-tō-jĕn'ĭk, spĕr"mă-tŏj'ĕ-nŭs)
spermatogeny (spĕr"mă-tŏj'ĕ-nē)
spermatogonium (sper"măt-ō-gō'nē-ŭm) [" + gone, generation]
spermatoid (spĕr'mă-toyd) [" + eidos, form, shape]
spermatology (spĕr"mă-tŏl'ō-jē) [" + logos, word, reason]
spermatolysin (spĕr"măt-ŏl'ĭ-sĭn) [" + lysis, dissolution]
spermatolysis (spĕr"măt-ŏl'ĭ-sĭs) [" + lysis, dissolution]
spermatolytic (spĕr"măt-ō-lĭt'ĭk)
spermatopathia, spermatopathy (spĕr"mă-tō-păth'ē-ă, spĕr-mă-tŏp'ă-

thē) [Gr. *spermatos*, seed, +
pathos, disease, suffering]
spermatophobia (spĕr″mă-tō-fō′bē-
ă) [″ + *phobos*, fear]
spermatopoietic (spĕr″măt-ō-poy-
ĕt′ĭk) [″ + *poiein*, to make]
spermatorrhea (spĕr″mă-tō-rē′ă)
[″ + *rhein*, to flow]
spermatoschesis (spĕr″măt-ŏs′kĕ-sĭs)
[″ + *schesis*, checking]
spermatospore (spĕr-măt′ō-spor)
[″ + *sporos*, seed]
spermatotoxin (spĕr′mă-tō-tŏk′sĭn)
[″ + *toxikon*, poison]
spermatovum (spĕr″măt-ō′vŭm)
[″ + L. *ovum*, egg]
spermatoxin (spĕr″mă-tŏks′ĭn) [″ +
toxikon, poison]
spermatozoa (spĕr″măt-ō-zō′ă)
spermatozoal (spĕr″mă-tō-zō′ăl)
[″ + *zoon*, life]
spermatozoicide (spĕr″mă-tō-zō′ĭ-
sīd) [″ + ″ + L. *caedere*, to kill]
spermatozoon (spĕr″măt-ō-zō′ŏn)
[″ + *zoon*, life]
spermaturia (spĕr″mă-tū′rē-ă) [″ +
ouron, urine]
spermectomy (spĕr-mĕk′tō-mē) [″ +
ektome, excision]
spermic (spĕr′mĭk)
spermicidal (spĕr″mĭ-sī′dăl) [″ + L.
cida fr. *caedere*, to kill]
spermicide (spĕr′mĭ-sīd)
spermidine (spĕr′mĭ-dīn)
spermiduct (spĕr′mĭ-dŭkt) [″ + L.
ductus, a duct]
spermine (spĕr′mĭn)
spermiogenesis (spĕr″mē-ō-jĕn′ĕ-sĭs)
spermiogram (spĕr′mē-ō-grăm)
[″ + *gramma*, letter, piece of writ-
ing]
spermoblast (spĕr′mō-blăst) [″ +
blastos, a germ]
spermolith (spĕr′mō-lĭth) [″ +
lithos, stone]
spermolysin (spĕr-mŏl′ĭ-sĭn)
spermolytic (spĕr-mō-lĭt′ĭk) [″ +
lysis, dissolution]

spermoneuralgia (spĕr″mō-nū-răl′jē-
ă) [″ + *neuron*, nerve, +
algos, pain]
spermophlebectasia (spĕr″mō-
flĕ″bĕk-tā′zē-ă) [″ + *phlebos*,
blood vessel, vein, + *ektasis*, dila-
tation]
spermoplasm (spĕr′mō-plăzm) [″ +
LL. *plasma*, form, mold]
spermosphere (spĕr′mō-sfēr) [″ +
sphaira, a circle]
spermospore (spĕr′mō-spor) [″ +
sporos, seed]
spermotoxin (spĕr″mō-tŏk′sĭn) [″ +
toxikon, poison]
sp. gr. *specific gravity*
sph. *spherical*
sphacelate (sfăs′ĕl-āt) [Gr. *sphakelos*,
gangrene]
sphacelation (sfăs″ĕl-ā′shŭn)
sphacelism (sfăs′ĕl-ĭzm) [″ +
-*ismos*, condition]
sphaceloderma (sfăs″ĕl-ō-dĕr′mă)
[″ + *derma*, skin]
sphacelotoxin (sfăs″ĕl-ō-tŏk′sĭn)
[″ + *toxikon*, poison]
sphacelous (sfăs′ĕl-ŭs) [Gr. *sphakelos*,
gangrene]
sphacelus (sfăs′ĕl-ŭs)
sphagiasmus (sfă″jē-ăz′mŭs) [Gr.
sphagiasmos, a slaying]
sphagitis (sfă-jī′tĭs) [Gr. *sphage*, throat,
+ *itis*, inflammation]
sphenethmoid (sfĕn-ĕth′moyd) [Gr.
sphen, wedge, + *ethmos*, sieve]
sphenion (sfē′nē-ŏn) [Gr. *sphen*,
wedge]
spheno- [Gr. *sphen*, wedge]
sphenobasilar (sfē″nō-băs′ĭ-lăr)
[″ + L. *basilaris*, basal]
sphenoccipital (sfē″nŏk-sĭp′ĭ-tăl)
[″ + L. *occipitalis*, occipital]
sphenocephalus (sfē″nō-sĕf′ă-lŭs)
[″ + *kephale*, head]
sphenoethmoid (sfē″nō-ĕth′moyd)
[″ + *ethmos*, sieve, + *eidos*,
form, shape]
sphenoethmoid recess

sphenofrontal (sfē″nō-frŭn'tăl) [″ + L. frontalis, frontal]

sphenoid (sfē'noyd) [″ + eidos, form, shape]

sphenoidal (sfē-noy'dăl)

sphenoid bone

sphenoid fissure

sphenoiditis (sfē″noy-dī'tĭs) [″ + ″ + itis, inflammation]

sphenoidostomy (sfē″noy-dŏs'tō-mē) [″ + ″ + stoma, mouth, opening]

sphenoidotomy (sfē″noyd-ŏt'ō-mē) [″ + ″ + tome, a cutting, slice]

sphenomalar (sfē″nō-mā'lăr) [″ + L. mala, cheek]

sphenomaxillary (sfē″nō-măk'sī-lā-rē) [″ + L. maxilla, jawbone]

spheno-occipital (sfē″nō-ŏk-sĭp'ĭ-tăl) [″ + L. occipitalis, occipital]

sphenopalatine (sfē″nō-păl'ă-tēn) [″ + L. palatum, palate]

sphenoparietal (sfē″nō-pă-rī'ĕ-tăl) [″ + L. paries, a wall]

sphenorbital (sfē″nor'bĭ-tăl) [″ + L. orbita, track]

sphenosis [Gr., wedging]

sphenosquamosal (sfē″nō-skwā-mō'săl) [Gr. sphen, wedge, + L. squamosa, scaly]

sphenotemporal (sfē″nō-tĕm'pō-răl) [″ + L. temporalis, temporal]

sphenotic (sfē-nŏt'ĭk) [Gr. sphen, wedge, + eidos, form, shape]

sphenotresia (sfē″nō-trē'zē-ă) [Gr. sphen, wedge, + tresis, boring]

sphenotribe (sfē'nō-trīb) [″ + tribein, to crush]

sphenoturbinal (sfē″nō-tŭr'bĭ-năl) [″ + turbo, whirl]

sphenovomerine (sfē″nō-vō'mĕr-ĭn) [″ + L. vomer, plowshare]

sphenozygomatic (sfē″nō-zī″gō-măt'ĭk) [″ + zygoma, cheekbone]

sphere (sfēr) [Gr. sphaira, a globe]
  s., attraction
  s., segmentation

spheresthesia (sfēr″ĕs-thē'zē-ă) [″ + aisthesis, feeling, perception]

spherical (sfĕr'ĭ-kăl) [Gr. sphairikos]

spherocylinder (sfē″rō-sĭl'ĭn-dĕr) [Gr. sphaira, globe, + kylindros, cylinder]

spherocyte (sfē'rō-sīt) [″ + kytos, cell]

spherocytosis (sfē″rō-sī-tō'sĭs) [″ + ″ + osis, condition]
  s., hereditary

spheroid (sfē'royd) [″ + eidos, form, shape]

spheroidal (sfē-roy'dăl)

spherolith (sfē'rō-lĭth) [″ + lithos, stone]

spheroma (sfē-rō'mă) [″ + oma, tumor]

spherometer (sfē-rŏm'ĕt-ĕr) [″ + metron, measure]

spheroplast (sfĕr'ō-plăst)

spherospermia (sfē″rō-spĕr'mē-ă) [″ + sperma, seed]

spherule (sfĕr'ul) [LL. sphaerula, little globe]

sphincter (sfĭngk'tĕr) [Gr. sphinkter, band]
  s. ampullae
  s. ani
  s., bladder
  s., cardiac
  s. choledochus
  s., ileocecal
  s. of Oddi
  s. pancreaticus
  s., pyloric

sphincteral (sfĭngk'tĕr-ăl)

sphincteralgia (sfĭngk″tĕr-ăl'jē-ă) [Gr. sphinkter, band, + algos, pain]

sphincterectomy (sfĭngk″tĕr-ĕk'tō-mē) [″ + ektome, excision]

sphincteric (sfĭngk-tĕr'ĭk)

sphincterismus (sfĭngk″tĕr-ĭz'mŭs) [″ + -ismos, condition]

sphincteritis (sfĭngk″tĕr-ī'tĭs) [″ + itis, inflammation]

sphincterolysis (sfĭngk″tĕr-ŏl'ĭ-sĭs) [″ + lysis, dissolution]

sphincteroplasty (sfĭngk'tĕr-ō-

plăs"tē) [" + *plassein*, to form]
sphincteroscope (sfĭngk'tĕr-ō-skōp")
[" + *skopein*, to examine]
sphincteroscopy (sfĭngk"tĕr-ŏs'kō-pē)
sphincterotome (sfĭngk'tĕr-ō-tōm")
[" + *tome*, a cutting, slice]
sphincterotomy (sfĭngk"tĕr-ŏt'ō-mē)
[" + *tome*, a cutting, slice]
sphingolipid (sfĭng"gō-lĭp'ĭd) [Gr.
sphingein, to bind, + *lipos*, fat]
sphingolipidosis [" + " +
osis, condition]
sphingolipodystrophy (sfĭng"gō-lĭp"
ō-dĭs'trō-fē) [" + *dys*, bad, difficult,
painful, disordered, + *trophe*, nu-
trition]
sphingomyelins (sfĭng"gō-mī'ĕl-ĭns)
sphingosine (sfĭng'gō-sĭn)
sphygmic (sfĭg'mĭk) [Gr. *sphygmikos*]
sphygmo- [Gr. *sphygmos*, pulse]
sphygmobolometer (sfĭg"mō-bō-
lŏm'ĕ-tĕr) [" + *bolos*, mass, +
metron, a measure]
sphygmocardiogram (sfĭg"mō-kăr'
dē-ō-grăm) [" + *kardia*, heart,
+ *gramma*, letter, piece of writing]
sphygmocardiograph (sfĭg"mō-kăr'
dē-ō-grăf) [" + " + *graphein*,
to write]
sphygmocardioscope (sfĭg"mō-kăr'
dē-ō-skōp) [" + " + *skopein*,
to examine]
sphygmochronograph (sfĭg"mō-krō'
nō-grăf) [" + *chronos*, time, +
graphein, to write]
sphygmogram (sfĭg'mō-grăm) [" +
gramma, letter, piece of writing]
sphygmograph (sfĭg'mō-grăf) [" +
graphein, to write]
sphygmography (sfĭg-mŏg'ră-fē)
sphygmoid (sfĭg'moyd) [Gr. *sphygmos*,
pulse, + *eidos*, form, shape]
sphygmology (sfĭg-mŏl'ō-jē) [" +
logos, word, reason]
sphygmomanometer (sfĭg"mō-măn-
ŏm'ĕt-ĕr) [" + *manos*, thin, +
metron, measure]
    s., random-zero

sphygmometer (sfĭg-mŏm'ĕt-ĕr)
[" + *metron*, measure]
sphygmopalpation (sfĭg"mō-păl-
pā'shŭn) [" + L. *palpatio*, palpa-
tion]
sphygmophone (sfĭg'mō-fōn) [Gr.
sphygmos, pulse, + *phone*, voice]
sphygmoplethysmograph (sfĭg"mō-
plĕth-ĭz'mō-grăf) [" + *plethysmos*,
to increase, + *graphein*, to write]
sphygmoscope (sfĭg'mō-skōp) [" +
skopein, to examine]
sphygmosystole (sfĭg"mō-sĭs'tō-lē)
[Gr. *sphygmos*, pulse, + *systole*,
contraction]
sphygmotonograph (sfĭg"mō-tō'nō-
grăf) [" + *tonos*, act of stretching,
tension, tone, + *graphein*, to
write]
sphygmotonometer (sfĭg"mō-tō-nŏm'
ĕt-ĕr) [" + " + *metron*, mea-
sure]
sphygmus (sfĭg'mŭs) [Gr. *sphygmos*,
pulse]
sphyrectomy (sfĭ-rĕk'tō-mē) [Gr.
sphyra, malleus, + *ektome*, exci-
sion]
sphyrotomy (sfĭ-rŏt'ō-mē) [" +
tome, a cutting, slice]
spica (spī'kă) [L., ear of grain]
spica hip cast
spicular (spĭk'ū-lar) [L. *spiculum*, a dart]
spicule (spĭk'ūl)
    s., bony
spiculed red cell
spiculum (spĭk'ū-lŭm) [L., a dart]
spider (spī'dĕr)
    s., black widow
    s., brown recluse
spider-burst
spider cells
spider fingers
spider nevus
Spielmeyer-Vogt disease [Walter
Spielmeyer, Ger. neurologist, 1879–
1935; Oskar Vogt, Ger. neurologist,
1870–1959]
spigelian line (spī-jē'lē-ăn) [Adrian van

der Spieghel, Flemish anatomist,
1578–1625]
spigelian lobe
spike
spikeboard
spill (spĭl) [AS. *spillan*, to squander]
   s., cellular
   s., radioactive
spillway (spĭl'way)
spiloma, spilus (spī-lō'mă, spī'lŭs) [Gr.
spiloma, spilos, spot]
spiloplania (spī"lō-plā'nē-ă) [" +
plane, a wandering about]
spiloplaxia (spī"lō-plăk'sē-ă) [" +
plax, plate]
spina (spī'nă) [L., thorn]
   s. bifida
   s. bifida occulta
   s. ventosa
spinal (spī'năl) [L. *spinalis*]
spinal accessory nerve
spinal anesthesia
spinal canal
spinal column
spinal cord
spinal curvature
spinal curvature, angular
spinal curvature, lateral
spinal fluid
spinal fusion
spinal ganglion
spinal nerves
spinal puncture
spinal reflex
spinal shock
spinalgia (spī-năl'jē-ă) [L. *spina*, thorn,
   + Gr. *algos*, pain]
spinalis (spī-nā'lĭs) [L.]
spinate (spī'nāt)
spindle (spĭn'dl) [AS. *spinel*]
   s., aortic
   s., enamel
   s., muscle
   s., neuromuscular
   s., neurotendinous
   s., sleep
spine (spīn)
   s., alar

   s., anterior nasal
   s., bifid
   s., fracture of
   s., frontal
   s., hemal
   s., Henle's
   s., iliac
   s., ischial
   s., mental
   s., nasal
   s., neural
   s. of pubis
   s. of scapula
   s. of sphenoid
   s., pharyngeal
   s., posterior nasal
   s., sciatic
   s., suprameatal
   s., typhoid
spinifugal (spī-nĭf'ū-găl) [L. *spina*,
thorn, + *fugare*, to flee]
spinipetal (spī-nĭp'ĕ-tăl) [" + *petere*, to seek]
spinnbarkeit (spĭn'băr-kīt) [Ger.]
spinobulbar (spī"nō-bŭl'băr) [" +
Gr. *bulbos*, a bulb]
spinocellular (spī"nō-sĕl'ū-lăr) [" +
cellula, little cell]
spinocerebellar (spī"nō-sĕr-ĕ-bĕl'ăr)
[" + *cerebellum*, little brain]
spinocortical (spī"nō-kor'tĭ-kăl) [" +
cortex, rind]
spinocostalis (spī"nō-kŏs-tā'lĭs) [" +
costa, rib]
spinoglenoid (spī"nō-glĕn'oyd) [" +
Gr. *glene*, socket, + *eidos*, form,
shape]
spinoglenoid ligament
spinose (spī'nōs) [L. *spina*, thorn]
spinotectal (spī"nō-tĕk'tăl) [" +
tectum, roof]
spinous (spī'nŭs) [L. *spina*, thorn]
spinous point
spinous process
spintherism (spĭn'thĕr-ĭzm) [Gr. *spinth-
erizein*, to emit sparks]
spintheropia (spĭn"thĕr-ō'pē-ă) [Gr.
spinther, spark, + *ops*, eye]

spiradenitis (spī″răd-ĕn-ī′tĭs) [Gr. *speira*, coil, + *aden*, gland, + *itis*, inflammation]

spiradenoma (spī″răd-ĕn-ō′mă) [" + " + *oma*, tumor]

spiral (spī′răl) [L. *spiralis*]
    s., Curschmann's

spiral bandage

spiral canal of cochlea

spiral canal of modiolus

spiral lamina

spiral organ of Corti

spirilla (spī-rĭl′ă) [L.]

spirillicidal (spī-rĭl″ĭ-sīd′ăl) [L. *spirillum*, coil, + *cida* fr. *caedere*, to kill]

spirillicide (spī-rĭl″ĭ-sīd)

spirillolysis (spī″rĭ-lŏl′ĭ-sĭs) [" + Gr. *lysis*, dissolution]

spirillosis (spī-rĭl-ō′sĭs) [" + Gr. *osis*, condition]

spirillotropic (spī″rĭ-lō-trŏp′ĭk) [" + Gr. *trope*, a turning]

spirillotropism (spī″rĭ-lŏt′rō-pĭzm) [" + " + *-ismos*, condition]

Spirillum (spī-rĭl′ŭm) [L., coil]
    S. minus

spirillum

spirit (spĭr′ĭt) [L. *spiritus*, breath]
    s. of ammonia
    s. of bitter almond
    s. of camphor
    s. of juniper
    s. of lavender
    s. of mustard
    s. of peppermint

spiritual therapy [L. *spiritus*, breath, + Gr. *therapeia*, treatment]

spirituous (spĭr′ĭt-ū-ŭs″) [L., *spiritus*, breath]

spiritus (spĭr′ĭ-tŭs) [L., breath]
    s. frumenti
    s. juniperi
    s. myrciae
    s. vini gallici

Spirochaeta (spī″rō-kē′tă) [Gr. *speira*, coil, + *chaite*, hair]
    S. icterohaemorrhagiae
    S. pallida

Spirochaetales (spī″rō-kē-tā′lēs)

spirochetal (spī″rō-kē′tăl) [" + *chaite*, hair]

spirochetalytic (spī″rō-kē″tă-lĭt′ĭk) [" + " + *lysis*, dissolution]

spirochete (spī′rō-kēt)

spirochetemia (spī″rō-kē-tē′mē-ă) [" + *chaite*, hair, + *haima*, blood]

spirocheticidal (spī″rō-kē″tĭ-sī′dăl) [" + " + L. *cida* fr. *caedere*, to kill]

spirocheticide (spī″rō-kē′tĭ-sīd)

spirochetolysis (spī″rō-kē-tŏl′ĭ-sĭs) [" + *chaite*, hair, + *lysis*, dissolution]

spirochetosis (spī″rō-kē-tō′sĭs) [" + " + *osis*, condition]

spirochetotic (spī″rō-kē-tŏt′ĭk)

spirocheturia (spī″rō-kē-tū′rē-ă) [Gr. *speira*, coil, + *chaite*, hair, + *ouron*, urine]

spirogram (spī′rō-grăm″) [L. *spirare*, to breathe, + Gr. *gramma*, letter, piece of writing]

spirograph (spī′rō-grăf) [" + Gr. *graphein*, to write]

spiroid (spī′royd) [Gr. *speira*, coil, + *eidos*, form, shape]

spirokinesis (spī″rō-kĭn-ē′sĭs) [" + *kinesis*, motion]

spiroma (spī-rō′mă) [" + *oma*, tumor]

spirometer (spī-rŏm′ĕt-ĕr) [L. *spirare*, to breathe, + Gr. *metron*, measure]

spirometry (spī-rŏm′ĕ-trē) [L. *spirare*, to breathe, + Gr. *metron*, measure]

spironolactone (spī-rō″nō-lăk′tōn)

spissated (spĭs′ăt-ĕd) [L. *spissatus*]

spissitude (spĭs′ĭ-tūd) [L. *spissitudo*]

spit (spĭt) [AS. *spittan*]

spittle [AS. *spatl*]

splanchna (splăngk′nă) [Gr.]

splanchnapophysis (splăngk″nă-pŏf′ĭ-sĭs) [Gr. *splanchnos*, viscus, + *apophysis*, offshoot]

splanchnectopia (splăngk″něk-tō′pē-ă) [″ + ektopos, out of place]

splanchnemphraxis (splăngk″něm-frăk′sĭs) [″ + emphraxis, stoppage]

splanchnesthesia (splăngk″něs-thē′zē-ă) [″ + aisthesis, feeling, perception]

splanchnesthetic (splăngk″něs-thět′ĭk)

splanchnic (splăngk′nĭk) [Gr. splanchnikos]

splanchnicectomy (splăngk″nē-sěk′tō-mē) [Gr. splanchnos, viscus, + ektome, excision]

splanchnic nerves

splanchnicotomy (splăngk″nī-kŏt′ō-mē) [″ + tome, a cutting, slice]

splanchnoblast (splăngk′nō-blăst) [″ + blastos, germ]

splanchnocele (splăngk′nō-sēl) [″ + koilos, a cavity]; [″ + kele, tumor, swelling]

splanchnocoele (splăngk′nō-sēl) [″ + koilos, a cavity]

splanchnocranium (splăngk″nō-krā′nē-ŭm) [″ + kranion, skull]

splanchnodiastasis (splăngk″nō-dī-ăs′tă-sĭs) [″ + diastasis, a separation]

splanchnodynia (splăngk-nō-dĭn′ē-ă) [Gr. splanchnos, viscus, + odyne, pain]

splanchnography (splăngk-nŏg′ră-fē) [″ + graphein, to write]

splanchnolith (splăngk′nō-lĭth) [″ + lithos, stone]

splanchnology (splăngk-nŏl′ō-jē) [″ + logos, word, reason]

splanchnomegaly (splăngk″nō-měg′ă-lē) [″ + megas, large]

splanchnomicria (splăngk″nō-mĭk′rē-ă) [″ + mikros, small]

splanchnopathia (splăngk″nō-păth′ē-ă) [″ + pathos, disease, suffering]

splanchnopleural (splăngk″nō-ploor′ăl) [″ + pleura, side]

splanchnopleure (splăngk′nō-plūr) [″ + pleura, side]

splanchnoptosia, splanchnoptosis

(splăngk″nō-tō′sē-ă, -sĭs) [″ + ptosis, fall, falling]

splanchnosclerosis (splăngk″nō-sklěr-ō′sĭs) [″ + sklerosis, a hardening]

splanchnoscopy (splăngk-nŏs′kō-pē) [″ + skopein, to examine]

splanchnoskeleton (splăngk″nō-skěl′ě-tŏn) [″ + skeleton, a dried-up body]

splanchnosomatic (splăngk″nō-sō-măt′ĭk) [″ + soma, body]

splanchnotomy (splăngk″nō-tŏt′ō-mē) [″ + tome, a cutting, slice]

splanchnotribe (splăngk″nō-trīb) [″ + tribein, to rub]

splayfoot [ME. splayen, to spread out, + AS. fot, foot]

spleen (splēn) [Gr. splen]
    s., accessory
    s., floating
    s., lardaceous
    s., sago

splenadenoma (splēn″ăd-ē-nō′mă) [Gr. splen, spleen, + aden, gland, + oma, tumor]

splenalgia (splē-năl′jē-ă) [″ + algos, pain]

splenceratosis (splēn″sěr-ă-tō′sĭs) [″ + keras, horn, + osis, condition]

splenectasia, splenectasis (splē″něk-tā′zē-ă, splē-něk′tă-sĭs) [″ + ektasis, dilatation]

splenectomy (splē-něk′tō-mē) [″ + ektome, excision]

splenectopia, splenectopy (splē″něk-tō′pē-ă, -něk′tō-pē) [″ + ektopos, out of place]

splenelcosis (splē″něl-kō′sĭs) [″ + helkosis, ulceration]

splenemia (splē-nē′mē-ă) [Gr. splen, spleen, + haima, blood]

splenemphraxis (splē″něm-frăk′sĭs) [″ + emphraxis, an obstruction]

spleneolus (splē-nē′ō-lŭs)

splenetic (splē-nět′ĭk)

splenetic cords

splenetic nodule

splenetic sinus
splenetic vein
splenial (splē'nē-ǎl) [Gr. *splen*, spleen]
splenic (splĕn'ĭk) [Gr. *splenikos*]
splenic flexure
splenicterus (splē-nĭk'tĕr-ŭs) [Gr. *splen*, spleen, + *ikteros*, jaundice]
splenification (splē"nĭ-fĭ-kā'shŭn) [" + L. *facere*, to make]
spleniform (splĕn'ĭ-form) [" + L. *forma*, form]
splenitis (splē-nī'tĭs) [" + *itis*, inflammation]
splenium (splē'nē-ŭm) [Gr. *splenion*, bandage]
    s. corporis callosi
splenius (splē'nē-ŭs)
splenization (splē"nī-zā'shŭn)
splenocele (splē'nō-sēl) [Gr. *splen*, spleen, + *kele*, tumor, swelling]
splenoceratosis (splē"nō-sĕr"ă-tō'sĭs) [" + *keras*, horn, + *osis*, condition]
splenocleisis (splē"nō-klī'sĭs) [" + *kleisis*, closure]
splenocolic (splē"nō-kŏl'ĭk) [" + *kolon*, colon]
splenocyte (splē'nō-sīt) [" + *kytos*, cell]
splenodynia (splē"nō-dĭn'ē-ă) [" + *odyne*, pain]
splenogenic, splenogenous (splē"nō-jĕn'ĭk, splē-nŏj'ĕn-ŭs) [" + *gennan*, to produce]
splenography (splē-nŏg'ră-fē) [" + *graphein*, to write]
splenohemia (splē"nō-hē'mē-ă) [Gr. *splen*, spleen, + *haima*, blood]
splenohepatomegaly (splē"nō-hĕp"ă-tō-mĕg'ă-lē) [" + *hepar*, liver, + *megas*, large]
splenoid (splē'noyd) [" + *eidos*, form, shape]
splenokeratosis (splē"nō-kĕr"ă-tō'sĭs) [" + *keras*, horn, + *osis*, condition]
splenolaparotomy (splē"nō-lăp"ă-rŏt'ō-mē) [" + *lapara*, flank, +

tome, a cutting, slice]
splenology (splē-nŏl'ō-jē) [" + *logos*, word, reason]
splenolymphatic (splē"nō-lĭm-făt'ĭk) [" + L. *lympha*, lymph]
splenolysin (splē-nŏl'ĭ-sĭn) [" + *lysis*, dissolution]
splenolysis (splē-nŏl'ĭ-sĭs)
splenoma (splē-nō'mă) [" + *oma*, tumor]
splenomalacia (splē"nō-mă-lā'shē-ă) [" + *malakia*, softening]
splenomedullary (splē"nō-mĕd'ū-lĕr"ē) [" + L. *medulla*, marrow]
splenomegalia, splenomegaly (splē"nō-mē-gā'lē-ă, -mĕg'ă-lē) [" + *megas*, large]
    s., congestive
    s., hemolytic
splenometry (splē-nŏm'ĕ-trē) [" + *metron*, measure]
splenomyelogenous (splē-nō-mī"ĕ-lŏj'ĕ-nŭs) [" + *myelos*, marrow, + *gennan*, to produce]
splenomyelomalacia (splē"nō-mī"ĕl-ō-mă-lā'shē-ă) [" + " + *malakia*, softening]
splenoncus (splē-nŏng'kŭs) [Gr. *splen*, spleen, + *onkos*, bulk, mass]
splenonephric (splē"nō-nĕf'rĭk) [" + *nephros*, kidney]
splenonephroptosis (splē"nō-nĕf"rŏp-tō'sĭs) [" + " + *ptosis*, fall, falling]
splenopancreatic (splē"nō-păn"krē-ăt'ĭk) [" + *pankreas*, pancreas]
splenopathy (splē-nŏp'ă-thē) [" + *pathos*, disease, suffering]
splenopexy (splē'nō-pĕk"sē) [" + *pexis*, fixation]
splenophrenic (splĕn-ō-frĕn'ĭk) [" + *phren*, diaphragm]
splenopneumonia (splē"nō-nū-mō'nē-ă) [" + *pneumonia*, inflammation of lung]
splenoportography (splē"nō-por-tŏg'ră-fē) [" + L. *porta*, gate, + Gr. *graphein*, to write]

splenoptosis (splē"nŏp-tō'sĭs) [" + ptosis, fall, falling]
splenorenal (splē"nō-rē'năl)
splenorenal shunt
splenorrhagia (splē"nō-rā'jē-ă) [" + rhegnynai, to burst forth]
splenorrhaphy (splē-nor'ă-fē) [" + rhaphe, seam]
splenotomy (splē-nŏt'ō-mē) [" + tome, a cutting, slice]
splenotoxin (splē"nō-tŏks'ĭn) [" + toxikon, poison]
splenulus (splĕn'ū-lŭs) [L., a little spleen]
splenunculus (splĕ-nŭng'kū-lŭs)
splint (splĭnt) [MD. splinte, a wedge]
  s., acrylic resin bite-guard
  s., Agnew's
  s., airplane
  s., anchor
  s., Ashhurst's
  s., Balkan
  s., banjo traction
  s., Bavarian
  s., blow-up
  s., Bond's
  s., Bowlby's
  s., bracketed
  s., Cabot's
  s., Carter's intranasal
  s., coaptation
  s., Denis Browne
  s., dental
  s., Dupuytren's
  s., dynamic
  s., Fox's
  s., functional
  s., Gibson walking
  s., Gordon's
  s., inflatable
  s., Jones' nasal
  s., Kanavel
  s., Levis'
  s., McIntire's
  s., permanent fixed
  s., Sayre's
  s., Stromeyer's
  s., temporary removable
  s., Thomas

  s., Thomas' knee
  s., Thomas' posterior
  s., Volkmann's
splinter (splĭn'tĕr) [MD. splinte, a wedge]
splinter hemorrhage
splinter skill
splinting
split (splĭt) [D. splitten, to divide]
split foot
split hand
split pelvis
splitting (splĭt'ĭng) [D. splitten, to divide]
split tongue
spodogenous (spō-dŏj'ĕn-ŭs) [Gr. spodos, ashes, + gennan, to produce]
spodophagous (spō-dŏf'ă-gŭs) [" + phagein, to eat]
spondee (spŏn-dē)
spondyl- (spŏn'dĭl) [Gr. spondylos, vertebra]
spondylalgia (spŏn"dĭl-ăl'jē-ă) [" + algos, pain]
spondylarthritis (spŏn"dĭl-ăr-thrī'tĭs) [" + arthron, joint, + itis, inflammation]
spondylarthrocace (splon"dĭl-ăr-thrŏk'ă-sē) [" + " + kake, badness]
spondylexarthrosis (spŏn"dĭl-ĕks"ăr-thrō'sĭs) [" + exarthrosis, dislocation]
spondylitic (spŏn"dĭ-lĭt'ĭk) [" + itis, inflammation]
spondylitis (spŏn-dĭl-ī'tĭs) [" + itis, inflammation]
  s., ankylosing
  s. deformans
  s., hypertrophic
  s., Kümmell's
  s., Marie-Strümpell
  s., rheumatoid
  s., tuberculous
spondylizema (spŏn"dĭl-ĭ-zē'mă) [Gr. spondylos, vertebra, + izema, depression]
spondylo- [Gr. spondylos, vertebra]

spondylocace (spŏn"dĭ-lŏk'ă-sē)
[" + kake, badness]

spondylodiagnosis (spŏn"dĭ-lō-dĭ"ăg-nō'sĭs) [" + dia, through, + gnosis, knowledge]

spondylodymus (spŏn"dĭ-lŏd'ĭ-mŭs) [" + didymos, twin]

spondylodynia (spŏn"dĭ-lō-dĭn'ē-ă) [" + odyne, pain]

spondylolisthesis (spŏn"dĭ-lō-lĭs"thē'sĭs) [" + oblisthesis, a slipping]

spondylolisthetic (spŏn"dĭ-lō-lĭs-thĕt'ĭk)

spondylolysis (spŏn"dĭ-lŏl'ĭ-sĭs) [" + lysis, dissolution]

spondylomalacia (spŏn"dĭ-lō-mă-lā'shē-ă) [" + malakia, softening]

spondylopathy (spŏn"dĭl-ŏp'ă-thē) [" + pathos, disease, suffering]

spondyloptosis (spŏn"dĭ-lō-tō'sĭs) [" + ptosis, fall, falling]

spondylopyosis (spon"dĭ-lō"pī-ō'sĭs) [" + pyosis, suppuration]

spondyloschisis (spŏn"dĭ-lŏs'kĭ-sĭs) [" + schisis, cleavage]

spondylosis (spŏn"dĭ-lō'sĭs) [Gr. spondylos, vertebra, + osis, condition]
  s., cervical or lumbar
  s., rhizomelic

spondylosyndesis (spŏn"dĭ-lō-sĭn'dē-sĭs) [" + syndesis, a binding together]

spondylotherapy (spŏn"dĭl-ō-thĕr'ă-pē) [" + therapeia, treatment]

spondylotomy (spŏn"dĭl-ŏt'ō-mē) [" + tome, a cutting, slice]

spondylous (spŏn'dĭ-lŭs) [Gr. spondylos, vertebra]

sponge (spŭnj) [Gr. sphongos, sponge]
  s., abdominal
  s., contraceptive
  s., gauze
  s., gelatin

sponge graft

spongia (spŏn'jē-ă) [Gr. sphongos, sponge]

spongiform (spŭn'jĭ-form) [Gr. sphongos, sponge, + L. forma, shape]

spongioblast (spŭn'jē-ō-blăst) [" + blastos, germ]

spongioblastoma (spŭn"jē-ō-blăs-tō'mă) [" + " + oma, tumor]

spongiocyte (spŭn'jē-ō-sīt") [" + kytos, cell]

spongioid (spŭn'jē-oyd) [" + eidos, form, shape]

spongioplasm (spŭn'jē-ō-plăzm) [Gr. sphongos, sponge, + LL. plasma, form, mold]

spongiosis (spŭn"jē-ō'sĭs) [" + osis, condition]

spongiositis (spŭn"jē-ō-sī'tĭs) [" + itis, inflammation]

spongy (spŭn'jē)

spontaneous (spŏn-tā'nē-ŭs) [L.]

spontaneous fracture

spontaneous version

spoon [AS. spon, a chip]

spoon nail

sporadic (spō-răd'ĭk) [Gr. sporadikos]

sporangiophore (spō-răn'jē-ō-for) [Gr. sporos, seed, + angeion, vessel, + phoros, a bearer]

sporangium (spō-răn'jē-ŭm)

spore (spor) [Gr. sporos, seed]

sporicidal (spor-ĭ-sī'dăl) [" + L. cida fr. caedere, to kill]

sporicide (spor'ĭ-sīd)

sporiferous (spor-ĭf'ĕr-ŭs) [" + L. ferre, to bear]

spork

sporoblast (spor'ō-blăst) [" + blastos, germ]

sporocyst (spor'ō-sĭst) [" + kystis, sac]

sporogenesis (spor"ō-jĕn'ĕ-sĭs) [Gr. sporos, seed, + genesis, generation, birth]

sporogenic (spor"ō-jĕn'ĭk) [" + gennan, to produce]

sporogenous (spor-ŏj'ĕ-nŭs) [" + gennan, to produce]

sporgeny (spor-ŏj'ĕ-nē)

sporogony (spor-ŏg'ō-nē) [" + goneia, generation]

sporophore (spor'ō-for) [" +

phoros, bearing]
sporophyte (spor′ō-fīt) [″ + *phyton*, plant]
sporoplasm (spor′ō-plăzm) [″ + LL. *plasma*, form, mold]
Sporothrix (spor′ō-thrĭks)
   S. schenckii
sporotrichin (spor-ō′trĭ-kĭn)
sporotrichosis (spor″ō-trĭ-kō′sĭs) [″ + *thrix*, hair, + *osis*, condition]
Sporotrichum (spō-rŏt′rĭ-kŭm)
   S. schenckii
Sporozoa (spor″ō-zō′ă) [″ + *zoon*, animal]
sporozoan
sporozoite (spor″ō-zō′īt) [″ + *zoon*, animal]
sporozoon
sport [ME. *sporten*, to divert]
sports medicine
sporular (spor′ū-lăr) [L. *sporula*, little spore]
sporulation (spor-ū-lā′shŭn) [L. *sporula*, little spore]
spot (spŏt) [MD. *spotte*]
   s., blind
   s., blue
   s., cherry-red
   s., cold
   s., corneal
   s.'s, Fordyce's
   s., genital
   s., hot
   s., hypnogenic
   s.'s, Koplik's
   s.'s, liver
   s., milk
   s., mongolian
   s.'s, rose
   s., ruby
   s., temperature
   s.'s, warm
   s.'s, white
   s., yellow
spotted fever
spotting
spp. *species*

sprain (sprān) [O. Fr. *espraindre*, to wring]
   s. of ankle or foot
   s. of back
   s., riders'
sprain fracture
spray (sprā) [MD. *spraeyen*, to sprinkle]
spray tube
spreader (sprĕd′ĕr)
   s., bladder-neck
   s., root canal
spreading (sprĕd′ĭng) [AS. *spraedan*, to strew]
spreading factor
spring [AS. *springan*, to jump]
spring conjunctivitis
spring fever
spring finger
spring ligament
sprue (sproo) [D. *sprouwe*]
spud (spŭd) [ME. *spudde*, short knife]
spur [AS. *spura*, a pointed instrument]
   s., calcaneal
   s., femoral
   s., scleral
spurious (spū′rē-ŭs) [L. *spurius*]
sputum (spū′tŭm) [L.]
   s., bloody
   s., nummular
   s., prune juice
   s., rusty
   s., septicemia
sputum specimen
sq. *subcutaneous*
squalene (skwăl′ēn)
squama (skwă′mă) [L.]
squamate (skwă′māt) [L. *squama*, scale]
squamatization (skwă″mă-tī-zā′shŭn) [L. *squama*, scale]
squame (skwăm) [L. *squama*, scale]
squamocellular (skwă″mō-sĕl′ū-lar) [L. *squama*, scale, + *cellula*, little cell]
squamofrontal (skwă″mō-frŏn′tăl) [″ + *frontalis*, frontal]
squamomastoid (skwă″mō-măs′toyd) [″ + Gr. *mastos*, breast, + *eidos*, form, shape]

squamo-occipital (skwā"mō-ŏk-sĭp'ĭ-tăl) [" + occipitalis, occipital]

squamoparietal (skwā"mō-pă-rī'ĕ-tăl) [" + paries, a wall]

squamopetrosal (skwā"mō-pē-trō'săl) [" + petrosus, stony]

squamosa (skwă-mō'să) [L., scaly]

squamosal (skwă-mō"săl) [L. squama, scale]

squamosphenoid (skwā"mō-sfē'noyd) [" + Gr. sphen, wedge, + eidos, form, shape]

squamous (skwā'mŭs) [L. squamosus]

squamous bone

squamous cell

squamous epithelium

squamous suture

squamozygomatic (sqwā"mō-zī"gō-măt'ĭk) [" + zygoma, cheekbone]

square knot

square lobe

squarrose, squarrous (skwăr'ōs, -ŭs) [L. squarrosus]

squatting position

squeeze-bottle

squill (skwĭl) [Gr. skilla]

squint (skwĭnt) [ME. asquint, sidelong glance]
   s., convergent
   s., divergent
   s., external
   s., internal

SR sedimentation rate

Sr strontium

SRF somatotropin releasing factor

sRNA soluble ribonucleic acid

SRS, SRS-A slow-reacting substance

SS saliva sample; soapsuds; sterile solution

ss [L.] semis, half; subjects

SSD source-skin distance

SSE soapsuds enema

SSS sterile saline soak

SSSS Society for the Scientific Study of Sex

ST sedimentation time

S.T. 37

stab (stăb) [ME. stob, stick]

stab culture

stabile (stā'bĭl) [L. stabilis, stable]

stabilization (stā"bĭl-ĭ-zā'shŭn) [L. stabilis, stable]

stable (stā'bl)

staccato speech (stă-kă'tō) [It. staccare, to detach]

stachyose

stactometer (stăk-tŏm'ĕt-ĕr) [Gr. staktos, dropping, + metron, measure]

stadium (stā'dē-ŭm) [Gr. stadion, alteration]
   s. acmes
   s. augmenti
   s. caloris
   s. decrementi
   s. fluorescentiae
   s. frigoris
   s. incrementi
   s. invasionis
   s. sudoris

Stadol

staff (stăf) [AS. staef, a stick]
   s., attending
   s., consulting
   s., house
   s. of Wrisberg

stage (stāj) [O. Fr. estage]
   s., algid
   s., amphibolic
   s., asphyxial
   s., cold
   s., defervescent
   s., eruptive
   s., expulsive, of labor
   s., first, of labor
   s., fourth, of labor
   s., hot
   s. of invasion
   s. of latency
   s., placental, of labor
   s., preeruptive
   s., pyrogenetic
   s., resting
   s., second, of labor
   s., sweating
   s., third, of labor

staggers (stăg'ĕrz)

staging
stagnation (stăg-nā'shŭn) [L. *stagnans*, stagnant]
stain (stān) [O. Fr. *desteindre*, deprive of color]
  s., acid
  s., acid-fast
  s., basic
  s., Commission Certified
  s., contrast
  s., counter
  s., dental
  s., differential
  s., double
  s., Giemsa
  s., Gram's
  s., hematoxylin-eosin
  s., intravital
  s., inversion
  s., metachromatic
  s., neutral
  s., nuclear
  s., port-wine
  s., substantive
  s., supravital
  s., tumor
  s., vital
  s., Wright's
staining (stān'ĭng) [O. Fr. *desteindre*]
staircase breaths
staircase phenomenon
stalagmometer (stăl-ăg-mŏm'ĕ-tĕr) [Gr. *stalagmos*, dropping, + *metron*, a measure]
stalk (stawk) [ME]
  s., belly
  s., body
  s., cerebellar
  s., infundibular
  s., optic
  s., yolk
stamina (stăm'ĭ-nă) [L., thread of the warp, thread of human life]
stammering (stăm'ĕr-ĭng) [AS. *stamerian*]
  s. of bladder
standard [O. Fr. *estandard*, marking rallying place]

  s., biological
standard deviation
standard error
standardization
standards of practice
standing orders
standstill
  s., atrial
  s., cardiac
  s., inspiratory
  s., respiratory
  s., ventricular
stannic (stăn'ĭk) [L. *stannum*, tin]
stannous (stăn'ŭs) [L. *stannum*, tin]
stannous fluoride
stannum (stăn'ŭm) [L.]
stanolone (stăn'ō-lōn)
stanozolol (stăn'ō-zō-lŏl″)
Stanton's disease
stapedectomy (stā″pē-dĕk'tō-mē) [L. *stapes*, stirrup, + Gr. *ektome*, excision]
stapedial (stā-pē'dē-ăl)
stapediotenotomy (stā-pē″dē-ō-tĕn-ŏt'ō-mē) [" + Gr. *tenon*, tendon, + *tome*, a cutting, slice]
stapediovestibular (stā-pē″dē-ō-vĕs-tĭb'ū-lar) [" + *vestibulum*, an antechamber]
stapedius (stā-pē'dē-ŭs) [L. *stapes*, stirrup]
stapes (stā'pēz) [L., stirrup]
Staphcillin
staphylagra (stăf″ĭ-lā'gră) [Gr. *staphyle*, a bunch of grapes, + *agra*, a way of catching]
staphyle (stăf'ĭ-lē) [Gr. *staphyle*, a bunch of grapes]
staphylectomy (stăf″ĭ-lĕk'tō-mē) [" + *ektome*, excision]
staphyledema (stăf″ĭl-ĕ-dē'mă) [" + *oidema*, swelling]
staphyline (stăf'ĭ-lĭn) [Gr. *staphyle*, a bunch of grapes]
staphylion (stăf-ĭl'ē-ŏn) [Gr., little grape]
staphylitis (stăf″ĭl-ī'tĭs) [Gr. *staphyle*, a bunch of grapes, + *itis*, inflamma-

stat. **733**

tion]
staphylo- [Gr. *staphyle*, a bunch of grapes]
staphyloangina (stăf"ĭl-ō-ăn'jĭ-nă) [" + L. *angina*, sore throat]
staphylococcal (stăf"ĭl-ō-kŏk'ăl) [" + *kokkos*, berry]
staphylococcal actinophytosis
staphylococcal food poisoning
staphylococcemia (stăf"ĭl-ō-kŏk-sē'mē-ă) [" + " + *haima*, blood]
staphylococci (stăf"ĭl-ō-kŏk'sē)
Staphylococcus (stăf"ĭl-ō-kŏk'ŭs) [Gr. *staphyle*, a bunch of grapes, + *kokkos*, berry]
   S. aureus
   S. epidermidis
   S. saprophyticus
staphylococcus (stăf"ĭl-ō-kŏk'ŭs)
staphyloderma (stăf"ĭ-lō-děr'mă) [" + *derma*, skin]
staphylodermatitis (stăf"ĭl-ō-derm"ă-tī'tĭs) [" + " + *itis*, inflammation]
staphylodialysis (stăf"ĭ-lō-dĭ-ăl'ĭ-sĭs) [" + *dia*, through, + *lysis*, dissolution]
staphylohemia (stăf"ĭ-lō-hē'mē-ă) [" + *haima*, blood]
staphylokinase (stăf"ĭ-lō-kī'nās)
staphylolysin (stăf"ĭ-lŏl'ĭ-sĭn) [" + *lysis*, dissolution]
staphyloma (stăf"ĭl-ō'mă) [Gr.]
   s., anterior
   s., ciliary
   s., corneae
   s., equatorial
   s., intercalary
   s., partial
   s., posterior
   s., total
   s. uveal
staphylomatous (stăf"ĭ-lōm'ă-tŭs)
staphyloncus (stăf"ĭ-lŏng'kŭs) [Gr. *staphyle*, a bunch of grapes, + *onkos*, bulk, mass]
staphylopharyngeus (stăf"ĭ-lō-făr-ĭn'jē-ŭs) [" + *pharynx*, throat]
staphylopharyngorrhaphy (stăf"ĭ-lō-făr"ĭn-gor'ă-fē) [" + " + *rhaphe*, seam]
staphyloplasty (stăf'ĭ-lō-plăs"tē) [" + *plassein*, to form]
staphyloptosia, staphyloptosis (stăf"ĭ-lŏp-tō'sē-ă, -sĭs) [" + *ptosis*, fall, falling]
staphylorrhaphy (stăf"ĭl-or'ă-fē) [" + *rhaphe*, seam]
staphyloschisis (stăf"ĭ-lŏs'kĭ-sĭs) [" + *schisis*, cleavage]
staphylotome (stăf'ĭ-lō-tōm) [" + *tome*, a cutting, slice]
staphylotomy (stăf"ĭ-lŏt'ō-mē)
staphylotoxin (stăf"ĭ-lō-tŏk'sĭn) [Gr. *staphyle*, a bunch of grapes, + *toxikon*, poison]
staple food
stapling
star [AS. *steorra*]
   s., lens
   s.'s of Verheyen
starch [AS. *stercan*]
   s., animal
   s., corn
starch glycerite
stare (stār) [AS. *starian*]
Starling's law of heart [Ernest Henry Starling, Brit. physiologist, 1866–1927]
Starling's law of intestine
starter
startle syndrome
starvation [AS. *steorfan*, to die]
stasibasiphobia (stā"sĭ-bā"sĭ-fō'bē-ă) [Gr. *stasis*, standing still, + *basis*, step, + *phobos*, fear]
stasimorphia, stasimorphy (stā"sĭ-mor'fē-ă, -fē) [" + *morphe*, form]
stasiphobia (stā"sĭ-fō'bē-ă) [" + *phobos*, fear]
stasis (stā'sĭs) [Gr. *stasis*, standing still]
   s., diffusion
   s., intestinal
   s., venous
stat. [L.] *statim*, immediately

state [L. *status*, condition]
  s., anxiety
  s., central excitatory
  s., central inhibitory
  s., dream
  s., excited
  s., fatigue
  s., ground
  s., refractory
  s., steady
static (stăt′ĭk) [Gr. *statikos*, causing to stand]
static electricity
static equilibrium
static pressure
static reflex
statics (stăt′ĭks)
static splint
statim (stăt′ĭm) [L.]
station (stā′shŭn) [L. *statio*, standing]
  s., aid
  s., dressing
  s., rest
stationary (stā′shŭn-ĕr-ē) [L. *stationarius*, belonging to a station]
statistical (stă-tĭs′tĭ-kăl)
statistical significance
statistics (stă-tĭs′tĭks) [LL. *statisticus*]
  s., medical
  s., morbidity
  s., vital
statoacoustic (stăt″ō-ă-koo′stĭk) [Gr. *statos*, placed, + *akoustikos*, acoustic]
statoconia (stăt″ō-kō′nē-ă) [" + *konos*, dust]
statokinetic (stăt″kō-kĭn-ĕt′ĭk) [" + *kinetikos*, moving]
statokinetic reflexes
statolith (stăt′ō-lĭth) [" + *lithos*, stone]
statometer (stă-tŏm′ĕt-ĕr) [" + *metron*, a measure]
statosphere (stăt′ō-sfēr) [" + *sphaira*, a globe]
stature (stăt′ūr) [L. *statura*]
  s., short
status (stā′tŭs) [L.]

  s. anginosus
  s. arthriticus
  s. asthmaticus
  s. dysgraphicus
  s. epilepticus
  s. parathyreoprivus
  s. praesens
  s. raptus
  s. sternuens
  s. verrucosus
  s. vertiginosus
staunch (stŏnch) [O. Fr. *estanche*, firm]
staurion (staw′rē-ŏn) [Gr. *stauros*, little cross]
stauroplegia (staw″rō-plē′jē-ă) [" + *plege*, stroke]
S.T.D. *skin test dose; sexually transmitted disease*
steal (stēl)
  s., subclavian
steam (stēm) [AS. *steam*, vapor]
steam tent
steapsin (stē-ăp′sĭn) [Gr. *stear*, fat, + *pepsis*, digestion]
stearate (stē′ă-rāt)
stearic acid (stē-ăr′ĭk) [Gr. *stear*, fat]
steariform (stē-ăr′ĭ-form) [" + *forma*, shape]
stearin (stē′ă-rĭn) [Gr. *stear*, fat]
stearodermia (stē″ă-rō-dĕr′mē-ă) [" + *derma*, skin]
stearopten(e) (stē″ă-rŏp′tēn) [" + *ptenos*, volatile]
stearrhea (stē″ă-rē′ă) [Gr. *stear*, fat, + *rhein*, to flow]
  s. flavescens
  s. nigricans
  s. simplex
steatadenoma (stē-ăt″ăd-ĕ-nō′mă) [Gr. *steatos*, fat, + *aden*, gland, + *oma*, tumor]
steatite (stē′ă-tīt)
steatitis (stē″ă-tī′tĭs) [" + *itis*, inflammation]
steato- [Gr. *steatos*, fat]
steatocele (stē-ăt′ō-sēl, stē′ăt-ō-sēl) [" + *kele*, tumor, swelling]
steatocryptosis (stē″ă-tō-krĭp-tō′sĭs)

[" + *krypte,* a sac, + *osis,* condition]

steatocystoma multiplex

steatogenous (stē″ă-tŏj′ĕn-ŭs) [Gr. *steatos,* fat, + *gennan,* to produce]

steatolysis (stē″ă-tŏl′ĭ-sĭs) [" + *lysis,* dissolution]

steatolytic (stē″ă-tō-lĭt′ĭk)

steatoma (stē″ă-tō′mă) [" + *oma,* tumor]

steatomatous (stē″ă-tō′mă-tŭs)

steatonecrosis (stē″ă-tō-nĕ-krō′sĭs) [" + *nekrosis,* state of death]

steatopathy (stē-ă-tŏp′ă-thē) [" + *pathos,* disease, suffering]

steatopygia (stē″ă-tō-pīj′ē-ă) [" + *pyge,* buttock]

steatopygous (stē″ă-tŏp′ĭ-gŭs) [" + *pyge,* buttock]

steatorrhea (stē″ă-tō-rē′ă) [Gr. *steatos,* fat, + *rhein,* to flow]
   s., idiopathic
   s. simplex

steatosis (stē″ă-tō′sĭs) [" + *osis,* condition]

stege (stē′jē) [Gr. *stegos,* roof]

stegnosis (stĕg-nō′sĭs) [Gr. *stegnosis,* obstruction]

stegnotic (stĕg-nŏt′ĭk)

Stegomyia (stĕg″ō-mī′ē-ă)

Steinert's disease (stīn′ĕrts) [Hans Steinert, Ger. physician, b. 1875]

Stein-Leventhal syndrome (stīn-lĕv′ĕn-thăl) [Irving F. Stein, Sr., U.S. gynecologist, b. 1887; Michael L. Leventhal, U.S. obstetrician and gynecologist, 1901 – 1971]

Steinmann's extension (stīn′mănz) [Fritz Steinmann, Swiss surgeon, 1872 – 1932]

Steinmann pin

Stelazine

stella [L.]
   s. lentis hyaloidea
   s. lentis iridica

stellate [L. *stellatus*]

stellate bandage

stellate cell

stellate fracture

stellate ganglion

stellate ligament

stellate veins

stellectomy (stĕl-lĕk′tō-mē) [" + *ektome,* excision]

Stellwag's sign (stĕl′văgs) [Carl Stellwag von Carion, Austrian oculist, 1823 – 1904]

stem [AS. *stemn,* tree trunk]
   s., brain

stem cell

stenion (stĕn′ē-ŏn) [Gr. *stenos,* narrow]

steno- [Gr. *stenos,* narrow]

stenobregmatic (stĕn″ō-brĕg-măt′ĭk) [" + *bregma,* front of head]

stenocardia (stĕn″ō-kăr′dē-ă) [" + *kardia,* heart]

stenocephaly (stĕn″ō-sĕf′ă-lē) [" + *kephale,* head]

stenochoria (stĕn″ō-kō′rē-ă) [" + *choros,* space]

stenocompressor (stĕn″ō-kŏm-prĕs′or) [" + L. *compressor,* that which presses together]

stenocoriasis (stĕn″ō-kō-rī′ă-sĭs) [" + *kore,* pupil, + *-iasis,* state or condition of]

stenocrotaphia (stĕn″ō-krō-tā′fē-ă) [" + *krotaphos,* the temple]

stenopaic, stenopeic (stĕn-ō-pā′ĭk, -pē′ĭk) [Gr. *stenos,* narrow, + *ope,* opening]

stenosal (stē-nō′săl) [Gr. *stenos,* narrow]

stenosed (stē-nōst′, stĕn′ōzd)

stenosis (stē-nō′sĭs) [Gr., act of narrowing]
   s., aortic
   s., cardiac
   s., cicatricial
   s., mitral
   s., pulmonary
   s., pyloric
   s., subaortic
   s., tricuspid

stenostomia (stĕn″ō-stō′mē-ă) [Gr.

stenos, narrow, + *stoma*, mouth, opening]

stenothermal (stĕn″ō-thĕr′măl) [″ + *therme*, heat]

stenothorax (stĕn″ō-thō′răks) [″ + *thorax*, chest]

stenotic [Gr. *stenosis*, act of narrowing]

Stensen's duct (stĕn′sĕns) [Niels Stensen, Danish anatomist, 1638 – 1686]

Stensen's foramina

stent [Charles R. Stent, Brit. dentist, 1845 – 1901]

step
    s., Rönne's

stephanion (stĕ-fā′nē-ŏn) [Gr. *stephanos*, crown]

steppage gait

stepping reflex

steradian (stē-rā′dē-ăn)

Sterane

sterco- [L. *stercus*, dung]

stercobilin (stĕr″kō-bī′lĭn) [″ + *bilis*, bile]

stercobilinogen (stĕr″kō-bī-lĭn′ō-jĕn)

stercolith (stĕr′kō-lĭth) [″ + Gr. *lithos*, stone]

stercoraceous (stĕr″kō-rā′shŭs) [L. *stercoraceus*]

stercoral (stĕr′kō-răl) [L. *stercus*, dung]

stercorin (stĕr′kō-rĭn)

stercorolith (stĕr′kō-rō-lĭth) [″ + Gr. *lithos*, stone]

stercoroma (stĕr″kō-rō′mă) [″ + Gr. *oma*, tumor]

stercorous (stĕr′kō-rŭs) [L. *stercorosus*]

stercus (stĕr′kŭs) [L.]

stere (stēr, stār) [Gr. *stereos*, solid]

stereoagnosis (stĕr″ē-ō-ŏg-nō′sĭs) [″ + *a-*, not, + *gnosis*, knowledge]

stereoanesthesia (stĕr″ē-ō-ăn″ĕs-thē′zē-ă) [″ + *an-*, not, + *aisthesis*, feeling, perception]

stereoarthrolysis (stĕr″ē-ō-ăr-thrŏl′ĭ-sĭs) [″ + *arthron*, joint, + *lysis*, dissolution]

stereoauscultation (stĕr″ē-ō-aws″kŭl-tā′shŭn) [″ + L. *auscultare*, listen to]

stereocampimeter (stĕr″ē-ō-kăm-pĭm′ĕ-tĕr) [″ + L. *campus*, field, + Gr. *metron*, measure]

stereochemical (stĕr″ē-ō-kĕm′ĭ-kăl) [″ + *chemeia*, chemistry]

stereochemistry (stĕr″ē-ō-kĕm′ĭs-trē)

stereocilia (stĕr″ē-ō-sĭl′ē-ă)

stereocinefluorography (stĕr″ē-ō-sĭn″ē-flū″or-ŏg′ră-fē)

stereoencephalotomy (stĕr″ē-ō-ĕn-sĕf″ă-lŏt′ō-mē) [″ + *enkephalos*, brain, + *tome*, a cutting, slice]

stereognosis (stĕr″ē-ŏg-nō′sĭs) [″ + *gnosis*, knowledge]

stereogram (stĕr′ē-ō-grăm) [″ + *gramma*, letter, piece of writing]

stereoisomer (stĕr″ē-ō-ī′sō-mĕr)

stereoisomerism (stĕr″ē-ō-ī-sō′mĕr-ĭzm)

stereology (stĕr″ē-ŏl′ō-jē) [Gr. *stereos*, solid, + *logos*, word, reason]

stereometer (stĕr″ē-ŏm′ĕ-tĕr) [″ + *metron*, measure]

stereometry (stĕr″ē-ŏm′ĕ-trē) [″ + *metron*, a measure]

stereo-ophthalmoscope (stĕr″ē-ō-ŏf-thăl′mō-skōp) [″ + *ophthalmos*, eye, + *skopein*, to examine]

stereo-orthopter (stĕr″ē-ō-or-thŏp′tĕr) [″ + *orthos*, straight, + *opsis*, sight, appearance, vision]

stereophantoscope (stĕr″ē-ō-făn′tō-skōp) [″ + *phantos*, visible, + *skopein*, to examine]

stereophorometer (stĕr″ē-ō-for-ŏm′ē-tĕr) [″ + *phoros*, a bearer, + *metron*, measure]

stereophotography (stĕr″ē-ō-fō-tŏg′ră-fē) [″ + *phos*, light, + *graphein*, to write]

stereophotomicrograph (stĕr″ē-ō-fō″tō-mī′krō-grăf) [″ + ″ + *mikros*, tiny, + *graphein*, to write]

stereopsis (stĕr″ē-ŏp′sĭs) [″ + *opsis*, sight, appearance, vision]

stereoradiography (stĕr″ē-ō-rā″dē-ŏg′ră-fē) [″ + L. *radius*, ray, + Gr. *graphein*, to write]

stereoroentgenography (stĕr"ē-ō-rĕnt"gĕn-ŏg'rȧ-fē) [" + roentgen, + Gr. graphein, to write]

stereoscope (stĕr'ē-ō-skōp) [" + skopein, to examine]

stereoscopic, stereoscopical

stereoscopic vision

stereospecific (stĕr"ē-ō-spĕ-sĭf'ĭk)

stereotactic (stĕr"ē-ō-tăk'tĭk)

stereotaxic (stĕr"ē-ō-tăk'sĭk) [Gr. stereos, solid, + taxis, arrangement]

stereotaxis (stĕr"ē-ō-tăk'sĭs) [" + taxis, arrangement]

stereotropic (stĕr"ē-ō-trŏp'ĭk) [" + trope, a turn]

stereotropism (stĕr"ē-ŏt'rō-pĭzm) [" + tropos, a turning, + -ismos, condition]

stereotypy (stĕr-ē-ō-tī'pē) [" + typos, type]

steric (stē'rĭk)

sterile (stĕr'ĭl) [L. sterilis, barren]

sterility (stĕr-ĭl'ĭ-tē) [L. sterilitas, barrenness]
s., absolute
s., acquired
s., female
s., male
s., primary
s., relative

sterilization (stĕr"ĭl-ĭ-zā'shŭn) [L. sterilis, barren]
s., dry heat
s., fractional
s., gas
s., intermittent
s., laparoscopic
s., steam

sterilize (stĕr'ĭ-līz) [L. sterilis, barren]

sterilizer (stĕr'ĭ-lī"zĕr)
s., steam

sternad (stĕr'năd) [Gr. sternon, chest]

sternal (stĕr'năl) [Gr. sternalis]

sternalgia (stĕr-năl'jē-ȧ) [Gr. sternon, chest, + algos, pain]

sternal puncture

Sternberg-Reed cell

sternebra (stĕr'nē-brȧ) [" + L. vertebra, vertebra]

sternen (stĕr'nĕn) [Gr. sternon, chest]

sterno- [Gr. sternon, chest]

sternoclavicular (stĕr"nō-klȧ-vĭk'ū-lȧr) [" + L. clavicula, little key]

sternocleidal (stĕr"nō-klī"dȧl) [" + clavis, key]

sternocleidomastoid (stĕr"nō-klī"dō-măs'toyd) [" + clavis, key, + mastos, breast, + eidos, form, shape]

sternocostal (stĕr"nō-kŏs'tăl) [" + L. costa, rib]

sternodymia (stĕr"nō-dĭm'ē-ȧ) [" + didymos, twin]

sternodynia (stĕr"nō-dĭn'ē-ȧ) [" + odyne, pain]

sternohyoid (stĕr"nō-hī'oyd) [" + hyoeides, U-shaped]

sternoid (stĕr'noyd) [" + eidos, form, shape]

sternomastoid (stĕr"nō-măs'toyd) [" + mastos, breast, + eidos, form, shape]

sternomastoid region

sternopagia (stĕr"nō-pā'jē-ȧ) [" + pagos, thing fixed]

sternopericardial (stĕr"nō-pĕr"ĭ-kăr'dē-ȧl) [" + peri, around, + kardia, heart]

sternoschisis (stĕr-nŏs'kĭ-sĭs) [" + schisis, cleavage]

sternothyroid (stĕr"nō-thī'royd) [" + thyreos, shield, + eidos, form, shape]

sternotomy (stĕr-nŏt'ō-mē [" + tome, a cutting, slice]

sternotracheal (stĕr"nō-trā'kē-ȧl) [" + tracheia, trachea]

sternotrypesis (stĕr"nō-trī-pē'sĭs) [" + trypesis, a boring]

sternovertebral (stĕr"nō-vĕr'tĕ-brȧl) [" + L. vertebra, vertebra]

sternum (stĕr'nŭm) [L.]
s., cleft

sternutament (stĕr-nū'tăm-ĕnt) [L. sternutare, to sneeze]

sternutatio (stĕr-nū-tā'shē-ō) [L.]
  s. convulsiva
sternutation (stĕr-nū-tā'shŭn)
  s., convulsive
sternutator (stĕr'nū-tā"tor) [L. *sternuta-torius*, causing sneezing]
sternutatory (stĕr-nū'tā-tō"rē)
steroid (stĕr'oyd)
steroidal withdrawal syndrome
steroid hormones
steroid hormone therapy
steroidogenesis (stē-roy"dō-jĕn'ē-sĭs)
sterol (stĕr'ŏl, stēr'ŏl) [Gr. *stereos*, solid, + L. *oleum*, oil]
stertor (stĕr'tor) [NL. *stertor*, to snore]
stertorous (stĕr'tō-rŭs)
stethalgia (stĕth-ăl'jē-ă)
stetho- [Gr. *stethos*, chest]
stethocyrtograph (stĕth"ō-sĕr'tō-grăf) [" + *kyrtos*, bent, + *graphein*, to write]
stethogoniometer (stĕth"ō-gō"nē-ŏm'ĕt-ĕr) [" + *gonia*, angle, + *metron*, measure]
stethogram (stĕth'ō-grăm) [" + *gramma*, letter, piece of writing]
stethograph (stĕth'ō-grăf) [" + *graphein*, to write]
stethokyrtograph (stĕth"ō-kĭr'tō-grăf) [" + *kyrtos*, bent, + *graphein*, to write]
stethometer (stĕth-ŏm'ĕt-ĕr) [" + *metron*, measure]
stethomyitis, stethomyositis (stĕth"ō-mī-ī'tĭs, -mī"ō-sī'tĭs) [" + *mys*, muscle, + *itis*, inflammation]
stethoparalysis (stĕth"ō-pă-răl'ĭ-sĭs) [" + *paralyein*, to loosen, disable]
stethophonometer (stĕth"ō-fō-nŏm'ĕt-ĕr) [" + *phone*, voice, + *metron*, measure]
stethoscope (stĕth'ō-skōp) [" + *skopein*, to examine]
  s., binaural
  s., compound
  s., double
  s., percussion
  s., single

stethoscopic (stĕth"ō-skŏp'ĭk)
stethoscopy (stĕth-ŏs'kō-pē) [" + *skopein*, to examine]
stethospasm (stĕth'ō-spăzm) [" + *spasmos*, a convulsion]
Stevens-Johnson syndrome (stē'vĕnz-jŏn'sŏn) [Albert M. Stevens, 1884–1945, Frank C. Johnson, 1894–1934, U.S. pediatricians]
STH *somatotropic hormone*
sthenia (sthē'nē-ă) [Gr. *sthenos*, strength]
sthenic (sthĕn'ĭk)
sthenometer (sthĕn-ŏm'ĕ-tĕr) [Gr. *sthenos*, strength, + *metron*, measure]
sthenometry (sthĕn-ŏm'ĕ-trē)
stibialism (stĭb'ē-ăl-ĭzm) [L. *stibium*, antimony, + Gr. *-ismos*, condition]
stibiated (stĭb'ē-āt"ĕd) [L. *stibium*, antimony]
stibium (stĭb'ē-ŭm) [L.]
stibophen (stĭb'ō-fĕn)
stichochrome (stĭk'ō-krōm) [Gr. *stichos*, row, + *chroma*, color]
stiff [AS. *stif*]
stiff joint
stiff man syndrome
stiff neck
stiff-neck fever
stigma (stĭg'mă) [Gr., mark]
  s., hysterical
  s. of degeneration
  s., psychic
stigmatic (stĭg-măt'ĭk) [Gr. *stigma*, mark]
stigmatism
stigmatization (stĭg"mă-tĭ-zā'shŭn)
stigmatometer (stĭg"mă-tŏm'ĕ-tĕr) [" + *metron*, measure]
stilbestrol (stĭl-bĕs'trŏl)
stilet, stilette (stī-lĕt') [Fr. *stilette*]
stillbirth [AS. *stille*, quiet, + Old Norse *burdhr*, birth]
stillborn [" + *boren*, to bring forth]
Still's disease [George F. Still, Brit. physician, 1868–1941]
stillicidium (stĭl"ĭ-sĭd'ē-ŭm) [L. *stilla*, drop, + *cadere*, to fall]

s. lacrimarum
s. narium
s. urinae
Stilphostrol
stimulant (stĭm'ū-lănt) [L. *stimulans*, goading]
stimulate (stĭm'ū-lāt) [L. *stimulare*, to goad on]
stimulation (stĭm″ū-lā'shŭn)
stimulator (stĭm″ū-lā'tor)
s., long-acting thyroid
stimulus (stĭm'ū-lŭs) [L., a goad]
s., adequate
s., chemical
s., conditioned
s., electric
s., homologous
s., iatrotropic
s., liminal
s., mechanical
s., minimal
s., nociceptive
s., subliminal
s., thermal
s., threshold
s., unconditioned
sting [AS. *stingan*]
stingray
S-T interval
stippling (stĭp'lĭng) [Dutch *stippelen*, to spot]
s., gingival
stirrup, stirrup bone (stĭr'ŭp) [AS. *stigrap*, a stirrup]
stitch (stĭch) [AS. *stice*, a pricking]
stitch abscess
stochastic model (stō-kăs'tĭk) [Gr. *stokastikos*, skillful in guessing]
stock (stŏk) [AS. *stocc*, tree trunk]
stock culture
stockinet
stocking
stoichiology (stoy″kē-ŏl'ō-jē) [Gr. *stoicheion*, element, + *logos*, word, reason]
stoichiometry (stoy″kē-ŏm'ĕ-trē) [" + *metron*, measure]
stoke (stōk) [Sir George Stokes, Brit.

physicist, 1819 – 1903]
Stokes-Adams syndrome (stōks-ăd'ăms) [William Stokes, Irish physician, 1804 – 1878; Robert Adams, Irish physician, 1791 – 1875]
Stokes' disease (stōks) [William Stokes]
Stokes' law (stōks) [William Stokes]
Stokes' lens [George Stokes]
stoma (stō'mă) [Gr., mouth]
stomach (stŭm'ăk) [Gr. *stomachos*, mouth]
s., bilocular
s., cardiac
s., cascade
s., cow horn
s., foreign bodies in
s., hourglass
s., leather-bottle
s., thoracic
s., water-trap
stomach ache
stomachal (stŭm'ă-kăl) [Gr. *stomachos*, mouth]
stomachalgia [" + *algos*, pain]
stomach cancer
stomachic (stō-măk'ĭk)
stomach intubation
stomachoscopy [" + *skopein*, to examine]
stomach pump
stomach tooth
stomach tube
stomal (stō'măl) [Gr. *stoma*, mouth, opening]
stomata
stomatal (stō'mă-tăl) [Gr. *stoma*, mouth, opening]
stomatalgia (stō″mă-tăl'jē-ă) [Gr. *stoma*, mouth, opening, + *algos*, pain]
stomatic
stomatitis (stō″mă-tī'tĭs)[" + *itis*, inflammation]
s., aphthous
s., catarrhal
s., corrosive
s., diphtheritic

s., follicular
s., herpetic
s., membranous
s., mercurial
s., mycotic
s. parasitica
s., simple
s., traumatic
s., ulcerative
s., vesicular
s., Vincent's
stomato- [Gr. *stoma*, mouth, opening]
stomatodynia (stō″mă-tō-dĭn′ē-ă) [Gr. *stoma*, mouth, opening, + *odyne*, pain]
stomatogastric (stō″mă-tō-găs′trĭk) [" + *gaster*, belly]
stomatognathic (stō″mă-tŏg-năth′ĭk) [" + *gnathos*, jaw]
stomatologist (stō″mă-tŏl′ō-jĭst) [" + *logos*, word, reason]
stomatology (stō″mă-tŏl′ō-jē)
stomatomalacia (stō″mă-tō-mă-lā′shē-ă) [" + *malakia*, softening]
stomatomenia (stō″mă-tō-mē′nē-ă) [" + *meniaia*, menses]
stomatomy (stō-măt′ō-mē) [" + *tome*, a cutting, slice]
stomatomycosis (stō″mă-tō-mī-kō′sĭs) [" + *mykes*, fungus, + *osis*, condition]
stomatonecrosis (stō″mă-tō-nĕ-krō′sĭs) [" + *nekrosis*, state of death]
stomatonoma (stō″mă-tō-nō′mă) [" + *nome*, a spreading]
stomatopathy (stō″mă-tŏp′ă-thē) [" + *pathos*, disease, suffering]
stomatoplasty (stō″mă-tō-plăs″tē) [" + *plassein*, to form]
stomatorrhagia (stō″mă-tō-rā′jē-ă) [" + *rhegnynai*, to burst forth]
stomatoscope (stō-măt′ō-skōp) [" + *skopein*, to examine]
stomatosis (stō″mă-tō′sĭs) [" + *osis*, condition]
stomatotomy (stō″mă-tŏt′ō-mē) [" + *tome*, a cutting, slice]
stomion (stō′mē-ŏn) [Gr., dim. of *stoma*, mouth, opening]

stomocephalus (stō″mō-sĕf′ă-lŭs) [Gr. *stoma*, mouth, opening, + *kephale*, head]
stomodeal (stō″mō-dē′ăl)
stomodeum (stō″mō-dē′ŭm) [" + *hodaios*, a way]
stone [AS. *stan*]
s., dental
s., red
s., salivary
stool (stool) [AS. *stol*, a seat]
s., bilious
s., fatty
s., lienteric
s., pea soup
s., rice water
stool softeners
stopcock (stŏp′kŏk)
stop needle
stoppage (stŏp′ăj) [AS. *stoppian*]
storax (stō′răks)
storm [AS.]
s., renal
s., thyroid
stout (stowt) [O. Fr. *estout*, bold]
Stoxil
STP *standard temperature and pressure*
STPD *standard temperature and pressure, dry*
Str. *Streptococcus*
strabismal (stră-bĭz′măl) [Gr. *strabismos*, a squinting]
strabismic (stră-bĭz′mĭk) [Gr. *strabismos*, a squinting]
strabismometer (stră-bĭz-mŏm′ĕt-ĕr) [" + *metron*, a measure]
strabismus (stră-bĭz′mŭs) [Gr. *strabismos*, a squinting]
s., accommodative
s., alternating
s., bilateral
s., concomitant
s., convergent
s. deorsum vergens
s., divergent
s., horizontal
s., intermittent

s., monocular
s., monolateral
s., nonconcomitant
s., paralytic
s., spastic
s. sursum vergens
s., vertical
strabometer (stră-bŏm'ĕt-ĕr) [Gr. *strabos*, squinting, + *metron*, a measure]
strabotome (strā'bō-tōm) [" + *tome*, a cutting, slice]
strabotomy (stră-bŏt'ō-mē) [" + *tome*, a cutting, slice]
strain (strān) [AS. *streon*, offspring; O. Fr. *estreindere*, to draw tight]
strainer (strān'ĕr)
strain x-ray
strait (strāt) [O. Fr. *estreit*, narrow]
s., inferior
s.'s of pelvis
s., superior
straitjacket
stramonium (stră-mō'nē-ŭm) [L.]
stramonium poisoning
strand
strangalesthesia (străng"găl-ĕs-thē'zē-ă) [L. *strangulare*, halter, + *aisthesis*, feeling, perception]
strangle (străng'gl) [L. *strangulare*, halter]
strangulated (străng'gū-lā"tĕd)
strangulation (străng"gū-lā'shŭn) [L. *strangulare*, halter]
s., internal
strangury (străng'gū-rē) [Gr. *stranx*, drop, squeezed out, + *ouron*, urine]
strap (străp) [Gr. *strophos*, a cord]
s., Montgomery
strapping (străp'ĭng)
stratification (străt"ĭ-fĭ-kā'shŭn) [L. *stratificare*, to arrange in layers]
stratified (străt'ĭ-fīd) [L. *stratificare*, to arrange in layers]
stratified epithelium
stratiform (străt'ĭ-form) [L. *stratum*, layer, + *forma*, shape]

stratum (strā'tŭm, străt'ŭm) [L.]
s. basale
s. compactum
s. corneum
s. disjunction
s. germinativum
s. granulosum
s. lucidum
s. malpighii
s. mucosum
s. papillare
s. reticulare
s. spinosum
s. spongiosum
s. submucosum
s. subserosum
s. supravasculare
s. vasculare
strawberry mark
strawberry tongue
straw itch
streak (strēk) [AS. *strica*]
s., angioid
s., medullary
s., meningitic
s., Moore's lightning
s., primitive
stream (strēm)
strength
s., breaking
s., compression
s., ego
s., impact
s., sheer
strephosymbolia (strĕf"ō-sĭm-bō'lē-ă) [Gr. *strephein*, to twist, + *symbolon*, symbol]
strepitus (strĕp'ĭ-tŭs) [L.]
Streptase
strepticemia (strĕp"tĭ-sē'mē-ă) [Gr. *streptos*, twisted, + *haima*, blood]
strepto- [Gr. *streptos*, twisted]
streptoangina (strĕp"tō-ăn'jĭ-nă) [" + L. *angina*, quinsy]
streptobacillus (strĕp"tō-bă-sĭl'ŭs)
streptococcal (strĕp"tō-kŏk'ăl) [" + *kokkos*, berry]
streptococcemia (strĕp"tō-kŏk-sē'mē-

ŏ) [" + " + *haima*, blood]
streptococci (strĕp"tō-kŏk'sī)
streptococcic (strĕp"tō-kŏk'sĭk) [" + *kokkos*, berry]
streptococcicosis (strĕp"tō-kŏk"sī-kō'sĭs) [" + " + *osis*, condition]
streptococcolysin (strĕp"tō-kŏk-kŏl'ĭ-sĭn) [" + " + *lysis*, dissolution]
Streptococcus (strĕp"tō-kŏk'ŭs) [" + *kokkos*, berry]
    Str. pneumoniae
    Str. pyogenes
    Str. thermophilus
    Str. viridans
streptococcus (strĕp"tō-kŏk'ŭs)
    s., β-hemolytic
streptocolysin (strĕp"tō-kŏl'ĭ-sĭn) [" + *lysis*, dissolution]
streptodermatitis (strĕp"tō-dĕr"mă-tī'tĭs) [" + *derma*, skin, + *itis*, inflammation]
streptodornase (strĕp"tō-dor'nās)
streptokinase (strĕp"tō-kī'nās)
streptokinase-streptodornase
streptoleukocidin (strĕp"tō-lū"kō-sī'dĭn) [" + *leukos*, white, + L. *caedere*, to kill]
streptolysin (strĕp-tŏl'ĭ-sĭn)
    s. O
    s. S
streptomycin   sulfate   (sterile) (strĕp"tō-mī'sĭn)
streptomycosis (strĕp"tō-mī-kō'sĭs) [" + *mykes*, fungus, + *osis*, condition]
streptosepticemia (strĕp"tō-sĕp"tĭ-sē'mē-ă) [" + *septikos*, putrid, + *haima*, blood]
streptothricin (strĕp"tō-thrī'sĭn)
streptothricosis (strĕp"tō-thrī-kō'sĭs) [Gr. *streptos*, twisted, + *thrix*, hair, + *osis*, condition]
stress (strĕs) [O. Fr. *estresse*, narrowness]
stress-breaker
stress fracture
stressor
    s., systemic
    s., topical

stress radiography
stress test
stress ulcer
stretch (strĕch) [AS. *streccan*, extend]
stretcher (strĕch'er)
stretching of contractures
stretch marks
stretch receptor
stretch reflex
stria (strī'ă) [L., a channel]
    striae acusticae
    s. atrophica
    striae cerebellares
    striae distensae
    s. gravidarum
    s. longitudinalis lateralis
    striae medullares
    s. of Retzius
    s. terminalis
striatal (strī-ā'tăl) [L. *striatus*, striped]
striate, striated (strī'āt, strī'ā-tĕd) [L. *striatus*]
striated arteries
striated body
striated muscle
striated veins, inferior
striation (strī-ā'shŭn) [L. *striatus*, striped]
striatum (strī-ā'tŭm) [L., grooved]
stricture (strĭk'chŭr) [LL. *strictura*, contraction]
    s., annular
    s., anorectal
    s., bridle
    s., cicatricial
    s., functional
    s., impermeable
    s., irritable
    s. of urethra
    s., spasmodic
stricturotome (strĭk'chŭr-ō-tōm) [L. *strictura*, contraction, + Gr. *tome*, a cutting, slice]
stricturotomy (strĭk"chŭr-ŏt'ō-mē)
stride length
strident (strī'dĕnt)
stridor (strī'dor) [L., a harsh sound]
    s., congenital laryngeal
    s. dentium
    s. serraticus

stridulous (strĭd'ū-lŭs) [L. *stridulus*]
string-of-pearls deformity
string sign
striocerebellar (strī"ō-sĕr"ĕ-bĕl'ăr) [L. *striatus*, striped, + *cerebellum*, little brain]
strip (strĭp) [AS. *striepan*, to plunder]
strobila (strō-bī'lă) [Gr. *strobilos*, anything twisted up]
strobiloid (strō'bī-loyd) [" + *eidos*, form, shape]
stroboscope (strō'bō-skōp) [Gr. *strobos*, whirl, + *skopein*, to examine]
stroke (strōk) [ME.]
　s., heat
　s., paralytic
stroke volume
stroking
stroma (strō'mă) [Gr., bed covering]
stromal, stromatic (strō'măl, strō-măt'ĭk)
stromatolysis (strō"mă-tŏl'ĭ-sĭs) [" + *lysis*, dissolution]
stromatosis (strō"mă-tō'sĭs) [" + *osis*, condition]
Stromeyer's splint (strō'mī-ĕrz) [Georg F. L. Stromeyer, Ger. surgeon, 1804 – 1876]
stromuhr (strō'moor) [Ger. *strom*, stream, + *uhr*, clock]
Strongyloides (strŏn"jĭ-loy'dēz)
　S. stercoralis
strongyloidosis (strŏn"jĭ-loy-dō'sĭs) [Gr. *strongylos*, compact, + *osis*, condition]
strongylosis (strŏn"jĭ-lō'sĭs)
Strongylus (strŏn'jĭ-lŭs)
strontium (strŏn'shē-ŭm) [Strontian, mining village in Scotland]
Strophanthus (strō-făn'thŭs) [Gr. *strophos*, twisted cord, + *anthos*, flower]
strophocephaly (strŏf"ō-sĕf'ă-lē) [" + *kephale*, head]
structural (strŭk'tū-răl) [L. *structura*, structure]
structure (strŭk'shŭr)
　s., denture-supporting

struma (stroo'mă) [L. *struma*, a mass]
　s. aberranta
　s., cast iron
　s. congenita
　s. lingualis
　s. lymphomatosa
　s. maligna
　s. ovarii
　s., Riedel's
strumectomy (stroo-mĕk'tō-mē) [" + *ektome*, excision]
strumiprivous (stroo"mī-prī'vŭs) [" + *privus*, deprived]
strumitis (stroo-mī'tĭs) [" + Gr. *itis*, inflammation]
strumous (stroo'mŭs) [L. *strumosus*]
Strümpell's disease (strĭm'pĕlz)
Strümpell-Marie disease [Adolf von Strümpell, Ger. physician, 1853 – 1925; Pierre Marie, Fr. neurologist, 1853 – 1940]
Strümpell's sign (strĭm'pĕlz)
struvite
strychnine (strĭk'nĭn, -nēn, -nĭn) [Gr. *strychnos*, nightshade]
strychnine poisoning
strychninism (strĭk'nĭn-ĭzm) [" + *-ismos*, condition]
strychnism (strĭk'nĭzm)
Stryker frame
STS *serological test for syphilis*
STU *skin test unit*
Stuart factor
study, case-control
stump
stump hallucination
stun (stŭn) [O. Fr. *estoner*, a blow]
stupe (stūp) [L. *stupa*, tow]
stupefacient (stū"pĕ-fā'shĕnt) [L. *stupefaciens*, stupefying]
stupefactive (stū"pĕ-făk'tĭv) [L. *stupefaciens*, stupefying]
stupemania (stū"pĕ-mā'nē-ă) [L. *stupor*, numbness, + Gr. *mania*, madness]
stupor (stū'por) [L.]
　s., anergic
　s., delusional
　s., epileptic

s., lethargic
s. melancholicus
stuporous
stuporous depression
Sturge-Weber syndrome [William Sturge, Brit. physician, 1850–1919; Frederick Weber, Brit. physician, 1863–1962]
sturine (stū'rĭn) [NL. *sturio*, sturgeon]
stutter (stŭt'ĕr) [ME. *stutten*, to stutter]
stuttering (stŭt'ĕr-ĭng)
s., urinary
sty(e) (stī) [AS. *stigan*, to rise]
s., meibomian
s., zeisian
style, stylet (stīl, stī'lĕt) [Gr. *stylos*, pillar]
styliform (stī'lĭ-form) [" + L. *forma*, form]
styliscus (stī-lĭs'kŭs) [Gr. *styliskos*, a pillar]
styloglossus (stī-lō-glŏs'ŭs) [Gr. *stylos*, pillar, + *glossa*, tongue]
stylohyal (stī"lō-hī'ăl) [" + *hyoeides*, hyoid]
stylohyoid (stī-lō-hī'oyd) [" + *hyoeides*, hyoid]
stylohyoideus (stī"lō-hī-oyd'ē-ŭs)
styloid (stī'loyd) [" + *eidos*, form, shape]
styloiditis (stī"loyd-ī'tĭs) [" + " + *itis*, inflammation]
styloid process
stylomandibular (stī"lō-măn-dĭb'ū-lar) [" + L. *mandibula*, lower jawbone]
stylomastoid (stī"lō-măs'toyd) [" + *mastos*, breast, + *eidos*, form, shape]
stylopharyngeus (stī"lō-făr-ĭn'jē-ŭs) [" + *pharynx*, throat]
stylostaphyline (stī"lō-stăf'ĭ-līn) [" + *staphyle*, bunch of grapes]
stylosteophyte (stī-lŏs'tē-ō-fīt)
stylus (stī'lŭs) [Gr. *stylos*, a pillar]
stype (stīp) [Gr., tow]
stypsis (stĭp'sĭs) [Gr., *styphein*, to contract]
styptic (stĭp'tĭk) [Gr. *styptikos*, contracting]

sub- [L. *sub*, under, below]
subabdominal (sŭb"ăb-dŏm'ĭ-năl) [L. *sub*, under, below, + *abdomen*, abdomen]
subabdominoperitoneal (sŭb"ăb-dŏm"ĭ-nō-pĕr"ĭ-tō-nē'ăl) [" + " + Gr. *peritonaion*, stretched around or over]
subacetate (sŭb-ăs'ĕ-tāt) [" + *acetum*, vinegar]
subacid (sŭb-ăs'ĭd) [" + *acidus*, sour]
subacromial (sŭb-ă-krō'mē-ăl) [" + Gr. *akron*, point, + *osmos*, shoulder]
subacute (sŭb"ă-kūt') [" + *acutus*, sharp]
subacute myelo-optic neuropathy
subacute sclerosing panencephalitis
subalimentation (sŭb"ăl-ĭ-mĕn-tā'shŭn) [" + *alimentum*, nourishment]
subanal (sŭb-ā'năl) [" + *analis*, anal]
subanconeus (sŭb"ăn-kō'nē-ŭs) [" + Gr. *ankon*, elbow]
subapical (sŭb-ăp'ĭ-kăl) [" + *apex*, tip]
subaponeurotic (sŭb"ăp-ō-nū-rŏt'ĭk) [" + Gr. *apo*, from, + *neuron*, sinew]
subarachnoid (sŭb"ă-răk'noyd) [" + Gr. *arachne*, spider, + *eidos*, form, shape]
subarachnoid cisternae
subarachnoid space
subarcuate (sŭb-ăr'kū-āt) [L. *sub*, under, below, + *arcuatus*, bowed]
subarcuate fossa
subareolar (sŭb"ă-rē'ō-lăr) [" + *areola*, a small space]
subastragalar (sŭb-ăs-trăg'ă-lăr) [" + Gr. *astragalos*, ball of the ankle joint]
subastringent (sŭb"ăs-trĭn'jĕnt) [" + *astringere*, to bind fast]
subatomic (sŭb"ă-tŏm'ĭk) [" + Gr. *atomos*, indivisible]
subaural (sŭb-aw'răl) [" + *auris*,

ear]

subauricular (sŭb"aw-rĭk'ū-lăr) [" + auricula, little ear]

subaxial (sŭb-ăk'sē-ăl) [" + axis, axis]

subaxillary (sŭb-ăk'sĭ-lĕr"ē) [" + axilla, armpit]

subbrachycephalic (sŭb"brā-kē-sĕ-făl'ĭk) [" + Gr. brachys, short, + kephale, head]

subcalcarine (sŭb-kăl'kăr-īn) [" + calcar, spur]

subcapsular (sŭb-kăp'sū-lăr) [" + capsula, little box]

subcarbonate (sŭb-kăr'bō-nāt) [" + carbo, carbon]

subcartilaginous (sŭb"kăr-tĭ-lăj'ĭn-ŭs) [" + cartilago, gristle]

subception (sŭb-sĕp'shŭn)

subchondral (sŭb"kŏn'drăl) [" + Gr. chondros, cartilage]

subchoroidal (sŭb"kō-roy'dăl) [" + Gr. chorioeides, skinlike]

subchronic (sŭb-krŏn'ĭk) [" + Gr. chronos, time]

subclass (sŭb'klăs)

subclavian (sŭb-klā'vē-ăn) [" + clavis, key]

subclavian artery

subclavian steal syndrome

subclavian triangle

subclavian vein

subclavicular (sŭb"klă-vĭk'ū-lăr) [L. sub, under, below, + clavicula, little key]

subclavius (sŭb-klā'vē-ŭs) [" + clavis, key]

subclinical (sŭb-klĭn'ĭ-kăl) [" + Gr. klinikos, pert. to a bed]

subcollateral (sŭb-kō-lăt'ĕr-ăl) [" + con, together, + lateralis, pert. to a side]

subconjunctival (sŭb"kŏn-jŭnk-tī'văl) [" + conjungere, to join together]

subconsciousness (sŭb-kŏn'shŭs-nĕs) [" + conscius, aware]

subcontinuous (sŭb"kŏn-tĭn'ū-ŭs) [" + continere, to hold together]

subcontinuous fever

subcoracoid (sŭb-kor'ă-koyd) [" + Gr. korakoeides, like a crow's beak]

subcortex (sŭb-kor'tĕks) [" + cortex, rind]

subcortical (sŭb-kor'tĭ-kăl)

subcostal (sŭb-kŏs'tăl) [" + costa, rib]

subcostalgia (sŭb"kŏs-tăl'jē-ă) [" + " + Gr. algos, pain]

subcranial (sŭb-krā'nē-ăl) [" + Gr. kranion, skull]

subcrepitant (sŭb-krĕp'ĭ-tănt) [" + crepitare, to rattle]

subcrureus (sŭb-kroo-rē'ŭs) [" + crus, leg]

subculture (sŭb-kŭl'chūr) [" + cultura, tillage]

subcutaneous (sŭb"kū-tā'nē-ŭs) [" + cutis, skin]

subcutaneous surgery

subcutaneous wound

subcuticular (sŭb"kū-tĭk'ū-lăr) [L. sub, under, below, + cuticula, little skin]

subcutis (sŭb-kū'tĭs)

subdelirium (sŭb"dē-lĭr'ē-ŭm) [" + de, away from, + lira, track]

subdeltoid (sŭb-dĕl'toyd) [" + Gr. delta, letter d, + eidos, form, shape]

subdental (sŭb-dĕn'tăl) [" + dens, tooth]

subdermal [" + Gr. derma, skin]

subdiaphragmatic (sŭb"dī-ă-frăg-măt'ĭk) [" + Gr. diaphragma, a partition]

subdorsal (sŭb-dor'săl) [" + dorsum, back]

subduct (sŭb-dŭkt') [" + ducere, to lead]

subdural (sŭb-dū'răl) [" + durus, hard]

subdural space

subendocardial (sŭb"ĕn-dō-kăr'dē-ăl) [" + Gr. endon, within, + kardia, heart]

subendothelial, subendothelium (sŭb"ĕn-dō-thē'lē-ăl, sŭb"ĕn-dō-thē-lē-ŭm) [" + Gr. endon, within, + thele, nipple]

subependymal (sŭb"ĕp-ĕn'dĭ-măl) [" + Gr. *ependyma,* an upper garment, wrap]

subepidermal (sŭb"ĕp-ĭ-dĕr'măl) [" + Gr. *epi,* upon, + *derma,* skin]

subepithelial (sŭb"ĕp-ĭ-thē'lē-ăl) [" + " + *thele,* nipple]

suberosis (sū"bĕr-ō'sĭs) [L. *suber,* cork, + Gr. *osis,* condition]

subfamily (sŭb-făm'ĭ-lē)

subfascial (sŭb-făsh'ē-ăl) [L. *sub,* under, below, + *fascia,* a band]

subfebrile (sŭb-fē'brĭl) [" + *febris,* fever]

subfertility (sŭb"fĕr-tĭl'ĭ-tē) [" + *fertilis,* fertile]

subflavous (sŭb-flā'vŭs) [" + *flavus,* yellow]

subflavous ligament

subfolium (sŭb-fō'lē-ŭm) [" + *folium,* leaf]

subfrontal (sŭb-frŏn'tăl) [" + *frontalis,* brow]

subgenus (sŭb-jē'nŭs)

subgingival (sŭb-jĭn'jĭ-văl) [" + *gingiva,* gum]

subglenoid (sŭb-glē'noyd) [" + Gr. *glene,* socket, + *eidos,* form, shape]

subglossal (sŭb-glŏs'ăl) [" + Gr. *glossa,* tongue]

subglossitis (sŭb-glŏs-sī'tĭs) [" + " + *itis,* inflammation]

subglottic (sŭb-glŏt'ĭk) [" + Gr. *glottis,* tongue]

subgranular (sŭb-grăn'ū-lăr) [" + *granulum,* little grain]

subgrondation, subgrundation (sŭb-grŏn-dā'shŭn, -grŭn-dā'shŭn) [Fr.]

subhepatic (sŭb"hĕ-păt'ĭk) [L. *sub,* under, below, + Gr. *hepatikos,* pert. to the liver]

subhyaloid (sŭb-hī'ă-loyd) [" + Gr. *hyalos,* glass, + *eidos,* form, shape]

subhyoid (sŭb-hī'oyd) [" + Gr. *hyoeides,* U-shaped]

subicteric (sŭb"ĭk-tĕr'ĭk) [" + Gr. *ikteros,* jaundice]

subicular (sū-bĭk'ū-lăr)

subiliac (sŭb-ĭl'ē-ăk) [" + *iliacus,* pert. to the ilium]

subilium (sŭb-ĭl'ē-ŭm)

subincision

subinfection (sŭb"ĭn-fĕk'shŭn) [" + *infectio,* a putting into]

subinflammation [" + *inflammare,* to flame within]

subinflammatory (sŭb"ĭn-flăm'ă-tō-rē)

subintimal (sŭb-ĭn'tĭ-măl) [" + *intima,* innermost]

subintrant (sŭb-ĭn'trănt) [L. *subintrans,* stealing into]

subintrant fever

subinvolution (sŭb"ĭn-vō-lū'shŭn) [L. *sub,* under, below, + *involutio,* a turning into]

subjacent (sŭb-jā'sĕnt) [" + *jacere,* to lie]

subject (sŭb'jĕkt) [L. *subjectus,* brought under]

subjective [L. *subjectivus*]

subjective sensation

subjective symptoms

subjugal (sŭb-jū'găl) [L. *sub,* under, below, + *jugum,* yoke]

sublatio (sŭb-lā'shē-ō) [L.]
    s. retinae

sublation (sŭb-lā'shŭn) [L. *sublatio,* elevation]

sublesional (sŭb-lē'shŭn-ăl) [L. *sub,* under, below, + *laesio,* wound]

sublethal (sŭb-lē'thăl) [" + Gr. *lethe,* oblivion]

sublethal dose

sublimate (sŭb'lĭ-māt) [L. *sublimare,* to elevate]

sublimation (sŭb"lĭ-mā'shŭn) [L. *sublimatio*]

Sublimaze

sublime (sŭb-līm') [L. *sublimis,* to the limit]

subliminal (sŭb-lĭm'ĭn-ăl) [L. *sub,* under, below, + *limen,* threshold]

subliminal self

sublimis (sŭb-lī'mĭs) [L.]

sublingual (sŭb-lĭng'gwăl) [L. *sub*, under, below, + *lingua*, tongue]

sublingual gland

sublinguitis (sŭb"lĭng-gwī'tĭs) [" + " + Gr. *itis*, inflammation]

sublobular (sŭb-lŏb'ū-lăr) [" + *lobulus*, small lobe]

sublumbar (sŭb-lŭm'băr) [" + *lumbus*, loin]

subluxation (sŭb"lŭks-ā'shŭn) [" + *luxatio*, dislocation]

submammary (sŭb-măm'ă-rē) [" + *mamma*, breast]

submandibular [" + *mandibula*, lower jawbone]

submandibular gland

submandibularitis

submarginal (sŭb-măr'jĭn-ăl) [" + *marginalis*, border]

submaxillary

submedial, submedian (sŭb-mē'dē-ăl, -ăn) [" + *medianus*, middle]

submembranous (sŭb-mĕm'bră-nŭs) [" + *membrana*, membrane]

submental [" + *mentum*, chin]

submerge (sŭb-mĕrj') [" + *mergere*, to immerse]

submetacentric (sŭb"mĕt-ă-sĕn'trĭk) [" + Gr. *meta*, beyond, + *kentron*, center]

submicron [" + Gr. *mikros*, tiny]

submicroscopic [" + " + *skopein*, to examine]

submorphous (sŭb-mor'fŭs) [" + Gr. *morphe*, form]

submucosa (sŭb"mū-kō'să) [L. *sub*, under, below, + *mucosus*, mucus]

submucous (sŭb-mū'kŭs) [" + *mucus*, mucus]

submucous resection

subnarcotic (sŭb-năr-kŏt'ĭk) [" + Gr. *narkotikos*, benumbing]

subnasal [" + *nasus*, nose]

subnasale (sŭb"nā-sā'lē) [" + *nasus*, nose]

subnasal point

subnasion (sŭb-nā'zē-ŏn) [" + *nasus*, nose]

subneural (sŭb-nū'răl) [" + Gr. *neuron*, nerve]

subnormal (sŭb-nor'măl) [" + *normalis*, accord. to pattern]

subnormality (sŭb"nor-măl'ĭ-tē) [" + *normalis*, accord. to pattern]

subnucleus (sŭb-nū'klē-ŭs) [" + *nucleus*, kernel]

suboccipital (sŭb"ŏk-sĭp'ĭ-tăl) [" + *occiput*, back of head]

suboperculum (sŭb"ō-pĕr'kū-lŭm) [" + *operculum*, a covering]

suboptimal (sŭb-ŏp'tĭ-măl) [" + *optimus*, best]

suborbital (sŭb-or'bĭ-tăl) [" + *orbita*, track]

suborder (sŭb-or'dĕr)

suboxides (sŭb-ŏk'sīdz)

subpapular (sŭb-păp'ū-lăr) [" + *papula*, pimple]

subparietal (sŭb"pă-rī'ĕ-tăl) [" + *paries*, a wall]

subpatellar (sŭb"pă-tĕl'ăr) [" + *patella*, a small pan]

subpectoral (sŭb-pĕk'tor-ăl) [" + *pectus*, chest]

subpeduncular (sŭb"pē-dŭn'kū-lăr) [" + *pedunculus*, a little foot]

subpeduncular lobe

subpelviperitoneal (sŭb-pĕl"vē-pĕr"ĭ-tō-nē'ăl) [L. *sub*, under, below, + *pelvis*, basin, + Gr. *peritonaion*, stretched around or over]

subpericardial (sŭb"pĕr-ĭ-kăr'dē-ăl) [" + Gr. *peri*, around, + *kardia*, heart]

subperiosteal (sŭb"pĕr-ē-ŏs'tē-ăl) [" + " + *osteon*, bone]

subperitoneal (sŭb"pĕr-ĭ-tō-nē'ăl) [" + Gr. *peritonaion*, stretched around or over]

subperitoneoabdominal (sŭb"pĕr-ĭ-tō-nē"ō-ăb-dŏm'ĭ-năl) [" + " + L. *abdomen*, belly]

subpharyngeal (sŭb"făr-ĭn'jē-ăl) [" + Gr. *pharynx*, throat]

subphrenic (sŭb-frĕn'ĭk) [" + Gr.

phren, diaphragm]
subphrenic abscess
subphylum (sŭb-fī'lŭm)
subpial (sŭb-pī'ăl) [" + pia, soft]
subplacenta (sŭb"plă-sĕn'tă) [" + placenta, a flat cake]
subpleural (sŭb-plū'răl) [" + Gr. pleura, side]
subpontine (sŭb-pŏn'tĭn, -tīn) [" + pons, bridge]
subpreputial (sŭb"prē-pū'shăl) [" + praeputium, prepuce]
subpubic (sŭb-pū'bĭk) [" + pubes, pubic region]
subpulmonary (sŭb-pŭl'mō-nă-rē) [" + pulmon, lung]
subpyramidal (sŭb"pī-răm'ĭ-dăl) [" + Gr. pyramis, a pyramid]
subretinal (sŭb-rĕt'ĭ-năl) [" + rete, a net]
subscapular (sŭb-skăp'ū-lăr) [" + scapula, shoulder blade]
subscleral (sŭb-sklē'răl) [" + Gr. skleros, hard]
subsclerotic (sŭb-sklē'rŏt-ĭk) [" + Gr. skleros, hard]
subscription (sŭb-skrĭp'shŭn) [L. subscriptas, written under]
subserous (sŭb-sē'rŭs) [L. sub, under, below, + serum, whey]
subsibilant (sŭb-sĭb'ĭ-lănt) [" + sibilans, hissing]
subsidence (sŭb-sīd'ĕns) [L. subsidere, to sink down]
subsistence
subspecies (sŭb'spē-sēz) [L. sub, under, below, + species, a kind]
subspinale (sŭb"spī-nă'lē) [" + spina, thorn]
subspinous (sŭb-spī'nŭs) [" + spina, thorn]
subspinous dislocation
substage (sŭb'stāj) [" + O. Fr. estage, position]
substance (sŭb'stăns) [L. substantia]
   s., anterior perforated
   s., anterior pituitary-like
   s., black

   s., chromophilic
   s., colloid
   s., gray
   s., ground
   s., ketogenic
   s., medullary
   s., Nissl
   s., posterior perforated
   s., pressor
   s., reticular
   s., slow-reacting
   s., specific soluble
   s., threshold, high
   s., threshold, low
   s., transmitter
   s., white
   s., white, of Schwann
substance P
substandard
substantia (sŭb-stăn'shē-ă) [L.]
   s. alba
   s., cinerea
   s. ferruginea
   s. gelatinosa
   s. grisea
   s. nigra
   s. propria membranae tympani
substernal (sŭb-stĕr'năl) [L. sub, under, below, + Gr. sternon, chest]
substernomastoid (sŭb-stĕr-nō-măs' toyd) [" + " + Gr. mastos, breast, + eidos, form, shape]
substituent
substitute (sŭb'stĭ-tūt)
   s., blood
substitution (sŭb-stĭ-tū'shŭn) [L. substitutio, replacing]
substitution products
substitution therapy
substitutive (sŭb'stĭ-tū"tĭv) [L. substitutivus]
substitutive therapy
substrate, substratum (sŭb'strāt, sŭb-strā'tŭm) [L. substratum, to lie under]
substructure (sŭb'strŭk-chŭr)
subsultus (sŭb-sŭl'tŭs) [L., to leap up]
   s. tendinum
subsylvian (sŭb-sĭl'vē-ăn)

subtarsal (sŭb-tăr′săl) [L. *sub,* under, below, + Gr. *tarsos,* flat of the foot, flat surface, edge of eyelid]
subtentorial
subterminal (sŭb-tĕr′mĭ-năl) [″ + *terminus,* a boundary]
subtetanic (sŭb″tĕ-tăn′ĭk) [″ + Gr. *tetanikos,* suffering from tetanus]
subthalamic (sŭb″thă-lăm′ĭk) [″ + Gr. *thalamos,* chamber]
subthalamic nucleus
subthalamus
subtile, subtle (sŭb′tĭl, sŭt′l) [L. *subtilis,* fine]
subtilin (sŭb′tĭl-ĭn)
subtotal (sŭb-tō′tăl) [L. *sub,* under, below, + *totus,* all]
subtraction
subtrapezial (sŭb″tră-pē′zē-ăl) [″ + Gr. *trapezion,* a little table]
subtribe (sŭb′trīb)
subtrochanteric (sŭb″trō-kăn-tĕr′ĭk) [″ + Gr. *trochanter,* to run]
subtrochlear (sŭb-trŏk′lē-ăr) [″ + Gr. *trokhileia,* system of pulleys]
subtuberal (sŭb-tū′bĕr-ăl) [″ + *tuber,* a swelling]
subtympanic (sŭb-tĭm-păn′ĭk) [″ + Gr. *tympanon,* drum]
subumbilical (sŭb″ŭm-bĭl′ĭ-kăl) [″ + *umbilicus,* navel]
subumbilical space
subungual, subunguial (sŭb-ŭng′gwăl, -gwē-ăl) [″ + *unguis,* nail]
subungual hematoma
subunit
suburethral (sŭb″ū-rē′thrăl) [″ + Gr. *ourethra,* urethra]
subvaginal (sŭb-văj′ĭn-ăl) [″ + *vagina,* sheath]
subvertebral (sŭb-vĕr′tĕ-brăl) [″ + *vertebra,* vertebra]
subvirile (sŭb-vĭr′ĭl, -vī′rĭl) [″ + *virilis,* masculine]
subvitrinal (sŭb-vĭt′rĭn-ăl) [″ + *vitrina,* vitreous body]
subvolution (sŭb″vō-lū′shŭn) [″ + *volutus,* turning]

subwaking (sŭb-wāk′ĭng)
subzonal (sŭb-zō′năl)
subzygomatic (sŭb″zī-gō-măt′ĭk) [″ + Gr. *zygoma,* cheekbone]
succagogue (sŭk′ă-gŏg) [L. *succus,* juice, + Gr. *agogos,* leading]
succedaneous (sŭk″sĕ-dā′nē-ŭs) [L. *succedaneus,* substituting]
succedaneum (sŭk″sĕ-dā′nē-ŭm) [L. *succedaneus,* substituting]
succenturiate (sŭk″sĕn-tū′rē-āt) [L. *succenturiare,* to substitute]
succi
succinate (sŭk′sĭ-nāt)
succinic acid
succinylcholine chloride (sŭk″sĭ-nĭl-kō′lēn)
succinylsulfathiazole (sŭk″sĭ-nĭl-sŭl″fă-thī′ă-zōl)
succorrhea (sŭk-kō-rē′ă) [L. *succus,* juice, + Gr. *rhein,* to flow]
succubus (sŭk′ū-bŭs) [L.]
succus (sŭk′ŭs) [L. *succus,* juice]
  s. entericus
  s. gastricus
  s. pyloricus
succussion (sŭ-kŭsh′ŭn) [L. *succussio,* a shaking]
suck [AS. *sucan,* to suck]
sucking pad
suckle
Sucostrin Chloride
sucrase (sū′krās) [Fr. *sucre,* sugar]
sucrose (sū′krōs) [Fr. *sucre,* sugar]
sucrosemia (sū″krō-sē′mē-ă) [″ + Gr. *haima,* blood]
sucrose polyester
sucrosuria (sū″krō-sū′rē-ă) [″ + Gr. *ouron,* urine]
suction [LL. *suctio,* sucking]
  s., post-tussive
suction abortion
suction biopsy
suction lipectomy
suctorial (sŭk-tō′rē-ăl) [LL. *suctio,* sucking]
Sudafed
sudamen (sū-dā′mĕn) [L., sweat]

sudamina (sū-dăm'ĭn-ă)
sudaminal (sū-dăm'ĭ-năl) [L. *sudamen*, sweat]
Sudan (sū-dăn')
sudanophil (sū-dăn'ō-fĭl) [*sudan* + Gr. *philein*, to love]
sudanophilia (sū-dăn"ō-fĭl'ē-ă)
sudanophilic (sū-dăn"ō-fĭl'ĭk)
sudation (sū-dā'shŭn) [L. *sudatio*]
sudatoria (sū"dă-tō'rē-ă) [L.]
sudatorium (sū"dă-tō'rē-ŭm) [L. *sudatorium*, a sweating room]
sudden death
sudden infant death syndrome
Sudeck's disease or atrophy (soo'dĕks) [Paul H. M. Sudeck, Ger. surgeon, 1866–1938]
sudokeratosis (sū"dō-kĕr"ă-tō'sĭs) [L. *sudor*, sweat, + Gr. *keras*, horn, + *osis*, condition]
sudomotor (sū"dō-mō'tor) [" + *motor*, a mover]
sudor (sū'dor) [L.]
  s. cruentus
sudoral (sū'dor-ăl)
sudoresis (sū"dō-rē'sĭs) [L.]
sudoriferous (sū-dor-ĭf'ĕr-ŭs) [" + *ferre*, to bear]
sudoriferous glands
sudorific (sū"dor-ĭf'ĭk) [L. *sudorificus*]
sudoriparous (sū"dor-ĭp'ă-rŭs) [L. *sudor*, sweat, + *parere*, to beget, produce]
suet (sū'ĕt) [Fr. *sewet*, suet]
suffocate (sŭf'ō-kāt) [L. *suffocare*]
suffocation (sŭf"ō-kā'shŭn)
suffusion (sū-fū'zhŭn) [L. *suffusio*, a pouring over]
sugar [O. Fr. *zuchre*]
  s., beet
  s., blood
  s., brain
  s., cane
  s., diabetic
  s., fruit
  s., grape
  s., invert
  s., liver

  s., malt
  s., milk
  s., muscle
  s., starch
  s., wood
suggestibility (sŭg-jĕs"tĭ-bĭl'ĭ-tē) [L. *suggestus*, suggested]
suggestible (sŭg-jĕs'tĭ-bl)
suggestion (sŭg-jĕs'chŭn) [L. *suggestio*]
  s., auto-
  s., hypnotic
  s., posthypnotic
suggestive (sŭg-jĕs'tĭv)
suggestive medicine
suggestive therapeutics
suggillation (sŭg-jĭl-ā'shŭn) [L. *suggillatio*]
suicide (sū'ĭ-sīd) [L. *sui*, of oneself, + *caedere*, to kill]
suicidology (soo"ĭ-sīd-ŏl'ō-jē) [" + " + Gr. *logos*, word, reason]
suint (swĭnt)
suit
  s., anti-G
sulcal (sŭl'kăl) [L.]
sulcal artery
sulcate, sulcated (sŭl'kāt, -ĕd) [L. *sulcatus*]
sulciform (sŭl'sĭ-form) [L. *sulcus*, groove, + *forma*, form]
sulculus (sŭl'kū-lŭs) [L.]
sulcus (sŭl'kŭs) [L., groove]
  s., alveololingual
  s., calcarine
  s. centralis
  s., collateral
  sulci cutis
  s., gingival
  s., hippocampal
  s., intraparietal
  s. precentralis
  s. pulmonalis
  s. spiralis cochleae
Sulf-10
sulfacetamide (sŭf"fă-sēt'ă-mīd)
  s., sodium
sulfadiazine (sŭl"fă-dī'ă-zēn)
  s., silver

sulfa drugs
sulfamerazine (sŭl″fă-mĕr′ă-zēn)
sulfameter (sŭl′fă-mē″tĕr)
sulfamethazine (sŭl″fă-mĕth′ă-zēn)
sulfamethizole (sŭl″fă-mĕth′ĭ-zōl)
sulfamethoxazole (sŭl″fă-mĕth-ŏks′ ă-zōl)
Sulfamylon
sulfanilamide (sŭl″făn-ĭl′ă-mīd)
sulfapyridine (sŭl″fă-pĭr′ĭ-dēn)
    s., sodium monohydrate
sulfarsphenamine (sŭlf″ăr-sfĕn′ă-mēn)
sulfasalazine (sŭl″fă-săl′ă-zēn)
sulfatase (sŭl′fă-tās)
sulfate (sŭl′fāt) [L. *sulphas*]
    s., cupric
    s., ferrous
    s., iron
    s., magnesium
sulfathiazole (sŭl″fă-thī′ă-zōl)
sulfatide (sŭl′fă-tīd)
sulfhemoglobin (sŭlf″hēm-ō-glō′bĭn)
sulfhemoglobinemia (sŭlf″hēm-ō-glō″bĭn-ē′mē-ă)
sulfhydryl (sŭlf-hī′drĭl)
sulfide (sŭl′fīd)
sulfinpyrazone (sŭl″fĭn-pī′ră-zōn)
sulfisoxazole (sŭl″fĭ-sŏk′să-zōl)
sulfmethemoglobin (sŭlf″mĕt-hē″mō-glō′bĭn)
sulfobromophthalein (sŭl″fō-brō″mō-thăl′ē-ĭn)
sulfonamides
sulfone (sŭl′fōn)
sulfourea (sŭl″fō-ū-rē′ă)
sulfoxide (sŭl-fŏk′sĭd)
sulfoxone sodium (sŭl-fŏks′ōn)
sulfur (sŭl′fŭr) [L.]
    s. dioxide
    s., precipitated
    s., sublimed
sulfurated, sulfureted (sŭl′fū-rā″tĕd, -rĕt″ ĕd)
sulfurated hydrogen
sulfuric acid (sŭl-fū′rĭk)
    s.a., dilute
sulfuric acid poisoning

sumac (soo′măk)
    s., poison
summation (sŭm-ā′shŭn) [L. *summatio*, adding]
summer (sŭm′ĕr) [AS. *sumer*]
Sumycin
sunburn [AS. *sunne*, sun, + *bernan*, to burn]
Sunday morning paralysis
sunflower eyes
sunglasses
sunscreen
sunscreen protective factor index
sunstroke (sŭn′strōk) [AS. *sunne*, sun, + *strake*, a blow]
super- [L., over, above, in addition]
superabduction (soo″pĕr-ăb-dŭk′shŭn) [L. *super*, over, above, in addition, + *abducens*, drawing away]
superacidity (soo″pĕr-ă-sĭd′ĭ-tē)
superacromial (soo″pĕr-ă-krō′mē-ăl)
superactivity (soo″pĕr-ăk-tĭv′ĭ-tē)
superacute (soo″pĕr-ă-kūt′) [″ + *acutus*, sharp]
superalimentation (soo″pĕr-ăl″ĭ-mĕn-tā′shŭn) [″ + *alimentum*, nourishment]
superalkalinity (soo″pĕr-ăl″kă-lĭn′ĭ-tē) [″ + *alkalinus*, alkaline]
superciliary (soo″pĕr-sĭl′ē-ĕr-ē) [L. *supercilium*, eyebrow]
supercilium (soo″pĕr-sĭl′ē-ŭm) [L.]
superclass (soo′pĕr-klăs)
superduct (soo″pĕr-dŭkt′) [L. *super*, over, above, in addition, + *ducere*, to lead]
superego (soo″pĕr-ē′gō) [″ + *ego*, I]
superexcitation (soo″pĕr-ĕk″sī-tā′shŭn) [″ + *excitatio*, excitation]
superextension (soo″pĕr-ĕks-tĕn′shŭn) [″ + *extensio*, extension]
superfamily (soo″pĕr-făm′ĭ-lē)
superfecundation (soo″pĕr-fē″kŭn-dă′shŭn) [″ + *fecundare*, to fertilize]
superfemale
superfetation (soo″pĕr-fē-tā′shŭn)

[" + *fetus,* fetus]

superficial (soo″pĕr-fish′ăl) [L. *superficialis*]

superficialis (soo″pĕr-fish-ē-ā′lĭs) [L.]

superficial reflex

superficies (soo″pĕr-fish′ē-ēz) [L.]

superflexion (soo″pĕr-flĕk′shŭn) [L. *super,* over, above, in addition, + *flexio,* flexion]

supergenual (soo″pĕr-jĕn′ū-ăl) [" + *genu,* knee]

superimpregnation (soo″pĕr-ĭm″rĕg-nā′shŭn) [" + *impregnare,* to make pregnant]

superinduce (soo″pĕr-ĭn-dūs′) [" + *in,* into, + *ducere,* to lead]

superinfection (soo″pĕr-ĭn-fĕk′shŭn) [" + *infectio,* a putting into]

superinvolution (soo″pĕr-ĭn-vō-lū′shŭn) [" + *involutus,* a turning]

superior (soo-pē′rē-or) [L. *superus,* upper]

superiority complex

superjacent (soo″pĕr-jā′sĕnt)

superlactation (soo″pĕr-lăk-tā′shŭn) [L. *super,* over, above, in addition, + *lactatio,* a sucking]

superlethal (soo″pĕr-lē′thăl) [" + Gr. *lethe,* oblivion]

supermedial (soo″pĕr-mē′dē-ăl) [" + *medium,* middle]

supermoron (soo″pĕr-mō′rŏn) [" + Gr. *moros,* stupid]

supermotility (soo″pĕr-mō-tĭl′ĭ-tē) [" + *motilis,* moving]

supernatant (soo″pĕr-nā′tănt) [" + *natare,* to float]

supernate (soo′pĕr-nāt)

supernumerary (soo″pĕr-nū′mĕr-ăr″ē) [L. *supernumerarius*]

supernumerary teeth

supernutrition (soo″pĕr-nū-trĭ′shŭn) [L. *super,* over, above, in addition, + *nutritio,* nourish]

superolateral (soo″pĕr-ō-lăt′ĕr-ăl) [" + *latus,* side]

superovulation (soo″pĕr-ŏv″ū-lā′shŭn) [" + *ovulum,* little egg]

superoxide

superoxide dismutase

superparasite (soo″pĕr-păr′ă-sīt) [" + Gr. *para,* alongside, past, beyond, + *sitos,* food]

superparasitism (soo″pĕr-păr′ă-sĭ″tĭzm) [" + " + *-ismos,* condition]

superphosphate (soo″pĕr-fŏs′fāt)

supersaturate

superscription (soo″pĕr-skrĭp′shŭn) [L. *super,* over, above, in addition, + *scriptio,* a writing]

supersecretion (soo″pĕr-sē-krē′shŭn) [" + *secretio,* separation]

supersensitiveness (soo″pĕr-sĕn′sĭ-tĭv″nĕs) [" + *sensitivus,* feeling]

supersoft (soo″pĕr-sŏft′) [" + AS. *softe,* soft]

supersonic (soo″pĕr-sŏn′ĭk) [" + *sonus,* sound]

superstructure (soo″pĕr-strŭk′chŭr)

supertension (soo″pĕr-tĕn′shŭn) [" + *tensio,* a stretching]

supervenosity (soo″pĕr-vē-nŏs′ĭ-tē)

supervention (soo″pĕr-vĕn′shŭn) [L. *superventio,* a coming over]

supervirulent (soo″pĕr-vĭr′ū-lĕnt) [L. *super,* over, above, in addition, + *virulentus,* full of poison]

supervisor (soo′pĕr-vīz″ĕr) [L. *supervisus,* having looked over]

supervitaminosis

supervoltage (soo′pĕr-vŏl″tĭj)

supinate (sū′pĭ-nāt) [L. *supinatus,* bent backward]

supination (sū″pĭn-ā′shŭn) [L. *supinatio*]

supinator (sū″pĭn-ā′tor) [L.]

supinator longus reflex

supine (sū-pīn′) [L. *supinus,* lying on the back]

suppedania (sŭp″ĕ-dā′nē-ă) [L. *sub,* under, + *pes,* foot]

supplemental (sŭp″lĕ-mĕn′tăl) [L. *supplementum,* an addition]

supplemental air

support (sŭp-port′)

suppository (sŭ-pŏz′ĭ-tō-rē) [L. *suppo-*

sitorium, something placed underneath]
suppression (sŭ-prĕsh'ŭn) [L. *suppressio*, a pressing under]
suppression of menses
suppurant (sŭp'ū-rănt) [L. *suppurans*]
suppurate (sŭp'ū-rāt) [L. *suppurare*]
suppuration (sŭp-ū-rā'shŭn) [L. *suppuratio*]
suppurative (sŭp'ū-rā"tĭv, -ră-tĭv) [L. *suppuratus*]
suppurative fever
supra- [L.]
supra-acromial (soo"pră-ă-krō'mē-ăl) [L. *supra*, above, on top, beyond, + Gr. *akron*, extremity + *omos*, shoulder]
supra-anal (soo-pră-ă'năl) [" + *analis*, anal]
supra-auricular (soo"pră-ŏ-rĭk'ū-lăr) [" + *auricula*, little ear]
supra-axillary (soo"pră-ăk'sĭ-lĕr"ē) [" + *axilla*, underarm]
suprabuccal (soo"pră-bŭk'ăl) [" + *bucca*, cheek]
suprabulge (soo'pră-bŭlj)
supracerebellar (soo"pră-sĕr"ĕ-bĕl'ăr) [" + *cerebellum*, little brain]
suprachoroid (soo"pră-kō'royd) [" + Gr. *chorioeides*, skinlike]
suprachoroidea (soo"pră-kō-roy'dē-ă)
suprachoroid lamina
supraciliary (soo"pră-sĭl'ē-ĕr"ē) [L. *supra*, above, on top, beyond, + *cilia*, eyelids]
supraclavicular (soo"pră-klă-vĭk'ū-lar) [" + *clavicula*, little key]
supraclavicular fossa
supraclavicular point
supracondylar (soo"pră-kŏn'dĭ-lăr) [" + Gr. *kondylos*, knuckle]
supracostal (soo"pră-kŏs'tăl) [" + *costa*, rib]
supracotyloid (soo"pră-kŏt'ĭ-loyd) [" + Gr. *kotyloeides*, cup-shaped]
supradiaphragmatic (soo"pră-dī"ă-frăg-măt'ĭk) [" + Gr. *dia*, across, + *phragma*, wall]

supraduction (soo"pră-dŭk'shŭn) [" + *ducere*, to lead]
supraepicondylar (soo"pră-ĕp"ĭ-kŏn'dĭ-lăr) [" + Gr. *epi*, upon, + *kondylos*, condyle]
supraglenoid (soo"pră-glē'noyd) [" + Gr. *glene*, socket, + *eidos*, form, shape]
supraglenoid tuberosity
supraglottic (soo"pră-glŏt'ĭk)
suprahepatic (soo"pră-hĕ-păt'ĭk) [" + Gr. *hepar*, liver]
suprahyoid (soo"pră-hī'oyd) [" + *hyoeides*, U-shaped]
suprahyoid muscles
suprainguinal (soo"pră-ĭn'gwĭn-ăl) [" + *inguinalis*, pert. to the groin]
supraintestinal (soo"pră-ĭn-tĕs'tĭ-năl) [" + *intestinum*, intestine]
supraliminal (soo"pră-lĭm'ĭ-năl) [L. *supra*, above, on top, beyond, + *limen*, threshold]
supralumbar (soo"pră-lŭm'băr) [" + *lumbus*, loin]
supramalleolar (soo"pră-mă-lē'ō-lăr) [" + *malleolus*, little hammer]
supramammary (soo"pră-măm'ă-rē) [" + *mamma*, breast]
supramandibular (soo"pră-măn-dĭb'ū-lăr) [" + *mandibula*, lower jawbone]
supramarginal (soo"pră-măr'jĭn-ăl) [" + *marginalis*, border]
supramarginal convolution
supramastoid (soo"pră-măs'toyd) [" + *mastos*, breast, + *eidos*, form, shape]
supramastoid crest
supramaxilla (soo"pră-măk-sĭl'ă) [" + Gr. *maxilla*, jawbone]
supramaxillary (soo"pră-măk'sĭ-lĕr-ē)
suprameatal (soo"pră-mē-ā'tăl) [" + *meatus*, passage]
suprameatal spine
suprameatal triangle
supramental (soo"pră-mĕn'tăl) [L. *supra*, above, on top, beyond, +

mentum, chin]
supranasal (soo″pră-nā′zăl) [″ +
nasus, nose]
supranuclear (soo″pră-nū′klē-lăr)
[″ + *nucleus*, little kernel]
supraoccipital (soo″pră-ŏk-sĭp′ĭ-tăl)
[″ + *occiput*, back of head]
supraocclusion (soo″pră-ŏ-kloo′zhŭn)
[″ + *occlusio*, occlusion]
supraorbital (soo″pră-or′bĭ-tăl) [″ +
orbita, track]
supraorbital neuralgia
supraorbital notch
supraorbital reflex
suprapatellar (soo″pră-pă-tĕl′ăr)
[″ + *patella*, a small pan]
suprapelvic (soo″pră-pĕl′vĭk) [″ +
pelvis, basin]
suprapontine (soo″pră-pŏn′tēn)
[″ + *pons*, bridge]
suprapubic (soo″pră-pū′bĭk) [″ +
NL. *(os) pubis*, bone of the groin]
suprapubic aspiration of urine
suprapubic catheter
suprapubic cystotomy
suprapubic reflex
suprarenal (soo″pră-rē′năl) [L. *supra*,
above, on top, beyond, + *ren*,
kidney]
suprarenalectomy (soo″pră-rē″năl-
ĕk′tō-mē) [″ + ″ + Gr. *ektome*, excision]
suprarenal gland
suprarenalopathy (soo″pră-rē-năl-
ŏp′ă-thē) [″ + ″ + Gr. *pathos*,
disease, suffering]
suprascapular (soo″pră-skăp′ū-lăr)
[″ + *scapula*, shoulder blade]
suprascleral (soo″pră-sklē′răl) [″ +
Gr. *skleros*, hard]
suprasegmental [″ + *segmentum*, segment]
suprasegmental brain
suprasellar (soo″pră-sĕl′ăr) [″ +
sella, saddle]
suprasonic, supersonic (soo″pră-
sŏn′ĭk) [″ + *sonus*, sound]
supraspinal (soo″pră-spī′năl) [″ +

spina, thorn]
supraspinous
supraspinous fossa
suprastapedial (soo″pră-stă-pē′dē-
ăl) [″ + *stapes*, stirrup]
suprasternal (soo″pră-stĕr′năl) [L.
supra, above, on top, beyond, +
Gr. *sternon*, chest]
suprasterol (soo″pră-stĕr′ŏl)
suprasylvian (soo″pră-sĭl′vē-ăn)
supratemporal (soo″pră-tĕm′pō-răl)
[″ + *temporalis*, temporal]
supratentorial (soo″pră-tĕn-tō′rē-ăl)
suprathoracic (soo″pră-thō-răs′ĭk)
[″ + Gr. *thorax*, chest]
supratonsillar (soo″pră-tŏn′sĭ-lăr)
[″ + *tonsilla*, almond]
supratrochlear (soo″pră-trŏk′lē-ăr)
[″ + *trochlea*, pulley]
supratympanic (soo″pră-tĭm-păn′ĭk)
[″ + *tympanon*, drum]
supravaginal (soo″pră-văj′ĭ-năl)
[″ + *vagina*, sheath]
supraventricular (soo″pră-vĕn-trĭk′ū-
lăr) [″ + *ventriculus*, a little belly]
supravergence (soo″pră-vĕr′jĕns)
[″ + *vergere*, to be inclined]
supraversion (soo″pră-vĕr′zhŭn)
[″ + *versio*, a turning]
sura (sū′ră) [L.]
sural (sū′răl)
suralimentation (sŭr″ăl-ĭ-mĕn-tā′shŭn)
[Fr. *sur*, above, + L. *alimentum*,
nourishment]
suramin sodium (soo′ră-mĭn)
surditas (sŭr′dĭ-tăs) [L.]
surdity (sŭr′dĭ-tē) [L. *surditas*, deafness]
surdomute (sŭr′dō-mūt″) [L. *surdus*,
deaf, + *mutus*, dumb]
surefooted
surface (sŭr′fĕs) [Fr. *sur*, above, +
L. *facies*, face]
s., body
surface tension
surfactant (sŭr-făk′tănt)
s., pulmonary
Surfak
surfer's knots

surgeon (sŭr'jŭn) [L. *chirurgia*]
  s., dental
surgeon general
surgery (sŭr'jĕr-ē) [L. *chirurgia*]
  s., aseptic
  s., aural
  s., conservative
  s., cosmetic
  s., major
  s., maxillofacial
  s., minor
  s., mucogingival
  s., oral
  s., orthopedic
  s., plastic
  s., radical
surgical (sŭr'jĭ-kăl)
surgical diathermy
surgical dressing
surgical fever
surgical neck
surgical resident
surgical suture, absorbable
surgical suture, nonabsorbable
Surgicel
Surital
Surmontil
surrogate (sŭr'ō-gāt) [L. *surrogatus*, substituted]
  s., sex
surrogate parenting
sursumduction (sŭr"sŭm-dŭk'shŭn) [L. *sursum*, upward, + *ducere*, to lead]
sursumvergence (sŭr"sŭm-vĕr'jĕns) [" + *vergere*, to turn]
sursumversion (sŭr"sŭm-vĕr'zhŭn) [" + *versio*, turning]
surveillance (sŭr-vāl'ăns)
  s., immunological
survivor guilt
susceptibility (sŭs-sĕp"tĭ-bĭl'ĭ-tē)
susceptible (sŭ-sĕp'tĭ-bl) [L. *susceptibilis*, capable of receiving]
suscitate (sŭs'ĭ-tāt) [L. *suscitare*, to rouse]
suscitation (sŭs"ĭ-tā'shŭn) [L. *suscitatio*, arousal]

sushi (soo'shē)
suspended (sŭs-pĕnd'ĕd) [L. *suspendere*, to hang up]
suspension (sŭs-pĕn'shŭn) [L. *suspensio*, a hanging]
  s., cephalic
  s., colloid
  s., tendon
suspensoid (sŭs-pĕn'soyd) [" + Gr. *eidos*, form, shape]
suspensory (sŭs-pĕn'sō-rē) [L. *suspensorius*, hanging]
suspensory bandage
suspensory ligament
Sus-Phrine
suspiration (sŭs"pĭr-ā'shŭn) [L. *suspiratio*]
suspirious (sŭs-pī'rē-ŭs) [L. *suspirare*, to sigh]
sustentacular (sŭs"tĕn-tăk'ū-lăr) [L. *sustentaculum*, support]
sustentacular cell
sustentacular fibers of Müller [Friedrich von Müller, Ger. physician, 1858 – 1941]
sustentaculum (sŭs"tĕn-tăk'ū-lŭm) [L.]
  s. hepatis
  s. lienis
  s. tali
susurrus (sū-sŭr'ŭs) [L., a whisper]
sutilains (soo'tĭ-lāns)
Sutton's disease (sŭt'ŏnz) [Richard L. Sutton, Sr., U.S. dermatologist, 1878 – 1952; Richard L. Sutton, Jr., U.S. dermatologist, b. 1908]
Sutton's law [Named for Willie Sutton, a U.S. bank robber]
sutura (sū-tū'ră) [L., a seam]
  s. dentata
  s., harmonia
  s. limbosa
  s. notha
  s. serrata
  s. squamosa
  s. vera
sutural (sū'tū-răl) [L. *sutura*, seam]
sutural joint
sutural ligament

suturation (sū"tū-rā'shŭn)
suture (sū'chŭr) [L. *sutura*, seam]
    s., absorbable surgical
    s., apposition
    s., approximation
    s., basilar
    s., bifrontal
    s., biparietal
    s.'s, buried
    s., button
    s., catgut
    s., coaptation
    s., cobbler's
    s., continuous
    s., coronal
    s.'s, cranial
    s., dentate
    s., ethmoidofrontal
    s., ethmoidolacrimal
    s., ethmosphenoid
    s., false
    s., figure-of-eight
    s., frontal
    s., frontolacrimal
    s., frontomalar
    s., frontomaxillary
    s., frontonasal
    s., frontoparietal
    s., frontotemporal
    s., glover's
    s., harmonic
    s., implanted
    s., intermaxillary
    s., internasal
    s., interparietal
    s., interrupted
    s., lambdoid
    s., longitudinal
    s., maxillolacrimal
    s., mediofrontal
    s., metopic
    s., nasomaxillary
    s., nonabsorbable
    s., nonabsorbable surgical
    s., occipital
    s., occipitomastoid
    s., occipitoparietal
    s., palatine

    s., palatine transverse
    s., parietal
    s., parietomastoid
    s., petro-occipital
    s., petrosphenoidal
    s., purse-string
    s., quilled
    s., relaxation
    s., relief
    s., right-angled
    s., sagittal
    s., serrated
    s., shotted
    s., silk
    s., silkworm gut
    s., sphenoparietal
    s., sphenosquamous
    s., sphenotemporal
    s., squamoparietal
    s., squamosphenoidal
    s., squamous
    s., subcuticular
    s., temporo-occipital
    s., temporoparietal
    s., twisted
    s., uninterrupted
    s., vertical mattress
    s., wire
suxamethonium chloride (sŭk"să-mĕ-thō'nē-ŭm)
SV 40 virus
swab (swăb) [Dutch *swabbe*, mop]
    s., test tube
    s., urethral
    s., uterine
swaddling
swage (swāj)
swallow (swăl'ō) [AS. *swelgan*]
swallowing (swăl'ō-ĭng)
    s., air
    s., tongue
swallow's nest
Swan-Ganz catheter [Harold James Swan, U.S. physician, b. 1922; Willian Ganz, U.S. physician, b. 1919]
swan neck deformity
swarming (sworm'ĭng)
sway-back (swā'băk)

sweat (swĕt) [AS. *sweatan*]
  s., bloody
  s., colliquative
  s., colored
  s., fetid
  s., night
  s., profuse
  s., scanty
sweat centers
sweat glands
sweating (swĕt'ĭng) [AS. *swat*, sweat]
  s., deficiency of
  s., excessive
  s., insensible
  s., sensible
  s., urinous
Swedish gymnastics
Swedish massage
sweet [AS. *swete*, sweet]
Sweet's syndrome [R. D. Sweet, contemporary Brit. physician]
swelling (swĕl'ĭng) [AS. *swellan*, swollen]
  s., albuminous
  s., Calabar
  s., cloudy
  s., fugitive
  s., glassy
  s., white
Swift's disease
swimmer's ear
swimmer's itch
switch (swĭch) [MD. *swijch*, bough]
  s., foot
  s., pole-changing
swoon [AS. *swogan*, to suffocate]
sycoma (sī-kō'mă) [Gr. *sykoma*]
sycophant (sĭk'ō-fănt)
sycosiform (sī-kō'sĭ-form) [Gr. *sykosis*, figlike disease, + L. *forma*, shape]
sycosis (sī-kō'sĭs) [Gr. *sykosos*, figlike disease]
  s., barbae
  s., lupoid
  s., vulgaris
Sydenham's chorea (sĭd'ĕn-hămz) [Thomas Sydenham, Brit. physician, 1624–1689]

syllabic utterance (sī-lăb'ĭk) [Gr. *syllabikos*]
syllable stumbling (sĭl'ă-bl) [Gr. *syllabe*, syllable]
syllabus (sĭl'ă-bŭs) [Gr. *syllabos*, table of contents]
syllepsis (sĭl-ĕp'sĭs) [Gr. *syllepsis*, conception]
sylvatic plague
sylvian aqueduct (sĭl'vē-ăn) [Jacobus Sylvius, Fr. anatomist, 1478–1555]
sylvian artery [François Sylvius, Fr. anatomist, 1614–1672]
sylvian fissure [François Sylvius]
sylvian line [François Sylvius]
sym- [Gr. *syn*, together]
symballophone (sĭm-băl'ō-fōn) [" + *ballein*, to throw, + *phone*, sound]
symbion, symbiont (sĭm'bē-ŏn, -bē-ŏnt) [Gr. *syn*, together, + *bios*, life]
symbiosis (sĭm"bē-ō'sĭs) [Gr.]
symbiote (sĭm'bī-ōt) [Gr. *syn*, together, + *bios*, life]
symbiotic (sĭm"bī-ŏt'ĭk)
symblepharon (sĭm-blĕf'ă-rŏn) [" + *blepharon*, eyelid]
symblepharopterygium (sĭm-blĕf"ă-rō-tĕr-ĭj'ē-ŭm) [" + " + *pterygion*, wing]
symbol (sĭm'bŏl) [Gr. *symbolon*, a sign]
  s., phallic
symbolia (sĭm-bō'lē-ă)
symbolism (sĭm'bŏl-ĭzm) [" + *-ismos*, condition]
symbolization
symbolophobia (sĭm"bŏl-ō-fō'bē-ă) [" + *phobos*, fear]
symbrachydactyly (sĭm-brăk"ē-dăk'tĭ-lē) [" + *brachys*, short, + *daktylos*, finger]
Syme's operation (sīmz) [James Syme, Scottish surgeon, 1799–1870]
symmelia (sĭm-mē'lē-ă) [Gr. *syn*, together, + *melos*, limb]
symmelus, symelus (sĭm'ĕ-lŭs, -ē-lŭs) [" + *melos*, limb]
Symmetrel
symmetromania (sĭm"ĕ-trō-mā'nē-ă)

[Gr. *symmetria*, symmetry, +
mania, madness]
symmetry (sĭm'ĕt-rē)
  s., bilateral
  s., radial
sympathectomize (sĭm"pă-
thĕk'tō-mīz)
sympathectomy (sĭm"pă-thĕk'tō-mē)
[Gr. *sympathetikos*, sympathy, +
ektome, excision]
  s., chemical
  s., periarterial
sympatheoneuritis (sĭm-păth"ē-ō-nū-
rī'tĭs) [" + *neuron*, nerve, +
itis, inflammation]
sympathetic (sĭm"pă-thĕt'ĭk)
sympatheticalgia (sĭm"pă-thĕt"ĭ-
kăl'jē-ă) [" + *algos*, pain]
sympathetic irritation
sympathetic nervous system
sympatheticoparalytic (sĭm"pă-thĕt"
ĭ-kō-păr"ă-lĭt'ĭk) [" + *paralytikos*]
sympatheticopathy (sĭm"pă-thĕt"ĭ-
kŏp'ă-thē) [" + *pathos*, disease,
suffering]
sympathetic ophthalmia
sympatheticotonia (sĭm"pă-thĕt"ĭ-kō-
tō'nē-ă) [" + *tonos*, act of stretching, tension, tone]
sympatheticotonic (sĭm"pă-thĕt"ĭ-kō-
tŏn'ĭk)
sympatheticotripsy
sympathetic plexuses
sympathetoblast (sĭm"pă-thĕt'ō-
blăst) [Gr. *sympathetikos*, sympathy,
+ *blastos*, germ]
sympathic (sĭm-păth'ĭk) [Gr. *sympathetikos*, sympathy]
sympathicectomy (sĭm-păth"ĭ-sĕk'tō-
mē) [" + *ektome*, excision]
sympathicoblast (sĭm-păth'ĭ-kō-blăst)
[" + *blastos*, a germ]
sympathicoblastoma (sĭm-păth"ĭ-kō-
blăs-tō'mă) [" + *oma*, tumor]
sympathicolytic (sĭm-păth"ĭ-kō-lĭt'ĭk)
[" + *lytikos*, dissolving]
sympathicomimetic (sĭm-păth"ĭ-kō-
mĭm-ĕt'ĭk) [" + *mimetikos*, imitating]

sympathiconeuritis (sĭm-păth"ĭ-kō-
nū-rī'tĭs) [" + *neuron*, nerve, +
itis, inflammation]
sympathicopathy (sĭm-păth"ĭ-kŏp'ă-
thē) [" + *pathos*, disease, suffer-
ing]
sympathicotonia (sĭm-păth"ĭ-kō-
tō'nē-ă) [" + *tonos*, act of stretching, tension, tone]
sympathicotripsy (sĭm-păth"ĭ-kō-
trĭp'sē) [" + *tripsis*, a rubbing, fric-
tion]
sympathicotropic (sĭm-păth"ĭ-kō-
trŏp'ĭk) [" + *tropos*, a turning]
sympathicus (sĭm-păth'ĭ-kŭs)
sympathism (sĭm'pă-thĭzm) [" +
-*ismos*, condition]
sympathist (sĭm'pă-thĭst) [" +
-*ismos*, condition]
sympathoadrenal (sĭm"păth-ō-ă-
drē'năl) [" + L. *ad*, to, + *ren*,
kideny]
sympathoblast (sĭm-păth'ō-blăst)
[" + *blastos*, germ]
sympathoblastoma (sĭm"păth-ō-
blăs-tō'mă) [" + " + *oma*,
tumor]
sympathoglioblastoma (sĭm"păth-ō-
glī"ō-blăs-tō'mă) [Gr. *sympathetikos*,
sympathy, + *glia*, glue, +
blastos, germ, + *oma*, tumor]
sympathogonia (sĭm"pă-thō-gō'nē-ă)
[" + *gone*, seed]
sympathogonioma (sĭm"pă-thō-
gō"nē-ō'mă) [" + " + *oma*,
tumor]
sympatholytic
sympathoma [" + *oma*, tumor]
sympathomimetic (sĭm"pă-thō-mĭm-
ĕt'ĭk) [" + *mimetikos*, imitating]
sympathy (sĭm'pă-thē) [Gr. *sympatheia*]
sympexion (sĭm-pĕks'ē-ŏn) [Gr. *sympexis*, concretion]
sympexis (sĭm-pĕks'ĭs)
symphalangism (sĭm-făl'ăn-jĭzm) [Gr.
syn, together, + *phalanx*, line of
battle]

symphyogenetic (sĭm″fē-ō-jĕ-nĕt′ĭk)
[Gr. *syn*, together, + *phyein*, to
grow, + *gennan*, to produce]
symphyseal (sĭm-fĭz′ē-ăl) [Gr. *symphysis*, growing together]
symphyseotomy (sĭm-fĭz″ē-ŏt′ō-mē)
[″ + *tome*, a cutting, slice]
symphysiectomy (sĭm-fĭz″ē-ĕk′tō-mē)
[″ + *ektome*, excision]
symphysion (sĭm-fĭz′ē-ŏn) [Gr. *symphysis*, growing together]
symphysiorrhaphy (sĭm-fĭz″ē-or′ă-
fē) [″ + *rhaphe*, seam]
symphysiotome (sĭm-fĭz′ē-ō-tōm)
[″ + *tome*, a cutting, slice]
symphysiotomy (sĭm-fĭz″ē-ŏt′ō-mē)
[″ + *tome*, a cutting, slice]
symphysis (sĭm′fĭ-sĭs) [Gr., growing to-
gether]
   s. cartilaginosa
   s. ligamentosa
   s. mandibulae
   s. menti
   s. of jaw
   s. pubis
symphysodactyly (sĭm″fĭ-sō-dăk′tĭ-lē)
[″ + *daktylos*, finger]
symplasm (sĭm′plăzm) [Gr. *syn*, together, + LL. *plasma*, form, mold]
sympodia (sĭm-pō′dē-ă) [″ +
pous, foot]
symporter (sĭm-por′tĕr)
symptom (sĭm′tŭm, sĭmp-) [Gr. *symptoma*, occurrence]
   s., accessory
   s., accidental
   s., assident
   s., cardinal
   s., concomitant
   s., constitutional
   s., delayed
   s., direct
   s., dissociation
   s., equivocal
   s., focal
   s., general
   s., indirect
   s., labyrinthine

   s., local
   s., negative pathognomonic
   s., objective
   s., passive
   s., pathognomonic
   s., presenting
   s.'s, prodromal
   s., rational
   s., signal
   s., static
   s., subjective
   s., sympathetic
   s.'s, withdrawal
symptomatic (sĭmp″tō-măt′ĭk) [Gr.
symptomatikos]
symptomatology (sĭmp″tō-mă-tŏl′ō-
jē) [Gr. *symptoma*, symptom, +
logos, word, reason]
symptomatolytic (sĭmp″tō-măt″ō-lĭt′ĭk)
[″ + *lysis*, dissolution]
symptom complex
symptomolytic (sĭmp″tō-mō-lĭt′ĭk)
[″ + *lysis*, dissolution]
symptosis (sĭmp-tō′sĭs) [Gr. *syn*, together, + *ptosis*, fall, falling]
sympus (sĭm′pŭs) [″ + *pous*, foot]
syn- [Gr., together]
synache
synactosis (sĭn″ăk-tō′sĭs) [Gr. *syn*, together, + L. *actio*, function, +
Gr. *osis*, condition]
synadelphus (sĭn″ă-dĕl′fŭs) [″ +
adelphos, brother]
Synalar
synalgia (sĭn-ăl′jē-ă) [″ + *algos*,
pain]
synalgic (sĭn-ăl′jĭk)
synapse (sĭn′ăps) [Gr. *synapsis*, point of
contact]
   s., axodendritic
   s., axodendrosomatic
   s., axosomatic
synapsis (sĭn-ăp′sĭs) [Gr., point of con-
tact]
synaptic
synaptic field
synaptolemma (sĭn-ăp″tō-lĕm′ă)
synaptology (sĭn″ăp-tŏl′ō-jē) [″ +

logos, word, reason]

synarthrodia (sĭn″ăr-thrō′dē-ă) [Gr. *syn*, together, + *arthron*, joint, + *eidos*, form, shape]

synarthrodial

synarthrophysis (sĭn″ăr-thrō-fĭ′sĭs) [″ + *arthron*, joint, + *physis*, growth]

synarthrosis [″ + *arthron*, joint, + *osis*, condition]

syncanthus (sĭn-kăn′thŭs) [″ + *kanthos*, corner of the eye]

syncaryon (sĭn-kăr′ē-ŏn)

syncephalus (sĭn-sĕf′ă-lŭs) [″ + *kephale*, head]

synchilia (sĭn-kī′lē-ă) [″ + *cheilos*, lip]

synchiria (sĭn-kī′rē-ă) [″ + *cheir*, hand]

synchondroseotomy (sĭn″kŏn-drō″sē-ŏt′ō-mē) [″ + *chondros*, cartilage, + *tome*, a cutting, slice]

synchondrosis (sĭn″kŏn-drō′sĭs) [″ + ″ + *osis*, condition]

synchondrotomy (sĭn-kŏn-drŏt′ō-mē) [″ + ″ + *tome*, a cutting, slice]

synchorial (sĭn-kō′rē-ăl) [″ + *chorion*, chorion]

synchronism (sĭn′krō-nĭzm) [″ + *chronos*, time, + *-ismos*, condition]

synchronous (sĭn′krō-nŭs)

synchrotron (sĭn′krō-trŏn)

synchysis (sĭn′kĭs-ĭs) [Gr., confound]
   s. scintillans

syncinesis (sĭn″sĭn-ē′sĭs) [″ + *kinesis*, motion]
   s., imitative
   s., spasmodic

synciput (sĭn′sĭ-pŭt)

synclinal (sĭn-klī′năl) [Gr. *synklinein*, to lean together]

synclitism (sĭn′klĭt-ĭzm) [Gr. *synklinein*, to lean together, + *-ismos*, condition]

synclonus (sĭn′klō-nŭs) [″ + *klonos*, turmoil]
   s. ballismus
   s. tremens

syncopal (sĭn′kō-păl) [Gr. *synkope*, fainting]

syncope (sĭn′kō-pē) [Gr. *synkope*, fainting]
   s. anginosa
   s., cardiac
   s., carotid sinus
   s., cough
   s., defecation
   s., hysterical
   s., laryngeal
   s., local
   s., micturition
   s., swallow
   s., vasovagal

syncopic (sĭn-kŏp′ĭk) [Gr. *synkope*, fainting]

syncretio (sĭn-krē′shē-ō) [L.]

syncytial (sĭn-sī′shăl)

syncytiolysin (sĭn″sĭt-ē-ŏl′ĭ-sĭn) [Gr. *syn*, together, + *kytos*, cell, + *lysis*, dissolution]

syncytioma (sĭn″sĭt-ē-ō′mă) [″ + ″ + *oma*, tumor]
   s. benignum
   s. malignum

syncytiotrophoblast (sĭn-sĭt″ē-ō-trō′fō-blăst) [″ + ″ + *trophe*, nourishment, + *blastos*, germ]

syncytium (sĭn-sĭsh′ē-ŭm) [″ + *kytos*, cell]

syndactylism (sĭn-dăk′tĭl-ĭzm) [″ + *daktylos*, finger, + *-ismos*, condition]

syndactylous (sĭn-dăk′tĭ-lŭs) [″ + *daktylos*, finger]

syndectomy (sĭn-dĕk′tō-mē) [″ + *dein*, to bind, + *ektome*, excision]

syndesis (sĭn-dē′sĭs) [″ + *desis*, binding]

syndesmectomy (sĭn″dĕs-mĕk′tō-mē) [Gr. *syndesmos*, ligament, + *ektome*, excision]

syndesmectopia (sĭn″dĕs-mĕk-tō′pē-ă) [″ + *ektopos*, out of place]

syndesmitis (sĭn″dĕs-mī′tĭs) [″ + *itis*, inflammation]

syndesmochorial (sĭn″dĕs″mō-kor'ē-ăl)

syndesmography (sĭn-dĕs-mŏg'ră-fē) [Gr. *syndesmos*, ligament, + *graphein*, to write]

syndesmologia (sĭn"dĕs-mō-lō'jē-ă) [" + *logos*, word, reason]

syndesmology (sĭn"dĕs-mŏl'ō-jē) [" + *logos*, word, reason]

syndesmoma (sĭn"dĕs-mō'mă) [" + *oma*, tumor]

syndesmopexy (sĭn-dĕs'mō-pĕk"sē) [" + *pexis*, fixation]

syndesmophyte (sĭn-dĕs'mō-fīt) [" + *phyton*, plant]

syndesmoplasty (sĭn-dĕs'mō-plăs"tē) [" + *plassein*, to form]

syndesmorrhaphy (sĭn"dĕs-mor'ă-fē) [" + *rhaphe*, seam]

syndesmosis (sĭn"dĕs-mō'sĭs) [Gr. *syndesmos*, ligament, + *osis*, condition]

syndesmotomy (sĭn"dĕs-mŏt'ō-mē) [" + *tome*, a cutting, slice]

syndrome (sĭn'drōm) [Gr., a running together]
  s., Adair-Dighton
  s., adiposogenital
  s., adrenogenital
  s., Angelucci's
  s., dumping
  s., Fröhlich's
  s., Gilles de la Tourette's
  s., Gradenigo's
  s., Horner's
  s., Korsakoff's
  s., Marfan's
  s., sick sinus
  s., skin-eye
  s., Stokes-Adams
  s., toxic shock
  s., Weber's

syndromic (sĭn-drŏm'ĭk) [Gr. *syndrome*, a running together]

synechia (sĭn-ĕk'ē-ă) [Gr. *synecheia*, continuity]
  s., annular
  s., anterior
  s., posterior

  s., total
  s., vulvae

synechotome (sĭn-ĕk'ō-tōm) [" + *tome*, a cutting, slice]

synechotomy (sĭn"ĕk-ŏt'ō-mē) [" + *tome*, a cutting, slice]

synechtenterotomy (sĭn"ĕk-tĕn"tĕr-ŏt'ō-mē) [" + *enteron*, intestine, + *tome*, a cutting, slice]

synecology (sĭn"ē-kŏl'ō-jē) [Gr. *syn*, together, + *oikos*, house, + *logos*, word, reason]

Synemol

synencephalocele (sĭn"ĕn-sĕf'ă-lō-sēl") [" + *enkephalos*, brain, + *kele*, tumor, swelling]

syneresis (sĭn-ĕr-ē'sĭs) [Gr. *synairesis*, drawing together]

synergetic (sĭn"ĕr-jĕt'ĭk) [Gr. *syn*, together, + *ergon*, work]

synergia (sĭn-ĕr'jē-ă)

synergic (sĭn-ĕr'jĭk) [" + *ergon*, work]

synergism (sĭn'ĕr-jĭzm) [" + " + *-ismos*, condition]

synergist (sĭn'ĕr-jĭst)

synergistic (sĭn"ĕr-jĭs'tĭk)

synergy (sĭn'ĕr-jē) [Gr. *synergia*]

synesthesia (sĭn"ĕs-thē'zē-ă) [Gr. *syn*, together, + *aisthesis*, feeling, perception]
  s. algica

synesthesialgia (sĭn"ĕs-thē-zē-ăl'jē-ă) [" + " + *algos*, pain]

synezesis (sĭn"ē-zē'sĭs) [Gr. *synizesis*, a sitting together]

Syngamus (sĭn'gă-mŭs)
  S. laryngeus

syngamy (sĭn'gă-mē) [Gr. *syn*, together, + *gamos*, marriage]

syngeneic

syngenesioplasty (sĭn"jē-nē"zē-ō-plăs'tē) [" + *genesis*, generation, birth, + *plassein*, to form]

syngenesious (sĭn"jē-nē'shŭs) [" + *genesis*, generation, birth]

syngenesis (sĭn-jĕn'ē-sĭs) [" + *genesis*, generation, birth]

syngnathia (sĭn-nā'thē-ă) [" + gnathos, jaw]

synhidrosis (sĭn"hī-drō'sĭs) [" + hidrosis, sweat]

synizesis (sĭn"ĭ-zē'sĭs) [Gr. synizesis]
  s. pupillae

synkaryon (sĭn-kăr'ē-ŏn) [Gr. syn, together, + karyon, nucleus]

synkinesis (sĭn"kĭ-nē'sĭs) [" + kinesis, motion]
  s., imitative

synnecrosis (sĭn"nĕ-krō'sĭs) [" + nekrosis, state of death]

synonym (sĭn'ō-nĭm) [Gr. synonymon]

synophrys (sĭn-ŏf'rĭs) [Gr. syn, together, + ophrys, eyebrow]

synophthalmus (sĭn"ŏf-thăl'mŭs) [" + ophthalmos, eye]

synopsia (sĭn'ŏp-sē-ă) [" + opsis, sight, appearance, vision]

synopsis (sĭn-ŏp'sĭs) [Gr.]

synoptophore (sĭn-ŏp'tō-for) [" + ops, sight, + phoros, bearing]

synoptoscope (sĭn-ŏp'tō-skōp) [" + " + skopein, to examine]

synorchidism, synorchism (sĭn-or'kĭd-ĭzm, -kĭzm) [" + orchis, testicle, + -ismos, condition]

synoscheos (sĭn-ŏs'kē-ŏs) [" + oscheon, scrotum]

synosteology (sĭn"ŏs-tē-ŏl'ō-jē) [" + " + logos, word, reason]

synosteosis (sĭn"ŏs-tē-ō'sĭs)

synosteotomy (sĭn"ŏs-tē-ŏt'ō-mē) [" + osteon, bone, + tome, a cutting, slice]

synostosis (sĭn"ŏs-tō'sĭs) [" + " + osis, condition]

synostotic (sĭn"ŏs-tŏt'ĭk) [" + " + osis, condition]

synotia (sĭn-ō'shē-ă) [" + ous, ear]

synotus (sĭ-nō'tŭs) [" + ous, ear]

synovectomy (sĭn"ō-vĕk'tō-mē) [L. synovia, joint fluid, + Gr. ektome, excision]

synovia (sĭn-ō'vē-ă) [L.]

synovial (sĭn-ō'vē-ăl)

synovial bursa

synovial crypt

synovial cyst

synovial fluid

synovial folds

synovial hernia

synovialis (sĭ-nō"vē-ā'lĭs) [L.]

synovial membrane

synovialoma (sĭ-nō"vē-ă-lō'mă) [L. synovia, joint fluid, + Gr. oma, tumor]

synovial tendon sheaths

synovial villi

synovioma (sĭn"ō-vē-ō'mă) [L. synovia, joint fluid, + Gr. oma, tumor]

synoviparous (sĭn"ō-vĭp'ă-rŭs) [" + parere, to beget, produce]

synovitis (sĭn"ō-vī'tĭs) [" + Gr. itis, inflammation]
  s., chronic
  s., dendritic
  s., dry
  s., purulent
  s., serous
  s., sicca
  s., simple
  s., tendinous
  s., vaginal
  s., vibration

synovium (sĭn-ō'vē-ŭm) [L. synovia, joint fluid]

syntactic (sĭn-tăk'tĭk)

syntasis (sĭn-tă'sĭs) [Gr. syn, together, + teinein, to stretch]

syntaxis (sĭn-tăk'sĭs) [" + taxis, arrangement]

syntectic (sĭn-tĕk'tĭk)

syntexis (sĭn-tĕk'sĭs) [Gr.]

synthase

synthermal (sĭn-thĕr'măl) [" + therme, heat]

synthesis (sĭn'thĕs-ĭs) [Gr.]

synthesize (sĭn'thĕ-sīz')

synthetase (sĭn-thĕ-tās)

synthetic (sĭn-thĕt'ĭk) [Gr. synthetikos]

synthorax (sĭn-thō'răks) [Gr. syn, together, + thorax, chest]

Synthroid

Syntocinon

syntone (sĭn'tōn) [" + *tonos,* act of stretching, tension, tone]

syntonic (sĭn-tŏn'ĭk)

syntonin (sĭn'tō-nĭn)

syntoxoid (sĭn-tŏk'soyd) [Gr. *syn,* together, + *toxikon,* poison, + *eidos,* form, shape]

syntripsis (sĭn-trĭp'sĭs) [Gr., destruction]

syntrophism (sĭn'trŏf-ĭzm) [" + *trophe,* nourishment, + *-ismos,* condition]

syntrophoblast (sĭn-trŏf'ō-blăst) [" + " + *blastos,* germ]

syntropic (sĭn-trŏp'ĭk) [" + *trope,* a turn]

syntropy (sĭn-trō-pē) [" + *trope,* a turn]

synulosis (sĭn"ū-lō'sĭs) [Gr. *synoulosis*]

synulotic (sĭn"ū-lŏt'ĭk)

syphilelcosis (sĭf-ĭl-ĕl-kō'sĭs) [*syphilis* + Gr. *helkosis,* ulceration]

syphilelcus (sĭf"ĭl-ĕl'kŭs) [" + Gr. *helkos,* ulcer]

syphilid(e) (sĭf"ĭl-ĭd) [Fr.]

syphilionthus (sĭf"ĭl-ē-ŏn'thŭs) [" + Gr. *ionthos,* eruption]

syphiliphobia (sĭf"ĭl-ĭ-fō'bē-ă) [" + Gr. *phobos,* fear]

syphilis (sĭf'ĭ-lĭs) [*Syphilis,* shepherd having the disease in a Latin poem]
  s., cardiovascular
  s., congenital
  s., extragenital
  s. insontium
  s., latent
  s., meningovascular
  s., neuro-
  s., nonvenereal
  s., prenatal
  s., visceral

syphilitic (sĭf"ĭ-lĭt'ĭk) [L. *syphiliticus*]

syphilitic fever

syphilitic macules

syphiloderm, syphiloderma (sĭf'ĭl-ō-dĕrm", sĭf"ĭl-ō-dĕr'mă) [" + Gr. *derma,* skin]

syphilogenesis, syphilogeny (sĭf"ĭl-ō-jĕn'ĕ-sĭs, sĭf"ĭl-ŏj'ĕn-ē) [" + Gr.

genesis, generation, birth]

syphilographer (sĭf"ĭl-ŏg'ră-fĕr) [" + Gr. *graphein,* to write]

syphilography (sĭf"ĭl-ŏg'ră-fē)

syphiloid (sĭf'ĭ-loyd) [" + Gr. *eidos,* form, shape]

syphilology (sĭf"ĭl-ŏl'ō-jē)

syphiloma (sĭf"ĭl-ō'mă) [" + Gr. *oma,* tumor]

syphilomania (sĭf"ĭl-ō-mā'nē-ă) [" + Gr. *mania,* madness]

syphilopathy (sĭf"ĭ-lŏp'ă-thē) [" + Gr. *pathos,* disease, suffering]

syphilophobia (sĭf"ĭl-ō-fō'bē-ă) [" + Gr. *phobos,* fear]

syphilophobic (sĭf"ĭl-ō-fō'bĭk)

syphilophyma (sĭf'ĭl-ō-fī'mă) [" + Gr. *phyma,* a growth]

syphilosis (sĭf"ĭ-lō'sĭs) [" + Gr. *osis,* condition]

syphilotherapy (sĭf"ĭl-ō-thĕr'ă-pē) [" + Gr. *therapeia,* treatment]

syphilotropic (sĭf"ĭl-ō-trŏp'ĭk) [" + Gr. *tropos,* a turning]

syphilous (sĭf"ĭl-ŭs)

syphionthus (sĭf"ē-ŏn'thŭs) [" + Gr. *ionthos,* eruption]

syr. [L.] *syrupus,* syrup

syrigmophonia (sĭr"ĭg-mō-fō'nē-ă) [Gr. *syrigmos,* a whistle, + *phone,* voice]

syrigmus (sĭr-ĭg'mŭs) [Gr. *syrigmos,* a whistle]

syringadenoma (sĭr-ĭng"ă-dĕ-nō'mă) [Gr. *syrinx,* pipe, + *aden,* gland, + *oma,* tumor]

syringe (sĭr-ĭnj', sĭr'ĭng) [Gr. *syrinx,* pipe]
  s., hypodermic
  s., oral

syringectomy (sĭr"ĭn-jĕk'tō-mē) [" + *ektome,* excision]

syringitis (sĭr"ĭn-jī'tĭs) [" + *itis,* inflammation]

syringoadenoma (sĭ-rĭng"gō-ăd"ĕ-nō'mă) [" + *aden,* gland, + *oma,* tumor]

syringobulbia (sĭr-ĭn"gō-bŭl'bē-ă) [" + *bulbos,* a bulb]

syringocarcinoma (sĭ-rĭng″gō-kăr″sĭ-nō′mă) [″ + *karkinos*, crab, + *oma*, tumor]

syringocele (sĭr-ĭn′gō-sēl) [″ + *koilia*, cavity, belly]

syringocystadenoma (sĭr-ĭn″gō-sĭs″tă-dĕ-nō′mă) [″ + *kystis*, bladder, sac, + *aden*, gland, + *oma*, tumor]

syringocystoma (sĭr-ĭn″gō-sĭs-tō′mă) [″ + ″ + *oma*, tumor]

syringoencephalomyelia (sĭ-rĭng″gō-ĕn-sĕf″ă-lō-mī-ē′lē-ă) [″ + *enkephalos*, brain, + *myelos*, marrow]

syringoid (sĭr-ĭn′goyd) [Gr. *syrinx*, pipe, + *eidos*, form, shape]

syringoma (sĭr″ĭn-gō′mă) [″ + *oma*, tumor]

syringomeningocele (sĭr-ĭn″gō-mĕn-ĭn′gō-sēl) [″ + *meninx*, membrane, + *kele*, tumor, swelling]

syringomyelia (sĭr-ĭn″gō-mī-ē′lē-ă) [″ + *myelos*, marrow]

syringomyelitis (sĭr-ĭn″gō-mī″ĕ-lī′tĭs) [″ + *myelos*, marrow, + *itis*, inflammation]

syringomyelocele (sĭr-ĭn″gō-mī″ĕl-ō-sēl) [″ + ″ + *kele*, tumor, swelling]

syringomyelus (sĭr-ĭn″gō-mī′ĕl-ŭs)

syringopontia (sĭr-ĭn″gō-pŏn′shē-ă) [″ + L. *pons*, bridge]

syringosystrophy (sĭr-ĭn″gō-sĭs′trō-fē) [″ + *systrophe*, a twist]

syringotome (sĭr-ĭn′gō-tōm) [″ + *tome*, a cutting, slice]

syringotomy (sĭr″ĭn-gŏt′ō-mē)

syrinx (sĭr′ĭnks) [Gr., pipe]

syrup (sĭr′ŭp) [L. *syrupus*]
    s., simple

syssarcosis (sĭs″ăr-kō′sĭs) [Gr. *syn*, together, + *sarkosis*, fleshy growth]

systaltic (sĭs-tăl′tĭk) [Gr. *systaltikos*, contracting]

system (sĭs′tĕm) [Gr. *systema*, a composite whole]
    s., alimentary

s., autonomic nervous
s., cardiovascular
s., centimeter-gram-second
s., central nervous
s., chromaffin
s., circulatory
s., conduction, of the heart
s., cytochrome
s., digestive
s., endocrine
s., extrapyramidal motor
s., genital
s., genitourinary
s., haversian
s., hematopoietic
s., heterogeneous
s., homogeneous
s., hypophyseoportal
s., impulse-conducting
s., integumentary
s., lymphatic
s., metric
s., muscular
s., nervous
S. of Units, International
s., osseous
s., parasympathetic nervous
s., peripheral nervous
s., portal
s., reproductive
s., respiratory
s., reticuloendothelial
s., skeletal
s., sympathetic nervous
s., urinary
s., urogenital
s., vascular
s., vasomotor
s., vegetative nervous
s., visceral efferent

systema (sĭs-tē′mă) [Gr., a composite whole]

systematic (sĭs″tĕ-măt′ĭk)

systematization (sĭs-tĕm″ă-tī-zā′shŭn)

systemic (sĭs-tĕm′ĭk)

systemic circulation

systemic remedies

systemoid (sĭs′tĕ-moyd) [″ +

eidos, form, shape]

systems theory

systole (sĭs'tō-lē) [Gr., contraction]
    s., aborted
    s., anticipated
    s., arterial
    s., atrial
    s., electrical
    s., extra-
    s., premature
    s., ventricular

systolic (sĭs-tŏl'ĭk) [Gr. *systole*, contraction]

systolic discharge

systolic murmur

systolic pressure

systremma (sĭs-trĕm'ă) [Gr. *systremma*, anything twisted together]

Sytobex

syzygial (sĭ-zĭj'ē-ăl) [Gr. *syzygia*, conjunction]

syzygiology (sĭ-zĭj"ē-ŏl'ō-jē) [" + *logos*, word, reason]

syzygium (sĭ-zĭj'ē-ŭm) [Gr. *syzygia*, conjunction]

syzygy (sĭz'ĭ-jē)

T

T temperature; time; intraocular tension

t. temporal; [L.] ter, three times

t₁/₂ T₁/₂

T₃ triiodothyronine

T₄ tetraiodothyronine

T-1824

T.A. toxin-antitoxin

Ta tantalum

tabacism (tăb'ă-sĭzm) [L. tabacum, tobacco, + Gr. -ismos, condition]

tabacosis (tăb"ă-kō'sĭs) [" + Gr. osis, condition]

tabacum (tă-bā'kum, tăb'ă-kum) [L.]

tabagism (tăb'ă-jĭzm) [" + Gr. -ismos, condition]

tabanid (tăb'ă-nĭd) [L. tabanus, horsefly]

Tabanidae (tă-băn'ĭ-dē) [L. tabanus, horsefly]

Tabanus (tă-bā'nŭs) [L., horsefly]

tabardillo (tăb"ăr-dē'lyō) [Sp.]

tabatière anatomique (tă-bă"tē-ār' ă-nă"tō-mēk') [Fr., anatomical snuffbox]

tabella (tă-bĕl'ă) [L., tablet]

tabes (tā'bēz) [L., wasting disease]
   t., diabetic
   t. dorsalis
   t. ergotica
   t. mesenterica

tabescent (tă-bĕs'ĕnt) [L. tabes, wasting disease]

tabetic (tă-bĕt'ĭk) [L. tabes, wasting disease]

tabetic crises

tabetic foot

tabetiform (tă-bĕt'ĭ-form) [" + forma, shape]

tabic, tabid (tăb'ĭk, tăb'ĭd)

tablature (tăb'lă-chūr)

table (tā'bl) [L. tabula, board]
   t.'s of skull

t., periodic
   t., tilt
   t., vitreous
   t., water

tablespoon (tā'bl-spoon)

tablet (tăb'lĕt) [O. Fr. tablete, a small table]
   t., buccal
   t., coated
   t., compressed
   t., dispensing
   t., enteric-coated
   t., fluoride
   t., hypodermic
   t., sublingual
   t. triturate

tablier (tă-blyā') [Fr., apron]

taboo [Polynesian tabu, tapu, inviolable]

taboparalysis (tā"bō-păr-ăl'ĭ-sĭs) [L. tabes, wasting disease, + Gr. paralyein, to loosen, disable]

taboparesis (tā"bō-păr-ē'sĭs, -păr'ĕ-sĭs) [" + Gr. parienai, let fall]

tabophobia (tā"bō-fō'bē-ă) [" + Gr. phobos, fear]

tabular (tăb'ū-lăr) [L. tabula, board]

tabular bone

tabun

Tacaryl Hydrochloride

TACE

tache (tŏsh) [Fr., spot]
   t. blanche
   t. bleuâtre
   t. cérébrale
   t. motrice
   t. noire

tachetic (tăk-ĕt'ĭk) [Fr. tache, spot]

tachistoscope (tă-kĭs'tō-skōp) [Gr. tachistos, swiftest, + skopein, to view]

tachogram (tăk′ō-grăm) [Gr. *tachos*, speed, + *gramma*, letter, piece of writing]

tachography (tăk-ŏg′ră-fē) [″ + *graphein*, to write]

tachy- [Gr. *tachys*, swift]

tachyarrhythmia (tăk″ē-ă-rĭth′mē-ă) [″ + *a*, not, + *rhythmos*, rhythm]

tachyauxesis (tăk″ē-awk-sē′sĭs) [″ + *auxesis*, increase]

tachycardia (tăk″ē-kăr′dē-ă) [″ + *kardia*, heart]
    t., atrial
    t., ectopic
    t., essential
    t., nodal
    t., paroxysmal atrial
    t., paroxysmal nodal
    t., paroxysmal ventricular
    t., polymorphic ventricular
    t., reflex
    t., sinus
    t. strumosa exophthalmica
    t., ventricular

tachycardiac (tăk″ē-kăr′dē-ăk) [Gr. *tachys*, swift, + *kardia*, heart]

tachylalia (tăk″ē-lā′lē-ă) [″ + *lalia*, chatter, prattle]

tachymeter (tăk-ĭm′ē-tĕr) [″ + *metron*, measure]

tachyphagia (tăk″ē-fā′jē-ă) [″ + *phagein*, to eat]

tachyphasia (tăk″ē-fā′zē-ă) [″ + *phasis*, utterance]

tachyphemia (tăk″ē-fē′mē-ă) [″ + *pheme*, speech]

tachyphrasia (tăk″ē-frā′zē-ă) [″ + *phrasis*, diction]

tachyphrenia (tăk″ē-frē′nē-ă) [″ + *phren*, mind]

tachyphylaxis (tăk″ē-fĭ-lăk′sĭs) [″ + *phylaxis*, guard]

tachypnea (tăk″ĭp-nē′ă) [″ + *pnoia*, breath]
    t., nervous

tachyrhythmia (tăk″ē-rĭth′mē-ă) [″ + *rhythmos*, rhythm]

tachysterol (tă-kĭs′tē-rŏl)

tachysystole (tăk″ē-sĭs′tō-lē) [″ + *systole*, contraction]

tachytrophism (tăk″ē-trō′fĭzm) [″ + *trophe*, nourishment, + *-ismos*, condition]

tactile (tăk′tĭl) [L. *tactilis*]

tactile corpuscles

tactile defensiveness

tactile discrimination

tactile disk

tactile localization

tactile system

taction (tăk′shŭn) [L. *tactio*]

tactometer (tăk-tŏm′ĕt-ĕr) [L. *tactus*, touch, + Gr. *metron*, measure]

tactor (tăk′tor)

tactual (tăk′tū-ăl) [L. *tactus*, touch]

tactus (tăk′tŭs) [L.]
    t. eruditus

taedium vitae (tē′dē-ŭm wē″tī) [L.]

Taenia (tē′nē-ă) [L., tape]
    T. echinococcus
    T. lata
    T. saginata
    T. solium

taenia (tē′nē-ă) [L., tape]
    t. coli
    t. fimbriae
    t. pontis
    t. semicircularis
    t. thalami
    t. ventriculi tertii

taeniacide (tē′nē-ă-sīd) [L. *taenia*, tapeworm, + *caedere*, to kill]

taeniafuge (tē′nē-ă-fūj″) [″ + *fugere*, to put to flight]

taeniasis (tē-nī′ă-sĭs) [″ + Gr. *-iasis*, state or condition of]

taeniform (tē′nĭ-form) [″ + *forma*, shape]

taenifuge (tē′nĭ-fūj) [″ + *fuga*, flight]

taeniophobia (tē″nē-ō-fō′bē-ă) [″ + Gr. *phobos*, fear]

tag
    t., hemorrhoidal
    t., radioactive

t., skin
Tagamet
tagging
tagliacotian operation (tă-lē-ă-kō'shē-ăn) [Gasparo Tagliacozzi, It. surgeon, 1546–1599]
tail (tāl) [AS. *taegel*]
tailgut (tāl'gŭt)
tailor's cramp
taint (tānt) [O. Fr. *teint*, color, tint]
Takayasu's arteritis (pulseless disease) [Michishige Takayasu, Japanese physician, b. 1872]
take
talalgia (tăl-ăl'jē-ă) [L. *talus*, heel, + Gr. *algos*, pain]
talar (tā'lăr) [L. *talaris*, of the ankle]
talbutal (tăl'bū-tăl)
talc (tălk) [Persian *talk*]
talcosis (tăl-kō'sĭs) [Persian *talk*, talc, + Gr. *osis*, condition]
talcum (tălk'ŭm) [L.]
tali (tā'lī)
talipedic (tăl"ĭ-pē'dĭk) [L. *talus*, ankle, + *pes*, foot]
talipes (tăl'ĭ-pēz) [L. *talus*, ankle, + *pes*, foot]
  t. arcuatus
  t. calcaneus
  t. cavus
  t. equinus
  t. percavus
  t. valgus
  t. varus
talipomanus (tăl"ĭp-ŏm'ăn-ŭs) [L. *talus*, ankle, + *pes*, foot, + *manus*, hand]
tallow (tăl'ō)
talocalcaneal (tā"lō-kăl-kā'nē-ăl) [" + *calcaneus*, heel]
talocrural (tā"lō-kroo'răl) [" + *crus*, leg]
talocrural articulation
talofibular (tā"lō-fĭb'ū-lăr) [" + *fibula*, pin]
talon (tăl'ŏn) [L.]
  t. noir
talonavicular (tā"lō-nă-vĭk'ū-lăr) [L.

talus, ankle, + *navicula*, boat]
talonid (tăl'ō-nĭd) [ME. *talon*, heel]
taloscaphoid (tā"lō-skăf'oyd) [L. *talus*, ankle, + Gr. *skaphe*, skiff, + *eidos*, form, shape]
talotibial (tā"lō-tĭb'ē-ăl) [" + *tibia*, shinbone]
talus (tā'lŭs) [L., ankle]
Talwin (tăl'wĭn)
tambour (tăm-boor') [Fr., drum]
Tamm-Horsfall mucoprotein
tamoxifen citrate (tă-mŏks'ĭ-fĕn)
tampon (tăm'pŏn) [Fr., plug]
  t., menstrual
  t., Mikulicz's
  t., nasal
tamponade (tăm"pŏn-ād') [Fr., plug]
  t., balloon
  t., cardiac
tamponage (tăm'pŏn-ŏj) [Fr., plug]
tamponing, tamponment (tăm'pŏn-ĭng, tăm-pŏn'mĕnt)
Tandearil
tang
Tangier disease (tăn-jēr') [Tangier Island, in Chesapeake Bay, where the disease was first discovered]
tank, Hubbard
tannase (tăn'ās)
tannate (tăn'āt)
tannic acid
tannin (tăn'ĭn) [Fr. *tanin*]
tantalum (tăn'tă-lŭm)
tantrum (tăn'trŭm)
TAO
tap (tăp) [AS. *taeppa*; O. Fr. *taper*]
Tapar
Tapazole (tăp'ă-zōl)
tape (tāp) [AS. *taeppe*]
  t., adhesive
tapeinocephalic (tăp"ĭ-nō-sĕ-făl'ĭk) [Gr. *tapeinos*, low-lying, + *kephale*, head]
tapeinocephaly (tăp"ĭ-nō-sĕf'ă-lē)
tapetum (tă-pē'tŭm) [NL., a carpet]
  t. choroideae
  t. lucidum
tapeworm [AS. *taeppe*, a narrow

band, + wyrm, worm]
t., armed
t., beef
t., broad
t., dog
t., dwarf
t., fish
t., hydatid
t., mouse
t., pork
t., rat
t., unarmed

taphephobia (tăf"ĕ-fō'bē-ă) [Gr. *taphos*, grave, + *phobos*, fear]

taphophilia (tăf"ō-fil'ē-ă) [" + *philos*, love]

Tapia syndrome (tā'pē-ă) [A. G. Tapia, Sp. physician, 1875–1950]

tapinocephalic (tăp"ĭn-ō-sĕf-ăl'ĭk) [Gr. *tapeinos*, lying low, + *kephale*, head]

tapinocephaly (tăp"ĭn-ō-sĕf'ă-lē)

tapiroid (tă'pĭr-oyd) [Amerind. *tapira*, tapir, + Gr. *eidos*, form, shape]

tapotement (tă-pōt-mŏn') [Fr.]

tapping (tăp'ĭng) [O. Fr. *taper*, of imitative origin; AS. *taeppa*, tap]

tar
t., coal
t., juniper
t., pine

Taractan

tarantism (tăr'ăn-tĭzm) [Taranto, seaport in southern Italy, + Gr. *-ismos*, condition]

tarantula (tă-răn'tū-lă)

Tardieu's spots (tăr-dyūz') [Auguste A. Tardieu, Fr. physician, 1818–1879]

tardive (tăr'dĭv) [Fr., tardy]

tare (tār)

tared

tarentism (tăr'ĕn-tĭzm)

target (tăr'gĕt) [O. Fr. *targette*, light shield]

target cell

target organ

tarichatoxin (tăr"ĭk-ă-tŏk'sĭn)

Tarnier's sign (tăr-nē-āz') [Etienne Sté-

phene Tarnier, Fr. obstetrician, 1828–1897]

tarnish

tarsadenitis (tăr"săd-ĕn-ī'tĭs) [Gr. *tarsos*, flat of the foot, flat surface, edge of eyelid, + *aden*, gland, + *itis*, inflammation]

tarsal (tăr'săl) [Gr. *tarsalis*]

tarsal arches

tarsal bones

tarsal cartilages

tarsalgia (tăr-săl'jē-ă) [Gr. *tarsos*, flat of the foot, flat surface, edge of eyelid, + *algos*, pain]

tarsal glands

tarsalia (tăr-sā'lē-ă) [L.]

tarsalis (tăr-sā'lĭs) [L.]

tarsal lacrimal glands

tarsal tunnel

tarsal tunnel syndrome

tarsectomy (tar-sĕk'tō-mē) [" + *ektome*, excision]

tarsectopia (tăr"sĕk-tō'pē-ă)

tarsi

tarsitis (tăr-sī'tĭs) [" + *itis*, inflammation]

tarso- [Gr. *tarsos*, flat of the foot, flat surface, edge of eyelid]

tarsocheiloplasty (tăr"sō-kī'lō-plăs"tē) [" + *cheilos*, lip, + *plassein*, to form]

tarsoclasia, tarsoclasis (tăr"sō-klă'sē-ă, tăr-sŏk'lăs-ĭs) [" + *klasis*, a breaking]

tarsomalacia (tăr"sō-mă-lā'sē-ă) [" + *malakia*, a softening]

tarsomegaly (tăr"sō-mĕg'ă-lē) [" + *megas*, large]

tarsometatarsal (tăr"sō-mĕt'ă-tăr'săl) [" + *meta*, between, + *tarsos*, flat of the foot, flat surface, edge of eyelid]

tarso-orbital (tăr"sō-or'bĭ-tăl) [" + L. *orbita*, track]

tarsophalangeal (tăr"sō-fă-lăn'jē-ăl) [" + *phalanx*, line of battle]

tarsophyma (tăr"sō-fī'mă) [" + *phyma*, a growth]

tarsoplasia, tarsoplasty (tăr″sō-plā′zē-ă, tăr′sō-plăs″tē) [″ + *plassein*, to form]

tarsoptosis (tăr″sŏp-tō′sĭs) [″ + *ptosis*, fall, falling]

tarsorrhaphy (tăr-sor′ă-fē) [″ + *rhaphe*, seam]

tarsotarsal (tăr″sō-tăr′săl) [″ + *tarsos*, flat of the foot, flat surface, edge of eyelid]

tarsotibial (tăr″sō-tĭb′ē-ăl) [″ + L. *tibia*, shinbone]

tarsotomy (tăr-sŏt′ō-mē) [″ + *tome*, a cutting, slice]

tarsus (tăr′sŭs) [Gr. *tarsos*, flat of the foot, flat surface, edge of eyelid]
   t. inferior palpebrae
   t. superior palpebrae

tartar [Gr. *tartaron*, dregs]
   t., cream of
   t. emetic

tartaric acid (tăr-tăr′ĭk)

tart cells

tartrate

tartrazine

taste (tāst) [O. Fr. *taster*, to feel, to taste]
   t., after

taste area

taste blindness

taste buds

taste cells

taster (tās′tĕr)

TAT thematic apperception test

T.A.T. *tetanus antitoxin; toxin-antitoxin*

tattooing (tă-too′ĭng) [Tahitian *tatau*]
   t., traumatic

taurine (taw′rĭn)

taurocholate (taw″rō-kō′lāt)

taurocholemia (taw″rō-kō-lē′mē-ă) [Gr. *tauros*, a bull, + *chole*, bile, + *haima*, blood]

taurocholic acid

taurodontism (taw″rō-dŏn′tĭzm) [″ + *odous*, tooth, + *-ismos*, condition]

Taussig-Bing syndrome (taw′sĭg-bĭng) [Helen B. Taussig, U.S. Pediatrician, b. 1898; Richard J. Bing, U.S. surgeon, b. 1909]

tauto- [Gr. *tautos*, identical]

tautomenial (taw″tō-mē′nē-ăl) [″ + *meniaia*, menses]

tautomer (taw′tō-mĕr) [″ + *meros*, a part]

tautomeral, tautomeric (taw-tŏm′ĕr-ăl, -tō-mĕr′ĭk) [″ + *meros*, a part]

tautomerase (taw-tŏm′ĕr-ās) [″ + ″ + *-ase*, enzyme]

tautomerism (taw-tŏm′ĕr-ĭzm) [″ + ″ + *-ismos*, condition]

tautorotation (taw″tō-rō-tā′shŭn) [″ + L. *rotare*, to turn round]

Tavist

taxis (tăk′sĭs) [Gr., arrangement]
   t., bipolar

taxon (tăk′sŏn) [Gr. *taxis*, arrangement]

taxonomic (tăk″sō-nŏm′ĭk)

taxonomy (tăks-ŏn′ō-mē) [″ + *nomos*, law]

Taylor brace (tā′lĕr) [C. F. Taylor, U.S. surgeon, 1827–1899]

Tay-Sachs disease [Warren Tay, Brit. physician, 1843–1927; Bernard Sachs, U.S. neurologist, 1858–1944]

Tay's spot

TB tuberculosis

Tb terbium

T.b. tubercle bacillus; tuberculosis

T bandage

T-bar

TBP thyroxine-binding protein

Tbs tablespoon

Tc technetium

T cells

TCID$_{50}$ tissue culture infective dose

t.d.s. [L.] *ter die sumendum*, to be taken three times a day

Te tellurium

tea (tē)
   t., black
   t., green
   t., Paraguay copper

TEAB tetraethylammonium bromide

TEAC tetraethylammonium chloride

tear (tăr, tēr) [AS. *taer*]

tear duct, test of patency of

tears (tērs) [AS. *tear*]
   t.'s, artificial
   t.'s, crocodile
tease (tēz) [AS. *taesan*, to pluck]
teaspoon (tē'spoon)
teat (tēt) [ME. *tete*, from AS. *tit*, teat]
teatulation (tēt″ū-lā'shŭn) [AS. *tit*, teat]
technetium (tĕk-nē'shē-ŭm)
technetium-99m
technetium Tc 99m albumin aggregated injection
technic (tĕk'nĭk) [Gr. *techne*, art]
technical (tĕk'nĭ-kăl) [Gr. *tekhnikos*, skilled]
technician (tĕk-nĭsh'ăn)
   t., biomedical engineering
   t., dental
   t., dialysis
   t., dietetic
   t., electrocardiographic
   t., electromyographic
   t., emergency medical, -paramedic
   t., environmental health
   t., histologic
   t., medical laboratory
   t., medical record
   t., orthopedic
   t., pharmacy
   t., psychiatric
   t., respiratory therapy
technique (tĕk-nēk') [Fr., Gr. *technikos*]
techno- [Gr. *techne*, art]
technologist (tĕk-nŏl'ō-jĭst)
   t., blood bank
   t., cardiovascular
   t., cyto-
   t., electroencephalographic
   t., histologic
   t., medical
   t., nuclear medicine
   t., radiation therapy
   t., radiologic
   t., surgical
technology (tĕk-nŏl'ō-jē) [″ + *logos*, word, reason]
tectocephalic (tĕk″tō-sĕ-făl'ĭk) [L. *tectum*, roof, + Gr. *kephale*, head]
tectocephaly (tĕk-tō-sĕf'ăl-ē)

tectorial (tĕk-tō'rē-ăl) [L. *tectum*, roof]
tectorium (tĕk-tō'rē-ŭm) [L. *tectorium*, a covering]
tectospinal (tĕk″tō-spī'năl) [L. *tectum*, roof, + *spina*, thorn]
tectospinal tract
tectum (tĕk'tŭm) [L., roof]
   t. mesencephali
T.E.D. *threshold erythema dose*
teenage
teeth (tēth) [AS. *toth*, tooth]
   t., anterior
   t., auditory
   t., charting and numbering
   t., deciduous
   t., Hutchinson's
   t., malacotic
   t., milk
   t., permanent
   t., reimplantation or repair of
   t., sclerotic
   t., secondary
   t., stained
   t., temporary
   t., wisdom
teething (tēth'ĭng) [AS. *toth*, tooth]
tegmen (tĕg'mĕn) [L. *tegmen*, covering]
   t. mastoideum
   t. tympani
   t. ventriculi quarti
tegmental (tĕg-mĕn'tăl) [L. *tegmentum*, covering]
tegmental nuclei
tegmentum (tĕg-mĕn'tŭm) [L. *tegmentum*, covering]
Tegopen (tĕg'ō-pĕn)
tegument (tĕg'ū-mĕnt)
tegumental, tegumentary (tĕg″ū-mĕn'tăl, -tă-rē)
teichopsia (tī-kŏp'sē-ă) [Gr. *teichos*, wall, + *opsis*, sight, appearance, vision]
teinodynia (tī″nō-dĭn'ē-ă) [Gr. *tenon*, tendon, + *odyne*, pain]
tel-, tele- [Gr. *telos*, end]
tela (tē'lă) [L. *tela*, web]
   t. choroidea
   t. conjunctiva

t. elastica

t. subcutanea

t. submucosa

telalgia (tĕl-ăl'jē-ă) [Gr. *tele*, distant, + *algos*, pain]

telangiectasia,   telangiectasis (tĕl-ăn"jē-ĕk-tā'zē-ă, -ĕk'tă-sĭs) [Gr. *telos*, end, + *angeion*, vessel, + *ektasis*, dilatation]

t., hereditary hemorrhagic

t. lymphatica

t., spider

telangiectatic (tĕl-ăn"jē-ĕk-tăt'ĭk)

telangiectodes (tĕl-ăn"jē-ĕk-tō'dēz)

telangiitis (tĕl-ăn"jē-ī'tĭs) [" + " + *itis*, inflammation]

telangioma (tĕl-ăn"jē-ō'mă) [Gr. *telos*, end, + *angeion*, vessel, + *oma*, tumor]

telangion (tĕl-ăn'jē-ŏn) [" + *angeion*, vessel]

telangiosis (tĕl"ăn-jē-ō'sĭs) [" + " + *osis*, condition]

telarche

Teldrin

telecanthus (tĕl"ē-kăn'thŭs) [Gr. *tele*, distant, + *kanthos*, corner of the eye]

telecardiogram (tĕl"ē-kăr'dē-ō-grăm) [" + *kardia*, heart, + *gramma*, letter, piece of writing]

telecardiography (tĕl"ē-kăr"dē-ŏg'ră-fē) [" + " + *graphein*, to write]

telecardiophone (tĕl"ē-kăr'dē-ō-fōn) [" + " + *phone*, voice]

teleceptive (tĕl-ē-sĕp'tĭv) [" + L. *ceptivus*, take]

teleceptor (tĕl'ē-sĕp"tor) [" + L. *ceptor*, a receiver]

telecinesia (tĕl"ē-sĭn-ē'zē-ă) [" + *kinesis*, motion]

telecurietherapy (tĕl-ē-kū"rē-thĕr'ă-pē) [" + *curie*, + Gr. *therapeia*, treatment]

teledendrite, teledendron (tĕl-ē-dĕn'drīt, -dĕn'drŏn) [Gr. *telos*, end, + *dendron*, a tree]

telediagnosis (tĕl"ē-dī"ăg-nō'sĭs) [Gr. *tele*, distant, + *diagignoskein*, to discern]

telediastolic (tĕl"ē-dī-ă-stŏl'ĭk) [Gr. *telos*, end, + *diastole*, a dilatation]

telefluoroscopy (tĕl"ē-floo"or-ŏs'kō-pē)

telekinesis (tĕl"ē-kī-nē'sĭs) [" + *kinesis*, motion]

telelectrocardiogram (tĕl"ē-lĕk"trō-kăr'dē-ō-grăm) [Gr. *tele*, distant, + *elektron*, amber, + *kardia*, heart, + *gramma*, letter, piece of writing]

telemeter (tĕl'ē-mē"tĕr) [" + *metron*, measure]

telemetry (tē-lĕm'ē-trē)

telemnemonic (tĕl"ē-nē-mŏn'ĭk) [" + *mnemonikos*, pert. to memory]

telencephalic (tĕl"ĕn-sĕf-ăl'ĭk) [Gr. *telos*, end, + *enkephalos*, brain]

telencephalization (tĕl"ĕn-sĕf"ăl-ī-zā'shŭn)

telencephalon (tĕl-ĕn-sĕf'ă-lŏn) [" + *enkephalos*, brain]

teleneurite (tĕl"ē-nū'rīt) [" + *neuron*, nerve]

teleneuron (tĕl"ē-nū'rŏn) [" + *neuron*, nerve]

teleo- [Gr. *teleos*, complete]

teleological (tē"lē-ō-lŏj'ĭ-kăl)

teleology (tĕl-ē-ŏl'ō-jē) [" + *logos*, word, reason]

teleomitosis (tĕl"ē-ō-mī-tō'sĭs) [" + *mitos*, thread, + *osis*, condition]

teleonomic (tĕl"ē-ō-nŏm'ĭk)

teleonomy (tĕl"ē-ŏn'ō-mē) [" + *nomos*, law]

teleopsia (tĕl-ē-ŏp'sē-ă) [Gr. *tele*, distant, + *ops*, eye]

teleorganic (tĕl"ē-or-găn'ĭk) [Gr. *teleos*, complete, + *organon*, organ]

teleotherapeutics (tĕl"ē-ō-thĕr-ă-pū'tĭks) [Gr. *tele*, distant, + *therapeutikos*, treating]

Telepaque (tĕl'ē-pāk)

telepathist (tē-lĕp'ă-thĭst) [" + *pathos*, disease, suffering]

telepathy (tĕ-lĕp'ă-thē)
teleradiography (tĕl"ĕ-rā-dē-ŏg'ră-fē) [Gr. *tele*, distant, + L. *radius*, ray, + Gr. *graphein*, to write]
teleradium (tĕl"ĕ-rā'dē-ŭm)
telergy (tĕl'ĕr-jē) [" + *ergon*, work]
teleroentgenogram (tĕl"ĕ-rĕnt-gĕn'ō-grăm) [" + *roentgen* + Gr. *gramma*, letter, piece of writing]
teleroentgenography (tĕl"ĕ-rĕnt"gĕn-ŏg'ră-fē) [" + " + Gr. *graphein*, to write]
telesthesia (tĕl-ĕs-thē'zē-ă) [" + *aisthesis*, feeling, perception]
telesystolic (tĕl"ĕ-sĭs-tŏl'ĭk) [Gr. *telos*, end, + *systole*, contraction]
teletactor (tĕl"ĕ-tăk'tor) [" + L. *tactus*, touch]
teletherapy (tĕl-ĕ-thĕr'ă-pē) [Gr. *tele*, distant, + *therapeia*, treatment]
teletypewriter
telluric (tĕ-lūr'ĭk) [L. *tellus*, earth]
tellurism (tĕl'ū-rĭzm) [" + Gr. *-ismos*, condition]
tellurium (tĕl-ū'rē-ŭm) [L. *tellus*, earth]
tellurium poisoning
telocentric (tĕl"ō-sĕn'trĭk) [Gr. *telos*, end, + *kentron*, center]
teloceptor
telodendron (tĕl-ō-dĕn'drŏn) [Gr. *telos*, end, + *dendron*, tree]
telogen (tĕl'ō-jĕn) [" + *genesis*, generation, birth]
teloglia (tĕl-ŏg'lē-ă)
telolecithal
telolemma (tĕl"ō-lĕm'mă) [" + *lemma*, rind]
telomere (tĕl'ō-mēr) [" + *meros*, part]
telophase (tĕl'ō-fāz) [" + *phasis*, appearance]
telophragma (tĕl"ō-frăg'mă) [" + *phragmos*, a fencing in]
telosynapsis (tĕl"ō-sĭ-năp'sĭs) [" + *synapsis*, point of contact]
telotism (tĕl'ō-tĭzm) [" + *-ismos*, condition]
TEM *triethylene melamine*

Temaril (tĕm'ă-rĭl)
tempeh
temper [AS. *temprian*, to mingle]
temperament (tĕm'pĕr-ă-mĕnt) [L. *temperamentum*, mixture]
temperate (tĕm'pĕr-ĭt)
temperature (tĕm'pĕr-ă-tūr) [L. *temperatura*, proportion]
   t., absolute
   t., ambient
   t., axillary
   t., body
   t. chart, basal
   t., core
   t., critical
   t., inverse
   t., maximum
   t., mean
   t., minimum
   t., normal
   t., optimum
   t., oral
   t., rectal
   t., room
   t., subnormal
temperature senses
temper tantrums
template (tĕm'plăt)
   t., occlusal
   t., wax
temple (tĕm'pl) [O. Fr. from L. *tempora*]
tempolabile (tĕm"pō-lā'bl) [L. *tempus*, period of time, + *labi*, to slip]
tempora (tĕm'pō-ră) [L.]
temporal (tĕm'por-ăl) [L. *temporalis*, period of time]
temporal bone
temporalis (tĕm"pō-rā'lĭs) [L.]
temporal line
temporal lobe
temporo- [L. *tempora*]
temporoauricular (tĕm"pō-rō-aw-rĭk'ū-lăr) [" + *auricula*, little ear]
temporohyoid (tĕm"pō-rō-hī'oyd) [" + Gr. *hyoeides*, U-shaped]
temporomalar (tĕm"pō-rō-mā'lăr) [" + *mala*, cheek]
temporomandibular (tĕm"pō-rō-

măn-dĭb′ū-lăr) [″ + *mandibula*, lower jawbone]

temporomandibular joint(s)

temporomandibular joint syndrome

temporomaxillary (tĕm″pō-rō-măk′sĭ-lĕr-ē) [″ + *maxilla*, jawbone]

temporo-occipital (tĕm″pō-rō-ŏk-sĭp′ĭ-tăl) [″ + *occipitalis*, pert. to the occiput]

temporoparietal (tĕm″pō-rō-pă-rī′ĕ-tăl) [″ + *paries*, wall]

temporopontine [″ + *pons*, bridge]

temporosphenoid (tĕm″pō-rō-sfē′noyd) [″ + Gr. *sphen*, wedge, + *eidos*, form, shape]

temporozygomatic (tĕm″pō-rō-zī″gō-măt′ĭk) [″ + Gr. *zygoma*, cheekbone]

tempostabile (tĕm″pō-stā′bĭl) [L. *tempus*, time, + *stabilis*, stable]

Tempra

tenacious (tĕ-nā′shŭs) [L. *tenax*]

tenacity (tĕ-năs′ĭ-tē)

tenaculum (tĕn-ăk′ū-lŭm) [L., a holder]

tenalgia (tĕn-ăl′jē-ă) [Gr. *tenon*, tendon, + *algos*, pain]

　t. crepitans

Tenckhoff peritoneal catheter

tenderizers

tenderness (tĕn′dĕr-nĕs)

　t., rebound

tendinitis (tĕn″dĭn-ī′tĭs) [L. *tendo*, tendon, + Gr. *itis*, inflammation]

tendinoplasty (tĕn′dĭ-nō-plăs″tē) [″ + Gr. *plassein*, to form]

tendinosuture (tĕn″dĭn-ō-sū′tūr) [″ + *sutura*, seam]

tendinous (tĕn′dĭ-nŭs) [L. *tendinosus*]

tendinous synovitis

tendo [L.]

tendolysis (tĕn-dŏl′ĭ-sĭs) [″ + Gr. *lysis*, dissolution]

tendon (tĕn′dŭn) [L. *tendo*, tendon]

　t., Achilles

　t., calcaneal

　t., central

　t. of Zinn

　t., superior, of Lockwood

tendon cells

tendonitis [″ + Gr. *itis*, inflammation]

tendon reflex

　t.r., patellar

tendon spindle

tendoplasty (tĕn′dō-plăs″tē) [″ + Gr. *plassein*, to mold]

tendosynovitis (tĕn″dō-sīn″ō-vī′tĭs) [″ + *synovia*, joint fluid, + Gr. *itis*, inflammation]

　t. crepitans

tendotome (tĕn′dō-tōm) [″ + Gr. *tome*, a cutting, slice]

tendotomy (tĕn-dŏt′ō-mē)

tendovaginal (tĕn″dō-văj′ĭ-năl) [L. *tendo*, tendon, + *vagina*, sheath]

tendovaginitis (tĕn″dō-văj″ĭn-ī′tĭs) [″ + ″ + Gr. *itis*, inflammation]

Tenebrio (tĕ-nĕb′rē-ō)

tenectomy [″ + *ektome*, excision]

　t., graduated

tenesmic (tĕn-ĕz′mĭk)

tenesmus (tĕ-nĕz′mŭs) [Gr. *teinesmos*, a stretching]

tenia (tē′nē-ă) [L. *taenia*, tape]

teniasis (tē-nī′ă-sĭs) [L. *taenia*, tapeworm, + Gr. -*iasis*, state or condition of]

tenicide (tĕn′ĭ-sīd) [″ + *caedere*, to kill]

tenifuge (tĕn′ĭ-fūj) [″ + *fuga*, flight]

tennis elbow

teno- [Gr. *tenon*]

tenodesis (tĕn-ŏd′ĕ-sĭs) [″ + *desis*, a binding]

tenodesis splint

tenodynia (tĕn″ō-dĭn′ē-ă) [″ + *odyne*, pain]

tenofibril (tĕn′ō-fī″brĭl) [″ + *fibrilla*, little fiber]

tenolysis (tĕn-ŏl′ĭ-sĭs) [″ + *lysis*, dissolution]

tenomyoplasty (tĕn″ō-mī′ō-plăs″tē) [″ + *mys*, muscle, + *plassein*, to form]

tenomyotomy (tĕn″ō-mī-ŏt′ō-mē) [″ + ″ + *tome*, a cutting, slice]

Tenon's capsule (tē′nŏns) [Jacques R. Tenon, Fr. surgeon, 1724–1816]

tenonectomy (tĕn″ō-nĕk′tō-mē) [″ + *ektome*, excision]

tenonitis (tĕn″ō-nī′tĭs) [″ + *itis*, inflammation]

tenonometer (tĕn″ō-nŏm′ĕ-tĕr) [Gr. *teinein*, to stretch, + *metron*, measure]

Tenon's space

tenontitis (tĕn″ŏn-tī′tĭs) [Gr. *tenontos*, tendon, + *itis*, inflammation]

tenontodynia (tĕn″ŏn-tō-dĭn′ē-ă) [″ + *odyne*, pain]

tenontography (tĕn″ŏn-tŏg′ră-fē) [″ + *graphein*, to write]

tenontolemmitis (tĕn-ŏn″tō-lĕm-mī′tĭs) [″ + *lemma*, rind, + *itis*, inflammation]

tenontology (tĕn″ŏn-tŏl′ō-jē) [″ + *logos*, word, reason]

tenontomyoplasty (tĕn-ŏn″tō-mī′ō-plăs″tē) [″ + *mys*, muscle, + *plassein*, to form]

tenontomyotomy (tĕn-ŏn″tō-mī-ŏt′ō-mē) [″ + ″ + *tome*, a cutting, slice]

tenontoplasty (tĕn-ŏn′tō-plăs″tē) [″ + *plassein*, to form]

tenontothecitis (tĕn-ŏn″tō-thē-sī′tĭs) [″ + *theke*, sheath, + *itis*, inflammation]

t. stenosans

tenophyte (tĕn′ō-fīt) [″ + *phyton*, a growth]

tenoplastic (tĕn″ō-plăs′tĭk)

tenoplasty (tĕn′ō-plăs″tē) [″ + *plassein*, to form]

tenoreceptor (tĕn″ō-rē-sĕp′tor) [″ + L. *receptor*, receiver]

tenorrhaphy (tĕn-or′ă-fē) [″ + *rhaphe*, seam]

tenositis (tĕn″ō-sī′tĭs) [″ + *itis*, inflammation]

tenostosis (tĕn″ŏs-tō′sĭs) [Gr. *tenon*, tendon, + *osteon*, bone, + *osis*, condition]

tenosuspension (tĕn″ō-sŭs-pĕn′shŭn) [″ + L. *suspensio*, a hanging under]

tenosuture (tĕn″ō-sū′chŭr) [″ + L. *sutura*, seam]

tenosynovectomy (tĕn″ō-sĭn″ō-vĕk′tō-mē) [″ + *synovia*, joint fluid, + Gr. *ektome*, excision]

tenosynovitis (tĕn″ō-sĭn″ō-vī′tĭs) [″ + ″ + ″ + Gr. *itis*, inflammation]

t. crepitans

t. hyperplastica

tenotome (tĕn′ō-tōm) [″ + *tome*, a cutting, slice]

tenotomist (tē-nŏt′ō-mĭst)

tenotomy (tē-nŏt′ō-mē)

tenovaginitis (tĕn″ō-văj″ĭn-ī′tĭs) [″ + L. *vagina*, sheath, + Gr. *itis*, inflammation]

TENS *transcutaneous electrical nerve stimulation*

tense (tĕns)

Tensilon

tensiometer (tĕn″sē-ŏm′ĕ-tĕr) [L. *tensio*, a stretching, + Gr. *metron*, measure]

tension (tĕn′shŭn) [L. *tensio*, a stretching]

t., arterial

t., intraocular

t., intravenous

t., muscular

t., premenstrual

t., surface

t., tissue

tension headache

tension of gases

tension pneumothorax

tension suture

tensometer (tĕn-sŏm′ĕ-tĕr) [L. *tensio*, a stretching, + Gr. *metron*, measure]

tensor (tĕn′sor) [L., a stretcher]

tent (tĕnt) [O. Fr. *tente*, from L. *tenta*, stretched out]

t., oxygen

t., sponge

tentacle (tĕn'tă-k'l)
tentative (tĕn'tă-tĭv) [L. _tentativus,_ feel, try]
tenth cranial nerve
tentorial (tĕn-tō'rē-ăl)
tentorial notch
tentorial pressure cone
tentorium (tĕn-tō'rē-ŭm) [L., tent]
   t. cerebelli
Tenuate
Tepanil
tephromalacia (tĕf"rō-măl-ā'shē-ă) [Gr. _tephros,_ gray, + _malakia,_ softening]
tephromyelitis (tĕf"rō-mī"ĕl-ī'tĭs) [" + _myelos,_ marrow, + _itis,_ inflammation]
tephrosis (tĕf-rō'sĭs) [" + _osis,_ condition]
tephrylometer (tĕf"rĭ-lŏm'ĕ-tĕr) [" + _hyle,_ matter, + _metron,_ measure]
tepid (tĕp'ĭd) [L. _tepidus,_ lukewarm]
tepidarium (tĕp"ĭd-ā'rē-ŭm) [L.]
tepor (tē'por) [L., lukewarmness]
TEPP _tetraethylpyrophosphate_
ter- [L., thrice]
teracurie (tĕr"ă-kū'rē)
teramorphous (tĕr-ă-mor'fŭs) [Gr. _teras,_ monster, + _morphe,_ form]
teras (tĕr'ăs) [Gr.]
teratic (tĕr-ăt'ĭk) [Gr. _teratikos,_ monstrous]
teratism (tĕr'ă-tĭzm) [Gr. _teratisma_]
   t., acquired
   t., atresic
   t., ceasmic
   t., ectogenic
   t., ectopic
   t., hypergenic
   t., symphysic
terato- [Gr. _teratos,_ monster]
teratoblastoma (tĕr"ă-tō-blăs-tō'mă) [" + _blastos,_ germ, + _oma,_ tumor]
teratocarcinoma (tĕr"ă-tō-kăr"sĭ-nō'mă) [" + _karkinos,_ cancer, + _oma,_ tumor]
teratogen (tĕr-ăt'ō-jĕn) [" + _gen-_

nan, to produce]
teratogenesis (tĕr"ă-tō-gĕn'ĕ-sĭs) [" + _genesis,_ generation, birth]
teratogenetic (tĕr"ă-tō-jĕ-nĕt'ĭk) [" + _genesis,_ generation, birth]
teratogenous (tĕr"ă-tŏj'ĕ-nŭs) [" + _gennan,_ to produce]
teratogeny (tĕr"ă-tŏj'ĕ-nē)
teratoid (tĕr'ă-toyd) [Gr. _teratos,_ monster, + _eidos,_ form, shape]
teratoid tumor
teratologic (tĕr"ă-tō-lŏj'ĭk)
teratology (tĕr-ă-tŏl'ō-jē) [" + _logos,_ word, reason]
teratoma (tĕr-ă-tō'mă) [" + _oma,_ tumor]
teratomatous (tĕr"ă-tō'mă-tŭs)
teratophobia (tĕr"ă-tō-fō'bē-ă) [" + _phobos,_ fear]
teratosis (tĕr"ă-tō'sĭs) [" + _osis,_ condition]
teratospermia (tĕr"ă-tō-spĕr'mē-ă) [" + _sperma,_ seed]
terbium (tĕr'bē-ŭm)
terbutaline sulfate
terchloride (tĕr-klō'rīd)
terebrant (tĕr'ĕ-brănt)
terebration (tĕr"ĕ-brā'shŭn) [L. _terebratio_]
teres (tē'rēz) [L., round]
tergal (tĕr'găl) [L. _tergum,_ back]
tergum (tĕr'gŭm) [L.]
ter in die (tĕr ĭn dē'ă) [L.]
term [L. _terminus,_ a boundary]
terminal (tĕr'mĭ-năl) [L. _terminalis_]
terminal arteriole
terminal bars
terminal cancer
terminal device
terminal ganglia
terminal illness
terminal infection
terminal veins
terminatio (tĕr"mĭ-nā'shē-ō) [L.]
termination [L. _terminatio,_ limiting]
terminology (tĕr-mĭ-nŏl'ō-jē) [L. _terminus,_ a boundary, + Gr. _logos,_ word, reason]

terminus (tĕr'mĭ-nŭs) [L.]
ternary (tĕr'nă-rē) [L. *ternarius*, triple]
teroxide (tĕr-ŏk'sīd)
terpene (tĕr'pēn)
terpin hydrate (tĕr'pĭn hī'drāt)
terra (tĕr'ă) [L.]
   t. alba
   t. fullonica
terracing (tĕr'ăs-ĭng) [O. Fr. *terrasse*]
Terramycin (tĕr"ă-mī'sĭn)
territoriality (tĕr"ĭ-tor"ē-ăl'ĭ-tē)
terror [L. *terrere*, to frighten]
   t., night
tertian (tĕr'shŭn) [L. *tertianus*, the third]
tertiary (tĕr'shē-ăr-ē) [L. *tertiarius*]
tertiary alcohol
tertiary care
tertiary syphilis
tertigravida (tĕr"shē-grăv'ĭ-dă) [" + *gravida*, pregnant]
tertipara (tĕr-shĭp'ă-ră) [L. *tertius*, third, + *parere*, to beget, produce]
Teslac
Tessalon
tessellated (tĕs'ĕ-lā"tĕd) [L. *tessella*, a square]
test [L. *testum*, earthen vessel]
   t., acetic acid
   t., acetone
   t., agglutination
   t., alkali denaturation
   t., Allen-Doisy
   t., aptitude
   t., Aschheim-Zondek
   t., association
   t., autohemolysis
   t., biuret
   t., challenge
   t., chromatin
   t., coin
   t., complement-fixation
   t., concentration
   t., conjunctival
   t., creatinine clearance
   t., double-blind
   t., finger-nose
   t., Friedman
   t., galactose tolerance

   t., glucose tolerance
   t., guaiac
   t., hardness
   t., histamine
   t., Huhner
   t., human repeated patch insult
   t., intracutaneous
   t., Kahn
   t., McMurray
   t., multiple-puncture
   t., neutralization
   t., patch
   t., precipitin
   t., pregnancy
   t., prothrombin consumption
   t., pulp vitality
   t., Rubin
   t., Schiller's
   t., Schwabach
   t., scratch
   t., serial sevens
   t., serologic
   t., sickling
   t., standardized
   t., thematic apperception
   t., three-glass
   t., tine
   t., tolerance
   t., tourniquet
   t., tuberculin
   t., urea balance
   t., Wassermann
testa (tĕs'tă) [L.]
testalgia (tĕs-tăl'jē-ă) [L. *testis*, testicle, + Gr. *algos*, pain]
testectomy (tĕs-tĕk'tō-mē) [" + Gr. *ektome*, excision]
testes (tĕs'tēs) [L.]
testicle (tĕs'tĭ-kl) [L. *testiculus*, a little testis]
   t., self-examination of
testicond (tĕs'tĭ-kŏnd) [L. *testis*, testicle, + *condere*, to hide]
testicular (tĕs-tĭk'ū-lăr)
testis (tĕs'tĭs) [L.]
   t., descent of
   t., displaced
   t., femoral

t., inverted
t., perineal
t., undescended
testis compression reflex
testitis (těs-tī'tĭs) [L. *testis*, testicle,   +
Gr. *itis*, inflammation]
testitoxicosis   (těs″tĭ-tŏk-sī-kō'sĭs)
[″   +   Gr. *toxikon*, poison,   +
osis, condition]
test meal
testoid (těs'toyd)
testolactone (těs-tō-lăk'tōn)
testopathy (těs-tŏp'ă-thē) [″   +
Gr. *pathos*, disease, suffering]
testosterone (těs-tŏs'tĕr-ōn) [L. *testis*,
testicle]
Testred
test tube baby
test type
tetanic (tě-tăn'ĭk) [Gr. *tetanikos*]
tetanic convulsion
tetaniform (tě-tăn'ĭ-form) [Gr. *tetanos*,
rigid, stretched,   +   L. *forma*, shape]
tetanigenous (tět″ă-nĭj'ě-nŭs) [″   +
gennan, to produce]
tetanilla (tět″ă-nĭl'ă) [L.]
tetanism (tět'ă-nĭzm) [″   +   *-ismos*,
condition]
tetanization (tět″ă-nī-zā'shŭn) [Gr. *tetanos*, rigid, stretched]
tetanize (tět'ă-nīz)
tetanode (tět'ă-nōd) [″   +   *eidos*,
form, shape]
tetanoid (tět'ă-noyd) [″   +   *eidos*,
form, shape]
tetanoid paraplegia
tetanolysin (tět″ă-nŏl'ĭ-sĭn)
tetanomotor (tět″ăn-ō-mō'tor) [″   +
L. *motor*, a mover]
tetanophil, tetanophilic (tět'ăn-ō-fĭl,
tět″ăn-ō-fĭl'ĭk) [″   +   *philein*, to love]
tetanospasmin (tět″ă-nō-spăs'mĭn)
[″   +   *spasmos*, a convulsion]
tetanus (tět'ă-nŭs) [Gr. *tetanos*, rigid,
stretched]
t. anticus
t., artificial
t., ascending

t., cephalic
t., cerebral
t., chronic
t., cryptogenic
t., descending
t. dorsalis
t., extensor
t., hydrophobic
t., idiopathic
t., imitative
t. infantum
t. lateralis
t., local
t. neonatorum
t. paradoxus
t., postoperative
t., puerperal
t., toxic
tetanus antitoxin
tetanus immune globulin
tetanus toxoid
tetany (tět'ă-nē) [Gr. *tetanos*, rigid,
stretched]
t., alkalotic
t., duration
t., epidemic
t., gastric
t., hyperventilation
t., hypocalcemic
t., latent
t., manifest
t., parathyroid
t., rachitic
t., thyreoprival
tetarcone (tět'ăr-kōn) [Gr. *tetartos*,
fourth,   +   *konos*, cone]
tetartanopia, tetartanopsia (tět″ăr-
tăn-ō'pē-ă, -ŏp'sē-ă) [″   +   *opsis*,
sight, appearance, vision]
tetartocone (tět-ăr'tō-kōn) [″   +
konos, cone]
tetra-, tetr- [Gr. *tetras*, four]
tetrabasic (tět″ră-bā'sĭk) [″   +
basis, base]
tetrablastic (tět″ră-blăs'tĭk) [″   +
blastos, germ]
tetrabrachius (tět″ră-brā'kē-ŭs) [″   +
brachion, arm]

tetrabromofluorescein (tĕt″ră-brōm″ō-flū-or-ĕs′ĭn, -ē-ĭn)
tetracaine hydrochloride
tetrachirus (tĕt″ră-kī′rŭs) [″ + cheir, hand]
tetrachlorethylene (tĕt″ră-klor-ĕth′ĭ-lēn)
tetrachloride (tĕt″ră-klō′rīd)
tetracid (tĕ-trăs′ĭd) [″ + L. acidus, sour]
Tetracoccus (tĕt″ră-kŏk′ŭs) [″ + kokkos, berry]
tetracrotic (tĕt″ră-krŏt′ĭk) [″ + krotos, beat]
tetracycline (tĕt″ră-sī′klēn)
tetrad (tĕt′răd) [Gr. tetras, four]
tetradactyly (tĕt″ră-dăk′tĭ-lē) [″ + daktylos, finger]
tetraethylammonium chloride (tĕt-ră-ĕth-ĭl-ăm-ō′nē-ŭm klō′rĭd)
tetraethylpyrophosphate (tĕt-ră-ĕth″ĭl-pī-rō-fŏs′făt)
tetragenous (tĕt-răj′ĕn-ŭs) [Gr. tetras, four, + gennan, to produce]
tetrahydrocannabinol (tĕt″ră-hī″drō-kă-năb′ĭ-nŏl)
tetrahydrozoline hydrochloride (tĕt″ră-hī-drō′zō-lēn)
tetraiodothyronine (tĕt″ră-ī″ō-dō-thī′rō-nēn)
tetralogy
  t. of Fallot
tetramastia, tetramazia (tĕt″ră-măs′tē-ă, tĕt″ră-mā′zē-ă) [″ + mastos, mazos, breast]
tetramastigote (tĕt″ră-măs′tĭ-gōt) [″ + mastix, lash]
tetrameric, tetramerous (tĕt″ră-mĕr′ĭk, tĕt-răm′ĕr-ŭs) [″ + meros, a part]
tetranopsia (tĕt″ră-nŏp′sē-ă) [″ + an-, not, + opsis, sight, appearance, vision]
tetraotus (tĕt″ră-ō′tŭs) [Gr. tetras, four, + otos, ear]
tetraparesis (tĕt″ră-păr′ĕ-sĭs) [″ + parienai, let fall]
tetrapeptide (tĕt″ră-pĕp′tĭd)

tetraplegia (tĕt″ră-plē′jē-ă) [″ + plege, a stroke]
tetraploid (tĕt′ră-ployd) [″ + ploos, a fold, + eidos, form, shape]
tetrapus (tĕt′ră-pŭs) [″ + pous, foot]
tetrasaccharide (tĕt″ră-săk′ă-rīd)
tetrascelus (tĕt-răs′ē-lŭs) [″ + skelos, leg]
tetrasomic (tĕt-ră-sō′mĭk) [″ + soma, body]
tetraster (tĕt-răs′tĕr) [″ + aster, star]
tetrastichiasis (tĕt″ră-stĭ-kī′ă-sĭs) [″ + stichos, row, + -iasis, state or condition of]
tetratomic (tĕt″ră-tŏm′ĭk) [″ + atcmos, indivisible]
tetravalent (tĕt″ră-vā′lĕnt)
Tetrex
tetrodotoxin (tĕt″rō-dō-tŏks′ĭn)
tetrotus (tĕt-rō′tŭs) [″ + otos, ear]
tetroxide (tĕ-trŏk′sīd)
texis (tĕk′sĭs) [Gr. tiktein, to give birth]
textiform (tĕks′tĭ-form) [L. textum, something woven, + forma, shape]
textoblastic (tĕks″tō-blăs′tĭk) [L. textus, tissue, + Gr. blastos, germ]
textural (tĕks′tū-răl) [L. textura, weaving]
texture (tĕks′tūr) [L. textura]
textus (tĕks′tŭs) [L.]
T fracture
T-group
Th thorium
thalamencephalon (thăl″ă-mĕn-sĕf′ă-lŏn) [Gr. thalamos, chamber, + enkephalos, brain]
thalamic (thăl-ăm′ĭk) [Gr. thalamos, chamber]
thalamic syndrome
thalamo- [Gr. thalamos, chamber]
thalamocele, thalamocoele (thăl′ăm-ō-sēl) [″ + koilia, cavity, belly]
thalamocortical (thăl″ăm-ō-kor′tĭ-kăl)

[" + L. *cortex*, rind]
thalamolenticular (thăl'ăm-ō-lĕn-tĭk'ū-lăr) [" + L. *lenticula*, lentil]
thalamotomy (thăl-ă-mŏt'ō-mē) [" + *tome*, a cutting, slice]
thalamus (thăl'ă-mŭs) [L.]
thalassemia (thăl-ă-sē'mē-ă) [Gr. *thalassa*, sea, + *haima*, blood]
    t. major
    t. minor
thalassophobia (thăl-ăs"ō-fō'bē-ă) [Gr. *thalassa*, sea, + *phobos*, fear]
thalassoposia (thăl-lăs"sō-pō'zē-ă) [" + *posis*, drinking]
thalassotherapy (thăl-ăs"sō-thĕr'ă-pē) [" + *therapeia*, treatment]
thalidomide (thă-lĭd'ō-mīd)
thallinization (thăl"ĭn-ĭ-zā'shŭn)
thallitoxicosis (thăl"ĭ-tŏk"sĭ-kō'sĭs)
thallium (thăl'ē-ŭm) [Gr. *thallos*, a young shoot]
    t. sulfate
thallium poisoning
thallotoxicosis (thăl"ō-tŏk"sĭ-kō'sĭs)
THAM
thamuria (thă-mū'rē-ă) [Gr. *thamys*, often, + *ouron*, urine]
thanato- [Gr. *thanatos*, death]
thanatobiological (thăn"ă-tō-bī-ō-lŏj'ĭ-kăl) [Gr. *thanatos*, death, + *bios*, life, + *logos*, word, reason]
thanatognomonic (thăn"ăt-ŏg-nō-mŏn'ĭk) [" + *gnomonikos*, knowing]
thanatoid (thăn'ă-toyd) [" + *eidos*, form, shape]
thanatology (thăn"ă-tŏl'ō-jē) [Gr. *thanatos*, death, + *logos*, word, reason]
thanatomania (thăn"ă-tō-mā'nē-ă) [" + *mania*, madness]
thanatophidia (thăn"ă-tō-fĭd'ē-ă) [" + *ophis*, snake]
thanatophobia (thăn"ă-tō-fō'bē-ă) [" + *phobos*, fear]
thanatophoric (thăn"ă-tō-for'ĭk) [" + *pherein*, to bear]
thanatophoric dwarfism
thaumato- [Gr. *thauma*, wonder]

thaumaturgic [" + *ergon*, work]
Thayer-Martin medium
theaism (thē'ă-ĭzm) [L. *thea*, tea, + Gr. *-ismos*, condition]
thebaic (thē-bā'ĭk) [L. *Thebaicus*, Theban, from Thebes, where opium was once prepared]
thebaine (thē-bā'ĭn)
thebesian foramina (thē-bē'zē-ăn) [Adam Christian Thebesius, Ger. physician, 1686–1732]
thebesian valve
thebesian veins
theca (thē'kă) [Gr. *theke*, sheath]
    t. cordis
    t. folliculi
thecal (thē'kăl) [Gr. *theke*, sheath]
thecitis (thē-sī'tĭs) [" + *itis*, inflammation]
theco- [Gr. *theke*, sheath]
thecodont (thē'kō-dŏnt) [" + *odous*, tooth]
thecoma (thē-kō'mă) [" + *oma*, tumor]
thecomatosis (thē"kō-mă-tō'sĭs) [" + *osis*, condition]
thecostegnosia, thecostegnosis (thē"kō-stĕg-nō'sē-ă, -nō'sĭs) [" + *stegnosis*, a narrowing]
Theelin
theine (thē'ĭn)
theinism (thē'ĭn-ĭzm)
thelalgia (thē-lăl'jē-ă) [Gr. *thele*, nipple, + *algos*, pain]
thelarche (thē-lăr'kē) [" + *arche*, beginning]
thelasis (thē-lăs'ĭs) [" + *-iasis*, state or condition of]
Thelazia (thē-lā'zē-ă) [Gr. *thelazo*, to suck]
thelaziasis (thē"lā-zī'ă-sĭs) [" + *-iasis*, state or condition of]
theleplasty (thē'lĕ-plăs"tē) [Gr. *thele*, nipple, + *plassein*, to form]
thelerethism (thēl-ĕr'ĕ-thĭzm) [" + *erethisma*, stimulation]
thelitis (thē-lī'tĭs) [" + *itis*, inflammation]
thelium (thē'lē-ŭm) [L.]

theloncus (thē-lòn'kŭs) [" + onkus, bulk, mass]

thelophlebostemma (thē"lō-flĕb"ō-stĕm'mă) [" + phelps, vein, + stemma, wreath]

thelorrhagia (thē"lō-rā'jē-ă) [" + rhegnynai, to burst forth]

thelothism (thē'lō-thĭzm) [" + erethisma, stimulation]

thelygenic (thē"lē-jĕn'ĭk) [Gr. thelys, female, + gennan, to produce]

thenad (thē'năd) [Gr. thenar, palm, + L. ad, toward]

thenal (thē'năl) [Gr. thenar, palm]

thenal aspect

thenar (thē'năr) [Gr. thenar, palm]

thenar cleft

thenar eminence

thenar fascia

thenar muscles

theobromine (thē-ō-brō'mēn) [Gr. theos, god, + broma, food]

theomania (thē-ō-mā'nē-ă) [Gr. theos, god, + mania, madness]

theophobia (thē"ō-fō'bē-ă) [" + phobos, fear]

theophylline (thē"ō-fĭl'ĕn, -ĭn) [L. thea, tea, + Gr. phyllon, plant]
   t. ethylenediamine
   t. olamine
   t. sodium glycinate

theorem (thē'ō-rĕm) [Gr. theorema, principle arrived at by speculation]
   t., Bayes

theory (thē'ō-rē) [Gr. theoria, speculation as opposed to practice]
   t., cell
   t., clonal selection, of immunity
   t., germ
   t., quantum
   t., recapitulation

theotherapy (thē"ō-thĕr'ă-pē) [Gr. theos, god, + therapeia, treatment]

thèque (tĕk) [Fr., a box]

Theralax

therapeusis (thĕr"ă-pū'sĭs)

therapeutic (thĕr-ă-pū'tĭk) [Gr. therapeutikos, treating]

therapeutic exercise

therapeutic recreation

therapeutics (thĕr"ă-pū'tĭks) [Gr. therapeutike, treatment]

therapia sterilisans magna (thĕr"ă-pē'ă stē-rĭl'ĭ-săns măg'nă) [L.]

therapist (thĕr'ă-pĭst) [Gr. therapeia, treatment]
   t., occupational
   t., physical
   t., radiation
   t., respiratory
   t., speech

therapy (thĕr'ă-pē) [Gr. therapeia, treatment]
   t., anticoagulant
   t., aversion
   t., behavior
   t., collapse
   t., electroconvulsive
   t., fever
   t., group
   t., immunosuppressive
   t., inhalation
   t., insulin shock
   t., light
   t., milieu
   t., nonspecific
   t., occupational
   t., opsonic
   t., photodynamic
   t., physical
   t., radiation
   t., replacement
   t., serum
   t., shock
   t., specific
   t., speech
   t., spiritual
   t., substitution
   t., vaccine

therapy putty

therm [Gr. therme, heat]

thermacogenesis (thĕr"mă-kō-jĕn'ĕs-ĭs) [Gr. therme, heat, + genesis, generation, birth]

thermaerotherapy (thĕr-mā"ĕr-ō-thĕr'ă-pē) [" + aer, air, + therapeia, treatment]

thermal (thĕr′măl) [Gr. *therme*, heat]

thermal death point

thermalgesia (thĕr″măl-jē′zē-ă) [" + *algesis*, sense of pain]

thermalgia (thĕr-măl′jē-ă) [" + *algos*, pain]

thermal radiation

thermal sense

thermanalgesia (thĕrm″ăn-ăl-jē′zē-ă) [" + *an-*, not, + *algesis*, sense of pain]

thermanesthesia (thĕrm″ăn-ĕs-thē′zē-ă) [" + " + *aisthesis*, feeling, perception]

thermatology (thĕr-mă-tŏl′ō-jē) [Gr. *therme*, heat, + *logos*, word, reason]

thermelometer (thĕr″mĕl-ŏm′ĕ-tĕr) [" + *elektron*, amber, + Gr. *metron*, a measure]

thermesthesia (thĕr″mĕs-thē′zē-ă) [" + *aisthesis*, feeling, perception]

thermesthesiometer (thĕrm″ĕs-thē-zē-ŏm′ĕt-ĕr) [" + *aisthesis*, feeling, perception, + *metron*, a measure]

thermhyperesthesia (thĕrm″hī-pĕr-ĕs-thē′zē-ă) [" + Gr. *hyper*, over, above, excessive, + *aisthesis*, feeling, perception]

thermhypesthesia (thĕrm″hī-pĕs-thē′zē-ă) [" + *hypo*, under, beneath, below, + *aisthesis*, feeling, perception]

thermic (thĕr′mĭk) [Gr. *therme*, heat]

thermic sense

thermistor (thĕr-mĭs′tor)

thermo- [Gr. *therme*, heat]

thermoalgesia (thĕr″mō-ăl-jē′zē-ă) [Gr. *therme*, heat, + *algesis*, sense of pain]

thermoanalgesia (thĕr″mō-ăn″ăl-jē′zē-ă) [" + *an*, not, + *algesis*, sense of pain]

thermoanesthesia (thĕr″mō-ăn″ĕs-thē′zē-ă) [" + " + *aisthesis*, feeling, perception]

thermobiosis (thĕr″mō-bī-ō′sĭs) [" + *biosis*, way of life]

thermobiotic (thĕr″mō-bī-ŏt′ĭk) [" + *bios*, life]

thermocauterectomy (thĕr″mō-kaw-tĕr-ĕk′tō-mē) [" + *kauterion*, branding iron, + *ektome*, excision]

thermocautery (thĕr″mō-kaw′tĕr-ē)

thermochemistry (thĕr″mō-kĕm′ĭs-trē)

thermochroic (thĕr″mō-krō′ĭk) [" + *chroa*, color]

thermochroism (thĕr-mŏk′rō-ĭzm) [" + *chroa*, color]

thermocoagulation (thĕr″mō-kō-ăg-ū-lā′shŭn) [" + L. *coagulatio*, clotting]

thermocouple (thĕr′mō-kŭ″pl) [" + L. *copula*, a bond]

thermocurrent (thĕr″mō-kŭr′ĕnt)

thermode

thermodiffusion (thĕr″mō-dĭ-fū′zhŭn)

thermodilution (thĕr″mō-dī-lū′shŭn)

thermoduric (thĕr″mō-dū′rĭk) [" + L. *durus*, resistant]

thermodynamics (thĕr″mō-dī-năm′ĭks) [" + *dynamis*, power]

thermoelectric (thĕr″mō-ē-lĕk′trĭk)

thermoelectricity (thĕr″mō-ē-lĕk-trĭs′ĭ-tē)

thermoesthesia (thĕr″mō-ĕs-thē′zē-ă) [Gr. *therme*, heat, + *aisthesis*, feeling, perception]

thermoexcitatory (thĕr″mō-ĕk-sī′tă-tor-ē) [" + L. *excitare*, to irritate]

thermogenesis (thĕr″mō-jĕn′ĕ-sĭs) [" + *genesis*, generation, birth]

thermogenics (thĕr″mō-jĕn′ĭks)

thermogram (thĕr′mō-grăm)

thermograph (thĕr′mō-grăf) [" + *graphein*, to write]

thermography

thermohyperalgesia (thĕr″mō-hī″pĕr-ăl-jē′zē-ă) [" + *hyper*, over, above, excessive, + *algesis*, sense of pain]

thermohyperesthesia (thĕr″mō-hī″pĕr-ĕs-thē′zē-ă) [" + *hyper*, over, above, excessive, + *aisthesis*, feeling, perception]

thermohypesthesia (thĕr″mō-hī″pĕs-thē'zē-ă) [" + *hypo*, under, beneath, below, + *aisthesis*, feeling, perception]

thermohypoesthesia (thĕr"mō-hī"pō-ĕs-thē'zē-ă) [" + " + *aisthesis*, feeling, perception]

thermoinhibitory (thĕr"mō-ĭn-hĭb'ĭ-tor"ē) [" + L. *inhibere*, to restrain]

thermolabile (thĕr"mō-lā'bĭl) [" + *labilis*, unstable]

thermolamp (thĕr'mō-lămp) [" + *lampe*, torch]

thermology (thĕr-mŏl'ō-jē) [" + *logos*, word, reason]

thermoluminescent dosimeter

thermolysis (thĕr-mŏl'ĭ-sĭs) [" + *lysis*, dissolution]

thermolytic (thĕr"mō-lĭt'ĭk) [" + *lytikos*, dissolving]

thermomassage (thĕr"mō-mă-săzh')

thermometer (thĕr-mŏm'ĕ-tĕr) [" + *metron*, measure]

   t., alcohol
   t., Celsius
   t., centigrade
   t., clinical
   t., differential
   t., Fahrenheit
   t., gas
   t., Kelvin
   t., mercury
   t., recording
   t., rectal
   t., self-registering
   t., spirit
   t., surface
   t., wet-and-dry-bulb

thermometer, disinfection of

thermometric (thĕr"mō-mĕt'rĭk) [Gr. *therme*, heat, + *metron*, measure]

thermometry (thĕr-mŏm'ĕ-trē)
   t., clinical

thermoneurosis (thĕr"mō-nū-rō'sĭs) [Gr. *therme*, heat, + *neuron*, nerve, + *osis*, condition]

thermonuclear (thĕr"mō-nū'klē-ăr)

thermopenetration (thĕr"mō-pĕn-ĕ-trā'shŭn) [" + L. *penetrare*, to go

within]

thermoperiodicity (thĕr"mō-pĕr-ē-ō-dĭs'ĭ-tē)

thermophagy (thĕr-mŏf'ă-jē) [" + *phagein*, to eat]

thermophilic (thĕr"mō-fĭl'ĭk) [" + *philein*, to love]

thermophils (thĕr'mō-fĭlz)

thermophobia (thĕr"mō-fō'bē-ă) [" + *phobos*, fear]

thermophore (thĕr'mō-for) [" + *phoros*, a bearer]

thermophylic (thĕr"mō-fĭ'lĭk) [" + *phylake*, guard]

thermopile (thĕr'mō-pĭl) [" + L. *pila*, pile]

thermoplacentography (thĕr"mō-plăs"ĕn-tŏg'ră-fē) [" + L. *placenta*, a flat cake, + Gr. *graphein*, to write]

thermoplastic (thĕr"mō-plăs'tĭk)

thermoplegia (thĕr"mō-plē'jē-ă) [" + *plege*, a stroke]

thermopolypnea (thĕr"mō-pŏl-ĭp-nē'ă) [" + *polys*, many, + *pnoia*, breath]

thermoradiotherapy (thĕr"mō-rā"dē-ō-thĕr'ă-pē) [" + L. *radius*, ray, + Gr. *therapeia*, treatment]

thermoreceptor (thĕr"mō-rē-sĕp'tor) [" + L. *receptor*, a receiver]

thermoregulation (thĕr"mō-rĕg"ū-lā'shŭn)

thermoregulatory (thĕr"mō-rĕg'ū-lă-tor"ē)

thermoregulatory centers

thermoresistant (thĕr"mō-rē-zĭs'tănt) [" + L. *resistentia*, resistance]

thermostabile (thĕr"mō-stā'bl) [" + L. *stabilis*, stable]

thermostasis (thĕr"mō-stā'sĭs) [" + *stasis*, standing still]

thermostat (thĕr'mō-stăt) [" + *statikos*, standing]

thermosteresis (thĕr"mō-stĕ-rē'sĭs) [" + *steresis*, deprivation]

thermosterilization

thermosystaltic (thĕr"mō-sĭs-tăl'tĭk)

[Gr. *therme*, heat, + *systellein*, to contract]

thermotactic, thermotaxic (thĕr″mō-tăk′tĭk, -tăks′ĭk) [″ + *taktikos*, regulating]

thermotaxis (thĕr″mō-tăks′ĭs) [″ + *taxis*, arrangement]

thermotherapeutics (thĕr″mō-thĕr-ă-pū′tĭks) [″ + *therapeutike*, treatment]

thermotherapy (thĕr″mō-thĕr′ă-pē) [″ + *therapeia*, treatment]

thermotics (thĕr-mŏt′ĭks)

thermotolerant (thĕr″mō-tŏl′ĕr-ănt) [″ + L. *tolerare*, to tolerate]

thermotonometer (thĕr″mō-tō-nŏm′ĕ-tĕr) [″ + *tonos*, act of stretching, tension, tone, + *metron*, measure]

thermotoxin (thĕr″mō-tŏks′ĭn) [″ + *toxikon*, poison]

thermotropism (thĕr-mŏt′rō-pĭzm) [″ + *trope*, turning, + *-ismos*, condition]

theroid (thē′royd) [Gr. *theriodes*, beastlike]

thesaurismosis (thē-să″rĭs-mō′sĭs) [Gr. *thesauros*, treasure, + *osis*, condition]

thesaurosis (thē″saw-rō′sĭs) [″ + *osis*, condition]

thiabendazole (thī″ă-bĕn′dă-zōl)

thiaminase (thī-ăm′ĭ-nās)

thiamine hydrochloride

thiamine mononitrate

thiamine pyrophosphate

thiamylal sodium for injection (thī-ăm′ĭ-lăl)

thiemia (thī-ē′mē-ă) [Gr. *theion*, sulfur, + *haima*, blood]

Thiersch's graft (tērsh′ĕz) [Karl Thiersch, Ger. surgeon, 1822–1895]

thiethylperazine malate (thī-ĕth″ĭl-pĕr′ă-zēn)

thigh (thī) [AS. *theoh*]

thigmesthesia (thĭg″mĕs-thē′zē-ă) [Gr. *thigma*, touch, + *aisthesis*, feeling, perception]

thigmotaxis (thĭg″mō-tăks′ĭs) [″ + *taxis*, arrangement]

thigmotropism (thĭg-mŏt′rō-pĭzm) [″ + *tropos*, a turning, + *-ismos*, condition]

thimerosal (thī-mĕr′ō-săl)

thinking

thin-layer chromatography

thio- [Gr. *theion*, sulfur]

thiocyanate (thī″ō-sī′ă-nāt)

thiogenic (thī″ō-jĕn′ĭk) [Gr. *theion*, sulfur, + *gennan*, to produce]

thioglucosidase (thī″ō-glū-kō′sĭ-dās)

thioguanine (thī″ō-gwă′nēn)

thioneine (thī′ō-nēn) [″ + *neos*, new]

thionic (thī′ō-nĭk)

thiopectic, thiopexic (thī-ō-pĕk′tĭk, -pĕks′ĭk) [″ + *pexis*, fixation]

thiopental sodium (thī″ō-pĕn′tăl)

thiopexy (thī″ō-pĕks′ē)

thiophil, thiophilic (thī′ō-fĭl, thī″ō-fĭl′ĭk) [Gr. *theion*, sulfur, + *philein*, to love]

thioridazine hydrochloride (thī″ō-rĭd′ă-zēn)

thiosulfate (thī″ō-sŭl′fāt)

Thiosulfil

thiotepa (thī″ō-tē′pă)

thiothixene (thī″ō-thĭks′ēn)

thiouracil (thī″ō-ū′ră-sĭl)

thiourea (thī″ō-ūr-ē′ă) [Gr. *theion*, sulfur, + *ouron*, urine]

thiram (thī′răm)

thiram poisoning

third cranial nerve

third intention

third ventricle

thirst [AS. *thurst*]

Thiry's fistula (tē′rēz) [Ludwig Thiry, Austrian physiologist, 1817–1897]

Thiuretic

thixolabile (thĭk″sō-lā′bĭl)

thixotropy (thĭks-ŏt′rō-pē) [Gr. *thixis*, a touching, + *trope*, turning]

thlipsencephalus (thlĭp″sĕn-sĕf′ă-lŭs) [Gr. *thlipsis*, pressure, + *enkephalos*, brain]

Thomas splint [Hugh O. Thomas, Brit. orthopedic surgeon, 1834–1891]

Thomas-White hypothesis [Clayton Thomas, b. 1921, U.S. physician; Arthur White, b. 1925, U.S. physician]

Thomsen's disease (tŏm'sĕnz) [Asmus Julius Thomsen, Danish physician, 1815–1896]

thoracalgia (thō"răk-ăl'jē-ă) [Gr. *thorakos*, chest, + *algos*, pain]

thoracectomy (thō"ră-sĕk'tō-mē) [" + *ektome*, excision]

thoracentesis (thō"ră-sĕn-tē'sĭs) [" + *kentesis*, a puncture]

thoracic (thō-răs'ĭk) [Gr. *thorax*, chest]

thoracic cage

thoracic cavity

thoracic duct

thoracic limbs

thoracicoabdominal (thō-răs"ĭ-kō-ăb-dŏm'ĭ-năl)

thoracicohumeral (thō-răs"ĭ-kō-hū'mĕr-ăl)

thoracic outlet compression syndrome

thoracic squeeze

thoracic surgery

thoraco- [Gr. *thorakos*, chest]

thoracoacromial (thō"ră-kō-ă-krō'mē-ăl)

thoracobronchotomy (thō"răk-ō-brŏn-kŏt'ō-mē) [" + *bronchos*, windpipe, + *tome*, a cutting, slice]

thoracocautery (thō"răk-ō-kaw'tĕr-ē) [" + *kauterion*, branding iron]

thoracoceloschisis (thō"răk-ō-sē-lŏs'kĭ-sĭs) [Gr. *thorakos*, chest, + *koilia*, cavity, belly, + *schisis*, cleavage]

thoracocentesis (thō"răk-ō-sĕn-tē'sĭs) [" + *kentesis*, a puncture]

thoracocyllosis (thō"răk-ō-sĭl-ō'sĭs) [" + *kyllosis*, crippling]

thoracocyrtosis (thō"răk-ō-sĭr-tō'sĭs) [" + *kyrtosis*, curvature]

thoracodelphus (thō"ră-kō-dĕl'fŭs) [" + *adelphos*, brother]

thoracodidymus (thō"ră-kō-dĭd'ĭ-mŭs) [" + *didymos*, twin]

thoracodynia (thō"răk-ō-dĭn'ē-ă) [" + *odyne*, pain]

thoracogastroschisis (thō"răk-ō-găs-trŏs'kĭ-sĭs) [" + *gaster*, belly, + *schisis*, cleavage]

thoracograph (thō-răk'ō-grăf) [" + *graphein*, to write]

thoracolaparotomy (thō"ră-kō-lăp"ă-rŏt'ō-mē) [" + *lapara*, loin, + *tome*, a cutting, slice]

thoracolumbar (thō"răk-ō-lŭm'bar) [" + L. *lumbus*, loin]

thoracolysis (thō"răk-ŏl'ĭ-sĭs) [" + *lysis*, dissolution]

thoracomelus (thō"ră-kŏm'ē-lŭs) [" + *melos*, limb]

thoracometer (thō"ră-kŏm'ē-tĕr) [Gr. *thorakos*, chest, + *metron*, measure]

thoracometry (thō"ră-kŏm'ĕt-rē) [" + *metron*, measure]

thoracomyodynia (thō"ră-kō-mī"ō-dĭn'ē-ă) [" + *mys*, muscle, + *odyne*, pain]

thoracopagus (thō"ră-kŏp'ă-gŭs) [" + *pagos*, fixed]

thoracoparacephalus (thō"ră-kō-păr"ă-sĕf'ă-lŭs) [" + *para*, alongside, past, beyond, + *kephale*, head]

thoracopathy (thō"răk-ŏp'ă-thē) [" + *pathos*, disease, suffering]

thoracoplasty (thō"ră-kō-plăs"tē, thō-rā'kō-plăs"tē) [" + *plassein*, to form]

thoracopneumoplasty (thō"ră-kō-nū'mō-plăs-tē) [" + *pneumon*, lung, + *plassein*, to form]

thoracoschisis (thō"ră-kŏs'kĭ-sĭs) [" + *schisis*, cleavage]

thoracoscope (thō-rā'kō-skōp, -răk'ō-skōp) [" + *skopein*, to examine]

thoracoscopy (thō"ră-kŏs'kō-pē)

thoracostenosis (thō"ră-kō-stĕn-ō'sĭs) [" + *stenosis*, act of narrowing]

thoracostomy (thō"răk-ŏs'tō-mē) [" + *stoma*, mouth, opening]

thoracotomy (thō"răk-ŏt'ō-mē) [" + *tome*, a cutting, slice]
thorax (thō'răks) [Gr., chest]
  t., barrel-shaped
  t., bony
  t. paralyticus
  t., Peyrot's
Thorazine
Thorel's bundle (tō'rĕlz) [Christen Thorel, Ger. physician, 1880–1935]
thorium (thō'rē-ŭm)
Thorn test [George W. Thorn, U.S. physician, b. 1906]
thoron (thō'rŏn)
thread (thrĕd)
threadworm
three-day fever
thremmatology (thrĕm"ă-tŏl'ō-jē) [Gr. *thremma*, nursling, + *logos*, word, reason]
threonine (thrē'ō-nīn)
threshold (thrĕsh'ōld) [AS. *therscold*]
  t., absolute
  t., auditory
  t., differential
  t., erythema
  t., ketosis
  t. of consciousness
  t., renal
  t., sensory
  t. stimulus
threshold dose
threshold substance
thrill (thrĭl) [ME. *thrillen*, to pierce]
  t., aneurysmal
  t., aortic
  t., arterial
  t., diastolic
  t., hydatid
  t., presystolic
  t., systolic
thrix
  t. annulata
-thrix [Gr. *thrix*, hair]
throat (thrōt) [AS. *throte*]
throat, foreign bodies in
throb (thrŏb) [ME. *throbben*, of imitative origin]

throbbing (thrŏb'ĭng)
Throckmorton's reflex (thrŏk'mor"tŭnz) [Thomas Bentley Throckmorton, U.S. neurologist, 1885–1961]
throe (thrō) [AS. *thruve*, paroxysm]
thrombase (thrŏm'bās)
thrombasthenia (thrŏm"băs-thē'nē-ă) [Gr. *thrombos*, clot, + *astheneia*, weakness]
thrombectomy (thrŏm-bĕk'tō-mē) [" + *ektome*, excision]
thrombi (thrŏm'bī)
thrombin (thrŏm'bĭn) [Gr. *thrombos*, clot]
thrombinogen (thrŏm-bĭn'ō-jĕn)
thromboangiitis (thrŏm"bō-ăn"jē-ī'tĭs) [Gr. *thrombos*, clot, + *angeion*, vessel, + *itis*, inflammation]
  t. obliterans
thromboarteritis (thrŏm"bō-ăr-tĕ-rī'tĭs) [" + *arteria*, artery, + *itis*, inflammation]
thromboclasis (thrŏm-bŏk'lă-sĭs) [" + *klasis*, a breaking]
thromboclastic (thrŏm"bō-klăs'tĭk)
thrombocyst (thrŏm'bō-sĭst) [Gr. *thrombos*, clot, + *kystis*, a sac]
thrombocyte (thrŏm'bō-sīt) [" + *kytos*, cell]
thrombocythemia (thrŏm"bō-sī-thē'mē-ă) [" + " + *haima*, blood]
thrombocytocrit (thrŏm"bō-sī'tō-krĭt) [" + " + *krinein*, to separate]
thrombocytolysis (thrŏm"bō-sī-tŏl'ĭ-sĭs) [" + " + *lysis*, dissolution]
thrombocytopathy (thrŏm"bō-sī-tŏp'ă-thē) [" + " + *pathos*, disease, suffering]
thrombocytopenia (thrŏm"bō-sī"tō-pē'nē-ă) [" + " + *penia*, lack]
thrombocytopoiesis (thrŏm"bō-sī"tō-poy-ē'sĭs) [" + " + *poiesis*, production]
thrombocytosis (thrŏm"bō-sī-tō'sĭs) [" + *kytos*, cell]
thromboembolism (thrŏm"bō-ĕm'bō-

lĭzm) [" + NL. *embolismus,* intercalary, + *-ismos,* condition]

thromboendarterectomy (thrŏm″bō-ĕnd″ăr-tĕr-ĕk′tō-mē) [" + *endon,* within, + *arteria,* artery, + *ektome,* excision]

thromboendarteritis (thrŏm″bō-ĕnd-ăr″tĕr-ī′tĭs) [" + " + " + *itis,* inflammation]

thromboendocarditis (thrŏm″bō-ĕn″dō-kăr-dī′tĭs) [" + *endon,* within, + *kardia,* heart, + *itis,* inflammation]

thrombogenesis (thrŏm″bō-jĕn′ĕ-sĭs) [" + *genesis,* generation, birth]

thrombogenic (thrŏm″bō-jĕn′ĭk) [" + *gennan,* to produce]

thromboid (thrŏm′boyd) [" + *eidos,* form, shape]

thrombokinase (thrŏm″bō-kīn′ās) [" + *kinesis,* motion]

thrombokinesis (thrŏm″bō-kĭ-nē′sĭs) [" + *kinesis,* motion]

thrombolymphangitis (thrŏm″bō-lĭm″făn-jī′tĭs) [" + L. *lympha,* lymph, + Gr. *angeion,* vessel, + *itis,* inflammation]

thrombolysis (thrŏm-bŏl′ĭ-sĭs) [" + *lysis,* dissolution]

thrombolytic (thrŏm-bō-lĭt′ĭk)

thrombon (thrŏm′bŏn) [Gr. *thrombos,* clot]

thrombopathy (thrŏm-bŏp′ă-thē) [" + *pathos,* disease, suffering]

thrombopenia (thrŏm-bō-pē′nē-ă) [" + *penia,* lack]

thrombophilia (thrŏm-bō-fĭl′ē-ă) [" + *philein,* to love]

thrombophlebitis (thrŏm″bō-flĕ-bī′tĭs) [" + *phleps,* blood vessel, vein, + *itis,* inflammation]

   t. migrans

   t., postpartum, iliofemoral

thromboplastic (thrŏm″bō-plăs′tĭk) [" + *plassein,* to form]

thromboplastid (thrŏm″bō-plăs′tĭd)

thromboplastin (thrŏm″bō-plăs′tĭn) [" + *plassein,* to form]

thromboplastinogen (thrŏm″bō-plăs-tĭn′ō-jĕn)

thrombopoiesis (thrŏm″bō-poy-ē′sĭs) [" + *poiesis,* production]

thrombosed (thrŏm′bōzd) [Gr. *thrombos,* a clot]

thrombosinusitis (thrŏm″bō-sī-nŭs-ī′tĭs) [" + L. *sinus,* a curve, hollow, + Gr. *itis,* inflammation]

thrombosis (thrŏm-bō′sĭs) [" + *osis,* condition]

   t., cardiac

   t., coagulation

   t., coronary

   t., embolic

   t., infective

   t., marasmic

   t., placental

   t., plate

   t., puerperal

   t., sinus

   t., traumatic

   t., venous

thrombostasis (thrŏm-bŏs′tă-sĭs) [" + *stasis,* standing still]

thrombosthenin (thrŏm″bō-sthē′nĭn) [" + *sthenos,* strength]

thrombotic (thrŏm-bŏt′ĭk) [Gr. *thrombos,* clot]

thrombus (thrŏm′bŭs) [Gr. *thrombos*]

   t., annular

   t., antemortem

   t., ball

   t., hyaline

   t., Laennec's

   t., lateral

   t., milk

   t., mural

   t., obstructing

   t., occluding

   t., parietal

   t., progressive

   t., stratified

   t., white

through-and-through drainage

through illumination

thrush (thrŭsh) [D. *troske,* rotten wood]

thrust

thrypsis (thrĭp′sĭs) [Gr., breaking in pieces]
thulium (thū′lē-ŭm)
thumb (thŭm) [AS. *thuma*, thumb]
    t., tennis
thumb sign
thumb sucking
thus (thŭs) [L.]
thylacitis (thī″lă-sī′tĭs) [Gr. *thylax*, pouch, + *itis*, inflammation]
thylakoid (thī′lă-koyd) [Gr. *thylakon*, a small sac, + *eidos*, form, shape]
thymectomize (thī-mĕk′tō-mīz)
thymectomy (thī-mĕk′tō-mē) [Gr. *thymos*, thymus gland, + *ektome*, excision]
thymelcosis (thī″mĕl-kō′sĭs) [″ + *helkosis*, ulceration]
-thymia [Gr. *thymos*, mind, spirit]
thymic (thī′mĭk) [L. *thymicus*]
thymicolymphatic (thī″mĭ-kō-lĭm-făt′ĭk)
thymidine (thī′mĭ-dēn)
thymine (thī′mīn)
thymion (thĭm′ē-ŏn) [Gr.]
thymitis (thī-mī′tĭs) [Gr. *thymos*, thymus gland, + *itis*, inflammation]
thymo- [Gr. *thymos*, thymus gland; mind, spirit]
thymocyte (thī′mō-sīt) [Gr. *thymos*, thymus gland, + *kytos*, cell]
thymokesis (thī″mō-kē′sĭs)
thymokinetic (thī″mō-kī-nĕt′ĭk) [″ + *kinesis*, motion]
thymol (thī′mōl) [Gr. *thumon*, thyme, + L. *oleum*, oil]
    t. iodide
thymolysis (thī-mōl′ĭ-sĭs) [Gr. *thymos*, thymus gland, + *lysis*, dissolution]
thymolytic (thī-mō-lĭt′ĭk)
thymoma (thī-mō′mă) [″ + *oma*, tumor]
thymopathy (thī-mŏp′ă-thē)
thymopexy (thī″mō-pĕks′ē) [″ + *pexis*, fixation]
thymopoietin (thī″mō-poy′ĕ-tĭn)
thymoprivic (thī″mō-prĭv′ĭk) [″ + L. *privus*, deprived of]
thymotoxic (thī″mō-tŏks′ĭk) [″ + *toxikon*, poison]
thymus (thī′mŭs) [Gr. *thymos*]
    t., accessory
    t. persistens hyperplastica
thymusectomy (thī″mŭs-ĕk′tō-mē) [Gr. *thymos*, thymus gland, + *ektome*, excision]
thyreo-, thyro- [Gr. *thyreos*, shield]
thyreoplasia
thyroadenitis (thī″rō-ăd-ĕ-nī′tĭs) [″ + *aden*, gland, + *itis*, inflammation]
thyroaplasia (thī″rō-ă-plā′zē-ă) [″ + *a-*, not, + *plasis*, a molding]
thyroarytenoid (thī″rō-ă-rĭt′ĕn-oyd) [″ + *arytaina*, ladle, + *eidos*, form, shape]
thyrocalcitonin (thī″rō-kăl″sĭ-tō′nĭn)
thyrocardiac (thī″rō-kăr′dē-ăk) [″ + *kardia*, heart]
thyrocele (thī′rō-sēl) [″ + *kele*, tumor, swelling]
thyrochondrotomy (thī″rō-kŏn-drŏt′ō-mē) [″ + *chondros*, cartilage, + *tome*, a cutting, slice]
thyrocolloid (thī″rō-kŏl′oyd)
thyrocricotomy (thī″rō-krī-kŏt′ō-mē) [″ + *krikos*, ring, + *tome*, a cutting, slice]
thyroepiglottic (thī″rō-ĕp″ĭ-glŏt′ĭk) [″ + *epi*, upon, + *glottis*, tongue]
thyroepiglottic muscle
thyroepiglottideus (thī″rō-ĕp″ĭ-glŏt-ĭd′ē-ŭs)
thyrofissure (thī″rō-fĭsh′ŭr)
thyrogenic, thyrogenous (thī-rō-jĕn′ĭk, thī-rŏj′ĕ-nŭs) [″ + *gennan*, to produce]
thyroglobulin (thī″rō-glŏb′ū-lĭn) [″ + L. *globulus*, globule]
thyroglossal (thī″rō-glŏs′săl) [″ + *glossa*, tongue]
thyroglossal duct
thyrohyal (thī″rō-hī′ăl)
thyrohyoid (thī″rō-hī′oyd) [″ + *hyoeides*, U-shaped]
thyroid (thī′royd) [″ + *eidos*, form, shape]

thyroid cachexia
thyroid cartilage
thyroid crisis
thyroidea accessoria; thyroidea ima (thī-roy'dē-ă)
thyroidectomized (thī"roy-dĕk'tō-mīzd) [" + *eidos*, form, shape, + *ektome*, excision]
thyroidectomy (thī"royd-ĕk'tō-mē)
thyroid function tests
thyroid gland
thyroidism (thī'royd-ĭzm)
thyroiditis (thī"royd-ī'tĭs) [" + *eidos*, form, shape, + *itis*, inflammation]
   t., giant cell
   t., Hashimoto's
thyroidomania (thī"royd-ō-mā'nē-ă) [" + " + *mania*, frenzy]
thyroidotomy (thī"royd-ŏt'ō-mē) [" + " + *tome*, a cutting, slice]
thyroidotoxin (thī"royd-ō-tŏk'sĭn)
thyroid-stimulating hormone
thyroid storm
Thyrolar
thyrolysin (thī-rŏl'ĭ-sĭn)
thyrolytic (thī"rō-lĭt'ĭk) [Gr. *thyreos*, shield, + *lysis*, dissolution]
thyromegaly (thī"rō-mĕg'ă-lē) [" + *megas*, large]
thyromimetic (thī"rō-mī-mĕt'ĭk)
thyroparathyroidectomy (thī"rō-păr"ă-thī"royd-ĕk'tō-mē) [" + *para*, alongside, past, beyond, + *thyreos*, shield, + *eidos*, form, shape, + *ektome*, excision]
thyropathy (thī-rŏp'ă-thē) [" + *pathos*, disease, suffering]
thyroprival (thī"rō-prī'văl) [" + L. *privus*, single, set apart]
thyroprivia (thī"rō-prĭv'ē-ă) [" + L. *privus*, single, set apart]
thyroptosis (thī"rŏp-tō'sĭs) [" + *ptosis*, fall, falling]
thyrosis (thī-rō'sĭs) [" + *osis*, condition]
thyrotherapy (thī"rō-thĕr'ă-pē) [" + *therapeia*, treatment]

thyrotome (thī'rō-tōm) [" + *tome*, a cutting, slice]
thyrotomy (thī-rŏt'ō-mē)
thyrotoxic (thī"rō-tŏks'ĭk) [" + *toxikon*, poison]
thyrotoxicosis (thī"rō-tŏks"ĭ-kō'sĭs) [" + " + *osis*, condition]
thyrotoxin (thī"rō-tŏk'sĭn)
thyrotrophic (thī"rō-trŏf'ĭk)
thyrotrophin (thī"rō-trŏf'ĭn)
thyrotropic (thī"rō-trŏp'ĭk) [" + *trope*, a turning]
thyrotropic hormone
thyrotropin (thī-rŏt'rō-pĭn)
thyrotropism (thī-rŏt'rō-pĭzm)
thyroxine (thī-rŏks'ĭn) [Gr. *thyreos*, shield]
Ti *titanium*
TIA *transient ischemic attack*
tibia (tĭb'ē-ă) [L. *tibia*, shinbone]
   t., saber-shaped
   t. valga
   t. vara
tibiad (tĭb'ē-ăd) [" + *ad*, to]
tibial (tĭb'ē-ăl) [L. *tibialis*]
tibialgia (tĭb"ē-ăl'jē-ă) [" + Gr. *algos*, pain]
tibialis (tĭb"ē-ā'lĭs) [L.]
tibioadductor reflex (tĭb"ē-ō-ăd-dŭk'tor) [L. *tibia*, shinbone, + *adducere*, to lead to]
tibiocalcanean (tĭb"ē-ō-kăl-kā'nē-ăn)
tibiofemoral (tĭb"ē-ō-fĕm'or-ăl) [" + L. *femur*, thigh]
tibiofibular (tĭb"ē-ō-fĭb'ū-lăr) [" + L. *fibula*, pin]
tibionavicular (tĭb"ē-ō-nă-vĭk'ū-lăr)
tibioperoneal (tĭb"ē-ō-pĕr"ō-nē'ăl)
tibioscaphoid (tĭb"ē-ō-skăf'oyd)
tibiotarsal (tĭb"ē-ō-tăr'săl) [" + Gr. *tarsos*, flat of the foot, flat surface, edge of eyelid]
tic (tĭk) [Fr.]
   t., convulsive
   t. douloureux
   t., facial
   t., habit
   t. rotatoire

t., spasmodic
Ticar
ticarcillin disodium, sterile (tī″kăr-sĭl′ĭn)
tick (tĭk) [ME. *tyke*]
tick bite
tick-borne rickettsiosis
tickle (tĭk′l) [ME. *tikelen*]
tickling (tĭk′lĭng)
t.i.d. [L.] *ter in die*, three times a day
tidal (tī′dăl)
tidal air
tidal drainage
tide [AS. *tid*, time]
t., acid
t., alkaline
t., fat
Tietze's syndrome (tēt′sĕz) [Alexander Tietze, Ger. surgeon, 1864–1927]
Tigan
tigering [Gr. *tigris*, tiger]
tigretier (tē-grĕt″ē-ā′) [Fr.]
tigroid (tī′groyd) [Gr. *tigroeides*, tiger-spotted]
tigroid bodies
tigrolysis (tĭg″rŏl′ĭ-sĭs)
tilmus (tĭl′mŭs) [Gr. *tilmos*, a plucking]
tiltometer (tĭl-tŏm′ĕ-tĕr)
timbre (tĭm′bĕr, tăm′br) [Fr., a bell to be struck with a hammer]
time (tīm) [AS. *tima*, time]
t., bleeding
t., clot retraction
t., coagulation
t., doubling
t., median lethal
t., prothrombin
t., reaction
t., setting
t., thermal death
time frame
time inventory
timer (tīm′ĕr)
Timoptic Solution
tin (tĭn) [AS.]
Tinactin
tinct. *tincture*

tinctable (tĭnk′tă-bl)
tinction (tĭnk′shŭn) [L. *tingere*, to dye]
tinctorial (tĭnk-tō′rē-ăl) [L. *tinctorius*, dyeing]
tinctura (tĭnk-tū′ră) [L., a dyeing]
tincturation (tĭnk″tū-rā′shŭn)
tincture (tĭnk′chŭr) [L. *tincture*, a dyeing]
tincture of iodine
tincture of iodine poisoning
Tindal
tinea (tĭn′ē-ă) [L., worm]
t. amiantacea
t. barbae
t. capitis
t. corporis
t. cruris
t. imbricata
t. kerion
t. nigra
t. nodosa
t. pedis
t. profunda
t. sycosis
t. unguium
t. versicolor
Tinel's sign (tĭn-ĕlz′) [Jules Tinel, Fr. neurologist, 1879–1952]
tine test
tingibility (tĭn″jĭ-bĭl′ĭ-tē)
tingible (tĭn′jĭ-bl) [L. *tingere*, to stain]
tingle (tĭng′gl)
tinnitus (tĭn-ī′tŭs) [L., a jingling]
t. aurium
tin poisoning
tintometer (tĭn-tŏm′ĕ-ter) [L. *tinctus*, a dyeing, + Gr. *metron*, a measure]
tintometric (tĭn″tō-mĕt′rĭk)
tintometry (tĭn-tŏm′ĕ-trē)
tip (tĭp) [ME]
tipped uterus
tipping (tĭp′ĭng)
tiqueur (tī-kĕr′) [Fr.]
tire (tīr) [AS. *teorian*, to tire]
tirefond (tēr-fŏn′) [Fr.]
tires (tīrz)
tiring (tīr′ĭng)
tissue (tĭsh′ū) [O. Fr. *tissu*, from L. *texere*, to weave]

t., adenoid
t., adipose
t., areolar
t., bony, bone
t., brown adipose, brown fat
t., cancellous
t., cartilage
t., chondroid
t., chordal
t.'s, chromaffin
t.'s, chromophil
t., cicatricial
t., connective
t., elastic
t., embryonic
t., endothelial
t., epithelial
t., erectile
t., extracellular
t., fatty
t., fibrous
t., gelatiginous
t., glandular
t., granulation
t., hard
t., indifferent
t., interstitial
t., lymphadenoid
t., lymphoid
t., mesenchymal
t., mucous
t., muscular
t., myeloid
t., nerve, nervous
t., osseous
t., reticular
t., scar
t., sclerous
t., skeletal
t., splenic
t., subcutaneous
t., subcutaneous adipose
t., white fibrous
t., white nervous
tissue bank
tissue culture
tissue factor
tissue macrophage

tissue plasminogen activator
tissue typing
tissular (tĭsh'ū-lăr)
titanium (tī-tā'nē-ŭm) [L. *titan*, the sun]
  t. dioxide
titer (tī'tĕr) [F. *titre*, standard]
  t., agglutination
titillation (tĭt″ĭl-ā'shŭn) [L. *titillatio*, a tickling]
titrate (tī'trāt)
titration (tī-trā'shŭn) [Fr. *titre*, a standard]
titre
titrimetric (tī″trī-mĕt'rĭk) [″ + Gr. *metron*, measure]
titrimetry (tī-trĭm'ĕ-trē) [*titration* + Gr. *metron*, measure]
titubation (tĭt″ū-bā'shŭn) [L. *titubatio*, a staggering]
  t., lingual
Tl *thallium*
TLC *thin-layer chromatography; tender loving care; total lung capacity*
T.L.R. *tonic labyrinthine reflex*
Tm *thulium; maximal tubular excretory capacity of the kidneys*
TMJ *temporomandibular joint*
Tn *normal intraocular tension*
TNM classification *tumor, nodes, metastases*
TNT *trinitrotoluene*
TO *old tuberculin*
toadskin (tōd'skĭn)
toadstool (tōd'stool)
toadstool poisoning
tobacco (tō-băk'ō) [Sp. *tabaco*]
tobramycin (tō″bră-mī'sĭn)
tocainide (tō-kāy'nīd)
toco- [Gr. *tokos*, birth]
tocodynagraph (tō″kō-dĭ'nă-grăf) [″ + *dunamis*, power, + *graphein*, to write]
tocodynamometer (tō″kō-dī″năm-ŏm'ĕ-tĕr) [″ + *dunamis*, power, + *metron*, a measure]
tocograph (tŏk'ō-grăf) [″ + *graphein*, to write]
tocography (tō″kŏg'ră-fē)

tocology (tō-kŏl'ō-jē) [" + *logos*, word, reason]

tocolysis (tō"kō-lĭ'sĭs) [" + *lysis*, dissolution]

tocometer (tō-kŏm'ĕt-ĕr) [" + *metron*, a measure]

tocopherol (tō-kŏf'ĕr-ŏl) [" + *pherein*, to carry, + L. *oleum*, oil]

tocophobia (tō"kō-fō'bē-ă) [" + *phobos*, fear]

tocus (tō'kŭs) [L.]

toe (tō) [AS. *ta*]
  t., claw
  t., dislocations of
  t.'s, fanning of
  t., hammer-
  t., Morton's
  t., pigeon
  t.'s, webbed

toe clonus

toe drop

toenail (tō'nāl)

toe reflex

Tofranil

Togaviridae [L. *toga*, coat, + *virus*, poison]

toilet (toy'lĕt) [Fr. *toilette*, a little cloth]

toilet training

tokodynagraph (tō"kō-dī'nă-grăf) [Gr. *tokos*, birth, + *dunamis*, power, + *graphein*, to write]

tolazamide (tŏl-ăz'ă-mīd)

tolazoline hydrochloride (tŏl-ăz'ō-lēn)

tolbutamide (tŏl-bū'tă-mīd)

Tolectin

tolerance (tŏl'ĕr-ăns) [L. *tolerantia*, tolerance]
  t., drug
  t., exercise
  t., glucose
  t., immunologic

tolerant

tolerogen (tŏl'ĕr-ō-jĕn)

tolerogenic (tŏl"ĕr-ō-jĕn'ĭk)

Toleron

Tolinase

tollwut (tŏl-voot') [Ger.]

tolnaftate (tŏl-năf'tāt)

tolu balsam

toluene

toluene poisoning

toluidine (tŏl-ū'ĭ-dĭn)

tomaculous neuropathy (tō-mă'cū-lŭs) [L. *tomaculum*, a kind of sausage]

tomatine (tō'mă-tēn)

-tome [Gr. *tome*, a cutting, slice]

tomo- [Gr. *tomos*, slice, section]

tomogram (tō'mō-grăm) [" + *gramma*, letter, piece of writing]

tomograph (tō'mō-grăf) [" + *graphein*, to write]

tomography (tō-mŏg'ră-fē)
  t., computerized axial

tonaphasia (tō"nă-fā'sē-ă) [L. *tonus*, tension, pitch, tone, + *a-*, not, + *phasis*, utterance]

tone (tōn) [L. *tonus*, tension, pitch, tone]
  t., muscular

tone deafness

tongs, Crutchfield

tongue (tŭng) [AS. *tunge*]
  t., bifid
  t., black hairy
  t., burning
  t., cleft
  t., coated
  t., deviation of
  t., dry
  t., fern-leaf
  t., filmy
  t., fissured
  t., forked
  t., furred
  t., geographic
  t., magenta
  t., parrot
  t., raspberry
  t., scrotal
  t., smoker's
  t., smooth
  t., strawberry
  t., trifid
  t., trombone

tongue-swallowing

tongue-tie

tonic (tŏn'ĭk) [Gr. *tonikos*, from *tonos*, act of stretching, tension, tone]

tonicity (tō-nĭs'ĭ-tē) [Gr. *tonos*, act of stretching, tension, tone]

tonic labyrinthine reflex

tonic neck reflex

tonicoclonic (tŏn"ĭ-kō-klŏn'ĭk)

tonic spasm

tonoclonic (tŏn"ō-klŏn'ĭk) [" + *klonos*, tumult]

tonofibril (tŏn'ō-fī"brĭl)

tonofilament (tŏn"ō-fĭl'ă-mĕnt)

tonogram (tō'nō-grăm) [" + *gramma*, letter, piece of writing]

tonograph (tō'nō-grăf) [" + *graphein*, to write]

tonography (tō-nŏg'ră-fē)

tonometer (tōn-ŏm'ĕ-tĕr) [" + *metron*, measure]

tonometry (tŏn-ŏm'ĕ-trē)
  t., digital
  t., non-contact

tonoplast (tŏn'ō-plăst) [" + *plassein*, to form]

tonsil (tŏn'sĭl) [L. *tonsilla*, almond]
  t., cerebellar
  t., faucial
  t., lingual
  t., Luschka's
  t., nasal
  t., palatine
  t., pharyngeal
  t., tubal

tonsilla (tŏn-sĭl'ă) [L.]

tonsillar (tŏn'sĭ-lăr)

tonsillar area

tonsillar crypt

tonsillar fossa

tonsillar ring

tonsillar sinus

tonsillectomy (tŏn-sĭl-ĕk'tō-mē) [L. *tonsilla*, almond, + Gr. *ektome*, excision]

tonsillith (tŏn'sĭ-lĭth) [" + Gr. *lithos*, stone]

tonsillitis (tŏn-sĭl-ī'tĭs) [" + Gr. *itis*, inflammation]
  t., acute

  t., follicular
  t., parenchymatous, acute

tonsilloadenoidectomy (tŏn"sĭl-ō-ăd"ĕ-noy-dĕk'tō-mē)

tonsillolith (tŏn'sĭl-ō-lĭth) [" + Gr. *lithos*, stone]

tonsillopathy (tŏn"sĭ-lŏp'ă-thē)

tonsilloscopy (tŏn"sĭl-lŏs'kō-pē) [" + Gr. *skopein*, to examine]

tonsillotome (tŏn-sĭl'ō-tōm)

tonsillotomy (tŏn"sĭl-ŏt'ō-mē) [" + Gr. *tome*, a cutting, slice]

tonus (tō'nŭs) [L., tension]

tooth [AS. *toth*]
  t., accessional
  t., impacted

toothache

toothbrush

topagnosis (tŏp"ăg-nō'sĭs) [Gr. *topos*, place, + *a*, not, + *gnosis*, knowledge]

topalgia (tō-păl'jē-ă) [" + *algos*, pain]

topectomy (tō-pĕk'tō-mē) [" + *ektome*, excision]

topesthesia (tŏp"ĕs-thē'zē-ă) [" + *aisthesis*, feeling, perception]

tophaceous (tō-fā'shŭs) [L. *tophaceus*, sandy]

tophus (tō'fŭs) [L., porous stone]

tophyperidrosis (tŏf"ĭ-pĕr"ĭ-drō'sĭs) [Gr. *topos*, place, + *hyper*, over, above, excessive, + *hidros*, sweat]

topical [Gr. *topos*, place]

Topicort

Topicycline

topoalgia (tō"pō-ăl'jē-ă) [" + *algos*, pain]

topoanesthesia (tō"pō-ăn"ĕs-thē'zē-ă) [" + *an-*, not, + *aisthesis*, feeling, perception]

topognosia, topognosis (tō"pŏg-nō'sē-ă, -sĭs) [" + *gnosis*, knowledge]

topographic (tŏp"ō-grăf'ĭk) [" + *graphein*, to write]

topographic anatomy

topography (tō-pŏg′rȧ-fē)
topology (tō-pŏl′ō-jē)
toponarcosis (tō″pō-nȧr-kō′sĭs) [″ + narkosis, action of benumbing]
toponeurosis (tō″pō-nū-rō′sĭs) [″ + neuron, nerve, + osis, condition]
toponym (tŏp′ō-nĭm)
toponymy (tō-pŏn′ĭ-mē) [″ + onoma, name]
topophobia (tō″pō-fō′bē-ȧ) [″ + phobos, fear]
topothermesthesiometer (tŏp″ō-thĕr″mĕs-thē-zē-ŏm′ĕ-ter) [″ + therme, heat, + aisthesis, feeling, perception, + metron, measure]
TOPS Take Off Pounds Sensibly
Topsyn
TOPV trivalent oral polio vaccine
torcular Herophili (tor′kū-lȧr)
toric (tō′rĭk)
tormina (tor′mĭn-ȧ) [L., twistings]
torose, torous (tō′rōs, -rŭs) [L. torosus, full of muscle]
torpent (tor′pĕnt) [L. torpens, numbing]
torpid (tor′pĭd) [L. torpidus, numb]
torpidity (tor-pĭd′ĭ-tē)
torpor [L. torpor, numbness]
   t. intestinorum
   t. peristalticus
   t. retinae
torque (tork) [L. torquere, to twist]
torr (tor)
torrefaction (tor″ĕ-făk′shŭn) [L. torrefactio]
torrefy (tor′ĕ-fī) [L. torrefacere]
Torsade de pointes
torsiometer (tor″sē-ŏm′ĕ-tĕr)
torsion (tor′shŭn) [L. torsio, a twisting]
torsionometer (tor″shŭn-ŏm′ĕ-tĕr) [″ + Gr. metron, measure]
torsive (tor′sĭv)
torsiversion (tor″sĭ-vĕr′zhŭn)
torso (tor′sō) [It.]
torsoclusion (tor″sō-kloo′zhŭn) [″ + L. occlusio, to occlude]
torticollar (tor″tĭ-kŏl′ȧr)
torticollis (tor″tĭ-kŏl′ĭs) [L. tortus, twisted, + collum, neck]

   t., fixed
   t., intermittent
   t., ocular
   t., rheumatic
   t., spasmodic
   t., spurious
   t., symptomatic
tortipelvis (tor″tĭ-pĕl′vĭs) [″ + pelvis, basin]
tortuous (tor′choo-ŭs) [L. tortuosus, fr. torqueo, to twist]
torture (tor′chŭr) [LL. tortura, a twisting]
Torula (tor′ū-lȧ)
toruloid (tor′ū-loyd) [L. torulus, a little bulge, + Gr. eidos, form, shape]
toruloma (tor-ū-lō′mȧ) [Torula, old name for Cryptococcus, + oma, tumor]
Torulopsis glabrata
torulosis (tor-ū-lō′sĭs)
torulus (tor′ū-lŭs) [L. torulus, a little elevation]
   t. tactiles
torus (tō′rŭs) [L., swelling]
   t. mandibularis
   t. palatinus
Totacillin
total allergy syndrome
total hip replacement
total parenteral nutrition
totipotency (tō″tē-pō′tĕn-sē)
totipotent (tō-tĭp′ō-tĕnt) [L. totus, all, + potentia, power]
touch (tŭch) [O. Fr. tochier]
   t., abdominal
   t., after-
   t., double
   t., rectal
   t., vaginal
   t., vesical
tour de maître (toor″ dĕ mā-tr′) [Fr., the master's turn]
Tourette's syndrome, disorder
Tournay's sign (tūr-nāz′) [Auguste Tournay, Fr. ophthalmologist, 1878–1969]
tourniquet (toor′nĭ-kĕt) [Fr., a turning instrument]

t., rotating
tourniquet paralysis
tourniquet test
Touton cells (toot'ŏn) [Karl Touton, Ger. dermatologist, 1858–1934]
towelette (tow"ĕl-ĕt') [ME. *towelle*, towel]
toxanemia (tŏks"ă-nē'mē-ă) [Gr. *toxikon*, poison, + *an-*, not, + *haima*, blood]
toxemia (tŏks-ē'mē-ă) [" + Gr. *haima*, blood]
t., alimentary
t., eclamptogenic
t. of pregnancy
toxenzyme (tŏks-ĕn'zīm) [" + Gr. *en*, in, + *zyme*, leaven]
toxic (tŏks'ĭk) [Gr. *toxikon*, poison]
toxic-allergic syndrome
toxicant (tŏks'ĭ-kănt) [L. *toxicans*, poisoning]
toxicemic
toxic erythema
toxicide (tŏks'ĭ-sīd) [Gr. *toxikon*, poison, + L. *caedere*, to kill]
toxicity (tŏks-ĭs'ĭ-tē)
toxico- [Gr. *toxikon*, poison]
Toxicodendron (tŏk"sī-kō-dĕn'drŏn)
toxicoderma (tŏks"ĭ-kō-dĕr'mă) [" + *derma*, skin]
toxicodermatitis (tŏks"ĭ-kō-dĕrm-ă-tī'tĭs) [" + " + *itis*, inflammation]
toxicodermatosis (tŏks"ĭ-kō-dĕrm-ă-tō'sĭs) [" + " + *osis*, condition]
toxicogenic (tŏks"ĭ-kō-jĕn'ĭk) [" + *gennan*, to produce]
toxicoid (tŏks'ĭ-koyd) [" + *eidos*, form, shape]
toxicologist (tŏks"ĭ-kŏl'ō-jĭst) [" + *logos*, word, reason]
toxicology (tŏks"ĭ-kŏl'ō-jē)
toxicomania (tŏks"ĭ-kō-mā'nē-ă) [" + *mania*, madness]
toxicopathic (tŏks"ĭ-kō-păth'ĭk) [" + *pathos*, disease, suffering]
toxicopathy (tŏks"ĭ-kŏp'ă-thē) [" + *pathos*, disease, suffering]

toxicopexy (tŏk'sī-kō-pĕk"sē) [" + Gr. *pexis*, fixation]
toxicophidia (tŏk"sī-kō-fĭd'ē-ă) [" + Gr. *ophis*, snake]
toxicophobia (tŏks"ĭ-kō-fō'bē-ă) [" + *phobos*, fear]
toxicosis (tŏks"ĭ-kō'sĭs) [" + *osis*, condition]
t., endogenic
t., exogenic
t., retention
toxic shock syndrome
toxic substance
toxidermitis (tŏks"ĭ-dĕr-mī'tĭs) [" + *derma*, skin, + *itis*, inflammation]
toxiferous (tŏks-ĭf'ĕr-ŭs) [" + L. *ferre*, to carry]
toxigenic (tŏks"ĭ-jĕn'ĭk) [" + *gennan*, to produce]
toxigenicity (tŏks"ĭ-jĕn-ĭs'ĭ-tē)
toxignomic (tŏks"ĭg-nŏm'ĭk) [" + *gnomikos*, knowing]
toxin (tŏks'ĭn) [Gr. *toxikon*, poison]
t., bacterial
t., botulinus
t., dermonecrotic
t., Dick
t., diphtheria
t., dysentery
t., erythrogenic
t., extracellular
t., fatigue
t., intracellular
t., plant
toxin-antitoxin (tŏks'ĭn-ăn"tĭ-tŏks'ĭn) [Gr. *toxikon*, poison, + *anti*, against, + *toxikon*, poison]
toxinicide (tŏks-ĭn'ĭs-īd) [" + *caedere*, to kill]
toxinology (tŏk"sĭn-ŏl'ō-jē) [" + Gr. *logos*, word, reason]
toxinosis (tŏk"sī-nō'sĭs) [" + Gr. *osis*, condition]
toxipathic
toxipathy (tŏks-ĭp'ă-thē) [" + Gr. *pathos*, disease, suffering]
toxiphobia (tŏks"ĭ-fō'bē-ă) [" + Gr. *phobos*, fear]

toxisterol (tŏk-sĭs'tĕr-ŏl)

toxitabellae (tŏks"ĭ-tăb-ĕl'ē) [" + *tabella,* tablet]

toxitherapy (tŏks"ĭ-thĕr'ă-pē) [" + Gr. *therapeia,* treatment]

toxituberculid (tŏks"ĭ-tū-bĕr'kū-lĭd)

toxoalexin (tŏks"ō-ăl-ĕks'ĭn) [" + *alexein,* to ward off]

toxocariasis (tŏks"ō-kăr-ī'ă-sĭs) [" + *kara,* head, + *-iasis,* state or condition of]

toxogenin (tŏks-ŏj'ĕn-ĭn) [Gr. *toxikon,* poison, + *gennan,* to produce]

toxoid (tŏks'oyd) [" + *eidos,* form, shape]
 t., alum-precipitated
 t., diphtheria
 t., tetanus

toxolecithin (tŏks"ō-lĕs'ĭ-thĭn) [" + *lekithos,* egg yolk]

toxolysin (tŏks-ŏl'ĭ-sĭn) [" + *lysis,* dissolution]

toxomucin (tŏks"ō-mū'sĭn) [" + L. *mucus,* mucus]

toxonosis (tŏks"ō-nō'sĭs) [" + *osis,* condition]

toxopeptone (tŏks"ō-pĕp'tōn) [" + *pepton,* digesting]

toxophil(e) (tŏks'ō-fĭl, -fīl) [" + *philein,* to love]

toxophilic (tŏk"sō-fĭl'ĭk) [" + *philein,* to love]

toxophore (tŏks'ō-for) [" + *phoros,* a bearer]

toxophorous (tŏk-sŏf'ō-rŭs)

toxophylaxin (tŏks"ō-fī-lăks'ĭn) [" + *phylax,* guard]

Toxoplasma (tŏks"ō-plăs'mă)
 T. gondii

toxoplasmin (tŏk"sō-plăs'mĭn)

toxoplasmosis (tŏks-ō-ō-plăs-mō'sĭs)

T.P.I. test *Treponema pallidum* immobilizing test

TPN *total parenteral nutrition; triphosphopyridine nucleotide*

TPR *temperature, pulse, respiration*

tr. [L.] *tinctura,* tincture

trabecula (tră-bĕk'ū-lă) [L., a little beam]

trabeculae carneae cordis

trabecular (tră-bĕk'ū-lăr)

trabecularism (tră-bĕk'ū-lăr-ĭzm)

trabeculate (tră-bĕk'ū-lāt)

trabs (trăbz) [L., a beam]
 t. cerebri

trace (trās) [O. Fr. *tracier*]
 t., primitive

trace elements

tracer

trachea (trā'kē-ă) [Gr. *tracheia,* rough]

tracheaectasy (trā"kē-ă-ĕk'tă-sē) [Gr. *tracheia,* rough, + *ektasis,* dilatation]

tracheal (trā'kē-ăl)

trachealgia (trā"kē-ăl'jē-ă) [" + *algos,* pain]

trachealis (trā"kē-ā'lĭs) [L.]

tracheal tugging

tracheitis (trā"kē-ī'tĭs) [Gr. *tracheia,* rough, + *itis,* inflammation]

trachelagra (trā"kĕl-ăg'ră) [Gr. *trachelos,* neck, + *agra,* seizure]

trachelectomopexy (trā"kĕ-lĕk'tŏm-ō-pĕk"sē) [" + *ektome,* excision, + *pexis,* fixation]

trachelectomy (trā"kĕl-ĕk'tō-mē) [" + *ektome,* excision]

trachelematoma (trā"kĕl-ĕm"ă-tō'mă) [" + *haima,* blood, + *oma,* tumor]

trachelism, trachelismus (trā'kĕ-lĭzm, trā-kĕ-lĭz'mŭs) [" + *-ismos,* condition]

trachelitis (trā-kĕ-lī'tĭs) [" + *itis,* inflammation]

trachelo- [Gr. *trachelos,* neck]

trachelobregmatic (trā"kĕ-lō-brĕg-măt'ĭk) [" + *bregma,* front of the head]

trachelocele (trăk'ĕ-lō-sēl) [" + *kele,* tumor, swelling]

trachelocyrtosis (trā"kĕ-lō-sĭr-tō'sĭs) [" + *kyrtos,* curved, + *osis,* condition]

trachelocystitis (trā"kĕl-ō-sĭs-tī'tĭs) [" + *kystis,* bladder, + *itis,* inflammation]

trachelodynia (trā"kĕ-lō-dĭn'ē-ă)

[" + *odyne*, pain]

trachelokyphosis (trā″kĕl-ō-kī-fō′sĭs)
[" + *kyphosis*, humpback]

trachelology (trā″kĕ-lŏl′ō-jē) [" +
logos, word, reason]

trachelomastoid (trā″kĕ-lō-măs′toyd)
[" + *mastos*, breast, + *eidos*,
form, shape]

trachelomyitis (trā″kĕ-lō-mī-ī′tĭs)
[" + *mys*, muscle, + *itis*, in-
flammation]

trachelopexy (trā′kĕl-ō-pĕks″ē)
[" + *pexis*, fixation]

tracheloplasty (trā′kĕl-ō-plăs″tē)
[" + *plassein*, to form]

trachelorrhaphy (trā″kĕl-or′ă-fē)
[" + *rhaphe*, seam]

tracheloschisis (trā″kĕ-lŏs′kĭ-sĭs)
[" + *schisis*, cleavage]

trachelotomy (trā″kĕl-ŏt′ō-mē) [" +
tome, a cutting, slice]

tracheo- [Gr. *tracheia*, rough]

tracheoaerocele (trā″kē-ō-ĕr′ō-sēl)
[Gr. *tracheia*, rough, + *aer*, air,
+ *kele*, tumor, swelling]

tracheobronchial (trā″kē-ō-
brŏng′kē-ăl)

tracheobronchomegaly (trā″kē-ō-
brŏng″kō-mĕg′ă-lē)

tracheobronchoscopy (trā″kē-ō-
brŏng-kŏs′kō-pē) [" + *bronchos*,
windpipe, + *skopein*, to examine]

tracheocele (trā′kē-ō-sēl) [" +
kele, tumor, swelling]

tracheoesophageal (trā″kē-ō-ē-
sŏf″ă-jē′ăl) [" + *oisophagos*,
gullet]

tracheolaryngeal (trā″kē-ō-lăr-
rĭn′jē-ăl)

tracheolaryngotomy (trā″kē-ō-
lăr″ĭn-gŏt′ō-mē) [" + *larynx*, larynx, + *tome*, a cutting, slice]

tracheomalacia

tracheopathia,   **tracheopathy**
(trā″kē-ō-păth′ē-ă, -ŏp′ă-thē) [" +
pathos, disease, suffering]

tracheopharyngeal (trā″kē-ō-făr-
ĭn′jē-ăl) [" + *pharynx*, throat]

tracheophonesia (trā″kē-ō-fōn-ē′zē-

ă) [" + *phonesis*, a sounding]

tracheophony (trā″kē-ŏf′ō-nē) [" +
phone, a sound]

tracheoplasty (trā′kē-ō-plăs″tē)
[" + *plassein*, to form]

tracheopyosis (trā″kē-ō-pī-ō′sĭs) ["
+ *pyon*, pus, + *osis*, condition]

tracheorrhagia (trā″kē-ō-rā′jē-ă) [Gr.
tracheia, rough, + *rhegnynai*, to
burst forth]

tracheoschisis (trā″kē-ŏs′kĭs-ĭs) [" +
schisis, cleavage]

tracheoscopy (trā″kē-ŏs′kō-pē)
[" + *skopein*, to examine]

tracheostenosis (trā″kē-ō-stĕn-ō′sĭs)
[" + *stenosis*, act of narrowing]

tracheostoma (trā″kē-ŏs′tō-mă)

tracheostomize (trā″kē-ŏs′tō-mīz)

tracheostomy (trā″kē-ŏs′tō-mē)
[" + *stoma*, mouth, opening]

tracheostomy care

tracheotome (trā′kē-ō-tōm) [" +
tome, a cutting, slice]

tracheotomy (trā″kē-ŏt′ō-mē)

trachitis (trā-kī′tĭs) [" + *itis*, inflam-
mation]

trachoma (trā-kō′mă) [Gr., roughness]
t., brawny
t. deformans
t., diffuse

trachomatous (trā-kō′mă-tŭs)

trachychromatic (trā″kī-krō-măt′ĭk)
[Gr. *trachys*, rough, + *chroma*,
color]

trachyphonia (trā″kī-fō′nē-ă) [" +
phone, voice]

tracing (trā′sĭng)

tract (trăkt) [L. *tractus*, extent]
t., afferent
t., alimentary
t., ascending
t., biliary
t., descending
t., digestive
t., dorsolateral
t., extrapyramidal
t., gastrointestinal
t., genitourinary
t., iliotibial

t., intestinal
t., motor
t., olfactory
t., optic
t., pyramidal
t., respiratory
t., rubrospinal
t., supraopticohypophyseal
t., urinary
t., uveal
tractellum (trăk-tĕl'ŭm) [L.]
traction (trăk'shŭn) [L. tractio]
t., axis
t., elastic
t., head
t., weight
tractor (trăk'tor) [L., drawer]
tractotomy (trăk-tŏt'ō-mē)
tractus (trăk'tŭs) [L.]
tragacanth (trăg'ă-kănth) [Gr. traga-kantha, a goat thorn]
tragal (trā'găl) [Gr. tragos, goat]
tragi (trā'jī)
tragicus (trăj'ĭk-ŭs) [L.]
tragion (trăj'ē-ŏn)
tragomaschalia (trăg"ō-măs-kāl'ē-ă) [Gr. tragos, goat, + maschale, the armpit]
tragophonia, tragophony (trăg"ō-fō'nē-ă, -ŏf'ŏ-nē) [" + phone, voice]
tragopodia (trăg"ō-pō'dē-ă) [" + pous, foot]
tragus (trā'gŭs) [Gr. tragos, goat]
train (trān)
trainable (trān'ă-bl)
training
t., assertiveness
trait (trāt)
t., acquired
t., inherited
trajector (tră-jĕk'tor) [L. trajectus, thrown across]
Tral
tramazoline hydrochloride (tră-măz'ō-lēn)
trance (trăns) [L. transitus, a passing over]

t., death
t., induced
Trancopal
tranquilizer (trăn"kwī-lĭz'ĕr) [L. tran-quillus, calm]
transabdominal (trăns"ăb-dŏm'ĭ-năl)
transacetylation (trăns-ăs"ĕ-tĭl-ā'shŭn)
transactional analysis
transamidination (trăns-ăm"ĭ-dĭn-ā'shŭn)
transaminase (trăns-ăm'ĭn-ās)
t., glutamic-oxaloacetic
t., glutamic-pyruvic
transamination (trăns"ăm-ĭ-nā'shŭn)
transanimation (trăns"ăn-ĭ-mā'shŭn) [L. trans, across, + anima, breath]
transaortic (trăns"ā-or'tĭk)
transatrial (trăns-ā'trē-ăl)
transaudient (trăns-aw'dē-ĕnt) [" + audire, to hear]
transaxial (trăns-ăk'sē-ăl)
transcalent (trăns-kā'lĕnt) [" + ca-lere, to be hot]
transcapillary (trăns"kăp'ĭl-lă-rē) [" + capillaris, relating to hair]
transcapillary exchange
transcervical (trăns-sĕr'vĭ-kăl)
transcortical (trăns-kor'tĭ-kăl)
transcortin (trăns-kor'tĭn)
transcriptase (trăns-krĭp'tās)
transcription (trăn-skrĭp'shŭn)
transcutaneous electrical nerve stimulation
transdermal infusion system
transducer (trăns-dū'sĕr) [L. trans, across, + ducere, to lead]
t., ultrasonic
transduction (trăns-dŭk'shŭn)
transection (trăn-sĕk'shŭn) [" + sectio, cutting]
transfection (trăns-fĕk'shŭn)
transfer, transference (trăns'fer, trăns-fĕr'ĕns) [" + ferre, to bear]
transferase (trăns'fĕr-ās)
transfer board
transfer factor
transferrin (trăns-fĕr'rĭn)

transferring
transfix (trăns-fĭks′) [″ + *figere*, to fix]
transfixion (trăns-fĭk′shŭn)
transforation (trăns″for-ā′shŭn) [″ + *forare*, to pierce]
transforator (trăns′for-ā″tor)
transformation (trăns″for-mā′shŭn) [″ + *formatio*, a forming]
transformer (trăns-form′er) [″ + *formare*, to form]
　t., step-down
　t., step-up
transfusion (trăns-fū′zhŭn) [″ + *fusio*, a pouring]
　t., cadaver blood
　t., direct
　t., exchange
　t., indirect
　t., replacement
　t., single unit
transfusion reactions
transfusion syndrome, multiple
Transgrow
transient ischemic attack
transiliac (trăns-ĭl′ē-ăk) [L. *trans*, across, + *iliacus*, pert. to ilium]
transilient (trăns-sĭl′ē-ĕnt)
transillumination (trăns″ĭl-lū″mĭ-nā′shŭn) [″ + *illuminare*, to light up]
transinsular (trăns-ĭn′sū-lăr)
transischiac (trăns-ĭs′kē-ăk)
transisthmian (trăns-ĭs′mē-ăn)
transition (trăn-zĭ′shŭn) [L. *transitio*, a going across]
transitional (trăn-zĭsh′ŭn-ăl)
translation (trăns-lā′shŭn) [L. *trans*, across, + *latus*, borne]
translocation (trăns″lō-kā′shŭn) [″ + *locus*, place]
translucent (trăns-lū′sĕnt) [″ + *lucens*, shining]
transmethylase (trăns-mĕth′ĭ-lās)
transmethylation (trăns″mĕth-ĭ-lā′shŭn)
transmigration (trănz″mī-grā′shŭn) [″ + *migrare*, to move from place to place]

　t., external
　t., internal
transmissible (trăns-mĭs′ă-bl) [L. *transmissio*, a sending across]
transmission (trăns-mĭsh′ŭn)
　t., biological
　t., duplex
　t., mechanical
　t., neuromyal
　t., placental
　t., synaptic
　t., transovarial
transmural (trăns-mū′răl) [L. *trans*, across, + *murus*, a wall]
transmutation (trăns″mū-tā′shŭn) [L. *transmutatio*, a changing across]
transocular (trăns-ŏk′ū-lăr) [″ + *oculus*, eye]
transonance (trăns′ō-năns) [L. *trans*, across + *sonans*, sounding]
transorbital (trăns-or′bĭ-tăl) [″ + *orbita*, track]
transovarial passage (trăns-ō-vā′rē-ăl)
transparent (trăns-păr′ĕnt) [″ + *parere*, to be visible, appear, show]
transparietal (trăns″pă-rī′ĕ-tăl) [″ + *paries*, a wall]
transpeptidase (trăns-pĕp′tĭ-dās)
transperitoneal (trăns″pĕr-ĭ-tō-nē′ăl)
transphosphorylase (trăns-fŏs-for′ĭ-lās)
transphosphorylation (trăns-fŏs″for-ĭ-lā′shŭn)
transpirable (trăns-pī′ră-bl) [″ + *spirare*, to breathe]
transpiration (trăns″pī-rā′shŭn) [″ + *spirare*, to breathe]
　t., cutaneous
　t., pulmonary
transplacental (trăns″plă-sĕn′tăl)
transplant (trăns-plănt′; trăns′plănt) [″ + *plantare*, to plant]
transplantar (trăns-plăn′tăr) [″ + *planta*, sole of the foot]
transplantation (trăns″plăn-tā′shŭn)
　t., autoplastic
　t., heteroplastic

t., heterotopic
t., homoplastic
t., homotopic
t., tenoplastic
transpleural (trăns-ploor'răl)
transport
    t., active
transportation of the injured
transposition (trănz"pō-zǐ'shŭn) [L. trans, across, + positio, a placing]
transposition of great vessels
transposon (trănz-pō'zŏn)
transsection (trăns-sĕk'shŭn)
transsegmental (trăns"sĕg-mĕn'tăl) [" + segmentum, a cutting]
transseptal (trăns-sĕp'tăl) [" + saeptum, partition]
transsexual (trăns-sĕks'ū-ăl) [" + sexus, sex]
transsexualism (trăns-sĕks'ū-ă-lĭzm)
transsexual surgery
transsphenoidal (trăns"sfē-noy'dăl)
transtemporal (trăns-tĕm'pō-răl) [" + temporalis, pert. to a temple]
transthalamic (trăns"thăl-ăm'ĭk) [" + Gr. thalamos, chamber]
transthermia (trăns-thĕr'mē-ă) [" + Gr. therme, heat]
transthoracic (trăns"thō-răs'ĭk) [" + Gr. thorax, chest]
transthoracotomy (trăns"thō-ră-kŏt'ō-mē) [" + Gr. thorax, chest, + tome, a cutting, slice]
transtracheal
transtympanic neurectomy
transubstantiation (trăn"sŭb-stăn"shē-ā'shŭn) [" + substantia, substance]
transudate (trăns'ū-dāt) [" + sudare, to sweat]
transudation (trăns-ū-dā'shŭn)
transureteroureterostomy (trăns"ū-rē"tĕr-ō-ū-rē"tĕr-ŏs'tō-mē)
transurethral (trăns"ū-rē'thrăl) [" + Gr. ourethra, urethra]
transvaginal (trăns-văj'ĭn-ăl) [" + vagina, sheath]
transvector (trăns-vĕk'tor)

transversalis (trăns"vĕr-să'lĭs) [" + vertere, to turn]
transversalis fascia
transverse (trăns-vĕrs') [L. transversus]
transversectomy (trăns"vĕr-sĕk'tō-mē) [" + Gr. ektome, excision]
transverse foramen
transverse plane
transversion (trăns-vĕr'zhŭn)
transversocostal (trăns-vĕr"sō-kŏs'tăl)
transversospinalis (trăns-vĕr"sō-spī-nă'lĭs) [L. transversus, turned across, + spina, thorn]
transversourethralis (trăns-vĕr"sō-ū"rē-thrā'lĭs)
transversus (trăns-vĕr'sŭs) [L.]
transvesical (trăns-vĕs'ĭ-kăl)
transvestism, transvestitism (trăns-vĕst'ĭzm, -ĭ-tĭzm) [L. trans, across, + vestitus, clothed, + Gr. -ismos, condition]
transvestite (trăns-vĕs'fīt)
Trantas' dots (trăn'tăs) [Alexios Trantas, Gr. ophthalmologist, 1867–1960]
Tranxene
tranylcypromine (trăn"ĭl-sī'prō-mēn)
trapeze bar
trapezial (tră-pē'zē-ăl)
trapeziform (tră-pē'zĭ-form)
trapeziometacarpal (tră-pē"zē-ō-mĕt"ă-kăr'păl)
trapezium (tră-pē'zē-ŭm) [Gr. trapezion, a little table]
trapezius (tră-pē'zē-ŭs)
trapezoid (trăp'ĕ-zoyd) [Gr. trapezoeides, table-shaped]
trapezoid body
trapezoid bone
trapezoid ligament
trauma (traw'mă) [Gr. trauma, wound]
    t., birth
    t., occlusal
    t., psychic
    t., toothbrush
traumatic (traw-măt'ĭk) [Gr. traumatikos]

traumatic psychosis
traumatism (traw′mă-tĭzm) [Gr. *trau-matismos*]
traumatology (traw-mă-tŏl′ō-jē) [Gr. *trauma*, wound, + *logos*, word, reason]
traumatonesis (traw″mă-tō-nē′sĭs)
traumatopathy (traw″mă-tŏp′ă-thē) [″ + *pathos*, disease, suffering]
traumatophilia (traw″mă-tō-fĭl′ē-ă) [″ + *philein*, to love]
traumatopnea (traw″mă-tŏp-nē′ă) [″ + *pnoia*, breath]
traumatopyra (traw″mă-tō-pī′ră) [″ + *pyr*, fever]
traumatotherapy (traw″mă-tō-thĕr′ă-pē)
travail (tră-vāl′)
Travase
travelers' diarrhea
tray (trā)
　　t., impression
Treacher Collins syndrome [Edward Treacher Collins, Brit. ophthalmologist, 1862–1919]
treacle (trē′kl) [Gr. *theriaka*]
treatment (trēt′mĕnt) [ME. *treten*, to handle]
　　t., active
　　t., causal
　　t., conservative
　　t., dental
　　t., dietetic
　　t., electric shock
　　t., empiric
　　t., expectant
　　t., Kenny
　　t., palliative
　　t., preventive
　　t., rational
　　t., shock
　　t., specific
　　t., starvation
　　t., supportive
　　t., surgical
　　t., symptomatic
treatment plan
Trecator SC

tree
　　t., bronchial
　　t., tracheobronchial
trehala (trē-hā′lă)
trehalase (trē-hā′lās)
trehalose (trē-hā′lōs)
Trematoda (trĕm″ă-tō′dă) [Gr. *tremaŧodes*, pierced]
trematode (trĕm′ă-tōd)
trematodiasis (trĕm″ă-tō-dī′ă-sĭs)
tremble (trĕm′bl) [O. Fr. *trembler*]
trembles (trĕm′blz)
tremelloid, tremellose (trĕm′ē-loyd, -lōs)
tremetol (trĕm′ē-tŏl)
Tremin
tremogram (trĕm′ō-grăm) [L. *tremere*, to shake, + Gr. *gramma*, letter, piece of writing]
tremograph (trĕm′ō-grăf) [″ + Gr. *graphein*, to write]
tremolabile (trē″mō-lā′bl) [″ + *labi*, to slip]
tremophobia (trē″mō-fō′bē-ă) [″ + Gr. *phobos*, fear]
tremor (trĕm′or, trē′mor) [L. *tremor*, a shaking]
　　t., action
　　t., alcoholic
　　t., cerebellar
　　t., coarse
　　t., continuous
　　t., enhanced physiologic
　　t., essential
　　t., fibrillary
　　t., fine
　　t., flapping
　　t., forced
　　t., Hunt's
　　t., hysterical
　　t., intention
　　t., intermittent
　　t., muscular
　　t., parkinsonian
　　t., physiologic
　　t., rest
　　t., senile
　　t., static

t., volitional
tremorgram (trĕm'or-grăm)
tremulor (trĕm'ū-lor)
tremulous (trĕm'ū-lŭs) [L. *tremulus*]
trench fever
trench foot
trench mouth
trend [ME. *trenden*, to revolve]
Trendelenburg position (trĕn-dĕl'ĕn-bŭrg) [Friedrich Trendelenburg, Ger. surgeon, 1844 – 1925]
trepan (trē-păn') [Gr. *trypanon*, a borer]
trepanation (trĕp"ă-nā'shŭn) [L. *trepanatio*]
t., corneal
trephination (trĕf"ĭn-ā'shŭn) [Fr. *trephine*, a bore]
trephine (trē-fīn')
trephining
trephocyte (trĕf'ō-sīt) [Gr. *trephein*, to feed, + *kytos*, cell]
trepidant (trĕp'ĭ-dănt) [L. *trepidans*, trembling]
trepidatio (trĕp"ĭ-dā'shē-ō) [L.]
t. cordis
trepidation (trĕp"ĭ-dā'shŭn) [L. *trepidatio*, a trembling]
Treponema (trĕp"ō-nē'mă) [Gr. *trepein*, to turn, + *nema*, thread]
T. carateum
T. pallidum
T. pertenue
Treponemataceae (trĕp"ō-nē"mă-tā'sē-ē)
treponematosis (trĕp"ō-nē-mă-tō'sĭs)
treponeme (trĕp'ō-nēm)
treponemiasis (trĕp"ō-nē-mī'ă-sĭs) [" + *nema*, thread, + *-iasis*, state or condition of]
treponemicidal (trĕp"ō-nē"mĭ-sī'dăl) [" + " + L. *cida* fr. *caedere*, to kill]
trepopnea (trĕp-ŏp'nē-ă) [" + *pnoia*, breath]
tresis (trē'sĭs) [Gr. *tresis*, perforation]
tretinoin (trĕt'ĭ-noyn)
TRF *thyrotropin releasing factor*

TRH *thyrotropin releasing hormone*
tri- [Gr. *treis*, three]
triacetate (trī-ăs'ĕ-tāt)
triacetin (trī-ăs'ĕ-tĭn)
triacetyloleandomycin (trī-ăs"ĕ-tĭl-ō"lē-ăn"dō-mī'sĭn)
triacylglycerols
triad (trī'ăd) [Gr. *trias*, group of three]
t., Hutchinson's
triage (trē-ăzh') [Fr., sorting]
triakaidekaphobia (trī"ă-kī"dĕk-ă-fō'bē-ă) [Gr. *treis*, three, + *kai*, and, + *deka*, ten, + *phobos*, fear]
triamcinolone (trī"ăm-sĭn'ō-lōn)
triamterene (trī-ăm'tĕr-ēn)
triangle (trī'ăng-gl) [L. *triangulum*]
t., anal
t., anterior, of neck
t., carotid, inferior
t., carotid, superior
t., cephalic
t., digastric
t., facial
t., femoral
t., frontal
t., Hesselbach's
t., inferior occipital
t., inguinal
t., Lesser's
t., lumbocostoabdominal
t., muscular
t., mylohyoid
t., occipital, of the neck
t. of elbow
t. of necessity
t. of Petit
t., omoclavicular
t., omohyoid
t., posterior cervical
t., pubourethral
t., Scarpa's
t., subclavian
t., submandibular
t., suboccipital
t., supraclavicular
t., suprameatal
t., urogenital

t., vesical
triangular
triangular bandage
triangularis (trī-ăng″gū-lā′rĭs) [L.]
triangular ligament
triangular nucleus of Schwalbe
Triatoma (trī-ăt′ō-mă)
triatomic (trī″ă-tŏm′ĭk)
tribadism (trĭb′ăd-ĭzm) [Gr. *tribein*, to rub, + *-ismos*, condition]
tribasic (trī-bā′sĭk) [Gr. *treis*, three, + L. *basis*, base]
tribasilar (trī-băs′ĭl-ăr) [″ + L. *basilaris*, base]
tribasilar synostosis
tribe (trīb) [L. *tribus*, division of the Roman people]
tribology (trī-bŏl′ō-jē)
triboluminescence (trī″bō-lū″mĭ-nĕs′ĕns) [Gr. *tribein*, to rub, + L. *lumen*, light, + O. Fr. *escence*, continuing]
tribrachia (trī-brā′kē-ă)
tribrachius (trī-brā′kē-ŭs)
tribromide (trī-brō′mīd) [Gr. *treis*, three, + *bromos*, stench]
tribromoethanol (trī-brō″mō-ĕth′ă-nŏl)
TRIC agents trachoma and inclusion conjunctivitis
tricarboxylic acid cycle
tricellular (trī-sĕl′ū-lăr)
tricephalus (trī-sĕf′ă-lŭs) [Gr. *treis*, three, + *kephale*, head]
triceps (trī′sĕps) [″ + L. *caput*, head]
triceps reflex
Tricercomonas (trī″sĕr-cŏm-ō′năs)
trichangiectasia, trichangiectasis (trĭk″ăn-jē-ĕk-tā′zē-ă, -ĕk′tă-sĭs) [Gr. *thrix*, hair, + *angeion*, vessel, + *ektasis*, dilatation]
trichatrophia (trĭk″ă-trō′fē-ă) [″ + *atrophia*, atrophy]
trichauxe, trichauxis (trĭk-awk′sē, -sĭs) [″ + *auxe*, increase]
trichi-, tricho- [Gr. *thrix*]
trichiasis (trĭk-ī′ă-sĭs) [Gr. *thrix*, hair, + *-iasis*, state or condition of]
trichilemmoma (trĭk″ĭ-lĕm-ō′mă)
Trichina (trĭk-ī′nă) [Gr. *trichinos*, of hair]
trichina (trī-kī′nă)
Trichinella (trĭk″ĭ-nĕl′lă)
    T. spiralis
trichinelliasis (trĭk″ĭ-nĕl-lī′ă-sĭs)
trichinellosis (trĭk″ĭ-nĕl-lō′sĭs) [Gr. *trichinos*, of hair, + *osis*, condition]
trichiniasis (trĭk″ĭ-nī′ă-sĭs)
trichiniferous (trĭk″ĭ-nĭf′ĕr-ŭs) [″ + L. *ferre*, to bear]
trichinization (trĭk″ĭn-ĭ-zā′shŭn)
trichinophobia (trĭk″ĭn-ō-fō′bē-ă) [Gr. *trichinos*, of hair, + *phobos*, fear]
trichinosis (trĭk″ĭn-ō′sĭs) [″ + *osis*, condition]
trichinous (trĭk′ĭn-ŭs) [Gr. *trichinos*, of hair]
trichinous myositis
trichion (trĭk′ē-ŏn) [Gr.]
trichitis (trĭk-ī′tĭs) [Gr. *thrix*, hair, + *itis*, inflammation]
trichloride (trī-klō′rīd)
trichlormethiazide (trī-klor″mĕ-thī′ă-zīd)
trichloroacetic acid
trichloroethylene (trī″klor-ō-ĕth′ĭl-ēn)
2,4,5-trichlorophenoxyacetic acid
tricho- [Gr. *thrix, trichos*, hair]
trichoanesthesia (trĭk″ō-ăn″ĕs-thē′zē-ă)
trichobacteria (trĭk″ō-băk-tē′rē-ă) [″ + *bakterion*, rod]
trichobezoar (trĭk″ō-bē′zor) [″ + Arabic *bazahr*, protecting against poison]
trichocardia (trĭk-ō-kăr′dē-ă) [″ + *kardia*, heart]
trichoclasia, trichoclasis (trĭk″ō-klā′zē-ă, -ŏk′lăs-ĭs) [″ + *klasis*, a breaking]
trichocryptosis (trĭk″ō-krĭp-tō′sĭs) [″ + *kryptos*, concealed]
trichocyst (trĭk′ō-sĭst) [″ + *kystis*, bladder]
Trichodectes (trĭk″ō-dĕk′tēz) [″ + *dektes*, biter]

trichoepithelioma (trĭk″ō-ĕp″ĭ-thē-lē-ō″mă) [″ + epi, upon, + thele, nipple, + oma, tumor]

trichoesthesia (trĭk″ō-ĕs-thē′zē-ă) [″ + aisthesis, feeling, perception]

trichoesthesiometer (trĭk″ō-ĕs-thē″zē-ŏm′ĕ-ter) [″ + ″ + metron, measure]

trichogen (trĭk′ō-jĕn) [″ + gennan, to produce]

trichogenous (trĭk-ŏj′ĕn-ŭs)

trichoglossia (trĭk″ō-glŏs′ē-ă) [″ + glossa, tongue]

trichohyalin (trĭk″ō-hī′ă-lĭn) [″ + hyalos, glass]

trichoid (trĭk′oyd) [″ + eidos, form, shape]

trichokryptomania (trĭk″ō-krĭp″tō-mā′nē-a) [″ + kryptos, hidden, + mania, madness]

tricholith (trĭk′ō-lĭth) [″ + lithos, stone]

trichologia (trĭk″ō-lō′jē-ă) [″ + legein, to pick out]

trichology (trĭk-ŏl′ō-jē) [″ + logos, word, reason]

trichoma (trĭk-ō′mă) [Gr., hairiness]

trichomadesis (trĭk″ō-mă-dē′sĭs)

trichomatosis (trĭk″ō-mă-tō′sĭs) [″ + osis, condition]

trichomatous (trī-kŏm′ă-tŭs)

trichome (trī′kōm) [Gr. trichoma, a growth of hair]

trichomegaly (trĭk″ō-mĕg′ă-lē) [Gr. trichos, hair, + megas, large]

trichomonacide (trĭk″ō-mō′nă-sīd)

trichomonad (trĭk″ō-mō′năd)

Trichomonas (trĭk″ō′mō′năs) [″ + monas, unit]

   T. hominis
   T. tenax
   T. vaginalis

trichomoniasis (trĭk″ō-mō-nī′ă-sĭs) [″ + ″ + -iasis, state or condition of]

trichomycosis (trĭk″ō-mī-kō′sĭs) [″ + mykes, fungus, + osis, condition]
   t. axillaris

   t. nodosa

trichonodosis (trĭk″ō-nō-dō′sĭs)

trichonosis, trichonosus (trĭk-ō-nō′sĭs, -ŏn′ō-sŭs) [Gr. trichos, hair, + nosos, disease]

trichopathic (trĭk″ō-păth′ĭk)

trichopathophobia (trĭk″ō-păth″ō-fō′bē-ă) [″ + pathos, disease, suffering, + phobos, fear]

trichopathy (trĭk-ŏp′ă-thē) [″ + pathos, disease, suffering]

trichophagia, trichophagy (trĭk-ō-fā′jē-ă, -ŏf′ă-jē) [″ + phagein, to eat]

trichophobia (trĭk″ō-fō′bē-ă) [″ + phobos, fear]

trichophytic (trĭk″ō-fĭt′ĭk) [″ + phyton, plant]

trichophytic granulosa (trĭk″ō-fĭt′ĭk)

trichophytid (trī-kŏf′ĭ-tĭd)

trichophytin (trī-kŏf′ĭ-tĭn)

trichophytobezoar (trĭk-ō-fī″tō-bē′zor) [″ + phyton, plant, + Arabic bazahr, protecting against poison]

Trichophyton (trī-kŏf′ĭt-ŏn)

   T. mentagrophytes
   T. schoenleinii
   T. tonsurans
   T. violaceum

trichophytosis (trĭk″ō-fī-tō′sĭs) [″ + phyton, plant, + osis, condition]

trichoptilosis (trĭk″ŏp-tĭl-ō′sĭs) [″ + ptilon, feather, + osis, condition]

trichorrhea (trĭk-or-ē′ă) [″ + rhein, to flow]

trichorrhexis (trĭk″ō-rĕks′ĭs) [″ + rhexis, a breaking]
   t. nodosa

trichorrhexomania (trĭk″ō-rĕks″ō-mā′nē-ă) [″ + ″ + mania, madness]

trichoschisis (trī-kŏs′kĭs-ĭs) [″ + schisis, cleavage]

trichoscopy (trĭk-ŏs′kō-pē) [″ + skopein, to examine]

trichosiderin (trĭk″ō-sĭd′ĕr-ĭn) [″ + sideros, iron]

trichosis (trī-kō'sĭs) [" + osis, condition]

t. decolor

t. setosa

Trichosporon (trī-kŏs'pō-rŏn) [" + sporos, seed]

T. beigelii

trichosporosis (trĭk"ō-spō-rō'sĭs) [" + " + osis, condition]

trichostasis spinulosa (trī-kŏs'tă-sĭs spīn"ū-lō'să) [" + stasis, standing still]

trichostrongyliasis (trĭk"ō-strŏn-jī-lī'ă-sĭs)

trichostrongylosis (trĭk"ō-strŏn"jī-lō'sĭs)

Trichostrongylus (trĭk"ō-strŏn'jī-lŭs)

Trichothecium (trĭk"ō-thē'sē-ŭm) [" + theke, a box]

T. roseum

trichotillomania (trĭk"ō-tĭl"ō-mā'nē-ă) [" + tillein, to pull, + mania, madness]

trichotomous (trī-kŏt'ō-mŭs) [Gr. tricha, threefold, + tome, a cutting, slice]

trichotomy (trī-kŏt'ō-mē)

trichotoxin (trĭk"ō-tŏks'ĭn) [Gr. trichos, hair, + toxikon, poison]

trichotrophy (trī-kŏt'rō-fē) [" + trophe, nourishment]

trichroic (trī-krō'ĭk) [Gr. treis, three, + chroa, color]

trichroism (trī'krō-ĭzm) [" + " + -ismos, condition]

trichromatic (trī"krō-măt'ĭk) [" + chroma, color]

trichromatism (trī-krō'mă-tĭzm)

trichromatopsia (trī"krō-mă-tŏp'sē-ă)

trichromic (trī-krō'mĭk)

trichterbrust (trĭch'tĕr-broost) [Ger.]

trichuriasis (trĭk"ū-rī'ă-sĭs) [Gr. trichos, hair, + oura, tail + -iasis, state or condition of]

Trichuris (trī-kū'rĭs)

T. trichiura

tricipital (trī-sĭp'ĭ-tăl) [Gr. treis, three, + L. caput, head]

tricitrates oral solution

triclofos sodium (trī'klō-fōs)

tricornic (trī-kor'nĭk) [" + L. cornu, horn]

tricornute (trī-kor'nūt) [" + L. cornutus, horned]

tricrotic (trī-krŏt'ĭk) [Gr. trikrotos, rowed with a triple stroke]

tricrotism (trī'krŏt-ĭzm) [" + -ismos, condition]

tricuspid (trī-kŭs'pĭd) [Gr. treis, three, + L. cuspis, point]

tricuspid area

tricuspid atresia

tricuspid murmur

tricuspid orifice

tricuspid tooth

tricuspid valve

trident, tridentate (trī'dĕnt, trī-dĕn'tāt) [L. tres, tria, three, + dens, tooth]

tridermic (trī-dĕr'mĭk) [Gr. treis, three, + derma, skin]

tridermoma (trī"dĕr-mō'mă) [" + " + oma, tumor]

Tridesilon

tridihexethyl chloride (trī"dī-hĕks-ĕth'ĭl)

Tridione

tridymite (trĭd'ĭ-mīt)

trielcon (trī-ĕl'kŏn) [" + helkein, to draw]

triencephalus (trī"ĕn-sĕf'ă-lŭs) [" + enkephalos, brain]

triethanolamine (trī"ĕth-ă-nōl'ă-mēn)

triethylenemelamine (trī-ĕth"ĭ-lĕn-mĕl'ă-mēn)

triethylenethiophosphoramide (trī-ĕth"ĭ-lĕn-thī"ō-fŏs-for'ă-mĭd)

trifacial (trī-fā'shăl) [L. trifacialis]

trifacial neuralgia

trifid (trī-fĭd) [L. trifidus, split thrice]

trifluoperazine hydrochloride (trī"floo-ō-pār'ă-zēn)

triflupromazine (trī"floo-prō'mă-zēn)

trifurcation (trī"fŭr-kā'shŭn) [Gr. treis, three, + L. furca, fork]

trigastric (trī-găs'trĭk) [Gr. treis, three,

+ *gaster*, belly]

trigeminal (trī-jĕm'ĭn-ăl) [L. *tres, tria,* three, + *geminus,* twin]

trigeminal cough

trigeminal nerve

trigeminal neuralgia

trigeminal pulse

trigeminus (trī-jĕm'ĭ-nŭs)

trigeminy (trī-jĕm'ĭ-nē)

trigenic (trī-jĕn'ĭk) [Gr. *treis,* three, + *gennan,* to produce]

trigger (trĭg'ĕr) [D. *trekker,* something pulled]

trigger action

trigger finger

trigger point or zone

trigger substance

trigger zone

triglycerides (trī-glĭs'ĕr-īds)

trigonal (trĭg'ō-năl) [Gr. *trigonon,* a three-cornered figure]

trigone (trī'gōn)
    t., carotid
    t. of bladder
    t., olfactory
    t., vesical

trigonectomy (trĭg"gōn-ĕk'tō-mē) [" + *ektome,* excision]

trigonid (trī-gō'nĭd)

trigonitis (trĭg"ō-nī'tĭs) [" + *itis,* inflammation]

trigonocephalic (trĭ"gō-nō-sĕ-făl'ĭk) [" + *kephale,* head]

trigonocephalus (trĭg"ō-nō-sĕf'ă-lŭs)

trigonocephaly (trī-gō"nō-sĕf'ă-lē)

trigonum (trī-gō'nŭm) [L.]
    t. lumbale

trihexyphenidyl hydrochloride (trī-hĕk"sē-fĕn'ĭ-dĭl)

trihybrid (trī-hī'brĭd) [Gr. *treis,* three, + L. *hybrida,* mongrel]

tri-iniodymus (trī"ĭn-ē-ŏd'ĭ-mŭs) [" + *inion,* nape of the neck, + *didymos,* twin]

triiodothyronine (trī"ī-ō"dō-thī'rō-nēn)

trikates

trilabe (trī'lāb) [Gr. *treis,* three, + *labe,* a handle]

Trilafon

trilaminar (trī-lăm'ĭ-năr)

trilateral (trī-lăt'ĕr-ăl) [" + L. *latus,* side]

trill (trĭl) [It. *trillare,* probably imitative]

trilobate (trī-lō'bāt) [" + *lobos,* lobe]

trilocular (trī-lŏk'ū-lăr) [" + L. *loculus,* cell]

trilogy (trĭl'ō-jē)

trimanual (trī-măn'ū-ăl) [" + *manualis,* by hand]

trimensual (trī-mĕn'shū-ăl) [" + *mensualis,* monthly]

trimeprazine tartrate (trī-mĕp'ră-zēn)

trimester (trī-mĕs'tĕr)
    t., first
    t., second
    t., third

trimethadione (trī"mĕth-ă-dī'ōn)

trimethaphan camsylate (trī-mĕth'ă-făn)

trimethidinium methosulfate (trī-mĕth"ĭ-dĭn'ē-ŭm)

trimethobenzamide hydrochloride (trī-mĕth"ō-bĕn'ză-mīd)

trimethoprim (trī-mĕth'ō-prīm)

trimethylene (trī-mĕth'ĭ-lēn)

trimmer
    t., gingival margin
    t., model

trimorphous (trī-mor'fŭs) [" + *morphe,* form]

Trimox

Trimpex

Trinitroglycerol (trī-nī"trō-glĭs'ĕr-ŏl)

trinitrophenol (trī"nī-trō-fē'nŏl)

trinitrotoluene (trī"nī-trō-tŏl'ū-ēn)

triocephalus (trī"ō-sĕf'ă-lŭs) [" + *kephale,* head]

triolein

triolism (trī'ō-lĭzm)

triophthalmos (trī"ŏf-thăl'mōs) [" + *ophthalmos,* eye]

triopodymus (trī"ō-pŏd'ĭ-mŭs) [" + *ops,* face, + *didymos,* twin]

triorchid, triorchis (trī-or'kĭd, -kĭs) [" + *orchis,* testicle]

triorchidism (trī-or'kĭd-īzm) [" + " + -ismos, condition]
triose (trī'ōs)
triotus (trī-ō'tŭs) [" + ous, ear]
trioxsalen (trī-ŏk'să-lĕn)
trip (trĭp)
tripara (trĭp'ă-ră) [L. tres, tria, three, + parere, to beget, produce]
tripelennamine citrate (trī"pĕ-lĕn'ă-mīn)
tripeptide (trī-pĕp'tĭd) [Gr. treis, three, + pepton, digested]
triphalangia (trī"fă-lăn'jē-ă) [" + phalanx, line of battle]
triphasic (trī-fā'sĭk) [" + phasis, appearance]
triphenylmethane (trī-fĕn"ĭl-mĕth'ān)
Tripier's amputation (trĭp-ē-āz') [Léon Tripier, Fr. surgeon, 1842–1891]
triple (trĭp'l) [L. triplus, threefold]
triplegia (trī-plē'jē-ă) [" + plege, stroke]
triple response
triplet (trĭp'lĕt) [L. triplus, threefold]
triplex (trī'plĕks, trĭp'lĕks) [Gr. triploos, triple]
triploblastic (trĭp"lō-blăst'ĭk) [" + blastos, germ]
triploid (trĭp'loyd)
triploidy (trĭp'loy-dē)
triplokoria (trĭp"lō-kor'ē-ă) [" + kore, pupil]
triplopia (trĭp-lō'pē-ă) [" + ope, vision]
tripod (trī'pŏd) [Gr. treis, three, + pous, foot]
　　t., Haller's
　　t., vital
tripodia (trī-pō'dē-ă)
tripoding (trī'pŏd-ĭng)
triprolidine hydrochloride (trī-prō'lĭ-dēn)
triprosopus (trī"prō-sō'pŭs) [" + prosopon, face]
tripsis (trĭp'sĭs) [Gr. tripsis, a rubbing, friction]
-tripsy (trĭp'sē) [Gr. tripsis, a rubbing, friction]

triquetral (trī-kwē'trăl) [L. triquetrus]
triquetral bone
triquetrous (trī-kwē'trŭs) [L. triquetrus, triangular]
triquetrum (trī-kwē'trŭm) [L.]
triradial, triradiate (trī-rā'dē-ăl, -āt) [Gr. treis, three, + L. radiatus, furnished with rays]
triradius (trī-rā'dē-ŭs)
trisaccharide (trī-săk'ă-rīd)
triskaidekaphobia (trī-skī-dĕk-ă-fō'bē-ă) [Gr. triskaideka, thirteen, + phobos, fear]
trismic (trĭz'mĭk)
trismoid (trĭz'moyd) [Gr. trismos, grating, + eidos, form, shape]
trismus (trĭz'mŭs) [Gr. trismos, grating]
　　t. nascentium
trisomic (trī-sōm'ĭk)
trisomy (trī'sō-mē)
　　t. 13
　　t. 18
　　t. 21
trisplanchnic (trī-splănk'nĭk) [Gr. treis, three, + splanchna, viscera]
tristichia (trī-stĭk'ē-ă) [" + stichos, row]
tristimania (trĭs"tĭ-mā'nē-ă) [L. tristis, sad, + Gr. mania, madness]
trisulcate (trī-sŭl'kāt) [L. tres, tria, three, + sulcus, groove]
trisulfapyrimidines oral suspension (trī-sŭl"fă-pī-rĭm'ĭ-dēnz)
trisulfate (trī-sŭl'fāt)
trisulfide (trī-sŭl'fĭd)
tritanomalopia (trī"tă-nŏm'ă-lō-pē-ă) [Gr. tritos, third, + anomalos, irregular, + ope, sight]
tritanomaly (trī"tă-nŏm'ă-lē)
tritanopia (trī"tă-nō'pē-ă) [Gr. tritos, third, + an-, not, + ope, vision]
Triten
tritiate (trĭt'ē-āt)
triticeous (trĭt-ĭsh'ŭs) [L. triticeus, of wheat]
　　t. cartilage
tritium (trĭt'ē-ŭm, trĭsh'ē-ŭm) [Gr. tritos, third]

triturable (trĭt′ū-ră-bl) [L. *triturare*, to pulverize]

triturate (trĭt′ū-rāt)

trituration (trĭt-ū-rā′shŭn) [LL. *triturare*, to pulverize]

trivalence (trĭv′ă-lĕns)

trivalent (trī-vā′lĕnt, trĭv′ăl-ĕnt) [Gr. *treis*, three, + L. *valens*, powerful]

trivalve (trī′vălv)

trivial name

trizonal (trī-zō′năl)

tRNA *transfer RNA*

Trobicin

trocar (trō′kăr) [Fr. *trois quarts*, three quarters]

troch

trochanter (trō-kăn′tĕr) [Gr. *trokhanter*, to run]
t., greater
t., lesser
t. major
t. minor
t. tertius
t., third

trochanterian,   trochanteric (trō″kăn-tē′rē-ăn, trō-kăn-tĕr′ĭk)

trochanterplasty (trō-kăn′tĕr-plăs″tē)

trochantin (trō-kăn′tĭn)

trochantinian (trō″kăn-tĭn′ē-ăn)

troche (trō′kē, trōk′) [Gr. *trokhiskos*, a small wheel]

trochiscus (trō-kĭs′kŭs) [L., Gr. *trochiskos*, a small disk]

trochlea (trŏk′lē-ă) [Gr. *trokhileia*, system of pulleys]

trochlea of the elbow

trochlear (trŏk′lē-ăr)

trochlear fovea

trochleariform (trŏk″lē-ăr′ĭ-form)

trochlearis (trŏk″lē-ā′rĭs) [L.]

trochlear nerve

trochocardia (trō″kō-kăr′dē-ă) [Gr. *trokhos*, a wheel, + *kardia*, heart]

trochocephalia,   trochocephaly (trō″kō-sē-fā′lē-ă, -sĕf′ă-lē) [″ + *kephale*, head]

trochoid (trō′koyd) [Gr. *trokhos*, a wheel, + *eidos*, form, shape]

trochoides (trō-koy′dēz)

Troglotrematidae (trŏg″lō-trē-măt′ĭ-dē)

Troisier's node (trwă-zē-āz′) [Charles E. Troisier, Fr. physician, 1844–1919]

trolamine (trō′lă-mēn)

troland (trō′lănd)

troleandomycin (trō″lē-ăn-dō-mī′sĭn)

trolnitrate phosphate (trŏl-nī′trāt)

Trombicula (trŏm-bĭk′ū-lă)
T. akamushi

trombiculiasis (trŏm-bĭk″ū-lī′ă-sĭs)

Trombiculidae (trŏm-bĭk′ū-lĭ″dē)

tromethamine (trō-mĕth′ă-mēn)

tromomania (trŏm″ō-mā′nē-ă) [Gr. *tromos*, a trembling, + *mania*, madness]

Tronothane Hydrochloride

troph-, tropho- [Gr. *trophe*]

trophectoderm (trŏf-ĕk′tō-dĕrm) [Gr. *trophe*, nourishment, + *ectoderm*]

trophedema (trŏf″ĕ-dē′mă) [Gr. *trophe*, nourishment, + *oidema*, a swelling]

trophic (trŏf′ĭk) [Gr. *trophikos*]

trophism (trŏf′ĭzm)

trophoblast (trŏf′ō-blăst) [Gr. *trophe*, nourishment, + *blastos*, germ]

trophoblastic (trŏf″ō-blăs′tĭk)

trophoblastoma (trŏf″ō-blăs-tō′mă) [″ + ″ + *oma*, tumor]

trophocyte (trŏf′ō-sīt)

trophoderm (trŏf′ō-dĕrm) [Gr. *trophe*, nourishment, + *derma*, skin]

trophodynamics (trŏf″ō-dī-năm′ĭks)

trophology (trō-fŏl′ō-jē) [″ + *logos*, word, reason]

trophoneurosis (trŏf″ō-nū-rō′sĭs) [″ + *neuron*, nerve, + *osis*, condition]
t., disseminated
t., facial
t., muscular

trophoneurotic (trŏf″ō-nū-rŏt′ĭk)

trophonosis (trŏf″ō-nō′sĭs) [″ + *nosos*, disease]

trophonucleus (trŏf″ō-nū′klē-ŭs) [″ + *nucleus*, kernel]

trophopathia (trŏf″ō-păth′ē-ă) [″ +
pathos, disease, suffering]
trophopathy (trŏf-ŏp′ă-thē)
trophotaxis (trŏf″ō-tăks′ĭs) [″ +
taxis, arrangement]
trophotherapy (trŏf″ō-thĕr′ă-pē)
trophotonus (trŏf-ŏt′ŏn-ŭs) [″ +
tonos, act of stretching, tension, tone]
trophotropism (trŏf-ŏt′rō-pĭzm) [″ +
tropos, a turning, + *-ismos*, condi-
tion]
trophozoite (trŏf″ō-zō′ĭt) [″ +
zoon, animal]
tropia (trō′pē-ă) [Gr. *trope*, turn]
tropical (trŏp′ĭ-kal) [Gr. *tropikos*, turn-
ing]
tropical immersion foot
tropical lichen
tropicamide (trō-pĭk′ă-mĭd)
-tropin [Gr. *tropos*, a turn]
tropine (trō′pĭn)
tropism (trō′pĭzm) [Gr. *trope*, turn, +
-ismos, condition]
tropocollagen (trō″pō-kŏl′ă-jĕn)
[″ + *collagen*]
tropometer (trŏp-ŏm′ĕ-ter) [″ +
metron, measure]
tropomyosin (trō″pō-mī′ō-sĭn)
troponin (trō′pō-nĭn)
trough (trŏf)
  t., gingival
  t., synaptic
Trousseau's sign (troo-sōz′) [Armand
Trousseau, Fr. physician, 1801 – 1867]
Trousseau's spots
Trousseau's symptom
troxidone (trŏk′sĭ-dōn)
troy weight
true (troo) [AS. *treowe*, faithful]
**true conjugate diameter of pelvic
inlet**
true pelvis
true ribs
truncal (trŭng′kăl) [L. *truncus*, trunk]
truncate (trŭng′kāt) [L. *truncare*, to
cut off]
truncus (trŭng′kŭs)
  t. arteriosus

  t. brachiocephalicus
  t. celiacus
  t. pulmonalis
trunk (trŭnk) [L. *truncus*, trunk]
  t., celiac
  t., lumbosacral
  t., sympathetic
trusion (troo′zhŭn) [L. *trudere*, to show]
truss (trŭs) [ME. *trusse*, a bundle]
truth serum
try-in
trypanocide, trypanocidal (trĭp-
ăn′ō-sīd, trĭp″ăn-ō-sī′dăl) [Gr. *trypanon*, a borer, + L. *cida* fr. *caedere*, to kill]
trypanolysis (trĭp-ăn-ŏl′ĭ-sĭs) [″ +
lysis, dissolution]
Trypanoplasma (trĭ″păn-ō-plăz′mă)
[″ + LL. *plasma*, form, mold]
Trypanosoma (trĭ″păn-ō-sō′mă)
[″ + *soma*, a body]
  T. brucei
  T. cruzi
  T. gambiense
  T. rhodesiense
trypanosomal (trĭ-păn-ō-sō′măl)
trypanosome (trĭ′păn-ō-sōm)
trypanosomiasis (trĭ-păn″ō-sō-mī′ă-
sĭs) [″ + *soma*, body, + *-iasis*,
state or condition of]
  t., African
  t., American
trypanosomic (trĭ-păn″ō-sō′mĭk)
trypanosomicide
trypanosomid (trĭ-păn′ō-sō-mĭd)
tryparsamide (trĭp-ărs′ă-mĭd, -mĭd)
trypsin (trĭp′sĭn) [Gr. *tryein*, to wear out]
  t., crystallized
trypsinized (trĭp′sĭ-nīzd)
trypsinogen (trĭp-sĭn′ō-jĕn) [″ +
gennan, to produce]
tryptic (trĭp′tĭk)
tryptolysis (trĭp-tĭk′ĭ-sĭs) [Gr. *tripsis*, a
rubbing, friction, + *lysis*, dissolu-
tion]
tryptone (trĭp′tōn)
tryptophan (trĭp′tō-făn)
tryptophanase (trĭp′tō-făn-ās)

tryptophanuria (trĭp"tō-fă-nū'rē-ă)
[*tryptophan* + Gr. *ouron*, urine]
T/S *thyroid:serum*
T.S. *test solution; triple strength*
TSD *target skin distance*
tsetse fly (tsĕt'sē) [S. African]
TSH *thyroid-stimulating hormone*
TSH-RF *thyroid-stimulating hormone re-leasing factor*
tsp *teaspoon*
TSTA *tumor-specific transplantation an-tigen*
tsutsugamushi disease (soot"soo-gă-moosh'ĭ) [Japanese, dangerous bug]
TT *transit time*
T-tube
T.U. *toxic unit; toxin unit*
tuaminoheptane sulfate (too-ăm"ĭ-nō-hĕp'tăn)
tub (tŭb) [ME. *tubbe*]
tuba (too'bă) [L. *tubus*, tube]
tubal (tū'băl) [L. *tubus*, tube]
tubal nephritis
tubal pregnancy
tubatorsion (tū"bă-tor'shŭn) [" + *torsio*, a twisting]
tubba, tubboe (tŭb'ă, -ō)
tube (tūb) [L. *tubus*, a tube]
    t., auditory
    t., Cantor
    t., cathode ray
    t., Coolidge
    t., Crookes'
    t., drainage
    t., endobronchial
    t., endotracheal
    t., esophageal
    t., eustachian
    t., fallopian
    t., fermentation
    t., hot-cathode
    t., hot cathode roentgen-ray
    t., intestinal decompression
    t., intubation
    t., Levin
    t., Miller-Abbott
    t., nasogastric

    t., neural
    t., otopharyngeal
    t., Sengstaken-Blakemore
    t., Southey's
    t., stomach
    t., test
    t., thoracostomy
    t., tracheotomy
    t., uterine
    t., ventilation
    t., Wangensteen
tubectomy (too-bĕk'tō-mē)
tube feeding
tuber (tū'bĕr) [L., a swelling]
    t. cinereum
tubercle (tū'bĕr-kl) [L. *tuberculum*, a little swelling]
    t., adductor
    t., articular
    t., condyloid
    t., dental
    t., deltoid
    t., fibrous
    t., genial
    t., genital
    t., lacrimal
    t., laminated
    t., Lisfranc's
    t., mental
    t., miliary
    t. of the upper lip
    t., pharyngeal
    t., pubic
    t., supraglenoid
    t., zygomatic
tubercula (tū-bĕr'kū-lă)
tubercular (tū-bĕr'kū-lăr) [L. *tuberculum*, a little swelling]
tuberculate, tuberculated (tū-bĕr'kū-lāt, -lāt"ĕd) [L. *tuberculum*, a small swelling]
tuberculation (tū-bĕr"kū-lā'shŭn)
tuberculid(e) (tū-bĕr'kū-lĭd, -lĭd) [L. *tuberculum*, a little swelling]
    t., follicular
    t., papulonecrotic
tuberculigenous (tū-bĕr-kū-lĭj'ĕn-ŭs) [" + Gr. *gennan*, to produce]

tuberculin (tū-bĕr'kū-lĭn) [L. *tuberculum*, a little swelling]
t., new
t., old
t., purified protein derivative
tuberculin test
tuberculin tine test
tuberculitis (tū″bĕr-kū-lī'tĭs)
tuberculocele (tū-bĕr'kū-lō-sēl″) [″ + *kele*, tumor, swelling]
tuberculocidal (tū-bĕr″kū-lō-sī'dăl)
tuberculoderma (tū-bĕr″kū-lō-dĕr'mă) [″ + Gr. *derma*, skin]
tuberculofibroid (tū-bĕr″kū-lō-fī'broyd) [″ + *fibra*, fiber, + Gr. *eidos*, form, shape]
tuberculofibrosis (tū-bĕr″kū-lō-fī-brō'sĭs) [″ + ″ + Gr. *osis*, condition]
tuberculoid (tū-bĕr'kū-loyd) [L. *tuberculum*, a little swelling, + Gr. *eidos*, form, shape]
tuberculoma (tū-bĕr″kū-lō'mă) [″ + Gr. *oma*, tumor]
tuberculophobia (tū-bĕr″kū-lō-fō'bē-ă) [″ + Gr. *phobos*, fear]
tuberculoprotein (tū-bĕr″kū-lō-prō'tē-ĭn)
tuberculosilicosis (tū-bĕr″kū-lō-sĭl″ĭ-kō'sĭs)
tuberculosis (tū-bĕr″kū-lō'sĭs) [″ + Gr. *osis*, condition]
t., avian
t., bovine
t., endogenous
t., exogenous
t., hematogenous
t., open
t. verrucosa
tuberculosis chemotherapy, short course
tuberculostatic (tū-bĕr″kū-lō-stăt'ĭk)
tuberculotic (tū-bĕr″kū-lŏt'ĭk)
tuberculous (tū-bĕr'kū-lŭs) [L. *tuberculum*, a little swelling]
tuberculum (tū-bĕr'kū-lŭm) [L. *tuberculum*, a little swelling]
t. acusticum

t. majus humeri
t. minus humeri
tuberin (tū'bĕr-ĭn) [L. *tuber*, a swelling]
tuberosis (tū″bĕr-ō'sĭs)
tuberositas (tū-bĕr-ŏs'ĭt-ăs) [L.]
tuberosity (tū-bĕr-ŏs'ĭ-tē) [L. *tuberositas*, tuberosity]
t., ischial
t., maxillary
tuberous (tū'bĕr-ŭs)
tuberous sclerosis
tubo- [L. *tubus*]
tuboabdominal (tū″bō-ăb-dŏm'ĭn-ăl) [L. *tubus*, tube, + *abdominalis*, pert. to the abdomen]
tuboabdominal pregnancy
tubocurarine chloride (tū″bō-kū-ră'rĭn klō'rīd)
tuboligamentous (tū″bō-lĭg-ă-mĕn'tŭs) [″ + *ligamentum*, a band]
tubo-ovarian (tū″bō-ō-vā'rē-ăn) [″ + NL. *ovarium*, ovary]
tubo-ovariotomy (tū″bō-ō-vā-rē-ŏt'ō-mē [″ + NL. *ovarium*, ovary, + Gr. *tome*, a cutting, slice]
tubo-ovaritis (tū″bō-ō″vă-rī'tĭs) [″ + ″ + Gr. *itis*, inflammation]
tuboperitoneal (tū″bō-pĕr-ĭ-tō-nē'ăl) [″ + Gr. *peritonaion*, stretched around or over]
tuboplasty (tū'bō-plăs″tē)
tuborrhea (tū-bor-rē'ă) [″ + Gr. *rhein*, to flow]
tubotorsion (tū″bō-tor'shŭn)
tubotympanal (tū″bō-tĭm'pă-năl) [″ + Gr. *tympanon*, a drum]
tubouterine (tū″bō-ū'tĕr-ĭn) [″ + *uterinus*, pert. to the uterus]
tubovaginal (tū″bō-văj'ĭ-năl)
tubular (tū'bū-lăr) [L. *tubularis*, like a tube]
tubule (tū'būl) [L. *tubulus*, a tubule]
t., collecting
t.'s, convoluted, of kidney
t.'s, convoluted seminiferous
t.'s, dentinal
t.'s, excretory
t.'s, galactophorous

t., Henle's
t., junctional
t.'s, lactiferous
t.'s, mesonephric
t.'s, metanephritic
t.'s, renal
t.'s, seminiferous
t.'s, uriniferous
tubulin (tū′bū-lĭn)
tubulization (too″bū-lĭ-zā′shŭn)
tubuloalveolar
tubulocyst (too′bū-lō-sĭst)
tubulodermoid (tū″bū-lō-dĕr′moyd) [″ + Gr. derma, skin, + eidos, form, shape]
tubuloracemose (too″bū-lō-răs′ĕ-mōs)
tubulorrhexis (too″bū-lō-rĕk′sĭs) [″ + rhexis, a breaking]
tubulous (too′bū-lŭs)
tubulus (tū′bū-lŭs) [L.]
tubus (too′bŭs) [L.]
    t. digestorius
tuft
    t., enamel
    t., malpighian
tugging
    t., tracheal
tularemia (tū-lăr-ē′mē-ă) [Tulare, part of California where disease was first discovered]
tumbu fly
tumefacient (tū-mē-fā′shĕnt) [L. tumefaciens, producing swelling]
tumefaction (tū″mē-făk′shŭn) [L. tumefactio, a swelling]
tumentia (tū-mĕn′shē-ă) [L.]
    t., vasomotor
tumescence (tū-mĕs′ĕns)
tumid (tū′mĭd) [L. tumidus]
tumor (tū′mor) [L. tumor, a swelling]
    t., carotid body
    t., connective tissue
    t., desmoid
    t., erectile
    t., Ewing's
    t., false
    t., fibroid

t., giant cell, of bone
t., giant cell, of tendon sheath
t., granulosa, granulosa cell
t., granulosa-theca cell
t., heterologous
t., homoiotypic, homologous
t., Hürthle cell
t., islet cell
t., Krukenberg's
t., lipoid cell, of the ovary
t., mast cell
t., melanotic neuroectodermal
t., mesenchymal mixed
t. of pregnancy
t., phantom
t., sand
t., turban
t., Wilms'
tumoraffin (tū′mor-ăf-ĭn) [L. tumor, a swelling, + affinis, related]
tumor angiogenesis factor
tumoricidal (too″mor-ĭ-sī′dăl)
tumorigenesis (too″mor-ĭ-jĕn′ĕ-sĭs)
tumorigenic (tū″mor-ĭ-jĕn′ĭk) [″ + Gr. genesis, generation, birth]
tumor markers, serum
tumor necrosis factor
tumorous (too′mor-ŭs)
tumor viruses
tumultus (tū-mŭl′tŭs) [L.]
    t. cordis
    t. sermonis
Tunga (tŭng′ă)
    T. penetrans
tungiasis (tŭng-gī′ă-sĭs)
tungsten (tŭng′stĕn)
tunic (tū′nĭk) [L. tunica, a sheath]
    t., Bichat's
tunica (tū′nĭ-kă) [L. tunica, a sheath]
    t. adventitia
    t. albuginea
    t. conjunctiva
    t. dartos
    t. externa
    t. interna
    t. intima
    t. media
    t. mucosa

t. muscularis
t. propria
t. serosa
t. vaginalis
t. vasculosa
tunicin (too'nĭ-sĭn)
tuning fork
tunnel (tŭn'ĕl)
t., carpal
t., flexor
t., inner
t., tarsal
tunnel vision
turbid (tŭr'bĭd) [L. turba, a tumult]
turbidimeter (tŭr-bĭ-dĭm'ĕ-ter) [L. turbidus, disturbed, + Gr. metron, measure]
turbidimetry (tŭr-bĭ-dĭm'ĕ-trē) [" + Gr. metron, measure]
turbidity (tŭr-bĭd'ĭ-tē) [L. turbiditas, turbidity]
turbinal, tubinate (tŭr'bĭ-nǎl, -nāt) [L. turbinalis, fr. turbo, a child's top]
turbinated (tŭr'bĭ-nā"tĕd) [L. turbo, whirl]
turbinectomy (tŭr-bĭn-ĕk'tō-mē) [" + Gr. ektome, excision]
turbinotome (tŭr-bĭn'ō-tōm) [" + Gr. tome, a cutting, slice]
turbinotomy (tŭr-bĭn-ŏt'ō-mē) [" + Gr. tome, a cutting, slice]
turgescence (tŭr-jĕs'ĕns) [L. turgescens, swelling]
turgescent (tŭr-jĕs'ĕnt) [L. turgescens, swelling]
turgid (tŭr'jĭd) [L. turgidus, swollen]
turgometer (tŭr-gŏm'ĕ-tĕr) [L. turgor, swelling, + Gr. metron, measure]
turgor [L., a swelling]
t., skin
t. vitalis
Turing test [Alan M. Turing, Brit. mathematician]
turista (tū-rēs'tǎ) [Sp.]
Turner's syndrome [H. H. Turner, U.S. physician, 1892–1970]
turning [AS. turnian, to turn]
turpentine (tŭr'pĕn-tĭn) [Gr. terebinthos, turpentine tree]
turpentine poisoning
turricephaly (tŭr"ĭ-sĕf'ǎ-lē)
turunda (tū-rŭn'dǎ) [L.]
tussal (tŭs'ǎl) [L. tussis, cough]
tussicular (tŭ-sĭk'ū-lǎr) [L. tussis, cough]
tussiculation (tŭ-sĭk"ū-lā'shŭn)
tussis (tŭs'ĭs) [L.]
t. convulsiva
t. stomachalis
tussive (tŭs'ĭv) [L. tussis, cough]
tussive syncope
tutamen (tū-tā'mĕn) [L.]
tutamina oculi
tutin (too'tĭn)
T.V.R. tonic vibration reflex
T wave
twelfth cranial nerve
twig
twilight sleep
twilight state
twin (twĭn) [AS. twinn]
t.'s, biovular
t.'s, conjoined
t.'s, dizygotic
t.'s, enzygotic
t.'s, fraternal
t.'s, identical
t.'s, impacted
t.'s, interlocked
t.'s, monozygotic
t., parasitic
t.'s, Siamese
t.'s, true
t.'s, unequal
t.'s, uniovular
twinge (twĭnj) [AS. twengan, to pinch]
twinning (twĭn'ĭng)
twitch (twĭch) [ME. twicchen]
twitching (twĭtch'ĭng)
two-point discrimination test
tybamate (tī'bǎ-māt)
tylectomy (tī-lĕk'tō-mē) [Gr. tylos, knot, + ektome, excision]
tylion (tĭl'ē-ŏn) [Gr. tyleion, knot]
tyloma (tī-lō'mǎ) [Gr. tylos, knot, + oma, tumor]
tylosis (tī-lō'sĭs) [" + osis, condition]

tyloxapol (tī-lŏks′ă-pōl)

tympanal (tĭm′păn-ăl) [Gr. *tympanon,* drum]

tympanectomy (tĭm″păn-ĕk′tō-mē) [″ + *ektome,* excision]

tympania (tĭm-păn′ē-ă)

tympanic (tĭm-păn′ĭk) [Gr. *tympanon,* drum]

tympanicity (tĭm″pă-nĭs′ĭ-tē)

tympanic membrane

tympanism (tĭm′păn-ĭzm) [Gr. *tympanon,* drum, + *-ismos,* condition]

tympanites (tĭm-păn-ī′tēz) [Gr., distention]

tympanitic (tĭm-păn-ĭt′ĭk)

tympanitic resonance

tympanitis (tĭm-păn-ī′tĭs) [Gr. *tympanon,* drum, + *itis,* inflammation]

tympano- [Gr. *tympanon,* drum]

tympanoeustachian (tĭm″pă-nō-ū-stā′kē-ăn)

tympanography

tympanohyal (tĭm″pă-nō-hī′ăl)

tympanomalleal (tĭm″pă-nō-măl′ē-ăl)

tympanomandibular (tĭm″pă-nō-măn-dĭb′ū-lăr)

tympanomastoiditis (tĭm″păn-ō-măs″toy-dī′tĭs) [″ + *mastos,* breast, + *eidos,* form, shape, + *itis,* inflammation]

tympanometry (tĭm″pă-nŏm′ĕ-trē)

tympanoplasty (tĭm″păn-ō-plăs′tē) [″ + *plassein,* to form]

tympanosclerosis (tĭm″pă-nō-sklĕ-rō′sĭs)

tympanosis (tĭm-pă-nō′sĭs) [″ + *osis,* condition]

tympanosquamosal (tĭm″pă-nō-skwă-mō′săl)

tympanostapedial (tĭm″pă-nō-stă-pē′dē-ăl)

tympanostomy tubes

tympanotemporal (tĭm″pă-nō-tĕm′pō-răl)

tympanotomy (tĭm″păn-ŏt′ō-mē) [″ + *tome,* a cutting, slice]

tympanous (tĭm′păn-ŭs) [Gr. *tympanon,* a drum]

tympanum (tĭm′păn-ŭm) [L., Gr. *tympanon*]

tympany (tĭm′pă-nē)

type (tīp) [Gr. *typos,* mark]
  t., asthenic
  t., athletic
  t., blood
  t., phage
  t., pyknic

typhlectasis (tĭf-lĕk′tă-sĭs) [Gr. *typhlon,* cecum, + *ektasis,* dilatation]

typhlectomy (tĭf-lĕk′tō-mē) [″ + *ektome,* excision]

typhlenteritis (tĭf″lĕn-tĕr-ī′tĭs) [″ + *enteron,* intestine, + *itis,* inflammation]

typhlitis (tĭf-lī′tĭs) [″ + *itis,* inflammation]

typhlodicliditis (tĭf″lō-dĭk-lĭ-dī′tĭs) [″ + *diklis,* door, + *itis,* inflammation]

typhloempyema (tĭf″lō-ĕm-pī-ē′mă) [″ + *en,* in, + *pyon,* pus, + *haima,* blood]

typhloenteritis (tĭf″lō-ĕn-tĕr-ī′tĭs) [″ + *enteron,* intestine, + *itis,* inflammation]

typhlolexia (tĭf″lō-lĕk′sē-ă) [Gr. *typhlos,* blind, + *lexis,* speech]

typhlolithiasis (tĭf″lō-lĭ-thī′ă-sĭs) [Gr. *typhlon,* cecum, + *lithos,* stone, + *-iasis,* state or condition of]

typhlology (tĭf-lŏl′ō-jē) [Gr. *typhlos,* blind, + *logos,* word, reason]

typhlomegaly (tĭf″lō-mĕg′ă-lē) [Gr. *typhlon,* cecum, + *megas,* large]

typhlon (tĭf′lŏn) [Gr.]

typhlopexy (tĭf′lō-pĕks″ē) [Gr. *typhlon,* cecum, + *pexis,* fixation]

typhlorrhaphy (tĭf-lor′ă-fē)

typhlosis (tĭf-lō′sĭs) [Gr. *typhlos,* blind, + *osis,* condition]

typhlospasm (tĭf′lō-spăsm)

typhlostenosis (tĭf″lō-stĕn-ō′sĭs) [Gr. *typhlon,* cecum, + *stenosis,* act of narrowing]

typhlostomy (tĭf-lŏs′tō-mē) [″ + *stoma,* mouth, opening]

typhlotomy (tǐf-lǒt′ō-mē) [Gr. *typhlon*, cecum, + *tome*, a cutting, slice]

typhloureterostomy (tǐf″lō-ū-rē″tĕr-ŏs′tō-mē) [″ + *oureter*, ureter, + *stoma*, mouth, opening]

typho- [Gr. *typhos*, fever]

typhohemia (tǐ″fō-hē′mē-ă) [″ + *haima*, blood]

typhoid (tǐ′foyd) [Gr. *typhos*, fever, + *eidos*, form, shape]

typhoidal (tǐ-foy′dăl)

typhoid carrier

typhoid fever

typhoid vaccine

typholysin (tǐ-fŏl′ǐ-sǐn) [″ + *lysis*, dissolution]

typhomalarial (tǐ″fō-mă-lā′rē-ăl) [″ + It. *malaria*, bad air]

typhomania (tǐ-fō-mā′nē-ă) [″ + *mania*, madness]

typhopneumonia (tǐ″fō-nū-mō′nē-ă) [″ + *pneumon*, lung, + *-ia*, condition, abnormal state]

typhous (tǐ′fŭs) [Gr. *typhos*, fever]

typhus (tǐ′fŭs) [Gr. *typhos*, fever]
  t., classic
  t., endemic
  t., epidemic
  t., flea-borne
  t., Mexican
  t., mite-borne
  t., murine
  t., recrudescent
  t., rural
  t., scrub
  t., shop
  t., urban

typhus vaccine

typical (tǐp′ǐ-kăl) [Gr. *typikos*, pert. to type]

typing (tǐp′ǐng)
  t., bacteriophage
  t., blood
  t., tissue

typo- [Gr. *typos*]

typoscope (tǐ′pō-skōp) [″ + *skopein*, to examine]

typus (tǐ′pŭs) [L.]

tyramine (tǐ′ră-mēn)

tyrannism (tǐr′ăn-ǐzm) [Gr. *tyrannos*, tyrant, + *-ismos*, condition]

tyrogenous (tǐ-rŏj′ĕn-ŭs) [Gr. *tyros*, cheese, + *gennan*, to produce]

Tyroglyphus (tǐ-rŏg′lǐ-fŭs) [Gr. *tyros*, cheese, + *glyphein*, to carve]

tyroid (tǐ′royd) [″ + *eidos*, form, shape]

tyroma (tǐ-rō′mă)

tyromatosis (tǐ″rō-mă-tō′sǐs) [″ + *oma*, tumor, + *osis*, condition]

tyrosinase (tǐ-rō′sǐn-ās) [Gr. *tyros*, cheese]

tyrosine (tǐ′rō-sǐn)

tyrosinemia (tǐ″rō-sǐ-nē′mē-ă)

tyrosinosis (tǐ″rō-sǐn-ō′sǐs) [″ + *osis*, condition]

tyrosinuria (tǐ″rō-sǐn-ū′rē-ă) [″ + *ouron*, urine]

tyrosis (tǐ-rō′sǐs) [″ + *osis*, condition]

tyrosyluria (tǐ″rō-sǐl-ū′rē-ă)

tyrothricin (tǐ″rō-thrǐ′sǐn)

tyrotoxism (tǐ″rō-tŏks′ǐzm) [″ + *toxikon*, poison, + *-ismos*, condition]

Tyrrell's fascia (tǐr′rĕlz) [Frederick Tyrrell, Brit. anatomist, 1797–1843]

Tyson's glands (tǐ′sŭnz) [Edward Tyson, Brit. physician and anatomist, 1649–1708]

tysonitis (tǐ″sŏn-ī′tǐs)

tyvelose (tǐ′vĕl-ōs)

Tyzine

Tzanck test (tsănk) [Arnault Tzanck, Russ. dermatologist in Paris, 1886–1954]

tzetze (sĕt′sē)

U

U *unit; uranium*
235U
UAO *upper airway obstruction*
uberous (ū'bĕr-ŭs) [L. *uber,* udder]
uberty (ū'bĕr-tē) [L. *uber,* udder]
ubiquinol (ū-bǐk'wǐ-nŏl)
ubiquinone (ū-bǐk'wǐ-nōn) [*ubiq*uitous + coenzyme *quinone*]
udder (ŭd'ĕr)
UDP *uridine diphosphate*
Uffelmann's test (oof'ĕl-mănz) [Jules Uffelmann, Ger. physician, 1837–1894]
U-Gencin
Uhthoff's sign (oot'hŏfs) [Wilhelm Uhthoff, Ger. ophthalmologist, 1853–1927]
ulaganactesis (ū-lăg"ă-năk'tĕ-sĭs) [Gr. *oulon,* gum, + *aganektesis,* irritation]
ulalgia (ū-lăl'jē-ă) [" + *algos,* pain]
ulatrophia (ū-lă-trō'fē-ă) [" + *atrophos,* ill-nourished]
ulcer (ŭl'sĕr) [L. *ulcus,* ulcer]
  u., amputating
  u., atonic
  u., callous
  u., chronic leg
  u., Curling's
  u., decubitus
  u., duodenal
  u., follicular
  u., fungus
  u., gastric
  u., Hunner's
  u., indolent
  u., peptic
  u., perforating
  u., phagedenic
  u., rodent
  u., serpiginous

  u., simple
  u., specific
  u., stasis
  u., stercoral
  u., stress
  u., trophic
  u., tropical
  u., varicose
  u., venereal
ulcera
ulcerate (ŭl'sĕr-āt) [L. *ulcerare,* to form ulcers]
ulcerated (ŭl'sĕr-ā"tĕd)
ulcerated tooth
ulceration (ŭl"sĕr-ā'shŭn)
ulcerative (ŭl'sĕr-ā-tǐv) [L. *ulcerare,* to form ulcers]
ulcerogangrenous (ŭl"sĕr-ō-găng'grĕ-nŭs)
ulcerogenic drugs
ulceromembranous (ŭl"sĕr-ō-mĕm'brăn-ŭs) [" + *membrana,* membrane]
ulceromembranous tonsillitis
ulcerous (ŭl'sĕr-ŭs)
ulcus (ŭl'kŭs) [L.]
  u. cancrosum
  u. induratum
  u. vulvae acutum
ulectomy (ū-lĕk'tō-mē) [Gr. *oule,* scar, + *ektome,* excision; *oulon,* gum, + *ektome,* excision]
ulegyria (ū"lĕ-jī'rē-ă) [Gr. *oule,* scar, + *gyros,* ring]
ulemorrhagia (ū"lĕm-ō-rā'jē-ă) [Gr. *oulon,* gum, + *rhegnynai,* to burst forth]
ulerythema (ū-lĕr-ĭ-thē'mă) [Gr. *oule,* scar, + *erythema,* redness]
  u. ophryogenes
  u. sycosiforme

uletic (ū-lĕt'ĭk) [Gr. *oulon, gum*]
uletomy (ū-lĕt'ō-mē) [Gr. *oule*, scar, + *tome*, a cutting, slice]
uliginous (ū-lĭj'ĭ-nŭs) [L. *uliginosus*, wet]
ulitis (ū-lī'tĭs) [Gr. *oulon*, gum, + *itis*, inflammation]
    u., interstitial
ulna (ŭl'nă) [L., elbow]
ulnad (ŭl'năd) [" + *ad*, to]
ulnar (ŭl'năr) [L. *ulna*, elbow]
ulnar drift
ulnaris (ŭl-nā'rĭs)
ulnocarpal (ŭl"nō-kăr'păl) [" + Gr. *karpos*, wrist]
ulnoradial (ŭl"nō-rā'dē-ăl) [" + *radius*, spoke of a wheel]
Ulo
ulocace (ū-lŏk'ă-sē) [Gr. *oulon*, gum, + *kake*, badness]
ulocarcinoma (ū"lō-kăr-sĭn-ō'mă) [" + *karkinos*, crab, + *oma*, tumor]
ulodermatitis (ū"lō-dĕrm-ă-tī'tĭs) [Gr. *oule*, scar, + *derma*, skin, + *itis*, inflammation]
uloglossitis (ū"lō-glŏs-ī'tĭs) [Gr. *oulon*, gum, + *glossa*, tongue, + *itis*, inflammation]
uloid (ū'loyd) [Gr. *oule*, scar, + *eidos*, form, shape]
uloncus (ū-lŏn'kŭs) [Gr. *oulon*, gum, + *onkos*, bulk, mass]
ulorrhagia (ū-lor-ā'jē-ă) [" + *rhegnynai*, to burst forth]
ulorrhea (ū"lor-rē'ă) [" + *rhein*, to flow]
ulosis (ū-lō'sĭs) [Gr. *oule*, scar, + *osis*, condition]
ulotic (ū-lŏt'ĭk) [Gr. *oule*, scar]
ulotomy (ū-lŏt'ō-mē) [" + *tome*, a cutting, slice; Gr. *oulon*, gum, + *tome*, a cutting, slice]
ulotrichous (ū-lŏt'rĭk-ŭs) [Gr. *oulos*, woolly, + *thrix*, hair]
ulotripsis (ū"lō-trĭp'sĭs) [Gr. *oulon*, gum, + *tripsis*, a rubbing, friction]
ultimate (ŭl'tĭm-ĭt) [L. *ultimus*, last]
ultimobranchial bodies (ŭl"tĭ-mō-brăng'kē-ăl)

ultrabrachycephalic (ŭl"tră-brăk"ĭ-sē-făl'ĭk) [L. *ultra*, beyond, + Gr. *brachys*, short, + *kephale*, head]
ultracentrifugation (ŭl"tră-sĕn-trĭf"ū-gā'shŭn)
ultracentrifuge (ŭl-tră-sĕn'trĭ-fūj) [" + *centrum*, center, + *fugere*, to flee]
ultradian (ŭl-trā'dē-ăn) [" + *dies*, day]
ultrafilter (ŭl-tră-fĭl'tĕr)
ultrafiltration (ŭl"tră-fĭl-trā'shŭn) [" + *filtrum*, a filter]
ultraligation (ŭl"tră-lĭ-gā'shŭn) [" + *ligare*, to bind]
ultramicrobe (ŭl"tră-mī'krōb) [" + Gr. *mikros*, small, + *bios*, life]
ultramicroscope (ŭl"tră-mī'krō-skōp) [" + " + *skopein*, to examine]
ultramicroscopy (ŭl"tră-mī-krŏs'kō-pē)
ultramicrotome (ŭl"tră-mī'krō-tōm)
ultrasonic (ŭl-tră-sŏn'ĭk) [" + *sonus*, sound]
ultrasonic cleaning
ultrasonics (ŭl-tră-sŏn'ĭks)
ultrasonogram (ŭl"tră-sŏn'ō-grăm)
ultrasonography (ŭl-tră-sŏn-ŏg'ră-fē)
ultrasound
    u., A-mode
ultrastructure (ŭl'tră-strŭk"chŭr)
ultraviolet (ŭl"tră-vī'ō-lĕt) [" + *viola*, violet]
ultraviolet rays
ultraviolet therapy
ululation (ŭl"ū-lā'shŭn) [L. *ululare*, to howl]
umbilical (ŭm-bĭl'ĭ-kăl) [L. *umbilicus*, navel]
umbilical artery catheter
umbilical cord
umbilical fissure
umbilical hernia
umbilical souffle
umbilical vesicle
umbilicate (ŭm-bĭl'ĭ-kāt) [L. *umbilicatus*, dimpled]
umbilication (ŭm-bĭl-ĭ-kā'shŭn) [L. *umbi-*

licatus, dimpled]

umbilicus (ŭm-bĭ-lī′kŭs, -bĭl′ĭ-kŭs) [L., a pit]

umbo (ŭm′bō) [L., boss of a shield]
 u. of tympanic membrane

umbra (ŭm′brŭ) [L., shade, shadow]

umbrella filter

UMP *uridine monophosphate*

un- [AS. *un-,* against]

uncal (ŭng′kăl)

uncal herniation

unciform (ŭn′sĭ-form) [L. *uncus,* hook, + *forma,* shape]

unciform bone

unciforme (ŭn″sĭ-for′mē) [L.]

unciform fasciculus

unciform process

uncinariasis (ŭn″sĭn-ă-rī′ă-sĭs)

uncinate (ŭn′sĭn-āt) [L. *uncinatus,* hooked]

uncinate bundle of Russell [J. S. R. Russell, Brit. physician, 1863–1939]

uncinate convolution

uncinate epilepsy

uncinate fasciculus

uncinate fits

uncinate gyrus

uncinatum (ŭn″sĭ-nā′tŭm) [L.]

uncipressure (ŭn′sĭ-prĕsh″ŭr) [L. *uncus,* hook, + *pressura,* pressure]

uncomplemented (ŭn-kŏm′plĕ-mĕnt″ĕd)

unconditioned reflex

unconscious (ŭn-kŏn′shŭs) [AS. *un,* not, + L. *conscius,* aware]
 u., collective

unconsciousness (ŭn-kŏn′shŭs-nĕs) [AS. *un,* not, + L. *conscius,* aware]

unco-ossified (ŭn″kō-ŏs′ĭ-fĭd)

uncovertebral (ŭn″kō-ver′tĕ-brăl)

unction (ŭnk′shŭn) [L. *unctio,* ointment]

unctuous (ŭnk′chū-ŭs) [L. *unctus,* an ointment]

uncus (ŭn′kŭs) [L. *uncus,* hook]

undecylenic acid

underachiever

undercut (ŭn′dĕr-kŭt)

undernutrition (ŭn″dĕr-nū-trĭsh′ŭn)

[AS. *under, beneath,* + LL. *nutritio,* nourish]

undertoe (ŭn′dĕr-tō) [″ + *ta,* toe]

underweight (ŭn′dĕr-wāt″)

undifferentiation (ŭn-dĭf″ĕr-ĕn-shē-ā′shŭn) [AS. *un,* not, + L. *differens,* bearing apart]

undine (ŭn′dĭn) [L. *unda,* wave]

undinism (ŭn′dĭn-ĭzm)

undulant (ŭn′dū-lănt) [L. *undulatio,* wavy]

undulant fever (ŭn′dū-lănt)

undulate (ŭn′dū-lāt) [L. *undulatio,* wavy]

undulation (ŭn-dū-lā′shŭn)
 u., jugular
 u., respiratory

unemployment

ung. [L.] *unguentum,* ointment

ungual (ŭng′gwăl) [L. *unguis,* nail]

ungual phalanx

ungual tuberosity

unguent (ŭng′gwĕnt) [L. *unguentum,* ointment]

unguentum (ŭn-gwĕn′tŭm) [L., ointment]

unguiculate (ŭng-gwĭk′ū-lāt)

unguinal

unguis (ŭng′gwĭs) [L., nail]
 u. incarnatus

ungula (ŭn′gū-lă) [L., claw]

uni- [L. *unus*]

uniarticular (ū″nē-ăr-tĭk′ū-lăr) [L. *unus,* one, + *articulus,* joint]

uniaxial (ū″nē-ăk′sē-ăl) [″ + *axis,* axis]

unibasal (ū″nē-bā′săl) [″ + *basis,* base]

unicameral (ū″nĭ-kăm′ĕr-ăl) [″ + Gr. *kamara,* vault]

unicellular (ū″nĭ-sĕl′ū-lăr) [″ + *cellula,* a little box]

unicentral (ū″nĭ-sĕn′trăl) [″ + *centrum,* center]

uniceps (ū′nĭ-sĕps) [″ + *caput,* head]

unicorn, unicornous (ū′nĭ-korn, ū-nĭ-kor′nŭs) [″ + *cornu,* horn]

unicuspid (ū″nĭ-kŭs′pĭd)

uniflagellate (ū″nĭ-flăj′ĕ-lāt)

uniforate (ū"nĭ-fō'rāt) [" + *foratus,* pierced]

unigerminal (ū"nĭ-jĕr'mĭ-năl)

uniglandular (ū"nĭ-glăn'dū-lăr)

unigravida (ū"nĭ-grăv'ĭ-dă) [" + *gravida,* pregnant]

unilaminar (ū"nĭ-lăm'ĭ-năr)

unilateral (ū"nĭ-lăt'ĕr-ăl) [" + *latus,* side]

unilobar (ū"nĭ-lō'băr)

unilocular (ū"nĭ-lŏk'ū-lăr) [" + *lo-culus,* a small space]

uninuclear (ū"nĭ-nū'klē-ăr) [" + *nu-cleus,* a kernel]

uninucleated (ū"nĭ-nū'klē-āt"ĕd)

uniocular (ū"nē-ŏk'ū-lăr) [" + *oculus,* eye]

union (ūn'yŭn) [L. *unio*]
    u., non-
    u., secondary
    u., vicious

unioval (ū"nē-ō'văl) [L. *unus,* one, + *ovum,* egg]

uniovular (ū"nē-ŏv'ū-lăr) [" + *ovum,* egg]

unipara (ū-nĭp'ă-ră) [" + *parere,* to beget, produce]

uniparous (ū-nĭp'ă-rŭs) [" + *par-ere,* to beget, produce]

Unipen

unipolar (ū"nĭ-pō'lăr) [" + *polus,* pole]

unipotent, unipotential (ū-nĭp'ō-tĕnt, ū"nĭ-pō-tĕn'shăl)

uniseptate (ū"nē-sĕp'tāt)

unisex

Unisom

unit (ū'nĭt) [L. *unus,* one]
    u., amboceptor
    u., angström
    u., antigen
    u., antitoxin
    u., atomic mass
    u., Bodansky
    u., British thermal
    u., cat
    u., complement
    u., dental

u., electrostatic
u., hemolytic
u., international
u., light
u., Mache
u., motor
u., mouse
u. of capacity
u., rat
u., SI
u., Todd
u., USP

unitarian (ū-nĭ-tār'ē-ăn) [L. *unitarius*]

unitary (ū'nĭ-tĕr-ē)

unit dose

United States Adopted Names

United States Pharmacopeia

uniterminal (ū"nĭ-tĕr'mĭn-ăl) [L. *unus,* one, + *terminus,* end]

univalence (ū"nĭ-vā'lĕns)

univalent (ū"nĭ-vā'lĕnt, ū-nĭv'ă-lĕnt) [" + *valens,* to be powerful]

universal (ū"nĭ-vĕr'săl) [L. *universalis,* combined into one whole]

universal antidote

universal cuff

universal donor

universal dressing

universal recipient

unmedullated (ŭn-mĕd'ū-lāt"ĕd)

unmyelinated (ŭn-mī'ĕ-lĭ-nāt"ĕd)

Unna's paste (oo'năz) [Paul G. Unna, Ger. dermatologist, 1850–1929]

Unna's (paste) boot

unofficial (ŭn-ō-físh'ăl) [AS. *un,* not, + L. *officialis,* doing work]

unorganized (ŭn-or'găn-īzd) [" + L. *organizare,* to form a structure]

unphysiological (ŭn-fĭz-ē-ō-lŏj'ĭk-ăl)

unrest

unsaturated (ŭn-săt'ū-rāt"ĕd) [" + L. *saturare,* to fill]

unsaturated compound

unsex (ŭn-sĕks') [" + L. *sexus,* sex]

unstriated (ŭn-strī'āt-ĕd) [" + *striatus,* striped]

Unverricht's disease, syndrome (oon'fĕr-ĭkts) [Heinrich Unverricht, Ger.

physician, 1853–1912]

unwell [" + *wel*, well]

upper airway obstruction

upper GI

upper motor neuron lesion

upper respiratory infection

upsiloid (ŭp′sĭ-loyd) [Gr. *upsilon*, letter U, + *eidos*, form, shape]

uptake (ŭp′tāk)

urachal (ū′ră-kăl) [Gr. *ourachos*, fetal urinary canal]

urachus (ū′ră-kŭs) [Gr. *ourachos*, fetal urinary canal]
    u., patent

uracil (ū′ră-sĭl)

uracil mustard

uracrasia (ū-ră-krā′sē-ă) [Gr. *ouron*, urine, + *akrasia*, bad mixture]

uracratia (ū-ră-krā′shē-ă) [" + *akratia*, incontinence]

uragogue (ū′ră-gŏg) [" + *agogos*, leading]

uranisconitis (ū-răn-ĭs″kŏn-ī′tĭs) [Gr. *ouraniskos*, palate, + *itis*, inflammation]

uraniscoplasty (ū-răn-ĭs′kō-plăs″tē) [" + *plassein*, to form]

uraniscorrhaphy (ū″răn-ĭs-kor′ră-fē) [" + *rhaphe*, seam]

uraniscus (ū-răn-ĭs′kŭs) [Gr. *ouraniskos*, palate]

uranium (ū-rā′nē-ŭm) [LL., planet Uranus]

uranoplasty (ū′răn-ō-plăs″tē) [Gr. *ouranos*, palate, + *plassein*, to form]

uranoplegia (ū″ră-nō-plē′jē-ă) [" + *plege*, stroke]

uranorrhaphy (ū-răn-or′ră-fē) [" + *rhaphe*, seam]

uranoschisis (ū-răn-ŏs′kĭs-ĭs) [" + *schisis*, cleavage]

uranostaphyloplasty (ū″răn-ō-stăf′ĭl-ō-plăs″tē) [" + *staphyle*, uvula, + *plassein*, to form]

uranostaphylorrhaphy (ū″răn-ō-stăf-ĭl-or′ă-fē) [" + " + *rhaphe*, seam]

uranostaphyloschisis (ū″ră-nō-stăf″ĭ-lŏs′kĭ-sĭs)

uranyl (ū′ră-nĭl)

urapostema (ū″ră-pŏs-tē′mă) [Gr. *ouron*, urine, + *apostema*, abscess]

uraroma (ū-ră-rō′mă) [" + *aroma*, spice]

urarthritis (ū″răr-thrī′tĭs)

urase (ū′rās)

urate (ū′rāt) [Gr. *ouron*, urine]

uratemia (ū″ră-tē′mē-ă) [" + *haima*, blood]

uratic (ū-răt′ĭk)

uratoma (ū″ră-tō′mă)

uratosis (ū″ră-tō′sĭs)

uraturia (ū″ră-tū′rē-ă) [Gr. *ouron*, urine]

urceiform (ŭr-sē′ĭ-form) [L. *urceus*, pitcher, + *forma*, shape]

urceolate (ŭr-sē′ō-lāt)

ur-defense(s) (ŭr″dē-fĕns′) [Ger. *ur*, ultimate, + *defense*]

urea (ū-rē′ă) [Gr. *ouron*, urine]

urea cycle

urea frost

ureagenetic (ū-rē″ă-jĕn-ĕt′ĭk) [" + *genesis*, generation, birth]

ureal (ū-rē′ăl)

ureameter (ū-rē-ăm′ĕt-er) [" + *metron*, measure]

ureametry (ū-rē-ăm′ĕt-rē)

urea nitrogen

Ureaphil

Ureaplasma urealyticum

ureapoiesis (ū-rē″ă-poy-ē′sĭs) [" + *poiesis*, forming]

urease (ū′rē-ās) [Gr. *ouron*, urine]

urecchysis (ū-rĕk′ĭs-ĭs) [" + *ekchysis*, a pouring out]

Urecholine

uredema (ū-rĕ-dē′mă) [" + *oidema*, swelling]

ureide (ū′rē-īd) [Gr. *ouron*, urine]

urelcosis (ū-rĕl-kō′sĭs) [" + *helkosis*, ulceration]

uremia (ū-rē′mē-ă) [" + *haima*, blood]
    u., extrarenal
    u., prerenal

uremic (ū-rē′mĭk)

uremigenic (ū-rē″mĭ-jĕn′ĭk) [Gr. *ouron*,

urine, + *haima*, blood, + *gennan*, to produce]

ureogenesis (ūr″ē-ō-jĕn′ē-sĭs) [″ + *genesis*, generation, birth]

ureometer (ū″rē-ŏm′ĕt-ĕr) [″ + *metron*, measure]

ureometry (ū-rē-ŏm′ĕt-rē)

ureotelic (ū″rē-ō-tĕl′ĭk) [*urea* + Gr. *telikos*, belonging to the completion]

uresiesthesia, uresiesthesis (ū-rē″sē-ĕs-thē′zē-ă, -sĭs) [Gr. *ouresis*, urination, + *aisthesis*, feeling, perception]

uresis (ū-rē′sĭs) [Gr. *ouresis*]

ureter (ū′rĕ-ter, ū-rē′tĕr) [Gr. *oureter*]

ureteral (ū-rē′tĕr-ăl)

ureteralgia (ū″rē-tĕr-ăl′jē-ă) [″ + *algos*, pain]

uretercystoscope (ū-rē″tĕr-sĭs′tō-skōp) [″ + *kystis*, bladder, + *skopein*, to examine]

ureterectasis (ū-rē″tĕr-ĕk′tă-sĭs) [″ + *ektasis*, dilatation]

ureterectomy (ū-rē″tĕr-ĕk′tō-mē) [″ + *ektome*, excision]

ureteric (ū″rĕ-tĕr′ĭk)

ureteritis (ū-rē″tĕr-ī′tĭs) [″ + *itis*, inflammation]

ureterocele (ū-rē′tĕr-ō-sēl) [″ + *kele*, tumor, swelling]

ureterocelectomy (ū-rē″tĕr-ō-sē-lĕk′tō-mē) [″ + ″ + *ektome*, excision]

ureterocervical (ū-rē″tĕr-ō-sĕr′vĭ-kăl) [″ + L. *cervicalis*, pert. to cervix]

ureterocolostomy (ū-rē″tĕr-ō-kō-lŏs′tō-mē) [″ + *kolon*, colon, + *stoma*, mouth, opening]

ureterocystanastomosis (ū-rē″tĕr-ō-sĭs″tă-năs″tō-mō′sĭs) [Gr. *oureter*, ureter, + *kystis*, bladder, + *anastomosis*, opening]

ureterocystoneostomy (ū-rē″tĕr-ō-sĭst″ō-nē-ŏs′tō-mē) [″ + *kystis*, bladder, + *neos*, new, + *stoma*, mouth, opening]

ureterocystoscope (ū-rē″tĕr-ō-sĭs′tō-skōp) [″ + ″ + *skopein*, to view]

ureterocystostomy (ū-rē″tĕr-ō-sĭs-tŏs′tō-mē) [″ + ″ + *stoma*, mouth, opening]

ureterodialysis (ū-rē″tĕr-ō-dī-ăl′ĭ-sĭs) [″ + *dia*, through, + *lysis*, dissolution]

ureteroenterostomy (ū-rē″tĕr-ō-ĕn-tĕr-ŏs′tō-mē) [″ + *enteron*, intestine, + *stoma*, mouth, opening]

ureterography (ū-rē″tĕr-ŏg′ră-fē) [″ + *graphein*, to write]

ureteroheminephrectomy (ū-rē″tĕr-ō-hĕm″ī-nĕ-frĕk′tō-mē) [″ + *hemi-*, half, + *nephros*, kidney, + *ektome*, excision]

ureterohydronephrosis (ū-rē″tĕr-ō-hī″drō-nĕ-frō′sĭs) [″ + *hydor*, water, + *nephros*, kidney, + *osis*, condition]

ureteroileostomy (ū-rē″tĕr-ō-ĭl″ē-ŏs′tō-mē) [″ + *ileum*, ileum, + *stoma*, mouth, opening]

ureterolith (ū-rē′tĕr-ō-lĭth) [″ + *lithos*, stone]

ureterolithiasis (ū-rē″tĕr-ō-lĭth-ī′ăs-ĭs) [″ + ″ + *-iasis*, state or condition of]

ureterolithotomy (ū-rē″tĕr-ō-lĭth-ŏt′ō-mē) [″ + ″ + *tome*, a cutting, slice]

ureterolysis (ū-rē″tĕr-ŏl′ĭ-sĭs) [″ + *lysis*, dissolution]

ureteroneocystostomy (ū-rē″tĕr-ō-nē″ō-sĭs-tŏs′tō-mē) [″ + *neos*, new, + *kystis*, bladder, + *stoma*, mouth, opening]

ureteroneopyelostomy (ū-rē″tĕr-ō-nē″ō-pī-ĕ-lŏs′tō-mē) [″ + ″ + *pyelos*, pelvis, + *stoma*, mouth, opening]

ureteronephrectomy (ū-rē″tĕr-ō-nĕf-rĕk′tō-mē) [″ + *nephros*, kidney, + *ektome*, excision]

ureteropathy (ū-rē″tĕr-ŏp′ă-thē) [″ + *pathos*, disease, suffering]

ureteropelvioplasty (ū-rē″tĕr-ō-pĕl′vē-ō-plăs″tē) [Gr. *oureter*, ureter, + L. *pelvis*, basin, + Gr. *plassein*, to mold]

ureterophlegma (ū-rē″tĕr-ō-flĕg′mă)
[″ + *phlegma*, phlegm]
ureteroplasty (ū-rē′tĕr-ō-plăs″tē)
[″ + *plassein*, to form]
ureteroproctostomy (ū-rē″tĕr-ō-prŏk-tŏs′tō-mē) [″ + *proktos*, anus, + *stoma*, mouth, opening]
ureteropyelitis (ū-rē″tĕr-ō-pī-ĕl-ī′tĭs) [″ + *pyelos*, pelvis, + *itis*, inflammation]
ureteropyeloneostomy (ū-rē″tĕr-ō-pī″ĕl-ō-nē-ŏs′tō-mē) [″ + ″ + *neos*, new, + *stoma*, mouth, opening]
ureteropyelonephritis (ū-rē″tĕr-ō-pī″ĕl-ō-nĕf-rī′tĭs) [″ + ″ + *nephros*, kidney, + *itis*, inflammation]
ureteropyeloplasty (ū-rē″tĕr-ō-pī′ĕl-ō-plăs″tē) [″ + ″ + *plassein*, to mold]
ureteropyelostomy (ū-rē″tĕr-ō-pī″ĕ-lŏs′tō-mē) [″ + ″ + *stoma*, mouth, opening]
ureteropyosis (ū-rē″tĕr-ō-pī-ō′sĭs) [″ + *pyon*, pus, + *osis*, condition]
ureterorectostomy (ū-rē″tĕr-ō-rĕk-tŏs′tō-mē) [″ + L. *rectum*, straight, + Gr. *stoma*, mouth, opening]
ureterorrhagia (ū-rē″tĕr-or-rā′jē-ă) [″ + *rhegnynai*, to burst forth]
ureterorrhaphy (ū-rē″tĕr-or′ră-fē) [″ + *rhaphe*, seam]
ureterosigmoidostomy (ū-rē″tĕr-ō-sĭg-moyd-ŏs′tō-mē) [″ + *sigma*, letter S, + *eidos*, form, shape, + *stoma*, mouth, opening]
ureterostegnosis (ū-rē″tĕr-ō-stĕg-nō′sĭs)
ureterostenosis (ū-rē″tĕr-ō-stĕn-ō′sĭs) [″ + *stenosis*, act of narrowing]
ureterostoma (ū″rē-tĕr-ŏs′tō-mă) [Gr. *oureter*, ureter, + *stoma*, mouth, opening]
ureterostomy (ū-rē″tĕr-ŏs′tō-mē) [″ + *stoma*, mouth, opening]
    u., cutaneous
ureterotomy (ū-rē″tĕr-ŏt′ō-mē) [″ +

tome, a cutting, slice]
ureterotrigonoenterostomy (ū-rē″tĕr-ō-trī-gō″nō-ĕn″tĕr-ŏs′tō-mē) [″ + *trigonon*, three-sided figure, + *enteron*, intestine, + *stoma*, mouth, opening]
ureteroureteral (ū-rē″tĕr-ō-ū-rē′tĕr-ăl) [″ + *oureter*, ureter]
ureteroureterostomy (ū-rē″tĕr-ō-ū-rē″tĕr-ŏs′tō-mē) [″ + ″ + *stoma*, mouth, opening]
ureterouterine (ū-rē″tĕr-ō-ū′tĕr-ĭn) [″ + L. *uterus*, womb]
ureterovaginal (ū-rē″tĕr-ō-văj′ĭ-năl) [″ + L. *vagina*, sheath]
ureterovesical (ū-rē″tĕr-ō-vĕs′ĭ-kăl) [″ + L. *vesica*, bladder]
ureterovesicostomy (ū-rē″tĕr-ō-vĕs″ĭ-kŏs′tō-mē) [″ + ″ + Gr. *stoma*, mouth, opening]
urethra (ū-rē′thră) [Gr. *ourethra*]
    u. muliebris
    u. virilis
urethral (ū-rē′thrăl) [Gr. *ourethra*, urethra]
urethralgia (ū-rē-thrăl′jē-ă) [″ + *algos*, pain]
urethral syndrome
urethrascope (ū-rē′thră-skōp)
urethratresia (ū-rē′thră-trē′zē-ă) [″ + *a-*, not, + *tresis*, a perforation]
urethrectomy (ū-rē-thrĕk′tō-mē) [″ + *ektome*, excision]
urethremphraxis (ū″rē-thrĕm-frăk′sĭs) [″ + *emphraxis*, an obstruction]
urethreurynter (ū-rēth″rūr-ĭn′tĕr) [″ + *eurynein*, to dilate]
urethrism, urethrismus (ū′rē-thrĭzm, ū″rē-thrĭz′mŭs) [″ + *-ismos*, condition]
urethritis (ū″rē-thrī′tĭs) [″ + *itis*, inflammation]
    u., anterior
    u., gonococcal
    u., nongonococcal
    u., nonspecific
    u., posterior

u., specific
urethro- [Gr. *ourethra*]
urethrobulbar (ū-rē″thrō-bŭl′băr)
urethrocele (ū-rē′thrō-sēl) [″ + *kele*, tumor, swelling]
urethrocystitis (ū-rē″thrō-sĭs-tī′tĭs) [″ + *kystis*, bladder, + *itis*, inflammation]
urethrocystopexy (ū-rē″thrō-sĭs′tō-pĕk″sē) [″ + *kystis*, bladder, + *pexis*, fixation]
urethrodynia (ū-rē″thrō-dĭn′ē-ă) [″ + *odyne*, pain]
urethrograph (ū-rē′thrō-grăf)
urethrography (ū-rē-thrŏg′ră-fē) [″ + *graphein*, to write]
u., voiding
urethrometer (ū-rē-thrŏm′ĕt-ĕr) [Gr. *ourethra*, urethra, + *metron*, measure]
urethropenile (ū-rē″thrō-pē′nīl) [″ + L. *penis*, penis]
urethroperineal (ū-rē″thrō-pĕr-ĭ-nē′ăl) [″ + *perinaion*, perineum]
urethroperineoscrotal (ū-rē″thrō-pĕr-ĭ-nē″ō-skrō′tăl) [″ + ″ + L. *scrotum*, a bag]
urethropexy (ū-rē′thrō-pĕks-ē) [″ + Gr. *pexis*, fixation]
urethrophraxis (ū-rē-thrō-frăks′ĭs) [″ + *phrassein*, to obstruct]
urethrophyma (ū-rē-thrō-fī′mă) [″ + *phyma*, growth]
urethroplasty (ū-rē′thrō-plăs″tē) [″ + *plassein*, to mold]
urethroprostatic (ū-rē″thrō-prŏs-tăt′ĭk)
urethrorectal (ū-rē″thrō-rĕk′tăl) [Gr. *ourethra*, urethra, + L. *rectus*, straight]
urethrorrhagia (ū-rē″thror-ā′jē-ă) [″ + *rhegnynai*, to burst forth]
urethrorrhaphy (ū-rē-thror′ăf-ē) [″ + *rhaphe*, seam]
urethrorrhea (ū-rē″thror-ē′ă) [″ + *rhein*, to flow]
u. ex libidine
urethroscope (ū-rē′thrō-skōp) [″ +

skopein, to examine]
urethroscopic (ū-rē″thrō-skŏp′ĭk)
urethroscopy (ū-rē-thrŏs′kō-pē)
urethrospasm (ū-rē′thrō-spăzm) [″ + *spasmos*, a convulsion]
urethrostaxis (ū-rē″thrō-stăks′ĭs) [″ + *staxis*, a dropping]
urethrostenosis (ū-rē″thrō-stĕn-ō′sĭs) [″ + *stenosis*, act of narrowing]
urethrostomy (ū-rē-thrŏs′tō-mē) [″ + *stoma*, mouth, opening]
urethrotome (ū-rē′thrō-tōm) [″ + *tome*, a cutting, slice]
urethrotomy (ū-rē-thrŏt′ō-mē)
urethrotrigonitis (ū-rē″thrō-trī″gō-nī′tĭs) [″ + *trigonon*, three-sided figure, + *itis*, inflammation]
urethrovaginal (ū-rē″thrō-văj′ĭ-năl) [″ + L. *vagina*, sheath]
urethrovesical (ū-rē″thrō-vĕs′ĭ-kăl) [″ + L. *vesica*, bladder]
urhydrosis (ūr″hī-drō′sĭs) [Gr. *ouron*, urine, + *hidros*, sweat]
URI upper respiratory infection
uric (ū′rĭk) [Gr. *ourikos*, urine]
uric acid
u.a., endogenous
u.a., exogenous
uricacidemia (ū″rĭk-ăs-ĭd-ē′mē-ă) [Gr. *ourikos*, urine, + L. *acidus*, sour, + Gr. *haima*, blood]
uricaciduria (ū″rĭk-ăs-ĭd-ū′rē-ă) [″ + ″ + Gr. *ouron*, urine]
uricase (ū′rĭ-kāz) [″ + -*ase*, enzyme]
uricemia (ū-rĭ-sē′mē-ă) [″ + *haima*, blood]
uricocholia (ū″rĭ-kō-kō′lē-ă) [″ + *chole*, bile]
uricolysis (ū-rĭ-kŏl′ĭ-sĭs) [″ + *lysis*, dissolution]
uricolytic (ū″rĭ-kō-lĭt′ĭk)
uricometer (ū″rĭk-ŏm′ĕ-ter) [″ + *metron*, measure]
uricopoiesis (ū″rĭ-kō-poy-ē′sĭs) [″ + *poiesis*, formation]
uricosuria (ū″rĭ-kō-sū′rē-ă) [″ + *ouron*, urine]

uricosuric (ū″rĭ-kō-sū′rĭk)
uricosuric agent
uricotelic (ū″rĭ-kō-tĕl′ĭk) [″ + te-likos, belonging to the completion]
uricoxidase (ū″rĭk-ŏks′ĭ-dās) [″ + oxys, sharp, + -ase, enzyme]
uridine (ūr′ĭ-dĭn)
  u. diphosphate
uridrosis (ū-rĭ-drō′sĭs) [″ + hidrosis, a sweating]
  u. crystallina
uriesthesis (ū-rē-ĕs-thē′sĭs) [″ + aisthesis, feeling, perception]
urina (ū-rī′nă) [L.]
  u. cibi
  u. galactodes
  u. hysterica
  u. jumentosa
urinaccelerator (ū″rĭn-ăk-sĕl′ĕr-ā″tor)
urinal (ū′rĭn-ăl) [L. urina, urine]
  u., condom
urinalysis (ū″rĭ-năl′ĭ-sĭs) [″ + Gr. ana, apart, + lysis, dissolution]
urinary (ū′rĭ-năr″ē) [L. urina, urine]
urinary bladder
urinary calculi
urinary casts
urinary director appliance
urinary incontinence
urinary infection
urinary organs
urinary pigments
urinary reflex
urinary sediment
urinary stammering
urinary system
urinary tract
urinate (ū′rĭ-nāt) [L. urinare, to discharge urine]
urination (ū″rĭ-nā′shŭn) [L. urinatio, a discharging of urine]
urine (ū′rĭn) [L. urina; Gr. ouron, urine]
  u., residual
urinemia (ū″rĭ-nē′mē-ă) [L. urina, urine, + Gr. haima, blood]
uriniferous (ū-rĭ-nĭf′ĕr-ŭs) [″ + ferre, to bear]
urinific (ū″rĭ-nĭf′ĭk)

uriniparous (ū-rĭ-nĭp′ă-rŭs) [″ + parere, to beget, produce]
urinogenital (ū″rĭ-nō-jĕn′ĭ-tăl) [″ + genitalia, genitals]
urinogenous (ū″rĭ-nŏj′ĭ-nŭs) [″ + Gr. gennan, to produce]
urinology (ū″rĭ-nŏl′ō-jē)
urinoma (ū″rĭ-nō′mă) [″ + Gr. oma, tumor]
urinometer (ū″rĭ-nŏm′ĕ-tĕr) [″ + Gr. metron, measure]
urinometry (ū″rĭ-nŏm′ĕ-trē)
urinophil (ū′rĭ-nō-fĭl) [″ + Gr. philein, to love]
urinoscopy (ū″rĭ-nŏs′kō-pē)
urinose, urinous (ū′rĭ-nōs, ū′rĭ-nŭs) [L. urina, urine]
urinosexual (ū″rĭ-nō-sĕks′ū-ăl)
uriposia (ū″rĭ-pō′zē-ă) [″ + posis, drinking]
urisolvent (ū″rĭ-sŏl′vĕnt) [″ + solvens, dissolving]
Urispas
uro- [Gr. ouron]
uroammoniac (ū″rō-ă-mō′nē-ăk)
uroanthelone (ū″rō-ăn′thĕ-lōn)
urobilin (ū″rō-bī′lĭn) [″ + L. bilis, bile]
urobilinemia (ū″rō-bī″lĭn-ē′mē-ă) [″ + ″ + Gr. haima, blood]
urobilinicterus (ū″rō-bī-lĭn-ĭk′tĕr-ŭs) [″ + L. bilis, bile, + Gr. ikteros, jaundice]
urobilinogen (ū″rō-bī-lĭn′ō-jĕn) [″ + ″ + Gr. gennan, to produce]
urobilinogenemia (ū″rō-bī″lĭn-ō-jĕn-ē′mē-ă) [″ + ″ + ″ + haima, blood]
urobilinuria (ū″rō-bī″lĭn-ū′rē-ă) [″ + ″ + Gr. ouron, urine]
urocele (ū′rō-sēl) [″ + kele, tumor, swelling]
urocheras (ū-rŏk′ĕr-ăs) [″ + cheras, gravel]
urochesia (ū-rō-kē′zē-ă) [″ + chezein, to defecate]
urochrome (ū′rō-krōm) [″ + chroma, color]

uroclepsia (ū-rō-klĕp'sē-ă) [" + kleptein, judge]

urocrisia (ū"rō-krīz'ē-ă) [" + krinein, to judge]

urocyanin (ū-rō-sī'ă-nĭn) [" + kyanos, blue]

urocyanogen (ū"rō-sī-ăn'ō-jĕn) [" + " + gennan, to produce]

urocyanosis (ū"rō-sī-ăn-ō'sĭs) [" + " + osis, condition]

urocyst (ū'rō-sĭst) [Gr. ouron, urine, + kystis, bladder]

urocystic (ū"rō-sĭs'tĭk)

urocystis (ū"rō-sĭs'tĭs)

urocystitis (ū"rō-sĭs-tī'tĭs)

urodynamics (ū"rō-dī-năm'ĭks)

urodynia (ū"rō-dĭn'ē-ă) [" + odyne, pain]

uroedema (ū"rō-ĕ-dē'mă) [" + oidema, swelling]

uroenterone (ū"rō-ĕn'tĕr-ōn)

uroerythrin (ū"rō-ĕr'ĭth-rĭn) [" + erythros, red]

uroflavin (ū"rō-flā'vĭn)

uroflowmeter

urofuscin (ū"rō-fūs'ĭn) [" + L. fuscus, dark brown]

urofuscohematin (ū"rō-fŭs"kō-hĕm'ăt-ĭn) [" + " + Gr. haima, blood]

urogastrone (ū"rō-găs'trōn) [" + gaster, belly]

urogenital (ū"rō-jĕn'ĭ-tăl) [" + L. genitalia, genitals]

urogenital fold

urogenous (ū-rŏj'ĕn-ŭs) [" + gennan, to produce]

uroglaucin (ū"rō-glaw'sĭn) [" + glaukos, gleaming, gray]

urogram (ū'rō-grăm) [" + gramma, letter, piece of writing]

urography (ū'rŏg'ră-fē) [Gr. ouron, urine, + graphein, to write]
　u., ascending; u., cystoscopic
　u., descending; u., excretion; u., excretory; u., intravenous
　u., retrograde

urohematin (ū"rō-hĕm'ăt-ĭn) [" + haima, blood]

urohematonephrosis (ū"rō-hĕm"ă-tō-nē-frō'sĭs) [" + " + nephros, kidney]

urohematoporphyrin (ū"rō-hĕm"ă-tō-por'fĭr-ĭn) [" + " + porphyra, purple]

urokinase (ū-rō-kī'nās)

urokinetic (ū"rō-kī-nĕt'ĭk) [" + kinesis, motion]

urolagnia (ū-rō-lăg'nē-ă) [" + lagneia, lust]

urolith (ū'rō-lĭth) [" + lithos, stone]

urolithiasis (ū"rō-lĭ-thī'ă-sĭs) [" + " + -iasis, state or condition of]

urolithic (ū"rō-lĭth'ĭk)

urolithology (ū"rō-lĭ-thŏl'ō-jē) [" + " + logos, word, reason]

urologic (ū-rō-lŏj'ĭk) [" + logos, word, reason]

urologist (ū-rŏl'ō-jĭst)

urology (ū-rŏl'ō-jē) [" + logos, word, reason]

urolutein (ū-rō-lū'tē-ĭn) [" + L. luteus, yellow]

uromancy (ūr'ō-măn"sē) [" + manteia, a divination]

uromelanin (ū-rō-mĕl'ăn-ĭn) [" + melas, black]

uromelus (ū-rŏm'ē-lŭs) [Gr. oura, tail, + melos, limb]

urometer (ū-rŏm'ĕt-ĕr) [Gr. ouron, urine, + metron, measure]

uroncus (ū-rŏn'kŭs) [" + onkos, bulk, mass]

uronephrosis (ū"rō-nĕf-rō'sĭs) [" + nephros, kidney, + osis, condition]

uronology (ū-rō-nŏl'ō-jē) [" + logos, word, reason]

uronophile (ū-rŏn'ō-fĭl) [" + philein, to love]

uropathogen (ū"rō-păth'ō-jĕn) [" + pathos, disease, suffering, + gennan, to produce]

uropathy (ū-rŏp'ă-thē)
　u., obstructive

uropenia (ū-rō-pē'nē-ă) [" + penia, lack]

uropepsin (ū″rō-pĕp′sĭn)
urophanic (ū-rō-făn′ĭk) [″ + *phain-ein*, to appear]
urophein (ū″rō-fē′ĭn) [″ + *phaios*, gray]
urophosphometer (ū″rō-fŏs-fŏm′ĕ-tĕr) [″ + L. *phosphas*, phosphorus]
uroplania (ū″rō-plā′nē-ă) [″ + *plane*, a wandering]
uropoiesis (ū″rō-poy-ē′sĭs) [Gr. *ouron*, urine, + *poiesis*, production]
uropoietic (ū″rō-poy-ĕt′ĭk) [″ + *poiein*, to form]
uroporphyria (ū″rō-por-fĭr′ē-ă)
uroporphyrin (ū″rō-por′fĭ-rĭn)
uroporphyrinogen (ū″rō-por″fĭ-rĭn′ō-jĕn)
　u. I
uropsammus (ū″rō-săm′ŭs) [″ + *psammos*, sand]
uropyonephrosis (ū″rō-pī-ō-nĕf-rō′sĭs) [″ + *pyon*, pus, + *nephros*, kidney, + *osis*, condition]
uropyoureter (ū″rō-pī″ō-ū-rē′tĕr) [″ + ″ + *oureter*, ureter]
urorosein (ū″rō-rō′zē-ĭn) [″ + L. *roseus*, rosy]
urorrhagia (ū-rō-ră′jē-ă) [″ + *rhegnynai*, to burst forth]
urorrhea (ū-rō-rē′ă) [″ + *rhein*, to flow]
urorrhodin (ū-rō-rō′dĭn) [″ + *rhodon*, rose]
urorrhodinogen (ū″rō-rō-dĭn′ō-jĕn) [Gr. *ouron*, urine, + *rhodon*, rose, + *gennan*, to produce]
urorubin (ū-rō-roo′bĭn) [″ + L. *ruber*, red]
urorubrohematin (ū″rō-rū″brō-hĕm′ă-tĭn) [″ + ″ + Gr. *haima*, blood]
urosacin (ū-rō′sā-sĭn)
uroscheocele (ū-rŏs′kē-ō-sēl) [″ + *oscheon*, scrotum, + *kele*, tumor, swelling]
uroschesis (ū-rŏs′kĕs-ĭs) [″ + *schesis*, a holding]
uroscopy (ū-rŏs′kō-pē) [″ + *sko-*

pein, to examine]
urosepsis (ū-rō-sĕp′sĭs)
urospectrin (ū-rō-spĕk′trĭn) [″ + L. *spectrum*, image]
urostealith (ū″rō-stē′ă-lĭth) [″ + *stear*, fat, + *lithos*, stone]
urotoxia (ū″rō-tŏk′sē-ă) [″ + *toxikon*, poison]
urotoxicity (ū″rō-tŏks-ĭs′ĭ-tē) [″ + *toxikon*, poison]
urotoxin (ū″rō-tŏk′sĭn)
uroureter (ū″rō-ū′rĕ-tĕr, ū″rō-ū-rē′tĕr) [″ + *oureter*, ureter]
urous (ū′rŭs) [Gr. *ouron*, urine]
uroxanthin (ū″rō-zăn′thĭn) [″ + *xanthos*, yellow]
uroxin (ū-rŏk′sĭn) [″ + *oxys*, sharp]
urtica (ŭr-tī′kă) [L., nettle]
urticant (ŭr′tĭ-kănt)
urticaria (ŭr-tĭ-kā′rē-ă) [L. *urtica*, nettle]
　u., aquagenic
　u. bullosa
　u., cold
　u. factitia
　u. gigantea
　u. haemorrhagica
　u. maculosa
　u. maritima
　u. medicamentosa
　u. papulosa
　u. pigmentosa
　u. pigmentosa juvenilis
　u. solaris
urticarial (ŭr″tĭ-kā′rē-ăl) [L. *urtica*, nettle]
urticate (ŭr′tĭ-kāt)
urtication (ŭr-tĭ-kā′shŭn)
urushiol (ū-roo′shē-ŏl″) [Japanese *urushi*, lac, + L. *oleum*, oil]
U.S. AEC U.S. Atomic Energy Commission
USAN United States Adopted Names
USAN and the USP Dictionary of Drug Names
Usher's syndrome [Charles H. Usher, Brit. physician, 1865–1942]
USP, U.S. Phar. United States Pharmacopeia

U.S.P.H.S. *United States Public Health Service*

ustilaginism (ŭs-tĭl-ăj'ĭn-ĭzm) [L. *ustulatus,* scorched, + Gr. *-ismos,* condition]

Ustilago (ŭs-tĭl-ā'gō)

ustion (ŭs'chŭn) [L. *ustio,* a burning]

ustulation (ŭs-tū-lā'shŭn) [L. *ustulare,* to scorch]

ustus (ŭs'tŭs) [L.]

uta (ū'tă)

ut dict. [L.] *ut dictum,* as directed

utend. [L.] *utendus,* to be used

uter-, utero- [L. *uterus,* womb]

uteralgia (ū"tĕr-ăl'jē-ă) [L. *uterus,* womb, + Gr. *algos,* pain]

uterectomy (ū"tĕr-ĕk'tō-mē) [" + Gr. *ektome,* excision]

uterine (ū'tĕr-īn, -ĭn) [L. *uterinus*]

uterine bleeding

uterine glands

uterine milk

uterine souffle

uterine subinvolution

uterine tube

uteroabdominal (ū"tĕr-ō-ăb-dŏm'ĭ-năl) [L. *uterus,* womb, + *abdomen,* belly]

uterocele (ū-tĕr'ō-sēl) [" + Gr. *kele,* tumor, swelling]

uterocervical (ū"tĕr-ō-sĕr'vĭ-kăl) [" + *cervix,* neck]

uterocystostomy (ū"tĕr-ō-sĭs-tŏs'tō-mē) [" + Gr. *kystis,* bladder, + *stoma,* mouth, opening]

uterofixation (ū"tĕr-ō-fĭks-ā'shŭn) [" + *fixatio,* a fixing]

uterogenic (ū"tĕr-ō-jĕn'ĭk)

uterogestation (ū"tĕr-ō-jĕs-tā'shŭn) [" + *gestare,* to bear]

uterography (ū"tĕr-ŏg'ră-fē) [" + Gr. *graphein,* to write]

uterolith (ū'tĕr-ō-lĭth) [" + Gr. *lithos,* stone]

uterometer (ū"tĕr-ŏm'ĕt-er) [" + Gr. *metron,* measure]

uteroovarian (ū"tĕr-ō-ō-vā'rē-ăn) [" + NL. *ovarium,* ovary]

uteropexia, uteropexy (ū"tĕr-ō-pĕks'ē-ă, ū'tĕr-ō-pĕks"ē) [" + Gr. *pexis,* fixation]

uteroplacental (ū"tĕr-ō-plă-sĕn'tăl) [" + *placenta,* a flat cake]

uteroplasty (ū"tĕr-ō-plăs'tē) [" + Gr. *plassein,* to form]

uterorectal (ū"tĕr-ō-rĕk'tăl)

uterosacral (ū"tĕr-ō-sā'krăl) [" + *sacralis,* pert. to the sacrum]

uterosalpingography (ū"tĕr-ō-săl-pĭng-ŏg'ră-fē) [" + Gr. *salpinx,* tube, + *graphein,* to write]

uteroscope (ū'tĕr-ō-skōp) [" + Gr. *skopein,* to examine]

uterotome (ū'tĕr-ō-tōm) [" + Gr. *tome,* a cutting, slice]

uterotomy (ū-tĕr-ŏt'ō-mē)

uterotonic (ū"tĕr-ō-tŏn'ĭk) [L. *uterus,* womb, + Gr. *tonos,* act of stretching, tension, tone]

uterotractor (ū"tĕr-ō-trăk'tor) [" + *tractor,* drawer]

uterotubal (ū"tĕr-ō-tū'băl) [" + *tuba,* tube]

uterotubography (ū"tĕr-ō-tū-bŏg'ră-fē) [" + " + Gr. *graphein,* to write]

uterovaginal (ū"tĕr-ō-văj'ĭ-năl) [" + *vagina,* sheath]

uteroventral (ū"tĕr-ō-vĕn'trăl)

uterovesical (ū"tĕr-ō-vĕs'ĭ-kăl) [" + *vesica,* bladder]

uterus (ū'tĕr-ŭs) [L.]
   u. acollis
   u. arcuatus
   u. bicornis
   u. biforis
   u. bilocularis
   u., bipartite
   u., cancer of
   u. cordiformis
   u., Couvelaire
   u. didelphys
   u. duplex
   u., fetal
   u., gravid
   u. masculinus

u. parvicollis
u., prolapse of
u., pubescent
u., rupture of, in pregnancy
u. septus
u., subinvolution of
u., tipped
u., tumors of
u. unicornis
Uticillin VK
Uticort
utilization review
Utimox
utricle (ū'trĭk'l) [L. *utriculus*, a little bag]
u. of urethra
u. of vestibule
u., prostatic
utricular (ū-trĭk'ū-lăr) [L. *utriculus*, a little bag]
utriculitis (ū-trĭk-ū-lī'tĭs) [" + Gr. *itis*, inflammation]
utriculoplasty (ū-trĭk'ū-lō-plăs"tē) [" + Gr. *plassein*, to form]
utriculosaccular (ū-trĭk"ū-lō-săk'ū-lăr) [" + NL. *sacculus*, small bag]
utriculosaccular duct
utriculus (ū-trĭk'ū-lŭs) [L., a little bag]
u. masculinus
u. prostaticus
utriform (ū'trĭ-form) [L. *uter*, a skin bag, + *forma*, shape]
uva (ū'vă) [L., grape]
uvea (ū'vē-ă) [L. *uva*, grape]
uveal (ū'vē-ăl)
uveitic (ū-vē-ĭt'ĭk) [" + Gr. *itis*, inflammation]
uveitis (ū-vē-ī'tĭs)
u., heterochromic
u., sympathetic

uveoparotitis (ū"vē-ō-păr-ō-tī'tĭs) [" + Gr. *para*, alongside, past, beyond, + *ous*, ear, + *itis*, inflammation]
uveoplasty (ū'vē-ō-plăs"tē) [" + Gr. *plassein*, to form]
uveoscleritis (ū"vē-ō-sklĕr-ī'tĭs)
uviform (ū'vĭ-form) [" + *forma*, form]
uviofast (ū'vē-ō-făst)
uviol (ū'vē-ŏl)
uviolize (ū'vē-ō-līz)
uviometer (ū"vē-ŏm'ĕ-tĕr)
uvioresistant (ū"vē-ō-rē-zīs'tănt)
uviosensitive (ū"vē-ō-sĕn'sĭ-tĭv)
uvula (ū'vū-lă) [L. *uvula*, a little grape]
u. fissa
u. of cerebellum
u. vermis
u. vesicae
uvulaptosis (ū"vū-lăp-tō'sĭs) [" + Gr. *ptosis*, fall, falling]
uvular (ū'vū-lăr) [L. *uvula*, little grape]
uvularis (ū-vū-lā'rĭs) [L.]
uvulatome (ū'vū-lă-tōm) [" + Gr. *tome*, a cutting, slice]
uvulatomy (ū-vū-lăt'ō-mē)
uvulectomy (ū"vū-lĕk'tō-mē) [" + Gr. *ektome*, excision]
uvulitis (ū"vū-lī'tĭs) [" + Gr. *itis*, inflammation]
uvulopalatopharyngoplasty
uvuloptosis (ū"vū-lŏp-tō'sĭs) [" + Gr. *ptosis*, fall, falling]
uvulotome (ū'vū-lō-tōm) [L. *uvula*, little grape, + Gr. *tome*, a cutting, slice]
uvulotomy (ū-vū-lŏt'ō-mē)
U wave

V

V *vanadium; Vibrio; vision; visual acuity*

v [L.] *vena*, vein; *volt*

vaccigenous (văk-sĭj′ĕn-ŭs) [L. *vaccinus*, pert. to cows, + Gr. *gennan*, to produce]

vaccina (văk-sī′nă)

vaccinable (văk-sĭn′ă-b′l)

vaccinal (văk′sĭn-ăl)

vaccinate (văk′sĭn-āt) [L. *vaccinus*, pert. to cows]

vaccination (văk″sĭ-nā′shŭn) [L. *vaccinus*, pert. to cows]

vaccinator (văk′sĭ-nā″tor)

vaccine (văk′sēn, văk-sēn′) [L. *vaccinus*, pert. to cows]

   v., aqueous

   v., autogenous

   v., bacterial

   v., BCG

   v., cholera

   v., DTP

   v., epidemic typhus fever

   v., heterologous

   v., homologous

   v., human diploid cell rabies (HDCV)

   v., humanized

   v., influenza

   v., killed

   v., measles virus, inactivated

   v., measles virus, live attenuated

   v., mixed

   v., multivalent

   v., mumps

   v., plague

   v., pneumococcal, polyvalent

   v., poliovirus, inactivated

   v., poliovirus, live oral

   v., polyvalent

   v., rabies

   v., Sabin

   v., Salk

   v., sensitized

   v., smallpox

   v., triple

   v., typhoid

   v., yellow fever

vaccinia (văk-sĭn′ē-ă) [L. *vaccinus*, pert. to cows]

   v. necrosum

vaccinia immune globulin

vaccinial (văk-sĭn′ē-ăl)

vacciniform (văk-sĭn′ĭ-form) [L. *vaccinus*, pert. to cows, + *forma*, shape]

vacciniola (văk″sĭn-ē-ō′lă) [L., little cows]

vaccinogen (văk-sĭn′ō-jĕn)

vaccinogenous (văk″sĭn-ŏj′ĕn-ŭs) [L. *vaccinus*, pert. to cows, + Gr. *gennan*, to produce]

vaccinoid (văk′sĭn-oyd) [″ + Gr. *eidos*, form, shape]

vaccinostyle (văk-sĭn′ō-stĭl)

vaccinotherapeutics (văk″sĭn-ō-thĕr″ă-pū′tĭks)

vaccinum (văk-sī′nŭm) [L.]

vacuolar (văk′ū-ō-lăr) [L. *vacuum*, empty]

vacuolar degeneration

vacuolated (văk′ū-ō-lāt″ĕd)

vacuolation (văk″ū-ō-lā′shŭn)

vacuole (văk′ū-ōl) [L. *vacuum*, empty]

   v., autophagic

   v., contractile

   v., heterophagous

   v., plasmocrine

   v., rhagiocrine

vacuolization (văk″ū-ō-lĭ-zā′shŭn) [L. *vacuum*, empty]

vacuome (văk′ū-ōm)

vacuum (văk′ū-ŭm) [L., empty]

vacuum aspiration

vacuum extractor
vacuum tube
vade mecum (wā"dē mē'kŭm) [L., go with me]
vagabond's disease
vagal (vā'găl) [L. *vagus*, wandering]
vagal attack
vagal escape
vagal tone
vagi (vā'gī)
vagina (vă-jī'nă) [L., sheath]
   v., bulb of
   v. fibrosa tendinis
   v. masculina
   v. mucosa tendinis
   v., septate
vaginal (văj'ĭn-ăl) [L. *vagina*, sheath]
vaginalectomy (văj"ĭn-ăl-ĕk'tō-mē) [" + Gr. *ektome*, excision]
vaginal hysterectomy
vaginalitis (văj-ĭn-ăl-ī'tĭs) [" + Gr. *itis*, inflammation]
vaginal vibrator
vaginapexy (văj"ĭn-ă-pĕk'sē) [" + Gr. *pexis*, fixation]
vaginate (văj'ĭn-āt) [L. *vaginatus*]
vaginectomy (văj-ĭn-ĕk'tō-mē) [L. *vagina*, sheath, + Gr. *ektome*, excision]
vaginismus (văj"ĭn-ĭz'mŭs) [L.]
   v., deep
   v., mental
   v., posterior
vaginitis (văj-ĭn-ī'tĭs) [L. *vagina*, sheath, + Gr. *itis*, inflammation]
   v. adhaesiva
   v., atrophic
   v., diphtheritic
   v., emphysematous
   v., Gardnerella vaginalis
   v., granular
   v., nonspecific
   v., postmenopausal
   v., senile
   v. testis
   v., Trichomonas vaginalis
vaginoabdominal (văj"ĭn-ō-ăb-dŏm'ĭn-ăl) [L. *vagina*, sheath, +

abdominalis, abdominal]
vaginocele (văj'ĭn-ō-sēl) [" + Gr. *kele*, tumor, swelling]
vaginodynia (văj"ĭn-ō-dĭn'ē-ă) [" + Gr. *odyne*, pain]
vaginofixation (văj"ĭn-ō-fĭks-ā'shŭn) [" + *fixatio*, a fixing]
vaginogenic (văj"ĭn-ō-jĕn'ĭk) [" + Gr. *gennan*, to produce]
vaginogram (văj'ĭn-ō-grăm) [" + gramma, letter, piece of writing]
vaginography (văj-ĭn-ŏg'ră-fē) [" + Gr. *graphein*, to write]
vaginolabial (văj"ĭn-ō-lā'bē-ăl) [" + *labium*, lip]
vaginometer (văj-ĭn-ŏm'ĕ-tĕr) [" + Gr. *metron*, measure]
vaginomycosis (văj"ĭn-ō-mī-kō'sĭs) [" + Gr. *mykes*, fungus, + *osis*, condition]
vaginopathy (văj"ĭ-nŏp'ă-thē) [" + Gr. *pathos*, disease, suffering]
vaginoperineal (văj"ĭn-ō-pĕr-ĭ-nē'ăl) [" + Gr. *perinaion*, perineum]
vaginoperineorrhaphy (văj"ĭn-ō-pĕr"ĭ-nē-or'ăf-ē) [" + " + *rhaphe*, seam]
vaginoperineotomy (văj"ĭn-ō-pĕr"ĭn-ē-ŏt'ō-mē) [" + " + *tome*, a cutting, slice]
vaginoperitoneal (văj"ĭn-ō-pĕr"ĭ-tō-nē'ăl)
vaginopexy (vă-jī'nō-pĕk"sē) [" + Gr. *pexis*, fixation]
vaginoplasty (vă-jī'nō-plăs"tē) [" + Gr. *plassein*, to form]
vaginoscope (văj'ĭn-ō-skōp) [" + Gr. *skopein*, to examine]
vaginoscopy (văj"ĭn-ŏs'kō-pē)
vaginosis, bacterial
vaginotome (vă-jī'nō-tōm) [" + Gr. *tome*, a cutting, slice]
vaginotomy (văj"ĭ-nŏt'ō-mē) [" + Gr. *tome*, a cutting, slice]
vaginovesical (văj"ĭ-nō-vĕs'ĭ-kăl) [" + *vesica*, bladder]
vaginovulvar (văj"ĭn-ō-vŭl'văr) [" + *vulva*, covering]

vagitis (vă-jī′tĭs) [L. *vagus*, wandering,
    + Gr. *itis*, inflammation]
vagitus (vă-jī′tŭs) [L. *vagire*, to squall]
    v. uterinus
    v. vaginalis
vagolysis (vā-gŏl′ĭ-sĭs) [L. *vagus*, wan-
    dering,   + Gr. *lysis*, dissolution]
vagolytic (vā″gō-lĭt′ĭk)
vagomimetic (vā″gō-mĭ-mĕt′ĭk) [″ +
    Gr. *mimetikos*, imitating]
vagosympathetic   (vā″gō-sĭm-pă-
    thĕt′ĭk) [″   + Gr. *sympathetikos*, suf-
    fering with]
vagotomy (vă-gŏt′ō-mē) [″   + Gr.
    tome, a cutting, slice]
    v., medical
vagotonia (vā″gō-tō′nē-ă) [″   +
    Gr. *tonos*, act of stretching, tension,
    tone]
vagotonic (vā″gō-tŏn′ĭk)
vagotropic (vā″gō-trŏp′ĭk) [″ +
    Gr. *tropos*, a turning]
vagotropism (vă-gŏt′rō-pĭzm) [″ +
    ″ + *-ismos*, condition]
vagovagal (vā″gō-vā′găl)
vagrant (vā′grănt) [L. *vagrans*]
vagus (vā′gŭs) [L., wandering]
vagus pulse
vagusstoff (vā′gŭs-stŏf) [″   + Ger.
    Stoff, substance]
Valadol
valence, valency (vā′lĕns, -lĕn-sē) [L.
    valens, powerful]
Valentin's ganglion   (văl′ĕn-tēnz)
    [Gabriel Gustav Valentin, Ger. physi-
    cian, 1810 – 1883]
valethamate bromide (văl-ĕth′ă-
    māt)
valetudinarian (văl″ē-tū″dĭn-ā′rē-ăn)
    [L., *valetudinarius*]
valgus (văl′gŭs) [L., bowlegged]
validity (vă-lĭd′ĭ-tē)
valine (văl′ēn, vā′lēn)
valinemia (văl″ĭ-nē′mē-ă)
Valisone
Valium
vallate (văl′āt) [L. *vallatus*, walled]
vallate papilla

vallecula (văl-lĕk′ū-lă) [L., a depression]
    v. cerebelli
    v. epiglottica
    v. ovata
    v. sylvii
    v. unguis
Valleix's points (văl-lāz′) [François L. I.
    Valleix, Fr. physician, 1807 – 1855]
valley fever
valley of cerebellum
vallis (văl′ĭs) [L., valley]
vallum unguis (văl′ŭm ŭng′gwĭs)
Valmid
Valpin 50
Valsalva's maneuver (văl-săl′văz)
    [Antonio Maria Valsalva, It. anatomist,
    1666 – 1723]
Valsalva's sinuses
value (văl′ū) [ME. from L. *valere*, to be of
    value]
valva (văl′vă) [sing. of L. *valvae*, leaf of
    folding doors]
valvate (văl′vāt) [L. *valva*, leaf of a fold-
    ing door]
valve (vălv) [L. *valva*, leaf of a folding
    door]
    v., aortic
    v., atrioventricular, left
    v., atrioventricular, right
    v., bicuspid
    v.'s, cardiac
    v., coronary
    v.'s, Houston's
    v., ileocecal
    v., mitral
    v. of Varolius
    v., pulmonary
    v., pyloric
    v., semilunar
    v., thebesian
    v., tricuspid
valvectomy
valvotomy (văl-vŏt′ō-mē) [″   + Gr.
    tome, a cutting, slice]
valvula (văl′vū-lă) [L., a small fold]
    v. bicuspidalis
    v. coli
    v. pylori

v. semilunaris
v. tricuspidalis
valvulae (văl′vū-lē)
v. conniventes
valvular (văl′vū-lăr) [L. *valvula*, a small fold]
valvulitis (văl″vū-li′tĭs) [″ + Gr. *itis*, inflammation]
valvuloplasty (văl′vū-lō-plăs″tē)
valvulotome (văl′vū-lō-tōm) [″ + Gr. *tome*, a cutting, slice]
valvulotomy (văl″vū-lŏt′ō-mē)
vanadium (vă-nā′dē-ŭm) [*Vanadis*, a Scandinavian goddess]
vanadiumism (vă-nā′dē-ŭm-ĭzm)
van Buren's disease (văn bū′rĕnz) [William Holme van Buren, U.S. surgeon, 1819–1883]
Vanceril
Vancocin Hydrochloride
vancomycin hydrochloride (văn′kō-mī″sĭn)
van den Bergh's test (văn″dĕn bŭrgz′) [A. A. Hymans van den Bergh, Dutch physician, 1869–1943]
van der Hoeve's syndrome [J. van der Hoeve, Dutch ophthalmologist, 1878–1952]
van der Waals forces [Johannes D. van der Waals, Dutch physicist, 1837–1923]
vanilla (vă-nĭl′ă) [Sp. *vainilla*, little sheath]
vanillin
vanillism (vă-nĭl′ĭzm)
vanillylmandelic acid
van't Hoff's rule [Jacobus Henricus van't Hoff, Dutch chemist, 1852–1911]
Vapo-Iso
vapor (vā′por) [L., steam]
vaporium (vă-pō′rē-ŭm) [L.]
vaporization (vā″por-ĭ-zā′shŭn) [L. *vapor*, steam]
vaporize (vā′por-īz)
vaporizer (vā′por-ī″zer)
vaporous (vā′por-ŭs) [L. *vapor*, steam]
vapor permeable membrane

vapotherapy (vā″pō-thĕr′ă-pē)
Vaquez's disease (vă-kāz′) [Louis Henri Vaquez, Fr. physician, 1860–1936]
variability (văr″ē-ă-bĭl′ĭ-tē)
variable (vā′rē-ă-b′l) [L. *variare*, to vary]
variance (văr′ē-ăns) [L. *variare*, to vary]
variant (văr′ē-ănt)
variate (vā′rē-āt)
variation (vā″rē-ā′shŭn)
v., continuous
v., meristic
varication (văr″ĭ-kā′shŭn)
variced
varicella (văr″ĭ-sĕl′ă) [L., a tiny spot]
v. gangrenosa
varicella-zoster immune globulin
varicelliform (văr″ĭ-sĕl′ĭ-form)
varicelloid (văr″ĭ-sĕl′oyd) [″ + Gr. *eidos*, form, shape]
varices (văr′ĭ-sēz) [L.]
variciform (văr-ĭs′ĭ-form) [L. *varix*, twisted vein, + *forma*, shape]
varicoblepharon (văr″ĭ-kō-blĕf′ă-rŏn) [″ + Gr. *blepharon*, eyelid]
varicocele (văr′ĭ-kō-sēl) [″ + Gr. *kele*, tumor, swelling]
v., ovarian
v., utero-ovarian
varicocelectomy (văr″ĭ-kō-sē-lĕk′tō-mē) [L. *varix*, twisted vein, + Gr. *kele*, tumor, swelling, + *ektome*, excision]
varicography (văr″ĭ-kŏg′ră-fē) [″ + Gr. *graphein*, to write]
varicoid (văr′ĭ-koyd) [″ + Gr. *eidos*, form, shape]
varicole (văr′ĭ-kōl)
varicomphalus (văr″ĭ-kŏm′fă-lŭs) [″ + Gr. *omphalos*, navel]
varicophlebitis (văr″ĭ-kō-flē-bī′tĭs) [″ + Gr. *phleps*, blood vessel, vein, + *itis*, inflammation]
varicose (văr′ĭ-kōs) [L. *varicosus*, full of dilated veins]
varicose ulcers
varicose veins

varicosis (văr″ĭ-kō′sĭs) [L.]
varicosity (văr″ĭ-kŏs′ĭ-tē) [L. *varix*, twisted vein]
varicotomy (văr″ĭ-kŏt′ō-mē) [" + Gr. *tome*, a cutting, slice]
varicula (văr-ĭk′ū-lă) [L., a tiny dilated vein]
variety (vă-rī′ĕ-tē) [L., *varietas*, variety]
variola (vă-rī′ō-lă) [L., pustule]
  v. minor
variolar (văr-ī′ō-lăr) [L. *variola*, pustule]
variolate (văr′ē-ō-lāt)
variolation, variolization (văr″ē-ō-lā′shŭn, văr″ē-ō-lĭ-zā′shŭn) [L. *variola*, pustule]
variolic (văr″ē-ŏl′ĭk)
varioliform (vă″rē-ŏl′ĭ-form)
varioloid (văr′ē-ō-loyd) [" + Gr. *eidos*, form, shape]
variolous (vă-rī′ō-lŭs)
varix (vā′rĭks) [L., twisted vein]
  v., aneurysmal
  v., arterial
  v., chyle
  varices, esophageal
  v., lymphaticus
  v., turbinal
varnish (văr′nĭsh)
varolian (vă-rō′lē-ăn) [Costanzo Varolio, It. surgeon, 1543 – 1575]
varolian bend
varus (vā′rŭs) [L.]
vas (văs) [L., vessel]
  v. aberrans
  v. afferens
  v. afferens glomeruli
  v. capillare
  v. deferens
  v. lymphaticum
  v. prominens
  v. spirale
vasa (vā′să) [L. *vas*, vessel]
  v. afferentia
  v. brevia
  v. efferentia
  v. praevia
  v. recta
  v. vasorum

  v. vorticosa
vasal (vā′săl) [L. *vas*, vessel]
vasalgia (vă-săl′jē-ă)
vascular (văs′kū-lăr) [L. *vasculum*, a small vessel]
vascularity (văs″kū-lăr′ĭ-tē)
vascularization (văs″kū-lăr-ĭ-zā′shŭn) [L. *vasculum*, a small vessel]
vascularize (văs′kū-lăr″ĭz) [L. *vasculum*, a small vessel]
vascular ring
vascular system
vascular tuft
vascular tumor
vasculature (văs′kū-lă-tūr″)
vasculitis (văs″kū-lī′tĭs) [" + *itis*, inflammation]
vasculogenesis (văs″kū-lō-jĕn′ĕ-sĭs) [" + Gr. *genesis*, generation, birth]
vasculomotor (văs″kū-lō-mō′tor)
vasculopathy (văs″kū-lŏp′ă-thē)
vasculum (văs′kū-lŭm) [L.]
vasectomy (văs-ĕk′tō-mē) [L. *vas*, vessel, + Gr. *ektome*, excision]
Vaseline
vasifactive (văs″ĭ-făk′tĭv) [" + *facere*, to make]
vasiform (văs′ĭ-form) [" + *forma*, shape]
vasitis (vă-sī′tĭs)
vaso- [L. *vas*, vessel]
vasoactive (văs″ō-ăk′tĭv)
vasoactive intestinal polypeptide
vasoconstriction (văs″ō-kŏn-strĭk′shŭn)
vasoconstrictive (văs″ō-kŏn-strĭk′tĭv) [" + *constrictus*, bound]
vasoconstrictor (văs″ō-kŏn-strĭk′tor) [" + *constrictor*, a binder]
vasodentin (văs″ō-dĕn′tĭn) [" + *dens*, tooth]
vasodepression (văs″ō-dē-prĕsh′ŭn) [" + *depressio*, a pressing down]
vasodepressor (văs″ō-dē-prĕs′or) [" + *depressor*, that which presses down]
Vasodilan
vasodilatation (văs″ō-dĭl-ă-tā′shŭn)

[" + *dilatare,* to enlarge]
v., antidromic
v., reflex
vasodilation (văs"ō-dĭ-lā'shŭn)
vasodilative (văs"ō-dĭ'lă-tĭv)
vasodilator (văs"ō-dĭ-lā'tor) [" +
dilatare, to enlarge]
vasoepididymostomy (văs"ō-ĕp"ĭ-
dĭd-ĭ-mŏs'tō-mē) [" + Gr. *epi,*
upon, + *didymos,* testicle, +
stoma, mouth, opening]
vasofactive (văs"ō-făk'tĭv) [" +
facere, to make]
vasoformative (văs"ō-for'mă-tĭv)
[" + *formare,* to form]
vasoganglion (văs"ō-găng'glē-ŏn)
vasography (văs-ŏg'ră-fē) [" +
Gr. *graphein,* to write]
vasohypertonic (văs"ō-hī"pĕr-tŏn'ĭk)
[" + Gr. *hyper,* over, above, excessive, + *tonikos,* pert. to tension]
vasohypotonic (văs"ō-hī"pō-tŏn'ĭk)
[" + Gr. *hypo,* under, beneath,
below, + *tonikos,* pert. to tension]
vasoinhibitor (văs"ō-ĭn-hĭb'ĭ-tor)
[" + *inhibere,* to restrain]
vasoinhibitory (văs"ō-ĭn-hĭb'ĭ-tor-ē)
vasoligation (văs"ō-lĭ-gā'shŭn) [" +
ligare, to bind]
vasomotion (văs"ō-mō'shŭn) [" +
motio, movement]
vasomotor (văs"ō-mō'tor) [" +
motor, a mover]
vasomotor epilepsy
vasomotor reflex
vasomotor spasm
vasoneuropathy (văs"ō-nū-rŏp'ă-
thē)
vasoneurosis (văs"ō-nū-rō'sĭs) [L. *vas,*
vessel, + Gr. *neuron,* nerve, +
osis, condition]
vaso-orchidostomy (văs"ō-or"kĭd-
ŏs'tō-mē) [" + Gr. *orchis,* testicle,
+ *stoma,* mouth, opening]
vasoparesis (văs"ō-păr-ē'sĭs) [" +
Gr. *parienai,* let fall]
vasopressin (văs"ō-prĕs'ĭn)
vasopressin injection

vasopressor (văs"ō-prĕs'or)
vasopuncture (văs'ō-pŭnk"chūr)
[" + *punctura,* prick]
vasoreflex (văs"ō-rē'flĕx)
vasorelaxation (văs"ō-rē-lăks-
ā'shŭn) [" + *relaxare,* to loosen]
vasorrhaphy (văs-or'ă-fē) [" +
Gr. *rhaphe,* seam]
vasosection (văs"ō-sĕk'shŭn) [" +
sectio, a cutting]
vasosensory (văs"ō-sĕn'sō-rē) [" +
sensorius, pert. to sensation]
vasospasm (văs'ō-spăzm) [" +
Gr. *spasmos,* a convulsion]
vasospastic (văs"ō-spăs'tĭk)
vasostimulant (văs"ō-stĭm'ū-lănt) [L.
vas, vessel, + *stimulans,* goading]
vasostomy (vă-sŏs'tō-mē) [" +
Gr. *stoma,* mouth, opening]
vasotomy (văs-ŏt'ō-mē) [" + Gr.
tome, a cutting, slice]
vasotonia (văs"ō-tō'nē-ă) [" +
Gr. *tonos,* act of stretching, tension,
tone]
vasotonic (văs"ō-tŏn'ĭk) [" + Gr.
tonikos, pert. to tone]
vasotribe (văs'ō-trīb) [" + Gr. *tribein,* to rub]
vasotripsy (văs'ō-trĭp"sē) [" + Gr.
tripsis, a rubbing, friction]
vasotrophic (văs"ō-trŏf'ĭk) [" +
Gr. *trophe,* nourishment]
vasotropic (văs"ō-trŏp'ĭk)
vasovagal (văs"ō-vā'găl)
vasovagal syncope
vasovasostomy (văs"ō-vă-sŏs'tō-mē)
[" + *vas,* vessel, + *stoma,*
mouth, opening]
vasovesiculectomy (văs"o-vĕ-sĭk"ū-
lĕk'tō-mē) [" + *vesicula,* a tiny
bladder, + Gr. *ektome,* excision]
vasovesiculitis (văs"ō-vĕ-sĭk"ū-lī'tĭs)
[" + *vesicula,* a tiny bladder, +
Gr. *itis,* inflammation]
Vasoxyl
vastus (văs'tŭs) [L., vast]
Vater's ampulla (fă'tĕrz) [Abraham
Vater, Ger. anatomist, 1684 – 1751]

Vater's corpuscles
Vater's papilla
vault (vawlt)
VC *vital capacity*
V-Cillin
V-Cillin K
VD *venereal disease*
VDH *valvular disease of the heart*
VDRL *Venereal Disease Research Laboratories*
vection (věk'shŭn) [L. *vectio*, a carrying]
vectis (věk'tĭs) [L., pole]
vector (věk'tor) [L., a carrier]
   v., biological
   v., mechanical
vectorcardiogram (věk"tor-kăr'dē-ō-grăm) [" + Gr. *kardia*, heart, + *gramma*, letter, piece of writing]
vectorcardiography
vectorial (věk-tō'rē-ăl) [L. *vector*, a carrier]
VEE *Venezuelan equine encephalitis*
vegan (věj'ăn)
veganism (věj'ă-nĭzm)
vegetable (věj'ě-tă-bl)
vegetal (věj'ě-tăl)
vegetarian (věj-ě-tā'rē-ăn) [from *vegetable*, coined 1847 by Vegetarian Society]
vegetarianism (věj-ě-tā'rē-ăn-ĭzm) [" + Gr. *-ismos*, condition]
vegetate (věj'ě-tāt) [LL. *vegetare*, to grow]
vegetation (věj-ě-tā'shŭn)
   v., adenoid
vegetative (věj'ě-tā"tĭv)
vegetoanimal (věj"ě-tō-ăn'ĭ-măl)
vehicle (vē'ĭ-kl) [L. *vehiculum*, that which carries]
veil (vāl) [L. *velum*, a covering]
vein (vān) [L. *vena*, vein]
velamen (vē-lā'měn) [L., veil]
   v. nativum
   v. vulvae
velamentous (věl"ă-měn'tŭs)
velamentum (věl"ă-měn'tŭm) [L., a cover]
velar (vē'lăr) [L. *velum*, a veil]

Velban
Velcro
veliform (věl'ĭ-form)
vellication (věl-ĭk-ā'shŭn) [L. *vellicare*, to twitch]
vellus (věl'ŭs) [L., fleece]
velopharyngeal (věl"ō-fă-rĭn'jē-ăl) [L. *velum*, veil, + Gr. *pharynx*, throat]
velosynthesis (věl"ō-sĭn'thěs-ĭs) [" + Gr. *synthesis*, a placing together]
Velpeau's bandage (věl-pōz') [Alfred Velpeau, Fr. surgeon, 1795–1867]
Velpeau's deformity
velum (vē'lŭm) [L., veil]
   v. palatinum
vena (vē'nă) [L.]
   v. cava inferior
   v. cava superior
venacavography (vē"nă-kā-vŏg'ră-fē)
venae comitantes [L.]
venation
venectasia (vē"něk-tā'zē-ă) [L. *vena*, a vein, + Gr. *ektasis*, dilation]
venectomy (vē-něk'tō-mē) [" + Gr. *ektome*, excision]
veneer
venenation (věn"ē-nā'shŭn) [L. *venenum*, poison]
venene (vē-nēn')
veneniferous (věn"ě-nĭf'ěr-ŭs) [" + *ferre*, to carry]
venenific (věn"ě-nĭf'ĭk) [" + *facere*, to make]
venenosalivary (věn"ě-nō-săl'ĭ-věr"ē)
venenosity (věn"ě-nŏs'ĭ-tē)
venenous (věn'ěn-ŭs) [L. *venenum*, poison]
venepuncture (věn'ē-pŭnk"chŭr) [L. *vena*, vein, + *punctura*, prick]
venereal (vē-nē'rē-ăl) [L. *venereus*]
venereal bubo
venereal collar
venereal disease
venereal sore
venereal urethritis
venereal wart
venereologist (vē-nēr"ē-ŏl'ō-jĭst)

[" + Gr. *logos*, word, reason]
venereology (vē-něr″ē-ŏl′ō-jē)
venereophobia (vē-něr″ē-ŏ-fō′bē-ă)
[L. *venereus*, pert. to sexual intercourse, + Gr. *phobos*, fear]
venery (věn′ěr-ē) [L. *venerus*, pert. to Venus]
venesection (věn″ē-sěk′shŭn) [L. *vena*, vein, + *sectio*, a cutting]
venin(e) (věn′ĭn) [L. *venenum*, poison]
venipuncture (věn′ĭ-pŭnk″chūr) [L. *vena*, vein, + *punctura*, prick]
venisection (věn″ĭ-sěk′shŭn)
venisuture (věn′ĭ-sū″chūr) [" + *sutura*, seam]
venoatrial (vē″nō-āt′rē-ăl) [" + *atrium*, corridor]
venoauricular (vē″nō-aw-rĭk′ū-lăr) [" + *auricula*, little ear]
venoclysis (vē-nŏk′lĭ-sĭs) [" + Gr. *klysis*, a washing]
venofibrosis (vē″nō-fĭ-brō′sĭs)
venogram (vē′nō-grăm) [" + Gr. *gramma*, letter, piece of writing]
venography (vē-nŏg′ră-fē) [" + Gr. *graphein*, to write]
venom (věn′ŏm) [L. *venenum*, poison]
  v., Russell's viper
  v., snake
venomization (věn″ŭm-ĭ-zā′shŭn)
venomosalivary (věn″ō-mō-săl′ĭ-věr″ē)
venomotor (vē″nō-mō′tor) [L. *vena*, vein, + *motus*, moving]
venomous (věn′ō-mŭs)
venomous snake
veno-occlusive (vē″nō-ŏ-kloo′sĭv)
venoperitoneostomy (vē″nō-pěr″ĭ-tō″nē-ŏs′tō-mē) [L. *vena*, vein, + Gr. *peritonaion*, stretched around or over, + *stoma*, mouth, opening]
venopressor (vē′nō-prěs″or) [" + *pressor*, that which squeezes]
venosclerosis (vē″nō-sklě-rō′sĭs) [" + Gr. *sklerosis*, a hardening]
venose (vē′nōs)
venosinal (vē″nō-sī′năl)
venosity (vē-nŏs′ĭ-tē) [L. *vena*, vein]

venospasm (vē′nō-spăzm) [" + Gr. *spasmos*, a convulsion]
venostasis (vē″nō-stā′sĭs) [" + Gr. *stasis*, standing still]
venostat (vē′nō-stăt) [" + Gr. *statikos*, standing]
venothrombotic (vē″nō-thrŏm-bŏt′ĭk)
venotomy (vē-nŏt′ō-mē) [" + Gr. *tome*, a cutting, slice]
venous (vē′nŭs) [L. *vena*, vein]
venous blood
venous hum
venous hyperemia
venous return
venous sinus
venous sinus of sclera
venous thrombosis
venovenostomy (vē″nō-vē-nŏs′tō-mē) [" + " + Gr. *stoma*, mouth, opening]
vent (věnt) [O. Fr. *fente*, slit]
  v., alveolar
venter (věn′těr) [L., belly]
ventilation (věn″tĭ-lā′shŭn) [L. *ventilare*, to air]
  v., continuous positive-pressure
  v., intermittent positive-pressure
  v., pulmonary
ventilation coefficient
ventilation rate
ventilation tube
ventilator
ventouse (věn-toos′) [Fr.]
ventrad (věn′trăd) [L. *venter*, belly, + *ad*, to]
ventral (věn′trăl) [L. *ventralis*, pert. to the belly]
ventral hernia
ventralis (věn-trā′lĭs) [L.]
ventricle (věn′trĭk-l) [L. *ventriculus*, a little belly]
  v., aortic
  v., fifth
  v., fourth
  v., lateral
  v., left
  v., Morgagni's
  v. of Arantius

v. of larynx
v., pineal
v., right
v., third

ventricornu (věn‴trĭ-kor′nū) [L. *venter*, belly, + *cornu*, horn]

ventricose (věn′trĭ-kōs) [L. *ventricosus*, big-bellied]

ventricular (věn-trĭk′ū-lăr) [L. *ventriculus*, a little belly]

ventricular assist pumping

ventricular compliance

ventricular folds

ventricular ligament

ventricular septal defect

ventriculitis (věn-trĭk″ū-lī′tĭs) [″ + Gr. *itis*, inflammation]

ventriculoatriostomy (věn-trĭk″ū-lō-ā″trē-ŏs′tō-mē) [″ + *atrium*, corridor, + Gr. *stoma*, mouth, opening]

ventriculocisternostomy (věn-trĭk″ū-lō-sĭs″tĕr-nŏs′tō-mē) [″ + *cisterna*, box, chest, + Gr. *stoma*, mouth, opening]

ventriculocordectomy (věn-trĭk″ū-lō-kor-děk′tō-mē) [″ + Gr. *khorde*, cord, + *ektome*, excision]

ventriculogram (věn-trĭk′ū-lō-grăm) [″ + Gr. *gramma*, letter, piece of writing]

ventriculography (věn-trĭk″ū-lŏg′ră-fē) [″ + Gr. *graphein*, to write]

ventriculometry (věn-trĭk″ū-lŏm′ě-trē) [″ + Gr. *metron*, measure]

ventriculonector (věn-trĭk″ū-lō-něk′tor) [L. *ventriculus*, a little belly, + *nector*, a joiner]

ventriculopuncture (věn-trĭk′ū-lō-pŭnk″tūr) [″ + *punctura*, prick]

ventriculoscopy (věn-trĭk″ū-lŏs′kō-pē) [″ + Gr. *skopein*, to examine]

ventriculostomy (věn-trĭk″ū-lŏs′tō-mē) [″ + Gr. *stoma*, mouth, opening]

ventriculosubarachnoid (věn-trĭk″ū-lō-sŭb″ă-răk′noyd)

ventriculotomy (věn-trĭk″ū-lŏt′ō-mē) [″ + Gr. *tome*, a cutting, slice]

ventriculus (věn-trĭk′ū-lŭs) [L., a little belly]

v. tertius

ventricumbent (věn‴trĭ-kŭm′běnt) [L. *venter*, belly, + *cumbere*, to lie]

ventriduct (věn′trĭ-dŭkt) [″ + *ducere*, to lead]

ventriduction (věn‴trĭ-dŭk′shŭn)

ventrimeson (věn‴trĭ-mēs′ŏn) [″ + Gr. *mesos*, middle]

ventripyramid (věn‴trĭ-pĭr′ă-mĭd) [″ + Gr. *pyramis*, a pyramid]

ventro- [L. *venter*, belly]

ventrocystorrhaphy (věn‴trō-sĭs-tor′ă-fē) [″ + Gr. *kystis*, sac, + *rhaphe*, seam]

ventrodorsal (věn‴trō-dor′săl) [″ + *dorsum*, back]

ventrofixation (věn‴trō-fĭks-ā′shŭn) [″ + *fixatio*, to fix]

ventrohysteropexy (věn‴trō-hĭs′tĕr-ō-pěks″ē) [″ + Gr. *hystera*, womb, + *pexis*, fixation]

ventroinguinal (věn‴trō-ĭng′gwĭ-năl) [″ + *inguen*, groin]

ventrolateral (věn‴trō-lăt′ĕr-ăl) [″ + *latus*, side]

ventromedial (věn‴trō-mē′dě-ăl) [″ + *medianus*, median]

ventroptosia, **ventroptosis** (věn‴trŏp-tō′sē-ă, -sĭs) [″ + Gr. *ptosis*, fall, falling]

ventroscopy (věn-trŏs′kō-pē) [L. *venter*, belly, + Gr. *skopein*, to examine]

ventrose (věn′trōs)

ventrosity (věn-trŏs′ĭ-tē)

ventrosuspension (věn‴trō-sŭs-pěn′shŭn) [″ + *suspensio*, a hanging]

ventrotomy (věn-trŏt′ō-mē) [″ + Gr. *tome*, a cutting, slice]

ventrovesicofixation (věn‴trō-věs″ĭ-kō-fĭks-ā′shŭn) [″ + L. *vesica*, bladder, + *fixare*, to fix]

Venturi mask [Giovanni Battista Venturi, It. scientist, 1746–1822]

venturimeter (věn‴tūr-ĭm′ě-ter)

venula (věn'ū-lă) [L., little vein]
venule (věn'ūl) [L., *venula*, little vein]
Venus, crown of
Venus, mount of
Venus's collar (vē'nŭs) [L., the Roman goddess of love]
verbigeration (věr-bĭj"ĕr-ā'shŭn) [L. *verbigerare*, to chatter]
verbomania (věr"bō-mā'nē-ă) [L. *verba*, word, + Gr. *mania*, madness]
Vercyte
verdigris (věr"dĭ-grĭs) [O. Fr. *vert de Grece*, green of Greece]
verdigris poisoning
verdohemoglobin (věr"dō-hēm'ō-glōb"ĭn)
Verga's ventricle (věr'găz) [Andrea Verga, It. neurologist, 1811–1895]
verge (věrj)
    v., anal
vergence (věr'jĕns) [L. *vergere*, to bend]
Verheyen's stars (fěr-hī'ĕns) [Philippe Verheyen, Flemish anatomist, 1648–1710]
vermicidal (věr"mĭ-sī'dăl) [L. *vermis*, worm, + *cida* fr. *caedere*, to kill]
vermicide (věr'mĭ-sīd)
vermicular (věr-mĭk'ū-lăr) [L. *vermicularis*]
vermicular movements
vermicular pulse
vermiculation (věr-mĭk"ū-lā'shŭn) [L. *vermiculare*, to wriggle]
vermicule (věr'mĭ-kūl) [L. *vermiculus*, a small worm]
vermiculose, vermiculous (věr-mĭk'ū-lōs, věr-mĭk'ū-lŭs) [L. *vermicularis*, wormlike]
vermiform (věr'mĭ-form) [L. *vermis*, worm, + *forma*, shape]
vermiform appendix
vermifugal (věr-mĭf'ū-găl) [" + *fugare*, to put to flight]
vermifuge (věr'mĭ-fūj)
vermilion border (věr-mĭl"yŏn) [ME. *vermilioun*, bright red]

vermilionectomy (věr-mĭl"yŏn-ĕk'tō-mē) [" + Gr. *ektome*, excision]
vermin (věr'mĭn) [L. *vermis*, worm]
verminal (věr'mĭ-năl)
vermination (věr"mĭn-ā'shŭn)
verminosis (věr"mĭn-ō'sĭs) [" + Gr. *osis*, condition]
verminous (věr'mĭn-ŭs)
vermiphobia (věr"mĭ-fō'bē-ă) [" + Gr. *phobos*, fear]
vermis (věr'mĭs) [L. worm]
    v. cerebelli
    v., inferior
    v., superior
Vermox
vernal (věr'năl) [L. *vernalis*, pert. to spring]
Vernet's syndrome (věr-nāz') [Maurice Vernet, Fr. physician, b. 1887]
vernix (věr'nĭks) [L.]
    v. caseosa
verruca (věr-roo'kă) [L., wart]
    v. acuminata
    v. digitata
    v. filiformis
    v. gyri hippocampi
    v. plana
    v. plantaris
    v. vulgaris
verruciform (vě-roo'sĭ-form) [L. *verruca*, wart, + *forma*, shape]
verrucose, verrucous (věr'roo-kōs, věr-roo'kŭs) [L. *verrucosus*, wartlike]
verrucosis (věr"oo-kō'sĭs) [L. *verruca*, wart, + Gr. *osis*, condition]
verruga peruana (vě-roo'gă pěr-wăn'ă) [Sp., Peruvian wart]
Versapen
Versapen K
Versed
Versene
versicolor (věr'sĭ-kŏl"or) [L., of changing colors]
version (věr'zhŭn) [L. *versio*, a turning]
    v., bipolar
    v., cephalic
    v., combined
    v., external

v., internal
v., pelvic
v., podalic
v., spontaneous
vertebra (vĕr'tĕ-bră) [L.]
v., basilar
v., cervical
v., coccygeal
v. dentata
v., false
v., fixed
v., flexion
v., lumbar
v. magnum
v., odontoid
v. prominens
v., rotation
v., sacral
v., sternal
v., thoracic
v., true
vertebral (vĕr'tĕ-brăl) [L. vertebra, vertebra]
vertebral arch
vertebral canal
vertebral column
vertebral foramen
vertebral groove
vertebral notch
vertebral ribs
vertebrarium (vĕr"tĕ-brā'rē-ŭm) [L.]
Vertebrata (vĕr"tĕ-brā'tă)
vertebrate (vĕr'tĕ-brāt) [L. vertebra, vertebra]
vertebrated (vĕr'tĕ-brāt"ĕd)
vertebrectomy (vĕr"tĕ-brĕk'tō-mē) [" + Gr. ektome, excision]
vertebroarterial (vĕr"tĕ-brō-ăr-tē'rē-ăl) [" + Gr. arteria, artery]
vertebrobasilar (vĕr"tĕ-brō-băs'ĭ-lăr) [" + basilaris, basilar]
vertebrochondral (vĕr"tĕ-brō-kŏn'drăl) [" + Gr. chondros, cartilage]
vertebrocostal (vĕr"tĕ-brō-kŏs'tăl) [" + costa, rib]
vertebrofemoral (vĕr"tĕ-brō-fĕm'or-ăl) [" + femur, thigh]

vertebroiliac (vĕr"tĕ-brō-ĭl'ē-ăk) [" + iliacus, pert. to ilium]
vertebromammary (vĕr"tĕ-brō-măm'mă-rē) [" + mamma, breast]
vertebrosacral (vĕr"tĕ-brō-sā'krăl) [" + sacrum, sacred]
vertebrosternal (vĕr"tĕ-brō-stĕr'năl) [" + Gr. sternon, chest]
vertex (vĕr'tĕks) [L., summit]
v. cordis
vertical (vĕr'tĭ-kăl) [L. verticalis, summit]
verticalis (vĕr"tĭ-kā'lĭs) [L.]
verticality
verticillate (vĕr-tĭs'ĭl-āt, -tĭs-ĭl'āt) [L. verticillus, a little whirl]
verticomental (vĕr"tĭ-kō-mĕn'tăl) [L. vertex, summit, + mentum, chin]
vertiginous (vĕr-tĭj'ĭ-nŭs) [L. vertiginosus, one suffering from dizziness]
vertigo (vĕr'tĭ-gō, vĕr-tī'gō) [L. vertigo, a turning round]
v., auditory
v., central
v., cerebral
v., epileptic
v., essential
v., gastric
v., hysterical
v., labyrinthine
v., laryngeal
v., objective
v., ocular
v., organic
v., peripheral
v., positional; v., postural
v., subjective
v., toxic
v., vestibular
verumontanitis (vĕr"ū-mŏn"tăn-ī'tĭs) [L. veru, spit, dart, + montanus, mountainous, + Gr. itis, inflammation]
verumontanum (vĕr"ū-mŏn-tā'nŭm) [L. veru, spit, dart, + montanus, mountainous]
very low density lipoproteins
vesalianum (vĕs-ā"lē-ā'nŭm) [Andreas Vesalius, Flemish anatomist and physi-

cian, 1514–1564]
Vesalius, foramen of   (vĕs-ā'lē-ŭs)
[Andreas Vesalius]
Vesalius, vein of
vesica   (vĕ-sī'kă) [L.]
  v. fellea
  v. prostatica
  v. urinaria
vesical   (vĕs'ĭ-kăl)
vesical reflex
vesicant   (vĕs'ĭ-kănt) [L. vesicare, to blister]
vesication   (vĕs"ĭ-kā'shŭn)
vesicatory   (vĕs'ĭ-kă-tor"ē)
vesicle   (vĕs'ĭ-kl) [L. vesicula, a tiny bladder]
  v., allantoic
  v., auditory
  v., blastodermic
  v.'s, brain
  v.'s, brain, primary
  v.'s, cerebral
  v., chorionic
  v., compound
  v.'s, encephalic
  v., lens
  v.'s, multilocular
  v.'s, optic
  v., otic
  v., seminal
  v., umbilical
vesico-   (vĕs'ĭ-kō) [L. vesica, bladder]
vesicoabdominal   (vĕs"ĭ-kō-ăb-dŏm'ĭ-năl) [" + abdomen, belly]
vesicocele   (vĕs'ĭ-kō-sēl") [L. vesica, bladder, + Gr. kele, tumor, swelling]
vesicocervical   (vĕs"ĭ-kō-sĕr'vĭ-kăl) [" + cervix, neck]
vesicoclysis   (vĕs"ĭ-kŏk'lĭ-sĭs) [" + Gr. klysis, a washing]
vesicoenteric   (vĕs"ĭ-kō-ĕn-tĕr'ĭk) [" + Gr. enteron, intestine]
vesicofixation   (vĕs"ĭ-kō-fĭks-ā'shŭn) [L. vesica, bladder, + fixatio, a fixing]
vesicointestinal   (vĕs"ĭ-kō-ĭn-tĕs'tĭ-năl)
vesicoprostatic   (vĕs'ĭ-kō-prŏs-tăt'ĭk) [" + Gr. prostates, prostate]

vesicopubic   (vĕs"ĭ-kō-pū'bĭk) [" + NL. (os) pubis, bone of the groin]
vesicopustule   (vĕs"ĭ-kō-pŭs'tūl) [" + pustula, blister]
vesicosigmoid   (vĕs"ĭ-kō-sĭg'moyd) [" + Gr. sigmoid, shaped like Gr. letter S]
vesicosigmoidostomy   (vĕs"ĭ-kō-sĭg"moy-dŏs'tō-mē) [" + " + stoma, mouth, opening]
vesicospinal   (vĕs"ĭ-kō-spī'năl) [" + spina, thorn]
vesicostomy   (vĕs"ĭ-kŏs'tō-mē) [" + Gr. stoma, mouth, opening]
vesicotomy   (vĕs"ĭ-kŏt'ō-mē) [" + Gr. tome, a cutting, slice]
vesicoumbilical   (vĕs"ĭ-kō-ŭm-bĭl'ĭ-kăl) [" + umbilicus, navel]
vesicoureteral   (vĕs"ĭ-kō-ū-rē'tĕr-ăl) [" + Gr. oureter, ureter]
vesicouterine   (vĕs"ĭ-kō-ū'tĕr-ĭn) [" + uterinus, pert. to the womb]
vesicouterine pouch
vesicouterovaginal   (vĕs"ĭ-kō-ū"tĕr-ō-văj'ĭ-năl) [" + uterus, womb, + vagina, sheath]
vesicovaginal   (vĕs"ĭ-kō-văj'ĭ-năl) [" + vagina, sheath]
vesicovaginorectal   (vĕs"ĭ-kō-văj"ĭ-nō-rĕk'tăl) [" + vagina, sheath, + rectum, straight]
vesicula   (vĕ-sĭk'ū-lă) [L.]
  v. seminalis
vesicular   (vĕ-sĭk'ū-lăr)
vesicular breathing
vesicular eczema
vesicular murmur
vesicular rale
vesicular resonance
vesiculase   (vĕ-sĭk'ū-lās)
vesiculated   (vĕ-sĭk'ū-lāt"ĕd)
vesiculation   (vĕ-sĭk"ū-lā'shŭn) [L. vesicula, a tiny bladder]
vesiculectomy   (vĕ-sĭk"ū-lĕk'tō-mē) [" + Gr. ektome, excision]
vesiculiform   (vĕ-sĭk'ū-lĭ-form) [" + forma, shape]
vesiculitis   (vĕ-sĭk"ū-lī'tĭs) [" + Gr.

itis, inflammation]

vesiculobronchial (vĕ-sĭk″ū-lō-brŏng′kĕ-ăl) [″ + Gr. *bronchos,* windpipe]

vesiculocavernous (vĕ-sĭk″ū-lō-kăv′ĕr-nŭs) [″ + *caverna,* a hollow]

vesiculogram (vĕ-sĭk′ū-lō-grăm) [″ + Gr. *gramma,* letter, piece of writing]

vesiculography (vĕ-sĭk″ū-lŏg′ră-fē) [″ + Gr. *graphein,* to write]

vesiculopapular (vĕ-sĭk″ū-lō-păp′ū-lăr) [″ + *papula,* pimple]

vesiculopustular (vĕ-sĭk″ū-lō-pŭs′tū-lăr) [″ + *pustula,* blister]

vesiculotomy (vĕ-sĭk″ū-lŏt′ō-mē) [″ + Gr. *tome,* a cutting, slice]

vesiculotubular (vĕ-sĭk″ū-lō-tū′bū-lăr) [″ + *tubularis,* like a tube]

vesiculotympanic (vĕ-sĭk″ū-lō-tĭm-păn′ĭk) [″ + Gr. *tympanon,* drum]

Vespidae [L. *vespa,* wasp]

Vesprin

vessel (vĕs′ĕl) [O. Fr. from L. *vascellum,* a little vessel]
  v.'s, absorbent
  v., blood
  v.'s, chyliferous
  v., collateral
  v.'s, great
  v., lacteal
  v.'s, lymphatic
  v.'s, nutrient
  v., radicular

vestibular (vĕs-tĭb′ū-lăr) [L. *vestibulum,* vestibule]

vestibular bulbs

vestibular nerve

vestibule (vĕs′tĭ-būl)
  v., aortic; v. of aorta
  v. of ear
  v. of larynx
  v. of mouth
  v. of nose
  v. of pharynx
  v. of vagina

vestibulocochlear nerve (vĕs-tĭb″ū-lō-kŏk′lē-ăr) [L. *vestibulum,* vestibule, + Gr. *kokhlos,* land snail]

vestibuloplasty (vĕs-tĭb′ū-lō-plăs″tē) [″ + Gr. *plassein,* to mold]

vestibulotomy (vĕs-tĭb″ū-lŏt′ō-mē) [″ + Gr. *tome,* a cutting, slice]

vestibulourethral (vĕs-tĭb″ū-lō-ū-rē′thrăl) [″ + Gr. *ourethra,* urethra]

vestibulum (vĕs-tĭb′ū-lŭm) [L.]

vestige (vĕs′tĭj) [L. *vestigium,* footstep]

vestigial (vĕs-tĭj′ē-ăl)

vestigium (vĕs-tĭj′ē-ŭm) [L., a footstep]

veta (vā′tă) [Sp.]

veterinarian (vĕt″ĕr-ĭ-nār′ē-ăn)

veterinary (vĕt′ĕr-ĭ-nār′ē)

veterinary medicine

VF *ventricular fibrillation; vocal fremitus*

V.H. *viral hepatitis*

via (vē′ă, vī′ă) [L.]

viability (vī″ă-bĭl′ĭ-tē) [L. *vita,* life, + *habilis,* fit]

viable (vī′ă-bl) [L. *vita,* life, + *habilis,* fit]

vial (vī′ăl) [Gr. *phiale,* a drinking cup]

vibex (vī′bĕks) [L. *vibix,* mark of a blow]

Vibramycin

vibrapuncture (vī″bră-pŭnk′tūr)

Vibra-Tabs

vibratile (vī′bră-tĭl) [L. *vibrare,* to shake]

vibration (vī-brā′shŭn)

vibrative (vī′bră-tĭv)

vibrator (vī′brā-tor) [L. *vibrator,* a shaker]
  v., vaginal
  v., whole body

vibratory (vī′bră-tō″rē) [L. *vibrator,* a shaker]

vibratory sense

Vibrio (vĭb′rē-ō)
  V. cholerae
  V. fetus

vibrio (vĭb′rē-ō)

vibriocidal (vĭb″rē-ō-sī′dăl)

vibrion (vē″brē-ŏn′) [Fr.]

vibriosis (vĭb″rē-ō′sĭs)

vibrissae (vī-brĭs′ē) [L. *vibrissa,* that which shakes]

vibromassage (vī″brō-mă-săj′)

vibromasseur (vī″brō-mă-sūr′)

vibrometer (vī-brŏm′ĕt-ĕr) [L. *vibrare,*

to shake,   +   Gr. *metron*, measure]
vibrotherapeutics   (vī″brō-thĕr″ă-
pū′tĭks) ["   +   Gr. *therapeutikos*,
treating]
vicarious   (vī-kā′rē-ŭs) [L. *vicarius*,
change, alternation]
vicarious learning
vicarious menstruation
vicarious respiration
Vicq d'Azyr's tract   (vĭk dă-zĕrz′) [Felix
Vicq d'Azyr, Fr. anatomist, 1748–
1794]
vidarabine   (vī-dăr′ă-bēn)
video display terminal
videognosis   (vĭd″ē-ŏg-nō′sĭs) [L. *vi-
dere*, to see,   +   Gr. *gnosis*, knowl-
edge]
vidian artery   (vĭd′ē-ăn) [Guido Guidi
(L. *Vidius*), It. physician, 1500–1569]
vidian canal
vidian nerve
vigil   (vĭj′ĭl) [L., awake]
    v., coma
vigilambulism   (vĭj″ĭl-ăm′bū-lĭzm) ["   +
ambulare, to walk,   +   Gr. *-ismos*,
condition]
vigilance   (vĭj′ĭ-lăns) [L. *vigilantia*, waste-
fulness]
vigintinormal   (vī-jĭn″tĭ-nor′măl) [L. *vi-
ginti*, twenty,   +   *normal*, rule]
vigor   (vĭg′or) [L.]
Villaret's syndrome   (vē-lăr-āz′)
[Maurice Villaret, Fr. neurologist,
1877–1946]
villi   (vĭl′ī) [L.]
    v., chorionic
villiferous   (vĭl-ĭf′ĕr-ŭs) ["   +   *ferre*, to
bear]
villoma   (vī-lō′mă) [L. *villus*, tuft of hair,
+   Gr. *oma*, tumor]
villose, villous   (vĭl′ōs, vĭl′ŭs) [L. *villus*,
tuft of hair]
villositis   (vĭl″ōs-ī′tĭs) ["   +   Gr. *itis*,
inflammation]
villosity   (vī-lŏs′ĭ-tē)
villus   (vĭl′ŭs) [L., tuft of hair]
    v., arachnoid
    v., chorionic

    v., intestinal
    v., synovial
villusectomy   (vĭl″ŭs-ĕk′tō-mē) ["   +
Gr. *ektome*, excision]
vinblastine sulfate   (vĭn-blăs′tēn)
vinca   (vĭn′kă)
Vincent's angina   (vĭn′sĕnts ăn-jī′nă)
[Henri Vincent, Fr. physician, 1862–
1950]
vincristine sulfate   (vĭn-krĭs′tēn)
vinculum   (vĭn′kū-lŭm) [L., to bind, tie]
    v. tendinum
vinegar   (vĭn′ē-găr) [ME. *vinegre*, from
Fr. *vin*, wine,   +   *aigre*, sour]
vinic   (vī′nĭk) [L. *vinum*, wine]
vinous   (vī′nŭs) [L. *vinum*, wine]
vinum   (vī′nŭm) [L.]
vinyl   (vī′nĭl)
    v. chloride
    v. cyanide
    v. ether
Vioform
violaceous   (vī″ē-lā′shŭs) [L. *violaceus*,
violet]
violate   (vī′ē-lāt″) [L. *violare*, to injure]
violence   (vī′ō-lĕnts) [L. *violentia*]
violet   (vī′ō-lĕt) [ME. *violett*, from L. *viola*,
violet]
    v., gentian
violet blindness
viomycin   (vī-ō-mī′sĭn)
viosterol   (vī-ŏs′tĕr-ōl)
viper   (vī′pĕr)
Vira-A
viraginity   (vĭr″ă-jĭn′ĭ-tē) [L. *virago*, an
amazon or manlike woman]
viral
viral interference
Virchow's node   (vēr′kōz) [Rudolf Virchow, Ger. pathologist, 1821–1902]
viremia   (vī″rēm′ē-ă)
vires   (vī′rēs)
virgin   (vĕr′jĭn) [L. *virgo*, a maiden]
virginal   (vĕr′jĭn-ăl) [L. *virgo*, a maiden]
virginal membrane
virginity   (vĕr-jĭn′ĭt-ē) [L. *virginitas*, maid-
enhood]
viricidal   (vī-rĭ-sī′dăl) [L. *virus*, poison,

+ *cida* fr. *caedere,* to kill]
viricide (vĭr'ĭ-sīd)
virile (vĭr'ĭl) [L. *virilis,* masculine]
virile reflex
virilescence (vĭr-ĭl-ĕs'ĕns) [L. *virilis,* masculine]
virilia (vĭr-ĭl'ē-ă) [L.]
virilism (vĭr'ĭl-ĭzm) [" + Gr. *-ismos,* condition]
virility (vĭr-ĭl'ĭ-tē) [L. *virilitas,* masculinity]
virilization (vĭr"ĭ-lĭ-zā'shŭn)
virion (vĭ'rē-ŏn, vī'rē-ŏn)
viripotent (vī-rĭp'ō-tĕnt) [L. *viripotens*]
viroids
virology (vī-rŏl'ō-jē) [L. *virus,* poison, + Gr. *logos,* word, reason]
viropexis (vī"rō-pĕk'sĭs) [" + Gr. *pexis,* fixation]
Viroptic
virose, virous (vī'rōs, vī'rŭs) [L. *virus,* poison]
virtual (vĕr'tū-ăl) [L. *virtus,* capacity]
virucidal (vĭr-ū-sī'dăl) [L. *virus,* poison, + *cida* fr. *caedere,* to kill]
virucide
virulence (vĭr'ū-lĕns) [LL. *virulentia,* stench]
virulent (vĭr'ū-lĕnt) [L. *virulentus,* poison]
viruliferous (vĭr-ū-lĭf'ĕr-ŭs) [L. *virus,* poison, + *ferre,* to bear]
viruria (vĭr-ūr'ē-ă) [" + Gr. *ouron,* urine]
virus (vī'rŭs) [L., poison]
  v., arbor
  v., attenuated
  v., bacterial
  v., chikungunya
  v., coxsackie
  v., cytomegalic
  v., defective
  v., EB
  v., ECHO *enteric cytopathogenic human orphan*
  v., enteric
  v., enteric orphan
  v., filtrable
  v. fixé, v., fixed
  v., helper

  v., hepadna-
  v., herpes
  v., human immunodeficiency
  v., latent
  v., lytic
  v., masked
  v.'s, neurotropic
  v.'s, orphan
  v., parainfluenza
  v., plant
  v., pox
  v., respiratory syncytial
  v., slow
  v., street
  v., tumor
virusemia (vī"rŭs-ēm'ē-ă) [" + Gr. *haima,* blood]
virustatic (vĭr"ū-stăt'ĭk) [" + Gr. *statikos,* bringing to a standstill]
vis (vĭs) [L., strength]
  v. afronte
  v. formativa
  v. medicatrix naturae
viscera (vĭs'ĕr-ă) [L.]
viscerad (vĭs'ĕr-ăd) [" + *ad,* toward]
visceral (vĭs'ĕr-ăl) [L. *viscera,* body organs]
visceral arches
visceral cavity
visceral clefts
visceralgia (vĭs"ĕr-ăl'jē-ă) [" + Gr. *algos,* pain]
visceral skeleton
viscerimotor (vĭs"ĕr-ĭ-mō'tor) [" + *motor,* mover]
viscero- (vĭs'ĕr-ō) [L. *viscera,* body organs]
viscerocranium (vĭs"ĕr-ō-krā'nē-ŭm)
viscerogenic (vĭs"ĕr-ō-jĕn'ĭk) [" + Gr. *gennan,* to produce]
visceroinhibitory (vĭs"ĕr-ō-ĭn-hĭb'ĭ-tō-rē) [" + *inhibere,* to restrain]
visceromegaly (vĭs"ĕr-ō-mĕg'ă-lē) [" + Gr. *megalos,* great]
visceromotor (vĭs"ĕr-ō-mō'tor) [L. *viscera,* body organs, + *motor,* a mover]

visceromotor reflex
visceroparietal (vĭs"ĕr-ō-pă-rī'ĕ-tăl)
[" + *paries*, wall]
visceroperitoneal (vĭs"ĕr-ō-pĕr"ĭ-tō-
nē'ăl) [" + Gr. *peritonaion*,
stretched around or over]
visceropleural (vĭs"ĕr-ō-ploo'răl)
[" + Gr. *pleura*, a side]
visceroptosis (vĭs"ĕr-ŏp-tō'sĭs) [" +
Gr. *ptosis*, fall, falling]
visceroreceptors (vĭs"ĕr-ō-rē-
sĕp'torz)
viscerosensory (vĭs"ĕr-ō-sĕn'sō-rē)
[" + *sensorius*, sensory]
viscerosensory reflex
visceroskeletal (vĭs"ĕr-ō-skĕl'ĕt-ăl)
[" + Gr. *skeleton*, a dried-up body]
viscerosomatic (vĭs"ĕr-ō-sō-măt'ĭk)
[" + Gr. *soma*, body]
viscerosomatic reaction
viscerotome (vĭs'ĕr-ō-tōm) [" +
Gr. *tome*, a cutting, slice]
viscerotonia (vĭs"ĕr-ō-tōn'ē-ă) [" +
Gr. *tonos*, act of stretching, tension,
tone]
viscerotrophic (vĭs"ĕr-ō-trŏf'ĭk) ["
+ Gr. *trophe*, nourishment]
viscerotropic (vĭs"ĕr-ō-trŏp'ĭk) ["
+ Gr. *tropos*, a turn]
viscerovisceral reaction (vĭs"ĕr-ō-
vĭs'ĕr-ăl)
viscid (vĭs'ĭd) [L. *viscum*, mistletoe, bird-
lime]
viscidity (vĭ-sĭd'ĭ-tē)
viscometer (vĭs-kŏm'ĕ-tĕr)
viscosimeter (vĭs"kŏs-ĭm'ĕ-tĕr) [LL. *viscosus*, viscous, + Gr. *metron*, mea-
sure]
viscosimetry (vĭs"kō-sĭm'ĕ-trē)
viscosity (vĭs"kŏs'ĭ-tē) [LL. *viscosus*, vis-
cous]
v., specific
viscous (vĭs'kŭs)
viscus (vĭs'kŭs) [L., body organ]
visibility (vĭz"ĭ-bĭl'ĭ-tē) [L. *visibilitas*]
visible (vĭz'ĭ-bl) [L. *visibilis*]
visile (vĭz'ĭl) [L. *visum*, seeing]
vision (vĭzh'ŭn) [L. *visio*, a seeing]

v., achromatic
v., artificial
v., binocular
v., central
v., day
v., dichromatic
v., double
v., field of
v., half
v., indirect
v., monocular
v., multiple
v., night
v., oscillating
v., peripheral
v., phantom
v., tunnel
visit
Visiting Nurse Association
Vistaril Pamoate
Vistaril Parenteral
visual (vĭzh'ū-ăl) [L. *visio*, a seeing]
visual acuity
visual angle
visual axis
visual cone
visual field
visual function
visualization (vĭzh"ū-ăl-ĭ-zā'shŭn)
visualize (vĭzh'ū-ăl-īz)
visual plane
visual point
visual yellow
visuoauditory (vĭzh"ū-ō-aw'dĭ-tor"ē)
[L. *visio*, a seeing, + *auditorius*,
pert. to hearing]
visuognosis (vĭzh"ū-ŏg-nō'sĭs) [" +
Gr. *gnosis*, knowledge]
visuopsychic (vĭzh"ū-ō-sī'kĭk) [" +
Gr. *psyche*, soul, mind]
visuosensory (vĭzh"ū-ō-sĕn'sō-rē) [L.
visio, a seeing, + *sensorius*, sen-
sory]
vita glass (vī'tă-glăs) [L. *vita*, life, +
AS. *glaes*, glass]
vital (vī'tăl) [L. *vitalis*, pert. to life]
vital capacity
vital capacity, timed

vital center

vitalism (vī'tăl-ĭzm) [" + Gr. -ismos, condition]

vitalist (vī'tăl-ĭst) [L. vitalis, pert. to life]

vitalistic (vī-tăl-ĭs'tĭk)

vitality (vī-tăl'ĭ-tē)

vitalize (vī'tăl-īz)

vital signs

vital statistics

vitamer (vī'tă-mĕr)

vitamin (vī'tă-mĭn) [L. vita, life, + amine]

   v., antiberiberi

   v., antidermatitis

   v., antihemorrhagic

   v., anti-infective

   v., antineuritic

   v., antipellagra

   v., antirachitic

   v., antiscorbutic

   v., antixerophthalmic

   v., coagulation

vitamin A

vitamin A_1

vitamin A_2

vitamin B complex

vitamin B_1

vitamin B_2

vitamin B_6

vitamin B_{12}

vitamin C

vitamin D

vitamin E

vitamin K

vitamin loss

vitaminoid (vī'tă-mĭn-oyd) [vitamin + Gr. eidos, form, shape]

vitaminology (vī'tă-mĭn-ŏl'ō-jē)

vitellary (vĭt'ĕl-ā-rē) [L. vitellus, yolk of an egg]

vitellin (vī-tĕl'ĭn)

vitelline (vī-tĕl'ēn)

vitelline circulation

vitelline duct

vitelline membrane

vitelline veins

vitellogenesis (vī'tĕl-ō-jĕn'ĕ-sĭs)

vitellointestinal (vī'tĕl-ō-ĭn-tĕs"tĭn-ăl)

vitellolutein (vī"tĕl-ō-lū'tē-ĭn) [L. vitellus, yolk, + luteus, yellow]

vitellorubin (vī"tĕl-ō-rū'bĭn) [" + ruber, red]

vitellose (vī-tĕl'ōs)

vitellus (vī-tĕl'ŭs) [L.]

vitiation (vĭsh"ē-ā'shŭn) [L. vitiare, to corrupt]

vitiligines (vĭt"ĭ-lĭj'ĭ-nēz)

vitiliginous (vĭt"ĭ-lĭj'ĭ-nŭs)

vitiligo (vĭt-ĭl-ī'gō) [L.]

   v. capitis

   v. perinevic

vitiligoidea (vĭt"ĭl-ĭg-oy'dē-ă) [" + Gr. eidos, form, shape]

vitium (vĭsh'ē-ŭm) [L., fault]

   v. cordis

vitrectomy (vī-trĕk'tō-mē) [L. vitreus, glassy, + Gr. ektome, excision]

vitreocapsulitis (vĭt"rē-ō-kăp"sū-lī'tĭs) [L. vitreus, glassy, + capsula, capsule, + Gr. itis, inflammation]

vitreodentin (vĭt"rē-ō-dĕn'tĭn)

vitreoretinal (vĭt"rē-ō-rĕt'ĭ-năl)

vitreous (vĭt'rē-ŭs) [L. vitreus, glassy]

vitreous body

vitreous chamber

vitreous degeneration

vitreous humor

vitreous membrane

vitreous table

vitrescence (vī-trĕs'ĕns)

vitreum (vĭt'rē-ŭm)

vitriol (vĭt'rē-ōl) [L. vitriolum]

   v., blue

   v., green

   v., oil of

   v., white

vitropression (vĭt"rō-prĕsh'ŭn) [L. vitrum, glass, + pressio, a squeezing]

vitrum (vĭt'rŭm) [L.]

Vivactil

vivi- (vĭv'ĭ) [L. vivus]

vividialysis (vĭv"ĭ-dī-ăl'ĭ-sĭs)

vividiffusion (vĭv"ĭ-dĭf-ū'zhŭn) [L. vivus, alive, + dis, apart, + fundere, to pour]

vivification (vĭv″ĭ-fĭ-kā'shŭn) [" + *facere*, to make]
viviparity (vĭv″ĭ-păr'ĭ-tē)
viviparous (vĭv-ĭp'ăr-ŭs) [" + *parere*, to beget, produce]
vivisect (vĭv'ĭ-sĕkt) [L. *vivus*, alive, + *sectio*, a cutting]
vivisection (vĭv″ĭ-sĕk'shŭn) [" + *sectio*, a cutting]
vivisectionist (vĭv″ĭ-sĕk'shŭn-ĭst)
vivisector (vĭv-ĭs-ĕk'tor) [" + *sector*, a cutting]
vivisepulture (vĭv″ĭ-sĕp'ŭl-tūr) [" + *sepultura*, buried]
VLDL *very low density lipoprotein*
Vleminckx's solution (flĕm'ĭnks) [Jean François Vleminckx, Belgian physician, 1800–1876]
VMA *vanillylmandelic acid*
V.N.A. *Visiting Nurse Association*
vocal (vō'kăl) [L. *vocalis*, talking]
vocal cord
vocal cords, false
vocal cords, true
vocal folds
vocal fremitus
vocal ligament
vocal lips
vocal muscle
vocal process
vocal resonance
vocal signs
voces (vō'sēz) [L.]
voice (voys) [L. *vox*]
   v., amphoric
   v., cavernous
   v., eunuchoid
voiceprint
voices (voys'ēz)
void (voyd) [O. Fr. *voider*, to empty]
vol. *volume*
vol.% *volume percent*
vola, volar (vō'lă, vō'lăr) [L.]
vola manus (vō'lă)
vola pedis
volaris (vō-lă'rĭs)
volatile (vŏl'ă-tĭl) [L. *volatilis*, flying]
volatilization (vŏl″ă-tĭl-ĭ-zā'shŭn)

volatilize (vŏl'ă-tĭl-īz)
vole (vōl)
volition (vō-lĭsh'ŭn) [L. *volitio*, will]
volitional (vō-lĭsh'ŭn-ăl)
Volkmann's canals (fōlk'mănz) [A. W. Volkmann, Ger. physiologist, 1800–1877]
Volkmann's contracture (fōlk'mănz) [Richard von Volkmann, Ger. surgeon, 1830–1899]
volley (vŏl'ē) [L. *volare*, to fly]
volsella (vŏl-sēl'ă) [L., tweezers]
volt (vōlt) [Count Alessandro Volta, It. physicist, 1745–1827]
voltage (vōl'tĭj)
voltaic (vōl-tā'ĭk)
voltaism (vŏl'tă-ĭzm)
voltammeter (vōlt-ăm'mē-tĕr)
voltampere (vōlt-ăm'pēr)
volubility (vŏl″ū-bĭl'ĭ-tē) [L. *volubilitas*, flow of discourse]
volume (vŏl'ūm)
   v., expiratory reserve
   v., inspiratory reserve
   v., mean corpuscular
   v., minute
   v., packed cell
   v., residual
   v., stroke
   v., tidal
volumenometer (vŏl″ūm-nŏm'ĕ-tĕr)
volume percent
volumetric (vŏl″ū-mĕt'rĭk) [L. *volumen*, a volume, + Gr. *metron*, measure]
volumometer (vŏl″ū-mŏm'ĕ-tĕr)
voluntary (vŏl'ŭn-tĕr″ē) [L. *voluntas*, will]
voluntary health agency
voluntary muscle
voluptuous (vō-lŭp'tū-ŭs) [L. *voluptas*, pleasure]
volupty (vŏl'ŭp-tē) [O. Fr. *volupte*, pleasure]
volute (vō-lūt') [L. *volutus*, rolled]
volvulosis (vŏl″vū-lō'sĭs)
volvulus (vŏl'vū-lŭs) [L. *volvere*, to roll]
vomer (vō'mĕr) [L., plowshare]
vomerine (vō'mĕr-īn)

vomerobasilar (vō″mĕr-ō-băs′ĭ-lăr)
vomeronasal (vō″mĕr-ō-nā′săl)
vomeronasal cartilages
vomeronasal organ
vomica (vŏm′ĭ-kă) [L., ulcer]
vomicose (vŏm′ĭ-kōs)
vomit (vŏm′ĭt) [L. vomere, to vomit]
   v., bilious
   v., black
   v., coffee-ground
vomiting (vŏm′ĭt-ĭng) [L. vomere, to vomit]
   v., cyclic
   v., dry
   v., epidemic
   v., incoercible
   v., induced
   v. of pregnancy
   v., pernicious
   v., projectile
   v., stercoraceous
vomitive (vŏm′ĭ-tĭv)
vomitory (vŏm′ĭ-tō-rē) [L. vomitorius, pert. to vomit]
vomiturition (vŏm″ĭ-tū-rĭsh′ŭn) [L. vomitus, vomit]
vomitus (vŏm′ĭ-tŭs)
   v., coffee-ground
   v. cruentus
   v. marinus
   v. matutinus
von Gierke disease (fŏn gēr′kĕz) [Edgar von Gierke, Ger. pathologist, 1877–1945]
von Graefe's sign (fŏn grā′fĕz) [Albrecht von Graefe, Ger. ophthalmologist, 1828–1870]
von Hippel's disease
von Jaksch's disease [Rudolf von Jaksch-Wartenhorst, Austrian physician, 1855–1947]
von Pirquet's test (fŏn pēr′kāz) [Clemens Freiherr von Pirquet, Austrian pediatrician, 1874–1929]
von Recklinghausen's canals
von Recklinghausen's disease
von Recklinghausen's tumor
Vontrol

von Willebrand's disease [E. A. von Willebrand, Finnish physician, 1870–1949]
voodoo [Creole Fr., voudou, a good or bad spirit or demon]
Voorhees' bag (voor′ēz) [James Ditmors Voorhees, U.S. obstetrician, 1869–1929]
voracious (vō-rā′shŭs) [L. vorare, to devour]
vortex (vor′tĕks) [L., a whirlpool]
   v., coccygeal
   v. lentis
   v. of heart
vortices (vor′tĭ-sēz) [L.]
   v. pilorum
vorticose (vor′tĭk-ōs) [L. vortices, whirlpools]
vorticose veins
vox (vŏks) [L.]
   v. abscissa
   v. capitus
   v. cholerica
   v. rauca
voyeur (voy-yĕr′) [Fr., one who sees]
voyeurism (voy′yĕr-ĭzm)
V.R. right vision; ventilation rate; vocal resonance
V.S. vesicular sound; vital signs; volumetric solution
vuerometer (vū″ĕr-ŏm′ĕ-tĕr) [Fr. vue, sight, + Gr. metron, measure]
vulgaris (vŭl-gā′rĭs) [L.]
vulnerable (vŭl′nĕr-ă-bl) [L. vulnerare, to wound]
vulnerant (vŭl′nĕr-ănt)
vulnerary (vŭl′nĕr-ār″ē)
vulnerate (vŭl′nĕr-āt)
vulnus (vŭl′nŭs) [L.]
Vulpian - Heidenhain - Sherrington phenomenon [E. F. A. Vulpian, Fr. physician, 1826–1887; R. P. H. Heidenhain, Ger. physiologist, 1834–1897; C. S. Sherrington, Brit. physiologist, 1856–1952]
vulsella, vulsellum (vŭl-sĕl′ă, vŭl-sĕl′ŭm) [L. vulsella, tweezers]
vulva (vŭl′vă) [L., covering]

v. connivens
v. hians
v., velamen
vulval, vulvar [L. *vulva,* covering]
vulvar leukoplakia
vulvar vestibulitis syndrome
vulvectomy (vŭl-vĕk'tō-mē) [" +
Gr. *ektome,* excision]
vulvismus (vŭl-vīz'mŭs) [" + Gr.
-ismos, condition]
vulvitis (vŭl-vī'tĭs) [L. *vulva,* covering,
+ Gr. *itis,* inflammation]
v., acute nongonorrheal
v., follicular
v., gangrenous
v., leukoplakic
v., mycotic
vulvo- [L. *vulva,* covering]

vulvocrural (vŭl"vō-kroo'răl) [" +
cruralis, pert. to the leg]
vulvopathy (vŭl-vŏp'ă-thē) [" +
Gr. *pathos,* disease, suffering]
vulvouterine (vŭl"vō-ū'tĕr-ĭn) [" +
uterinus, pert. to the uterus]
vulvovaginal (vŭl"vō-văj'ĭ-năl) [" +
vagina, a sheath]
vulvovaginal glands
vulvovaginitis (vŭl"vō-văj"ĭ-nī'tĭs)
[" + " + Gr. *itis,* inflammation]
v., diabetic
vv *veins*
v/v *volume of dissolved substance per
volume of solvent*
V.W. *vessel wall*
v/w *volume of a substance per unit of
weight of another component*

W

W *tungsten* (wolfram)

w. *watt; week; wife; with*

Waardenburg syndrome [Petrus Johannes Waardenburg, Dutch ophthalmologist, 1886–1979]

Wachendorf's membrane (vŏk'ĕn-dorfs) [Eberhard J. Wachendorf, Dutch physician, 1703–1758]

wafer (wā'fĕr) [Ger. *wafel*]

Wagstaffe's fracture (wăg'stăfs) [William Warwick Wagstaffe, Brit. surgeon, 1843–1910]

waist (wāst) [ME. *wast,* growth]

wakeful (wāk'fŭl) [AS. *wacian,* to be awake, + *full,* complete]

Walcher's position (vŏl'kĕrz) [Gustav Adolf Walcher, Ger. gynecologist, 1856–1935]

Wald, Lillian (wăld) [U.S. nurse, 1867–1940]

Wald cycle

Waldenström's disease (văl'dĕn-strĕmz) [Johann Henning Waldenström, Swedish surgeon, b. 1877]

Waldeyer's gland (vŏl'dī-ĕrz) [Wilhelm von Waldeyer, Ger. anatomist, 1836–1921]

Waldeyer's neuron

Waldeyer's ring

walk

walker

walking [AS. *wealcan,* to roll]
   w., sleep-

walking cast

walking system

walking typhoid

walking well

walking wounded

wall [AS. *weall*]

Wallenberg's syndrome (vŏl'ĕn-bĕrgz) [Adolf Wallenberg, Ger. physi-

cian, 1862–1949]

wallerian degeneration (wŏl-ē'rē-ăn) [Augustus Volney Waller, Brit. physician, 1816–1870]

walleye [ME. *wawil-eghed*]

Walthard's islets or inclusions [Max Walthard, Swiss gynecologist, 1867–1933]

wandering (wăn'dĕr-ĭng) [AS. *wandrian*]

wandering abscess

wandering kidney

wandering mind

wandering spleen

Wangensteen tube (wăn'gĕn-stēn) [Owen H. Wangensteen, U.S. surgeon, 1898–1981]

Warburg apparatus [Otto H. Warburg, Ger. biochemist, 1883–1970]

ward [AS. *weard,* watching over]
   w., accident
   w., psychiatric

Wardrop's disease (wăr'drŏps) [James Wardrop, Brit. surgeon, 1782–1869]

Wardrop's operation

warehousemen's itch

warfarin poisoning

warfarin potassium

warfarin sodium [name derived from initials of Wisconsin Alumni Research Foundation]

war gases

wart (wort) [AS. *wearte*]
   w., fig
   w., genital
   w., plantar
   w., seborrheic
   w., senile
   w., venereal

wash (wŏsh) [AS. *wacsan*]

w., eye
washerwoman's itch
washout, nitrogen
wasp [AS. *waesp*]
wasp sting
Wassermann-fast (wäs'ĕr-mǎn) [August Paul von Wassermann, Ger. bacteriologist, 1866 – 1925]
Wassermann reaction
waste (wāst) [L. *vastus*, empty]
waste products
    w.p., metabolic
wasting (wāst'ĭng) [L. *vastare*, to devastate]
wasting palsy
water (wǎ'tĕr) [AS. *waeter*]
    w., bound
    w., deionized
    w., distilled
    w., emergency preparation of safe drinking
    w., hard
    w., heavy
    w., lime
    w., purified
    w., pyrogen-free
    w., soft
water bed
water brash
water cure
water for injection
waterhammer pulse
Waterhouse-Friderichsen syndrome [Rupert Waterhouse, Brit. physician, 1873 – 1958; Carl Friderichsen, Danish physician, b. 1886]
water intoxication
water on brain
waters
Watson-Crick helix [James Dewey Watson, U.S. biochemist, b. 1928; Francis Harry Compton Crick, Brit. biochemist, b. 1916]
Watson-Schwartz test (wŏt'sŏn-shwärts) [Cecil J. Watson, U.S. physician, b. 1901; Samuel Schwartz, U.S. physician, b. 1916]
watt [James Watt, Scottish engineer,

1736 – 1819]
wattage (wŏt'ĭj)
wave (wāv) [ME. *wave*]
    w., a
    w., alpha
    w., beta
    w., brain
    w., c
    w., delta
    w., electromagnetic
    w., excitation
    w.'s, hertzian
    w.'s, light
    w., P
    w., pulse
    w., Q
    w., R
    w.'s, radio
    w., S
    w.'s, sound
    w., T
    w.'s, theta
    w., ultrashort
    w., ultrasonic
wavelength (wāv'lĕngth)
wax [AS. *weax*]
    w., dental
waxing-up
waxy (wǎks'ē) [AS. *weax, wax*]
waxy cast
waxy degeneration
WBC *white blood cells; white blood count*
weak (wēk) [Old Norse *veikr*, flexible]
wean (wēn) [AS. *wenian*]
weanling
weanling diarrhea
web
    w., esophageal
    w., terminal
webbed (wĕbd) [AS. *webb*, a fabric]
Weber-Christian disease (wĕb'ĕr-krĭs'chĕn) [Friedrich Weber, Brit. physician, 1863 – 1962; Henry A. Christian, U.S. physician, 1876 – 1951]
Weber's glands (vā'bĕrz) [Moritz I. Weber, Ger. anatomist, 1795 – 1875]
Weber's paralysis (wĕb'ĕrz) [Sir Her-

mann David Weber, Brit. physician, 1824–1918]
Weber test [Friedrich Eugen Weber, Ger. otologist, 1823–1891]
Wechsler Intelligence Scale for Children
wedge pressure
WEE *western equine encephalomyelitis*
weeping [AS. *wepan*, to lament]
weeping eczema
weeping sinew
Wegener's granulomatosis or syndrome [F. Wegener, 20th century Ger. pathologist]
Weidel reaction (vī'dĕl) [Hugo Weidel, Austrian chemist, 1849–1899]
Weigert's law (vī'gĕrts) [Karl Weigert, Ger. pathologist, 1843–1904]
weight (wāt) [AS. *gewiht*]
  w., apothecaries'
  w., atomic
  w., avoirdupois
  w., equivalent
  w., molecular
  w., set point
weightlessness
weights and measures
Weil-Felix reaction, test (vīl-fā'lĭks) [Edmund Weil, Ger. physician, 1880–1922; Arthur Felix, Ger. bacteriologist, 1887–1956]
Weil's disease (vīlz) [Adolf Weil, Ger. physician, 1848–1916]
Weir Mitchell's treatment (wĕr mĭt'chĕlz) [S. Weir Mitchell, U.S. neurologist, 1829–1914]
weismannism (wīs'măn-ĭzm) [August F. L. Weismann, Ger. biologist, 1834–1914]
Weitbrecht's foramen (vīt'brĕkts) [Josias Weitbrecht, Ger.-born Russian anatomist, 1702–1747]
Weitbrecht's ligament
Welch's bacillus (wĕlsh'ĕz) [William Henry Welch, U.S. pathologist, 1850–1934]
welding
welt [ME. *welte*]

wen (wĕn) [AS.]
Wenckebach's period, pauses, or phenomenon (vĕn'kĕ-bŏks) [Karel F. Wenckebach, Dutch-born Aust. internist, 1864–1940]
Werdnig-Hoffmann disease (vĕrd'nĭg-hŏf'măn) [Guido Werdnig, Austrian neurologist, 1844–1919; Johann Hoffmann, Ger. neurologist, 1857–1919]
Werdnig-Hoffmann paralysis
Werdnig-Hoffmann syndrome
Werlhof's disease (vĕrl'hŏfs) [Paul G. Werlhof, Ger. physician, 1699–1767]
Wermer's syndrome [Paul Wermer, U.S. physician, d. 1975]
Wernicke's encephalopathy (vĕr'nĭ-kēz) [Karl Wernicke, Ger. neurologist, 1848–1905]
Wernicke's syndrome
western blotting
Westphal-Edinger nucleus [Karl Westphal, Ger. neurologist, 1833–1890; Ludwig Edinger, Ger. neurologist, 1855–1918]
Westphal-Stümpell pseudosclerosis (vĕst'fàl-strĭm'p'l) [K. Westphal; Ernst A. G. G. von Strümpell, Ger. physician, 1853–1925]
wet (wĕt) [AS. *waet*]
wet brain
wet cup
wet dream
wet-dry dressing or pack
wet nurse
wet pack
Wetzel grid (wĕt'sĕl) [Norman C. Wetzel, U.S. pediatrician, b. 1897]
Wharton's duct (hwăr'tŏnz) [Thomas Wharton, Brit. anatomist, 1614–1673]
Wharton's jelly
wheal (hwēl) [AS. *hwele*; ME. *wale*, a stripe]
wheat (hwēt) [AS. *hwaete*]
wheatstone bridge
wheel

w., carborundum
w., diamond
w., polishing
w., wire
wheelchair
wheeze (hwēz) [ME. *whesen*]
wheezing
whelk (hwĕlk) [AS. *hwylca*]
whiff
whinolalia (wĭn″ō-lā′lē-ă) [AS. *whinan*, whine, + Gr. *lalia*, chatter, prattle]
whiplash injury
Whipple's disease (hwĭp′ĕlz) [George Hoyt Whipple, U.S. pathologist, 1878–1976]
whipworm
whirl (hwŭrl) [Old Norse *hvirfla*]
whirlbone
whirlpool bath
whiskey, whisky (hwĭs′kē)
whisper (hwĭs′pĕr) [AS. *hwisprian*]
w., cavernous
whistle (hwĭs′ĕl)
whistling face syndrome
white (hwīt) [AS. *hwit*]
white cell
white gangrene
whitehead (hwīt′hĕd)
white leg
white line
white lotion
white matter
white of egg
white of eye
white ointment
whitepox (hwīt′pŏks)
white precipitate
white softening
whitlow (hwĭt′lō) [ME. *whitflawe*, white flow]
Whitmore's disease [Alfred Whitmore, Brit. surgeon, 1876–1946]
W.H.O. *World Health Organization*
whole body counter
wholism
wholistic health
whoop (hoop) [AS. *hwopan*, to threaten]

whooping cough
whorl (hwŭrl) [ME. *whorle*]
Widal's reaction or test (vē-dŏlz′) [Georges Fernand Isidore Widal, Fr. physician, 1862–1929]
wild cherry
will [AS.]
Willis' circle (wĭl′ĭs) [Thomas Willis, Brit. anatomist, 1621–1675]
Willis' cords
Wilms' tumor (vĭlmz) [Marx Wilms, Ger. surgeon, 1867–1918]
Wilson's disease (wĭl′sŭnz) [Samuel A. K. Wilson, Brit. internist, 1877–1937]
Wilson-Mikity syndrome [Miriam G. Wilson, U.S. pediatrician, b. 1922; Victor G. Mikity, U.S. radiologist, b. 1919]
Winckel's disease (vĭng′kĕlz) [Franz von Winckel, Ger. gynecologist, 1837–1911]
windburn
windchill
windchill factor
windchill index
winding sheet
window [Old Norse *vindauga*]
w., aortic
w., cochlear
w., oval
w., round
w., vestibular
windpipe
wine (wīn) [L. *vinum*, wine]
wineglass
wine sores
wing [Old Norse *vaengi*]
wink [AS. *wincian*]
winking
w., jaw
w., jaw-, syndrome
Winslow, foramen of (wĭnz′lō) [Jakob B. Winslow, Fr. anatomist, 1669–1760]
Winslow, ligament of
Winslow, pancreas of
Winstrol
wintergreen oil
winter itch

wire (wīr)
  w., arch
  w., Kirschner
  w., ligature
  w., separating
wiring (wīr'ĭng)
  w., circumferential
  w., continuous loop
  w., craniofacial suspension
  w., Gilmer
  w., Ivy loop
  w., perialveolar
  w., pyriform
  w., Stout's
Wirsung, duct of (vēr'soong) [Johann Georg Wirsung, Ger. physician, 1600–1643]
wisdom tooth (wĭz'dŏm)
Wiskott-Aldrich syndrome [Alfred Wiskott, Ger. pediatrician, b. 1898; Robert A. Aldrich, U.S. pediatrician, b. 1917]
witches' milk
withdrawal
withdrawal syndrome
witkop (wĭt'kŏp) [Afrikaans, white scalp]
witzelsucht (vĭt'sĕl-zookt) [M. Jastrowitz, Ger. physician, b. 1839]
  w., primary affective
Wohlfahrtia (vōl-fär'tē-ă)
  W. magnifica
  W. opaca
  W. vigil
wolffian body (wool'fē-ăn) [Kaspar Friedrich Wolff, Ger. anatomist, 1733–1794]
wolffian cyst
wolffian duct
wolffian tubules
Wolff-Parkinson-White syndrome [L. Wolff, U.S. physician, 1898–1972; Sir John Parkinson, Brit. physician b. 1885; Paul Dudley White, U.S. cardiologist, 1886–1974]
Wolfina 100
wolfram (wool'frăm)
wolfsbane (wŏlfs'bān)
Wolhynia fever

Wolman's disease [M. Wolman, Israeli physician, b. 1914]
womb (woom) [AS. wamb]
wood alcohol
Wood's rays [Robert Williams Wood, U.S. physicist, 1868–1955]
wood tick
wool fat
woolsorter's disease
word blindness
word salad
work [Ger. wirken]
work and mental health
working through
work-up
World Health Organization
worm (wŭrm) [AS. wyrm]
wormian bones (wŭr'mē-ăn) [Olaus Worm, Dan. anatomist, 1588–1654]
wormseed (wĕrm'sēd)
  w., American
wormwood (wĕrm'wood)
worried well
wound (woond) [AS. wund]
  w., abdominal
  w., bullet
  w., cellulitis of
  w., contused
  w., crushing
  w., fishhook
  w., incised
  w., lacerated
  w., nonpenetrating
  w., open
  w., penetrating
  w., perforating
  w., puncture
  w., subcutaneous
  w., tunnel
W-plasty
wreath (rēth)
Wright's stain [James H. Wright, U.S. pathologist, 1871–1928]
Wright's technique
wrinkle (rĭng'kl) [AS. gewrinclian, to wind]
Wrisberg's cardiac ganglion (rĭs'bŭrgz) [Heinrich August Wrisberg,

Ger. anatomist, 1739 – 1808]
Wrisberg's cartilages
Wrisberg's ganglion
Wrisberg's nerve
wrist (rĭst) [AS]
wrist bones
wrist drop
wrist unit
writer's cramp
writing
    w., dextrad
    w., mirror
writing hand
wrongful birth or wrongful life
wryneck (rī'nĕk)

w.s. *water soluble*
wt *weight*
Wuchereria (voo"kĕr-ē'rē-ă) [Otto Wucherer, Ger. physician, 1820 – 1873]
    W. bancrofti
    W. malayi
wuchereriasis (voo"kĕr-ē-rī'ă-sĭs)
w/v *weight in volume*
w/w *weight in weight*
Wyamine Sulfate
Wyamycin S
Wyamycin Liquid
Wycillin
Wydase

X

X *Kienböck's unit of x-ray dose; xanthine*
Xanax
xanchromatic (zăn″krō-măt′ĭk)
xanthelasma (zăn″thĕl-ăz′mă) [Gr.
   xanthos, yellow, + *elasma,* plate]
xanthelasmoidea (zăn″thĕl-ăz-
   moy′dē-ă) [″ + ″ + *eidos,*
   form, shape]
xanthematin (zăn-thĕm′ă-tĭn)
xanthemia (zăn-thē′mē-ă) [″ +
   haima, blood]
xanthene (zăn′thēn)
xanthic (zăn′thĭk) [Gr. *xanthos,* yellow]
xanthic calculus
xanthine (zăn′thĭn, -thēn)
   x., dimethyl-
xanthine base
xanthinuria (zăn″thĭn-ū′rē-ă) [″ +
   ouron, urine]
xanthiuria (zăn″thē-ū′rē-ă)
xanthochroia (zan″thō-krō′ē-ă)
   [″ + *chroia,* skin]
xanthochromatic (zăn″tho-krō-măt′ĭk)
xanthochromia (zăn″thō-krō′mē-ă)
   [″ + *chroma,* color]
xanthochromic (zăn″thō-krō′mĭk)
xanthochroous (zăn-thŏk′rō-ŭs) [Gr.
   xanthochroos]
**xanthocyanopia, xanthocyanop-
   sia** (zăn″thō-sī-ăn-ō′pē-ă, -ŏp′sē-ă)
   [Gr. *xanthos,* yellow, + *kyanos,*
   blue, + *opsis,* sight, appearance,
   vision]
xanthocyte (zăn′thō-sīt) [″ +
   kytos, cell]
xanthoderma (zăn″thō-dĕr′mă)
   [″ + *derma,* skin]
xanthodont (zăn′thō-dŏnt) [″ +
   odous, tooth]
xanthoerythrodermia   perstans
   (zăn″thō-ĕ-rĭth″rō-dĕr′mē-ă)
xanthogranuloma (zăn″thō-grăn″ū-
   lō′mă) [″ + L. *granulum,* grain, +

oma, tumor]
   x., juvenile
xanthokyanopy (zăn″thō-kī-ăn′ō-pē)
   [″ + *kyanos,* blue, + *opsis,*
   sight, appearance, vision]
xanthoma (zăn-thō′mă) [Gr. *xanthos,*
   yellow, + *oma,* tumor]
   x., diabetic
   x. disseminatum
   x. multiplex
   x. palpebrarum
   x. tuberosum
xanthomatosis (zăn″thō-mă-tō′sĭs)
   [″ + ″ + *osis,* condition]
xanthomatous (zăn-thō′mă-tŭs)
xanthophose (zăn′thō-fōz) [″ +
   phos, light]
xanthophyll (zăn′thō-fĭl) [″ +
   phyllon, leaf]
xanthoprotein (zăn″thō-prō′tē-ĭn)
xanthopsia (zăn-thŏp′sē-ă) [″ +
   opsis, sight, appearance, vision]
xanthopsin (zăn-thŏp′sĭn)
xanthopsis (zăn-thŏp′sĭs)
xanthorrhea (zăn″thō-rē′ă) [″ +
   rhein, to flow]
xanthosine (zăn′thō-sēn)
xanthosis (zăn-thō′sĭs) [″ + *osis,*
   condition]
xanthous (zăn′thŭs) [Gr. *xanthos,* yel-
   low]
xanthurenic acid
xanthuria (zăn-thū′rē-ă) [″ +
   ouron, urine]
X chromosome
x-disease
Xe *xenon*
xeno- [Gr. *xenos,* stranger]
xenobiotic (zĕn″ō-bī-ŏt′ĭk)
xenogeneic (zĕn″ō-jĕn-ā′ĭk) [″ +
   gennan, to produce]
xenogenesis (zĕn″ō-jĕn′ĕ-sĭs)
xenogenous (zĕn-ŏj′ĕn-ŭs) [Gr. *xenos,*

stranger, + *gennan,* to produce]
xenograft (zĕn′ō-grăft) [″ + L.
graphium, stylus]
xenology (zĕn-ŏl′ō-jē) [″ + *logos,*
word, reason]
xenomenia (zĕn-ō-mē′nē-ă) [″ +
meniaia, menses]
xenon (zē′nŏn) [Gr. *xenos,* stranger]
xenon-133
xenoparasite (zĕn″ō-păr′ă-sīt)
xenophobia (zĕn″ō-fō′bē-ă) [″ +
phobos, fear]
xenophonia (zĕn″ō-fō′nē-ă) [″ +
phone, voice]
xenophthalmia (zĕn″ŏf-thăl′mē-ă)
[″ + *ophthalmia,* eye inflamma-
tion]
Xenopsylla (zĕn″ŏp-sĭl′ă) [″ +
psylla, flea]
X. cheopis
xenorexia (zĕn″ō-rĕk′sē-ă) [″ +
orexis, appetite]
xerantic (zē-răn′tĭk) [Gr. *xeros,* dry]
xerasia (zē-rā′sē-ă) [Gr. *xeros,* dry]
xero- [Gr. *xeros*]
xerocheilia (zē″rō-kī′lē-ă) [″ +
cheilos, lip]
xeroderma (zē″rō-dĕr′mă) [″ +
derma, skin]
x. pigmentosum
xerography (zē-rŏg′ră-fē)
xeroma (zē-rō′mă) [″ + *oma,*
tumor]
xeromammography (zē″rō-măm-
mŏg′ră-fē)
xeromenia (zē″rō-mē′nē-ă) [″ +
meniaia, menses]
xeromycteria (zē″rō-mĭk-tē′rē-ă)
[″ + *mykter,* nose]
xeronosus (zē-rŏn′ō-sŭs) [″ +
nosos, disease]
xerophagia (zē″rō-fā′jē-ă) [″ +
phagein, to eat]
xerophagy (zē-rŏf′ă-jē)
xerophthalmia (zē-rŏf-thăl′mē-ă)
[″ + *ophthalmos,* eye]
xerophthalmus (zē″rŏf-thăl′mŭs)
xeroradiography (zē″rō-rā″dē-
ŏg′ră-fē)

xerosis (zē-rō′sĭs) [Gr.]
xerostomia (zē″rō-stŏ′mē-ă) [″ +
stoma, mouth, opening]
xerotes (zē′rō-tēz) [Gr.]
xerotic (zē-rŏt′ĭk) [Gr. *xeros,* dry]
xerotocia (zē″rō-tō′sē-ă) [″ +
tokos, birth]
xerotripsis (zē″rō-trĭp′sĭs) [″ +
tripsis, a rubbing, friction]
xiphi-, xipho- [Gr. *xiphos,* sword]
xiphisternum (zĭf″ĭ-stĕr′nŭm) [Gr.
xiphos, sword, + *sternon,* chest]
xiphocostal (zĭf″ō-kŏs′tăl) [″ + L.
costa, rib]
xiphocostal ligament
xiphodynia (zĭf″ō-dĭn′ē-ă) [″ +
odyne, pain]
xiphoid (zĭf′oyd) [Gr. *xiphos,* sword,
+ *eidos,* form, shape]
xiphoid process
xiphoiditis (zĭf″oyd-ī′tĭs) [″ + ″
+ *itis,* inflammation]
xiphopagotomy (zī-fŏp″ă-gŏt′ō-mē)
xiphopagus (zī-fŏp′ă-gŭs) [″ +
pagos, thing fixed]
X-linked
X-linked disorders
x radiation
x-ray
x-r., bitewing
x-r., strain
x-ray dermatitis
xylene (zī′lēn, zī-lēn′)
xylene poisoning
xylenin (zī′lē-nĭn) [Gr. *xylon,* wood]
xylenol (zī′lĕ-nŏl)
xylo- [Gr. *xylon,* wood]
Xylocaine
xylol (zī′lŏl)
xylometazoline   hydrochloride
(zī″lō-mĕt″ă-zō′lēn)
xylose (zī′lōs) [Gr. *xylon,* wood]
xylulose (zī′lū-lōs)
xylyl (zī′lĭl)
xyrospasm (zī′rō-spăzm) [Gr. *xyron,*
razor, + *spasmos,* a convulsion]
xysma (zĭz′mă) [Gr. *zysma,* filings]
xyster (zĭs′tĕr) [Gr., scraper]

Y

Y *yttrium*
yard [AS. *gerd*, a rod]
yaw (yaw)
   y., mother
yawn (yawn) [AS. *geonian*]
yawning (yawn'ĭng)
yaws (yawz)
Yb *ytterbium*
Y cartilage
Y chromosome
yeast (yēst) [AS. *gist*]
   y., brewer's
   y., dried
yellow (yĕl'ō) [AS. *geolu*]
   y., visual
yellow body
yellow fever
yellow ointment
yellow spot
yellow vision
yerba (yĕr'bä) [Sp.]
   y. maté
Yersin's serum (yĕr'sĭnz) [Alexandre Emil Jean Yersin, Swiss bacteriologist, 1863–1943]
Yersinia (yĕr-sĭn'ē-ä) [Yersin]
   Y. enterocolitica

Y. pestis
Y. pseudotuberculosis
yersiniosis (yĕr-sĭn"ē-ō'sĭs)
yin-yang
-yl [Gr. *hyle*, matter, substance]
Y ligament
Yodoxin
yoga [Sanskrit, union]
yogurt, yoghurt (yōg'hŭrt) [Turkish]
yohimbine (yō-hĭm'bēn)
yoke (yōk)
yolk (yōk) [AS. *geolca*]
   y. sac
   y. stalk
Young-Helmholtz theory (yŭng-hĕlm'hōlts) [Thomas Young, Brit. physician, 1773–1829; H. L. F. Helmholtz, Ger. physician, 1821–1894]
Young's rule (yŭngz) [Thomas Young]
youth (yooth) [AS. *geoguth*]
ypsiliform (ĭp-sĭl'ĭ-form)
y.s. *yellow spot*
ytterbium (ĭ-tŭr'bē-ŭm)
yttrium (ĭt'rē-ŭm)
yushi
Yutopar

Z

Z [Ger.] *Zuckung,* contraction; *atomic number*

z zero; zone

Zaglas' ligament (ză'glŭs)

Zahn's lines (zŏnz) [Frederick W. Zahn, Ger. pathologist, 1845–1904]

Zang's space (zăngz) [Christoph B. Zang, Ger. surgeon, 1772–1835]

Zaroxolyn

Z disk

zeatin (zē'ă-tĭn)

zeaxanthin (zē″ă-zăn'thĭn)

zein (zē'ĭn) [Gr. *zeia,* a kind of grain]

Zeis' glands [Edvard Zeis, Ger. surgeon, 1807–1868]

zeisian (zī'sē-ăn)

zelotypia (zē″lō-tĭp'ē-ă) [Gr. *zelos,* zeal, + *typtein,* to strike]

Zenker, Friedrich Albert von (zĕng'kĕr) [Ger. pathologist, 1825–1898]
    Z.'s degeneration
    Z.'s diverticulum

zenkerism (zĕng'kĕr-ĭzm)

Zephiran chloride

zero (zē'rō) [It.]
    z., absolute
    z., limes

zero population growth

zestocausis (zĕs″tō-kŏw'sĭs) [Gr. *zestos,* boiling hot, + *kausis,* burning]

Zide

Ziehl-Neelsen method (zēl-nēl'sĕn) [Franz Ziehl, Ger. bacteriologist, 1857–1926; Friedrich K. A. Neelsen, 1854–1894]

Zieve's syndrome [L. Zieve, U.S. physician, b. 1915]

Zim jar opener

zinc (zĭnk) [L. *zincum*]

z. acetate
z. bacitracin
z. cadmium sulfide
z. carbonate
z. chloride
z. gelatin
z. oxide
z. oxide and eugenol
z. peroxide
z. salts
z. stearate
z. sulfate
z. undecylenate
z. white

zinc-eugenol cement

zinciferous (zĭng-kĭf'ĕr-ŭs)

zincoid (zĭng'koyd) [L. *zincum,* zinc, + Gr. *eidos,* form, shape]

zinc ointment

zinc salts poisoning

Zinn's ligament (zĭnz) [Johann G. Zinn, Ger. anatomist, 1727–1759]

zipper pull

zirconium (zĭr-kō'nē-ŭm)

Zn zinc

zoacanthosis (zō″ăk-ăn-thō'sĭs)

zoanthropy (zō-ăn'thrō-pē) [Gr. *zoon,* animal, + *anthropos,* man]

zoescope (zō'ĕ-skōp) [Gr. *zoe,* life, + *skopein,* to view]

zoetic (zō-ĕt'ĭk) [Gr. *zoe,* life]

zoic (zō'ĭk)

Zollinger-Ellison syndrome [Robert M. Zollinger, b. 1903, and Edwin H. Ellison, b. 1918, U.S. surgeons]

Zolyse

Zomax

zona (zō'nă) [L., a girdle]
    z. ciliaris
    z. facialis
    z. fasciculata

z. glomerulosa
z. ophthalmica
z. pellucida
z. radiata
z. reticularis
z. striata
zonae
zonal (zō'năl) [L. *zonalis*]
zonary (zō'năr-ē) [L. *zona*, a girdle]
zonary placenta
Zondek-Aschheim test (zŏn'děk-ăsh'hīm) [Bernhard Zondek, Ger. gynecologist, 1891 – 1966; Selmar Aschheim, Ger. gynecologist, 1878 – 1965]
zone (zōn) [L. *zona*, a girdle]
z., cell-free
z., cell-rich
z., ciliary
z., comfort
z., epileptogenic
z., erogenous
z., hypnogenic, hypnogenous
z., transitional
zonesthesia (zōn"ĕs-thē'zē-ă) [" + *aisthesis*, feeling, perception]
zonifugal (zō-nĭf'ū-găl) [" + *fugere*, to flee]
zoning
zonipetal (zō-nĭp'ĕt-ăl) [" + *petere*, to seek]
zonoskeleton (zōn"ō-skĕl'ĕ-tŏn)
zonula (zōn'ū-lă) [L.]
z. adherens
z. ciliaris
z. occludens
zonular (zōn'ū-lăr)
zonular cataract
zonular fibers
zonular spaces
zonule (zōn'ūl) [L. *zonula*, small zone]
z. of Zinn
zonulitis (zōn-ū-lī'tĭs) [" + Gr. *itis*, inflammation]
zonulolysis (zōn"ū-lōl'ĭ-sĭs) [" + Gr. *lysis*, dissolution]
zonulotomy (zōn"ū-lŏt'ō-mē) [" + Gr. *tome*, a cutting, slice]
zonulysis (zōn"ū-lī'sĭs)

zoobiology (zō"ō-bī-ŏl'ō-jē) [Gr. *zoon*, animal, + *bios*, life, + *logos*, word, reason]
zooblast (zō'ō-blăst) [" + *blastos*, germ]
zoochemistry (zō"ō-kĕm'ĭs-trē)
zoodermic (zō"ō-dĕr'mĭk) [" + *derma*, skin]
zoodynamics (zō"ō-dī-năm'ĭks) [" + *dynamis*, power]
zooerasty (zō"ō-ē'răs-tē)
zoofulvin (zō"ō-fŭl'vĭn)
zoogenesis (zō"ō-jĕn'ĕ-sĭs)
zoogenous (zō-ŏj'ĕn-ŭs) [" + *gennan*, to produce]
zoogeny (zō"ŏj'ĕ-nē) [" + *gennan*, to produce]
zoogeography (zō"ō-jē-ŏg'ră-fē)
zooglea (zō"ō-glē'ă) [" + *gloios*, sticky]
zoogonous (zō-ŏg'ō-nŭs)
zoogony (zō-ŏg'ō-nē) [" + *gone*, offspring]
zoograft (zō'ō-grăft) [" + L. *graphium*, stylus]
zoografting (zō"ō-grăft'ĭng)
zooid (zō'oyd) [" + *eidos*, form, shape]
zoolagnia (zō"ō-lăg'nē-ă) [" + *lagneia*, lust]
zoologist (zō-ŏl'ō-jĭst) [" + *logos*, word, reason]
zoology (zō-ŏl'ō-jē)
zoomania (zō"ō-mā'nē-ă) [Gr. *zoon*, animal, + *mania*, madness]
zoonoses (zō-ō-nō'sēz) [" + *nosos*, disease]
zoonotic (zō"ō-nŏt'ĭk)
zooparasite (zō"ō-păr'ă-sīt) [" + *para*, alongside, past, beyond, + *sitos*, food]
zoopathology (zō"ō-păth-ŏl'ō-jē) [" + *pathos*, disease, suffering, + *logos*, word, reason]
zoophagous (zō-ŏf'ă-gŭs) [" + *phagein*, to eat]
zoophile (zō'ō-fīl) [" + *philein*, to love]

zoophilism (zō-ŏf'ĭl-ĭzm) [" + " + -ismos, condition]

zoophobia (zō"ō-fō'bē-ă) [" + phobos, fear]

zoophyte (zō'ō-fīt) [" + phyton, plant]

zooplankton (zō"ō-plănk'tŏn) [" + planktos, wandering]

zooplasty (zō'ō-plăs"tē) [" + plassein, to form]

zoopsia (zō-ŏp'sē-ă) [" + opsis, sight, appearance, vision]

zoopsychology (zō"ō-sī-kŏl'ō-jē)

zoosadism (zō"ō-sā'dĭzm)

zooscopy (zō-ŏs'kō-pē) [" + skopein, to examine]

zoosmosis (zō"ŏs-mō'sĭs) [Gr. zoe, life, + osmos, impulsion]

zoospore (zō'ō-spor) [" + sporos, seed]

zoosterol (zō"ō-stē'rŏl)

zootechnics (zō"ō-tĕk'nĭks) [Gr. zoon, animal, + techne, art]

zootic (zō-ŏt'ĭk)

zootomy (zō-ŏt'ō-mē) [" + tome, a cutting, slice]

zootoxin (zō"ō-tŏks'ĭn) [" + toxikon, poison]

zootrophic (zō"ō-trŏf'ĭk) [" + trophe, nutrition]

zoster (zŏs'tĕr) [Gr. zoster, girdle]
    z. auricularis
    z. ophthalmicus

zosteriform (zŏs-tĕr'ĭ-form) [" + L. forma, shape]

zosteroid (zŏs'tĕr-oyd) [" + eidos, form, shape]

ZPG zero population growth

Z-plasty

Zr zirconium

Z-track

zwitterions (tsvĭt'ĕr-ī"ŏns)

zygal (zī'găl) [Gr. zygon, yoke]

zygapophyseal (zī"gă-pō-fĭz'ē-ăl)

zygapophysis (zī"gă-pŏf'ĭ-sĭs) [" + apo, from, + physis, growth]

zygion (zĭj'ē-ŏn) [Gr. zygon, yoke]

zygocyte

zygodactyly (zī"gō-dăk'tĭl-ē) [" + daktylos, finger]

zygoma (zī-gō'mă) [Gr., cheekbone]

zygomatic (zī"gō-măt'ĭk)

zygomatic arch

zygomatic bone

zygomaticoauricularis (zī"gō-măt"ĭ-kō-ăw-rĭk"ū-lā'rĭs) [L.]

zygomaticofacial (zī"gō-măt"ĭ-kō-fā'shăl)

zygomaticofrontal (zī"gō-măt"ĭ-kō-frŏn'tăl)

zygomaticomaxillary (zī"gō-măt"ĭ-kō-măk'sĭ-lĕr"ē)

zygomatico-orbital (zī"gō-măt"ĭ-kō-or'bĭ-tăl)

zygomaticosphenoid (zī"gō-măt"ĭ-kō-sfē'noyd)

zygomaticotemporal (zī"gō-măt"ĭ-kō-tĕm'por-ăl)

zygomatic process

zygomatic reflex

zygomaticum (zī"gō-măt'ĭ-kŭm) [L.]

zygomaticus (zī"gō-măt'ĭk-ŭs) [L.]

zygomaxillary (zī"gō-măks'ĭl-ār-ē) [Gr. zygoma, cheekbone, + L. maxilla, jawbone]

zygomaxillary point

zygomycosis

zygon (zī'gŏn) [Gr.]

zygopodium (zī"gō-pō'dē-ŭm)

zygosis (zī-gō'sĭs) [Gr. zygosis, a balancing]

zygosity (zī-gŏs'ĭ-tē) [Gr. zygon, yoke]

zygosperm (zī'gō-spĕrm)

zygospore (zī'gō-spor)

zygote (zī'gŏt) [Gr. zygotos, yoked]

zygotene (zī'gō-tēn) [Gr. zygotos, yoked]

zygotic (zī-gŏt'ĭk)

zygotoblast (zī-gō'tō-blăst) [" + blastos, germ]

zygotomere (zī-gō'tō-mēr) [" + meros, part]

Zyloprim

zymase (zī'mās) [Gr. zyme, leaven, + -ase, enzyme]

zyme (zīm) [Gr. zyme, leaven]

zymic (zī'mĭk)
zymogen (zī'mō-jĕn) [" + gennan, to produce]
zymogene (zī'mō-jēn)
zymogen granules
zymogenic (zī"mō-jĕn'ĭk)
zymogenous (zī-mŏj'ĕ-nŭs)
zymogram (zī'mō-grăm)
zymohexase (zī"mō-hĕk'sās)
zymohydrolysis (zī"mō-hī-drŏl'ĭ-sĭs) [" + hydor, water, + lysis, dissolution]
zymoid (zī'moyd) [" + eidos, form, shape]
zymologic (zī"mō-lŏ'jĭk) [" + logos, word, reason]
zymologist (zī-mŏl'ō-jĭst)
zymology (zī-mŏl'ō-jē)
zymolysis (zī-mŏl'ĭ-sĭs) [Gr. zyme, leaven, + lysis, dissolution]
zymolyte (zī'mō-līt")
zymolytic (zī"mō-lĭt'ĭk) [" + lytikos, dissolved]
zymometer (zī-mŏm'ĕ-ter) [" + metron, measure]

Zymonema (zī"mō-nē'mă) [" + nema, thread]
zymophore (zī'mō-for) [" + phoros, a bearer]
zymophoric, zymophorous (zī"mō-for'ĭk, zī-mŏf'or-ŭs)
zymophyte (zī'mō-fīt) [" + phyton, growth]
zymoplastic (zī"mō-plăs'tĭk) [" + plassein, to form]
zymoprotein (zī"mō-prō'tē-ĭn)
zymosan (zī'mō-săn)
zymoscope (zī'mō-skōp) [" + skopein, to examine]
zymose (zī'mōs)
zymosis (zī-mō'sĭs) [Gr. zymosis, fermentation]
z. gastrica
zymosterol (zī-mŏs'tĕr-ŏl)
zymosthenic (zī-mōs-thĕn'ĭk) [Gr. zyme, leaven, + sthenos, strength]
zymotic (zī-mŏt'ĭk)
Z.Z.'Z." increasing strengths of contraction

Appendix

Appendix 1

Latin and Greek Nomenclature

Greek Alphabet

Name of letter	Capital	Lower case	Trans-literation	Name of letter	Capital	Lower case	Transliteration
alpha	A	α	a	nu	N	ν	n
beta	B	6 or β	b	xi	Ξ	ξ	x
gamma	Γ	γ	g	omicron	O	o	o short
delta	Δ	δ	d	pi	Π	π	p
epsilon	E	ϵ	e short	rho	P	ρ	r
zeta	Z	ζ	z	sigma	Σ	σ or ς	s
eta	H	η	e long	tau	T	τ	t
theta	Θ	θ	th	upsilon	Υ	υ	y
iota	I	ι	i	phi	Φ	ϕ or φ	f
kappa	K	κ	k, c	chi	X	χ	ch as in German echt
lambda	Λ	λ	l	psi	Ψ	ψ	ps
mu	M	μ	m	omega	Ω	ω	o long

English with Latin and Greek Equivalents

acid. [L.] acidum
afternoon. [L.] post meridiem
age. [L.] aetas; maturas; adultus; impubis
ague. [L.] febris
and. [L.] et
arm. [L.] brachium; [Gr.] brachion
artery. [L.] arteria
attachment. [L.] adhesio
autumn. [L.] autumnus
back. [L.] tergum; dorsum
backbone. [L.] spina
backward. [L.] retro
bath. [L.] balneum
beef. [L.] bubula
belly. [L.] venter; abdomen
bend. [L.] flexus
bile. [L.] bilis; [Gr.] chole
birth. [L.] partus; natales
bitter. [L.] acerbus
black. [L.] niger; nigra; nigrum
bladder. [L.] vesica

bleed. [L.] fluere
blind. [L.] obscurus
blister. [L.] pustulo; vesicatorium
bloat. [L.] tumeo
blood. [L.] sanguis; [Gr.] haima
blood vessel. [L.] vena
blue. [L.] caeruleus; cyaneus; lividus
body. [L.] corpus; [Gr.] soma
boiling up. [L.] effervescens
bone. [L.] os; [Gr.] osteon
bony. [L.] osseus
bowels. [L.] intestina; viscera
bowlegged. [L.] valgus
brain. [L.] cerebrum; [Gr.] enkephalos
breach. [L.] ruptura
breakfast. [L.] prandium
breast. [L.] mamma; [Gr.] mastos
breath. [L.] halitus
brown. [L.] fulvus
bubble. [L.] pustula
bulb. [L.] bulbus
buttock. [L.] clunis; [Gr.] gloutos

Adapted from Thomas, C. L. (ed.): *Taber's Cyclopedic Medical Dictionary*, ed. 16, F. A. Davis, Philadelphia, 1989, p. 2213.

English with Latin and Greek Equivalents (cont'd)

calcareous. [L.] calci similis
canal. [L.] canalis
cartilage. [L.] cartilago; [Gr.] chondros
catarrh. [L.] coryza
cavity. [L.] caverna
change. [L.] mutatio
chest. [L.] thorax; [Gr.] thorax
child. [L.] infans; puer; filius
chill. [L.] friguscolum
chin. [L.] mentum; [Gr.] geneion
choke. [L.] strangulo
clavicle. [L.] clavicula
cold. [L.] frigidus
confinement. [L.] puerperium
congestion. [L.] conglobatio
consumption. [L.] phthisis, pulmonaria
convulsion. [L.] convulsio
copper. [L.] cuprum; cuprinus
cord. [L.] corda
corn. [L.] callus-clavus
cornea. [L.] cornu; [Gr.] keras
costive. [L.] astrictus
cough. [L.] tussio
countenance. [L.] vultus
cramp. [L.] spasmus
crimson. [L.] coccum; coccineus
crisis. [L.] dies crisimus
cup. [L.] poculum
cure. [L.] sano
curvature. [L.] curvatura
cuticle. [L.] cuticula
daily. [L.] diurnus
dandruff. [L.] furfures capitas
date. [L.] status dies
dawn. [L.] prima lux
day. [L.] dies
dead. [L.] mortuus; defunctus
deadly. [L.] lethalis
deafness. [L.] surditas
death. [L.] mors
decompose. [L.] dissolvo
dental. [L.] dentalis
depression. [L.] depressio
digestive. [L.] digestorius; pepticus
dilute. [L.] dilutus
dinner. [L.] cena
discharge. [L.] eluvies; effluens

disease. [L.] morbus
dorsal. [L.] dorsalis
dose. [L.] potio
dram. [L.] drachma
drink. [L.] bibo; potis
dropsy. [L.] hydrops; opis
drug. [L.] medicamentum
dry. [L.] aridus
duct. [L.] ductus
dull. [L.] stupidus; hebes
dysentery. [L.] dysenteria
ear. [L.] auris; [Gr.] ous
eat. [L.] edo; [Gr.] phagos
egg. [L.] ovum
elbow. [L.] cubitum; [Gr.] ankon
embryo. [L.] partus immaturus
emission. [L.] emmissio
entrails. [L.] viscera
epidemic. [L.] epidemus
epilepsy. [L.] morbus comitalis; epilepsia
epileptic. [L.] epilepticus
erection. [L.] erectio
erotic. [L.] amatorius
eunuch. [L.] eunuchus
evening. [L.] vesper
every. [L.] omnis
excrement. [L.] excrementum
excretion. [L.] excrementum; excretio
exhalation. [L.] exhalatio
exhale. [L.] exhalo
expel. [L.] expello
expire. [L.] expiro
external. [L.] externus
extract. [L.] extractum
eye. [L.] oculus; [Gr.] ophthalmos
eyeball. [L.] pupula
eyebrow. [L.] supercilium
eyelid. [L.] palpebra
eyetooth. [L.] dens caninus
face. [L.] facies
faculty. [L.] facultas
faint. [L.] collabor
faintness. [L.] languor
fat. [L.] adeps; obesus; pinguis; [Gr.] lipos
feature. [L.] lineomentum

English with Latin and Greek Equivalents (cont'd)

febrile. [L.] febriculosus
fecundity. [L.] fecunditas
feel. [L.] tactus
fever. [L.] febris
film. [L.] membranula
filter. [L.] percolo
finger. [L.] digitus; [Gr.] daktylos
fistula. [L.] fistula putris
fit. [L.] accessus
flesh. [L.] carnis; [Gr.] sarx
fluid. [L.] fluidus
food. [L.] cibus
foot. [L.] pes, pedis; [Gr.] pous
forearm. [L.] brachium
forehead. [L.] frons
freckle. [L.] lentigo
gall. [L.] bilis
gangrene. [L.] gangraena
gargle. [L.] gargarizo
gland. [L.] glandula
gleet. [L.] ichor
gold. [L.] aurum; aureus
gout. [L.] morbus articularis; (in feet) podagra
grain. [L.] granum
gravel. [L.] calculus
gray. [L.] cinereus
green. [L.] viridis
grinder tooth. [L.] dens maxillaris
gullet. [L.] gula
gum. [L.] gingiva
gut. [L.] intestinum
hair. [L.] capillus; [Gr.] thrix
half. [L.] dimidus
hand. [L.] manus; [Gr.] cheir
harelip. [L.] labrum fissum
haunch. [L.] clunis
head. [L.] caput; [Gr.] kephale
heal. [L.] sano
healer. [L.] medicus
healing. [L.] salutaris
health. [L.] sanitas
healthful. [L.] salutaris; saluber
healthy. [L.] sanus
hear. [L.] audio
hearing. [L.] auditio; (sense of) auditus

heart. [L.] cor; [Gr.] kardia
heartburn. [L.] redundatio stomachi
heat. [L.] calor; ardor; fervor
heavy. [L.] gravis; ponderosus
hectic. [L.] hecticus
heel. [L.] calx, talus
hirsute. [L.] hirsutus
homeopathic. [L.] homeopathicus
hot. [L.] calidus; fervens; candens
hour. [L.] hora
hysterics. [L.] hysteria
illness. [L.] morbus
incisor. [L.] dens acutus
infant. [L.] infans; puerilis
infect. [L.] inficio
infectious. [L.] contagiosus
infirm. [L.] infirmus; debilis
inflammation. [L.] inflammatio; (of
  lungs) inflammatio pulmonaria
injection. [L.] injectio
insane. [L.] insanus
intellect. [L.] intellectus
intercourse. [L.] congressus
internal. [L.] intestinus
intestine. [L.] intestinum; [Gr.] enteron
iron. [L.] ferrum; ferreus
itch. [L.] scabies
itching. [L.] pruritus
jaw. [L.] maxilla
joint. [L.] artus; [Gr.] arthron
jugular vein. [L.] vena jugularis
kidney. [L.] ren; [Gr.] nephros
knee. [L.] genu; [Gr.] gonu
kneepan. [L.] patella
knuckle. [L.] condylus
labor. [L.] partus
labyrinth. [L.] labyrinthus
lacerate. [L.] lacero
larynx. [L.] guttur
lateral. [L.] lateralis
leech. [L.] sanguisuga
leg. [L.] tibia
lemon. [L.] citreum
leprosy. [L.] leprosus
ligament. [L.] ligamentum; [Gr.] syndesmos

English with Latin and Greek Equivalents (cont'd)

ligature. [L.] ligatura
light. [L.] levis
limb. [L.] membrum
lime. [L.] calx
liquid. [L.] liquidus
listen. [L.] ausculto
liver. [L.] jecur; [Gr.] hepar
livid. [L.] lividus
loin. [L.] lumbus; [Gr.] lapara
looseness. [L.] laxitas
lotion. [L.] lotio
lukewarm. [L.] tepidus
lung. [L.] pulmo; [Gr.] pneumon
lymph. [L.] lympha
mad. [L.] insanus
malady. [L.] morbus
male. [L.] masculinus
malignant. [L.] malignus
maternity. [L.] conditio matris
maturity. [L.] maturitas; aetas matura
meal. [L.] epulae
medicated. [L.] medicatus
medicine. [L.] (remedy) medicamentum
midnight. [L.] media nox
midsummer. [L.] media aestas
milk. [L.] lac
mind. [L.] animus
mix. [L.] misceo
mixture. [L.] mistura
moist. [L.] humidus; uvidus
molar. [L.] dens molaris
moment. [L.] punctum
month. [L.] mensis; mens
monthly. [L.] menstruus
morbid. [L.] morbidus
morning. [L.] matutinum
mouth. [L.] os; [Gr.] stoma
mucous. [L.] mucosus
muscle. [L.] musculus; [Gr.] mys
mustard. [L.] sinapis
nail. [L.] unguis
navel. [L.] umbilicus; [Gr.] omphalos
neck. [L.] cervix; collum; [Gr.] trachelos
nerve. [L.] nervus; [Gr.] neuron
night. [L.] nox; noctis
nipple. [L.] papilla

no, none. [L.] nullus
noon. [L.] meridies
normal. [L.] normalis
nose. [L.] nasus; [Gr.] rhis
nostril. [L.] naris
not. [L.] non
nourish. [L.] nutrio
nourishment. [L.] alimentus
now. [L.] nunc
nudity. [L.] nudatio
nurse. [L.] nutrix
obesity. [L.] obesitas
ocular. [L.] ocularis
oculist. [L.] ocularis medicus
oil. [L.] oleum
ointment. [L.] unguentum
old. [L.] antiquus
operator. [L.] manus curatio
opiate. [L.] medicamentum somnificum
optics. [L.] optice
orifice. [L.] foramen
pain. [L.] dolor
palate. [L.] palatum
palm. [L.] palma
parasite. [L.] parasitus
part. [L.] pars
patient. [L.] patiens
pectoral. [L.] pectoralis
pedal. [L.] pedale
phlegm. [L.] pituita
pill. [L.] pilus
pimple. [L.] pustula
pink. [L.] rosaceus
plaster. [L.] emplastrum
poison. [L.] venenum
poultice. [L.] cataplasma
powder. [L.] pulvis
pregnant. [L.] gravida
prepare. [L.] paro
prescribe. [L.] praescribo
prescription. [L.] praescriptum
puberty. [L.] pubertas
pubic bone. [L.] os pubis; [Gr.] pecten
pulverize. [L.] pulvero
pupil. [L.] pupilla
purgative. [L.] purgativus

English with Latin and Greek Equivalents (cont'd)

purple. [L.] purpura; purpureus
putrid. [L.] putridus
quinsy. [L.] cynanche; angina
rash. [L.] exanthema
recover. [L.] convalesco
recumbent. [L.] recumbens
recur. [L.] recurro
red. [L.] ruber
redness. [L.] rubor
remedy. [L.] remedium
respiration. [L.] respiratio
rheum. [L.] fluxio
rib. [L.] costa
rigid. [L.] rigidus
ringing. [L.] tinnitus
rupture. [L.] hernia
saliva. [L.] sputum
sallow. [L.] salix
salt. [L.] sal
salve. [L.] unguentum
sane. [L.] sanus
scab. [L.] scabies
scalp. [L.] pericranium
scaly. [L.] squamosus
scar. [L.] cicatrix
scarlet. [L.] coccineus
sciatica. [L.] ischias
scruple. [L.] scrupulum
second. [L.] secundum
seed. [L.] semen
senile. [L.] senilis
serum. [L.] sanguinis pars equosa
sharp. [L.] acutus
sheath. [L.] vagina
shin. [L.] tibia
shock. [L.] concussio; (of electricty) ictus electricus
short. [L.] brevis
shoulder. [L.] humerus; [Gr.] omos
shoulder blade. [L.] scapula
shudder. [L.] tremor
sick. [L.] aegrotus
side. [L.] latus
silver. [L.] argentum; argenteus
sinew. [L.] nervus
skeleton. [Gr.] skeleton

skin. [L.] cutis; [Gr.] derma
skull. [L.] cranium; [Gr.] kranion
sleep. [L.] somnus
smallpox. [L.] variola
smell. [L.] odoratus
soap. [L.] sapo
socket. [L.] cavum
soft. [L.] mollis
solid. [L.] solidus
solution. [L.] dilutum
soporific. [L.] soporus
sore. [L.] ulcus
sour. [L.] acidus
spasm. [L.] spasmus
spinal. [L.] dorsalis; spinalis
spine. [L.] spina
spirit. [L.] spiritus
spittle. [L.] sputum
spleen. [L.] lien
spoon. [L.] cochleare
sprain. [L.] luxatio
spring. [L.] ver; veris
stomach. [L.] stomachus; [Gr.] gaster
stone. [L.] calculus
stricture. [L.] strictura
sugar. [L.] saccharum
summer. [L.] aestas
sunrise. [L.] solis ortus
sunset. [L.] solis occasus
supper. [L.] cena
suture. [L.] sutura
swallow. [L.] glutio
sweat. [L.] sudor; [Gr.] hidros
sweet. [L.] dulcis
symptom. [L.] symptoma
system. [L.] systema
tail. [L.] cauda
take. [L.] sumo
tall. [L.] longus; celsus; procerus
tapeworm. [L.] taenia
taste. [L.] gustatus
tear. [L.] lacrima
teeth. [L.] dentes
tendon. [L.] tendo; [Gr.] tenon
testicle. [L.] testis; [Gr.] orchis
thick. [L.] densus

English with Latin and Greek Equivalents (cont'd)

thigh. [L.] femur
thin. [L.] tenuis; macer
throat. [L.] fauces; [Gr.] pharynx
throb. [L.] palpito
thumb. [L.] pollex
time. [L.] tempus
tin. [L.] stannum; plumbum album
tongue. [L.] lingua; [Gr.] glossa
tonsil. [L.] tonsilla
tooth. [L.] dens; [Gr.] odous
troche. [L.] trochiscus
tube. [L.] tuba
twin. [L.] geminus
twitching. [L.] subsultus
ulcer. [L.] ulcus
unless. [L.] nisi
urine. [L.] urina
uterine. [L.] uterinus
vaccine. [L.] vaccinum
vagina. [L.] vagina; [Gr.] kolpos
valve. [L.] valvula
vein. [L.] vena; [Gr.] phleps
vertebra. [L.] vertebra; [Gr.] spondylos
vessel. [L.] vas

violet. [L.] violaceus
warm. [L.] calidus
warmth. [L.] calor
wash. [L.] lavo
water. [L.] aqua
wax. [L.] cera
waxed dressing. [L.] ceratum
weary. [L.] lassus; languidus; fatigatus
wet. [L.] humidus
white. [L.] albus
windpipe. [L.] arteria aspera
wine. [L.] vinum
winter. [L.] hiems; hiemis
woman. [L.] femina
womb. [L.] uterus; [Gr.] hystera
worm. [L.] vermis
wound. [L.] vulnus
wrist. [L.] carpus; [Gr.] karpos
year. [L.] annus
yellow. [L.] flavus; luteus; croceus
yolk. [L.] luteum
young. [L.] parvus; infans
youth. [L.] adolescentia

Appendix 2

Abbreviations

Principal Medical Abbreviations

Abbreviation	Latin (unless indicated)	English Definition
ad	ad	to; up to
ad lib.	ad libitum	freely; at pleasure
ALT		alanine aminotransferase (formerly SGPT)
AQ	aqua	water
AST		aspartate aminotransferase (formerly SGOT)
AV		atrioventricular
av.	(French)	avoirdupois
		average
B.P.		British Pharmacopeia
BUN		blood urea nitrogen
C		Calorie (kilocalorie)
		Celsius
		centigrade
C	congius	gallon
ca.	circa	about
CBC		complete blood count
cc.	(French)	cubic centimeter
CDC		Centers for Disease Control
cg	(French)	centigram
cm	(French)	centimeter
comp.	compositus	compound
CNS		central nervous system
cong.	congius	gallon
CSF		cerebrospinal fluid
CV		cardiovascular
d	dexter	right
	dies	day (24 hours)
/d		per day
D&C		dilatation and curettage
DPT		diphtheria-pertussis-tetanus
dr.	drachma	dram
ECG		electrocardiogram
ECT		electroconvulsive therapy
EEG		electroencephalogram
elix.	(Arabic)	elixir
EMG		electromyogram
emp.	emplastrum	a plaster
ENT		ear, nose, and throat
ESR		erythrocyte sedimentation rate
F	(proper name)	Fahrenheit
f		female
FDA		Food and Drug Administration
FEV		forced expiratory volume
Fld	fluidus	fluid

From Thomas, C. L. (ed.): *Taber's Cyclopedic Medical Dictionary*, ed. 16, F. A. Davis Company, Philadelphia, 1989, pp. 2207–2212.

Principal Medical Abbreviations *(cont'd)*

Abbreviation	Latin (unless indicated)	English Definition
fl. dr.	fluidrachma	fluidram
fl. oz.	fluidus uncia	fluidounce
FSH		follicle-stimulating hormone
GI		gastrointestinal
Gm; gm	gramme (French)	gram
gr	granum	grain
Gtt, gtt	guttae	drops
h.	hora	hour
hgb		hemoglobin
I.M.		intramuscular
inf.	infusum	infusion
inhal.	inhalatio	inhalation
inj.	injectio	injection
instill.		instillation
IQ		intelligence quotient
I.U.		international unit
IUD		intrauterine device
I.V.		intravenously
kg	(French)	kilogram
l	litre (French)	liter
lab.		laboratory
lb.	libra	pound
LD_{50}		lethal dose, median
liq.	liquor	liquid; fluid
m		male
	(French)	meter
	minimum	minim
MED		minimum effective dose
mEq		milliequivalent
mg		milligram
ml		milliliter
mM		millimole
mm	(French)	millimeter
mol. wt.		molecular weight
mph		miles per hour
MPN		most probable number
μEq		microequivalent
μg		microgram
no.	numerus	number
NPN		nonprotein nitrogen
O	octarius	pint
OC		oral contraceptive
C.D.	oculus dexter	right eye
O.L.	oculus laevus	left eye
O.S.	oculus sinister	left eye
oz.	uncia	ounce
paren.		parenterally
PBI		protein-bound iodine
pH		hydrogen ion concentration
ppm		parts per million
pt	pinte (French)	pint
qt	quartina	quart
rad		radiation absorbed dose
s	sans	without
s̄	sine	without
S	signa	mark

Principal Medical Abbreviations (cont'd)

Abbreviation	Latin (unless indicated)	English Definition
s.c.	sub cutis	subcutaneously
s.cut.		subcutaneously
SGOT		serum glutamic oxaloacetic transaminase (see AST)
SGPT		serum glutamic pyruvic transaminase (see ALT)
sp. gr.	gravitus	specific gravity
spt.	spiritus	spirit
s.q.		subcutaneously
stat.	statim	immediately
syr.	syrupus	syrup
top.		topically
tr., tinct.	tinctura	tincture
UHF		ultrahigh frequency
ung.	unguentum	ointment
UV		ultraviolet
vin.	vinum	wine
Vo_2		maximum oxygen consumption
vol. %		volume per cent
WBC		white blood count
Wt.	wiht (Old English)	weight
w/v.		weight in volume
x		multiplied by

Charting: Abbreviations and Their Meanings

Some of these abbreviations are used rarely if at all. They are recorded for their historical interest. See also *Principal Medical Abbreviations* above.

Abbreviation	Latin Phrase	English Definition
abs. feb.	absente febre	without fever
a.c.	ante cibum	before a meal
ad effect.	ad effectum	to effect
adhib.	adhibendus	to be administered
ad lib.	ad libitum	at pleasure
ad part. dolent.	ad partes dolentes	to the aching parts
adst. feb.	adstante febre	when fever is present
ad us.	ad usum	according to custom
ad us. ext.	ad usum externum	for external use
ag. feb.	aggrediente febre	when the fever increases
alt. dieb.	alternis diebus	every other day
alt. hor.	alternis horis	every other hour
alt. noc.	alterna nocte	every other night
aq.	aqua	water
bal.	balneum	bath
bal. sin.	balneum sinapis	mustard bath
bis in 7d.	bis in septem diebus	twice a week
BP		blood pressure

Charting: Abbreviations and Their Meanings *(cont'd)*

Abbreviation	Latin Phrase	English Definition
c̄	cum	with
cat.	cataplasma	a poultice
cito disp.	cito dispensetur	let it be dispensed quickly
c.m.	cras mane	tomorrow morning
c.m.s.	cras mane sumendus	to be taken tomorrow morning
c.n.	cras nocte	tomorrow night
cont. rem.	continuentur remedia	let the medicine be continued
c.v.	cras vespere	tomorrow evening
cyath.	cyathus	ladle (wineglass)
cyath. vinos.	cyathus vinosus	wineglassful
d	da	give
d	dies	day
/d		per day
decub.	decubitus	lying down
donec. alv. sol. ft.	donec alvus soluta fuerit	until the bowels are open
dur. dolor.	durante dolore	while pain lasts
en., enem.		enema
exhib.	exhibeatur	let it be displayed
h.n.	hoc nocte	tonight
hor. som, h.s.	hora somni	bedtime
in d.	in dies	daily
mod. praesc.	modo praescripto	as prescribed
mor. dict.	more dicto	in the manner directed
mor. sol.	more solito	in the usual manner
n.b.	nota bene	note well
noct.	nocte	of the night
n.p.o.		nothing by mouth
p̄	post	after
p.a.a.	parti affectae applicetur	let it be applied to the affected region
post. cib. or p. c.	post cibos	after meals
p.r.	per rectum	through the rectum
p.r.n.	pro re nata	as needed
p.v.	per vaginam	through the vagina
Q.h.	quaque hora	every hour
Q. 2h.		every two hours
Q. 3h.		every three hours
q.i.d.	quater in die	four times a day
q.l.	quantum libet	as much as wanted
q.p.	quantum placeat	as much as desired
q.s.	quantum sufficiat	as much as may be needed
quotid.	quotidie	daily
s̄	sine	without
s.a. or sec. a.	secundum artem	by skill
semih.	semihora	half an hour
s.o.s.	si opus sit	if necessary
st.	stet, stent	let it (them) stand
sum.	sumat, sumendum	let him take; to be taken
s.v.	spiritus vini	alcoholic spirit
s.v.v.	spiritus vini vitus	brandy
T		temperature
ter.	tere	rub
t.i.d.	ter in die	three times a day
t.i.n.	ter in nocte	three times a night
ur.		urine

Prescription Writing: Abbreviations and Their Meanings

Some of these abbreviations are used rarely if at all. They are recorded for their historical interest. See also *Principal Medical Abbreviations* on previous pages.

Abbreviation	Latin (unless indicated)	English Definition
āā or a	ana (Greek)	of each
add.	adde	add
adhib.	adhibendus	to be administered
admov.	admove	apply
ad sat.	ad saturandum	to saturation
aeq.	aequales	equals
agit.	agita	shake; stir
agit. ante sum.	agita ante sumendum	shake before taking
alb.	albus	white
aq. bull.	aqua bulliens	boiling water
aq. cal.	aqua calida	hot water
aq. dest.	aqua destillata	distilled water
aq. ferv.	aqua fervens	boiling water
aq. font.	aqua fontis	spring water
aq. frig.	aqua frigida	cold water
aq. menth. pip.	aqua menthae piperitae	peppermint water
aq. pur.	aqua pura	pure water
bib.	bibe	drink
b.i.d.	bis in die	twice daily
b.i.n.	bis in noctus	twice a night
bol.	bolus	a pill
bull.	bulliat	let it boil
c̄	cum	with
cap.	capsula	a capsule
chart. or cht.	chartula	a small medicated paper
coch. mag.	cochleare magnum	a large spoonful
coch. med	cochleare medium	a half spoonful
coch. parv.	cochleare parvum	a teaspoonful
collyr.	collyrium	an eyewash
comp.	compositus	compounded of
cuj. lib.	cujus libet	of any you please
D	dosis	dose
d.	da	give
d.d. in d.	de die in diem	from day to day
dec.	decanta	pour off
dent. tal. dos.	dentur tales doses	give of such doses
det.	detur	let it be given
dieb. alt.	diebus alternis	every other day
dieb. tert.	diebus tertiis	every 3rd day
dil.	dilue, dilutus	dilute, diluted
dim.	dimidius	halved
div.	dividatur	divide
div. in p. aeq.	dividatur in partes aequales	let it be divided into equal parts
donec alv. sol. ft.	donec alvus soluta fuerit	until the bowels are open
dos.	dosis	dose
dur. dolor.	durante dolore	while pain lasts
e.m.p.	ex modo praescripto	as directed
emp.	emplastrum	a plaster
emuls.	emulsio	an emulsion
epistom.	epistomium	a stopper
ext.	extendere	to spread
	extractum	extract

Prescription Writing: Abbreviations and Their Meanings (cont'd)

Abbreviation	Latin (unless indicated)	English Definition
ferv.	fervens	boiling
f.h.	fiat hastus	let a draught be made
filt.	filtra	filter
f.m.	fiat mistura	let a mixture be made
f.p.	fiat potio	let a potion be made
f. pil.	fiat pilula	let a pill be made
ft.	fiat	let it be made
garg.	gargarisma	a gargle
grad.	gradatim	by degrees
gtt	guttae	drops
guttat.	guttatim	drop by drop
haust.	haustus	a draught
hor. decub.	hora decubitus	at bedtime
hor. som. or h. s.	hora somni	at bedtime
hor. 1 spat.	horae unius spatio	one hour's time
inf.	infusum	an infusion
int.	intime	to the innermost
lin.	linimentum	a liniment
liq.	liquor	a solution
lot.	lotio	a lotion
M	misce	mix
mac.	macera	soften
man. prim.	mane primo	first thing in the morning
mas.	massa	a mass
med.	medicamentum	a medicine
m. et n.	mane et nocte	morning and night
mist.	mistura	a mixture
mitt.	mitte	let go
mitt. x tal.	mitte decem tales	send 10 like this
mod.	modicus	moderate-sized
mod. praesc.	modo praescripto	in the manner prescribed
moll.	mollis	soft
mor. dict.	more dicto	in the manner directed
mor. sol.	more solito	as accustomed
ne tr. s. num.	ne tradas sine nummo	deliver not without the money
no.	numerus	number
noct. maneq.	nocte maneque	night and morning
non. rep., n. r.	non repetatur	do not repeat
omn. bid.	omni bidendis	every 2 days
omn. bih.	omni bihoris	every 2 hours
omn. hor.	omni hora	every hour
omn. noct.	omni nocte	every night
om. ¼ h.	omni quadranta hora	every 15 minutes
om. mane vel. noc.	omni mane vel nocte	every morning or night
part. aeq.	partes aequales	equal parts
part. vic.	partitis vicibus	in divided doses
p.c.	post cibos	after meals
pil.	pilula	a pill
p.o.	per os	by mouth
p. p. a.	phiala prius agitata	the bottle having first been shaken
pro. rat. aet.	pro ratione aetatis	according to patient's age
pulv.	pulvis	powder
red. in pulv.	redactus in pulverem	reduced to powder

Prescription Writing: Abbreviations
and Their Meanings *(cont'd)*

Abbreviation	Latin (unless indicated)	English Definition
repetat., rep.	repetatur	let it be repeated
rub.	ruber	red
sig.	signa	write
	signetur	let it be labeled
sing.	singulorum	of each
sol.	solutio	a solution
solv.	solve	dissolve
ss.	semi- or semisse	a half
subind.	subinde	immediately after
sum.	sume	take
sum. tal.	sumat talem	take 1 like this
suppos.	suppositorium	a suppository
s.v.r.	spiritus vini rectificatus	rectified spirit of wine
tab.	tabella	a medicated tablet
tinct.	tinctura	a tincture
trit.	tritura	triturate or grind
ult. praes.	ultimus praescriptus	the last ordered
ung.	unguentum	ointment
ut dict.	ut dictum	as directed
vitel.	vitellus	yolk of an egg

PREFIXES AND SUFFIXES

a-, an. Negative
a-, ab-, abs-. Away from
ad-, -ad. Toward
-aemia. Blood
aer-. Air
-aesthesia. Sensation
-algesia, algia. Suffering; pain
algi-. Pain
all-. Other
amb-. Both; on both sides
amph-. Around; on both sides
ana-, an-. Up
angio-. Relating to blood or lymph vessels
ante-. Before
anti-. Against
apo-. From; opposed
-ase. Enzyme
aut-, auto-. Self
bi, bis-. Twice; double
brachy-. Short
brady-. Slow
cac-, caco-. Bad; evil
cat, cata, cath-. Down
-cele. A tumor; a cyst; a hernia
cent-. Hundred
cephal-. Relating to a head
chrom-, chromo-. Color
-cide. Causing death
circum-. Around
co, com, con-. Together
contra-. Against
cyst-, -cyst. Bag; bladder
-cyte. A cell
dacry-. Tears
dactyl-. Fingers
de-. From; not
deca-. Ten
deci-. Tenth
demi-. Half
dent-. Relating to the teeth
derma-. The skin
di-. Double; apart from
dia-. Through; between; asunder
dipla, diplo-. Double
dis-. Negative; double; apart; absence of
-dynia. Pain
dys-. Difficult; bad
ec, ecto-. Out; on the outside
-ectomy. A cutting out
ef, es, ex, exo-. Out
-emesis. Vomiting

-emia. Blood
en-. In; into
endo-. Within
entero-. Relating to the intestine
ento-. Within
epi-. Upon
-esthesia. Sensation
eu-. Well
ex-, exo-. Out
extra-. On the outside; beyond
fore-. Before; in front of
-form. Form
-fuge. to drive away
galact, galacto-. Milk
gaster, gastro-. The stomach; the belly
-gene, -genesis, -genetic, -genic. Production; origin; formation
glosso-. Relating to the tongue
-gog, gogue. To make flow
-gram. A tracing; a mark
-graphy. A writing; a record
hem, hemato-. Relating to the blood
hemi-. Half
hepa-, hepar-, hepato-. Liver
hetero-. Other; indicating dissimilarity
holo-. All
homo, homeo-. Same; similar
hydra, hydro-. Relating to water
hyp, hyph, hypo-. Under
hyper-. Over; above; beyond
hypo-. Under
-iasis. Condition; pathological state
idio-. Peculiar to the individual or organ
ileo-. Relating to the ileum
in-. In; into; not
infra-. Beneath
inter-. Between
intra, intro-. Within
-ism. Condition; theory
iso-. Equal
-itis. Inflammation
-ize. To treat by special method
juxta-. Near
karyo-. Nucleus; nut
kata-, kath-. Down
kera-. Horn; indicates hardness
kinesi-. Movement
-kinesis. Motion
lact-. Milk
laparo-. The loin; relating to the loin or abdomen

Adapted from Thomas, C. L. (ed.): *Taber's Cyclopedic Medical Dictionary*, ed. 15, F. A. Davis, Philadelphia, 1985, p. 1937.